AMERICAN ASSOCIATION OF CRITICAL-CARE NURSES

Acute Care Nurse Practitioner

Clinical Curriculum and Certification Review

EDITED BY

Anna Gawlinski, RN, DNSc, CS-ACNP
Clinical Nurse Specialist
University of California, Los Angeles,
 Medical Center
Assistant Clinical Professor
University of California, Los Angeles,
 School of Nursing
Los Angeles, California

Deborah Hamwi, RN, MSN, NP
Assistant Clinical Professor
Department of Family Medicine
University of California, Irvine
Irvine, California
Nurse Practitioner
Kaiser Permanente
Bellflower, California

AACN
CRITICAL CARE

W.B. SAUNDERS COMPANY
A Division of Harcourt Brace & Company
Philadelphia   London   Toronto   Montreal   Sydney   Tokyo

W.B. SAUNDERS COMPANY
A Division of Harcourt Brace & Company

The Curtis Center
Independence Square West
Philadelphia, Pennsylvania 19106

Library of Congress Cataloging-in-Publication Data

Acute care nurse practitioner : clinical curriculum and certification
review / [edited by] Anna Gawlinski, Deborah Hamwi.—1st ed.
    p.   cm.
    "American Association of Critical Care Nurses."
    ISBN 0–7216–7311–2
    1. Intensive care nursing.—2. Intensive care nursing-
-Examinations, questions, etc.   I. Hamwi, Deborah.   II. American
Association of Critical-Care Nurses.
    [DNLM: 1. Acute Disease—nursing.   2. Acute Disease—nursing
examination questions.   3. Nurse Practitioners.   4. Nurse
Practitioners examination questions.   WY 150 A189 1999]
RT120.I5A3385   1999
610.73′61—dc21
DNLM/DLC   98-4059

ACUTE CARE NURSE PRACTITIONER   ISBN 0–7216–7311–2

Printed in the United States of America

Last digit is the print number: 9   8   7   6   5   4   3   2   1

To acute care nurse practitioners who are in the forefront of delivering health care in the acute care setting. We hope this book will serve as a valuable resource in the care of the acute and critically ill.

To our husbands
Ronald Philip Ramus
and
Steve Hamilton Truax
for their endless support and love throughout the development of this book.

Contributors

Barbara M. Bates-Jensen, RN, MN, CETN
Assistant Professor of Clinical Nursing
University of Southern California
Los Angeles, California
Infections and Common Problems in Acute Care

Randy M. Caine, RN, EdD, CS, ANP-C, CCRN
Professor of Nursing
Coordinator, Adult-Geriatric Practitioner
 Nurse Program
California State University
Long Beach, California;
Adjunct Professor of Education
Pepperdine University
Graduate School of Education and Psychology
Culver City, California
Test-Taking Strategies

Deborah Caswell, RN, MN, ANP-C, CCRN
Assistant Director
Gunda Vascular Center
University of California, Los Angeles,
 Medical Center
Assistant Clinical Professor
University of California, Los Angeles,
 School of Nursing;
Los Angeles, California
Cardiovascular Disorders; Gastrointestinal Disorders

Suzanne Clark, RN, MSN, MA, NP
Nurse Practitioner
Department of Care Management
Kaiser Permanente
Los Angeles, California
Mental Health Disorders

Joan E. Davies, RN, MSN, NP

Clinical Preceptor Faculty
School of Nursing
College of New Jersey
Ewing, New Jersey;
School of Nursing
Seton Hall University
West Orange, New Jersey;
Supervisor, Nurse Practitioner
Sexuality, Education, Counseling, and Health
Princeton University
Princeton, New Jersey
Infections and Common Problems in Acute Care

Anna Gawlinski, RN, DNSc, CS-ACNP, CCRN

Clinical Nurse Specialist
University of California, Los Angeles,
 Medical Center
Assistant Clinical Professor
University of California, Los Angeles,
 School of Nursing;
Los Angeles, California
Cardiovascular Disorders

Paula Gull, RN, MSN, CS, ANP, CCTC

Renal Transplant Coordinator–Nurse
 Practitioner
St Joseph Hospital
Orange, California
Urology

Deborah Hamwi, RN, MSN, NP

Assistant Clinical Professor
Department of Family Medicine
University of California, Irvine
Irvine, California
Nurse Practitioner
Kaiser Permanente
Bellflower, California
  Endocrine Disorders

Maryann T. Hardesty, RN, MSN, ANP

Adult Nurse Practitioner
Geriatrics/Extended Care and Hospice
Veteran's Administration Medical Center
Boise, Idaho
  *Infections and Common Problems in Acute
  Care*

**Cydney G. Hirsch, RN, MN, CS-ANP,
CCRN**

Nurse Practioner III
University of California, Los Angeles,
  Medical Center
Los Angeles, California
  Gastrointestinal Disorders

**Dorothy Anderle Johnson, RN, DNSc,
FNP**

Nurse Practitioner
University of Southern California Medical
  Center
Los Angeles, California
  *Musculoskeletal and Connective Tissue
  Disorders*

**Megan M. Keiser, RN, MS, CS,
ANP-C, CNRN**

Orthopedic/Neuroscience Outcomes Manager
St Jude Medical Center
Fullerton, California
  Neurologic Disorders

**Ruth M. Kleinpell, RN, PhD, CS-ACNP,
CCRN**

Associate Professor/Teacher Practitioner
Rush University College of Nursing;
Clinical Nurse
Surgical Intensive Care Unit
University of Illinois Hospital
Chicago, Illinois
  Roles, Issues, Policies, and Trends

Diana I.G. Lithgow, RN, MSN, FNP

Professor, Western University
Pomona, California;
Professor, University of California, Irvine
Irvine, California;
Nurse Practitioner
Laguna Beach Community Clinic
Laguna Beach, California
  Roles, Issues, Policies, and Trends

Mary Pat Lynch, RN, MSN, CRNP, AOCN

Clinical Faculty
Oncology Advanced Practice Nurse Program
University of Pennsylvania School of Nursing
Oncology Nurse Practitioner
Graduate School, University of Pennsylvania
Philadelphia, Pennsylvania
  Hematologic and Oncologic Disorders

Kathy McCloy, RN, MSN, CS-ACNP

Acute Care Nurse Practitioner
Interventional Cardiology
University of California, Los Angeles,
  Medical Center
Assistant Clinical Professor
University of California, Los Angeles,
  School of Nursing;
Los Angeles, California
  Cardiovascular Disorders

Nancy M. Oldham, RN, MN, FNP

Lecturer, Department of Nursing
California State University Long Beach
University of California, Los Angeles,
  School of Nursing
Los Angeles, California;
Director of Disease Management
Bristol Park Medical Group Inc.
Irvine, California
  Health Promotion and Health Protection

William J. Quiñones-Baldrich, MD

Professor of Surgery
Section of Vascular Surgery
University of California, Los Angeles,
  School of Medicine;
Attending Staff
Section of Vascular Surgery
University of California, Los Angeles,
  Medical Center
Los Angeles, California
  Cardiovascular Disorders

Kathy Stull Rodgers, RN, MSN, CCRN, CEN

Trauma Coordinator
St Elizabeth Hospital
Beaumont, Texas
*Review Questions for Infections and
Common Problems in Acute Care*

Vickie Ruch, RN, MSN, CS, FNP, ANP

Clinical Faculty, Division of Nursing
California State University
Carson, California;
Emergency Department Nurse Practitioner
Robert F. Kennedy Medical Center
Emergency Department
Hawthorne, California
Pulmonary Disorders

Mary B. Sherman, MD

Leisure World Medical Group
Seal Beach, California;
Los Alamitos Medical Center
Los Alamitos, California
Renal Disorders

Mary K. Shook, RN, BSN, NP

Administrative Supervisor
Martin Luther Medical Center
Anaheim, California
Ethical and Legal Issues

Eileen Simpson, RN, MSN, ANP, GNP, PNP

Affiliate Faculty Nurse Practitioner Program
Long Beach State University and
Nurse Practitioner Urgent Care
Long Beach Community Medical Center
Long Beach, California
*Musculoskeletal and Connective Tissue
Disorders*

Debra L. Tribett, RN, MS, CS, LNP

Clinical Instructor
Acute Care Nurse Practitioner Program
Georgetown University School of Nursing
Washington, DC;
Adult and Acute Care Nurse Practitioner
Infectious Diseases Physicians Inc.
Annandale, Virginia
*Infections and Common Problems in Acute
Care*

Dat Vo, MD

Internal Medical
Cove Health Care
Fountain Valley, California
Endocrine Disorders

Kim Wilkins, MS, RD, CNSD

Critical Care Dietitian
University of California, Los Angeles,
Medical Center
Los Angeles, California
*Infections and Common Problems in Acute
Care*

Reviewers

Diane Beuerle, RN, MS, NP
Private Practice
Corona del Mar, California

James E. Branahl, MD
University of Washington School of Medicine
Veterans Affairs Medical Center
Boise, Idaho

Annette Galassi, RN, MA, CANP, AOCN
Division of Hematology/Oncology
Vincent T. Lombardi Cancer Center
Georgetown University Medical Center
Washington, District of Columbia

Hugh A. Gelabert, MD
Associate Professor of Surgery
University of California, Los Angeles,
   School of Medicine
Los Angeles, California

Philip M. Gold, MD
Director, Division of Critical Care Medicine
Loma Linda University Medical Center
Loma Linda, California

Jennifer M. Grossman, MD
Fellow, Rheumatology Department
University of California, Los Angeles
Los Angeles, California

Antoine Hage, MD
Division of Cardiology
University of California, Los Angeles,
   Medical Center
Los Angeles, California

Janie Heath, RN, MS, CS-ACNP, ANP, CCRN
Adjunct Clinical Faculty, School of Nursing
Medical College of Georgia
Nurse Practitioner
Veterans Administration Medical Center
Augusta, Georgia

Edwin Jacobson, MD
Clinical Professor of Medicine
University of California, Los Angeles, School
   of Medicine
Los Angeles, California

Ruth M. Kleinpell, RN, PhD, CS-ACNP, CCRN
Rush University College of Nursing
Chicago, Illinois

Mary D. Knudtson, RN, MN, FNP, PNP, CS
Division of Infectious Diseases
University of California, Los Angeles,
   Medical Center
Los Angeles, California;
University of California, Irvine
Irvine, California

Bernard M. Kubak, MD
Atending Physician and Assistant Clinical
   Professor
Division of Infectious Diseases
University of California, Los Angeles,
   Medical Center
Los Angeles, California

Norma D. McNair, RN, MSN, CS, CCRN, CNRN
University of California, Los Angeles, Medical Center
Los Angeles, California

Petrea Monson, MS, RD, CNSD
University of California, San Diego, Medical Center
San Diego, California

Barbara Natterson, MD
Division of Cardiology
University of California, Los Angeles, Medical Center
Los Angeles, California

Son Nguyen, MD
Orange Coast Memorial Medical Center
Fountain Valley, California

Anna Omery, RN, DNSc
Kaiser Permanente Medical Center
Pasadena, California

Gretchen Pitti, RN, CETN
ET Nursing Enterprises, Inc.
Huntington Beach, California

Ervin Ruzics, MD
University of California, Irvine, Medical Center
Orange, California

Barbara Schaefer, RN, MS, CS-ACNP, CCRN
Department of Neurosurgery
Kaiser Permanente Medical Center
Anaheim, California

Preface

The purpose of this book is twofold. This text can be used as a clinical curriculum and review guide for acute care nurse practitioners who are responsible for caring for patients in the acute care setting; and can assist individuals engaged in self study preparation for the acute care nurse practitioner certification examination.

Many nurses preparing for certification examinations find that reviewing an extensive body of scientific knowledge requires a difficult search of many sources that must be synthesized to provide a review base for the examination. This book is developed especially for acute care nurse practitioners preparing to take the certification examination. It brings together much of what is the essence of acute care nurse practitioner practice by well known experts in the field. This text will provide a succinct, yet comprehensive review of core acute care material as well as study questions.

Organization of the Text

This book is organized into 15 chapters based on content. The first chapter provides the reader with test-taking strategies. In addition there are 10 chapters which address common disorders and diseases found in acute care practice. These are organized under organ systems. These chapters provide succinct summaries of the following: definitions, pathophysiology and etiology, signs and symptoms, physical findings, differential diagnoses, diagnostic tests, therapeutic management/treatment and patient education. The next chapter addresses common problems found in acute care (e.g., fever, pain management, nutrition, wound care). The following chapter addresses health promotion and health protection of the acutely ill patient. A chapter on the ethical issues in the care of the acutely ill patient follows. The final chapter addresses role issues in advanced nursing practice and current issues and trends for acute care nurse practitioners.

REVIEW QUESTIONS

Within each chapter are **review questions** which serve as an introduction to the process of test taking. These review questions can help the reader study content and simulate a test taking arena. Test questions examine knowledge at several levels, such as memory (or recall), comprehension (or application) and critical thinking. There are several questions for each disorder. Short case scenarios are frequently used to test the applicants' decision making ability, diagnostic reasoning and ability to develop the correct management plan. Correct answers and rationales are provided on a separate page. In this way the learner can practice test taking similar to the actual exam. In addition, a bibliography is included for those who need more in-depth explanation of the subject matter in each chapter. These references can serve as additional instructional material for the acute care nurse practitioner.

It is assumed that the reader of this review guide has completed a course of study in an acute care nurse practitioner or adult nurse practitioner program. *Acute Care Nurse Practitioner: Clinical Curriculum and Certification Review* is not intended to be a basic learning tool.

Target Audience and Goals

This book will be of value to ACNPs preparing for the certification examination but will also serve as a curriculum and review guide for the following groups:

- practicing acute care nurse practitioners
- graduate nursing students (current and potential)
- graduate school of nursing faculty
- physicians working with ACNPs
- medical staff office utilizing ACNPs

The goals of this book:

1. Provide an authoritative resource for acute care nurse practitioners preparing to take the national certification examination.
2. Provide a reference for all levels of ACNPs and other advanced practice nurses from novice to expert.
3. Provide a reference for nurses in graduate nursing education for ACNP and serve as a tool to stimulate knowledge and professional growth.

Contributors and Reviewers

The philosophy of collaborative practice is reflected in this book. Contributors and reviewers of the text are practicing nurse practitioners and advanced practice nurses in the acute care setting and physicians with whom nurse practitioners work. The contribution of the professionals in this book reflects the philosophy of collaborative yet independent practice of the acute care nurse practitioner.

Contents

CHAPTER 4

CHAPTER 5

CHAPTER **6**

CHAPTER **7**

CHAPTER **8**

CHAPTER **9**

CHAPTER **10**

CHAPTER **11**

CHAPTER **1 2**

CHAPTER **1 3**

CHAPTER **14**

CHAPTER **1 5**

CHAPTER 1

Test-Taking Strategies

Randy M. Caine, RN, EdD, CS, ANP-C, CCRN

Certification as an acute care nurse practitioner (ACNP) is granted after nurses who have met specific eligibility criteria take and pass an examination that is based on nationally recognized standards of nursing practice beyond those required for licensure. The ACNP certification examination is administered by the American Nurses Credentialing Center and the ACCN Certification Corporation; the credential is CS. The intent of this chapter is to provide information about the ACNP examination as well as provide strategies for test taking.

You have embarked on a professional trajectory that has taken you from your basic nursing education to this moment in your career. By this point in your professional life, you have spent many years learning and understanding facts, applying them to practice, and integrating them into your clinical performance. During your basic program in nursing, you took tests. On completion of that program you took and passed your National Council Licensure Examination for Registered Nurses (NCLEX). Passing that examination marked the beginning of your professional career. Since that time you may have taken and passed certification examinations in critical care (CCRN), oncology (OCN), or emergency (CEN) nursing. You have now completed additional education as a nurse practitioner. Incorporated in that program you again spent time learning and understanding facts, applying them to practice, and integrating them into your performance as an ACNP. During that program you, again, took many tests. It is now time to take yet another examination, one that you have been preparing for since entering your nurse practitioner program.

Eligibility for the Examination

In 1995, the American Nurses Credentialing Center and the AACN Certification Corporation established a joint venture certification program for ACNPs. To be eligible for the ACNP examination, specific requirements in a clinical or functional area beyond the basic preparation in nursing have been established. Registered nurses who meet these requirements are eligible to sit for certification examinations that articulate nationally recognized practice standards.

The *Standards of Clinical Practice and Scope of Practice for the Acute Care Nurse Practitioner* were developed collaboratively by the American Association

1

of Critical-Care Nurses and the American Nurses Association. The standards define the acute care nurse practitioner as a registered nurse who holds a graduate degree in nursing and is prepared for advanced practice in acute care. This practice includes providing direct services to individuals who are acutely or critically ill in a variety of settings, using a collaborative model. The key elements of direct care include diagnostic reasoning, advanced therapeutic interventions, and education.

Individuals are eligible to sit for this examination if they currently hold an active license to practice as a registered nurse (RN) in the United States or its territories. Individuals must hold a master's degree or higher in nursing, and either have been prepared as an adult acute care nurse practitioner in an ACNP master's degree program in nursing or have completed a formal postgraduate acute care nurse practitioner program within a school of nursing granting graduate-level academic credit. Individuals who meet the following criteria may also be considered:

- completed a master's degree as an adult nurse practitioner with a minimum of 500 hours of post-master's practice within the past 2 years in an advanced practice role providing direct services to patients who are acutely or critically ill; or
- completed a formal postgraduate adult nurse practitioner program within a school of nursing granting graduate level academic credit; or
- completed a formal postgraduate ACNP program within a school of nursing granting graduate level academic credit and a minimum of 500 hours of post-master's practice within the past 2 years in an advanced practice role providing direct services to patients who are acutely or critically ill after completion of an adult nurse practitioner program.

Potential candidates for the examination who have *not* completed an ACNP program but have met the other requirements will be eligible to sit for the exam only until the year 2000. After that time applicants must have graduated from an ACNP program.

Programs must be accredited by a nationally recognized regional accrediting body. Foreign graduates must have their transcripts evaluated by a foreign credential evaluation service. Submission of verification of completion of the program by the program director, nurse practitioner and master's or higher degree in nursing transcripts, and a completed application form are usually required by at least 1–1½ months prior to the examination date.

Description of the Examination

The examination for certification as an ACNP is an objective test of knowledge, skills, and abilities of professional nursing practice that has been developed by the Board on Certification for Acute Care Nursing Practice. The items have been developed by a committee composed of experts representative of certification based on system-specific health problems, common problems in acute care, professionalism in advanced practice issues, and trends in health promotion and risk assessment that are to be covered on the examination. After each item has been submitted, there is a period of review and critique of the item as well as a rating of its accuracy and relevancy. The psychometric properties of reliability and validity are ensured and representative items are selected for each printed examination. Currently this examination is administered three times a year, generally February, June, and October.

Candidates are reminded that they must arrive early for the examination for check-in and processing before they are admitted to the examination room, and that they must bring their own sharpened #2 pencils. Beginning in January 1999, all nurse practitioner examinations administered by the American Nurses Credentialing Center will be computer based. You will be asked to turn off all pagers, telephones, and watches that make sounds during the examination. In addition, you may not bring any food, beverages, or water into the examination room. If you need to get a drink of water or use the restroom during the examination, you will be required to sign out according to instructions that will be provided on the day of the examination. Arrangements for special testing can be made for candidates with medical needs who cannot comply with these rules.

The total time for the actual examination is 4 hours, generally in the morning. There is usually sufficient time for examination candidates to complete all test items with additional time at the end for review. However, each candidate manages time differently; therefore, it is recommended to proceed quickly and carefully through the examination, avoiding excessive time on any one question until all have been responded to.

Needless to say, you may not bring books, papers, reading material, calculators, or scratch paper into the examination room, so you should probably leave them home. Nor may you ask anyone questions about the examination, or give or receive help from other examination candidates.

There will be some items on the examination that are being pretested for subsequent examinations. Since there is no possible way to know which questions they are, you are encouraged to answer each question on the examination. Your final score will be based only on the regular questions that have been selected for this examination and will exclude these pretest items.

Measurement of Learning Outcomes

The ACNP examination has been developed based on a taxonomy of cognitive learning. Cognitive learning occurs in a sequential pattern, from simple to complex. For example, recall of information involves the least complex behavior, while higher levels where critical thinking is involved require more complex cognitive ability. In general, mastery of lower levels must occur before the learner is able to progress to and demonstrate competency at the next level; thus, the levels represent a taxonomy of cognitive ability. Items on this examination have been developed according to this taxonomy and incorporate leveling of items based on the type of cognitive mental activity necessary to answer the question correctly. The taxonomy has six levels of cognitive mental activity.

The lowest level of the taxonomy is *knowledge (level I)*. It is the ability to recall facts about principles, discrete bits of information, facts, concepts, theories, terminology, or procedures. Recall learning is the most basic component of the learning process. Test items written at this level will ask you to define, identify, indicate, state, match, or select the best response from the possible options. The following is an example of this type of question.

A *standard of care* may be defined as:
A. Community criteria used to measure whether negligence has occurred
B. Community expectations of practice given the current available technology
C. Doing no harm
D. The most recent data written on a practice issue

Comprehension (level II) represents the lowest level of understanding. It requires translation, interpretation, and extrapolation of data. Items written at this level will ask you to interpret, explain, classify, describe, estimate, expand, recognize, suggest, summarize, compare, distinguish, or predict. The following is an example of this type of question.

Which of the following statements is correct about reimbursement for nurse practitioner services to Medicare patients?
A. The nurse practitioner must possess a master of science degree.
B. The RN must meet nurse practitioner qualifications in the state in which he or she practices.
C. Nurse practitioners may not receive reimbursement under federal guidelines.
D. Nurse practitioners are not required to work in collaboration with a physician.

Items written at the *application (level III)* level involve the use of abstractions in particular and concrete situations. The abstractions may be in the form of general ideas, rules of procedures, or generalized methods. The abstractions may be technical principles, ideas, and theories that must be remembered and applied. At this level, test takers are expected to solve problems, modify plans, manipulate data, apply principles, differentiate among choices, and demonstrate appropriate use of the information provided. The following is an example of this type of question.

Initial therapy for a patient with duodenal ulcers includes all of the following EXCEPT:
A. Cimetidine (Tagamet)
B. Ranitidine (Zantac)
C. Omeprazole (Prilosec)
D. Metoclopramide (Reglan)

Analysis (level IV) requires the candidate to recognize relationships among several parts. It involves dissection or breakdown into elements or parts so that the relative hierarchy of ideas is made clear or the relationship between the ideas is made clear or both. Items at this level require the test taker to analyze, determine, form generalizations, deduce, draw conclusions, make inferences, or interpret data from a variety of sources. The following is an example of this type of question.

You are the acute care nurse practitioner for a patient you suspect has thyrotoxicosis. Which of the following cardiac changes would you anticipate finding that most characterizes this disorder?
A. Atrial fibrillation
B. Pericardial effusion
C. Systolic murmur
D. Bradycardia

The next level of the cognitive domain is *synthesis (level V)*. It is at this level that items will require the candidate to put together elements and parts in more complex interrelationships to form a whole. This requires the examinee to arrange and combine elements to constitute a pattern or structure not clearly present before and in new and meaningful ways. The following is an example of this type of question.

A 62-year-old man with a history of chronic alcohol ingestion is admitted with acute alcohol intoxication and lobar pneumonia. Physical examination reveals pallor, a large tender liver, and consolidation of the right lower lobe. Laboratory data indicate a Hgb of 7 gm, WBC of 4000, and a platelet count of 85,000. The most likely cause of anemia in this patient is:
   A. Bone marrow suppression
   B. Gastrointestinal bleeding
   C. Vitamin D deficiency
   D. Presence of von Willibrand's disease

Finally, the highest level is *evaluation (level VI)*. This level requires a quantitative and qualitative appraisal of the data in order to make judgments about its value. The following is an example of this type of question.

Which of the following is the most likely set of laboratory values you will see in a female patient with iron-deficiency anemia?
   A. Serum iron increased, total iron-binding capacity (TIBC) normal, ferritin increased
   B. Serum iron normal, total iron-binding capacity (TIBC) normal, ferritin normal
   C. Serum iron decreased, total iron-binding capacity (TIBC) increased, ferritin decreased
   D. Serum iron decreased, total iron-binding capacity (TIBC) decreased, ferritin increased

It is important for the examinee to know that items will be written to test at each level within the cognitive domain. It is most likely, however, that the ACNP examination items will be written to test *levels III and IV, application* and *analysis* of nurse practitioner knowledge.

The test is constructed based on an analysis of job-related common health care situations that ACNPs are likely to encounter in clinical practice. Each item represents aspects of the ACNP's role.

The questions for the examination are contained in a booklet that will be given to you on the day of the examination and your answers will be recorded on a separate computer-graded test answer form. You will be responsible for verifying that you have been given the correct booklet for the examination you are eligible to take. These instructions will be repeated on the day of the examination and you are encouraged to listen carefully to the proctors as they review the instructions for the examination.

Scoring of the Examination

Scoring of the examination is based on one of the two major approaches to testing development and testing performance, *norm-referenced* or *criterion-referenced evaluation*. Norm-referenced evaluations provide information about how examinees perform relative to other examinees, while criterion-referenced evaluations provide information about how examinees perform relative to a specified standard or criterion of performance. Norm-referenced tests are useful when it is appropriate to sort individuals into groups. Because the purpose of a norm-referenced test is not only to compare people but to view their achievement in relation to other individuals, test scores are graphed and subsequent test takers are compared to the norm established by the initial group. It is easy to see how this type of approach is not a measure of an examinee's overall performance with respect to the content, but of his or her reference to the norm group.

Criterion-referenced testing, on the other hand, helps ascertain what, if anything, individuals have learned with respect to the given content area. Since these tests are used to determine whether individuals have demonstrated mastery of specific objectives, the tests are called *criterion-referenced*. Examinee's pass these tests by achieving or surpassing the score predetermined as the *criterion* of satisfactory knowledge or skill. One advantage of using such a test is that it provides a clear means of generalizing what an examinee knows. In addition, *equating*, a statistical method of scoring, is used to adjust the passing standard score to ensure comparability from test to test. Most certification examinations use these methods of scoring because they are clearly advantageous to the examinee.

The actual number of items on the examination varies from time to time; however, there are approximately 225 questions to be answered during the timed portion of the test. Of these questions, approximately 200 are scored questions while 25 are nonscored items that are undergoing pretesting. These items are pretested to determine how well they perform before they are used in the scored portion of the examination. You will not be able to distinguish nonscored from scored items; therefore, it is important to answer all questions. Your score will be based only on the number of items you answered correctly out of the 200 scored items, and so since there is no penalty for guessing, you are encouraged to answer every question. Your performance on the nonscored items has no effect on your passing score. You can expect your scores to be sent to you about 6–8 weeks after the examination and will include your total raw and percentage score on the entire test as well as the total raw score required to pass the examination. The report usually will also include your scores on each of the major content areas of the examination. For example, your scores may be as reported in the following manner:

	Passing Score	Your Scores	Percent Scores	Maximum Scores
Total Score	140	144	72.0	200
I. System-Specific Health Problems		52	67.5	77
II. Common Problems in Acute Care		47	71.2	66
III. Professionalism in Advanced Practice		16	80.0	20
IV. Issues and Trends		14	82.4	17
V. Health Promotion & Risk Assessment		15	75.0	20

Item Type Examples

Measurement of performance may be accomplished in many ways. The ACNP examination uses an objective paper and pencil measurement instrument from which you will select responses to items from among various choices. Most common in this category of evaluation instruments is selected response tests. The multiple choice, or forced-choice, item is one type of selected response test. Multiple choice tests are the most widely used type of objective examination. The multiple choice test is particularly useful when many examinees must be evaluated under standardized conditions; therefore, the ACNP examination has been developed using this format because of the ease of administering and scoring the test.

In multiple choice exam tests, the question is referred to as the *stem*. The stem is either an introductory statement in which a question may be asked, a problem may be posed, a statement left uncompleted, or a scenario presented. The following is an example of a stem:

The most common depressive experience in the hospitalized patient is

The stem is usually followed by four alternative possible options, one that is the correct option and three that are *distracters*. Examples of distracters that might go with the stem above include:

A. Delirium
B. Alcohol withdrawal
C. Digitalis toxicity
D. Grief

While these distracters may be completely wrong, partially wrong, or less comprehensive than the intended answer, their primary intent is to distract the examinee's attention from selecting the best/correct answer. The following is a guide to help you prepare for studying for this type of test and is intended to help you become better equipped and more test-wise when responding to various stems, and to more appropriately confront test items.

Preparation for Studying

This book delineates a curriculum for the ACNP and is intended primarily for the individual preparing for the certification examination for ACNPs. Others may choose to use the text as a basic review guide. Regardless, you should prepare for any studying with a comprehensive plan. Anyone preparing for an examination undergoes a variety of responses from anxiety to anticipation to optimism to confidence. Factors that differentiate the anxious test taker from the confident one are found in knowing how to prepare for and take examinations such as this. This preparation must begin with a plan for taking the examination. The following may be used to assist you in developing your own personal plan.

KNOW YOURSELF

Identify if anxiety is a factor for you when you are going to take an examination. If so, you have a lot of company, because most people experience anxiety in this situation. Some anxiety is beneficial, while some is detrimental. Effectiveness in taking a test is learned, and that effectiveness contributes to exam success. Channeling the negative energy created by anxiety could be put to better use in your plan for studying. Ways to do this include identifying what has and what hasn't worked for you and knowing what test-taking skills have worked for you in the past. Reviewing the test-taking skills you have used in the past makes you confident about taking the test, for example. Ask yourself what your feelings are before an exam situation, during an exam situation, or afterwards. It helps to review these strategies, and capitalize on these positive strategies while trying to eliminate the negative ones. Consider adding some of the ones presented in this chapter to your repertoire.

INCREASE YOUR SKILLS IN THINKING

Remember that cognitive learning occurs in a sequential pattern, from simple to complex. You must learn to master the preceding cognitive learning level before mastery of the next level can occur. Remember that the first level is *knowledge*, being able to recall information. Next is *comprehension* or the ability to understand. This level is followed by *application* to a clinical situation, followed by *analysis* which requires recognition of relationships among data. *Synthesis*, the next level is the ability to form interrelationships. Finally, the highest level of learning to be mastered is *evaluation*. Begin studying each section with an overview that focuses on general information and then moves to the specific information. For example, review general assessment and management principles the ACNP would consider when managing any cardiac patient, then review more specific information related to a patient with coronary artery disease, then to a patient with myocardial infarction, and then to a patient with congestive failure. Finally, prioritize your treatment plans as well as determine which situations are appropriate to consult and/or refer. Through this process—movement from general to specific and simple to complex information that requires prerequisite knowledge—you will be able to identify your strengths and areas where additional review and study may be necessary.

ORGANIZE YOUR TIME AND STUDY MATERIALS

It is important to develop good study habits. In your basic nursing program you learned that discipline related to study was necessary in order to achieve success. This discipline included the development of study habits that enhance learning and involve organization of both time and study materials. Decisions that you make about studying should be realistic. Make time for regular study knowing that last-minute "cramming" is not the key to success on an examination, but just creates additional anxiety, thus creating a "study calendar" may prove helpful. You may also find it helpful to study with a partner or in a group. You may know if this technique has worked for you in the past. Systematic studying, begun at least a month before the examination, should incorporate small blocks of study time. These study blocks should each exceed no more than 1–2 hours at a time, since there is only so much that the mind can absorb at any one time. You should select no more than two study references. Selecting numerous books and relying on countless resources only promote confusion and increase anxiety. Begin to study material that is less familiar or material in which you consider yourself weak. Once the review of these areas is completed, you can move more quickly through content with which you are more familiar thus having time to return for reinforced review of those weaker content areas. Finally, you should include a simulated or mock test situation in which you answer sample test questions in a timed setting.

REINFORCE LEARNED CONTENT

A comprehensive study plan should include the opportunity to reinforce that which has been learned. The value of personal discipline and study cannot be stressed enough, and should be the central focus of your study plan; however, there is also an added value to cooperative group study. Individual review of content will assist the examinee to recall important relevant facts and concepts prior to taking the ACNP examination, but when small study groups of two to three individuals subsequently review each section and present different parts to each other this ultimately enhances individual learning.

Basic Rules for Test Taking

ACNP examination candidates who know how to take a timed multiple choice test have conquered one of the major hurdles of the examination. It is as important as the content being tested. The "how" of test taking, also called "test-wiseness," can be learned and used to improve test scores. Examinees are encouraged to become test-wise. That is, ACNP examination candidates should develop the skills necessary to choose correct responses to a stem when presented with a set of alternative options. The following are some suggestions for building a repertoire of effective test-taking strategies:

READ EACH WORD IN THE STEM CAREFULLY

Each item on the examination is a client-based scenario that presents data necessary for you to answer each question correctly. As you respond to each item, relate each of the options to the data that have been provided. Is there congruency? Is the stem asking for the most common or least common response? Is the stem asking for you to choose the one exception in the alternatives? Is the stem asking for the highest or the lowest priority? Is the stem asking you for subjective or objective data, diagnosis, therapeutic management, or patient education? Is the question asking for a response requiring independent, interdependent collaborative, or referral functions of the ACNP? Finally, is the stem requiring you to know, understand, apply, analyze, synthesize, or evaluate information presented?

AVOID READING INTO THE MEANING OF OR SEARCHING FOR HIDDEN MEANINGS IN AN ITEM

Reliable and valid test items are direct and to the point. Each item has only one correct response and you should not try to reinterpret what the question is asking, nor should you read additional significance into the item. You must ask yourself, "What is this question asking?" Test items will have key words or phrases that are intended to assist you in understanding what has been asked. Read the following stem for an example of this.

Third party reimbursement is the traditional method of health care provider payment in the United States. An advantage of this system includes which of the following?

The first sentence of the stem intends to assist the test taker in clarifying the question. By maintaining clarity of the item, your ability to eliminate distracters will be easier. Do not assume information that has not been provided. Just as you do not put words into your patient's mouth, do not add words to the test item.

REPHRASE THE STEM IN YOUR OWN WORDS

In a particularly complex item, it is helpful to put the stem into your own words. This may assist you in selecting the best response from the alternatives provided. For example, you might say to yourself "this item is asking me to distinguish between an iatrogenic and insulin-dependent diabetes mellitus."

ELIMINATE INCORRECT RESPONSES

Construction of multiple choice test items requires there to be one correct and three incorrect alternatives. A formula that can be used to assist the examinee in selecting from among the alternatives is to ask yourself if each possible alternative is correct or incorrect with respect to the stem. If your choice for the answer is correct/true and it answers the question, while the others are incorrect, then you have most likely selected the best alternative. In a well-constructed examination, all options (including the distracters) should be plausible; however, the examinee must remember that the correct response is unequivocally correct while the distracters are unequivocally wrong. Another method of rejecting incorrect responses is to rule options in or out in a process of elimination. Eliminating those you know to be incorrect from those you are not sure are correct increases the likelihood of a correct response.

USE YOUR EXPERIENCE TO GUIDE IN THE SELECTION OF THE BEST RESPONSE

If you are faced with a difficult item or have not managed a patient with the diagnosis presented in the question, and you are not able to immediately identify the correct answer, you should draw on your comprehensive experience and education to identify what you do know about the situation. If you are not sure of exactly what you would do, you may be sure of what you would not do. It is no surprise that you possess a wealth of knowledge in your unconscious upon which you can draw.

BEWARE OF ANSWERS THAT CONTAIN SPECIFIC QUALIFIERS

Options that contain the words "always" or "never" are rarely the correct response. They usually do not fit within a reasonable framework of practice since, for example, few things always or never occur. However, there are sometimes exceptions, so read the stem carefully.

LOOK FOR INCOMPATIBLE STEMS AND OPTIONS

Options that are grammatically or otherwise different from all of the others are often not the correct response. Avoid choosing that alternative because it is different from the others. For example, if the item requires that you select the medication most likely to be prescribed for a patient with a bacterial pneumonia and three of the options are antibiotics and one is a non-steroidal anti-inflammatory, the most plausible answer will be one of the three antibiotic choices. This may seem obvious to you, but many examination candidates select the option that is different because they are "distracted" from what they know to be true.

SELECT THE MOST INCLUSIVE/COMPREHENSIVE ANSWER

If, after using the test-taking strategies presented, you find that two or more of the response options are correct, then you must select the one that is the most comprehensive. If two of the response options are reasonable but one answer includes the other or has greater detail, then that answer would be the best option. For example, if the stem asks you to choose between the following vital sign changes that which is most likely to occur in increased intracranial pressure—bradycardia and increased systolic blood pressure or bradycardia and widened pulse pressure—you would choose the latter because it is a more inclusive and comprehensive response.

CHECK RESPONSES AFTER SELECTING YOUR BEST ANSWER

Because distracters are intended to divert the attention of the examinee, you must make an attempt to check each response following your selection of the best answer from each of the alternatives. Keep in mind that an answer, in and of itself, may be correct on its own, but incorrect in terms of what the item seeks. After selecting your best response, avoid changing your answer if, upon reflection, it just doesn't seem right. On the other hand, if information is provided later in the examination that now assists you to make more complex cognitive connections and you believe your previous answer is now incorrect, do change your answer.

LEAVE NO ANSWER BLANK

Every question should be answered. By leaving a question unanswered, there is virtually no possibility that you will get the question right. Remember, even an "off-the-wall" guess gives you a 25% chance of choosing a correct response. Short of tossing a coin (which only has two sides) or saying "eenie meanie miney mo," there are some tried-and-true, non–research-based methods for guessing (i.e., when the examination candidate is not able to use any of the above strategies for answering a question). Some of these include: selecting the correct response from either option B or C from the four alternatives presented; selecting an option that is a direct opposite of another option (e.g., if the stem asks for a common side effect of a particular medication and the options include diarrhea and constipation); or selecting the longest-worded option.

MANAGE YOUR TIME JUDICIOUSLY

The ACNP examination is a timed test, so you should avoid spending too much time on one item. On the other hand, you should also avoid rushing through the test. Generally, allowing about 1 minute per question is reasonable. When you have completed the entire test, go back over it to answer any items you did not answer the first time, reconsider those questions of which you were unsure, and review your previous selections.

Sample Study Plan

IDENTIFY CONTENT AREAS FOR REVIEW

Begin your study with an analysis of the content presented in your nurse practitioner program. Ask yourself which content areas you were most comfortable with, and those you were least comfortable with. What was easy for you to learn and what required additional time and practice? What were your strengths and what were your weaknesses? What content was taught early in the program and what was taught later? Use this analysis to study the content that was least comfortable, areas needing additional practice, weak areas, and content taught early in your program first.

ORGANIZE YOUR TIME AND MATERIAL

Identify a special place for study that is quiet and has room for your books, papers, and you. Select a place that is convenient and comfortable. This should be an area that permits uninterrupted study time. Decide on a regular time for study and ensure that you maintain a regular commitment to it. Some people require absolute quiet, while others prefer music. Some people identify a greater attention to learning in the morning while others prefer afternoon or evenings. Some people must eat while studying, others have to outline, underline, or take notes. There are no rules other than to know what works best for you in order to enhance your plan of study.

USE EFFECTIVE MEMORY DEVICES TO INCREASE RETENTION OF INFORMATION

Memorization of information based on repetitiveness is rarely imprinted in long-term memory. Everyone has their personal favorite mechanism to assist in memorizing information. This may include the use of acronyms or mnemonics to remember lists of things (e.g., the mnemonic everyone learned to memorize the names of each of the 12 pairs of cranial nerves). In addition to acronyms or mnemonics, individuals can develop other skills that are intended to facilitate rapid recall of information such as creating mental pictures or using rhymes, songs, and limericks. Some have found that transcribing these memory devices onto small index cards that can be reviewed during short breaks during the day or making an audiotape to listen to while driving to and from work can be extremely helpful.

EVALUATE YOUR PROGRESS

Periodically, it is important to survey your progress. Make a checklist that outlines your study plan and identifies specific content areas to be reviewed. Keep track of your progress noting content you have mastered, attainment of higher scores on the practice exam questions, or in areas with which you feel confident. Be sure to also review your progress in areas needing additional review. Another way to evaluate your progress is to validate your knowledge by simulating a timed test situation to provide additional reinforcement of learning. For example, you might take the practice test items in this text in a specified time frame as previously described. Use a #2 pencil to practice filling in bubbles on a sheet of paper. Evaluate your results after completing the test questions following each section of study and again upon completion of all study. If on average, you answered more than 75% of the items in a section correctly, you will likely be effective in answering items in that content area on the ACNP examination. If, however, you answered less than 75% correctly, you must identify the reason for the incorrect response. For example, ask yourself if your answer was incorrect because you did not know the content or because you did not read the item carefully to determine what it was asking? The answer regarding your reason for an incorrect response will prove invaluable as you study for the examination. It will tell you if additional study time is required in content areas or on test-wiseness.

KNOW THE DETAILS ABOUT THE TEST ADMINISTRATION SITE

Ensure that you have received your admission ticket to the examination. It will confirm the time, date, and place the examination will be administered. It may be helpful to drive to the test administration site about a week ahead on the same day of the week that the examination will be administered so you are familiar with traffic patterns and parking. After you park on this preliminary dry run, actually walk to the examination administration site so you can visualize where the test will be given. On the day of the examination, allow ample time to arrive early so that you can have time to relax. Room temperatures at test administration sites vary so you should dress comfortably in layers of clothing so that you can adjust to your personal comfort level. If you have particular medical or other needs that you are aware of prior to the examination, you must contact the ANCC for them to accommodate your request for additional time, etc.

BE PHYSICALLY PREPARED TO TAKE THE EXAMINATION

Plan to complete your studying a week before the examination. Make sure you are well rested prior to the examination since fatigue impairs concentration ability. Request the day off prior to the exam to relax. Do not take on any stressful activities for about a week prior to the exam such as a move. If you work alternative shifts, adjust your work schedule to avoid sleep deprivation. Your diet prior to the exam should be well balanced, avoiding foods or beverages you do not normally consume (such as coffee, tea, caffeinated beverages, or chocolate). On the other hand, if you are a coffee drinker, the day before the exam is not the day to decide to quit.

MANAGE ANY TEST ANXIETY YOU MAY EXPERIENCE

All test takers experience some anxiety. A certain amount of anxiety is motivating, but be prepared to control unwanted anxiety. Develop and practice the following stress-reduction techniques and use them during the exam as needed.

- *Mental rehearsal* involves anticipating activities and the environment during the examination. Ask yourself how you will feel, what the room will be like, what you will wear, how you will take the exam, what you will say to yourself during the exam, and what you will do if you have test anxiety.

- *Relaxation exercises* involve contracting and relaxing various muscle groups to relieve the physical effects of anxiety. By practicing these exercises ahead of time, systematically contracting and relaxing muscle groups from your toes to your neck to release energy for concentration, you will be able to do these exercises during the exam to promote relaxation.
- *Deep breathing exercises* that require you to take deep cleansing breaths in through your nose slowly while counting to five and then exhaling slowly through your mouth while counting to ten increase oxygen flow to the lungs and brain. Deep breathing also decreases tension and helps manage anxiety by causing you to focus on your breathing.
- *Clear your mind of negative or self-destructive talk* such as "I'm going to fail." Eliminate all negative thoughts and focus on the positive ones repeatedly saying to yourself that you can do this because you are prepared for the experience.
- *Remove distractions from your mind.* Do not allow distractions from those around you or the environment to break your concentration. You must focus all your energy on concentrating on the examination.

REWARD YOURSELF AS YOU STUDY

Determine ahead of time how you will reward yourself following a successful study session and after the examination.

BECOME YOUR OWN BEST CHEERLEADER

Build your confidence through self-talk. Give yourself that all important pep talk or find someone else to do it. Knowing that you have support from a significant other who is confident of your ability to succeed, and more importantly, your own belief in that ability, is one of the most important factors in achieving success on the ACNP examination. *Remember, you can make it happen!*

References

American Association of Critical-Care Nurses and American Nurses' Association. *Standards of Clinical Practice and Scope of Practice for the Acute Care Nurse Practitioner.* Washington, DC: American Nurses Publishing, 1995.

AACN Certification Corporation and American Nurses Credentialing Center. *Recommended Study Reference List for the ACNP Examination.* Aliso Viejo, CA: AACN, 1996.

American Nurses Credentialing Center. (1996). *Nurse Practitioner Certification Examinations.* Washington, DC: American Nurses Credentialing Center.

Bloom, B. (1956). *Taxonomy of Educational Objectives: The Classification of Educational Goals. Handbook I: Cognitive Domain.* New York: David McKay Co., Inc.

Cummings, A. (1995). Test review made easy. *Learning 23*, (5), 68.

Dickinson-Hazard, N. (1989). Making the grade as a test-taker. *Pediatr Nurs 15*, 302–304.

Dickinson-Hazard, N. (1990). The psychology of successful test taking. *Pediatr Nurs 16*, 66–67.

Dickinson-Hazard, N. (1990). Study smart. *Pediatr Nurs 16*, 314–316.

Dickinson-Hazard, N. (1990). Develop your thinking skills for improved test taking. *Pediatr Nurs 16*, 480–481.

Gronlund, N.E. (1988). *How to Construct Achievement Tests.* New York: Prentice-Hall.

Morris, L.L., Fitz-Gibbon, C.T., & Lindheim, E. (1987). *How to Measure Performance and Use Tests.* Newbury Park, CA: Sage Publications.

National Council of State Boards of Nursing, Inc. (1987). *NCLEX-RN: Test Plan for the National Council Licensure Exam—NCLEX/CAT.* Chicago: National Council Of State Boards of Nursing, Inc.

Sides, M., & Cailles, N.B. (1994). *Nurse's Guide to Successful Test Taking* (2nd ed.). Philadelphia: J.B. Lippincott Co.

CHAPTER 2

Pulmonary Disorders

Vickie Ruch, RN, MSN, CS, FNP, ANP

Pneumonia

DEFINITION

An acute infection of lung parenchyma including alveolar spaces and interstitial tissue; involvement may be confined to an entire lobe, a segment of a lobe, alveoli contiguous to bronchi, or interstitial tissue. These distinctions are generally based upon x-ray findings.

ETIOLOGY/INCIDENCE

1. Up to 6 million annual episodes in the United States, with up to 1 million of those patients requiring hospitalization.
2. First-ranked cause of death from infectious disease and the sixth-ranked cause of death overall in the United States.
3. Fourth leading cause of death in those >65 years, and the most common cause of death in those >100 years old.
4. Mortality risk from pneumonia is three to five times greater in those >65 years old than in younger patients.
5. The most common cause of transfer from a skilled nursing facility (SNF) to a hospital.
6. About $1 billion per year are spent to treat pneumonia.
7. Over 275,000 cases per year of nosocomial, institutional/hospital-acquired pneumonia (HAP), usually in seriously ill patients.
   A. Second most common nosocomial infection in the United States but has the highest morbidity and mortality.
   B. Increases hospital length of stay by an average of 7–9 days per patient.
   C. Occurs in approximately 5–10 cases per 1000 hospital admissions.
   D. Ventilator-associated pneumonia (VAP) is correlated with a 6–20 times increased incidence of HAP among patients being mechanically ventilated.
   E. Approximately one third to one half of all HAP deaths are the direct result of infection, with a higher attributable mortality if presence of bacteremia and/or virulent pathogen such as *Pseudomonas aeruginosa* or *Acinetobacter* species.

PATHOPHYSIOLOGY

1. Infection by any of a variety of microbes can lead to pneumonia.
   A. Viruses
      1) Influenzas A and B
      2) Parainfluenza viruses
      3) Respiratory syncytial viruses (RSV)
      4) Adenovirus
   B. Bacteria
      1) Hospital-acquired
         a. *Escherichia coli*
         b. *Klebsiella pneumoniae*
         c. *Enterobacter* spp.
         d. Enterobacteriaceae
         e. *Pseudomonas aeruginosa*
         f. *Staphylococcus aureus*
         g. *Serratia* spp.
      2) Community-acquired
         a. *Streptococcus pneumoniae*
         b. *Haemophilus influenzae*
         c. *Staphylococcus aureus*
         d. Anaerobic bacteria
         e. *Moraxella catarrhalis*
         f. *Klebsiella pneumoniae*
         g. *Legionella* spp.
         h. *Bacteroides* spp.
         i. *Peptococcus* spp.
         j. *Peptostreptococcus* spp.
         k. *Fusobacterium* spp.
   C. Fungi
      1) Hospital-acquired
         a. *Candida*
         b. *Aspergillus* spp.
      2) Community-acquired
         a. *Blastomyces dermatitidis*
         b. *Histoplasma capsulatum*
         c. *Cryptococcus neoformans*
         d. *Coccidioides immitis*
   D. Other causative microbes
      1) Mycobacteria
         a. *Mycobacterium tuberculosis* (TB)
      2) Rickettsia
      3) Protozoa
      4) Parasites
         a. *Pneumocystis carinii* pneumonia (PCP)
      5) *Chlamydia pneumoniae* (TWAR agent)
      6) *Mycoplasma pneumoniae*
2. Bacteria often reach the lower airway without leading to disease, due to defense by the host's intact, complex immune system. For pneumonia to occur, therefore, requires:
   A. Virulent pathogen
   B. Large exposure to pathogen *and/or*
   C. Immunocompromised host

3. Patients with community-acquired pneumonia (CAP) may have pathogens reach the lung via:
   A. Inhaling airborne pathogens
   B. Aspiration from a colonized upper airway
   C. Hematogenous spread of pathogens
   D. Direct inoculation from adjacent sites of infection
4. Institutional, nosocomial/HAP is generally defined as that occurring ≥48 hours after admission and excludes any infection that is incubating at the time of admission. Such critically ill, hospitalized patients often acquire pneumonia from:
   A. Colonized gastrointestinal (GI) tract (i.e., via nasogastric [NG] tube which presents pathogens from the gut to the oropharynx, microaspiration of such pathogens down small leaks around endotracheal tube [ETT]
   B. Contaminated hospital environment (i.e., directly via ETT, mechanical ventilator tubing, lack of handwashing by health care workers)
5. Risk factors to develop pneumonia include several factors.
   A. Primary medical status associated with increased infection risks
      1) Other lung disease
      2) Diabetes mellitus (DM)
      3) Elderly
      4) Acquired immunodeficiency syndrome (AIDS)
      5) Adult respiratory distress syndrome (ARDS)
      6) Cardiac disease
   B. Comorbid/associated illnesses that may impair lower airway defenses
      1) Cancer (CA)
      2) Cerebrovascular accident (CVA)
      3) Hypotension
      4) Alcoholism
      5) Hypoxia
      6) Head trauma
      7) Sepsis
      8) Hypophosphatemia
   C. Therapeutic interventions
      1) ETT
      2) NG tube
   D. Medications that may interfere with how the patient's lungs may handle bacteria
      1) β-Blockers
      2) Calcium channel blockers
      3) Oxygen
      4) Acetylsalicylic acid (ASA)
      5) Digoxin
      6) Morphine
      7) Antibiotics
      8) Antacids
      9) Corticosteroids
      10) Cimetidine
   E. Poor nutritional status
      1) Interferes with humoral and cell-mediated immunity in the lung
      2) Increases epithelial cell receptivity to bacteria
6. Certain conditions may predispose to pneumonia from specific pathogenic microbes.

A. SNF residents and/or the elderly are associated with pneumonia from:
   1) Methicillin-resistant *Staphylococcus aureus* (MRSA)
   2) Respiratory viruses
   3) TB
   4) Enterobacteriaceae
   5) *Haemophilus influenzae*
   6) Pneumococcus
   7) Enteric gram-negative bacilli
B. Patients with immunocompromise are associated with pneumonia from:
   1) TB
   2) PCP
   3) Cytomegalovirus
   4) *Cryptococcus neoformans*
   5) *Mycobacterium avium* complex (MAC)
   6) *Nocardia* spp.
   7) *Salmonella*
C. Chronic obstructive pulmonary disease (COPD) patients are associated with pneumonia from:
   1) *Haemophilus influenzae*
   2) *Streptococcus pneumoniae*
   3) *Moraxella catarrhalis*
   4) *Branhamella catarrhalis*
   5) *Pneumococcus*
D. Influenza epidemics are associated with pneumonia from *Staphylococcus aureus*. Post influenza also may be associated with:
   1) *Pneumococcus*
   2) *Haemophilus influenzae*
E. Altered level of consciousness (ALOC) and/or suspected gastric aspiration are associated with pneumonia from anaerobic pathogens.
F. Mechanical ventilation and/or ARDS are associated with pneumonia from:
   1) *Pseudomonas aeruginosa*
   2) Enteric gram-negative bacilli (EGNB).
G. Alcoholic patients are associated with pneumonia from:
   1) TB
   2) *Haemophilus influenzae*
   3) *Klebsiella pneumoniae*
   4) *Pneumococcus*
H. Cardiac patients are associated with pneumonia from:
   1) Gram-negative bacilli
   2) *Pneumococcus*

SIGNS AND SYMPTOMS

Clinical manifestations of pneumonia were traditionally thought to be manifested as typical and atypical presentations, which were believed to correlate patterns of signs and symptoms with specific pathogens. Recent data suggest that these distinctions may be less distinct than were once thought, however.

1. Acute bacterial pneumonia (*Streptococcus pneumoniae* most common)
   A. Sudden onset: Fever, chills, pleuritic chest pain, cough, purulent sputum.

       B. Evidence of consolidation on examination of the chest.

       C. Leukocytosis with leftward shift; leukopenia in some patients.

       D. Patchy or lobar infiltrates on chest x-ray (CXR).

       E. Arterial blood-gas abnormalities due to hypoxia.

          1) May show hypoxemia, with $P_{O_2} < 80$ mm Hg

       F. Gram's stain typically shows gram-positive diplococci in *S. pneumoniae*.

2. Atypical pneumonia (*Mycoplasma pneumoniae, Legionella, Chlamydia pneumoniae, Pneumocystis carinii*)

       A. Constitutional symptoms, including headache, myalgia, malaise, low-grade fever; cough, minimal chest pain, scanty sputum production.

       B. Minimal physical findings; usually no respiratory distress.

       C. Mucoid sputum (rather than purulent) that lacks a predominant bacterial organism on Gram's stain.

       D. Normal or slightly elevated white blood cell (WBC) count.

       E. Segmental or subsegmental opacities on chest x-ray.

       F. Almost 50% of AIDS patients initially present with pulmonary disease. The most common pulmonary infection is PCP. Chest x-ray often demonstrates diffuse interstitial or alveolar infiltrates.

3. Anaerobic pneumonia (*Bacteroides melaninogenicus*, anaerobic streptococci, and *Fusobacterium nucleatum*)

       A. Predisposition to aspiration

       B. Poor dental hygiene

       C. Fever, weight loss, malaise

       D. Foul-smelling sputum

       E. Infiltrate in dependent lung zone, with single or multiple areas of cavitation or pleural effusion

4. Pulmonary tuberculosis

       A. Fatigue, weight loss, fever, night sweats

       B. Productive cough; pulmonary infiltrates on CXR

       C. Positive tuberculin skin test reaction (in most cases)

       D. Acid-fast bacilli on sputum smear

       E. Sputum culture positive for *Mycobacterium tuberculosis*

5. Viral pneumonia (influenza types A and B and adenoviruses)

       A. Nonproductive cough.

       B. Constitutional symptoms, often including malaise, headache, myalgia.

       C. Fever

       D. WBC count is often low, but may be normal or moderately elevated.

       E. Gram-stained sputum smears reveal neutrophils or mononuclear cells but no predominant bacterial pathogens.

       F. Chest x-ray may show an interstitial pneumonia or peribronchial thickening.

PHYSICAL FINDINGS

1. Physical examination may be normal in early stages.
2. Bacterial pneumonia.

       A. Evidence of consolidation

          1) Dullness to percussion

          2) Bronchial breath sounds, egophony

          3) Increased fremitus

          4) Whispered pectoriloquy

       B. Crackles

3. Dyspnea.
4. Elderly patients may fail to manifest expected clinical findings of pneumonia.
   A. May only be heralded by confusion and/or altered mental status
5. May see worsening of underlying disease such as COPD or congestive heart failure (CHF).
6. Atypical pneumonia.
   A. No physical findings of consolidation
7. Viral pneumonia.
   A. No physical findings of consolidation

DIFFERENTIAL DIAGNOSIS

1. Acute bronchitis
2. Primary tuberculosis
3. CHF
4. Pulmonary thromboembolism
5. Lung tumor
6. Atelectasis
7. Drug reactions
8. Pulmonary hemorrhage (more often as a result of mechanical ventilation)
9. ARDS
10. Chemical, noninfectious pneumonitis (from aspiration)
11. Lung contusion (in trauma patients)

DIAGNOSTIC TESTS/FINDINGS

1. CXR: Typical findings for pneumonia are likely to include patchy or lobar infiltrates. The radiographic pattern is not pathognomonic of a specific cause of pneumonia, however.
2. Gram's stain/sputum smear may reveal the predominant organism.
3. Sputum culture and sensitivity (C&S).
   A. Induce for specimen if unable to obtain an adequate sputum specimen by spontaneous cough.
   B. To review effective technique for successful sputum induction, refer to the references following this section.
4. The presence of bacteria within polymorphonuclear leukocytes (PMNs) is highly suggestive of infection.
5. Obtain complete blood count (CBC) with differential, electrolytes.
6. Pulse oximetry/arterial oxygen saturation.
7. Consider arterial blood gases (ABGs) (especially for HAP patients).
   A. To review ABG interpretation, refer to the references following this section.
8. Before antimicrobial therapy is started, obtain blood cultures in patients who appear especially ill.
   A. Obtain two sets of blood cultures from separate sites in hospitalized patients.
   B. When blood cultures do isolate a pathogen, other sites of infection must be excluded.
   C. Up to 50% of patients with severe HAP have an additional source of infection present (e.g., sinusitis, vascular catheter-related infection, pseudomembraneous enterocolitis, urinary tract infection.)

9. Patients with a pleural effusion may need to have a diagnostic thoracentesis to rule out complications (e.g., empyema, especially if large effusion present or patient appears toxic). (See "Pleural Effusion" in the following section.)

MANAGEMENT/TREATMENT

Referrals and Admissions

1. Several factors enter into the decision to admit a patient with CAP to an acute care unit, rather than to manage CAP on an outpatient basis. The frequency and importance of these factors may differ somewhat between types of treatment settings and medical providers. Depending upon the setting, the acute care nurse practitioner (ACNP) may be called upon to arrange hospital admission and to manage the patient with physician collaboration.
   A. Hospital admission criteria frequently include:
      1) Comorbid medical problems (especially alcohol abuse, asthma, coronary artery disease, CHF, COPD, CA, or diabetes mellitus)
      2) Lung involvement (>1 lobe)
      3) Clinical appearance (looks very sick)
      4) Arterial P_{O_2} <60 mm Hg on room air, or arterial P_{CO_2} >50 mm Hg on room air
      5) Respiratory distress (especially tachypnea >30 breaths/min)
      6) Inability to maintain oral intake
      7) Low estimation of patient reliability
   B. Additional criteria often cited
      1) The need for mechanical ventilation
      2) Moderately to severely abnormal vital signs (including blood pressure [BP] <90/60 mm Hg, or heart rate [HR] >140 bpm)
      3) Inadequate home care support
      4) Confusion and/or altered mental status
      5) Fever (> 101°F)
      6) Abnormal WBC (WBC $<4 \times 10^9$/L or $>30 \times 10^9$/L, or an absolute neutrophil count $<1 \times 10^9$/L)
      7) Suspected virulent microbiologic cause
      8) Immunocompromise (AIDS, postsplenectomy state, etc.)
      9) Suspected aspiration (gastric or oropharyngeal secretions)
      10) Elderly (age >65 years old)
      11) Failure of outpatient management
   C. Additional admission factors
      1) Other coexisting illnesses or conditions (malnutrition, chronic renal failure, any chronic liver disease, or previous hospitalization for pneumonia within the previous year)
      2) Extrapulmonary sites of disease (meningitis, septic arthritis, etc.)
      3) Abnormal renal function (serum creatinine >1.2 mg/dL, or blood urea nitrogen [BUN] >20 mg/dL [>7 mmol/L])
      4) Other unfavorable CXR findings (presence of a cavity, pleural effusion, or rapid CXR spreading)
      5) Hematocrit (Hct) <30%, or hemoglobin (Hgb) <9 gm/dL
      6) Other signs of sepsis or organ dysfunction (metabolic acidosis, increased prothrombin time (PT), increased partial thromboplastin time (PTT), decreased platelets, or fibrin split products >1:40)

2. *Patients with severe community-acquired pneumonia may need prompt admission to intensive care unit (ICU).* Depending upon the setting, the ACNP may be called upon to help arrange hospital admit/ICU transfer with physician consult. A physician needs to manage the patient, while the ACNP may collaborate with the physician. *Referral to a pulmonary/critical care MD specialist is also advisable to follow the patient through this potentially life-threatening course. Any of these may be indicators for ICU admit*:
   A. Tachypnea (>30 breaths/min)
   B. Acute respiratory failure (PaO_2/FIO_2 ratio <250 mm Hg)
   C. The need for mechanical ventilation
   D. Marked CXR abnormalities (bilateral involvement, multiple lobe infiltrates, or infiltrate increase by ≥50% within 2 days of hospital admission)
   E. Shock (BP <90/60 mm Hg)
   F. The need for vasopressors for >4 hours
   G. Oliguria (urinary output <20 mL/hr, or total urinary output <80 mL/4 hr—unless another explanation is available), or acute renal failure (necessitating renal dialysis)
3. *Patients with HAP need to be managed by a physician, while the ACNP may collaborate with the physician. Those patients with severe HAP need to be followed through this potentially life-threatening course by a pulmonary/ infectious disease specialist MD. Depending upon the setting, the ACNP may be called upon to arrange ICU transfer and/or physician specialist referral.*

Pharmacologic and Treatment Plans

1. Antimicrobial therapy: General principles
   A. Duration of therapy needs to be individualized and is gauged by severity of illness, rapidity of clinical response, infecting pathogen, and choice of antimicrobial agent(s). Treatment durations commonly range from 10–14 days. Longer courses may be needed on occasion (e.g., *Legionella* species may require a 21-day course).
   B. Optimal treatment can better be directed by sputum Gram's stain and C&S results (i.e., from sputum, blood, and possibly pleural fluid), once available (within 48–72 hours). These results may be more useful in the treatment of HAP, however.
   C. Empiric treatment (pending clinical response and/or results of C&S and Gram's stain)
      1) May be applied to the two basic categories of pneumonia
         a. CAP
         b. Institutional, nosocomial/HAP
      2) Needs to take into account local bacterial spectra and patterns of antimicrobial resistance.
      3) Empiric approach attempts to categorize patients based on likelihood of certain organisms and their anticipated sensitivities and possible resistance. This method relies on assessments of:
         a. Disease severity
         b. Presence of risk factors for specific organisms
      4) Empiric antibiotic (ABX) choice can be guided more effectively by placing the patient into one of the 4 CAP categories or one of the 3 HAP categories identified in the 1993 and 1996 American Thoracic

Sociey (ATS) consensus statements on CAP and HAP, respectively (Niederman et al., 1993; Campbell et al., 1996). These classifications include the above-listed assessments, in addition to:

a. Age and comorbidity (for CAP)

b. Expected outpatient versus inpatient management (for CAP)

c. Time of onset (for HAP).

5) ATS consensus statements on CAP and HAP are empiric treatment guidelines that use generalized categories, excluding patients with immunosuppression. Such patients need additional considerations in the appropriate choice of pharmacologic intervention, and may well benefit from referral to an infectious disease or immunology physician specialist.

a. Depending upon the setting, the ACNP may be called upon to collaborate with the patient's attending physician to manage such patient's care and/or to make referral to a physician specialist.

b. Refer to the references following this section, as well as the sections of this ACNP review book which address the medical management of patients with immunocompromise.

2. Antimicrobial therapy for CAP

A. Outpatient CAP treatment: Younger adult (≤60 years) without comorbidity (Niederman et al., 1993)

1) Macrolide (i.e., erythromycin 250–500 mg PO qid × 10–14 days, or clarithromycin 250 mg PO q12 h × 10–14 days, or azithromycin 500 mg PO on day 1 and then 250 mg PO qd on days 2–5); or

2) Tetracycline (e.g., tetracycline 250–500 mg PO qid × 10–14 days, or doxycycline 100 mg PO bid × 10–14 days)

3) *Note:* Avoid tetracyclines or clarithromycin in pregnancy

B. Outpatient CAP treatment: Older adult (≥60 years) and/or comorbidity (Niederman et al., 1993)

1) Second-generation cephalosporin (e.g., cefuroxime axetil 250–500 mg PO bid × 10 days, or cefaclor 500 mg PO q8h × 10 days, or cefixime 400 mg PO qd × 10 days); or

2) Trimethoprim-sulfamethoxazole (TMP-SMX) (e.g., 160/800 mg, one DS tab PO q12h × 10–14 days); or

3) β-Lactam/β-lactamase inhibitor (e.g., amoxicillin-clavulanate 500 mg PO q8h × 10 days)—*plus*, may need to *add* erythromycin or other macrolide, especially if suspect *Legionella* species (e.g., erythromycin 250–500 mg PO qid × 10–14 days, or clarithromycin 250 mg PO q12h × 7–14 days, or azithromycin 500 mg PO on day 1 and then 250 mg PO qd on days 2–5).

4) *Note:* Avoid clarithromycin in pregnancy.

C. Treatment of patients hospitalized with CAP (Niederman et al., 1993)

1) Second-generation cephalosporin (e.g., cefuroxime sodium 0.75–1.5 gm IV q8h × 5–10 days); or

2) Third-generation cephalosporin (e.g., ceftriaxone sodium 1–2 gm IV q12–24h, up to 4 gm/day × 5–10 days); or

3) β-Lactam/β-lactamase inhibitor (e.g., amoxicillin-clavulanate 500 mg PO q8h × 10 days)—*plus*, may need to *add* erythromycin or other macrolide, especially if suspect *Legionella* species (e.g., erythromycin 250–500 mg PO qid × 10–14 days, or clarithromycin 250

mg PO q12h × 10–14 days, or azithromycin 500 mg PO on day 1 and then 250 mg PO on days 2–5).

4) *Note:* Avoid clarithromycin in pregnancy.

D. Treatment of patients hospitalized with severe CAP, usually requiring ICU admit (Niederman et al., 1993)

1) Severe CAP especially benefits from C&S results (i.e., from sputum, blood, and possibly pleural fluid) to help guide appropriate pharmacologic intervention.

2) Combination therapy is advised with a macrolide (e.g., erythromycin 15–20 mg/kg/day divided into q6h doses), *plus:*

a. *Either:* Third-generation cephalosporin with antipseudomonas coverage (i.e., ceftazidime sodium 1–2 gm IV q8–12h, up to 6 gm/day × 7–10 days); *or*

b. Other agent with antipseudomonas coverage, such as

i. Imipenem-cilastin (250–500 mg IV/IM q6–8h); *or*

ii. Ciprofloxacin (200–400 mg IV q12h, or 250–500 mg PO bid)

iii. *Note:* Avoid ciprofloxacin for teens or in pregnancy.

E. Empiric CAP treatment: Younger adult

1) Other authors cite general, empiric CAP treatment in younger adults:

a. Erythromycin (15–20 mg/kg/day IV divided into q6h doses), *plus, either*

i. Second-generation cephalosporin (e.g., cefuroxime sodium 0.75–1.5 gm IV q8h × 5–10 days); *or*

ii. Third-generation cephalosporin (e.g., ceftriaxone sodium 1–2 gm IV q12–24 h, up to 4 gm/day × 5–10 days)

b. If allergic to penicillin, may use doxycycline (100 mg PO bid). (*Note:* Avoid tetracyclines for teens or in pregnancy.)

F. Empiric CAP treatment: Older adult

1) Other authors cite general, empiric CAP treatment in older adults

a. Ceftriaxone (1–2 gm IV/IM qd, may divide into q12h doses, if preferred); *or*

b. Ampicillin-sulbactam (1.5 gm IV q8h)

3. Antimicrobial therapy for institutional, nosocomial/HAP

A. Empiric treatment, pending C&S results: general principles

1) Opinions vary at present as to the best empiric ABX treatment of HAP. Certain principles apply to all regimens cited, however. Initial treatment must be broad-spectrum and appropriate to the specific clinical setting. After C&S results are back from sputum, blood, and possibly pleural fluid (usually within 48–72 hours), it may be possible to switch to a more narrow-spectrum treatment. Duration of therapy is usually 10–14 days, even up to 21 days (e.g., gram-negative bacillary pneumonia is treated for at least 14 days, and *Legionella* species may require a 21-day course).

2) The 1996 ATS consensus statement (Campbell et al., 1996) on treatment of HAP discusses how ABX choice can be guided more effectively by placing the HAP patient into one of the three categories identified:

a. *Category 1:* Patients with mild-to-moderate HAP, without unusual risk factors, onset anytime; or patients with severe HAP, early onset

      b. *Category 2:* Patients with mild-to-moderate HAP, with risk factors, onset anytime.

      c. *Category 3:* Patients with severe HAP, with risk factors, early onset; or patients with severe HAP, late onset

    3) Other authors cite a more general approach to the initial management of HAP that includes using *both* a third-generation cephalosporin, *plus* antipseudomonas coverage (e.g., imipenem or aminoglycoside).

B. HAP Treatment: Category 1 (Campbell et al., 1996)

    1) Definition

      a. Patients with mild-to-moderate HAP, without unusual risk factors, onset anytime; or patients with severe HAP, early onset

    2) Discussion

      a. Mild-to-moderate HAP is most often influenced by presence or absence of risk factors for specific pathogens. A shorter length of hospital stay (<5 days) is often associated with *H. influenzae, S. pneumoniae, S. aureus,* in addition to enteric EGNB.

    3) Core organisms (most likely to be present)

      a. EGNB

      b. Nonpseudomonal *Enterobacter* series

      c. *Escherichia coli*

      d. *Klebsiella* series

      e. *Proteus* series

      f. *Serratia marcescens*

      g. *Haemophilus influenzae*

      h. Methicillin-sensitive *Staphylococcus aureus*

      i. *Streptococcus pneumoniae*

    4) Core ABX (most likely to be effective)

      a. Cephalosporin

        i. Second-generation (e.g., β-lactam such as cefuroxime sodium 0.75–1.5 gm IV q8h); *or*

        ii. Nonantipseudomonal third-generation (e.g., ceftriaxone sodium 1–2 gm IV q12–24 h, up to 4 gm/day); *or*

      b. β-lactam/β-lactamase inhibitor combination (e.g., imipenem-cilastin 250–500 mg IV q6–8 h, or ampicillin-sulbactam 1.5–3 gm IV q6h).

      c. If PCN-allergic, consider:

        i. Fluoroquinolone (e.g., ciprofloxacin 200–400 mg IV q12h, or 250–500 mg PO bid); *or*

        ii. clindamycin (600–900 mg IV q8h), *plus* aztreonam (2 gm IV q8h)

        iii. *Note:* Avoid fluoroquinolones in teens or pregnancy.

C. HAP treatment: Category 2 (Campbell et al., 1996)

    1) Definition

      a. Patients with mild-to-moderate HAP, with risk factors, onset anytime

    2) Discussion

      a. The likely pathogens in patients with mild-to-moderate HAP can be changed by specific risk factors. Core organisms (previously listed for Category 1), plus other bacteria dependent upon risk factors, are frequently seen in mild-to-moderate HAP. When multiple risk factors exist, the spectrum of potential pathogens is expanded to include the same microbes as are seen in severe HAP. Pneumonia caused by certain pathogens is associated with specific comorbidities and/or therapeutic interventions.

3) Core organisms (most likely to be present) from Category 1, *plus:*
   a. Anaerobes (e.g., witnessed aspiration or recent abdominal surgery)
   b. *Staphylococcus aureus* (e.g., coma, head trauma, DM, chronic renal failure [CRF])
   c. *Legionella* species (e.g., high-dose steroids)
   d. *Pseudomonas aeruginosa* (e.g., prolonged ICU course, steroids, previous ABX, structural lung disease)

4) Core ABX (most likely to be effective) from Category 1, *plus*
   a. Clindamycin (600–900 mg IV q8h), *or* β-lactam/β-lactamase inhibitor (e.g., imipenem-cilastin 250–500 mg IV q6–8h, or ampicillin-sulbactam 1.5–3 gm IV q6h) *(alone)*
      i. use against suspected anaerobes
   b. ± Vancomycin (1 gm IV q12h)
      i. use against *Staphylococcus aureus* (until MRSA is ruled out)
   c. Erythromycin (500 mg IV q6h)
      i. Use against *Legionella* species
   d. Treat as if HAP Treatment: Category 3 (Campbell et al., 1996)
      i. If suspect *Pseudomonas aeruginosa*

D. HAP treatment: Category 3 (Campbell et al., 1996)
   1) Definition
      a. Patients with severe HAP, with risk factors, early onset; or patients with severe HAP, late onset.
   2) Discussion
      a. Severe HAP occurs in ICU patients (especially those on mechanical ventilation/VAP), or else may prompt admission to ICU. Severe HAP often results from the presence of multiple, specific risk factors and/or from virulent pathogen(s). In addition to core organisms frequently isolated in this setting, additional pathogens also may be present, usually if specific risk factors exist and/or if the patient has been hospitalized for ≥5 days.
   3) Criteria for severe HAP definition (any of these may qualify):
      a. ICU admission; *or*
      b. Acute respiratory failure (i.e. needs mechanical ventilation and/or needs FIO_2 >35% to keep SaO_2 >90%); *or*
      c. Multilobar pneumonia, rapid CXR progression, or lung infiltrate which shows cavitation; *or*
      d. Severe sepsis with end-organ dysfunction and/or hypotension:
         i. Shock (BP <90/60 mm Hg); or
         ii. Vasopressors are needed >4 hours; or
         iii. Acute renal failure, resulting in need for dialysis; or
         iv. Urine output <20 mL/hr in 4 hours, or total urine output <80 mL in 4 hours (unless can be explained otherwise)
   4) Core organisms (most likely to be present) from Category 1, *plus:*
      a. *Pseudomonas aeruginosa*
      b. *Actinobacter* series
      c. Consider MRSA presence
   5) ABX therapy
      a. *Key:* Use combination of ABX against most virulent pathogens, especially *P. aeruginosa, Acinetobacter*, and *Enterobacter*.

b. Use *one* of the following:
   i. Broad-spectrum β-lactam; an antipseudomonal penicillin (e.g., piperacillin, mezlocillin, piperacillin-tazobactam, ticarcillin, or ticarcillin-clavulanate); *or* a third-generation antipseudomonal cephalosporin (e.g., ceftazidime sodium 1–2 gm IV q8–12 h, up to 6 gm/day × 7–10 days); or *imipenem-cilastin* (250–500 mg IV q6–8 h); *or*
   ii. *β-Lactam/β-lactamase* inhibitor (e.g., imipenem-cilastin 250–500 mg IV q6–8h, or ampicillin-sulbactam 1.5–3 gm IV q6h); *or*
   iii. Ceftazidime (2 gm IV q8h), or cefoperazone (2–4 gm IV q12h—*Caution:* cefoperazone can lead to clotting impairments); *or*
   iv. Imipenem (500 mg IV q6h); *or*
   v. Aztreonam (2 gm IV q8h—*Caution:* Use only if suspect EGNB; do not use in combination with an aminoglycoside if gram-positive or if *Haemophilus influenzae* infection is suspected.); *or*
   vi. ± Vancomycin (1 gm IV q12h—*Note:* Consider if suspect *S. aureus* and patient is at risk for MRSA)
c. *Plus, add either*:
   i. An aminoglycoside (gentamycin or tobramycin 5 mg/kg/day IV divided into q8h doses); *or*
   ii. Ciprofloxacin (200–400 mg IV q12h, or 250–500 mg PO bid).
   iii. *Note:* Do not use fluoroquinolones for teens or in pregnancy.
d. *Then, once C&S results are back,* a fluoroquinolone to which the responsible pathogen is susceptible may be considered to simplify treatment and allow earlier discharge from hospital (e.g., ciprofloxacin 500–750 mg PO q12h).
   i. *Note:* Do not use fluoroquinolones for teens or in pregnancy.

4. Empiric therapy for atypical pneumonia
   A. Some authors cite general, empiric treatment for atypical pneumonia.
      1) Erythromycin (500 mg IV q8h); *or*
      2) Ampicillin-sulbactam (1.5 gm IV q6h)
5. Empiric therapy for anaerobic pneumonia
   A. Some authors cite general, empiric treatment for anaerobic pneumonia.
      1) Clindamycin (600 mg IV q8h); *or*
      2) Ampicillin-sulbactam (1.5 gm IV q6h)
6. Antimicrobial therapy for viral pneumonia
   A. Amantadine given as prophylactic or within 48 hours of the onset of symptoms (200 mg/day in most adults, and 100 mg/day in those >65 years old).
7. Additional supportive measures
   A. IV hydration and oxygen
   B. Acetaminophen for fever and headaches (650 mg PO or PR q 4h, prn)
   C. Hand-held nebulizer (HHN) or meter dose inhaler (MDI) treatments for relief of bronchospasm (e.g., with history of asthma, COPD)
      1) Albuterol (Proventil, Ventolin)
         a. HHN: 2.5 mg/3 mL normal saline, usually q4h, prn
         b. MDI: 2 puffs, usually q4h, prn (may consider greater frequency/prn acute exacerbation; more effective when used with prescription spacer device)

2) Ipratropium bromide (Atrovent)
   a. HHN: 0.5 mg/3 mL normal saline, usually q4h, prn
   b. MDI: 2 puffs, usually q4h, prn (may consider greater frequency/prn acute exacerbation; more effective when used with prescription spacer device)
D. Pulmonary hygiene, deep breathing and coughing
E. Antitussives are unnecessary unless continued coughing exhausts the patient
F. Monitor intake and output
G. Follow-up CXR (results may lag behind clinical findings)

8. Invasive procedures (such as transtracheal aspiration, transthoracic needle aspiration, bronchial brushings, transbronchial biopsy) are only indicated in CAP when the patient is seriously ill and the diagnosis is uncertain. This may include patients who fail to respond to therapy, are immunocompromised, or are likely to have a nonbacterial etiology for their infiltrate.
   A. When these procedures are indicated, the ACNP consults with the physician. Depending upon the setting, the ACNP may be called upon to make a referral to a specialist as needed to perform these.

9. Prevention of HAP
   A. Vigilant handwashing between patient contacts by health care workers.
   B. Respiratory isolation of patients with multiply resistant respiratory pathogens (e.g., MRSA)
   C. Influenza and pneumonia vaccination for specific at-risk populations. (Health care workers, SNF residents, those with chronic lung disease, etc.)

10. Follow-up
    A. Multiple factors may impede a favorable response to empiric drug treatment of pneumonia. Consider misdiagnosis, wrong medication, adverse reaction, complication, or compromised host defenses.

PATIENT EDUCATION

1. Explain the definition of pneumonia and possible cause.
2. Review probable course of recovery.
3. Inform patient about influenza and pneumonia vaccines.
4. Discuss treatment plan, including tests, antibiotics (and the need to complete the full course of antibiotics), and the importance of hydration.
5. Discuss discharge plans with patient and family.
6. Explain importance of follow-up after discharge.
7. Reiterate the importance of avoiding exposure to cigarette smoke. Quit-smoking tips and other useful community resources are offered through:
   A. American Lung Association
   B. American Thoracic Society (which is the medical section of the American Lung Association)
   C. American Cancer Society
   D. American Heart Association
   E. Centers for Disease Control (CDC)
   F. National Institutes of Health (NIH)

Review Questions

2.1. Mr. GM is a symptomatic, 43-year-old COPD patient whom you have admitted to the acute care unit. He has tachypnea and CXR confirms that he has patchy, lobar infiltrates consistent with pneumonia. On an F_{IO_2} of 21%, his ABGs are:

   pH: 7.58
   P_{CO_2}: 45 mm Hg
   P_{O_2}: 38 mm Hg
   Sa_{O_2}: 83%
   Bicarb: 40 mEq/L
   BE: +5 mEq/L
   Your interpretation of his ABG results:

   A. Acute metabolic acidosis without hypoxemia
   B. Chronic metabolic acidosis with hypercapnia
   C. Both A and B
   D. Acute alveolar hyperventilation (respiratory alkalosis), superimposed upon chronic ventilatory failure (respiratory acidosis)

2.2 In the elderly patient, which one of the following is most likely to be seen with early pneumonia?
   A. Leukocytosis
   B. Diarrhea
   C. Mental status changes
   D. Fever <101°F

2.3 Miss SH is a 64-year-old woman in whom you suspect CAP. She is otherwise healthy and denies any comorbidities. Medications that would be appropriate for the outpatient management of her pneumonia include any one of these, EXCEPT:
   A. Amantadine
   B. Second-generation cephalosporin
   C. Trimethoprim-sulfamethoxazole
   D. β-Lactam/β-lactamase inhibitor (plus, may need to add erythromycin or other macrolide)

2.4 Considerations for hospital admission of a patient with CAP are likely to include all, EXCEPT:
   A. Arterial P_{O_2} <60 mm Hg on room air, or arterial P_{CO_2} >50 mm Hg on room air
   B. Lung involvement (>1 lobe)
   C. Inability to maintain oral intake
   D. Fever <101°F

2.5 Mrs. SB is a 79-year-old woman who is a direct admit from her SNF to your acute care unit, after suffering a new-onset CVA with right-sided weakness. You are managing her care. On exam you hear crackles in the right lung base and notice that she is pooling her oral secretions. Her temperature is 99.2°F orally, and the WBC count is 13,000 despite being on ceftriaxone (Rocephin) IV for the past 4 days. Based upon the above, what antibiotic would you consider adding to this patient's treatment regimen?
   A. Vancomycin
   B. Clindamycin
   C. TMP-SMX
   D. Erythromycin

Answers and Rationales

2.1 **D** Acute alveolar hyerventilation (respiratory alkalosis), superimposed upon chronic ventilatory failure (respiratory acidosis). The increased pH indicates alkalosis, while the history of tachypnea in a COPD patient suggests that he may be blowing off his CO_2 via hyperventilation. Acute alveolar hyperventilation or respiratory alkalosis may then result. PCO_2 of 45 is in the normal range, but may represent lower PCO_2 than baseline for a COPD patient who may be a chronic CO_2 retainer. Chronic ventilatory failure (as in COPD) can predispose to such ongoing CO_2 retention and chronic respiratory acidosis. Mr. GM may have developed an elevated bicarbonate level as a means of compensating for this over the long term.

2.2 **C** Mental status changes may often be the only sign of an early pneumonia, especially in the elderly.

2.3 **A** Choices B, C, and D are all consistent with the American Thoracic Society guidelines for the outpatient treatment of CAP in patients >60 years old without comorbidities. Choice A, amantadine, is not consistent with these.

2.4 **D** Fever >101°F may be an additional, less frequently cited criteria for admission of a patient with CAP. Answer D, however, listed fever <101°F, which is a consideration for outpatient management of CAP, not for hospital admit. Frequently cited considerations for hospital admission of a patient with CAP include
arterial PO_2 <60 mm Hg on room air, or arterial PCO_2 > 50 mm Hg on room air; lung involvement (>1 lobe); and/or inability to maintain oral intake.

2.5 **B** In a patient you suspect to be aspiration-prone, cover for anaerobic organisms with a drug such as clindamycin.

References

Campbell, G.D., Jr., Niederman, M.S., Broughton, W.A., et al. (1996). Hospital-acquired pneumonia in adults: Diagnosis, assessment of severity, initial antimicrobial therapy, and preventative strategies: A consensus statement. ("Official Statement of the American Thoracic Society," medical section of the American Lung Association.) *Am J Respir Crit Care Med 153*, 1711–1725.

Fine, M.J., Hough, L.J., Medsger, A.R., et al. (1997). The hospital admission decision for patients with community-acquired pneumonia: Results from the pneumonia patient outcomes research team cohort study. *Arch Intern Med 157*, 36–44.

Levison, M.E. (1994). Pneumonia, including necrotizing pulmonary infections (lung abscess). In K.J. Isselbacher, E. Braunwald, & D.L. Kasper (eds.). *Harrison's Principles of Internal Medicine* (13th ed., Vol. 2), New York: McGraw-Hill, pp. 1184–1191.

Niederman, M.S., Bass, J.B., Campbell, G.D., et al. (1993). Guidelines for the initial management of adults with community-acquired pneumonia: Diagnosis, assessment of severity, and initial antimicrobial therapy. ("Official Statement of the American Thoracic Society," medical section of the American Lung Association.) *Am Rev Respirat Dis 148*, 1418–1426.

Niederman, M.S., & Fein, A.M. (1993). Bacterial pneumonia. In R.E. Rakel (ed.). *Conn's Current Therapy*. Philadelphia: W.B. Saunders Co.

Niederman, M.S., & Sarosi, G.A. (1995). Parenchymal lung infections/pathogenesis of pneumonia. In R.B. George, R.W. Light, M.A. Mathay, & R.A. Mathay (eds.). *Chest Medicine: Essentials of Pulmonary and Critical Care Medicine* (3rd ed.). Baltimore, MD: Williams & Wilkins, pp. 433–457.

Reves, R.R. (1996). Acute infectious pneumonia. In J.M. Rippe, R.S. Irwin, M.P. Fink, & F.B. Cerra (eds.). *Intensive Care Medicine* (3rd ed., Vol. 1). Boston: Little, Brown & Co., pp. 903–922.

Stauffer, J.L. (1997). Pneumonia. In L.M. Tierney, Jr., S.J. McPhee, & M.A. Papadakis (eds.). *Current Medical Diagnosis and Treatment, 1997* (36th ed.). Stamford, CT: Appleton & Lange, pp. 260–268.

Swisher, J.W. (1996). Pneumonia. In R.E. Rakel (ed.). *Saunders Manual of Medical Practice*. Philadelphia: W.B. Saunders Co., pp. 135–137.

Additional Recommended References

Anup, A.B. (1996). *Arterial Blood Gas Analysis Made Easy*. Valhalla, NY: Author, pp. 11–93.

Benjamin, G.C. (1996). Aspiration pneumonia, empyema and lung abscess. In J.E. Tintinalli, R.L. Krome, & E. Ruiz (eds.). *Emergency Medicine: A Comprehensive Study Guide* (4th ed.). New York: McGraw-Hill, pp. 419–421.

Benjamin, G.C. (1996). Bacterial pneumonias. In J.E. Tintinalli, R.L. Krome, & E. Ruiz (eds.). *Emergency Medicine: A Comprehensive Study Guide* (4th ed.). New York: McGraw-Hill, pp. 405–409.

Fein, A.M., & M.S. Niederman. (1995). Clinical commentaries: Guidelines for the initial management of community-acquired pneumonia: Savory recipe or cookbook for disaster? *Am J Respir Crit Care Med 152*, 1149–1153.

Moroney, C., & M.A. Fitzgerald. (1996). Pharmacologic update: Management of pneumonia in elderly people. *J Am Acad Nurse Pract 8*(5), 237–241.

Papadakis, M.A. (1997). Acid-base disorders. In L.M. Tierney, Jr., S.J. McPhee, & M.A. Papadakis (eds.). *Current Medical Diagnosis and Treatment, 1997* (36th ed.). Stamford, CT: Appleton & Lange, pp. 815–825.

Ravikrishnan, K.P. (1996). Viral and mycoplasma pneumonias. In J.E. Tintinalli, R.L. Krome, & E. Ruiz (eds.). *Emergency Medicine: A Comprehensive Study Guide* (4th ed.). New York: McGraw-Hill, pp. 409–413.

Thompson, G.A., & S. Sheehan. (1997). Drug consults: Rifampin therapy of Legionnaires' disease. *DRUGDEX®, Micromedex, Inc., Vol. 91, Expiration Date: 2/28/97*. Englewood, CO: Medical Economics Co.

Turkeltaub, M. (1994). Pneumonia. In V.L. Millonig (ed.). *Adult Nurse Practitioner Certification Review Guide* (2nd ed.). Potomac, MD: Health Leadership Associates, Inc., pp. 146–149.

Weinberger, S.E., and J.M. Drazen. (1994). Disturbances of respiratory function. In K.J. Isselbacher, E. Braunwald, and D.L. Kasper (eds.). *Harrison's Principles of Internal Medicine* (13th ed., Vol. 2). New York: McGraw-Hill, pp. 1152–1159.

Wilson, R.F., & C. Barton. (1996). Blood gases: Pathophysiology and interpretation. In J.E. Tintinalli, R.L. Krome, & E. Ruiz (eds.). *Emergency Medicine: A Comprehensive Study Guide* (4th ed.). New York: McGraw-Hill, pp. 108–117.

Zaman, M.K. (1996). Procedure: Technique of sputum induction. In R.E. Rakel (ed.). *Saunders Manual of Medical Practice*, Philadelphia: W.B. Saunders Co., pp. 187–188.

Zwanger, M. (1996). Pneumonias in immunocompromised patients. In J.E. Tintinalli, R.L. Krome, & E. Ruiz (eds.). *Emergency Medicine: A Comprehensive Study Guide* (4th ed.). New York: McGraw-Hill, pp. 413–418.

COPD: Emphysema and Chronic Bronchitis

DEFINITION

Chronic obstructive pulmonary disease refers to a group of disorders, including emphysema and chronic bronchitis, characterized by progressive airway obstruction of lung parenchyma. With emphysema this leads to permanent lung parenchymal damage. Most COPD patients have symptoms of both diseases, and most COPD patients have been smokers.

In the past, asthma has been included in discussions of COPD. However, asthma's increasing prevalence and significance have led to it commonly being discussed separately, as is the case here. (See "Asthma" in the following section.)

ETIOLOGY/INCIDENCE

1. About 10–14 million Americans are affected by COPD (depending on definitions used).
2. Cigarette smoking is by far the most important cause of COPD, even though only 10–15% of smokers develop COPD.
3. Risk is also increased by age, by air pollution exposure through work or the environment, and occasionally by heredity.
4. COPD death rates are increasing, with COPD currently ranked fifth among leading causes of death in the United States (75,000 annually). When COPD and asthma are statistically combined, they represent the fourth leading cause of death (90,000 annually), or 4.2% of all deaths in 1991, surpassing the numbers of deaths due to accidents.
5. COPD is the second-most frequent cause of permanent disability (exceeded only by coronary artery disease) in those over 40 years of age, with estimated costs for associated health care and time lost from work at $7 billion and $8 billion, respectively.

PATHOPHYSIOLOGY

1. Both
   A. When the airways are damaged, the amount of oxygen in the blood is limited, and carbon dioxide may not be adequately eliminated.
   B. Pathophysiologic consequences of COPD also include reduced minute ventilation, a ventilation-perfusion ($\dot{V}/\dot{Q}$) mismatch, and increased work of breathing.
2. Emphysema
   A. Emphysema involves permanent destruction of the alveoli due to irreversible destruction of elastin, a lung protein important to maintain alveolar wall strength. When elastin is lost, the smallest air passages, or bronchioles, may narrow and collapse, while alveoli stretch out of shape and become abnormally large. These developments limit air flow out of the lung. Approximately 2 million Americans have emphysema.
   B. Emphysema has also been defined in terms of permanent, abnormal enlargement of air spaces distal to the terminal bronchiole, with destruction of such walls and without obvious fibrosis.
   C. Destruction of alveolar walls causes loss of elastic recoil and subsequent expiratory airflow limitation. Functional airway narrowing or bronchoconstriction also occurs due to an inflammatory response that includes edema, excessive mucus, and glandular hypertrophy.

   D. Approximately 1–3% of emphysemics are affected by a genetic deficiency
       of the blood component AAT (α_1-antitrypsin or α_1-antiprotease). Recent
       research suggests that those with AAT deficiency may have a greater
       inflammatory and destructive response to certain aspects of cigarette
       smoke, resulting in excessive lysis of elastin and other structural pro-
       teins in the lung matrix by elastase and other proteases formed from
       lung neutrophils, macrophages, and mononuclear cells.
3. Chronic Bronchitis
   A. Chronic bronchitis involves irritation, inflammation, and edema of the
       airway lining. In response to such irritation and inflammation, excess
       mucus is produced which, in combination with the edema, can then nar-
       row the airways further and interfere with the previously normal air
       flow.
   B. A productive cough, especially after a respiratory tract infection, may
       develop and last for weeks to months, especially in the mornings.
       Chronic bronchitis is considered to have developed when a productive
       cough with excessive mucus occurs for at least 6 months in 1 year, or
       else 3 months in each of 2 consecutive years in the absence of any other
       condition that could account for this symptom.
   C. Cardinal features include:
       1) Increased number and size of mucus-secreting glands in airways
       2) Overproduction of mucus
       3) Obstruction of small airways by mucus
       4) Narrowing and inflammation of small airways
       5) "Mucous pits" (dilated mucous gland openings/diverticula visible
           during bronchoscopy)
       6) Bacterial colonization of normally sterile airways (i.e., often with
           S. pneumoniae, *H. influenzae*, and/or *M. catarrhalis*)

SIGNS AND SYMPTOMS

1. Both
   A. Most COPD patients have features of both emphysema and chronic bron-
       chitis.
   B. Impaired exercise performance, progressing to dyspnea on exertion (usu-
       ally sooner with emphysema).
   C. See Table 2–1 for a comparison of clinical, CXR, and laboratory results
       for emphysema versus chronic bronchitis.
2. Emphysema
   A. Occasionally referred to as type A COPD or "pink puffer"
   B. Hallmark symptom: Dyspnea on exertion (especially with activities that
       previously did not bring on shortness of breath [SOB]); May become
       progressive, constant, and severe
   C. Early stage: Fatigue, little cough, mild dyspnea on exertion
   D. Later state: Thin, pursed-lip breathing, marked dyspnea at rest
   E. Cough with clear mucus
3. Chronic Bronchitis
   A. Occasionally referred to as type B COPD or "blue bloater"
   B. Hallmark symptoms: Daily morning cough (progressing to chronic, per-
       sistent, severe cough) with copious, thick sputum production (progress-
       ing to mucopurulent or purulent sputum)
   C. Constitutional signs: Fever, chills, fatigue

TABLE 2–1. Emphysema Versus Chronic Bronchitis: Clinical, Roentgenographic, and Laboratory Findings*†

	Emphysema	Chronic Bronchitis
History		
Onset of symptoms	After age 50	After age 35
Dyspnea	Progressive, constant, severe	Intermittent, mild or moderate
Cough	Absent or mild	Persistent, severe
Sputum production	Absent or mild	Copious
Sputum appearance	Clear, mucoid	Mucopurulent or purulent
Other features	Weight loss‡	Airway infections, right heart failure, obesity
Physical Examination		
Body habitus	Thin, wasted‡	Stocky, obese
Central cyanosis	Absent	Present‡
Plethora	Absent	Present
Accessory respiratory muscles	Hypertrophied	Unremarkable
Anteroposterior chest diameter	Increased	Normal
Percussion note	Hyperresonant	Normal
Auscultation	Diminished breath sounds	Wheezes, rhonchi
Chest X-Ray		
Bullae, blebs	Present	Absent
Overall appearance	Decreased markings periphery	Increased markings ("dirty lungs")
Hyperinflation	Present	Absent
Heart size	Normal or small vertical	Large, horizontal
Hemidiaphragms	Low, flat	Normal, rounded
Laboratory studies		
Hematocrit	Normal	Increased
ECG	Normal	Right axis deviation, right ventricular hypertrophy, "P" pulmonate‡
Hypoxemia	Absent, mild	Moderate, severe
Hypercapnia	Absent	Moderate, severe
Respiratory acidosis	Absent	Present
Total lung capacity	Increased	Normal
Static lung compliance	Increased	Normal
Diffusing capacity	Decreased	Normal

* From Celli, B.R., Snider, G.L., Heffner, J., et al., (1995). Standards for the diagnosis and care of patients with chronic obstructive pulmonary disease. ("Official Statement of the American Thoracic Society," medical section of the American Lung Association.) *Am Rev Respir Dis 152*(Suppl.), S72–S120, with permission.

† As noted in the text, most patients with COPD have features of both emphysema and chronic bronchitis.

‡ In advanced disease.

    D. Airway infections become more frequent

    E. Right heart failure and leg edema

PHYSICAL FINDINGS

1. Both
    A. Most COPD patients have features of both emphysema and chronic bronchitis and often show a combination of physical findings related to both diseases.
    B. Prolonged expiration.

2. Emphysema
    A. Hypertrophied accessory respiratory muscles and unique "tripod" posture (leaning forward onto elbows)
    B. Thin, wasted appearance
    C. Barrel chest (increased anteroposterior [AP] diameter)
    D. May have flushed coloring
    E. Decreased breath sounds to auscultation
    F. Hyperresonant percussion notes
    G. Occasional wheezes (usually expiratory) by later stages of disease
    H. Late stage: Cor pulmonale/right heart failure may develop, with occasional leg edema
3. Chronic Bronchitis
    A. Stocky, obese appearance.
    B. Wheezes (often) and occasional rhonchi and/or crackles may be auscultated.
    C. Central cyanosis and/or plethora may be present.
    D. Lungs may be resonant to percussion (or dull, if consolidation is present).
    E. Cor pulmonale may be present. (Check for jugular venous distention [JVD], leg edema, right ventricular heave with a loud pulmonic valve component of S_2, tricuspid insufficiency, and ascites.)
    F. Occasional hemoptysis during bronchitic exacerbations (bronchoscopy may be needed to confirm absence of lung cancer).

DIFFERENTIAL DIAGNOSIS

1. If suspect emphysema, also rule out chronic bronchitis
2. If suspect chronic bronchitis, also rule out emphysema
3. For both diseases, rule out:
    A. Asthma
    B. Acute bronchitis
    C. Pneumonia
    D. TB
    E. Lung cancer
    F. Bronchiectasis
    G. Congestive heart failure
    H. Cystic fibrosis (in young adults)

DIAGNOSTIC TESTS/FINDINGS

1. Both
    A. Pulmonary function testing (PFT) best provides objective data about the severity of pulmonary dysfunction and can be used to assess results of therapy.
        1) Decreased forced expiratory volume at 1 second (FEV_1) to forced vital capacity (FVC) is hallmark of obstruction and can help diagnose mild to marked COPD. May be some reversibility after bronchodilator therapy (especially in asthmatic bronchitis).
        2) Increased FEV_1 >3 seconds.
        3) Decreased vital capacity (VC) and expiratory flow rates.
        4) Increased total lung capacity (TLC), static lung compliance, residual volume (RV), and functional residual capacity (FRC).

TABLE 2–2. **Results of Pulmonary Function Tests in Obstructive and Restrictive Pulmonary Dysfunction***

Tests	Obstructive	Restrictive
Spirometry		
FVC (L)	N or ↓	↓
FEV_1 (L)	↓	N or ↓
FEV_1/FVC (%)	↓	N or ↑
FEF_{25-75} (L/sec)	↓	N or ↓
PEFR (L/sec)	↓	N or ↑
MVV (L/min)	↓	N or ↓
Lung volumes		
SVC (L)	N or ↓	↓
TLC (L)	N or ↑	↓
FRC (L)	↑	N or ↓
ERV (L)	N or ↓	N or ↓
RV (L)	↑	N, ↓ or ↑
RV/TLC ratio	↑	N or ↑

* From Stauffer, J. (1997). Lung. In L. Tierney, S. McPhee, & M. Papadakis (eds). *Current Medical Diagnosis and Treatment,* (36th ed.). Stamford, CT: Appleton & Lange, pp. 317–318, with permission.

N, normal; ↓, less than predicted; ↑, greater than predicted; FVC, forced vital capacity; FEV_1, forced expiratory volume in 1 second; FEF_{25-75}, forced expiratory flow, mid–expiratory phase; PEFR, peak expiratory flow rate; MVV, maximum voluntary ventilation; SVC, slow vital capacity; TLC, total lung capacity; FRC, functional residual capacity; ERV, expiratory reserve volume; RV, residual volume.

    B. See Table 2–2 for results of PFTs in obstructive versus restrictive pulmonary dysfunction.

    C. To review PFT interpretation, refer to the references listed following this section.

2. Emphysema

    A. Diffusing capacity: Decreased

3. Chronic Bronchitis

    A. Diffusing capacity: Normal

Arterial Blood Gases

1. Both

    A. Useful to diagnose severity of associated acute respiratory failure.

    B. Hypoxemia usually found in advanced COPD.

    C. Exercise caution in relying solely upon pulse oximetry (oxyhemoglobin saturation) rather than partial pressure of oxygen in blood (available with ABG determination). As a review, pulse oximetry is readily available, noninvasive, and well tolerated by patients, yet may be somewhat misleading. For example, some authors define hypoxemia at Po_2 <60 mm Hg. Yet a low Po_2 of 63 mm Hg correlates with a relatively benign appearing Sao_2 of 92%, due to the nonlinearity of their two scales. Order ABGs when indicated and appropriate.

    D. To review ABG interpretation, refer to the references listed following this section.

2. Emphysema

    A. May show normocapnia (possible Pco_2 of 35–45 mm Hg)

    B. May show mild to moderate hypoxemia (possible Po_2 of 70–80 mm Hg)

3. Chronic Bronchitis
    A. May show hypercapnia (possible P_{CO_2} >45 mm Hg)
    B. May show hypoxemia (possible P_{O_2} of 60–80 mm Hg)

Chest X-Ray

1. Both
    A. Routine CXR may not be as helpful as CXR done during exacerbation to exclude reversible conditions (i.e., pneumonia, pneumothorax, pleural effusion, atelectasis, and pulmonary edema).
2. Emphysema
    A. Bullae, blebs.
    B. Hyperinflation with flattened diaphragmatic domes.
    C. Decreased peripheral markings (vascular attenuation).
    D. Increased AP diameter.
    E. High-resolution computed tomography (CT) scan is the most objective diagnostic tool.
3. Chronic Bronchitis
    A. Large, horizontal heart (especially with right heart enlargement)
    B. "Dirty lungs": Increase in and thickening of bronchial (bronchovascular) markings

Tuberculosis Skin Testing (PPD)

1. Rule out TB
2. Useful for all COPD patients

Complete Blood Count

1. Hemoglobin and hematocrit may be elevated.
2. May be useful for patients with chronic bronchitis

α_1-Antitrypsin or α_1-Antiprotease

1. Blood levels may be decreased in 1–3% of emphysemic patients who have inherited a genetic deficiency of this enzyme.
2. As AAT replacement therapy begins to show promise, this lab measurement may help identify suitable candidates who could benefit from its use and for whom it is available.

MANAGEMENT/TREATMENT

1. Both
    A. Several factors enter into the decision to admit a patient with COPD exacerbation to an acute care unit, rather than to manage COPD on an outpatient basis. The frequency and importance of these factors may differ somewhat between types of treatment settings and medical practitioners. Depending upon the setting, the ACNP may be called upon to arrange hospital admission and to manage the patient with Physician collaboration. Hospital admission criteria often include:
        1) Patient has acute COPD exacerbation with increased cough, dyspnea, and/or sputum production, *plus* at least one of the following:
            a. Failure of outpatient treatment

  b. Dyspnea so severe that it limits eating or sleeping, or walking across a room (if patient previously able to do so)

  c. Delay in seeking emergency medical care, with prolonged symptoms that progressively worsen

  d. Altered mental status

  e. Worsening hypoxemia

  f. New-onset or worsening hypercarbia

  g. Low estimation of patient reliability, and/or inadequate home care resources and support

  h. High-risk comorbid medical condition, either pulmonary (e.g., pneumonia) or other (e.g., DM, CHF, CAD, CA, unstable psychiatric illness)

  i. Theophylline toxicity, fever, or inability to maintain oral intake

 2) Additional considerations

  a. New or worsening cor pulmonale, unresponsive to outpatient treatment

  b. Planned surgical or diagnostic procedure which may worsen PFTs (e.g., due to need for analgesics and/or sedatives)

  c. Comorbid condition that has worsened PFTs (e.g., severe steroid myopathy, or acute vertebral compression fractures)

B. *Patients with severe COPD exacerbation may need prompt admission to the ICU.* Depending upon the setting, the ACNP may be called upon to arrange ICU transfer or admit, along with referral to a pulmonary/critical care MD specialist who needs to follow the patient. Any of these may be indicators for ICU admit:

 1) Continuing or worsening hypoxemia, despite supplemental O_2

 2) Severe or worsening respiratory acidosis (pH <7.30)

 3) Mechanical ventilation is needed, via ETT or noninvasive technique

 4) Severe dyspnea, unresponsive to initial emergency therapy

 5) Confusion, lethargy, or respiratory muscle fatigue (i.e., paradoxical diaphragmatic motion).

C. Bronchodilators/drugs of choice

 1) β-Agonists: Albuterol or metaproterenol, 2 puffs q4h prn via MDI; may also be given via HHN, oral, or parenteral routes.

 2) Anticholinergic: Ipratropium bromide via MDI, 2 puffs q4h prn via MDI; may also be given via HHN

 3) More effective when used with prescription spacer device.

D. Alternative drugs

 1) Theophylline PO or aminophylline IV

  a. Calculate dose using lean body mass; Need to check serum theophylline levels to keep in the therapeutic range, between 10 and 20 μg/mL.

  b. Theophylline: 200 mg PO q12h to start, then 200–600 mg PO q8–12h.

  c. Aminophylline: Load at 2.5–5 mg/kg via IV over 30 minutes. Maintenance dose is given by constant infusion via IV pump at 0.7 mg/kg/hr. Decrease maintenance dose accordingly if patient has CHF or liver disease, or is taking cimetidine or erythromycin.

 2) Diuretics: Only if cor pulmonale is present.

 3) Corticosteroids: Only of limited usefulness for COPD. May be useful if there is an asthmatic component in a patient with responsiveness

---

TABLE 2–3
Step-by-Step Pharmacologic Therapy for COPD*

1. For mild, variable symptoms:
   Selective β_2-agonist MDI aerosol, 1–2 puffs q2–6 h prn not to exceed 8–12 puffs/day
2. For mild to moderate continuing symptoms:
   Ipratropium MDI aerosol, 1–4 puffs as required qid for rapid relief, when needed or as regular supplement.
3. If response to step 2 is unsatisfactory, or there is a mild to moderate increase in symptoms:
   Add sustained-release theophylline, 200–400 mg bid 400–800 mg at qhs for nocturnal bronchospasm; *and/or*
   consider use of mucokinetic agent
4. If control of symptoms is suboptimal:
   Consider course of oral steroids (e.g. prednisone), up to 40 mg/day for 10–14 days
   • If no improvement occurs, wean to low daily or alternate-day dose (e.g., 7.5 mg)
   • If no improvement occurs, stop abruptly
   • If steroid appears to help, consider possible use of aerosol MDI, particularly if patient has evidence of bronchial hyperactivity
5. For severe exacerbation:
   Increase β_2-agonist dosage, e.g., MDI with spacer 6–8 puffs every ½–2 hr or inhalant solution, unit dose every ½–2 hr or SQ administration of epinephrine or terbutaline, 0.1–0.5 mL; *and/or*
   Increase ipratropium dosage, e.g., MDI with spacer 6–8 puffs q3–4 h or inhalant solution of ipratropium 0.5 mg q4–8 hs; *and*
   Provide theophylline dosage IV with calculated amount to bring serum level to 10–12 μg/mL; *and*
   Provide methylprednisolone dosage IV giving 50–100 mg immediately, then q6–8 hs; taper as soon as possible; *and add*
   An antibiotic, if indicated
   A mucokinetic agent if sputum is very viscous

---

* From Celli, B.R., Snider, G.L., Heffner, J., et al., (1995). Standards for the diagnosis and care of patients with chronic obstructive pulmonary disease. ("Official Statement of the American Thoracic Society," medical section of the American Lung Association.) *Am Rev Respir Dis 152*(Suppl.), S77–S120, with permission.
COPD, chronic obstructive pulmonary disease; MDI, metered dose inhaler.

to β-agonist therapy. Given by oral, parenteral, or inhaled routes. Reduce to the lowest possible dose as soon as reasonable. (See "Asthma.")

E. See also Table 2–3 for COPD medication management.

F. Supplemental, low-flow *oxygen* therapy (usually 1–3 L/min), to achieve Pao_2 >55 mm Hg may be indicated, especially for acute exacerbations.
   1) O_2 is the standard of care for COPD patients whose Pao_2 is <55 mm Hg at rest, with exercise, or nocturnally.
   2) COPD patients with cor pulmonale whose Pao_2 is <59 mm Hg also need O_2.
   3) To review O_2 management for COPD patients, refer to the Celli et al. reference listed following this section.

G. See Figure 2–1 to review the American Thoracic Society (ATS) suggested algorithm for correcting hypoxemia in the acutely ill COPD patient.

H. Short-term antibiotic therapy
   1) May be useful in exacerbations, especially with fever, purulent sputum, and increasing dyspnea.
   2) *H. influenzae, S. pneumoniae, M. catarrhalis* are the organisms usually responsible, and are often β-lactamase producing, and are therefore resistant to amoxicillin.

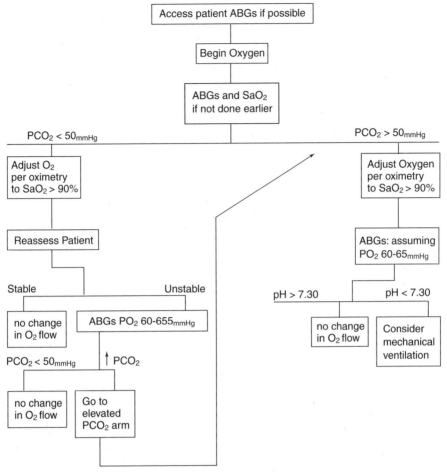

FIGURE 2–1. Algorithm for correcting hypoxemia in the acutely ill COPD patient. (From Celli, B.R., Snider, G.L., Heffner, J., et al. [1995]. Standards for the diagnosis and care of patients with chronic obstructive pulmonary disease. ["Official Statement of the American Thoracic Society," medical section of the American Lung Association.] *Am Rev Respir Dis 152* [Suppl.], S77–S120, with permission.)

         3) Suitable antibiotic choices may include ampicillin-clavulanate, second- or third-generation cephalosporins, trimethoprim-sulfamethoxazole, quinolones, tetracyclines, and clarithromycin.

  I. Help liquefaction of sputum
     1) Encourage patient to drink 2 L or more of fluids daily.
     2) Measures of limited usefulness:
        a. Routine home humidifier use
        b. Expectorant/mucolytics (e.g., guaifenesin)
        c. Periodic use of vaporizer and steam from bath or shower, as needed

  J. Avoid airway irritants
     1) Smoking (primary risk factor)
     2) Air pollutants and inhaled occupational irritants
     3) Certain medications (β-blockers)
     4) Temperature extremes (particularly cold, dry air at higher altitudes)

  K. Smoking cessation aids
     1) Prescriptions for nicotine gum or transdermal patches

      2) Referral to quit-smoking classes, especially those that emphasize behavioral change and self-management
      3) Quit-smoking tips and other useful community resources are offered through:
        a. American Lung Association
        b. American Thoracic Society (which is the medical section of the American Lung Association)
        c. American Cancer Society
        d. American Heart Association
        e. CDC
        f. NIH

L. Immunizations
    1) Annual influenza vaccinations
    2) Lifetime pneumococcal vaccination

M. Referral to a pulmonary rehabilitation program to provide:
    1) Exercise training (upper-extremity exercise, stair climbing, progressive walking)
    2) Physical and occupational therapy (how to conserve energy)
    3) Education sessions (disease process, inspiratory muscle training, rationale for medications and how to optimize their use)
    4) Support group sessions with the patient's loved ones and fellow pulmonary rehab patients

N. Follow-up with periodic PFTs, ABGs, and CXR (annually), and observe for any concomitant development of cor pulmonale or bronchogenic carcinoma

2. Emphysema
  A. If patient is deficient in α_1-antitrypsin or α_1-antiprotease, consider AAT replacement via IV, if available.

3. Chronic Bronchitis
  A. Do not use cough suppressants.
  B. Chest percussion and postural drainage can be helpful.

PATIENT EDUCATION

1. Both
  A. Review disease process, medication use, community resources available, how to manage exacerbations, and the need to notify the medical provider early when exacerbations occur.
  B. Strongly encourage smoking cessation by patients and those with whom they live.
  C. Teach effective cough technique: Deep breathe, lean forward, huff repeatedly, intersperse with relaxed breaths.
  D. Teach deep breathing and accessory respiratory muscle exercises.
  E. Review signs and symptoms of respiratory infections, CHF, and peptic ulcer disease (which can occur concurrently with and exacerbate COPD), and how to minimize and manage these.

2. Emphysema
  A. Teach pursed-lip exhalation.
  B. Encourage adequate nutrition (and supplements, as needed), especially for thin, malnourished patients.

3. Chronic Bronchitis
   A. A lower carbohydrate and higher calorie diet may lessen the degree of hypercapnia (i.e., >2000 calories, 50% carbohydrates.) For obese bronchitics, encourage carbohydrate reduction to attempt a decrease in hypercapnia.

Review Questions

2.6 Mr. AA is a stocky, 69-year-old man who has chronic dyspnea, productive cough, and mucopurulent sputum. Although an ex-smoker now, he has a 40-pack-year smoking history. Review of his old chart reveals PFT results that help support the diagnosis of COPD/chronic bronchitis:
   A. Increased: FRC, FEV_1, RV, compliance
      Decreased: None of these parameters
   B. Increased: FEV_1, TLC
      Decreased: RV, compliance
   C. Increased: Compliance, RV
      Decreased: FEV_1, FRC
   D. Increased: None of these parameters
      Decreased: RV, FEV_1, compliance, FRC

2.7 Ms. Generation X is a slim, 25-year-old woman who lives in a smoggy suburb of Los Angeles, and has an 18-pack-year smoking history. Because she exercises regularly and eats prudently it is hard for her to accept that as a young adult she may have developed a chronic disease based upon her lifestyle choices. Yet when you read her routine CXR you can already detect signs which may indicate COPD/emphysema. When she asks you to show her the films, they are likely to reveal any or all of the following, EXCEPT:
   A. Bullae, blebs
   B. Hyperinflation with flattened diaphragmatic domes
   C. Decreased peripheral markings (vascular attenuation)
   D. Hilar cavitation

2.8 Which test routinely provides the best, most objective data about the severity of pulmonary dysfunction in COPD and can be used to assess results of maintenance therapy?
   A. PFTs/spirometry
   B. ABGs
   C. CXR
   D. CBC

2.9 Mrs. LR is a cachectic, 54-year-old woman who is admitted to the hospital for acute COPD exacerbation. She has a 76-pack-year smoking history. Prior to this latest exacerbation, her ABGs showed pH of 7.40 and P_{CO_2} of 50. Admission ABGs revealed:
   pH: 7.33
   P_{O_2}: 59
   P_{CO_2}: 60
   Sa_{O_2}: 89%
   Bicarb: 30

Your interpretations of her admission ABGs include (circle all that apply):
A. Acute respiratory alkalosis with hypoxemia
B. Acute on chronic respiratory acidosis with hypoxemia
C. Acute respiratory alkalosis with normocapnia
D. Partially compensated respiratory acidosis with hypoxemia

2.10 The drugs of choice to routinely treat COPD may include all, EXCEPT:
A. Albuterol (Proventil, Ventolin) MDI, 2 puffs qid/prn
B. Ipratropium bromide (Atrovent) MDI, 2 puffs qid/prn
C. Flunisolide (AeroBid) MDI, 2 puffs, bid/prn
D. Metaproterenol (Alupent, Metaproterenol) MDI, 2 puffs qid/prn

---

Answers and Rationales

2.6   **A** COPD/chronic bronchitis is characterized by PFTs that reveal obstruction. These typically include increases in FRC, FEV_1, RV, and compliance.

2.7   **D** Answer **D**, hilar cavitation, is a post–primary disease CXR finding in TB. The other three findings listed are characteristics found on routine CXRs of patients with COPD/emphysema.

2.8   **A** PFTs routinely provide the best, most objective data about the severity of pulmonary dysfunction in COPD and can be used to assess results of maintenance therapy.

2.9   **B, D** Hypoxemia is shown by the decreased Po_2 and decreased percentage of O_2 saturation. Acute respiratory acidosis is indicated by the decreased pH and increased Pco_2. Partial compensation by elevation of bicarbonate reveals concomitant chronic respiratory acidosis.

2.10 **C** Bronchodilators are the drugs of choice to routinely treat COPD. Examples include β-agonists (albuterol or metaproterenol) or anticholinergics (ipratropium bromide). Answer **C**, flunisolide (AeroBid), is an inhaled steroid; however it is not a bronchodilator. Also it is taken bid as a routine maintenance medication, not prn.

References

Bellencourt, P.E. (1996). Chronic obstructive pulmonary disease. In R.E. Rakel (ed.). *Saunders Manual of Medical Practice* Philadelphia: W.B. Saunders Co., pp. 124–125.

Celli, B.R., Snider, G.L., Heffner, J., et al. (1995). Standards for the diagnosis and care of patients with chronic obstructive pulmonary disease. ("Official Statement of the American Thoracic Society," medical section of the American Lung Association.) *Am Rev Resp Dis 152*(Suppl.), S77–S120.

Lapinsky, S.E., & Grossman, R.F. (1996). Chronic obstructive pulmonary disease. In J.M. Rippe, R.S. Irwin, M.P. Fink, & F.B. Cerra (eds.). *Intensive Care Medicine.* (3rd ed., Vol. 1). Boston: Little, Brown & Co., pp. 618–627.

National Institutes of Health/U.S. Department of Health and Human Services. (1995). *Chronic Obstructive Pulmonary Disease* (NIH Publication No. 95-2020). Bethesda, MD: Author.

Stauffer, J.L. (1997). Chronic obstructive pulmonary disease. In L.M. Tierney, Jr., S.J. McPhee, & M.A. Papadakis (eds.). *Current Medical Diagnosis and Treatment, 1997* (36th ed.). Stamford, CT: Appleton & Lange, pp. 250–255.

Stoller, J.K., & Aboussouan, L.S. (1995). Chronic obstruction lung diseases. In R.B. George, R.W. Light, M.A. Matthay, & R.A. Matthay (eds.). *Chest Medicine: Essentials of Pulmonary and Critical Care Medicine* (3rd ed.). Baltimore, MD: Williams & Wilkins, pp. 201–246.

Turkeltaub, M. (1994). Chronic bronchitis. In V.L. Millonig (ed.). *Adult Nurse Practitioner Certification Review Guide* (2nd ed.). Potomac, MD: Health Leadership Associates, Inc., pp. 144–145.

Turkeltaub, M. (1994). Chronic obstructive pulmonary disease. In V.L. Millonig (ed.). *Adult Nurse Practitioner Certification Review* (2nd ed.). Potomac, MD: Health Leadership Associates, Inc., pp. 153–156.

Additional Recommended References

Anup, A.B. (1996). *Arterial Blood Gas Analysis Made Easy*. Valhalla, NY: Author, pp. 11–93.

Cropp, A. (1994). Chronic obstructive pulmonary disease and emphysema. In H.W. Griffith, & M.R. Dambro (eds.). *The Five Minute Clinical Consult. 1994* Philadelphia: Lea & Febiger, pp. 212–213.

Ingram, R.H., Jr. (1994). Chronic bronchitis, emphysema, and airways obstruction. In K.J. Isselbacher, E. Braunwald, J.D. Wilson, et al. (eds.). *Harrison's Principles of Internal Medicine.* (13th ed. Vol. 2) New York: McGraw-Hill, pp. 1197–1206.

Papadakis, M.A. (1997). Acid-base disorders. In L.M. Tierney, Jr., S.J. McPhee, & M.A. Papadakis (eds.). *Current Medical Diagnosis and Treatment, 1997* (36th ed.). Stamford, CT: Appleton & Lange, pp. 815–825.

Sanford, J.P., D.N. Gilbert, & M.A. Sande. (1997). *Sanford Guide: 27th Edition Guide to Antimicrobial Therapy, 1997.* Dallas: Antimicrobial Therapy, Inc.

Seidman, J. (1996). Chronic obstructive pulmonary disease. In J.E. Tintinalli, R.L. Krome, & E. Ruiz (eds.). *Emergency Medicine: A Comprehensive Study Guide* (4th ed.). New York: McGraw-Hill, pp. 438–442.

Stauffer, J.L. (1997). Lung: diagnostic tests: Pulmonary function tests, pulmonary exercise stress testing, and bronchoscopy. In L.M. Tierney, Jr., S.J. McPhee, & M.A. Papadakis (eds.) *Current Medical Diagnosis and Treatment, 1997* (36th ed.). Stamford, CT: Appleton & Lang, pp. 238–241.

Weinberger, S.E., & J.M. Drazen. (1994). Disturbances of respiratory function. In K.J. Isselbacher, E. Braunwald, J.D. Wilson, et al. (eds.). *Harrison's Principles of Internal Medicine.* (13th ed., Vol. 2). New York: McGraw-Hill, pp. 1152–1159.

Wilson, R.F., & C. Barton. (1996). Blood gases: Pathophysiology and interpretation. In J.E. Tintinalli, R.L. Krome, & E. Ruiz (eds.). *Emergency Medicine: A Comprehensive Study Guide* (4th ed.). New York: McGraw-Hill, pp. 108–117.

Asthma

DEFINITION

Asthma is a chronic, hyperreactive lung disease subject to intermittent bouts of widespread, reversible tracheobronchial airways obstruction. Airway inflammation and edema, smooth-muscle spasm, bronchoconstriction, and mucous plugging are its hallmarks. Successful treatment to prevent and manage acute exacerbations requires reversing these pathogenic conditions.

ETIOLOGY/INCIDENCE

1. Over 15 million Americans (including 4–5% of all adults) suffer from asthma. Half the cases develop after age 10 and another one third occur

before age 40. Young men are affected more often, but this equalizes with women by age 30. Adult women are more likely to have new-onset and more severe asthma. African Americans/blacks are proportionately more likely to be affected.

2. Morbidity and mortality are significant and continue to climb. In 1990, $6.2 billion (almost 1% of all U.S. health care costs) were spent on asthma-related illness. Of these outlays, 43% involved emergency department use, hospitalization, and death. Inpatient hospitalization alone accounted for $1.6 billion. Each year, 5000 U.S. deaths are attributed to asthma and the mortality rate is increasing worldwide. In the past 15 years, asthma prevalence and severity have risen in the United States and most other Western nations. Numerous theories have been advanced for this phenomenon, including increasing environmental pollution and overuse of β_2-agonists.

3. Asthma is characterized by reversible tracheobronchial inflammation, smooth-muscle hypertrophy and spasm, bronchoconstriction, mucosal edema, and plugging of airways by copious, thick mucus. This combination leads to widespread airflow obstruction. Severe airflow obstruction that cannot be relieved can lead to $\dot{V}/\dot{Q}$ mismatch, acute hypoxemic respiratory failure, and even death.

4. Current consensus is that asthma is a hyperreactivity syndrome of many overlapping etiologies with a final common pathway of reversible airways obstruction. Ongoing, subacute airways inflammation plays a primary role in the pathogenesis of asthma. Numerous accepted references (including the 1991 and 1993 NIH guidelines on asthma) have addressed this key aspect, and treatment to include early and aggressive use of anti-inflammatory medication in acute exacerbations is gaining more widespread clinical acceptance.

5. Most asthmatics (perhaps two thirds) have an allergic component to their disease also. Nearly all of these patients have an immediate airway obstruction response within minutes of exposure to an allergenic trigger. A late reaction occurs as well in 30–50% of these patients, in which a second wave of bronchoconstriction develops 6–10 hours later.

6. There are many proposed mechanisms of the pathogenesis of asthma. A number of these center on the key role played by sensitized lung tissue mast cells. Through their degranulation and release of various biochemical mediators, combined with neural factors, local and then widespread airway narrowing occurs. Histamine, bradykinin, chemotactic factors, platelet-activating factor, and arachidonic acid metabolites such as prostaglandins and leukotrienes are the major mast cell mediators involved. The familiar bronchoconstriction, cellular infiltration, platelet activation, increased vascular permeability, edema, and increased mucus secretion then result. Infiltration of the lung mucosa and submucosa by eosinophils and other inflammatory cells (such as lymphocytes and neutrophils), plus epithelial damage and denuding, are also important in the immunopathogenesis of asthma.

7. Although there is no agreed-upon genetic pattern, there does seem to be a familial association of reactive airway disease (asthma and bronchospasm), allergic rhinitis, and eczema/atopic dermatitis.

8. Asthmatic exacerbations may occur spontaneously or from various trigger factors, including:
   A. Respiratory infections (the most common asthmatic exacerbation trigger)
   B. Allergens; very common overall—seasonal (pollens) or nonseasonal (especially dust mites, animal dander, feathers, mold)

    C. Exercise/exertion (one of the most common triggers)

    D. Certain drugs (nonsteroidal anti-inflammatory drugs [NSAIDs], ASA, sulfite food preservatives, and especially β-blockers—even in eyedrops)

    E. Environment (air pollution, thermal inversions, or cold, dry air)

    F. Occupational exposure (may occur immediately or may take weeks to months after initial exposure to a sensitizing chemical or other triggering agent)

    G. Smoking (especially before and during an acute exacerbation)

    H. Emotional stress (complex interaction with vagal efferent activity, endorphins, and psychological factors of perceived stress; up to one half of asthmatics may have these overlapping pathways)

9. Prognosis

    A. Generally excellent outlook, despite small increase in mortality over the past 10–15 years.

    B. Appropriate medical regimens used with motivated, compliant patients can reduce hospitalization rates for exacerbations and can significantly improve such patients' level of function in their daily lives.

SIGNS AND SYMPTOMS

1. Signs and symptoms vary with the severity of the exacerbation.
2. Symptoms of an exacerbation may include any or all of these:

    A. Wheezing

    B. Cough

    C. Dyspnea

    D. Exercise intolerance

    E. Nocturnal attacks

    F. Diffuse chest tightness (important later symptom)

    G. Fatigue (important late symptom that may signal need for more critical interventions, such as intubation and mechanical ventilation)

3. Signs of an exacerbation may include any or all of these:

    A. Tachypnea

    B. Wheezing (expiratory alone or combined with inspiratory wheezes)

    C. Prolonged expiration

    D. Cough

    E. Moderate or no sputum production

    F. Tachycardia

    G. Increased work of breathing (important later signs)

        1) Accessory respiratory muscle use

        2) Sitting up and leaning forward onto elbows to aid breathing ("tripod" position)

        3) Difficulty speaking

        4) Hypoxemic signs of air hunger:

            a. Restlessness

            b. Anxiety and/or fearfulness

            c. Sweating

            d. Possible irritability and/or confusion

PHYSICAL FINDINGS

1. See also asthma signs listed above.
2. Wheezing (inspiratory usually is a later finding than expiratory wheezing)

3. Decreased breath sounds (often correlate with patient's sense of chest tightness and can be an important later finding)
4. Hyperresonance to percussion
5. Flattened diaphragms (seen on CXR, consistent with hyperresonance)
6. Cyanosis (important later finding)
7. Pulsus paradoxus (systolic BP decline $\geq$10 mm Hg with inspiration—important late finding that may signal need for more critical interventions, such as intubation and mechanical ventilation)

DIFFERENTIAL DIAGNOSIS

1. Wheezes alone do not distinguish asthma. Consider other diseases or conditions that could cause wheezing, cough and/or dyspnea.
2. Cardiac disease, including CHF.
3. COPD.
4. Pulmonary embolism.
5. Pneumonia.
6. Foreign body or tumor obstruction of upper or lower airway.
7. TB.
8. Other respiratory infection.
9. Cough due to *B*-blocker or angiotensin converting enzyme (ACE) inhibitor medications.
10. Acute asthmatic exacerbation can resemble an anaphylactic reaction.

DIAGNOSTIC TESTS/FINDINGS

1. Airflow limitation can be measured in a convenient, widely available manner using a peak flow meter (PFM). This simple, inexpensive hand-held device measures peak expiratory flow rate (PEFR), which indicates the severity of airway obstruction.
   A. PFMs have the advantage in the emergency department, acute care, and critical care settings of showing earlier, more subtle signs of respiratory decompensation before the onset of oxygen desaturation would be registered on measurements such as pulse oximetry.
   B. Predicted values vary according to height, sex, and age. Adult men normally can forcefully exhale 450–640 L/min, while adult women typically reach 350–500 L/min. It is useful for patients to monitor their PEFR over time to establish their own personal best readings (highest PEFR after a period of maximum therapy). As a general rule of thumb:
      1) With 80–100% of personal best or predicted PEFR, maintain current therapy.
      2) With 60–80% of personal best or predicted PEFR, treat the acute exacerbation and adjust maintenance program.
      3) With <60% of personal best or predicted PEFR, patient must seek immediate medical aid for bronchodilator and other acute exacerbation therapy.
   C. PEFR <200 means an acute exacerbation that needs immediate medical attention. *PEFR <100 is a grave sign that may indicate impending acute respiratory failure and must be treated emergently.*
   D. It is important to properly instruct patients in how to use PFMs and to observe their PEFR results in order to avoid overtreating a poorly obtained measurement.

E. PFMs also allow patients to identify (and thereby help avoid and/or minimize) environmental, occupational, and other triggers to their asthma exacerbations.

2. PFTs are useful in outpatient settings to demonstrate reversible obstruction, which could be diagnostic of asthma. Look for decreases in FEV_1. FVC also may be <1 L. Obstruction that improves after inhaled bronchodilator (FEV_1 increases by at least 15%) is consistent with reversible bronchospasm. Conversely, the absence of PFT improvement after bronchodilator does not prove irreversibility of airway obstruction.

A. The ACNP may choose to recommend this for follow-up after the patient is discharged from the acute care setting.

3. On an outpatient basis it is sometimes helpful to diagnose asthma using nonspecific bronchial provocation testing with inhaled histamine or methacholine, or with exercise challenge. This can be most useful when asthma is suspected with unexplained cough, despite normal baseline spirometry. (A positive test correlates with FEV_1 decrease of $\geq 20\%$ after challenges.)

A. The ACNP may choose to recommend this for follow-up after the patient is discharged from the acute care setting.

4. Routine CXRs show hyperinflation and flattened diaphragms in asthma. In acute exacerbation, however, consider CXR if febrile, or if signs and/or symptoms are sudden onset or first-time onset. CXR during asthma attack can help rule out pneumonia, pneumothorax, foreign body obstruction, or other disorders which could exacerbate and/or mimic asthma.

5. Labs

A. CBC: May be normal, or may have increased eosinophils related to an allergic asthmatic response

B. Sputum exam: Thick, viscous mucus that may be positive for eosinophilia

C. Nasal secretion stain: May be positive for eosinophilia

D. Allergy skin patch testing or in vitro methods: May determine allergic component (not done often)

E. Immunoglobulins: Screen for immunodeficiency, and check for elevated IgE (not done often)

6. ABGs

A. Measurements may be normal during a mild asthma attack.

B. Mild hypoxemia and respiratory alkalosis (blowing off CO_2) occur with moderate asthma attack.

C. In more severe cases, respiratory muscle fatigue can lead to worsened hypoxemia and disappearance of respiratory alkalosis.

D. The need to consider emergent intubation and mechanical ventilation exists when P_{CO_2} normalizes or respiratory acidosis develops in the face of worsening hypoxemia.

E. To review ABG interpretation, refer to the references listed following this section.

7. Electrocardiogram (ECG)

A. Not routinely done in asthmatics, unless otherwise indicated

B. During acute exacerbation, especially if severe, may show:

1) Dysrhythmias, including supraventricular tachycardia

2) Right-axis deviation or right bundle branch block (RBBB)

MANAGEMENT/TREATMENT

Pharmacologic

1. A host of pharmacologic agents and other treatments (including precautions for ventilator management of asthma-induced acute respiratory failure) are available and are supported by standard references, including the aforementioned 1991 and 1993 NIH asthma guidelines.
   A. For further information, the reader is referred to any of the several excellent references listed.
   B. A selected list of drugs commonly encountered is included below, along with the usual adult doses for stable patients.
2. Basic categories of drug management for asthma include:
   A. Oxygen
   B. Bronchodilators
   C. Corticosteroids
   D. Antimediators
   E. Prescription devices
   F. Rehydration measures
3. Oxygen therapy: Unless more aggressive measures are immediately needed, low-flow O_2 (1–3 L/min, as needed and tolerated) should be begun on all patients in asthmatic exacerbation who present to the emergency room (ER) or other acute care settings.
4. Bronchodilators (all relax bronchial smooth muscle)
   A. Sympathomimetics
      1) Albuterol (Proventil, Ventolin)
         a. *Note*: Selective B_2-agonist. The most frequently used drug in emergency department treatment of acute exacerbations. Similar clinical effect as metaproterenol but longer duration of effect. Relatively inexpensive.
         b. MDI: 1–4 puffs q4–6h/prn. (May consider greater frequency/prn acute exacerbation. More effective when used with prescription spacer device.)
         c. HHN solution (0.5%): 0.5 mL (2.5 mg) + 2.5 mL NS via HHN, q4–6h/prn. (May consider 5-mg HHN dose and/or a greater frequency/prn acute exacerbation.)
         d. HHN unit dose (0.083%) solution: One 3-mL ampule dose via HHN, q4–6h/prn. (May consider greater frequency prn/acute exacerbation.)
         e. Tablets (2 or 4 mg) or syrup (2 mg/5 mL): 2–4 mg PO, q6–8h/prn.
      2) Salmeterol (Serevent)
         a. *Note*: Caution patient *not* to use this for acute exacerbations due to delayed onset of action. The longest-acting and also most expensive B_2-agonist. May be used for maintenance therapy. Especially useful for nocturnal asthma. More effective when used with prescription spacer device.
         b. MDI: 2 puffs q12h/prn.
      3) Metaproterenol (Alupent, Metaprel)
         a. *Note*: MDI is the preferred formulation in most cases. Selective B_2-agonist. Similar clinical effect as albuterol but somewhat shorter duration of effect. More effective when used with prescription spacer device.

      b. MDI: 1–4 puffs q3–4h prn. (May consider greater frequency/prn acute exacerbation).

    4) Terbutaline (Brethine, Bricanyl)

      a. *Note*: Oral formulations not recommended due to side effects commonly found: tremor, anxiety, palpitations. SQ route has slow onset of effect (30 minutes). Stimulation not limited to B_2-adrenergic effect.

      b. SQ injection (1 mg/mL): 0.25 mg SQ, may repeat $\times$ 1 after 30 minutes.

    5) Epinephrine (variety of brands)

      a. *Note*: Epinephrine SQ has similar effects as inhaled B_2-agonists. Use epinephrine only with caution if must be given to older patients or to those with cardiac abnormalities (tachycardia, hypertension [HTN], dysrhythmias). MDI is available over the counter but is not very useful due to α and B_1-stimulation.

      b. SQ injection (0.1%, or 1:1000); 0.3–0.5 mL (0.3–0.5 mg) SQ. May repeat $\times$ 1 after 30 minutes.

  B. Anticholinergics

    1) Ipratropium bromide (Atrovent)

      a. *Note*: Few side effects. More helpful in COPD exacerbations than are sympathomimetics. Useful for asthmatics with an overlapping COPD component.

      b. MDI: 2–4 puffs q6h/prn. (More effective when used with prescription spacer device.)

      c. HHN unit dose (0.02%) solution: One 2.5-mL ampule dose via HHN, 6–8h/prn.

  C. Methylxanthines

    1) Aminophylline

      a. *Note*: Seldom indicated except in certain refractory asthma exacerbations. Theophylline-dependent patients whose serum theophylline levels are subtherapeutic are good candidates for IV aminophylline, however.

      b. Calculate dose using lean body mass. Need to check serum theophylline levels to keep between range of 10 and 20 μg/mL.

      c. Load at 5.6 mg/kg via IV over 30 minutes for patient not using PO theophylline. Maintenance dose is given by constant infusion via IV pump at 0.7 mg/kg/hr. Decrease maintenance dose accordingly if patient has CHF or liver disease, or is taking cimetidine or erythromycin.

    2) Oral theophylline (variety of brands)

      a. *Note*: Theophylline has generally lost favor in asthma treatment, especially for routine maintenance. β_2-selective agonists have largely replaced it as the drugs of choice to treat bronchospasm. Serum theophylline levels are needed to guide maintenance dosing. Dose it to maintain therapeutic serum levels at 10–20 μg/mL.

      b. Sustained-release tablets and bead-filled capsules: 200 mg PO, q12h to start; then change to 200–600 mg PO, q8–12h.

5. Corticosteroids (the most effective anti-inflammatory agents)

  A. Methylprednisolone sodium succinate (Solu-Medrol, Medrol)

    1) *Note*: Onset of effective response may take several hours. Commonly used in emergent treatment of asthma attacks.

        2) IV injection (vials of 40, 125, 500, 1000, and 2000 mg): Load 125 mg or 1–2 mg/kg IV; then 0.5–1 mg/kg IV, q6h/prn. May also give same doses IM, as alternate route.

        3) PO tablets (2, 4, 8, 16, 24 and 32 mg): 4–48 mg PO qd, generally given as a taper-down therapy over 7–10 days.

        4) Medrol Dosepack: Tapers 24 mg to 0 mg over 7 days.

    B. Hydrocortisone sodium succinate (Solu-Cortef)

        1) *Note*: Onset of effective response may take several hours.

        2) IV injection (vials of 100, 250, 500, and 1000 mg): 4 mg/kg IV, q6h/prn.

    C. Prednisone (variety of brands)

        1) *Note*: Generally given as taper-down therapy over 7–14 days. Caution with systemic side effects and steroid dependence if on long-term therapy.

        2) Tablets (2.5, 5, 10, 20, or 50 mg) or elixir (5 mg/5 mL)

           a. For acute bronchospasm: 1 mg/kg or 40–60 mg PO, q24h to load, then taper down (some advocate dividing qd dose in half and giving bid).

           b. For chronic bronchospasm: 5–40 mg PO qd to qod.

    D. Inhaled corticosteroids

        1) These have *no* use in acute exacerbations. Helpful for chronic maintenance therapy, as locally absorbed and minimal systemic side effects. Rinse mouth after use to prevent oral candidiasis. Use of prescription spacer devices improves delivery and minimizes side effect of oral candidiasis or cough/wheeze after inhalation.

        2) Flunisolide (AeroBid).

           a. MDI: 2–4 puffs q12h

        3) Triamcinolone acetonide (Azmacort).

           a. MDI: 2–6 puffs q6–12h

        4) Beclomethasone dipropionate (Beclovent, Vanceril).

           a. MDI: 2–4 puffs q6–12h

6. Antimediators

    A. Neither of these has use in acute exacerbations. These exert a nonsteroidal, anti-inflammatory effect by stabilizing mast cells. Advantages include no corticosteroid side effects, but may not be quite as effective as inhaled corticosteroids in the maintenance therapy of moderate to more severe asthma. May take 2–4 weeks of treatment for onset of effective response. Cromolyn has the advantage that it may also be used 15–30 minutes before exercise or exposure to allergens or cold air as a prophylactic against bronchospasm. MDIs are more effective when used with prescription spacer devices.

    B. Cromolyn sodium (Intal)

        1) MDI: 2–4 puffs qid

        2) HHN (20 mg/2 mL ampule) solution: 20 mg qid by HHN

    C. Nedocromil sodium (Tilade)

        1) MDI: 2 puffs qid

7. Prescription devices

    A. Prescription spacer devices

        1) These small, convenient, and relatively inexpensive chambers improve MDI effectiveness by up to 50%, as shown by radioisotope uptake studies.

        2) Variety of brands, including Aerochamber and others. A mask is available as well that can accommodate the elderly, infants, or others who may need help providing a tight seal across the mouth.

   B. PFMs

      1) These small, convenient, and relatively inexpensive devices measure PEFR, giving patients and their medical providers quicker, more accurate feedback on how open versus constricted a patient's airways are at any given time. With a motivated, compliant patient, such information provides greater personal control by decreasing exacerbations, and by allowing early, appropriate intervention when warranted.

      2) Measurement of PEFR is a more sensitive early indicator of an impending asthma attack than is pulse oximetry. It is also far more accurate than relying upon clinical signs and symptoms to judge the severity of an acute exacerbation. For these reasons many hospital clinics and emergency departments have begun to use PFMs. Perhaps this may become a useful trend for other acute care settings as well.

      3) Variety of brands, including Peak, Mini-Wright, and others.

   C. Powered nebulizers

      1) These larger, bulky, expensive devices are used to aerosolize liquid solutions (e.g., bronchodilators such as albuterol, anticholinergics such as ipratropium bromide, or antimediators such as cromolyn sodium).

      2) Variety of brands. Home units such as PulmoAid use room air via a compressor. Hospital units are usually HHNs connected to an oxygen source, offering the advantages of simultaneous bronchodilation along with the supplemental O_2 recommended for acute asthma attacks.

8. Rehydration measures include IV fluids, PO liquids, and aerosolized saline (as part of HHN treatments).

Classifications of Severity, Referrals and Admissions, and Treatment Plans

1. *Consider physician specialist referral (i.e., pulmonologist or allergist/immunologist)* for:

   A. New-onset asthmatics

   B. Geriatric patients

   C. Patients who are not responding to therapy

   D. Patients whose conditions during an exacerbation are deteriorating

2. Classification of asthma managed on an outpatient basis

   A. The reader is referred to National Asthma Education Program. (1991). *Executive Summary: Guidelines for the Diagnosis & Management of Asthma.* (Publication No. 91-3042A) for several useful algorithms for the management of asthma, including outpatient (chronic, mild, moderate, or severe) emergent, and inpatient evaluation and treatment.

   B. Mild stage

      1) Defined for adults as one or more of these:

         a. Periodic, limited symptoms (<1 hour) at ≤2 times per week

         b. Limited symptoms (<1/2 hour) with physical exertion

         c. No symptoms between exacerbations

         d. Infrequent nighttime symptoms (once or less per month)

      2) Baseline PEFR or FEV_1 values are usually ≥80% of personal best or predicted value

         a. Variability ≥20% with symptoms/mild asthma attacks

3) Treatment plan
   a. Short-acting β_2-agonist MDI (such as albuterol, etc.) at 1–2 puffs, as directed/prn to relieve symptoms, or prior to trigger exposure or exercise/exertion
   b. Other than identifying and avoiding triggers, no daily maintenance program needed at this stage

4) The reader is referred to: National Asthma Education Program. (1991). *Executive Summary: Guidelines for the Diagnosis and Management of Asthma.* (Publication No. 91-3042A) for algorithm for the management of chronic, mild adult asthma.

C. Moderate stage
   1) Defined for adults as one or more of these:
      a. Symptoms once or less per week
      b. Longer symptoms (asthma attack may last many days)
      c. Asthma attacks begin to limit activity and affect sleep
      d. Patient occasionally requires emergency medical treatment
   2) Baseline PEFT or FEV_1 values are usually only 60–80% of personal best or predicted values
      a. Variability: 20–30% with mild to moderate attacks
      b. Variability: >30% with the worst asthma attacks
   3) *The ACNP may collaborate with a physician until the patient is stabilized. Depending upon the setting and the patient's needs, referral to a physician specialist, such as a pulmonologist or allergist/immunologist may be advisable.*
   4) Treatment plan
      a. Daily maintenance program with
         i. Avoidance of triggers
         ii. MDI of cromolyn sodium or nedocromil (for more stable cases), or MDI corticosteroids (for less stable cases)
      b. Use short-acting β_2-agonist MDI or HHN (such as albuterol, etc.) as directed at ≤ tid–qid/prn to relieve symptoms
      c. If symptoms continue to persist despite above measures, either:
         i. Increase dose of MDI steroids; or
         ii. Add another drug to the regimen
            • PO β_2-agonist
            • Long-acting β_2-agonist MDI (salmeterol)
            • PO theophylline, sustained-release
            • Any of these three drugs is longer-acting and may help relieve nighttime asthma symptoms
            • Finally, MDI anticholinergic (ipratropium bromide) can be added prn. (Can be helpful, especially for asthmatics with an overlapping COPD component.)

D. Severe stage
   1) Defined for adults as one or more of these:
      a. Symptoms are continual
      b. Physical activities have become limited or curtailed
      c. Frequent asthma attacks
      d. Frequent nighttime asthma symptoms
      e. Patient occasionally requires emergency medical treatment
   2) Baseline PEFR or FEV_1 values are usually <60% of personal best or predicted values.
      a. Variability: 20–30% even with routine medication program
      b. Variability: ≥30–50% with the worst asthma attacks

3) *Referral is advised to a physician specialist, such as a pulmonologist or allergist/immunologist.*
4) Treatment plan
   a. Daily maintenance program with:
      i. Avoidance of triggers
      ii. Pacing of activities (to help conserve energy)
      iii. MDI corticosteroids at higher doses and greater frequency
      iv. A long-acting drug:
         • PO β_2-agonist
         • Long-acting β_2-agonist MDI (salmeterol)
         • PO theophylline, sustained release
         • Any of these three drugs is longer acting and may help relieve nighttime asthma symptoms
         • Finally, MDI anticholinergic (ipratropium bromide) can be added & prn. (Can be helpful, especially for asthmatics with overlapping COPD component.)
   b. Use short-acting β_2-agonist MDI or HHN (such as albuterol, etc.), as directed, at ≤tid-qid/prn breakthrough symptoms. (*Caution*: Advise patient *not* to use this as part of daily maintenance therapy. If patient needs this frequently, in addition to daily maintenance program listed above, inform patient to visit medical provider promptly to adjust regimen or arrange other medical care.)
   c. If symptoms continue to persist despite above measures:
      i. Add qd or qod PO corticosteroids. (*Caution*: Can cause systemic side effects and foster steroid dependence.)
5) Categories of drugs used in severe asthma stage
   a. Sympathomimetics: Inhaled and PO
   b. Corticosteroids: Inhaled and PO
   c. Antimediators: Inhaled
   d. Anticholinergics: Inhaled
   e. Theophylline: PO
   f. Antimicrobial agents
      i. Not routinely needed, but may be useful with bacterial tracheobronchitis concurrent with asthma attack
      ii. Consider amoxicillin, amoxicillin-clavulanate, tetracycline, or TMP-SMX
   g. Avoid drugs that trigger asthma symptoms
      i. Key offenders are β-blockers, even in eyedrops
      ii. ACE-inhibitors also worsen cough in asthmatics
      iii. ASA, NSAIDs, and various others
   h. Desensitization therapy
      i. Rarely used
      ii. Better to try environmental control, trigger avoidance, and compliance with daily maintenance program.
3. Emergency treatment and hospitalization
   A. *Depending upon the setting, the ACNP may be called upon to collaborate with an emergency medicine physician and/or to make a referral to a physician specialist, such as a pulmonologist or allergist/immunologist for immediate follow-up and possible hospital admission.*
   B. NIH summaries provide the following information:
      1) ER indices of acutely severe adult asthma

2) Algorithm of ER management for acute exacerbations of adult asthma

3) Algorithm of hospital management for acute exacerbations of adult asthma

C. Objective air flow measurements (PEFR/PFM) are vital, yet patient may be unable to cooperate.
   1) PEFR <200 L/min: severe asthma attack
   2) PEFR <100 L/min: very severe asthma attack.

D. Monitor with pulse oximetry.

E. Start all patients with acute, severe asthma on supplemental O_2.
   1) Low-flow (1–3 L/min) via nasal cannula is appropriate.

F. Give inhaled β_2-agonist drugs (HHN or MDI if tolerated).
   1) Up to three HHN treatments may be given over 1 to 1½ hr.
   2) Best to use PEFR/PFM as guide, although pulse oximetry may also be used to guide therapy.

G. Order ABGs, as appropriate (particularly if patient is not responding to therapy).

H. Patients with an acute, severe asthma attack appear fatigued, irritable, and anxious.

I. Rehydration and attention to toxic side effects from overuse of medications are needed.

J. IV aminophylline is not often indicated for the emergency treatment of asthma, except in certain refractory exacerbations. Theophylline-dependent patients whose serum theophylline levels are subtherapeutic are good candidates for IV aminophylline, however.
   1) Calculate dose using lean body mass. Need to check serum theophylline levels to keep in the therapeutic range, between 10 and 20 μg/ml.
   2) Load at 2.5–5 mg/kg via IV over 30 minutes. Maintenance dose is given by constant infusion via IV pump at 0.7 mg/kg/hr. Decrease maintenance dose accordingly if patient has CHF or liver disease, or is taking cimetidine or erythromycin.

K. Terbutaline SQ (up to three doses of 0.25 mg each, over 1 to 1½ hr). May be useful in younger or middle-aged patients.
   1) Alternative sympathomimetic therapy

L. IV corticosteroids, if patient does not improve with sympathomimetic therapy, or if has severe, acute asthma.
   1) Lag time of 4–6 hours before clinical effect is noted
   2) PO corticosteroids: Possibly useful alternative for less severe attacks
   3) Inhaled corticosteroids: No place in emergency treatment

M. Ipratropium bromide HHN:
   1) Controversial in acute, severe attack
   2) Possibly may help overlapping COPD component

4. *Depending upon the setting, the ACNP may be called upon to arrange hospital admission and pulmonary physician specialist referral during an acute, severe asthma exacerbation.*

A. Hospital admission is indicated for more than one of these:
   1) Emergency treatment: No objective improvement after vigorous ER treatment
   2) Severity of airflow restriction: PEFR or FEV_1 remain persistently low (<40% of personal best or predicted value)

3) BP: Pulsus paradoxus

4) ABGs: Respiratory acidosis and/or worsening hypoxemia, unresponsive to supplemental O_2

5) ECG: Supraventricular dysrhythmias (e.g., multifocal atrial tachycardia; ventricular ectopy; and/or conduction disturbances)

6) CXR: Pneumomediastinum; pneumothorax; or suspected airway infection that cannot be managed well as an outpatient

7) Severity of clinical symptoms: Patient exhaustion or fatigue of respiratory muscles; or confusion, lethargy, or altered mental status

8) History: Patient in status asthmaticus, previous intubation for acute respiratory failure, or previous hospitalizations for severe asthma attacks

B. Additional considerations for hospital admission

1) Low estimation of patient reliability and/or inadequate home care resources and support

2) Delay in seeking emergency medical care, with prolonged symptoms that progressively worsen

3) High-risk co-morbid medical condition, either pulmonary (e.g., pneumonia or COPD) or other (e.g., DM, CHF, CAD, CA, unstable psychiatric illness)

4) Theophylline toxicity; fever; or inability to maintain oral intake

C. *Patients with severe asthmatic exacerbation/status asthmaticus may need prompt admission to the ICU.* Depending upon the setting, the ACNP may be called upon to arrange ICU transfer or admit, along with referral to a pulmonary/critical care physician specialist who needs to follow the patient. *Any of these may be indicators for ICU admit:*

1) Continuing or worsening hypoxemia, despite supplemental O_2

2) Severe respiratory acidosis (pH $\leq$ 7.30)

3) Mechanical ventilation is needed, via ETT or noninvasive technique

4) Severe dyspnea, unresponsive to initial emergency therapy

5) Confusion, lethargy, or respiratory muscle fatigue (i.e., paradoxical diaphragmatic motion).

5. Follow-up

A. Ensure patient has prescriptions.

B. Adjust medications as needed.

C. Monitor patient's PFM readings regularly and during asthma attacks.

D. For those patients taking theophylline:

1) Check serum levels as appropriate.

2) Instruct patient to report conditions that could affect theophylline levels (fever, liver disease, cimetidine, erythromycin).

E. See patient as needed to promptly and vigorously treat exacerbations.

PATIENT EDUCATION

1. Key to proper management of this chronic and potentially life-threatening disease. Include patient's family in treatment plan when possible. Written plans help patient and family to better comanage exacerbations.

2. Emphasize that prevention is vital to remain either symptom-free, or else to minimize the impact of symptoms upon normal, daily activities.

3. Identify and eliminate or minimize asthmatic triggers (e.g., quit smoking; and for patients with exercise-induced symptoms, premedicate before exercise).

4. Emphasize allergy control measures for those asthmatics with an allergic component. (e.g., minimize or eliminate what are identified as an individual patient's known allergenic triggers. Common examples include dust-proofing the home against dust mites, and avoiding pets such as dogs and cats.)

   A. Refer also to the excellent NIH guidelines listed in the following reference section for assessing the possible role of allergy in patients with asthma, as well as effective house-dust mite control measures.

5. Have backup plans in place with family, work site, and/or school to make it easier to identify and promptly manage an asthmatic exacerbation.

6. Educate the patient about asthma pathophysiology, drug use and side effects, and the need to comply with long-term, daily maintenance program (when ordered).

7. Reiterate the importance of avoiding exposure to cigarette smoke. Inform patient of quit-smoking tips and other community resources offered through:

   A. Asthma and Allergy Foundation of America

      1) Especially helpful for information about dust-proofing the home and other hypoallergenic measures, as well as useful diagrams and diaries for use with PFMs

   B. American Lung Association

   C. American Thoracic Society (which is the medical branch of the American Lung Association)

   D. American Cancer Society

   E. American Heart Association

   F. CDC

   G. NIH

8. Advise patient that early, appropriate therapy for asthma attacks significantly improves prognosis. Tell patient to notify medical provider promptly for new or increasing symptoms, or any failure to respond to therapy.

9. Strongly encourage smoking cessation by patients and those with whom they live. Decrease exposure to other sources of air pollution.

10. Demonstrate how to properly use PFMs and encourage their use along with a symptom diary in order for patient to regain maximum control over his or her life.

11. Demonstrate how to correctly use HHNs or MDIs. Prescribe MDI spacer devices (such as Aerochamber) and show patient how to use these, emphasizing that they may improve medication delivery by up to 50%.

12. Encourage stress management, both for patient and for their family members.

13. For patients with exercise-induced asthma, encourage pretreatment with medications before exercise, or moderation of activities when needed.

14. Review with patient where he or she can go for emergency treatment, especially if medical provider is unavailable or if patient experiences an acute asthma attack.

15. Instruct patient to avoid use of medications that may exacerbate asthma (β-blockers, ASA, etc.).

16. Instruct patient to keep up to date on immunizations (pneumovax and annual flu vaccine).

17. The ACNP may refer patient for stress reduction class.

Review Questions

2.11 Asthma is characterized by:
   A. Irreversible bronchoconstriction
   B. Smooth muscle wasting
   C. Tracheobronchial inflammation
   D. Paucity of mucus

2.12 Use of these prescription treatments and devices can help improve asthma outcomes, especially during acute exacerbations:
   A. Oxygen low-flow therapy
   B. Peak flow meters
   C. Spacer chamber devices (for use with MDIs)
   D. All of the above

The following three-part case scenario is for asthma Questions 2.13–2.15 listed below.

Mr. RR is a 43-year-old man who presents to ER with wheezing, dry cough, diffuse chest tightness, and increasing dyspnea over the past 45 minutes. After work today he had decided to jog along the Potomac River to enjoy seeing all the spring cherry blossoms. Midway through his run he became breathless and stopped at the nearest ER.

   Meds: None. PMH: Asthma (rare exacerbations); URI Sx and mild fever × past 3 days.
   FSH: Rare cigarette use; no ETOH intake; no IVDA. Works as a laborer at a dusty job site.
   Vital signs: RR, 28; HR, 102; BP, 128/80; T, 100.8°F
   Pulse oximetry: 95%, room air

On exam, Mr. RR has scattered expiratory wheezes, lungs otherwise clear, occasional dry cough, clear nasal discharge, injected pharynx, and no accessory muscle use.

2.13 As you quickly complete Mr. RR's H&P, you note that he still is able to speak in short sentences. He asks you, "What sets off an asthma attack?" You briefly reply that asthmatic exacerbations may occur spontaneously or from various trigger factors. Of the possible asthmatic exacerbation trigger factors listed above, the most common category is:
   A. Allergens (seasonal and nonseasonal)
   B. Exercise/exertion
   C. Respiratory infection
   D. Occupational exposure

2.14 You diagnose Mr. RR as having a mildly acute asthmatic exacerbation. At your ER, patients in mildly acute exacerbation may be given either HHN or MDI treatment. Mr. RR prefers to try MDI. As you write your medication orders, you recall that the drugs of choice to treat acute asthmatic exacerbations may include all, EXCEPT:
   A. Albuterol (Proventil, Ventolin) MDI, 2 puffs q4h/prn
   B. Ipratropium bromide (Atrovent) MDI, 2 puffs q4h/prn
   C. Beclomethasone dipropionate (Beclovent, Vanceril) MDI, 2 puffs q4h/prn
   D. Metaproterenol (Alupent, Metaproterenol) MDI, 2 puffs q4hr/prn

2.15 After three treatments over 1½ hours, Mr. RR has improved well enough
to be discharged home: RR, 22; HR, 88; pulse oximetry, 98%, room air.
His lungs are clear without wheezes, and he ambulates easily and speaks
in complete, lengthy sentences now. Among the discharge prescriptions
you write, you include a bronchodilator and additional medication to treat
his exacerbation. This category of medication was often omitted during
previous years' treatments for acute exacerbations, yet now is considered
mainstay therapy during an acute asthma attack:

A. Corticosteroids—PO, IM, or IV
B. Corticosteroids—MDI
C. Bronchodilators/sympathomimetics—MDI, HHN, SQ, or PO
D. Bronchodilators/methylxanthines—PO or IV

Answers and Rationales

2.11 **C** Asthma is characterized by tracheobronchial inflammation. It also
is characterized by reversible bronchoconstriction, smooth muscle
hypertrophy, and increased mucus production.

2.12 **D** Oxygen low-flow therapy, peak flow meters, and spacer chamber devices (for use with MDIs) are prescription treatments and devices
that all help improve outcomes, especially during acute exacerbations.

2.13 **C** Respiratory infections are the most common asthmatic exacerbation
trigger. Exercise/exertion is also quite common as an asthmatic trigger, as are allergens (seasonal and nonseasonal). Occupational exposure, while important, is not nearly as widespread or common an
asthmatic trigger.

2.14 **C** Bronchodilators are the drugs of choice to treat acute asthmatic exacerbations. Examples include β_2-agonists (albuterol or metaproterenol) or anticholinergics (ipratropium bromide). Answer **C**, beclomethasone dipropionate (Beclovent, Vanceril), is an inhaled steroid;
however, it is not a bronchodilator. Also it is taken regularly as a
routine maintenance medication (such as 2–4 puffs bid–qid), not prn.
MDI corticosteroids are not used in the treatment of acute asthmatic
exacerbations.

2.15 **A** Corticosteroids are the most effective anti-inflammatory agents during an acute asthmatic exacerbation, ideally given IV or IM, or else
PO. Inhaled corticosteroids have no use in acute asthmatic exacerbation. The widespread tracheobronchial inflammatory process during
acute asthma attacks has been better recognized in recent years.
Some investigators note that the small annual increase in asthma
deaths could be due to overuse of β_2-agonists without adding anti-
inflammatory therapy when needed.

References

Kavuru, M.S., & H.P. Wiedeman. (1995). Asthma. In R.B. George, R.W. Light, M.A.
Matthay, & R.A. Matthay (eds.). *Chest Medicine: Essentials of Pulmonary and Critical Care Medicine* (3rd ed.). Baltimore, MD: Williams & Wilkins, pp. 163–200.

National Asthma Education Program. (1991). *Executive Summary: Guidelines for the Diagnosis and Management of Asthma.* (Publication No. 91-3042A). Bethesda, MD: National Institutes of Health/U.S. Department of Health and Human Services.

Sherman, S. (1996). Acute asthma in adults. In J.E. Tintinalli, R.L., Krome, & E. Ruiz (eds.). *Emergency Medicine: A Comprehensive Study Guide* (4th ed.). New York: McGraw-Hill, pp. 430–438.

Stauffer, J.L. (1997). Asthma. In L.M. Tierney, Jr., S.J. McPhee, & M.A. Papadakis (eds.). *Current Medical Diagnosis and Treatment, 1997* (36th ed.). Stamford, CT: Appleton & Lange, pp. 241–250.

Tronchale, J.A. (1996). Asthma. In R.E. Rakel (ed.). *Saunders Manual of Medical Practice.* Philadelphia: W.B. Saunders Co., pp. 117–119.

Turkeltaub, M. (1994). Asthma. In V.L. Millonig (ed.). *Adult Nurse Practitioner Certification Review Guide* (2nd ed.). Potomac, MD: Health Leadership Associates, Inc., pp. 149–153.

Additional Recommended References

Anup, A.B. (1996). *Arterial Blood Gas Analysis Made Easy.* Valhalla, NY: Author, pp. 11–93.

Asthma. (1992). In C.S. Rivers, D.E. Weber, M.K. Schuda, & E.R. Vaughn (eds.). *Preparing for the Written Board Exam in Emergency Medicine.* Milford, OH: Emergency Medicine Educational Enterprises, Inc., pp. 199–207.

Global Initiative For Asthma. (1996). *Global Strategy for Asthma Management and Prevention: NHLBI/WHO Workshop Report.* (Publication No. 95-3659). Bethesda, MD: National Institutes of Health/U.S. Department of Health and Human Services.

Madison, J.M., & R.S. Irwin. (1996). Status asthmaticus. In J.M. Rippe, R.S. Irwin, M.P. Fink, & F.B. Cerra (eds.). *Intensive Care Medicine* (3rd ed., Vol. I). Boston: Little, Brown & Co., pp. 605–617.

McFadden, E.R. (1994). Asthma. In K.J. Isselbacher, E. Braunwald, & D.L. Kasper (eds.). *Harrison's Principles of Internal Medicine, (13th ed., Vol. 2).* New York: McGraw-Hill, pp. 1167–1172.

Papadakis, M.A. (1997). Acid-base disorders. In L.M. Tierney, Jr., S.J. McPhee, & M.A. Papadakis (eds.). *Current Medical Diagnosis and Treatment, 1997 (36th ed.).* Stamford, CT: Appleton & Lange, pp. 815–825.

Sokolove, P.E. (1997). Emergency treatment of asthma. In J. Hizon (Chair), *Essentials in Emergency Medicine and Urgent Care*, proceedings syllabus. Symposium presented by Continuing Medical Education Associates, Inc., San Diego, CA, pp. 62–69.

Status asthmaticus. (1995). In K.M. Baldwin, C.S. Garza, R.N. Martin, et al. (eds.). *Davis's Manual of Critical Care Therapeutics.* Philadelphia: F.A. Davis Co., pp. 25–35.

Weinberger, S.E., & J.M. Drazen. (1994). Disturbances of respiratory function. In K.J. Isselbacher, E. Braunwald, J.D. Wilson, et al. (eds.). *Harrison's Principles of Internal Medicine. (13th ed., Vol. 2)* New York: McGraw-Hill, pp. 1152–1159.

Wilson, R.F., & C. Barton. (1996). Blood gases: Pathophysiology and interpretation. In J.E. Tintinalli, R.L. Krome, & E. Ruiz (eds.). *Emergency Medicine: A Comprehensive Study Guide* (4th ed.). New York: McGraw-Hill, pp. 108–117.

Acute Bronchitis

DEFINITION

Acute bronchitis can be defined as an acute infection and inflammation of the large bronchi of the tracheobronchial tree, usually by viruses or bacteria. This acute condition often follows an upper respiratory infection.

ETIOLOGY/INCIDENCE

1. Viruses cause >40% of cases. Rhinovirus is most common and is usually associated with shorter, less febrile episodes. Other viral agents may include coronavirus, adenovirus, influenza A and B viruses, herpes simplex, respiratory syncytial virus (RSV), and parainfluenza virus.
2. Bacteria play a variable and somewhat unclear role, particularly in those with chronic bronchitis, as pre-existing colonization of normally sterile air passageways may be hard to distinguish from infection. Bacterial agents may include *H. influenzae, M. catarrhalis, M. pneumoniae,* and *S. pneumoniae.*
3. Atypical organisms such as *Mycoplasma* and *Chlamydia pneumoniae* (TWAR agent) are other infectious agents, more recently identified in young adults. *Moraxella* spp. may also be present, especially in those with abnormal host defenses, including smokers and those with chronic cardiopulmonary disease. Previously thought to be "normal flora," these *Neisseria*-like organisms are now recognized as pathogens that often are β-lactamase producers (as are 20–40% of *H. influenzae*), and thus are resistant to such antibiotics as amoxicillin.
4. One of the most common and often self-limiting diagnoses in primary care, acute bronchitis may have further implications in an acute care setting. When superimposed upon other medical or surgical conditions, especially in a compromised host (such as the geriatric, human immunodeficiency virus (HIV)-positive, or COPD patient), acute bronchitis can develop into a more serious entity.
5. Cigarette smokers (both active and passive) and patients with chronic lung disease often have more frequent, severe episodes. Those with chronic bronchitis tend to experience acute bronchitis episodes every 20–36 weeks.
6. Episodes also are more frequent among the young and the elderly, especially during the winter months.
7. Postinfectious bronchospasm often develops, which may lead to a lingering, dry cough and wheezing for 4–6 weeks after the acute infection abates. In the young, this transient airway hyperactivity sometimes is persistent and may become a risk factor to develop asthma.

SIGNS AND SYMPTOMS

1. Cough, usually worse in the morning.
2. Purulent sputum.
3. Low-grade fever, usually without chills.
4. Chest burning and substernal discomfort.
5. Mild dyspnea on exertion.
6. Systemic symptoms (including myalgias, lethargy, headache, rhinorrhea, postnasal drip, pharyngeal injection, and cervical lymphadenopathy).
7. Hemoptysis may occur. (Acute bronchitis is the most common cause of this symptom, although other, more serious factors such as lung cancer may need to be ruled out.)
8. Wheezes and possibly rhonchi or crackles.
9. In COPD patients, dyspnea, sputum purulence, and increased amounts of sputum are the three cardinal symptoms that correlate with the severity of acute infectious bronchitis episodes.
10. Lung auscultation may be normal, or wheezes may be present, especially with forced exhalation.

PHYSICAL FINDINGS

1. See "Signs," above.

DIFFERENTIAL DIAGNOSIS

1. Cough with upper respiratory tract infections
   A. Influenza
   B. Acute or chronic sinusitis
   C. Nasopharyngitis
2. Cough with lower respiratory tract infections
   A. Pneumonia
   B. Pertussis/whooping cough (infrequent in adults)
3. Noninfectious causes of cough
   A. Postnasal drip
   B. Asthma
   C. Allergens
   D. Medications (e.g., NSAIDs, β-blockers, ACE inhibitors)
   E. Neoplasm
   F. Gastroesophageal reflux

DIAGNOSTIC TESTS/FINDINGS

1. CXR: Normal. Diagnosis can be made by the presence of clinical signs and symptoms and the absence of a lung infiltrate.
2. Sputum Gram's stain and C&S: Usually not done, nor useful. If done, these are likely to show many PMNs and possibly bacteria.
3. CBC: Not generally done, nor useful. WBC may be normal or slightly elevated.

MANAGEMENT/TREATMENT

1. Antibiotics
   A. These are *not* usually indicated for otherwise healthy persons, as many acute bronchitis episodes are viral. Nonetheless, antibiotics are often prescribed, particularly for smokers and others with pre-existing lung disease.
      1) While their use is controversial, many patients who receive antibiotics do seem to improve faster, particularly COPD patients with two or three of the cardinal exacerbation symptoms (dyspnea, increased sputum, and sputum purulence).
      2) Also, by reducing the bacterial load, antibiotics can help modulate the host inflammatory response to such pathogens. This can interrupt the vicious cycle of infection, inflammation, and further infection, more often seen in acute bronchitic exacerbations of chronic bronchitis and other chronic lung disease.
   B. With the increasing prevalence of β-lactamase–producing pathogens (e.g., *M. catarrhalis* and *H. influenzae*), appropriate regimens may include:
      1) Amoxicillin-clavulanate (500 mg PO q8h $\times$ 10 days); *or*
      2) Erythromycin (500 mg PO qid $\times$ 10 days); *or*
      3) A newer macrolide

a. Azithromycin (500 mg PO on day 1, then 250 mg PO qd on days 2–5); *or*

b. Clarithromycin (250 mg PO q12h × 10 days) (*Caution*: Avoid clarithromycin in pregnancy); *or*

4) TMP-SMX DS (1 tab PO bid × 10 days); *or*

5) Tetracycline (500 mg PO qid × 10 days) (*Caution*: Avoid tetracycline in pregnancy); *or*

6) A fluoroquinolone

a. Ciprofloxacin (250–500 mg PO bid × 10 days); *or*

b. Ofloxacin (200–400 mg PO bid × 10 days)

c. *Note*: Avoid fluoroquinolones in teens or pregnancy.

2. Symptomatic Relief

A. Cough suppressants: Codeine preparations may be especially helpful for night cough (e.g., guaifenesin and codeine, 2 tsp q4h/prn).

B. Encourage fluids (e.g., drink 2 or more L/day).

C. Use of vaporizer may be helpful (e.g., cool mist or steam inhalations).

D. Antipyretics, as needed (e.g., Acetaminophen).

E. Bronchodilators, if wheezing is present (e.g., β_2-agonists, such as albuterol MDI, 1 to 2 puffs q4–6h/prn).

F. Expectorants: Not generally useful.

G. Antihistamines: Avoid, as these dry secretions and make it harder to clear infections.

H. Corticosteroids: Only for severely bronchospastic patients. (See "Asthma.")

3. Physician Consultation

A. If symptoms do not begin to improve in 3 days, or if condition worsens.

PATIENT EDUCATION

1. Reiterate the importance of avoiding exposure to cigarette smoke. Quit-smoking tips and other useful community resources are offered through:

A. American Lung Association

B. American Thoracic Society (which is the medical section of the American Lung Association)

C. American Cancer Society

D. American Heart Association

E. CDC

F. NIH

2. Avoid other air pollutants.

3. Rest.

4. Review disease process, medication use, resources available, and the need to notify the medical provider early if condition worsens.

Review Questions

2.16 Postinfectious bronchospasm may develop after a bout of acute bronchitis abates. This sequela is NOT associated with:

A. Brief, productive cough

B. Presence of wheezing

C. Lasts 4–6 weeks after acute infection abates
D. None of the above

2.17 Acute bronchitis is the second most common cause of hemoptysis.
A. True
B. False

2.18 Mr. DA is a 41-year-old man who presents to the ER with A.M. cough, purulent sputum, low-grade fever without chills, mild dyspnea on exertion, and rare hemoptysis × 4 days. He is a nonsmoker who denies wheezes, chest pain, or TB exposure. Your differential diagnosis includes acute bronchitis, which can be diagnosed by the presence of clinical signs and symptoms and the results of lab test(s):
A. Sputum Gram's stain and C&S: Usually show gram-negative diplococci
B. CBC: Usually shows elevated WBC with acute bronchitis
C. CXR: Usually shows pleural effusion that layers out in lateral decubitus position
D. CXR: Usually shows absence of a lung infiltrate

2.19 Ms. Generation X is a young adult, nonsmoker, with no COPD risk factors. During her bout of acute bronchitis you recommend:
A. No antibiotics, initially.
B. Amoxicillin PO 500 mg tid × 10 days
C. Amoxicillin-clavulanate PO 500 mg q8h × 10 days
D. Erythromycin PO 500 mg qid × 10 days

2.20 Mr. DM is a 29-year-old harried sales representative who has just flown into town for a major presentation that he must give in the morning. He feels ill but does not know any local medical providers, so he has come to your ER for treatment. You diagnose acute bronchitis and order minimal medication, with a number of symptomatic relief measures. Mr. DM becomes insistent that he wishes, "Lots of medicines to get well fast," as he feels that tomorrow's presentation will be crucial to his annual bonus. He also asks about taking an over-the-counter medication "To help me sleep tonight." Although you respect the patient's concerns, you advise him that for symptomatic relief during acute bronchitis, the drug category to avoid is:
A. Bronchodilators, if wheezing is present
B. Cough suppressants
C. Antihistamines
D. Antipyretics, as needed

Answers and Rationales

2.16 **A** Postinfectious bronchospasm often develops, which may lead to a lingering, dry cough and wheezing for 4–6 weeks after the acute infection abates in acute bronchitis.

2.17 **B** False. Acute bronchitis is the most common cause of hemoptysis; although other, more serious factors such as lung CA may need to be ruled out.

2.18 **D** Diagnosis of acute bronchitis can be made by the presence of clinical signs and symptoms and the absence of a lung infiltrate on CXR.

2.19   **A**   Antibiotics are usually not indicated for otherwise healthy persons, as many acute bronchitis episodes are viral (40%). For patients who are smokers and others with pre-existing lung disease, however, antibiotics may reduce the bacterial load and thus help modulate the host inflammatory response to such pathogens. This can interrupt the vicious cycle of infection, inflammation, and further infection, more often seen in acute bronchitic exacerbations of chronic bronchitis and other chronic lung disease. The last two drug regimens listed are reasonable choices for patients in this latter category.

2.20   **C**   Avoid antihistamines when possible during acute bronchitis, as these dry secretions and make it harder to clear infections.

References

Jacobs, R.A., & J. Guglielmo. (1997). Anti-infective chemotherapeutic and antibiotic agents. In L.M. Tierney, Jr., S.J. McPhee, & M.A. Papadakis (eds.). *Current Medical Diagnosis and Treatment, 1997* (36th ed.). Stamford, CT: Appleton & Lange, p. 1372.

Niederman, M.S., & G.A. Sarosi. (1995). Respiratory tract infections. In R.B. George, R.W. Light, M.A. Matthay, & R.A. Matthey (eds.). *Chest Medicine: Essentials of Pulmonary and Critical Care Medicine* (3rd ed.). Baltimore: Williams & Wilkins, p. 424 and pp. 430–431.

Stauffer, J.L. (1997). Acute bronchitis. In L.M. Tierney, Jr., S.J. McPhee, & M.A. Papadakis (eds.). *Current Medical Diagnosis and Treatment, 1997* (36th ed.). Stamford, CT: Appleton & Lange, p. 260.

Turkeltaub, M. (1994). Acute bronchitis. In V.L. Millonig (ed.). *Adult Nurse Practitioner Certification Review Guide* (2nd ed.). Potomac, MD: Health Leadership Associates, Inc., pp. 142–144.

Weller, K.A. (1996). Bronchitis. In R.E. Rakel (ed.). *Saunders Manual of Medical Practice*. Philadelphia: W.B. Saunders Co., pp. 120–121.

Additional Recommended References

Cropp, A., & R. Fleming. (1994). Bronchitis, acute. In H.W. Griffith, & M.R. Dambro (eds.). *The 5 Minute Clinical Consult, 1994*. Philadelphia: Lea & Febiger, pp. 138–139.

Koster, F. (1991). Respiratory tract infections. In L.R. Barker, J.R. Burton, & P.D. Zieve (eds.). *Principles of Ambulatory Medicine* (3rd ed.) Baltimore: Williams & Wilkins, pp. 303–319.

Sanford, J.P., D.N. Gilbert, & M.A. Sande. (1998). *Sanford Guide: 28th Edition Guide to Antimicrobial Therapy, 1998*. Dallas: Antimicrobial Therapy, Inc.

Lung Cancer

DEFINITION

Bronchogenic carcinoma is a primary malignant neoplasm arising from the lung itself. The cell types of bronchogenic carcinoma typically include small cell carcinoma (SCC) (including oat cell) and non–small cell carcinoma (NSCC) (including squamous/epidermoid cell carcinoma, adenocarcinoma, and large cell carcinoma). Cancer within the lung may also occur due to metastases from other sites.

ETIOLOGY/INCIDENCE

1. Lung carcinoma is now the leading cause of cancer death for both American men (33%) and women (24%), and causes 6% of all U.S. deaths.
2. Men are affected more often than women but the death rate in women is increasing, due largely to smoking trends.
3. Older patients are at higher risk, particularly those between ages 50 and 70 years.
4. Dose-related occurrence, directly proportional to number of pack-years of cigarette smoking. Approximately 85–90% of cases involve active smoking, while many cases have been attributed to passive smoking.
5. Occupational exposure (especially to asbestos and radiation) is additive and often synergistic with tobacco in increasing lung cancer risk. Other occupational exposures that place workers at risk include chromium, nickel, hydrocarbons, and chloromethyl ether. Nonsmokers exposed to the same occupational risks are far less likely to become afflicted with lung cancer.
6. Dietary deficiencies of vitamins A and E are a less well-established risk.
7. U.S. lung cancer—associated medical costs are more than $10 billion, or 1.5% of the nation's total cost of illnesses. Of this expense, 20% is for direct health care. Lost productivity and wages comprise the other 80%.
8. Most lung cancer patients will die within 1 year of diagnosis.

PATHOPHYSIOLOGY

1. Over 20 malignant and benign primary lung neoplasms are classified histologically. Of all malignant lung cancers, 90% are either SCC or NSCC. These are types of bronchogenic carcinoma, or primary malignant tumors of the airway epithelium.
2. SCC (oat cell, intermediate, and combined) accounts for about 20–25% of bronchogenic carcinoma. This type occurs centrally, narrows bronchi by extrinsic compression, and commonly metastasizes widely.
3. NSCC comprises mainly adenocarcinoma, squamous cell/epidermoid carcinoma, and large cell carcinoma.
   A. Adenocarcinoma is the most prevalent lung cancer in both sexes, and accounts for about 35% of cases. This type tends to occur in the lung periphery and, therefore, is not easily detected by sputum cytology. It often metastasizes to distant organs.
   B. Squamous cell/epidermoid carcinoma is the second most prevalent lung cancer and accounts for about 30% of cases. This type occurs centrally as an intraluminal growth in bronchi and can therefore often be detected earlier via sputum cytology. Squamous cell carcinoma is likely to metastasize to regional lymph nodes, and about 10% of these squamous cell carcinomas cavitate.
   C. Large cell carcinoma accounts for about 15% of bronchogenic carcinoma. This type tends to occur in the lung periphery and is therefore not easily detected by sputum cytology. It often metastasizes to distant organs.
4. Treatment decisions are based in large part on the histologic typing of a tumor as SCC or NSCC, as well as by tumor staging.
5. Primary lung cancer carries a generally grim prognosis, despite treatment. When diagnosed, 20% of lung cancer patients have localized disease, 25% have disease spread to regional lymph nodes, and 55% have cancer that has

already metastasized to distant sites. Most lung cancer patients die within a year of diagnosis. Patients fortunate enough to have only localized disease still have a 5-year survival rate of 30% among men and 50% among women.

6. Remote effects may also occur from paraneoplastic syndromes. These often result from the tumor's peptide hormone secretion and/or an immunologic cross-reaction between tumor and normal tissue antigens.

SIGNS AND SYMPTOMS

1. Signs and symptoms of lung cancer correlate with:
   A. The primary cancer type and size
   B. Its metastatic spread to lymph nodes and other organs
   C. Systemic effects
   D. Paraneoplastic syndromes
2. Signs and symptoms vary and may be absent.
   A. Approximately 5–25% of patients may be asymptomatic when diagnosed with lung cancer.
   B. Those who are symptomatic at the time of diagnosis often have advanced lung cancer that is not resectable.
   C. Most bronchogenic cancer is diagnosed because of the appearance of new or increasing symptoms, or by an abnormality noted on CXR.
3. Symptoms
   A. Cough: The most common early symptom, especially "smoker's cough." (May present in 40–75% of patients.)
   B. Unintentional weight loss. (May present in 70% of patients.)
   C. Dyspnea, related to obstruction of major bronchus, is often an early symptom. (May present in 60% of patients.)
   D. Chest pain, related to extension beyond parenchyma, or inflammation of parietal pleura and chest wall. (May present in 50–60% of patients.)
   E. Sputum production. (May present in 45% of patients.)
   F. Hemoptysis. (May present in 20–60% of patients.)
   G. Wheezing, dyspnea, and even stridor, due to partial to nearly complete airway obstruction.
   H. Fever, secondary to atelectasis and infection of distal lung parenchyma. (May present in one third of patients.)
   I. Fatigue.
   J. Anorexia.
   K. Hoarseness. (May present in 5% of patients.)
   L. Shoulder or arm pain.
   M. Bone pain.
   N. Dysphagia.
4. Signs
   A. Hemoptysis
   B. Hoarseness (often from recurrent laryngeal nerve palsy)
   C. Fever
   D. Stridor
   E. Clubbing
   F. Superior vena cava syndrome
   G. Adenopathy
   H. Horner's syndrome

I. Paraneoplastic syndromes or ectopic hormone production
    1) Endocrine and metabolic
    2) Neuromuscular
    3) Cardiovascular and hematologic
    4) Other
       a. Skeletal
       b. Dermatologic
       c. Renal
J. Anemia
K. Hypertrophic pulmonary osteoarthropathy
L. Swelling in face or neck
M. Recurring pneumonia or bronchitis
N. Phrenic nerve palsy

PHYSICAL FINDINGS

1. Physical findings vary and may be absent unless a major bronchus has been obstructed, leading to wheezing or stridor associated with sudden onset of dyspnea.
2. Clinical findings confined to the chest include bronchopulmonary and extra-pulmonary intrathoracic categories. Manifestations may include:
   A. Stridor
   B. Hoarseness
   C. Atelectasis with related changes on physical exam
   D. Consolidation
   E. Superior vena cava obstruction syndrome (an oncologic emergency) that may present with:
      1) Cyanosis
      2) Swelling of neck and/or face
      3) Neck vein engorgement and absent pulsations
3. Clinical findings associated with regional or distant involvement include extrathoracic metastatic and extrathoracic nonmetastatic categories. Manifestations may include:
   A. Lymphadenopathy (especially supraclavicular or scalene)
   B. Horner's syndrome (miosis, ptosis, anhidrosis from supracervical ganglia involvement)
   C. Clinical findings specific to the affected organ(s) (e.g., neurologic impairments from central nervous system [CNS] metastases, especially to the brain)
4. Clinical evidence of paraneoplastic syndromes or ectopic hormone production. Approximately 15% of patients (especially those with SCC) first present with a paraneoplastic syndrome before any other signs or symptoms of lung cancer are recognized.

DIFFERENTIAL DIAGNOSIS

1. Other diseases with similar CXR or clinical appearances:
   A. Granulomatous diseases
      1) Mycobacterial disease
         a. TB
         b. MAC

        2) Fungal diseases
        3) Sarcoidosis
    B. Hamartoma (the most common benign lung tumor)
    C. Pneumonia
    D. Lung abscess
    E. Bronchitis
    F. Carcinoid tumors
2. Cancer that has metastasized to the lung from extrapulmonary sites:
    A. Breast
    B. Head and neck
    C. Gastrointestinal (GI) tract
    D. Genitourinary (GU) tract
    E. Germ cell
    F. Melanoma

DIAGNOSTIC TESTS/FINDINGS

1. CXR, sputum cytology, and biopsy are key to diagnosing lung cancer.
    A. CXR may be positive 85% of the time, and directs the need for and sequence of additional testing.
    B. Definitive diagnosis requires cytologic or histologic evidence, with biopsy most often considered the "gold standard" to diagnose lung cancer.
2. Typical tests may include:
    A. Serial CXRs, comparing old and new. Abnormal CXR is not necessarily specific, but common patterns include:
        1) Central lesions: SCC or NSCC (squamous cell)
        2) Peripheral lesions: NSCC (adenocarcinoma, large cell carcinoma, and/or bronchoalveolar cell carcinoma)
        3) Cavitation: NSCC (squamous cell and/or large cell)
        4) Early hilar and/or mediastinal involvement: SCC or NSCC (squamous cell carcinoma)
        5) General: Atelectasis, infiltrates, pleural effusion, enlarging masses
    B. Fiberoptic bronchoscopy is usually the first step after abnormal CXR, in many medical centers. This permits biopsies, needle aspiration and/or lavage, and is most useful when:
        1) Sputum cytology is nondiagnostic.
        2) Occult cancer is suspected (i.e., negative CXR but positive sputum cytology).
    C. Sputum cytology, especially serial, may be positive 40–60% of the time, depending on cancer type and locale. Central, endobronchial tumors are more likely to be detected by sputum cytologies.
    D. Chest CT scan or magnetic resonance imaging (MRI) are often done now for staging; other CT scans are ordered as needed (e.g., brain, GI, bone).
    E. Percutaneous, fine-needle aspiration biopsy can be useful for peripheral lesions with negative cytology.
    F. Pleural fluid samples (when present): Send for cytology, pH, cell counts, lactic dehydrogenase (LDH), and protein.
    G. On occasion, lymph node biopsy may be needed: Scalene, supraclavicular and/or cervical.
    H. Mediastinoscopy or pleural biopsy are done rarely.
    I. Laboratory—consider:
        1) CBC (check for anemia and platelet count).

2) Chemistries and serum electrolytes (to include Na^+, K^+, Ca^{2+}, bone alkaline phosphatase, and liver function tests).
3) PT, PTT.
    J. Consider PPD to rule out TB.
3. Lung cancer staging
    A. The individual diagnostic sequence chosen needs to render accurate histologic diagnosis and clinical staging. Such information is key for planning of appropriate treatment and to better understand the prognosis. A crucial aspect of staging is to evaluate whether or not mediastinal involvement has occurred.
    B. Staging consists of two parts:
        1) Anatomic staging (tumor size, locale, and extent of involvement)
        2) Physiologic staging (patient's ability to withstand treatment options)
    C. NSCC utilizes TNM classification (the new international staging system for lung cancer):
        1) Primary tumor (T)
        2) Nodal involvement (N)
        3) Distant metastasis (M)
    D. SCC utilizes Veterans Administration Lung Cancer Study Group classification:
        1) Limited-stage disease (about 30% of SCC patients)
        2) Extensive-stage disease (about 70% of SCC patients)
    E. The more extensive and severe the staging, the worse the anticipated prognosis. Despite treatment, prospects remain generally grim.
        1) Patients with only localized disease treated early may survive 5 years, up to half of the time.
        2) When all stages of lung cancer are considered, however, 85–90% of patients will not survive 5 years after diagnosis.

MANAGEMENT/TREATMENT

1. The ACNP will consult with collaborating physician as soon as carcinoma is suspected, in order to make a timely referral to a physician pulmonologist.
2. In general, a patient would not be hospitalized strictly because of a newly diagnosed lung CA. Depending upon the patient's condition and the setting, however, the ACNP may be called upon to make arrangements for hospital admission. Admit criteria vary on a case-by-case basis. Suggested considerations for hospital admit may include:
    A. Surgical resection of lung is anticipated
    B. Hemorrhage, secondary to lung CA
    C. Complicating illnesses
    D. Chemotherapy that cannot be managed on an outpatient basis
3. Treatment depends upon cell type, disease staging, underlying lung function, and the patient's overall condition (including age and any pre-existing disease, especially COPD and coronary artery disease [CAD]). Current options may include one or more of the following:
    A. Surgical resection (for approximately 25% of patients)
    B. Chemotherapy
        1) Radiation therapy
        2) Laser therapy
        3) Immunotherapy/other:
            a. New chemical agents

b. Biologic agents

c. Gene therapies

C. SCC, regardless of staging, is usually treated with chemotherapy. A three-drug combination therapy is superior to single-agent chemotherapy. By the time of diagnosis, SCC is usually metastatic and spreads rapidly. Radiation therapy may be used in conjunction with chemotherapy. If a solitary pulmonary nodule exists, excision may be done first and then chemotherapy may be given.

D. NSCC treatment depends on the disease staging.

1) Surgical resection is the treatment of choice for localized disease or a solitary pulmonary nodule. Ideally, the surgical candidate would have stage I to IIIA disease, along with adequate pulmonary reserve. Recurrences may be common. Radiation therapy is an alternate for patients not suitable for surgery.

2) More advanced cases, such as stage IIIB or IV, are not usually treated by surgery. Such patients may require palliative radiation, combination chemotherapy, and/or laser therapy as an alternate to or occasionally before surgery.

E. Malignant pleural effusions may be treated with therapeutic thoracentesis. Pleurodesis may be considered for recurrences.

F. Pain control management.

G. Recurrence or progression of disease needs to be closely monitored by periodic clinical examinations and serial CXRs.

PATIENT EDUCATION

1. Review disease process, treatment options, medication use, community resources available, how to manage uncomfortable side effects of disease and/or treatment, and the need to notify the medical provider promptly concerning any new or increasing signs and symptoms.

2. Encourage adequate nutrition.

3. Reiterate the importance of avoiding exposure to cigarette smoke. Quit-smoking tips and other useful community resources are offered through:

A. American Lung Association

B. American Thoracic Society (which is the medical section of the American Lung Association)

C. American Cancer Society

D. American Heart Association

E. CDC

F. NIH

4. Decrease exposure to other pollutants.

5. Advise patient of additional community resources that may be available, including:

A. The Wellness Community

B. National Cancer Institute (NCI) Cancer Information Service

1) Telephone: 1-800-4CANCER

2) Extensive CA information database via "Physician Data Query" (PDQ) is available via Internet or CD-ROM

C. CANCERLIT feature of MEDLINE (which can be accessed by author or by subject words)

6. Help maintain hope in the face of generally poor prognosis:

A. There is a 10–15% overall 5-year survival rate for lung cancer patients.

   B. NSCC patients—Squamous cell carcinoma: 5-year survival rate of
      35–40% after "curative resection."
   C. SCC patients rarely survive to 5 years following diagnosis.
7. Hospice referral may be indicated.

Review Questions

The following three-part case scenario is for lung cancer Questions 2.21–2.23 listed below

Miss MG is a 51-year-old business associate working in the ER. Recently she
and other ER personnel were exposed to a patient with active TB disease, and
were asked to follow-up with periodic PPD testing. She remains PPD-negative.
Over the next 6–8 weeks co-workers become concerned that she may have active
TB when she begins to note chronic productive cough, mild dyspnea, occasional
pleuritic type chest pain, and periodic hemoptysis. Miss MG is given repeat
PPD testing, which continues negative at 8 weeks following exposure. She has
no HIV risk factors that might suggest an anergic response to PPD testing.
She becomes too fatigued to work and misses two shifts. Unable to schedule
an appointment with her physician's office before the following Monday (3 days
away), she presents to the ER for evaluation and treatment. She has become
anorexic and has experienced an unintentional weight loss of 12 lbs during the
8 weeks since initial TB exposure.

   PMH: Right breast CA, successfully treated 10 years previously with
        lumpectomy and follow-up chemotherapy. (Pt. does monthly breast
        self-exams and has regular follow-up visits with her physician. No
        CA recurrence has been noted to date.) Negative for asthma.
   FSH: Ex-smoker with a 34-pack-year smoking history; no ETOH intake;
        no IVDA. She lives alone and has no family or close friends nearby.

As the ACNP on-duty in the ER when she presents for evaluation and treatment, you note her mild dyspnea, slight hoarseness, generalized weakness,
low-grade fever, and an occasional loose cough. Her lungs are essentially clear
and without wheezes. Lymphadenopathy is noted to supraclavicular and
scalene lymph nodes (LNs). Pulse oximetry is 97% on room air. As part of her
work-up a CXR is performed, which is negative for evidence of TB. Anecdotally,
however, three small to medium sized, central lung lesions are found on CXR
that show early hilar and mediastinal involvement.

2.21 Promptly you obtain a physician pulmonologist consult and the decision
     is made to admit Miss MG at least overnight for further evaluation and
     treatment. SCC is initially suspected. When your patient asks you about
     SCC you explain that it:
     A. Occurs peripherally
     B. Accounts for 20–25% of bronchogenic carcinoma
     C. Seldom metastasizes
     D. None of the above

2.22 As an ACNP, you recall that most lung CA patients die within a year of
     diagnosis. To avoid dashing hope in your co-worker, you spare Miss MG

this grim statistic and are brief in your explanations about lung CA. She insists that, as your co-worker, she wants to know more about what she can expect during her work-up. You describe that definitive diagnosis of lung CA requires:
A. Fiberoptic bronchoscopy, and possible CT of the chest
B. CBC, ABGs, PT, PTT, PPD, sputum cytology, and CEA
C. Sputum cytology, lung biopsy/histology
D. Both A and C

2.23 When you go to visit Miss MG in the acute care unit in days to come, you learn from her attending pulmonologist that SCC has just been confirmed. Her physician requests that you come with her to the bedside as she shares this diagnosis with your patient and co-worker. Miss MG is upset to have to face CA again, after having been in successful remission from breast CA for 10 years. She had become so ill from the chemotherapy used to save her life back then that she wants to be reassured that other options exist now to treat lung CA. In collaboration with her physician, the two of you explain that SCC, regardless of staging, is usually treated with:
A. Triple-drug combination chemotherapy
B. Radiation therapy alone
C. Surgical resection alone
D. Surgical resection with single drug chemotherapy

2.24 Signs and symptoms of lung CA correlate with the primary CA type and size, and:
A. Its metastatic spread to lymph nodes and other organs
B. Systemic effects
C. Paraneoplastic syndromes
D. All of the above

2.25 Superior vena cava obstruction syndrome (an oncologic emergency) may present with:
A. Flushing
B. Gauntness about the neck and/or face
C. Neck vein engorgement and absent pulsations
D. Absence of pericardial tamponade

Answers and Rationales

2.21   **B** SCC (oat cell, intermediate, and combined) accounts for about 20–25% of bronchogenic carcinoma. This type occurs centrally, narrows bronchi by extrinsic compression, and commonly metastasizes widely.

2.22   **D** Definitive diagnosis of lung CA requires fiberoptic bronchoscopy, lung biopsy/histology, sputum cytology, and possible CT of the chest.

2.23   **A** SCC, regardless of staging, is usually treated with chemotherapy. A three-drug combination therapy is superior to single-agent chemotherapy.

2.24   **D** Signs and symptoms of lung CA correlate with the primary CA type and size, its metastatic spread to lymph nodes and other organs, systemic effects, and paraneoplastic syndromes.

2.25 **C** Superior vena cava obstruction syndrome (an oncologic emergency) may present with cyanosis, swelling of the neck and/or face, and neck vein engorgement and absent pulsations.

References

Matthay, R.A., & D.C. Carter. (1996). Lung neoplasms. In R.B. George, R.W. Light, M.A. Matthay, & R.A. Matthay (eds.). *Chest Medicine: Essentials of Pulmonary and Critical Care Medicine.* (3rd ed.). Baltimore: Williams & Wilkins, pp. 393–422.

McLemore, T.L., & P.L. Smith. (1991). Lung cancer. In L.R. Barker, J.R. Burton, & P.D. Zieve (eds.). *Principles of Ambulatory Medicine* (3rd ed.). Baltimore: Williams & Wilkins, pp. 636–645.

Minna, J.D. (1994). Neoplasms of the lung. In K.J. Isselbacher, E. Braunwald, J.D. Wilson, et al. (eds.). *Harrison's Principles of Internal Medicine: Vol. 2* (13th ed.). New York: McGraw-Hill, pp. 1221–1229.

Stauffer, J.L. (1997). Lung: Neoplastic and related diseases. In L.M. Tierney, Jr., S.J. McPhee, & M.A. Papadakis (eds.). *Current Medical Diagnosis and Treatment, 1997* (36th ed.). Stamford, CT: Appleton & Lange, pp. 276–284.

Turkeltaub, M. (1994). Lung cancer. In V.L. Millonig (ed.). *Adult Nurse Practitioner Certification Review Guide* (2nd ed.). Potomac, MD: Health Leadership Associates, Inc., pp. 159–161.

Willsie, S.K. (1996). Cancers of the larynx and lung. In R.E. Rakel (ed.). *Saunders Manual of Medical Practice.* Philadelphia: W.B. Saunders Co., pp. 173–175.

Additional Recommended References

Joshi, J.H. (1996). Metastatic Cancer of Unknown origin. In R.E. Rakel (ed.). *Saunders Manual of Medical Practice.* Philadelphia: W.B. Saunders Co., pp. 176–179.

Miller, J. (1994). Lung primary malignancies. In H.W. Griffith, M.R. Dambro, & J. Griffith (eds.). *The Five Minute Clinical Consult, 1994* (pp. 590–591). Philadelphia: Lea & Febiger, pp. 590–591.

Rosen, M.J. (1996). Acquired immunodeficiency syndrome: Pulmonary complications and intensive care. In J.M. Rippe, R.S. Irwin, M.P. Fink, & F.B. Cerra (eds.). *Intensive Care Medicine: Vol. I* (3rd ed.). Boston: Little, Brown & Co., p. 878.

Rugo, H.S. (1997). Cancer. In L.M. Tierney, Jr., S.J. McPhee, & M.A. Papadakis (eds.). *Current Medical Diagnosis and Treatment, 1997* (36th ed.). Stamford, CT: Appleton & Lange, pp. 69–105.

Smith, P.L., E.J. Britt, & P.B. Terry. (1991). Common pulmonary problems: Cough, hemoptysis, dyspnea, chest pain, and the abnormal chest x-ray. In L.R. Barker, J.R. Burton, & P.D. Zieve (eds.). *Principles of Ambulatory Medicine* (3rd ed.). Baltimore: Williams & Wilkins, pp. 587–592, 599–600.

What You Need to Know About Cancer. [Special issue.] (September 1996). *Sci Am 275* (3).

Tuberculosis

DEFINITION

Chronic infectious disease caused by tuberculosis complex mycobacteria, most often *Mycobacterium tuberculosis* (MTB). Lungs primarily affected, but MTB can also be disseminated throughout the body or can be localized to lymph nodes, bones, meninges, kidneys or skin. This section will cover primary pulmonary TB. Further discussions of this and other sites are available in other texts, including the references listed herein.

ETIOLOGY/INCIDENCE

1. Worldwide: One billion persons infected, 16 million TB cases, 3 million deaths per year.
2. United States: 25,000 cases reported per year, 90% are due to reactivation of previously infected persons, while 10% are newly infected.
3. Increasing number of cases since 1988 due in part to:
   A. Incompletely treated cases promoting multidrug-resistant (MDR) TB.
   B. Rise in numbers of immunocompromised hosts, such as AIDS and HIV-positive patients.
   C. Lax TB control measures at hospitals, prisons, nursing homes, and other institutions.
4. High risk/higher incidence among:
   A. AIDS and HIV-positive persons
   B. Close contacts of patients infected with TB
   C. Nursing home and other long-term care facility residents
   D. Prison inmates
   E. Foreign-born persons (most often immigrants from Southeast Asia, Africa, Latin America, Oceania, and the Caribbean)
   F. Alcoholics and IV drug users
   G. Low socioeconomic groups and the homeless
   H. Chronically debilitated patients
   I. Elderly (>60 years), nonwhites, and males
5. Threat to emergency room (ER) and other hospital personnel.
   A. TB cases may not be isolated until after admitted for hospitalization. By then, numerous ER and other hospital personnel may have been exposed.
   B. Examples from major, urban medical centers:
      1) Olive View/Los Angeles County Medical Center, CA (1994)—Mean time from patient registration to isolation for TB was 6.5 hours; 46% of TB cases were first isolated on the hospital wards.
      2) Parkland Memorial/Dallas County Medical Center, TX (1983)—15 PPD conversions and six cases of active TB in ER personnel; baseline PPD conversion of 3% per year.
      3) Harbor-UCLA/Los Angeles County Medical Center, CA (1993)— During a community epidemic of TB, 31% of ER personnel were found to have converted PPD during employment; Kaplan-Meier estimate of PPD conversion risk:
         a. 6% after 1 year of employment
         b. 14% after 2 years
         c. 27% after 4 years
         d. 40% after 5 years

PATHOPHYSIOLOGY

1. Primary TB infection
   A. Transmitted via infectious, airborne droplet nuclei 1–5 μm in size. Droplet nuclei that reach host alveoli may initiate TB infection. The tubercle bacilli multiply in alveolar macrophages initially. A small number may

spread via lymphatic channels to regional lymph nodes and then through the bloodstream to reach more distant, extrapulmonary sites.

B. MTB replication is usually stopped by host defenses within 2–10 weeks after infection.

C. Cellular immunity arises by 2–4 weeks, but before that TB may be spread via blood or lymph, leading to miliary TB, meningeal TB or TB adenitis.

D. Infected individual then enters latent TB infection period when he or she feels well, is not infectious, and CXR either shows no infiltrate or shows hilar cavitation or peripheral granuloma. PPD reactivity may develop.

E. Immunocompromised adults may not contain the initial infection site, leading to progressive, primary TB disease. (Pleural effusion, cavitation, adenopathy, pneumonitis, or pericarditis may develop.)

2. Tuberculin skin testing is used to identify those who have been infected with MTB. PPD will be positive with active disease or prior TB exposure.

A. Most of those with TB infection have a positive reaction to tuberculin skin testing within 2–10 weeks after infection.

B. Those with TB infection but who do not have active TB disease are not infectious to others.

C. TB infection without active TB disease is often referred to as latent TB infection, and is not considered a case of TB.

3. Active TB disease or reactivation

A. When cell-mediated immunity decreases, reactivation of TB may occur. Latent TB infection can progress to active TB disease when MTB overcome host immune system defenses and begin multiplying. This progression can occur very quickly or many years after infection.

1) In the United States, approximately 5% of those recently infected by MTB will develop active TB disease within 1–2 years after infection. In another 5%, active TB disease will develop >2 years after infection.

2) Approximate lifetime risk is 10% for progression from latent TB infection to active TB disease. The other 90% of those with latent TB infection are most likely to remain infected but free of active TB disease for the rest of their lives.

B. Active TB disease may be heralded by such symptoms as cough, night sweats, unintentional weight loss, hemoptysis, fever, fatigue, or anorexia.

C. Do not assume a patient could not have TB because of previous TB treatment.

D. Various medical conditions can increase the risk that latent TB infection will progress to active TB disease.

1) Per the CDC (1994), two quantified examples of greater risk that TB infection will progress to active TB disease are:
   a. HIV-positive infection (>100 times greater risk)
   b. Diabetes mellitus (3 times greater risk)

2) Other conditions that can increase the risk of progression from latent TB to active TB disease include:
   a. Recent MTB infection (within the past 2 years)
   b. CXR results suggestive of previous TB (in a patient who received inadequate treatment or none at all)
   c. Substance abuse (especially IVDA)

        d. CA (especially of the head and neck)

        e. Chemotherapy or other immunosuppressive therapy

        f. Prolonged corticosteroid therapy

        g. Silicosis

        h. Renal failure, end-stage renal disease

        i. Malnutrition and/or low body weight ($\geq$10% below the ideal)

        j. Hematologic and reticuloendothelial diseases (i.e., leukemia and Hodgkin's disease)

        k. Intestinal bypass or gastrectomy

        l. Chronic malabsorption syndromes

4. Clinical classification system for TB

    A. This CDC-recommended TB classification system is based upon the pathogenesis of the disease. Any patient suspected to have TB (class # 5) should have a diagnosis made within 3 months. All of those with class # 3 (current, active TB disease) or class # 5 should be reported promptly to state or local health departments. Medical providers need to comply with state and local laws and regulations that require the reporting of TB.

    B. Class # 0: No TB exposure; not infected with TB

        1) No history of exposure to TB; and

        2) PPD-negative

    C. Class # 1: TB exposure; no evidence of TB infection

        1) History of exposure to TB; and

        2) PPD-negative

    D. Class # 2: TB latent infection; no active TB disease

        1) PPD-positive; and

        2) Bacteriologic studies for TB (if done) are negative; and

        3) Clinical evidence of TB is negative; and

        4) CXR evidence of TB is negative

    E. Class # 3: Current, active TB disease

        1) *M. tuberculosis* culture (if done) is positive; *or*

        2) PPD-positive, plus clinical or CXR evidence of current, active TB disease

    F. Class # 4: Previous TB disease

        1) PMH of previous episode(s) of TB; *or*

        2) Abnormal but stable CXR findings, PPD-positive, bacteriologic studies for TB (if done) are negative, and no clinical or CXR evidence of current TB disease

    G. Class # 5: TB suspected

        1) Diagnosis is pending.

5. Extrapulmonary TB occurrence

    A. Reactivation: 85% localize to lungs, while 15% localize to extrapulmonary sites.

    B. Extrapulmonary sites, listed by decreasing frequency: Lymph nodes, pleura, kidneys, joints and bones, meninges.

    C. Unless in open skin lesions (such as PO or at abscess), extrapulmonary TB is not infectious.

6. Patients likely to have increased infectivity:

    A. Greater number of MTB coughed into the air.

    B. Pulmonary TB, laryngeal TB, active cough (from any reason), acid-fast bacilli (AFB) in sputum smear, CXR cavitation, noncompliant patient, incomplete and/or inadequate treatment.

7. AIDS and HIV-positive persons
    A. HIV is a large contributor to the resurgence of TB.
    B. One million HIV-positive cases in the United States, while 10% are also infected with TB.
    C. Those infected with HIV are also more likely to develop active TB disease. (>100 times greater risk, per the CDC, 1994.)
    D. About 40% of HIV-positive close contacts exposed to TB may develop active TB disease within 4–8 weeks of exposure to TB.
    E. Patients who are both HIV-positive and PPD-positive carry a risk of 7–10% per year to develop active TB disease. This contrasts with an approximate lifetime risk of 10% for PPD-positive, HIV-negative patients to develop active TB disease.
        1) In the United States, approximately 5% of those recently infected by MTB will develop active TB disease within 1–2 years after infection. In another 5%, active TB disease will develop >2 years after infection.
        2) Approximate lifetime risk is 10% for progression from latent TB infection to active TB disease. The other 90% of those with latent TB infection are most likely to remain infected but free of active TB disease for the rest of their lives.
8. Multidrug-resistant TB (MDR-TB)
    A. MDR-TB is considered to be present when a patient shows resistance to two or more of the five primary antituberculous drugs:
        1) Isoniazid (INH)
        2) Rifampin (RIF)
        3) Pyrazinamide (PZA)
        4) Ethambutol (EMB)
        5) Streptomycin (SM)
    B. About 14% of TB cases may be resistant to at least one anti-TB drug.
    C. Majority of cases reported in seven major cities (New York, Newark, Dallas, Oakland, Sacramento, Chicago, and Los Angeles), with New York reporting an estimated 61% of cases.
    D. Likely to be seen in previously treated patients, usually if patient was noncompliant. Noncompliance with medication therapy is a major problem in TB control.
    E. Higher incidence in hospitals, prisons, HIV-positive persons, foreign countries (especially Southeast Asia, Central and South America, and Africa).
    F. MDR-TB takes longer to treat, is harder to treat, and can be infectious for an extended period of time if treated inadequately.

SIGNS AND SYMPTOMS

1. Fatigue.
2. Unintentional weight loss.
3. Night sweats with fever.
4. Cough, often productive of purulent sputum.
5. Hemoptysis (as disease progresses).
6. Pleuritic chest pain.
7. Dyspnea on exertion (with advancing disease or large pleural effusion).

8. Lymphadenopathy.
9. Anorexia.
10. Elderly patients may have more subtle symptoms that may be discounted as part of aging or attributed to associated conditions.

PHYSICAL FINDINGS

1. Patient may appear weak, cachectic, chronically ill.
2. Chest exam
   A. Crackles
   B. Increased tactile fremitus to palpation over areas of consolidation
   C. Dullness to percussion
3. Fever of unknown origin may often be from TB, especially in the elderly.
4. In patients who are also HIV positive, TB often:
   A. Occurs early
   B. Progresses rapidly from exposure to infection to active disease
   C. Disseminates and involves extrapulmonary sites (include in physical exam)
   D. Is hard to separate from other HIV-related pulmonary complications. (Thus, hospital personnel and others may be exposed to TB when only PCP is being considered, for example.)
   E. Carries a high mortality rate if accurate diagnosis and effective treatment are delayed

DIFFERENTIAL DIAGNOSIS

1. TB can be confused with many other diseases, including other pulmonary complications of AIDS or HIV-positive patients (e.g., PCP).
2. Other pneumonias, including PCP. (Consider TB for any patient with CXR infiltrate, regardless of locale.)
3. Other infections. (e.g., Atypical *Mycobacteria* or *Nocardia* or fungi. MAC causes 10% of mycobacterial infections seen in clinical practice.) It is common as an opportunistic infection in advanced HIV cases and often does not respond well to anti-TB drugs.
4. Lymphomas.
5. Bronchogenic cancer.
6. Pleurisy.

DIAGNOSTIC TESTS/FINDINGS

1. CXR
   A. Primary pulmonary disease
      1) Consolidation/infiltrates
      2) Lymphadenopathy (especially hilar)
      3) Pleural effusion
   B. Postprimary disease
      1) Cavitation or fibrosis of parenchyma of apical or posterior segments of upper lobes
   C. Additional
      1) CXR cannot be relied upon to establish activity of disease.
      2) HIV-positive patients may have atypical CXR. (10% normal, 25% lymphadenopathy only, 75% of infiltrates not at the usually expected

upper lobes.) Therefore, a negative CXR does not rule out TB in AIDS or HIV-positive patients.

3) "Millet seed" appearance possible with diffuse miliary pattern.

4) Useful to repeat periodically and follow clinical signs and symptoms in high-risk patients and health care personnel who work in high-risk areas.

2. PPD

A. Mantoux skin test: 5 U intermediate strength, 0.1 mL intradermally (intracutaneously) to volar forearm. Read diameter of induration/wheal at 48–72 hours afterwards.

B. Tuberculin skin testing is used to identify those who have been infected with MTB. PPD will be positive with active disease or prior TB exposure.

1) Most of those with TB infection have a positive reaction to tuberculin skin testing within 2–10 weeks after infection.

2) Those with TB infection but who do not have active TB disease are not infectious to others.

3) TB infection without active TB disease is often referred to as latent TB infection, and is not considered a case of TB.

C. Greater than 5-mm induration is considered PPD-positive for patients who:

1) Are HIV-positive

2) Have radiographic evidence of inactive TB disease

3) Have had recent close contact with a TB infected person

D. Greater than 10-mm induration is considered PPD-positive for nearly all other cases, including:

1) Those with chronic illnesses (cancer, diabetes, end-stage renal disease, etc.)

2) Foreign immigrants (especially from Asia, Latin America and Africa)

3) Institutionalized patients (prisons, nursing homes, other long-term care facilities)

4) High-risk minorities and lower socioeconomic groups

E. Greater than 15-mm induration is considered PPD-positive for all cases.

F. Patients or health care workers from TB-endemic areas may have received bacille Calmette-Guérin (BCG) vaccine. BCG can cause a false-positive PPD, particularly when the BCG vaccine has been applied recently. Yet studies show that BCG may not be 100% effective against TB, even initially, and that its protective effect often wanes over the years.

1) While current CDC guidelines state that BCG recipients may be tested with PPD, some authorities decline to do so if the BCG recipient has had a medically documented, previously positive PPD.

2) In certain cases, however, a positive PPD in a BCG recipient may represent the presence of active TB that may need further evaluation and treatment, particularly if:

a. Recent exposure to active TB; and/or

b. BCG was received many years ago

3) For further discussion, refer to the latest CDC guidelines as to use of PPD skin testing in those known to have had BCG vaccine.

4) Ongoing updates on these and other aspects of TB management are reported via the CDC's *Morbidity and Mortality Weekly Report*

(MMWR) and other literature. (*MMWR* is available free of charge in electronic format and on a paid subscription basis for paper copy.)

G. AIDS or HIV-positive patients may have negative PPD skin tests due to anergy or diminished reactivity.

H. For the elderly, consider recommending baseline PPD prior to entering a long-term care facility.

I. It is useful to repeat PPD periodically for higher risk patients in whom TB may be suspected, and for health care personnel who work in higher risk areas.

J. Adequacy of ER triage and ER/hospital-wide respiratory isolation procedures can better be assessed and improved by systematic monitoring and follow-up of PPD conversion rates among health care personnel (especially those who work in the ER).

3. Bacteriology studies of sputum and gastric/tracheal culture.

A. Bacteriology is the key to diagnosing active TB disease.

B. CDC recommends drug susceptibility testing on the first sputum isolate in all patients in whom MTB is isolated. Best to submit three specimens for AFB sputum smear, all from early morning (in order to increase diagnostic yield).

C. Sputum induction procedure and/or bronchoscopy may be needed for difficult cases.

D. Conventional mycobacterial cultures can take 6–12 weeks to obtain results, while more rapid methods may give results in 1–3 weeks. (Meanwhile, missed TB diagnosis and/or lax TB control measures can lead to undue exposure of the TB patient's close contacts and/or health care personnel.)

E. HIV-positive patients may show decreased sensitivity of AFB smear staining.

F. MDR-TB patients often do show AFB-positive smears.

G. Even if patient was recently hospitalized and showed one or two negative AFB smears, do not assume patient could not be infectious now.

MANAGEMENT/TREATMENT

1. *Physician referral is advised at the time treatment is begun for PPD-positive patients, while follow-up may be managed through collaboration by ACNP and physician. Depending upon the patient's condition and the setting, the ACNP may be called upon to make a referral to an infectious disease specialist physician.*

2. Admission to an acute care unit for TB is not often indicated, but is typically decided on a case-by-case basis. Depending upon the patient's condition and the setting, the ACNP may be called upon to arrange such hospital admission for the patient with TB. *Suggested considerations for hospital admit may include:*

A. Severity of illness (including whether patient has TB meningitis or acute respiratory failure).

B. Protection of the TB patient's immediate contacts (including patients who reside at SNFs, or who are homeless or otherwise noncompliant with treatment regimens).

C. Comorbid conditions (including AIDS or HIV-positive status).

D. Hospital admission, when indicated, can provide an opportunity to initially get control over the patient's TB condition and to effectively implement medication and infection control measures.

3. *TB is a reportable disease that must be reported to local and state health departments.*
   A. Contact tracing is vital.
4. Nearly all properly treated TB patients can be cured.
5. HIV-positive patients also respond well to TB therapy and should not have such treatment withheld. Maintaining a high index of suspicion for TB in HIV-positive patients can help in earlier diagnosis and treatment, and more successful outcomes.
6. Refer to ongoing CDC guideline updates for the latest recommendations on anti-TB drugs and treatment regimens.
7. If positive-PPD converter *without* active TB disease:
   A. Do history and physical (H&P), and CXR. Look for source and patterns of susceptibility. Consider using INH.
   B. Balance risk of developing active TB against risk of developing drug-induced hepatitis (especially in older patients).
   C. Usually treat with INH, including if:
       1) Recent positive PPD converter
       2) HIV-positive
       3) Close contact of TB patient
       4) On chronic steroids
       5) IV drug use
       6) Under 35 years old
   D. INH: 5 mg/kg up to 300 mg PO qd × 6–12 months (12 months for HIV-positive patients).
   E. Pyridoxine/vitamin B_6: 50 mg PO qd × 6–12 months may also be added to help prevent or reduce INH hypersensitivity reactions and/or peripheral neuritis.
8. The therapeutic regimen for *active TB* needs to be guided by sputum culture and smear results. Empiric treatment is begun until these results are available and then is modified accordingly.
   A. Currently recommended therapy is to use two or more drugs to which the TB organism has demonstrated sensitivity.
   B. Initial empiric adult regimen includes four drugs (INH + RIF + PZA, and either EMB or SM) × 2 months and then two or more drugs to which organism is known to be sensitive (usually INH + RIF) × ≥4 months more (≥6 months total). (Per 1993 CDC and American Thoracic Society recommendations.)
       1) INH: 5 mg/kg (300 mg max) PO qd
           a. Give with vitamin B_6: 50 mg PO qd.
           b. Side effects can include peripheral neuritis, hepatitis, and hypersensitivity. Hepatitis is more likely with alcohol use.
           c. Monitor with periodic liver function tests (LFTs).
       2) RIF: 10 mg/kg (600 mg max) PO qd
           a. Side effects can include hepatitis; thrombocytopenia; nausea; vomiting; acute renal failure (rare); and orange discoloration of urine, secretions, and tears (which can permanently stain contact lenses). Can inactivate birth control pills.
           b. Monitor with periodic LFTs.

   c. Use with caution for the following drugs metabolized by the liver, as RIF accelerates their clearance: Anticonvulsants, Coumadin, digitalis, oral hypoglycemics, estrogen.

  3) PZA: 15–30 mg/kg (2 gm max) PO qd

   a. Side effects can include hepatotoxicity, rash, hyperuricemia, GI distress and arthralgias.

   b. Monitor with periodic LFTs and BUN.

  4) EMB: 15–25 mg/kg PO qd

   a. Side effects can include GI distress and possibly optic neuritis.

   b. Monitor with periodic visual acuity and color testing.

   c. If pregnant patient has active TB, can only use EMB after first trimester.

  5) SM: 15 mg/kg (1 gm max) IM qd

   a. Side effects can include ototoxicity and nephrotoxicity. Therefore, never use longer than 12 weeks.

   b. Do not use in pregnant women because of risk of ototoxicity to the fetus.

   c. May need to reduce dosage in elderly patients over age 60 and in patients with renal insufficiency.

9. Adults with active pulmonary disease but who have negative AFB smear and sputum culture should continue all four drugs for 4 months.

10. For *resistant* TB, *in addition* to above, give the following until drug sensitivities of bacilli are known:

 A. EMB for first 2 months if suspect INH resistance (EMB 15–20 mg/kg PO qd); *or*

 B. PZA for 2 months (15–30 mg/kg PO qd, to a maximum of 2 gm PO qd); *or*

 C. SM for 2 months (20–40 mg/kg IM qd, to a maximum of 1 gm IM qd)

11. HIV-positive patients with active TB need treatment with three or more anti-TB drugs to which the TB organism has shown sensitivity. Treat for 9 months and at least 6 months beyond culture conversion.

12. PPD-negative persons who have repeated exposure to TB may need to consider BCG vaccine. (Refer to the latest CDC guidelines.)

13. For additional treatment options, including directly observed therapy (DOT) to permit intermittent administration, refer to the latest CDC guidelines.

14. Follow-up

 A. Order sputums for AFB smear and culture q1–2mo until conversion can be documented.

 B. For standard treatment, continue Rx for ≥6 months and 3 months beyond conversion of sputum culture.

 C. For HIV-positive patients with TB, continue Rx for 9 months and ≥6 months beyond conversion of sputum culture.

 D. Re-evaluate patient q2–3 mo for duration of TB treatment.

 E. Repeat CXR q2–3mo during TB treatment and also if symptoms change.

 F. Order baseline values of LFTs, bilirubin, creatinine, BUN, and CBC. If PZA is used, also order serum uric acid level. If EMB is used, also document visual acuity.

 G. If symptoms of liver disease arise, recheck LFTs and modify Rx as needed.

 H. If a drug regimen is failing, do not add only a single drug.

I. If drug susceptibility lab results cannot be obtained, EMB or SM are recommended for the entire course of TB treatment (in addition to the standard INH and RIF regimen mentioned above).

PATIENT EDUCATION

1. General
   A. Review disease process, medication use and potential toxic side effects, treatment options, community resources available, and the need to notify the medical provider promptly concerning any new or increasing signs and symptoms.
   B. Encourage nutritious diet and advise patients taking INH to also take vitamin B_6 (as previously directed).
   C. Activity as tolerated is permitted.
   D. Noncompliance with medication therapy is a major problem in TB control. As a result, treatment failure, drug resistance, continuing transmission of infection, increasing disability, and even death may occur. To help prevent these outcomes it is important for all medical providers to learn how to prevent, recognize, and manage noncompliant behavior.
   E. Patients with a high risk of noncompliance may do better on an alternate DOT regimen, if such can be arranged through hospital, clinic, or medical provider's office. (Refer to the latest CDC guidelines.)
   F. Reiterate the importance of avoiding exposure to cigarette smoke. Quit-smoking tips and other useful community resources are offered through:
       1) American Lung Association
       2) American Thoracic Society (which is the medical section of the American Lung Association)
       3) American Cancer Society
       4) American Heart Association
       5) CDC
       6) NIH
   G. Additional educational resources for the medical provider and interested patients include:
       1) TB materials disseminated through the CDC (*MMWR* is available free of charge in electronic format and on a paid subscription basis for paper copy)
       2) State or local public health departments
       3) American Lung Association
2. Infection control
   A. Stress the vital importance of contact tracing and of the need for strict compliance with the treatment regimen.
   B. For the elderly, consider recommending baseline PPD or CXR prior to entering a long-term care facility. Baseline CXR may be more accurate, given that a certain number of elderly patients show anergy or false-negative PPD tests.
   C. It is useful to repeat PPD periodically for higher risk patients in whom TB may be suspected, and for health care personnel who work in higher risk areas.
   D. Ensure adequate hospital ventilation (including "negative pressure" airflow in AFB/respiratory isolation rooms), high-efficiency particulate air (HEPA) filters, UV germicidal irradiation, and particulate

respirators/HEPA filter masks or U-95 TB masks for health care workers and patients.
   E. Develop a TB screening protocol for your hospital or clinic setting, if only to catch the most likely cases. (Refer to the latest CDC guidelines.)
      1) Typical risk factors, symptoms, or complaints to be considered for TB screening might include:
         a. Generally higher risk factors:
            i. Current or previously active TB, even if on TB medications
            ii. AIDS or HIV-positive with pulmonary complaints
            iii. Hemoptysis
            iv. Chronic cough with fever, night sweats, or weight loss
         b. Generally less high risk factors:
            i. PPD-positive conversion within past 2 years, or history of recent TB exposure
            ii. Foreign-born, or male homosexual, or IVDA
            iii. Homeless, or in shelter or jail within past 2 years
      2) Consider placing TB masks on suspected TB patients prior to obtaining CXR, especially if AFB/respiratory isolation room is not immediately available.
      3) Consider TB in differential diagnosis of any patient with CXR infiltrate, regardless of locale.
   F. Adequacy of ER triage and ER/hospital-wide respiratory isolation procedures can better be assessed and improved by systematic monitoring and follow-up of PPD conversion rates among health care personnel (especially those who work in the ER).

Review Questions

2.26 The CDC-recommended clinical classification system for TB is based upon the pathogenesis of the disease. Describe components of this classification system (circle all that apply):
   A. Evidence for Class # 2 (TB latent infection; no active disease) includes:
      1) PPD-positive; *and*
      2) Bacteriologic studies for TB (if done) are negative; *and*
      3) Clinical evidence of TB is negative; *and*
      4) CXR evidence of TB is negative
   B. Evidence for Class # 3 (Current, active TB disease) includes:
      1) *M. tuberculosis* culture (if done) is positive; *or*
      2) PPD-positive, plus clinical or CXR evidence of current, active TB disease
   C. Class # 5 (TB suspected) is designated when the diagnosis is pending; diagnosis must be made within 3 months, however.
   D. All of those with Class # 3 or Class # 5 designations should be reported promptly to state or local health departments. Medical providers need to comply with state and local laws and regulations that require the reporting of TB.

2.27. With regard to MDR-TB:
   A. 14% of TB cases may be resistant to at least one anti-TB therapy.
   B. It is less likely to be seen in previously treated patients.

    C. It is considered to be present when the patient shows resistance to two or fewer of the three primary antituberculous drugs.

    D. Higher incidence occurs in institutions, foreign countries, and HIV-negative persons.

The following 3-part case scenario is for tuberculosis Questions 2.28–2.30 listed below.

Mr. MT is a 62-year-old man admitted to the acute care unit with increasing dyspnea, fevers with night sweats, and hemoptysis for the past 2 weeks. Because of his marked weakness and fatigue, he asks you to obtain the rest of his history from his roommate and longtime companion, Mr. SG, who is at the bedside with the patient. The visitor mentions their concerns about the patient's increasing anorexia, productive cough, pleuritic type chest pain, and unintentional weight loss of 15 lb over the past 6 weeks.
PMH: NIDDM; HIV-positive; previous TB (treated 10 years ago abroad).
FSH: Nonsmoker; moderate social intake of ETOH; no IVDA. Retiree, who also has been a longtime community volunteer. Both the patient and his visitor have volunteered regularly at a homeless shelter that serves a number of refugees among its clientele.

2.28 In accordance with your hospital's TB screening protocol, you arrange admission to an AFB/respiratory isolation room and promptly order CXR for patient. The patient and his visitor express surprise at these routine infection control measures, as Mr. MT previously had been treated for TB. You mention that the increasing number of TB cases since 1988 is due in part to:
    A. Completely treated cases promoting MDR-TB
    B. Increased surveillance and TB control measures at hospitals, prisons, nursing homes, and other institutions
    C. Rise in numbers of immunocompromised hosts, such as AIDS and HIV-positive patients.
    D. A decrease in the reactivation rates of previously infected persons

2.29 Mr. MT's random blood sugar and other routine lab results are within normal limits. CXR results are obtained, however, that indicate presence of active TB disease. Sputum specimens are obtained and sent to lab for culture and sensitivity, Gram's stain, and AFB stain/smear. Mr. MT and his visitor request further information with regard to the likelihood of TB reactivation. You explain that:
    A. It is reasonable to assume that a previously treated TB patient does not now have active TB.
    B. Lifetime risk of reactivation is approximately 5% within the first 10 years after PPD-conversion, and 5% more after that.
    C. Patients who are both HIV-positive and PPD-positive carry a risk of 7–10% per year to develop active TB disease.
    D. When cell-mediated immunity increases, reactivation of TB may occur.

2.30 In collaboration with the patient's attending physician, the decision is made to begin Mr. MT on TB treatment. Empiric TB treatment is to be initiated until sputum culture and smear results are available, and then will be modified accordingly. Per 1993 CDC and American Thoracic Society recommendations, initial standard empiric adult TB regimen in-

cludes _____ for 2 months, and then treatment with two or more drugs
to which organism is known to be sensitive for ≥4 months more (≥6
months total). *In addition, HIV-positive patients with active TB need treat-*
ment with three or more drugs to which the TB organism has shown sensi-
tivity for 9 months more (and ≥6 months beyond culture conversion).
A. Two drugs (INH and PZA)
B. Three drugs (INH, RIF, and EMB)
C. Three drugs (INH, RIF, and SM)
D. Four drugs (INH, RIF, PZA; and either EMB or SM).

Answers and Rationales

2.26 **All** The CDC recommended clinical classification system for TB is based
upon the pathogenesis of the disease. The components of this classification system which are listed here all apply:
  A. Evidence for Class # 2 (TB latent infection; no active disease)
  includes:
    1) PPD-positive; *and*
    2) Bacteriologic studies for TB (if done) are negative; *and*
    3) Clinical evidence of TB is negative; *and*
    4) CXR evidence of TB is negative
  B. Evidence for Class # 3 (Current, active TB disease) includes:
    1) *M. tuberculosis* culture (if done) is positive; *or*
    2) PPD-positive, plus clinical or CXR evidence of current, active
    TB disease
  C. Class # 5 (TB suspected) is designated when the diagnosis is pending; diagnosis must be made within 3 months, however.
  D. All of those with Class # 3 or Class # 5 designations should be
  reported promptly to state or local health departments. Medical
  providers need to comply with state and local laws and regulations
  which require the reporting of TB.

2.27 **A** About 14% of TB cases may be resistant to at least one anti-TB drug.
MDR-TB is likely to be seen in previously treated patients, usually
if patient was noncompliant. Higher incidence is noted in institutions,
foreign countries, and HIV-positive persons. MDR-TB is considered
to be present when patient show resistance to two or more of the five
primary antituberculous drugs (INH, RIF, PZA, EMB, or SM).

2.28 **C** The increasing number of TB cases since 1988 is due in part to: incompletely treated cases promoting MDR-TB; the rise in numbers of immunocompromised hosts such as AIDS and HIV-positive patients;
and lax TB control measures at hospitals, prisons, nursing homes,
and other institutions. About 25,000 cases are reported annually in
the United States, with 90% of those due to reactivation of previously
infected persons.

2.29 **C** TB reactivation may occur when cell-mediated immunity decreases.
Lifetime risk of reactivation is approximately 5% within the first 2
years after PPD-positive conversion, and 5% more after that. Patients
who are both HIV-positive and PPD-positive carry a risk of 7–10%
per year to develop active TB disease. (This contrast with a 5%–10%

lifetime risk for PPD-positive, HIV-negative patients.) Do not assume that a patient could not have TB because of previous TB treatment.

2.30 **D** Per 1993 CDC and American Thoracic Society recommendations, initial standard empiric adult TB treatment regimen includes four drugs (INH, RIF, PZA; and either EMB or SM) for 2 months, and then two or more drugs to which organism is known to be sensitive (usually INH and RIF) for ≥4 months more (≥6 months total). In addition, HIV-positive patients with active TB need treatment with three or more drugs to which the TB organism has shown sensitivity for 9 months more (and ≥6 months beyond culture conversion).

References

Abou-Shala, N. (1996). Tuberculosis. In R.E. Rakel (ed.). *Saunders Manual of Medical Practice*. Philadelphia: W.B. Saunders Co., pp. 183–186.

Centers for Disease Control and Prevention/U.S. Department of Health and Human Services. (1994). *Core Curriculum on Tuberculosis: What the Clinician Should Know* (3rd ed.). Atlanta, GA: Author.

Chambers, H.F. (1997). Mycobacterium Tuberculosis infections. In L.M. Tierney, Jr., S.J. McPhee, & M.A. Papadakis (eds.). *Current Medical Diagnosis and Treatment, 1997* (3rd ed.). Stamford, CT: Appleton & Lange, pp. 1268–1271.

Daniel, T.M. (1994). Tuberculosis. In K.J. Isselbacher, E. Braunwald, J.D. Wilson, et al. (eds.). *Harrison's Principles of Internal Medicine: Vol. 2* (13th ed.). New York: McGraw-Hill, pp. 710–718.

Niederman, M.S., & Sarosi, G.A. (1995). Tuberculosis. In R.B. George, R.W. Light, M.A. Mathay, & R.A. Mathay (eds.). *Chest Medicine: Essentials of Pulmonary and Critical Care Medicine* (3rd ed.). Baltimore, MD: Williams & Wilkins, pp. 457–462.

Reves, R.R. (1996). Tuberculosis. In J.M. Rippe, R.S. Irwin, M.P. Fink, & F.B. Cerra (eds.). *Intensive Care Medicine: Vol. I* (3rd ed.). Boston: Little, Brown & Co., pp. 1210–1224.

Sokolove, P.E. (1997). Tuberculosis—It's back. In J. Hizon (Chair). *Essentials in Emergency Medicine and Urgent Care*. Proceedings syllabus. Symposium presented by Continuing Medical Education Associates, Inc., San Diego, CA, pp. 71–82.

Sokolove, P.E., Mackey, D., Wiles, J., & R.J. Lewis. (1994). Exposure of emergency department personnel to tuberculosis: PPD testing during an epidemic in the community. *Ann Emerg Med 24* (3), 418–421.

Stauffer, J.L. (1997). Lung: Pulmonary tuberculosis. In L.M. Tierney, Jr., S.J. McPhee, & M.A. Papadakis (eds.). *Current Medical Diagnosis and Treatment, 1997* (36th ed.). Stamford, CT: Appleton & Lange, pp. 269–276.

Welch, R. (1996). Tuberculosis. In J.E. Tintinalli, R.L. Krome, & E. Ruiz (eds.). *Emergency Medicine: A Comprehensive Study Guide* (4th ed.). New York: McGraw-Hill, pp. 422–425.

Additional Recommended References

Bass, J., Farer, L., Hopewell, P., et al. (1992). Control of tuberculosis in the United States. ("Official Statement of the American Thoracic Society," medical section of the American Lung Association.) *Am Rev Respir Dis 146*(6), 1623–1633.

Bass, Jr., J.B., Farer, L.S., Hopewell, P.C., et al. (1994). Treatment of tuberculosis and tuberculosis infection in adults and children. ("Official Statement of the American Thoracic Society," medical section of the American Lung Association.) *Am J Respir Crit Care Med 149*, 1359–1374.

Essential components of a tuberculosis prevention and control program/screening for tuberculosis and tuberculosis infection in high-risk populations. (1995). *MMWR Morb Mortal Wkly Rep 44* (RR-11).

Guidelines for preventing the transmission of mycobacterium tuberculosis in health-care facilities, 1994. (1994). *MMWR Morb Mortal Wkly Rep 43* (RR-13).

Hardy, K. (1994). Tuberculosis. In H.W. Griffith, M.R. Dambro, & J. Griffith (eds.). *The Five Minute Clinical Consult, 1994*, Philadelphia: Lea & Febiger, pp. 1038–1039.

The role of BCG vaccine in the prevention and control of tuberculosis in the United States. (1996). *MMWR Morb Mortal Wkly Rep 45* (RR-4).

Tuberculosis. (1992). In C.S. Rivers, D.E. Weber, M.K. Schuda, & E.R. Vaughn (eds.). *Preparing for the Written Board Exam in Emergency Medicine.* Milford, OH: Emergency Medicine Educational Enterprises, Inc., pp. 199–207.

Zaman, M.K. (1996). Procedure: Technique of sputum induction. In R.E. Rakel (ed.). *Saunders Manual of Medical Practice.* Philadelphia: W.B. Saunders Co., pp. 187–188.

Pulmonary Embolism

DEFINITION

A pulmonary embolism (PE) refers to a blood clot (thromboembolism), tumor fragment (from tumors invading venous circulation), or other embolic material (fat, air, amniotic fluid, infected tissue, bone marrow, calcium, or foreign IV material—e.g., sheared catheter tip) that has lodged in the lung circulation and blocked blood flow to an area of lung tissue.

ETIOLOGY/INCIDENCE

1. Associated with approximately 650,000 cases, 250,000 hospitalizations, and over 50,000 deaths annually in the United States.
2. Death within the first hour occurs in 10% of victims.
3. Difficulty in diagnosis (especially if not considered early in the differential work-up) is underscored by the fact that 90% of patients who die of PE have not received treatment for the condition.
4. The most common embolic material is thrombus from a distant site, particularly from deep veins of the legs and pelvis (90–95%). Risk of thromboembolism is related to Virchow's triad: Venous stasis, hypercoagulability, vascular wall damage.
5. Thromboembolism can occasionally arise from the right side of the heart.
6. Less than 10% of PEs result in death. Clinical findings, morbidity, and mortality depend on the size of the pulmonary embolism, extent of obstruction, and the patient's pre-existing cardiopulmonary status.
   A. In massive PE (clot obstructs more than two thirds of pulmonary circulation), acute right ventricular failure and systemic hypotension often develop, and cardiovascular collapse may occur. A major cause of sudden, unexpected death is massive PE.
   B. It is more difficult to recognize PE in a patient with pre-existing cardiopulmonary disease, especially since signs or symptoms are nonspecific.
7. PE may be manifest as three syndromes:
   A. Acute onset of unexplained dyspnea (the most common presentation)
   B. Acute cor pulmonale (due to massive obstruction of more than two thirds of pulmonary circulation)

T A B L E 2–4. **Predisposing Factors for Thromboembolism***

Cardiopulmonary disease
Congestive heart failure
Myocardial infarction
Chronic obstructive pulmonary disease
Stasis of blood flow
Pregnancy and parturition
Prolonged immobilization
History of DVT or PE
Marked obesity
Alterations in coagulation
Malignancy
Estrogen use
Other†
Trauma
Surgery within 3 months
Lower extremity injury

* From Hockberger, R.S. (1996). Pulmonary embolism. In J.E. Tintinalli, R.L. Krome, & E. Ruiz (eds.) *Emergency Medicine: A Comprehensive Study Guide* (4th ed.). New York: McGraw-Hill, pp. 370–374, with permission.
† Deficiencies of antithrombin III, protein C, protein S: presence of lupus anticoagulant; and homocystinuria.
DVT, deep venous thrombosis; PE, pulmonary embolism.

C. Pulmonary infarction (more rare, occurs with complete occlusion of a distal branch of pulmonary circulation without usual pulmonary collateral circulation, resulting in death of lung tissue)
8. See Table 2–4 for a summary of predisposing risk factors for thromboembolism.
9. Physiologic risk factors.
   A. Deep vein thrombosis (DVT)/phlebitis of legs and pelvis (especially thighs) account for 90–95% of pulmonary thromboembolism cases.
   B. Hypercoagulability (CA, oral contraceptives, antithrombin III deficiency, protein C or S deficiency, lupus anticoagulant, nephrotic syndrome, and polycythemia).
   C. Elderly (more common and more often fatal in geriatric population).
10. Clinical risk factors.
   A. Immobilization or prolonged bed rest
   B. CA (often occult CA, especially of the lungs, breast, GI tract/viscera, uterus, prostate)
   C. Trauma (especially fractures of legs, pelvis, hips)
   D. Surgery (especially major abdominal or orthopedic)
   E. Pregnancy and childbirth
   F. Obesity
   G. Cardiac disease (especially CHF, myocardial infarction [MI], atrial fibrillation)
   H. CVA
   I. Diabetes mellitus
   J. Smoking
   K. Previous pulmonary embolism
   L. Varicose veins
11. In situ thrombosis without embolism rarely occurs in pulmonary arteries. Risk factors for this less common scenario include:
   A. Chest trauma

    B. Sickle cell anemia
    C. Various congenital heart abnormalities
12. Emboli involve right lung more than left, lower lobes more than upper, and may travel through venous or arterial systems.
13. Emboli >7–8 mm diameter are the most rapidly fatal, while those <4 mm diameter cause far fewer clinical problems.
14. Hemodynamic effects of PE:
    A. Mechanical blockage of pulmonary circulation leads to increased pulmonary vascular resistance. Pulmonary hypertension and acute right ventricular failure may result from massive obstruction.
    B. Vasoconstriction due to neurohumoral reflexes. (Release of serotonin, thromboxane, and other chemical mediators from platelets surrounding the embolism can lead to bronchoconstriction and vasospasm.)
15. Respiratory effects of PE:
    A. Reflex bronchoconstriction in the area of lung embolism.
    B. Increased pulmonary dead space/wasted ventilation.
    C. Loss of alveolar surfactant (leading to alveolar collapse, atelectasis, blood shunting, and hypoxemia) within 2–15 hours after blood flow interruption.
    D. Atelectasis leads to further decrease in lung volume within 24–48 hours after blood flow interruption.
    E. Arterial hypoxemia often results (due to $\dot{V}/\dot{Q}$ mismatch, greater arteriovenous difference with cardiac failure, decreased mixed venous P_{O_2}).

SIGNS AND SYMPTOMS

1. Clinical findings generally depend on the size of the PE, extent of obstruction, and the patient's pre-existing cardiopulmonary status.
2. Symptoms may seem vague and nonspecific, often resulting in misdiagnosis.
    A. Acute onset dyspnea is the most frequent symptom.
    B. Chest pain (especially pleuritic) occurs in 80–90% of cases, especially with a large PE.
    C. History of risk factors for thromboembolism.
    D. Other symptoms may include apprehension, cough, hemoptysis, palpitations, or sweats.
    E. Syncope may present occasionally (in cases of massive PE).
3. Signs of PE are nonspecific and may lead to misdiagnosis. Such signs may range from none (with small PE) to cardiovascular collapse, shock, and sudden, unexpected death (with massive PE). On the other hand, PEs of intermediate size and blockage may have signs and symptoms that differ little, despite wide ranges of severity.
    A. Tachypnea (RR >16/min) in most cases (>90%).
    B. Nonspecific lung crackles.
    C. Other lung findings include localized consolidation or wheezing, pleural friction rub, and/or pleural effusion.
    D. Accentuated S_2P.
    E. Tachycardia (HR >100 bpm).
    F. Phlebitis.
    G. Ventricular gallop and/or atrial dysrhythmias.
    H. Edema (especially of legs).
    I. Heart murmur (especially over lung field).
    J. Cough (may include hemoptysis).

TABLE 2-5. Incidence of Symptoms and Signs of Angiographically Proved Pulmonary Thromboembolism in 327 Patients*,†

	(%)
Symptoms	
Chest pain	88%
Pleuritic	74%
Nonpleuritic	14%
Dyspnea	84%
Apprehension	59%
Cough	53%
Hemoptysis	30%
Sweats	27%
Syncope	13%
Signs	
Respiratory rate >16/min	92%
Crackles	58%
Accentuated S_2P	53%
Pulse >100/min	44%
Temperature >37.8°C	43%
Phlebitis	32%
Gallop	34%
Diaphoresis	36%
Edema	24%
Murmur	23%
Cyanosis	19%

* From Stauffer, J. (1997). Lung. In L. Tierney, S.M. Phee, & M. Papadakis (eds.), *Current Medical Diagnosis and Treatment* (36th ed.). Stamford, CT: Appleton & Lange, pp. 317–318, with permission.

† Data from Bell, W.R., Simon, T.L., & DeMets, D.L. (1977). The clinical features of submassive and massive pulmonary emboli. *Am J Med 62*, 355.

K. Patient may have dullness to percussion over involved lung site and/or splinting of the affected side.

L. Nonspecific signs, often related to hypoxemia (apprehension, anxiety, restlessness, weakness, and/or possibly nausea and vomiting).

M. Signs of right ventricular failure (right sided S_4, JVD, edema, and/or hepatosplenomegaly).

N. Fat embolism signs may present within hours to 3–4 days following long bone fracture. These usually include petechial rash on chest, shoulders, and/or axilla.

O. A notable air embolism sign is a churning sound auscultated over right ventricle.

P. More ominous signs may range from syncope, cyanosis, and hypotension to shock and cardiopulmonary arrest.

4. Table 2–5 shows a summary for the incidence of signs and symptoms in angiographically proven PE.

PHYSICAL FINDINGS

1. In addition to the signs listed above, check all patients suspected of PE for signs of DVT (most common cause). Check patients' legs for pain (especially calf pain with dorsiflexion/positive Homan's sign), edema, erythema, and/or palpable vein cords. To be thorough, check arms, abdomen, and pelvis as well.

DIFFERENTIAL DIAGNOSIS

1. CV disease (MI, CHF, pericarditis, dissecting aortic aneurysm)
2. Other lung pathology (pneumonia, pleural effusion, pleuritis, pneumothorax)
3. Other chest wall pathology (rib fractures, other trauma)
4. GI pathology that may produce atypical chest pain (esophageal rupture, gastritis, ulcers, hiatal hernia)
5. Other conditions with signs and/or symptoms similar to DVT (cellulitis, muscle strain or rupture, lymphangitis, Baker's cyst rupture).

DIAGNOSTIC TESTS/FINDINGS

1. A high index of suspicion is required to avoid missing PE.
2. Figures 2–2 and 2–3 provide useful algorithms for the initial and further evaluation of patients with suspected PE.
3. $\dot{V}/\dot{Q}$ scan.
    A. $\dot{V}/\dot{Q}$ scan should be the first test done when PE is suspected. This allows comparison of pulmonary ventilation and perfusion, with few likely complications. Patterns suggesting PE include normal ventilation with multiple segmental or lobar perfusion defects.
    B. Other diseases (asthma, COPD, pneumonia, CHF) may result in $\dot{V}/\dot{Q}$ scan abnormalities, but the test results can still be used to direct pulmonary angiography and to reduce the amount of contrast dye needed.
    C. Normal $\dot{V}/\dot{Q}$ scan results rule out clinically significant PE, and no further diagnostic tests are needed.

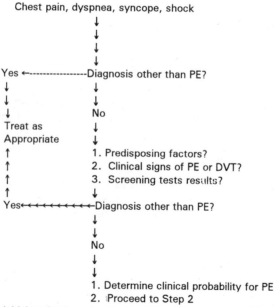

Step 1: The initial evaluation of patients with symptoms suggestive of PE

FIGURE 2–2. Chest pain, dyspnea, syncope, shock. (From Hockberger, R.S. [1996]. Pulmonary embolism. In J.E. Tintinalli, R.L. Krome, & E. Ruiz [eds.]. *Emergency Medicine: A Comprehensive Study Guide* [4th ed.]. New York: McGraw-Hill, pp. 370–374, with permission.)

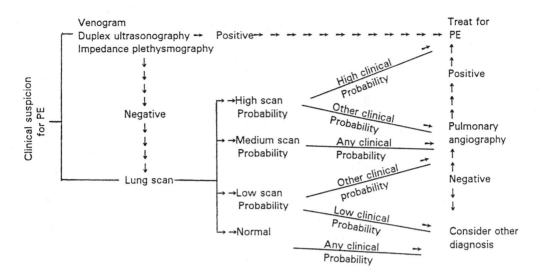

Step 2: **The further evaluation of patients with suspected PE.**

    FIGURE 2–3. Step 2: The further evaluation of patients with suspected PE. (From Hockberger, R.S. [1996]. Pulmonary embolism. In J.E. Tintinalli, R.L. Krome, & E. Ruiz [eds.]. *Emergency Medicine: A Comprehensive Study Guide* [4th ed.]. New York: McGraw-Hill, pp. 370–374, with permission.)

    D. Low or intermediate (also called nondiagnostic) V̇/Q̇ scan results must be correlated with clinical data, as many of these patients still are at significant risk for PE (especially those with DVT). The 1990 Prospective Investigation of Pulmonary Embolism Diagnosis (PIOPED) study outlined diagnostic criteria for PE and V̇/Q̇ scan. In this benchmark investigation, 12–33% of nondiagnostic V̇/Q̇ scan results still correlated with positive pulmonary angiography results (the gold standard to diagnose PE), representing PEs that could have been missed by V̇/Q̇ scan alone.

    E. About 88% of high-probability V̇/Q̇ scan results correlated with positive pulmonary angiography results.

  4. Venous thrombosis/lower extremity studies.

    A. By and large, PE results from DVT of lower extremities (>90%). Acute venous thromboembolism is a term that combines both diagnoses appropriately, as approximately 40% of patients with DVT, but without symptoms of PE, do have PE demonstrated radiographically.

    B. Doppler studies are highly reliable.

    C. Duplex ultrasonography may exceed 95% for sensitivity and specificity.

    D. Impedance plethysmography may be used and repeated serially.

    E. Venography is both sensitive and specific but carries small risks of allergic dye reaction and/or venous thrombosis. Though not done as often, it remains the gold standard to test for venous thrombosis. It is still used when Doppler studies or impedance plethysmography are unavailable or unreliable.

  5. Pulmonary angiography/arteriography.

    A. The gold standard to diagnose PE.

    B. For nondiagnostic and some high-probability V̇/Q̇ scan results, pulmonary angiography is needed to make the definite diagnosis because of its high sensitivity and specificity.

    C. Pulmonary angiography is advised when PE must be diagnosed with certainty, as when anticoagulation would be risky for an individual patient, or prior to surgical intervention to prevent recurrent thromboemboli (such as inferior vena cava interruption).

    D. Patterns indicative of PE include arterial cutoffs and/or intraluminal filling defects.

    E. Complications may include dysrhythmias, allergic dye reactions, or renal failure.

    F. Relative contraindications to the use of angiography may include severe pulmonary hypertension (HTN), left bundle branch block (LBBB), ventricular dysrhythmias, and/or renal failure.

6. Baseline PT, PTT, and CBC are important to guide anticoagulation therapy if PE is diagnosed.

7. Routine lab tests are not helpful to diagnose PE. Rather, because PE is so frequently misdiagnosed and has potentially grave consequences, these associated tests are used to rule out other possible causes.

    A. ABGs

      1) Commonly show hypoxia—90% of PE patients have Po_2 <80 mm Hg.

      2) May also show decreased Pco_2, respiratory alkalosis, and/or increased A-a gradient.

      3) On the other hand, ABGs may be normal, and therefore not diagnostic of PE.

      4) To review ABG interpretation, refer to the references listed following this section.

    B. CXR

      1) Usually nonspecific abnormalities in PE. May show pleural effusion or parenchymal infiltrate. CXR is useful to rule out other causes of shortness of breath (SOB) and chest pain.

    C. ECG

      1) May be normal with PE, or may show nonspecific ST- or T-wave changes.

      2) Tachycardia is common in PE.

      3) Occasionally may see right heart strain, incomplete RBBB, or $S_1/Q_3/T_3$ pattern. ECG is useful mostly to rule out cardiac causes of chest pain and SOB.

8. In certain settings, it also may be useful to evaluate for hypercoagulability, including tests of antithrombin III, proteins C and S, and anticardiolipin antibody.

MANAGEMENT/TREATMENT

1. *Patients suspected to have PE require timely hospital admission for further evaluation and treatment. Depending upon the setting, the ACNP may be called upon to help arrange hospital admission/ICU transfer with physician consult. A physician needs to manage the patient, while the ACNP may collaborate. Referral to a pulmonary/critical care physician specialist is also advisable to follow the patient through this potentially life-threatening course.*

2. Prevention.

    A. Prevention of DVT and PE is essential. Appropriate antithrombotic prevention should be used whenever patients are at risk:

      1) Intermittent external pneumatic leg compression (especially during

and after neurosurgery, urology surgery, or major knee or hip surgery).

2) Early ambulation after any surgery, as tolerated and appropriate.
3) Immobilized patients should have legs elevated and begin range-of-motion exercises when stable.
4) Elastic support stockings are less useful than external pneumatic leg compression.
5) Prophylactic low-dose heparin, low-molecular-weight heparin, or warfarin therapy.

3. Oxygen therapy, as needed.
4. Anticoagulation therapy.
   A. For an excellent summary table of standard heparin and warfarin/Coumadin treatment guidelines the reader is referred to p. 337-S of the *Fourth ACCP Consensus Conference on Antithrombotic Therapy*. (1995). In J.E. Dalen & J. Hirsh (eds.). Chest 108(4).
   B. Standard heparin is the drug of choice to initially treat PE. While heparin treatment does not affect thrombi that have already formed, it does stop propagation and allow fibrinolysis to occur. Heparin does so by binding to antithrombin III and increasing its antithrombotic activity, which prevents further thrombosis and extension of the clot. If there are no contraindications to anticoagulation (such as no recent or active bleeding or known hemostatic defect), heparin should be started promptly (i.e., at the ER or ICU) as soon as PE or DVT are suspected.
      1) If DVT is strongly suspected (and there are no contraindications to anticoagulation) begin standard regimen heparinization while ordering venous thrombosis leg studies. If results are positive, continue therapy. If negative, repeat test serially (q 2days × 7–10 days). If results remain negative, treatment may be discontinued.
      2) For PE, a large IV bolus of standard heparin at 50–75 U/kg to load (5000–20,000 U) is usually given to stop the aggregation and release reaction of platelets that have adhered to the embolus. Then one of the standard regimens (also used for DVT) may be begun immediately.
      3) The most popular standard regimen is continuous IV infusion heparin at 20–30 µg/kg/hr (or approximately 1000 U/hr). The activated partial thromboplastin time (aPTT) is checked 6 hours after infusion begins and then rechecked at least daily.
      4) Heparin doses are begun empirically, and usually adjusted to keep aPTT or clotting time (CT) at ≥1.5 times baseline (measured just before next intermittent dose), or at 1.5–2.0 (some sources state up to 2.5) times control with continuous IV infusion for 5–7 days. (Heparin therapy for 10 days may be necessary on occasion, such as for patients with massive PE or extensive iliofemoral thrombosis.)
         a. Platelet counts should be checked q 2–3 days (because heparin can cause thrombocytopenia).
      5) Prolonged prophylactic therapy is usually begun by initiating a prothrombogenic drug (warfarin/Coumadin) on day 1 of heparin therapy. Alternatively, self-injected heparin at 7500–10,000 U q12h SQ is well tolerated and effective. Dose is adjusted to maintain a PTT of 1.5 times control value at the mid-dosing interval. This is preferable for patients in whom warfarin is contraindicated (as in pregnancy).

C. Warfarin/Coumadin has long been considered the drug of choice to treat PE over the long term.
    1) Warfarin is given concurrently with heparin on day 2 or day 3 (or even on day 1). This allows the 6–7 days for the slower onset warfarin to achieve full effect. Its mechanism of action is to alter the synthesis of vitamin K–dependent procoagulants (factors II, VII, IX, and X) and proteins C and S.
    2) Warfarin dosing is begun empirically at 5–10 mg PO qd (usually for 3–5 days), until the PT is 1.3–1.5 times control, or international normalized ratio (INR) of 2.0–3.0. Maintenance therapy varies widely from 2–15 mg PO qd.
    3) Warfarin is contraindicated in pregnancy.
    4) The PT is affected by a variety of drugs, requiring close PT monitoring.
        a. A partial list of drugs that increase PT includes: Alcohol (if concomitant liver disease), ASA, cimetidine, ciprofloxacin, erythromycin, Flu-Vax, INH, metronidazole, phenylbutazone, phenytoin, propranolol, quinidine, sulfinpyrazone, tamoxifen, tetracycline, trimethoprim-sulfamethoxazole.
        b. A partial list of drugs that decrease PT includes: Barbiturates, carbamazepine, chlordiazepoxide, cholestyramine, griseofulvin, nafcillin, oral contraceptives, dicloxacillin, rifampin, sucralfate, vitamin K (including that in multivitamin supplements and high vitamin K content foods/enteral feedings).

D. Low-molecular-weight heparin (LMWH) is a newer alternative for antithrombotic maintenance therapy that seems to offer promise. Although more expensive than standard heparin, LMWH can provide simple, safe, effective treatment, especially for patients with proximal DVT, which can help prevent PE. LMWH is given SQ and does not require routine PTT monitoring, thereby facilitating the convenience of outpatient management and potentially decreasing overall costs. LMWH appears to be as effective (some studies indicate more effective) in appropriate candidates than is standard heparin, while offering somewhat decreased bleeding complications.
    1) Mechanism: LMWH prevents formation or extension of venous thrombi, primarily via inhibition of factor Xa (and, to a lesser extent, inhibition of thrombin).
    2) Onset: Immediate.
    3) Administration: One common formulation is enoxaparin sodium/Lovenox, which is dosed at 30 mg SQ, q12h for maintenance therapy.
    4) Contraindications: Do not use in patients with major active bleeding, thrombocytopenia, or known hypersensitivity to heparin or pork products.
    5) Warnings: Use only with extreme caution for any conditions with increased risk of hemorrhage. Bleeding can occur at any site during enoxaparin therapy; therefore, search for a site of bleeding in any patient with an unexplained fall in Hct or BP.
    6) Drug interactions: Advisable to discontinue hemostatic agents prior to enoxaparin therapy to reduce risk of hemorrhage (i.e., oral anticoagulants and/or platelet inhibitors, such as ASA, salicylates,

NSAIDs, dipyridamole, or sulfinpyrazone). If these agents must be given concomitantly, use close clinical and lab value monitoring.

E. Hemorrhage is always a possibility with anticoagulation (with standard heparin, LMWH, or warfarin/Coumadin), but the risk is lower when PTT or PT are appropriately adjusted. When possible, minimize venipuncture, arterial puncture, and IM injections during heparin therapy to help prevent hematoma formation. Risk factors include comorbid disorders of heart, liver, or kidneys; elderly patients (>60 years); and those taking ASA.

F. A minimum of 3 months of anticoagulant therapy (using standard heparin, LMWH, or warfarin) is common, with shorter or longer regimens depending upon PE or DVT risk factors, venous thrombosis leg study results, $\dot{V}/\dot{Q}$ lung scan results, and risks of continued therapy. Lifetime maintenance therapy is sometimes warranted.

5. Thrombolytic therapy.

A. Lysis of PE in situ is the definitive medical treatment, yet this potentially promising therapy remains somewhat controversial and has not achieved wide usage. Only 10% of U.S. patients with acute PE currently receive thrombolysis.

B. Most medical authorities reserve such use for massive, acute PE with hemodynamic compromise, and for those patients who fail to improve hemodynamically after standard heparin therapy. The consideration as to whether or not to use thrombolytics needs to be made relatively early in the clinical course.

C. Thrombolytic therapy is expensive, carries extra risks of bleeding (including intracranial), and does not improve overall survival rates better than does standard heparin alone.

D. Recombinant tissue plasminogen activator (t-PA), streptokinase (SK), and urokinase (UK) are the three drugs approved for thrombolysis of PE or DVT. The thromboembolic agent of choice may be given by continuous IV infusion into a peripheral vein.

E. These agents promote endogenous fibrinolysis by activating plasminogen. This generates plasmin, which lyses thrombi in the pulmonary artery (PA) and the venous circulation, and which also has a secondary anticoagulant effect.

F. Thrombolytic therapy appears to accelerate PE resolution, reduce PA and right heart pressures, and improve right and left ventricular function in those patients with established PE.

G. Cautious monitoring of therapy, management of bleeding, and control of subsequent anticoagulation are required.

1) When possible, minimize venipuncture, arterial puncture, and IM injections during thrombolytic therapy to help prevent hematoma formation.

2) Important contraindications include:

a. Active internal bleeding

b. Recent CVA (within 2 months)

c. Severe HTN

d. Recent GI bleed

e. Recent trauma

f. Major obstetric (OB) or surgical procedures.

H. Since standard heparin is often begun prior to initiating thrombolytic therapy, if the decision is made to use thrombolytics, stop the heparin

IV infusion. Thrombolytic IV infusion may be started when the aPTT or thrombin time (TT) is ≤1.5 times control.

I. Thrombolytic therapy is given in one of the following three regimens:
   1) t-PA 100 mg (56 million IU) via IV over 2 hours; *or*
   2) Streptokinase 250,000 IU via IV over 30 minutes to load, then 100,000 IU/h continuous IV maintenance dose for 24–72 hours; *or*
   3) Urokinase 4400 IU/kg via IV over 10 minutes to load, then 4400 IU/kg/h continuous IV maintenance dose for 12–24 hours

J. The thrombolytic doses are fixed; therefore, no coagulation tests are needed during therapy. At the end of thrombolytic therapy, resume standard heparin IV infusion without a loading dose or with a small loading dose when the aPTT or TT is ≤1.5 times control.

6. *Informed consent is important, both for patient safety and as an educational tool. The patient ill enough to require antithrombotic treatment is likely to be at risk for serious complications such as CVA, both with or without undergoing such treatment.* However small, the potential exists for a disastrous occurrence as a result of either the disease process itself or of the therapy used to protect the patient from that disease:
   A. Possible hemorrhagic CVA, when antithrombotic treatment is used
   B. Possible embolic CVA, when antithrombotic treatment is withheld

7. Additional measures requiring referral to surgeon
   A. Surgical interruption and possible insertion of intraluminal filters into the inferior vena cava are options reserved for patients with life-threatening PE who have major contraindications to anticoagulants, or failure of or complications from anticoagulants or thrombolytics.
   B. Pulmonary embolectomy is an emergency procedure for patients with life-threatening hemodynamic compromise or cardiac arrest after massive PE. This emergency surgery is rarely performed and its outcome is nearly always dismal.

PATIENT EDUCATION

1. Encourage bed rest for only the first 2–3 days of PE therapy, and then initiate the leg exercises and other PE/DVT preventive measures mentioned previously.

2. Inform patient about risk factors for PE and DVT, and encourage modification of those risk factors within the patient's control.
   A. Eliminate oral contraceptive use, smoking, and prolonged immobility after a bone fracture.
   B. Avoid prolonged sitting in a chair, such as during long airliner or automobile trips.
   C. Do get up and walk for brief but regular periods (including on trips).

3. Reiterate the importance of avoiding exposure to cigarette smoke. Quit-smoking tips and other useful community resources are offered through:
   A. American Lung Association
   B. American Thoracic Society (which is the medical section of the American Lung Association)
   C. American Cancer Society
   D. American Heart Association
   E. CDC
   F. NIH

4. Educate patient about PE pathophysiology, drug use and side effects, and the need to comply with long-term anticoagulant therapy.
   A. Patient compliance is vital to safe and effective anticoagulation.
   B. Practice safety precautions by avoiding contact sports or trauma that could put patient at risk of serious injury during anticoagulation therapy.
   C. Patients need to notify their medical provider if they experience unusual bleeding:
      1) Bloody gums, nose, urine, stools, or vagina; *or*
      2) Excessive bruising
   D. Female patients also need to alert their medical provider if they are planning to become pregnant or have already become pregnant (especially since certain medications such as warfarin are contraindicated in pregnancy).
5. Remind patient of the importance of ongoing medical provider follow-up to monitor for recurrence. If occurrences of PE continue, the patient requires evaluation for underlying hypercoagulability or occult CA.
6. Advise patient that prompt, appropriate therapy for PE significantly improves prognosis. While PE may cause sudden death, those patients who survive to reach medical attention and who receive heparin can have good prospects of further survival, often without morbidity or mortality.
7. Caution the patient of the ongoing need for PE/DVT prevention measures, as ≥30% of patients with undiagnosed PE die.

Review Questions

2.31 Signs and symptoms may not be specific to PE and may lead to misdiagnosis unless PE is initially considered in the differential diagnosis work-up. Clinical findings, morbidity, and mortality depend on:
   A. Size of the PE
   B. Extent of obstruction
   C. Patient's pre-existing cardiopulmonary status
   D. All of the above

2.32 The most common embolic material is thrombus from a distant site, particularly from:
   A. Tumor fragments invading venous circulation
   B. Deep veins of the legs and pelvis
   C. Fat embolism
   D. Infected tissue

The following three-part case scenario is for pulmonary embolism Questions 2.33–2.35 listed below.

Ms. JM is a 46-year-old woman brought in by ambulance to the ER with an acute onset of unexplained dyspnea and pleuritic type chest pain. She had noted increasing cough, apprehension, and occasional hemoptysis over the past 2 hours, culminating in a near-syncopal episode that prompted a call to 911. Ms. JM has been on bed rest at home for the past 8 days after right foot surgery. Her job requires her to be on her feet and there are no light-duty options, so she has taken time off to recuperate. Although her surgeon had encouraged early ambulation with crutches, she has "preferred to rest instead." She has occasionally worn elastic support hose since surgery.

> PMH: Varicose veins; negative for asthma; no recent fever or URI symptoms
> Medications: Oral contraceptive pills for 27 years including at present.
> FSH: 48-pack-year smoking history; moderate social intake of ETOH; no IVDA. Vital Signs: RR, 28/min; HR, 120 pm; BP, 90/58; T, 98.6°F
> Pulse Oximetry: 95%, room air.

On exam you note a thin, slightly anxious patient who has scattered, faint lung crackles without wheezes. Ms. JM coughs in your presence and expectorates a small amount of foamy white sputum, tinged with blood. She has scattered varicosities throughout both lower extremities. Her right lower extremity has edema, erythema, and palpable vein cords; no pus, and the affected sites are nonfluctuant. Ms. JM also has right calf tenderness to dorsiflexion/positive Homan's sign.

2.33 For your differential diagnosis you now suspect right lower extremity phlebitis, and possible PE. A high index of suspicion is needed to avoid missing a pulmonary embolism. Which test(s) would be least helpful for you to accurately diagnose PE?
A. $\dot{V}/\dot{Q}$ scan that demonstrates $\dot{V}/\dot{Q}$ mismatch
B. Lower-extremity Doppler/duplex studies that show venous thrombosis
C. Pulmonary angiography/arteriography that reveals arterial cutoffs and/or intraluminal filling defects
D. ABG interpretation of hypoxemia with acute respiratory alkalosis

2.34 Results of Ms. JM's tests confirm thromboembolism of her right lower extremity, and arrangements are made to further confirm PE. The patient is concerned that someone like herself, in apparently good health, could have the sudden onset of a potentially life-threatening condition like PE. You explain to her that prevention of DVT and PE is essential, and that appropriate antithrombotic prevention should be used whenever patients are at risk. Which of these commonly used interventions is less likely to achieve this purpose?
A. Early ambulation after surgery, as tolerated and appropriate.
B. Immobilized patients should have legs elevated and begin range-of-motion exercises when stable.
C. Elastic support stockings (preferably thigh-high).
D. Intermittent external leg compression.

2.35 You discuss Ms. JM's case with her attending physician, who asks you to have the patient admitted to the telemetry unit now. As a monitored bed is being arranged for her admission, standard heparinization therapy is initiated at the ER. All of the following apply to standard heparinization therapy, EXCEPT:
A. Standard heparin is the drug of choice to treat PE over the long term.
B. The risk of hemorrhage may be greater in elderly patients (>60 years), and those with comorbid disorders (of heart, liver, or kidneys), or who are taking ASA.
C. For PE, a large IV bolus of 50–75 U/kg to load (5000–20,000 U) is usually given. Then one of the standard regimens (also used for DVT) may be begun immediately.

D. The most popular standard regimen is continuous IV infusion heparin at 20–30 μg/kg/hr (or approximately 1000 U/hr). The aPTT is checked 6 hours after infusion begins and then rechecked at least daily.

Answers and Rationales

2.31   **D**   In general, clinical findings depend on size of the PE, extent of obstruction, and patient's pre-existing cardiopulmonary status.

2.32   **B**   The most common embolic material is thrombus from a distant site, particularly from deep veins of the legs and pelvis (90–95%), especially from clots at the thigh.

2.33   **D**   Routine lab tests are not helpful to diagnose PE. Rather, because PE is so frequently misdiagnosed, these associated tests (i.e., ABGs, CXR, ECG) are used to rule out other possible causes. The diagnosis of PE is supported by $\dot{V}/\dot{Q}$ scan, which should be the first test done when PE is suspected. Patterns suggesting PE include normal ventilation with multiple segmental or lobar perfusion defects. Over 90% of PEs result from DVT of lower extremities; therefore, lower-extremity Doppler/duplex studies play an increasing role in accurately diagnosing PEs. Acute venous thromboembolism is a term that combines both diagnoses appropriately, as approximately 40% of patients with DVT, but without symptoms of PE, do have PE demonstrated radiographically. Pulmonary angiography/arteriography, despite morbidity and mortality risks, remains the gold standard to diagnose PE. Patterns indicative of PE include arterial cutoffs and/or intraluminal filling defects.

2.34   **C**   In the prevention of DVT and PE, elastic support stockings may offer some benefit but are less useful than are the other interventions listed.

2.35   **A**   All of these statements apply to standard heparinization therapy, except for the first one. Standard heparin is the drug of choice to initially treat PE. Warfarin/Coumadin has long been considered the drug of choice to treat PE over the long term, however.

References

Arroliga, A.C., Mathay, M.A., & Mathay, R.A. (1995). Pulmonary thromboembolism and other pulmonary vascular diseases. In R.B. George, R.W. Light, M.A. Mathay, & R.A. Mathay (eds.). *Chest Medicine: Essentials of Pulmonary and Critical Care Medicine* (3rd ed.). Baltimore, MD: Williams & Wilkins, pp. 271–302.

Dalen, J. (1994). Pulmonary embolism. In H.W. Griffith, M.R. Dambro, & J. Griffith (eds.). *The Five Minute Clinical Consult, 1994*, Philadelphia: Lea & Febiger, pp. 838–839.

Dietzen, D.L. (1996). Pulmonary embolus. In R.E. Rakel (ed.). *Saunders Manual of Medical Practice.* Philadelphia: W.B. Saunders Co., pp. 142–144.

Fourth ACCP Consensus Conference on Antithrombotic Therapy. (1995). In J.E. Dalen & J. Hirsh (eds.). *Chest 108* (4), 225S–522S.

Moser, K.M. (1994). Pulmonary thromboembolism. In K.J. Isselbacher, E. Braunwald, J.D. Wilson, et al. (eds.). *Harrison's Principles of Internal Medicine: Vol. 2* (13th ed.). New York: McGraw-Hill, pp. 1214–1220.

Pulmonary Embolism. (1995). In K.M. Baldwin, C.S. Garza, R.N. Martin, et al. (eds.). *Davis's Manual of Critical Care Therapeutics.* Philadelphia: F.A. Davis Co., pp. 36–48.

Stauffer, J.L. (1997). Pulmonary thromboembolism. In L.M. Tierney, Jr., S.J. McPhee, & M.A. Papadakis (eds.). *Current Medical Diagnosis and Treatment, 1997* (36th ed.). Stamford, CT: Appleton & Lange, pp. 290–297.

Additional Recommended References

Anup, A.B. (1996). *Arterial Blood Gas Analysis Made Easy.* Valhalla, NY: Author, pp. 11–93.

Feldman, A.J. (1996). Acute extremity ischemia and thrombophlebitis. In J.E. Tintinalli, R.L. Krome, & E. Ruiz (eds.). *Emergency Medicine: A Comprehensive Study Guide* (4th ed.). New York: McGraw-Hill, pp. 389–394.

Hockberger, R.S. (1996). Pulmonary embolism. In J.E. Tintinalli, R.L. Krome, & E. Ruiz (eds.). *Emergency Medicine: A Comprehensive Study Guide* (4th ed.). New York: McGraw-Hill, pp. 370–374.

Papadakis, M.A. (1997). Acid-base disorders. In L.M. Tierney, Jr., S.J. McPhee, & M.A. Papadakis (eds.). *Current Medical Diagnosis and Treatment, 1997* (36th ed.). Stamford, CT: Appleton & Lange, pp. 815–825.

Tierney, L.M., Jr., & L.M. Messina. (1997). Thrombophlebitis. In L.M. Tierney, Jr., S.J. McPhee, & M.A. Papadakis (eds.), *Current Medical Diagnosis and Treatment, 1997* (36th ed.). Stamford, CT: Appleton & Lange, pp. 451–455.

Weg, J.G. (1996). Pulmonary embolism and deep vein thrombosis. In J.M. Rippe, R.S. Irwin, M.P. Fink, & F.B. Cerra (eds.). *Intensive Care Medicine: Vol. I* (3rd ed.). Boston: Little, Brown & Co., pp. 660–679.

Weinberger, S.E., & J.M. Drazen. (1994). Disturbances of respiratory function. In K.J. Isselbacher, E. Braunwald, J.D. Wilson, et al. (eds.). *Harrison's Principles of Internal Medicine: Vol. 2* (13th ed.). New York: McGraw-Hill, pp. 1152–1159.

Wilson, R.F., & C. Barton. (1996). Blood gases: Pathophysiology and interpretation. In J.E. Tintinalli, R.L. Krome, & E. Ruiz (eds.). *Emergency Medicine: A Comprehensive Study Guide* (4th ed.). New York: McGraw-Hill, pp. 108–117.

Acute Respiratory Failure

DEFINITION

1. Acute respiratory failure (ARF)
   A. ARF may be defined as relatively rapid respiratory dysfunction leading to acute hypoxemia and/or acute hypercapnia, severe enough to compromise the function of vital organs.
   B. Generally, ARF is considered present when ABGs reveal:
      1) Hypoxemia (Pao_2 of $\leq$50–60 mm Hg)
      2) Hypercapnia ($Paco_2$ of $\geq$50 mm Hg)
   C. Both pulmonary and nonpulmonary disorders may cause ARF.
   D. Acute hypoxemic respiratory failure is most commonly seen with:
      1) Increased permeability pulmonary edema
         a. Noncardiogenic.
         b. Normal pressure.
         c. Adult respiratory distress syndrome (ARDS) is the prototype for this type of pulmonary edema.

2) Cardiogenic pulmonary edema
   a. Normal permeability.
   b. High-pressure.
   c. Heart failure is the prototype for this type of pulmonary edema.
3) For further discussion of these differences, see also the references following this section, as well as the Chapter on Cardiovascular disorders in this text.

E. Acute hypercapnic respiratory failure is most commonly seen with:
   1) Neuromuscular disease/trauma/respiratory muscle fatigue/certain drug overdoses
   2) Exacerbation of obstructive pulmonary diseases (i.e., COPD)

F. This section will emphasize ARDS (adult respiratory distress syndrome/acute respiratory distress syndrome) as an example of a clinically significant pulmonary disorder in the critically ill patient.
   1) Synonyms for ARDS include stiff lung, shock lung, traumatic wet lung, and adult hyaline membrane syndrome.
   2) For additional discussions of ARDS and other types of ARF (including the use of mechanical ventilation), see the references listed at the end of this section.

2. ARDS
   A. ARDS may be defined as a clinical syndrome of severe, acute lung injury involving diffuse alveolar damage and noncardiogenic pulmonary edema:
      1) Due to increased permeability of the pulmonary microvasculature.
      2) Resulting in acute, refractory hypoxemia.
      3) Increased permeability, noncardiogenic pulmonary edema can develop as a progressive syndrome of mild, moderate, or severe acute lung injury.
      4) Recent proposals try to quantify scoring of the physiologic and radiographic abnormalities involved, including presence or absence of organ failure (besides that of the lung itself) and of the associated clinical disorders.
         a. ARDS is defined as:
            i. CXR: Bilateral infiltrates present
            ii. Pao_2: FIo_2 ratio: <200–300
            iii. Exclude clinical evidence of:
               • Left atrial HTN from intravascular volume overload or left ventricular failure
               • Pneumonia
      5) Use of a flow-directed, thermodilution pulmonary artery (PA) catheter can identify normal pulmonary capillary wedge pressure (PCWP) (<15–18 mm Hg) and cardiac index (>3.5 L/min/m^2) which would exclude cardiogenic pulmonary edema (heart failure).
         a. The ACNP consults with the collaborating physician or makes referral to pulmonary/critical care physician specialist for PA catheter insertion.
      6) Prognosis depends upon the cumulative insult of nonpulmonary factors, plus the extent of acute lung injury.
         a. Concomitant multisystem organ failure (MSOF) or pre-existing liver, renal, or chronic GI disease with malnutrition greatly increase morbidity and mortality with ARDS.

ETIOLOGY/INCIDENCE

1. Pathogenesis of ARF in adults
   A. Caused by a variety of pulmonary and systemic insults:
      1) Pulmonary vascular disorders
         a. Pulmonary embolism
         b. Fluid overload
      2) Parenchymal lung disorders
         a. ARDS
         b. Aspiration (especially gastric, also near-drowning)
         c. Pneumonia
         d. Cardiogenic pulmonary edema
         e. Hypersensitivity pneumonitis
      3) Airway disorders
         a. Acute exacerbation of COPD (emphysema and/or chronic bronchitis)
         b. Status asthmaticus
         c. Partial airway obstruction (including food or other foreign body lodged in airways)
      4) Chest and pleural derangements
         a. Pneumothorax
         b. Flail chest
      5) Neuromuscular disorders
         a. Certain drug overdoses (especially narcotic, sedative, and/or hypnotic overdose)
         b. Cervical spinal cord injury
         c. Stroke/CVA
         d. Severe electrolyte disorders
         e. Heavy metal intoxication
         f. Amyotrophic lateral sclerosis (ALS)
         g. Guillain-Barré syndrome
         h. Myasthenia gravis
         i. Botulism
         j. Sleep apnea syndrome
   B. Mechanisms of injury
      1) Acute hypoxemic respiratory failure
         a. Caused by:
            i. Increased permeability (noncardiogenic) pulmonary edema/ARDS
         b. Respiratory failure due to arterial hypoxemia
            i. Anatomic aspects:
               • Alveolar filling
               • Microatelectasis
               • Diffusion impairment
            ii. Physiologic aspects:
               • $\dot{V}/\dot{Q}$ mismatch
               • Right-to-left intrapulmonary shunting
               • Decreased lung compliance ("stiff lung")
      2) Acute hypercapnic respiratory failure
         a. Caused by chest trauma, airway obstruction/disorders, and neuromuscular disorders

   b. Respiratory failure due to arterial hypercapnia:
      i. Increased work of breathing and respiratory muscle fatigue
      ii. Insufficient central ventilatory drive (ventilatory failure)
      iii. Impaired neuromuscular transmission of the respiratory drive
2. Etiology/incidence of ARDS
   A. Estimated 150,000 cases per year of ARDS
   B. All ages affected
   C. Men and women affected equally
   D. Patients at greatest risk to develop ARDS are those with:
      1) Systemic sepsis/septic shock/systemic inflammatory response syndrome (SIRS)
      2) Direct lung injury/gastric aspiration
3. Pathogenesis of ARDS in adults
   A. Caused by a wide variety of catastrophic pulmonary and systemic/nonpulmonary insults:
      1) Sepsis: Sepsis from any cause (often due to pneumonia)
      2) Shock: Shock of any etiology, but especially SIRS. (One third of all ARDS patients initially have septic shock.)
      3) Liquid aspiration: Gastric contents (very often), near-drowning/fresh and saltwater (often), liquid hydrocarbons
      4) Trauma: Lung contusion (often), head injury/other nonthoracic trauma (often), burns, fat embolism, snake bite
      5) Toxic gas inhalation (often): Smoke, oxygen toxicity, corrosive chemicals, NO_2, CI_2, NH_3, phosgene
      6) Drug overdose or poisoning: Especially narcotics/barbiturates
      7) Hematologic disorders: Multiple blood transfusions (often), disseminated intravascular coagulation (DIC)
      8) Metabolic disorders: Acute pancreatitis, uremia, diabetic ketoacidosis
      9) Miscellaneous: CA, high altitude pulmonary edema (HAPE), pulmonary embolism, bowel infarct, amniotic fluid embolism, eclampsia

SIGNS AND SYMPTOMS OF ARDS

1. Patients demonstrate similar signs and symptoms, regardless of the associated clinical condition or precipitating cause of ARDS. Typical findings:
   A. Severe hypoxemia that does not improve with low-flow oxygen therapy
   B. CXR: Fluffy bilateral infiltrates
   C. Decreased static lung compliance
      1) Manifested by high ventilator pressures needed to deliver adequate tidal volume
2. Symptoms
   A. Dyspnea is the cardinal symptom, and precedes development of CXR abnormalities.
      1) Rapid onset of profound SOB, usually by 12–48 hours after a serious precipitating event (e.g., gastric aspiration, septic shock, auto accident)
   B. As ARDS progresses, patients develop:
      1) Labored breathing
      2) Tachypnea
      3) Anxiety and restlessness
      4) Fatigue and exhaustion

3. Signs
   A. Early and ongoing signs
      1) Tachypnea (RR >20/min, and often >30/min)
      2) Increased work of breathing
         a. Accessory respiratory muscle use
         b. Intercostal retractions
         c. Nasal flaring
      3) Tachycardia (HR >100 bpm)
   B. Later signs may include any or all of these:
      1) Diaphoresis
      2) Hypotension
      3) Cyanosis
      4) Altered mental status
      5) Breath sounds may be normal initially, but later patients may develop:
         a. Signs of consolidation
         b. Diffuse crackles

CLINICAL COURSE OF ARDS

1. ARDS is a progressive syndrome whose clinical presentation may initially appear benign. This may delay the early recognition of ARDS and the prompt institution of appropriate therapy. Within several hours, ARDS can become a full-blown emergency and life-threatening condition. Therefore, be alert to any clinical changes in patients with predisposing causes of ARDS.
2. Four phases are generally recognized in ARDS:
   A. Phase 1: Acute insult/injury
      1) Tachypnea, tachycardia, respiratory alkalosis
      2) Physical exam and CXR may be normal
   B. Phase 2: Latent period
      1) Develops by 6–48 hours following initial insult/injury
      2) Hyperventilation and increased work of breathing
      3) Hypocapnia and widening alveolar-arterial oxygen gradient
      4) CXR may be normal or may show early infiltrates
   C. Phase 3: Acute hypoxemic respiratory failure
      1) Tachypnea, dyspnea
      2) Diffusely scattered crackles
      3) Decreasing lung compliance
      4) CXR: Diffuse infiltrates bilaterally
   D. Phase 4: Severe abnormalities
      1) Severe hypoxemia, no longer responsive to therapy
      2) Increased intrapulmonary shunting
      3) Metabolic and respiratory acidosis
      4) Inability to deliver adequate tidal volume, even with higher ventilator pressures

DIFFERENTIAL DIAGNOSIS OF ARDS

1. It is important to rule out cardiogenic pulmonary edema, or heart failure, because this can be effectively treated with specific therapy when correctly diagnosed, especially early in the clinical course.
   A. Clinical differentiation between ARDS and cardiogenic pulmonary edema (heart failure) may be accurate in only 60–80% of cases.

B. Use of a flow-directed, thermodilution PA catheter can identify normal PCWP (<15–18 mm Hg) and cardiac index (>3.5 L/min/m^2), which would exclude cardiogenic pulmonary edema (heart failure).
   1) The ACNP consults with the collaborating physician or makes referral to pulmonary/critical care physician specialist for PA catheter insertion.
2. Although ARF is often categorized as acute hypoxemic or acute hypercapnic respiratory failure, overlapping conditions may require the application of differing treatments.
3. Sources of overlap syndromes may include:
   A. Other causes of pulmonary edema
   B. Acute inflammatory processes (e.g., pneumonia)
   C. Alveolar hemorrhage syndromes

DIAGNOSTIC TESTS/FINDINGS WITH ARDS

1. ABGs.
   A. Change over course of illness
      1) Pao_2 continues to decline, despite treatment with increasingly high concentrations of inspired oxygen.
      2) $Paco_2$ initially decreases, then may normalize or even increase.
      3) Respiratory alkalosis initially, then may change to acidosis.
      4) Widening Pao_2–Pao_2.
      5) To review ABG interpretation, refer to the references listed following this section.
2. CXRs.
   A. Change over course of illness
      1) May initially be normal
      2) Bilateral interstitial infiltrates then develop, which are patchy and fluffy, and have irregular borders
      3) May eventually progress to total white-out of the lung due to diffuse bilateral interstitial and alveolar infiltrates.
3. Hemodynamic monitoring.
   A. Cardiac output (CO)
      1) Initially increases
      2) May decrease with positive end-expiratory pressure (PEEP)
   B. PCWP may be normal or decreased
   C. PAP increases
4. PFTs.
   A. FRC decreases markedly
   B. Respiratory effort and rate always increase
   C. Tidal volume (TV) decreases
   D. Compliance decreases
   E. Dead space ventilation increases (often ≥60%)
   F. Right-to-left intrapulmonary shunt develops (with shunt fraction often ≥30%)
   G. Peak inspiratory pressures increase
5. $S\bar{v}o_2$ decreases
6. Capnography shows $\dot{V}/\dot{Q}$ mismatch.
   A. Increased end-tidal Pco_2.
7. Pulse oximetry shows decreased O_2 saturation.

MANAGEMENT/TREATMENT OF ARDS

1. *Patients suspected of having ARDS or other types of ARF require prompt hospital admission to a monitored bed in a critical care unit for further evaluation and treatment. Depending upon the setting, the ACNP may be called upon to help arrange hospital admission/ICU transfer with physician consult. A physician needs to manage the patient, while the ACNP may collaborate. Timely referral to a pulmonary/critical care physician specialist is also imperative to follow the patient through this life-threatening course.*
2. At this time there is no clinically proven, widely accepted curative treatment for ARDS. The two principle approaches at present are to:
   A. Treat the initiating process or precipitating event
   B. Provide aggressive and appropriate supportive management
3. Maintain tissue oxygenation and perfusion by improving gas exchange and blood flow via:
   A. Supplemental O_2
   B. Improvement of CO_2
   C. Mechanical ventilation:
      1) Benefits:
         a. Increases alveolar size, leading to increased lung volume.
         b. Alveolar liquid is spread out over a greater surface area, leading to easier gas entry into alveolus.
         c. Increases FRC, leading to better compliance.
      2) Potential pitfalls:
         a. May precipitate pneumothorax or other barotrauma.
         b. To review pneumothorax and mechanical ventilation, refer to the references listed following this section.
4. PEEP may be added to mechanical ventilation to help improve gas exchange in ARDS.
   A. The principal benefit of PEEP is that it decreases shunt fraction by improving FRC.
   B. A potential pitfall of PEEP is that it may decrease cardiac output (CO).
      1) Patient may require CO monitoring via flow-directed, thermodilution PA catheter. (The ACNP consults with physician or makes referral to pulmonary/critical care physician specialist for PA catheter insertion.)
   C. Attempt to reduce PEEP once patient stabilizes with:
      1) F_{IO_2}: <40%
      2) Pa_{O_2}: Adequate
      3) Effective compliance: >25
5. General guidelines as to when it is appropriate to increase F_{IO_2} versus increasing PEEP in the treatment of ARDS.
   A. Increase F_{IO_2} first when:
      1) F_{IO_2} <60% and patient is also on PEEP; *or*
      2) There are concerns about the potential for PEEP-related consequences
         a. Hypotensive state, despite adequate volume and vasopressors (i.e., dopamine); *or*
         b. Barotrauma concerns (i.e., chest tube in place, due to pneumothorax)
   B. Increase PEEP when:
      1) Patient has already been on F_{IO_2} 100% without improvement; *or*

2) There are concerns about the potential for oxygen toxicity (especially after initial 1–3 days)

6. Additional ventilator management issues. Once intubated, a patient can no longer protect his or her airway and is completely dependent upon medical caregivers to provide:

A. Patency of endotracheal tube (ET-T) and airway
B. A means for the patient to call for help
C. Vigilant infection control
D. Effective cough/pulmonary toilet/suction of secretions
E. Humidified inspired air
F. Measures to prevent aspiration
  1) Elevate the head of the bed (HOB) $\geq$ 30 degrees.
  2) Consider NG tube insertion.

7. Maintain effective fluid balance with ARDS.

A. Keep patient as dry as possible and avoid fluid volume overload via:
  1) Effective IV fluid management
  2) Judicious use of diuretic therapy when indicated

PATIENT EDUCATION

1. Educate patient about:
A. ARF or ARDS pathogenesis and probable cause
B. Drug, ventilator, and other therapy use and side effects
C. The need to comply with potentially uncomfortable therapies during the acute phase of illness

2. Depending upon how quickly a patient's condition deteriorates, give psychological preparation by briefly informing conscious patient of need for ET intubation and what to expect. Limit teaching to simple, focused explanations:
A. Need to intubate to help patient breathe better
B. What to expect, immediately and once connected to ventilator
C. Need to comply once intubation drugs wear off
D. How to summon help

3. Help foster hope, in spite of generally poor prognosis
A. Overall mortality approximately 60%
B. Greater morbidity and mortality with MSOF
C. Most patients who do recover from ARDS have few ongoing sequelae

---

Review Questions

The following three-part case scenario is for ARF/ARDS Questions 2.36–2.38 listed below.

Mr. MK is a 22-year-old triathlete brought to the ER by his buddies after a near-drowning episode when he was caught in a strong current. He complains of increasing dyspnea and demonstrates accessory muscle use. Initial RR, 36; HR, 110; BP, 90/50. Initial CXR: clear. Interpretation of initial ABGs: Respiratory alkalosis with moderately severe hypoxemia. He is transferred to the ICU, intubated, and placed on a mechanical ventilator with these settings:

FIO_2	1.0 (100%)
Mode:	Assist control (AC)
V_T	800 mL
Rate:	15/min
PEEP:	5 cm

At 12 hours following injury, repeat CXR shows bilateral fluffy infiltrates. Mr. MK is becoming obtunded and his PaO_2: FIO_2 ratio is now 220. ABGs drawn on FIO_2 of 100% now show:

PH:	7.30
PO_2:	220
PCO_2:	35
SaO_2:	99%
Bicarb:	16

2.36 Your interpretation of Mr. MK's present ABG results:
   A. Acute metabolic acidosis. Significant PAO_2–PaO_2 indicates a right-to-left intrapulmonary shunt.
   B. Acute respiratory acidosis. Significant PAO_2–PaO_2 indicates a left-to-right intrapulmonary shunt.
   C. Chronic respiratory alkalosis with hypercapnia. No significant intrapulmonary shunt is indicated by the above values.
   D. Chronic metabolic alkalosis. Significant PAO_2–PaO_2 indicates a left-to-right intrapulmonary shunt.
2.37 As you review Mr. MK's case with his treating pulmonary/critical care physician specialist, you note that all of the current approaches to ARDS treatment are being utilized. These include all of the following, EXCEPT:
   A. Treat the initiating process or precipitating event.
   B. Provide conservative and incremental supportive management.
   C. Maintain tissue oxygenation and perfusion by improving gas exchange and blood flow.
   D. PEEP may be added to mechanical ventilation to help improve gas exchange.
2.38 Mr. MK is not improving on FIO_2 of 100% along with 5 cm of PEEP. The decision is made to increase PEEP to 10 cm. Describe when it is appropriate to increase FIO_2 versus increasing PEEP in the treatment of ARDS. Any of these guidelines could apply, EXCEPT:
   A. When on both FIO_2 >70% and PEEP, increase FIO_2 first.
   B. When there are concerns about the potential for PEEP related consequences (e.g., hypotension, barotrauma), increase FIO_2 first.
   C. When there are concerns about the potential for oxygen toxicity (especially after initial 1–3 days), increase PEEP.
   D. If patient is already on FIO_2 of 100% without improvement, increase PEEP.
2.39 ARF may be caused by (circle all that apply):
   A. Acute COPD exacerbation
   B. Flail chest
   C. Aspiration pneumonia
   D. Pulmonary embolism

2.40 Which of these may help to identify ARDS? (circle all that apply):
   A. CXR: Presence of unilateral fluffy infiltrate
   B. Pao_2: Fio_2 ratio >300
   C. Pao_2 ≤50–60 mm Hg, and/or $Paco_2$ ≥50 mm Hg
   D. Relatively rapid respiratory dysfunction, severe enough to compromise the function of vital organs

---

Answers and Rationales

2.36 **A** Acute metabolic acidosis. Significant Pao_2–Pao_2 indicates a right-to-left intrapulmonary shunt.

2.37 **B** All of these are current approaches to ARDS treatment EXCEPT answer **B,** which states to provide conservative and incremental supportive management. An important aspect of current ARDS treatment is to provide aggressive and appropriate supportive management, such as via supplemental oxygen, improvement of CO_2, and mechanical ventilation.

2.38 **A** Any of these guidelines EXCEPT answer **A** could apply to the decision-making process of when to increase Fio_2 versus increasing PEEP in the treatment of ARDS. Answer **A** incorrectly states to increase Fio_2 first when the patient is on PEEP and also has Fio_2 of >70%. An important guideline is to increase Fio_2 first when the patient is on PEEP and also has Fio_2 of <60%.

2.39 **All** All of these are correct. ARF may be caused by a host of pulmonary and/or systemic insults, including acute COPD exacerbation, flail chest, aspiration pneumonia, or pulmonary embolism.

2.40 **C,D** The diagnosis of ARDS is supported by answers **C** (Pao_2 ≤50–60 mm Hg, and/or $Paco_2$ ≥50 mm Hg) and **D** (relatively rapid respiratory dysfunction, severe enough to compromise the function of vital organs). Answer A incorrectly states that the CXR is likely to show presence of a unilateral fluffy infiltrate. Bilateral fluffy infiltrates are a hallmark of ARDS, however. Answer B incorrectly states that the Pao_2: Fio_2 ratio is >300 in ARDS. In fact, the Pao_2: Fio_2 ratio is <200–300 in ARDS.

References

Acute respiratory failure type I: Adult respiratory distress syndrome. (1995). In K.M. Baldwin, C.S. Garza, R.N. Martin, et al. (eds.). *Davis's Manual of Critical Care Therapeutics*. Philadelphia: F.A. Davis Co., pp. 1–14.

Acute respiratory failure type II: Acute exacerbation of chronic obstructive pulmonary disease. (1995). In K.M. Baldwin, C.S. Garza, R.N. Martin, et al. (eds.). *Davis's Manual of Critical Care Therapeutics*. Philadelphia: F.A. Davis Co., pp. 15–24.

Ingram, R.H., Jr. (1994). Adult respiratory distress syndrome. In K.J. Isselbacher, E. Braunwald, J.D. Wilson, et al. (eds.). *Harrison's Principles of Internal Medicine, Vol. 2* (13th ed.). New York: McGraw-Hill, pp. 1240–1243.

Ingram, R.H., Jr. (1994). Acute respiratory failure. In K.J. Isselbacher, E. Braunwald, J.D. Wilson, et al. (eds.). *Harrison's Principles of Internal Medicine, Vol. 2*, (13th ed.). New York: McGraw-Hill, pp. 1203–1205.

Lapinsky, S.E., and Grossman, R.F. (1996). Chronic obstructive pulmonary disease/respiratory failure. In J.M. Rippe, R.S. Irvin, M.P. Fink, & F.B. Cerra (eds.). *Intensive Care Medicine* (3rd ed., Vol. I). Boston: Little, Brown & Co., pp. 591–605.

Matthay, M.A. (1995). Acute hypercapnic respiratory failure: Neuromuscular and obstructive disease. In R.B. George, R.W. Light, M.A. Matthay, & R.A. Matthay (eds.). *Chest Medicine: Essentials of Pulmonary and Critical Care Medicine* (3rd ed.). Baltimore, MD: Williams & Wilkins, pp. 578–592.

Matthay, M.A. (1995). Acute hypoxemic respiratory failure: Pulmonary edema and ARDS. In R.B. George, R.W. Light, M.A. Matthay, & R.A. Matthay (eds.). *Chest Medicine: Essentials of Pulmonary and Critical Care Medicine* (3rd ed.). Baltimore, MD: Williams & Wilkins, pp. 593–608.

Matthay, M.A. (1995). General principles of managing the patient with respiratory insufficiency. In R.B. George, R.W. Light, M.A. Matthay, & R.A. Matthay (eds.). *Chest Medicine: Essentials of Pulmonary and Critical Care Medicine* (3rd ed.). Baltimore, MD: Williams & Wilkins, pp. 563–577.

Schuster, D.P., & Kollef, M.H. (1996). Acute respiratory distress syndrome. In J.M. Rippe, R.S. Irvin, M.P. Fink, & F.B. Cerra (eds.). *Intensive Care Medicine* (3rd ed., Vol. I). Boston: Little, Brown & Co., pp. 591–605.

Stauffer, J.L. (1997). Acute respiratory distress syndrome (ARDS). In L.M. Tierney, Jr., S.J. McPhee, & M.A. Papadakis (eds.). *Current Medical Diagnosis and Treatment, 1997* (36th ed.). Stamford, CT: Appleton & Lange, pp. 311–313.

Stauffer, J.L. (1997). Acute respiratory failure. In L.M. Tierney, Jr., S.J. McPhee, & M.A. Papadakis (eds.). *Current Medical Diagnosis and Treatment, 1997* (36th ed.). Stamford, CT: Appleton & Lange, pp. 309–311.

Stauffer, J.L. (1997). Chronic obstructive pulmonary disease/acute exacerbation of COPD. In L.M. Tierney, Jr., S.J. McPhee, & M.A. Papadakis (eds.). *Current Medical Diagnosis and Treatment, 1997* (36th ed.). Stamford, CT: Appleton & Lange, pp. 254–255.

Steinberg, E. (1996). Acute respiratory distress syndrome. In R.E. Rakel (ed.). *Saunders Manual of Medical Practice*, Philadelphia: W.B. Saunders Co., pp. 145–147.

Additional Recommended References

Anup, A.B. (1996). *Arterial Blood Gas Analysis Made Easy.* Valhalla, NY: Author, pp. 11–93.

Benditt, J. (1996). Pneumothorax. In R.E. Rakel (ed.). *Saunders Manual of Medical Practice.* Philadelphia: W.B. Saunders Co., pp. 160–161.

Cairns, C. (1996). Heart failure and pulmonary edema. In J.E. Tintinalli, R.L. Krome, & E. Ruiz (eds.). *Emergency Medicine: A Comprehensive Study Guide* (4th ed.). New York: McGraw-Hill, pp. 354–358.

Haupt, M.T., & Carlson, R.W. (1992). Permeability pulmonary edema and the adult respiratory distress syndrome. In J.E. Tintinalli, R.L. Krome, & E. Ruiz (eds.). *Emergency Medicine: A Comprehensive Study Guide* (3rd ed.). New York: McGraw-Hill, pp. 287–288.

Ingenito, E.P., & J.M. Drazen. (1994). Mechanical ventilatory support. In K.J. Isselbacher, E. Braunwald, J.D. Wilson, et al. (eds.). *Harrison's Principles of Internal Medicine, Vol. 2* (13th ed.). New York: McGraw-Hill, pp. 1244–1248.

Kennedy, J.I., Jr. (1996). Ventilator support. In R.E. Rakel (ed.). *Saunders Manual of Medical Practice.* Philadelphia: W.B. Saunders Co., pp. 154–156.

Papadakis, M.A. (1997). Acid-base disorders. In L.M. Tierney, Jr., S.J. McPhee, & M.A. Papadakis (eds.). *Current Medical Diagnosis and Treatment, 1997* (36th ed.). Stamford, CT: Appleton & Lange, pp. 815–825.

Plummer, D. (1996). Dyspnea, hypoxia, and hypercapnia. In J.E. Tintinalli, R.L. Krome, & E. Ruiz (eds.). *Emergency Medicine: A Comprehensive Study Guide* (4th ed.). New York: McGraw-Hill, pp. 194–196.

Seidman, J.C. (1996). Chronic obstructive pulmonary disease/decompensated chronic airflow obstruction. In J.E. Tintinalli, R.L. Krome, & E. Ruiz (eds.). *Emergency Medicine: A Comprehensive Study Guide* (4th ed.). New York: McGraw-Hill, pp. 440–442.

Weinberger, S.E., & J.M. Drazen. (1994). Disturbances of respiratory function. In K.J. Isselbacher, E. Braunwald, J.D. Wilson, et al. (eds.). *Harrison's Principles of Internal Medicine: Vol. 2* (13th ed.) New York: McGraw-Hill, pp. 1152–1159.

Wilson, R.F., & C. Barton. (1996). Blood gases: Pathophysiology and interpretation. In J.E. Tintinalli, R.L. Krome, & E. Ruiz (eds.). *Emergency Medicine: A Comprehensive Study Guide* (4th ed.). New York: McGraw-Hill, pp. 108–117.

Pleural Effusion

DEFINITION

Excess accumulation (>25 mL) of fluid in the pleural space. Over 1 million cases occur annually in the United States. Prognosis depends upon the prognosis of the underlying disease/trauma.

ETIOLOGY/INCIDENCE

1. Exudates result from alterations in local factors that determine formation and absorption of pleural fluid.
    A. Typical mechanisms include pleural disease in combination with:
        1) Increased permeability of capillaries
            a. Bacterial pneumonia causes 300,000 U.S. cases per year.
            b. Viral infections cause 100,000 U.S. cases per year.
        2) Decreased lymphatic drainage
            a. Blockage by malignancy causes approximately 300,000 U.S. cases per year.
            b. Blockage by TB is the most common cause in many countries, although less common in the United States.
    B. Pathogenesis/additional categories
        1) Postoperative
        2) Iatrogenic
        3) Immunologic
        4) Inflammatory
    C. Pathogenesis/additional types
        1) Pulmonary embolism
            a. Causes 75,000 U.S. cases per year
            b. The most commonly missed underlying cause of pleural effusions
            c. Can be an exudate or a transudate, and nothing characterizes its pleural fluid
            d. More likely to cause exudate than transudate
            e. More likely to be identified by lung scan and/or pulmonary arteriography
        2) Other infections
            a. Empyema
            b. Fungi

       c. Rickettsia
       d. Parasites
     3) GI disease
       a. Postsurgical
       b. Pancreatic disease
     4) Collagen-vascular/connective tissue disease
     5) Following cardiac injury/Dressler's syndrome
     6) Drug induced
     7) Hemothorax
     8) Chylothorax
     9) Electrical burns
     10) Uremia
     11) Asbestos exposure
     12) Iatrogenic injury
     13) Radiation therapy

2. Transudates result from alterations in systemic factors which determine formation and absorption of pleural fluid.

  A. Typical mechanisms include:
     1) Increased hydrostatic pressure
       a. CHF and left ventricular failure cause approximately 500,000 U.S. cases per year.
     2) Decreased oncotic pressure
       a. Hypoalbuminemia and nephrotic syndrome
     3) Greater negative intrapleural pressure
       a. Acute atelectasis
  B. Pathogenesis/additional types
     1) Pulmonary embolism
       a. Less likely to cause transudate than exudate
     2) Cirrhosis
       a. Causes approximately 50,000 U.S. cases per year
     3) Pericardial disease/constrictive pericarditis
     4) Peritoneal dialysis
     5) Superior vena cava obstruction

3. Classification as transudate or exudate helps in differential diagnosis:

  A. Pleural fluid analysis from thoracentesis is the definitive test for pleural effusions.
  B. Exudates are pleural fluid with one or more of:
     1) Ratio >0.5 for pleural fluid protein divided by serum protein
     2) Ratio >0.6 for pleural fluid LDH divided by serum LDH
     3) Pleural fluid LDH above two thirds the upper normal limit for serum LDH (>200 IU)
  C. Transudates are pleural fluid without these characteristics.
  D. *Note:* CHF patients on diuretics may have unreliable pleural fluid values, as protein is removed from pleural space more slowly during diuresis.

4. Other pleural effusion types

  A. Empyema
     1) Often associated with exudative pneumonia, this direct infection of the pleural space causes pleural fluid to:
       a. Have turbid or purulent appearance from pus
       b. Be gram-positive

B. Fluid entry from sources outside the pleura
   1) Hemothorax or hemorrhagic pleural effusion
      a. Caused by trauma, CA, pulmonary embolism, or TB
      b. Grossly bloody pleural fluid results
   2) Chylous or chyliform effusion
      a. Caused by thoracic duct rupture
      b. Milky appearance pleural fluid results
   3) Effusion from IV fluids
      a. Misplaced central line
5. Prognosis depends upon prognosis of the underlying disease/trauma.
   A. Approximately 20% mortality with exudates.
   B. Worse prospects for the elderly and/or those with serious underlying disease/trauma.
   C. Prognosis is poor for CA-related pleural effusions.

SIGNS AND SYMPTOMS

1. Often asymptomatic if small effusion (<200–300 mL)
2. SOB and tachypnea
3. Pleuritic chest pain
4. Dry cough
5. Symptoms related to associated illnesses/underlying causes
   A. Fever
   B. Chills
   C. Night sweats
   D. Hemoptysis
   E. Weight loss

PHYSICAL FINDINGS

1. Small effusions (<200–300 mL) are usually undetectable.
2. Splinting with a pleural friction rub is associated with pleurisy/pleuritis.
3. Larger pleural effusions demonstrate decreased breath sounds, dullness to percussion, and decreased tactile fremitus over the effusion itself.
4. Bronchial breath sounds with egophony are associated with atelectasis.
5. A large effusion that compresses the lung may have egophony and breath sounds accentuation just above the effusion.
6. A very large effusion (one with high intrapleural pressure) may have intercostal space bulging and contralateral tracheal shift.

DIFFERENTIAL DIAGNOSIS

1. Atelectasis.
2. Pneumonia: To review pneumonia, see "Pneumonia."
3. Pneumothorax: To review pneumothorax, refer to the references listed following this section.
4. MI.

DIAGNOSTIC TESTS/FINDINGS

1. CXR
   A. Upright PA view

        1) Blunted costophrenic angle, with possible meniscus sign (faint, if early and small effusion)

        2) Misses smaller effusions (<250 mL).

  B. Lateral decubitus view

        1) Can detect smaller effusions (even <50 mL).

        2) Fluid layers out along dependent part of chest wall.

        3) A pleural effusion that is loculated will not change position.

  C. Moderate effusion

        1) Lung field has ground glass appearance.

        2) Absence of air bronchograms.

  D. Pseudotumor/phantom tumor: Fissure containing pleural fluid

2. Ultrasound: Helpful to localize site for thoracentesis with loculated pleural effusions

3. CT scan: Rarely used, but loculated effusions can be found and aspirated using ultrasound guidance

4. Pleural fluid analysis from thoracentesis

  A. Definitive test for pleural effusions.

  B. Classification as transudate or exudate helps in differential diagnosis.

  C. Exudates are pleural fluid with one or more of:

        1) Ratio >0.5 for pleural fluid protein divided by serum protein

        2) Ratio >0.6 for pleural fluid LDH divided by serum LDH

        3) Pleural fluid LDH above two thirds the upper normal limit for serum LDH (>200 IU)

  D. Transudates are pleural fluid without these characteristics.

  E. Exception: CHF patients on diuretics may have unreliable pleural fluid values, as protein is removed from pleural space more slowly during diuresis.

  F. These pleural fluid tests may be helpful, especially if exudate is found.

        1) Description/general appearance

          a. Pus from empyema

          b. Milky appearance from chylothorax

          c. Clear yellow liquid from transudates and some exudates

        2) Protein: Protein leakage into intrapleural space from inflammation

        3) LDH

        4) Glucose

          a. Low (<60) from empyema or rheumatoid arthritis/pleuritis

          b. Low from TB or parapneumonic effusions

        5) pH

          a. Low (<7.1) in empyema

          b. Low in CA, CT disease, TB, or esophageal rupture

        6) Culture and sensitivity, and Gram's stain/acid-fast stain

          a. Distinguish bacterial, mycobacterial, AFB, and fungal sources.

        7) Cytology

          a. Check for tumor cells.

        8) CBC with differential

  G. See Table 2–6 for a summary of characteristics of important exudative pleural effusions.

  H. For thoracentesis, the ACNP consults with physician and makes referral as needed. The ACNP may assist with procedure and must be knowledgeable. Depending upon the setting, the ACNP may be called upon to perform the procedure based upon NP protocols and clinical competencies.

TABLE 2–6. Characteristics of Important Exudative Pleural Effusions*

Etiology or Type of Effusion	Gross Appearance	White Blood Cell Count (cells/L)	Differential	Red Blood Cell Count (cells/L)	Glucose	Comments
Malignant effusion	Turbid to bloody; occasionally serous	1000–<100,000	M	100 to several hundred thousand	Equal to serum levels; <60 mg/dL in 15% of cases	Eosinophilia uncommon; positive results on cytologic examination
Uncomplicated parapneumonic effusion	Clear to turbid	5000–25,000	P	<5000	Equal to serum levels	Tube thoracostomy unnecessary
Empyema	Turbid to purulent	25,000–100,000	P	<5000	Less than serum levels; often very low	Drainage necessary; putrid odor suggests anaerobic infection
Tuberculosis	Serous to serosanguineous	5000–10,000	M	<10,000	Equal to serum levels; occasionally <60 mg/dL	Protein may exceed 5 g/dL; eosinophils (>10%) or mesothelial cells (<5%) make diagnosis unlikely
Rheumatoid effusion	Turbid; greenish yellow	1000–20,000	M or P	<1000	<40 mg/dL	Secondary empyema common; high LDH, low complement, high rheumatoid factor, cholesterol crystals are characteristic
Pulmonary infarction	Serous to grossly bloody	1000–50,000	M or P	100–>100,000	Equal to serum levels	Variable findings; no pathognomonic features
Esophageal rupture	Turbid to purulent; red-brown	<5000–>50,000	P	1000–10,000	Usually low	High amylase level (salivary origin); pneumothorax in 25% of cases; effusion usually on left side; pH <6.0 strongly suggests diagnosis
Pancreatitis	Turbid to serosanguineous	100–50,000	P	1000–10,000	Equal to serum levels	Usually left-sided; high amylase level

* From Stauffer, J. (1997). Lung. In L. Tierney, S. McPhee, & M. Papadakis (eds). *Current Medical Diagnosis and Treatment*, (36th ed.). Stamford, CT: Appleton & Lange, pp. 317–318, with permission.

M, mononuclear cell predominance; P, polymorphonuclear leukocyte predominance.

> 1) To review effective technique for successful thoracentesis, refer to the references listed following this section.

5. Less helpful: CBC (to check for leukocytosis and/or anemia)

MANAGEMENT/TREATMENT

Therapeutic

1. Primary goal is treatment of the underlying disease process or trauma.
2. Depending upon the size of the pleural effusion and the patient's underlying condition, medical management may be accomplished at clinic, ER, or inpatient settings. *Physician referral is advised at the time treatment is begun for pleural effusion patients, while follow-up may be managed through collaboration by ACNP and physician.*
3. Admission to an acute care unit may be indicated on occasion, but is typically decided on a case-by-case basis. Depending upon the patient's condition and the setting, the ACNP may be called upon to arrange such hospital admission for the patient with pleural effusion. While criteria vary on a case-by-case basis, suggested considerations for hospital admit may include:
   A. Large-sized pleural effusion
   B. Chronic effusion, warranting investigation of underlying cause(s)
   C. Complicating illnesses or comorbid conditions
4. Patients with severe SOB and who appear unstable may need therapeutic thoracentesis, plus treatment of the underlying cause.
   A. Remove ≤1.5 L of pleural fluid per single thoracentesis to reduce risk of re-expansion pulmonary edema.
   B. For thoracentesis, the ACNP consults with physician and makes referral as needed. The ACNP may assist with procedure and must be knowledgeable. Depending upon the setting, the ACNP may be called upon to perform the procedure based upon NP protocols and clinical competencies.
5. May need drainage by chest tubes or tube thoracostomy (e.g., for empyema).
   A. When chest tube insertion or tube thoracostomy is indicated, the ACNP consults with physician. Depending upon the setting, the ACNP may be called upon to make referral to physician specialist as needed to perform this procedure.
      1) To review effective technique for successful chest tube insertion, refer to the references listed following this section.
6. Pleurodesis performed by physician specialist may benefit recurrent, symptomatic pleural effusions in which treatment of underlying disease process is ineffective or inadequate (e.g., for CA). Depending upon the setting, the ACNP may be called upon to make referral to physician specialist as needed to perform this procedure.
7. In addition to treating the underlying disease/trauma, specific treatment may be necessary, such as:
   A. Transudates (especially from CHF) may not need to be drained unless massive effusion causes SOB.
   B. CA-related effusions may need chemotherapy, radiation therapy, chemical pleurodesis, or possibly surgical resection.
   C. Parapneumonic effusions of bacterial origin respond well to antibiotics

and require early intervention for successful treatment. Low pH parapneumonic effusions require chest tube insertion.
  D. Empyema requires antibiotics, chest tube insertion, and possible decortication.
  E. Chylothorax may need radiation therapy (if from CA), or surgical ligation of thoracic duct (if from trauma).
  F. Hemothorax nearly always requires chest tubes for drainage.

Patient Education

1. Educate patient as to need for periodic follow-up (perhaps q 3mo) for serial CXRs and possibly PFTs until patient is well.
2. Reiterate the importance of avoiding exposure to cigarette smoke. Quit-smoking tips and other useful community resources are offered through:
   A. American Lung Association
   B. American Thoracic Society (which is the medical section of the American Lung Association)
   C. American Cancer Society
   D. American Heart Association
   E. CDC
   F. NIH
3. Emphasize that appropriate follow-up is based upon the underlying disease/trauma.
4. Advise patient that prognosis depends upon prognosis of the underlying disease/trauma.

Review Questions

2.41 Describe the relationship between pleural effusion and pulmonary embolism.
   A. Pulmonary embolism is the most commonly missed underlying cause of pleural effusion.
   B. Pulmonary embolism causes 10,000 cases of pleural effusion per year.
   C. Pulmonary embolism is more likely to cause pleural effusion transudates than exudates.
   D. Pulmonary embolism is more likely to be identified as a cause of pleural effusion via initial CXR than by lung scan and/or pulmonary arteriography.

2.42 Describe pleural effusion exudates.
   A. Viral infections and bacterial pneumonia can cause pleural effusion exudates via decreased capillary permeability.
   B. Typical mechanisms of pleural effusion exudate formation include systemic disease with decreased capillary permeability and/or decreased lymphatic drainage.
   C. Pleural effusion exudates may result from alterations in local factors that determine formation and absorption of pleural fluid.
   D. Lymph blockage by malignancy causes 20,000 cases of pleural effusion exudates per year.

The following three-part case scenario is for pleural effusion Questions 2.43–2.45 listed below

Mrs. LR is a 54-year-old woman with a history of breast CA, brought to the ER via ambulance with complaints of progressive dyspnea, dry cough, and chest pain every time she coughs. She denies syncope, sweats, palpitations, fever, mucus, or trauma. Past medical history (PMH) and family history are negative for cardiovascular disease.

On exam you note that she has tachypnea, occasional dry cough, and pleuritic type chest pain—reproducible only when she coughs. Her stat 12-lead ECG and pulse oximetry are normal, and serum cardiac enzyme panel is unremarkable. As part of your differential diagnosis, pleural effusion is now being considered.

2.43 As the ACNP, you order CXRs for Mrs. LR to help diagnose her condition. Radiographic results reveal a moderate sized pleural effusion. While you are examining the films, her daughter (who is an RN) requests that you interpret the results to her. You describe that for pleural effusions (circle all that apply):
  A. The upright PA view shows a blunted costophrenic angle, which could be missed with a smaller effusion (<250 mL).
  B. The lateral decubitus view can detect smaller effusions (even <50 mL).
  C. The lateral decubitus view shows fluid layering out along the dependent part of the chest wall.
  D. The lung field has a ground glass appearance for moderate effusions.

2.44 In collaboration with your attending physician, you arrange for thoracentesis to be performed on Mrs. L.R. When you discuss informed consent with the patient and her daughter, they are interested to learn more about the purpose and anticipated results of this procedure. You explain that (circle all that apply):
  A. Pleural fluid analysis from thoracentesis permits classification as transudate or exudate, which helps in differential diagnosis.
  B. Transudates show ratio >0.5 for pleural fluid protein divided by serum protein.
  C. Transudates show ratio >0.6 for pleural fluid LDH divided by serum LDH.
  D. Exudates show pleural fluid LDH more than two thirds the upper normal limit for serum LDH (>200 IU).

2.45 Eventually, 850 mL of pleural fluid are removed during thoracentesis and Mrs. L.R. states, "I can breathe better now." Lab analysis confirms that this is an exudate. Considerations for your disposition of her case include (circle all that apply):
  A. Marked SOB from pleural effusion can be relieved by therapeutic thoracentesis alone.
  B. Remove <500 mL of pleural fluid per single thoracentesis to reduce the risk of hypotension.
  C. The primary goal with pleural effusion is treatment of the underlying disease process or trauma. CA can cause exudates. Given the patient's PMH of breast CA, this warrants further investigation.
  D. CA-related effusions may need chemotherapy, radiation therapy, chemical pleurodesis, or possible surgical resection.

Answers and Rationales

2.41   **A** Pulmonary embolism *is* the most commonly missed underlying cause of pleural effusion, therefore answer A is correct. The other answers are incorrect because: (B) Pulmonary embolism causes *75,000* cases of pleural effusion per year—not 10,000 cases; (C) pulmonary embolism is more likely to cause pleural effusion *exudates* than transudates—not vice versa; and (D) pulmonary embolism is more likely to be identified as a cause of pleural effusion by lung scan and/or pulmonary arteriography—not via initial CXR.

2.42   **C** Pleural effusion exudates result from alterations in *local* factors that determine formation and absorption of pleural fluid, therefore answer C is correct. The other answers are incorrect because: (A) viral infections and bacterial pneumonia can cause pleural effusion/ exudates via *increased* capillary permeability—not decreased; (B) typical mechanisms of pleural effusion/exudate formation include *pleural* disease (not systemic disease) with *increased* capillary permeability (not decreased permeability) and/or decreased lymphatic drainage; and (D) lymph blockage by malignancy causes *300,000* cases of pleural effusion exudates per year—not 20,000.

2.43 **All** All four answers are correct. The CXR considerations for pleural effusions include: (A) the upright PA view shows a blunted costophrenic angle, which could be missed with a smaller effusion (<250 mL); (B) the lateral decubitus view can detect smaller effusions (even <50 mL); (C) the lateral decubitus view shows fluid layering out along the dependent part of the chest wall; and (D) the lung field has a ground glass appearance for moderate effusions.

2.44 **A, D** Both answers A and D are correct, as pleural fluid analysis from thoracentesis permits *classification* as transudate or exudate, which *helps* in *differential diagnosis*. Also, *exudates do* show pleural fluid LDH greater than two thirds the upper normal limit for serum LDH (>200 IU). The other answers are incorrect because: (B) *Exudates* (not transudates) show ratio >0.5 for pleural fluid protein divided by serum protein; and (C) *Exudates* (not transudates) show ratio >0.6 for pleural fluid LDH divided by serum LDH.

2.45 **C, D** Both answers C and D are correct, as CA-related effusions may need chemotherapy, radiation therapy, chemical pleurodesis, or possible surgical resection. Also, the primary goal with pleural effusion is treatment of the underlying disease process or trauma; CA can cause exudates; therefore, given the patient's PMH of breast CA, this warrants further investigation. The other answers are incorrect because: (A) marked SOB from pleural effusion can be relieved by therapeutic thoracentesis, *plus treatment of the underlying cause*; and (B) Remove <1.5 L (not only 500 mL) of pleural fluid per single thoracentesis to reduce the risk of re-expansion pulmonary edema (not hypotension).

References

Kuribayashi, L. (1996). Pleural effusions. In R.E. Rakel (ed.). *Saunders Manual of Medical Practice*. Philadelphia: W.B. Saunders Co., pp. 164–165.

Light, R.W. (1995). Diseases of the pleura. In R.B. George, R.W. Light, M.A. Mathay, & R.A. Mathay (eds.). *Chest Medicine: Essentials of Pulmonary and Critical Care Medicine* (3rd ed.). Baltimore, MD: Williams & Wilkins, pp. 501–518.

Light, R.W. (1994). Disorders of the pleura. In K.J. Isselbacher, E. Braunwald, J.D. Wilson, et al. (eds.). *Harrison's Principles of Internal Medicine: Vol. 2* (13th ed.). New York: McGraw-Hill, pp. 1229–1232.

Pleural Effusion. (1992). In C.S. Rivers, D.E. Weber, M.K. Schuda, & E.R. Vaughn (eds.). *Preparing for the Written Board Exam in Emergency Medicine.* Milford, OH: Emergency Medicine Educational Enterprises, Inc., pp. 188–190.

Stauffer, J.L. (1997). Pleural effusion. In L.M. Tierney, Jr., S.J. McPhee, & M.A. Papadakis (eds.). *Current Medical Diagnosis and Treatment, 1997* (36th ed.). Stamford, CT: Appleton & Lange, pp. 313–317.

Additional Recommended References

Barry, K.C. (1996). Procedure: Chest tube insertion. In R.E. Rakel (ed.). *Saunders Manual of Medical Practice.* Philadelphia: W.B. Saunders Co., pp. 162–163.

Benditt, J. (1996). Pneumothorax. In R.E. Rakel (ed.). *Saunders Manual of Medical Practice.* Philadelphia: W.B. Saunders Co., pp. 160–161.

Grogan, D.R., & R.S. Irwin. (1996). Thoracentesis. In J.M. Rippe, R.S. Irwin, M.P. Fink, & F.B. Cerra (eds.). *Intensive Care Medicine: Vol. I* (3rd ed.). Boston: Little, Brown & Co., pp. 156–164.

Hadeed, S. (1994). Pleural effusion. In H.W. Griffith, M.R. Dambro, & J. Griffith (eds.). *The Five Minute Clinical Consult, 1994.* Philadelphia: Lea & Febiger, pp. 766–767.

Johnson, R.L. (1996). Procedure: Thoracentesis. In R.E. Rakel (ed.). *Saunders Manual of Medical Practice.* Philadelphia: W.B. Saunders Co., pp. 166–167.

Artificial Airway Management

AIRWAY MANAGEMENT

Overview

1. Proper airway management in the emergency department, acute care and critical care settings is essential to provide optimal ventilation and oxygenation to acutely ill patients.
2. A variety of airway adjuncts are available to improve ventilation and provide supplemental O_2 delivery. These should be used initially in an attempt to oxygenate without intubating the patient.
3. Prolonged airway management, however, will usually require ETT placement. Endotracheal (ET) intubation should be done *only* by those medical providers who are properly trained in the procedure and who are familiar with the pharmacologic agents (such as IV anesthetics and muscle relaxants) that may be needed. Given the frequency with which patients are intubated in the emergency and critical care settings, medical providers working in this environment should obtain specialized training to become skilled in airway management, ET intubation, and management of intubated patients.
4. For intubation, the ACNP promptly consults with physician and makes referral as needed. The ACNP may assist with procedure and must be knowl-

edgeable. Depending upon the setting, the ACNP may be called upon to perform intubation, based upon NP protocols and clinical competencies.

5. *This brief review is no substitute for specialized training or procedural skill.* Due to space limitations, the reader is referred to the several excellent references which follow this section for more in-depth coverage of airway management, ET intubation, and mechanical ventilation of intubated patients.

ENDOTRACHEAL INTUBATION

Indications for Intubation

1. Provides patent airway for patients with or at risk of airway obstruction:
   A. Trauma
   B. Laryngeal edema
   C. Massive burns (especially smoke inhalation)
2. Facilitates mechanical ventilation in patients with ARF:
   A. Hypoxemia with intrapulmonary blood shunting, such that external adjuncts cannot provide adequate FIO_2
   B. Progressive alveolar hypoventilation, leading to respiratory acidosis
   C. Barely adequate gas exchange with high work of breathing
3. Protects bronchial tree from aspiration of GI contents when airway reflexes are impaired (e.g., obtunded patient)
4. Promotes easier route for tracheal suctioning of copious, thick mucus secretions (e.g., COPD exacerbation, pneumonia)
5. Provides mechanical ventilation for patients who require:
   A. General anesthetic during surgery
   B. Heavy sedation for diagnostic and/or therapeutic interventions
   C. Prophylactic ventilatory support following cardiac, thoracic, or GI surgery

CONTRAINDICATIONS TO INTUBATION

1. Lack of specialized training and procedural skill of the medical provider.
2. Airway can be managed appropriately without ET intubation.

PREPARATION

1. Special considerations are needed for patients with:
   A. Full stomach/aspiration risk
   B. History of prior difficult intubations
   C. Limited cervical mobility
   D. Anatomical abnormalities of head and/or neck
2. Warnings
   A. Extensive head and neck trauma may render conventional orotracheal ET intubation potentially dangerous, such as with:
      1) Cervical spine instability
      2) Injuries of oropharynx, larynx, and/or face
   B. Such trauma requires a very skillful ET intubation, ideally with a fiberoptic scope.
3. Prepare airway
   A. Clear away foreign material (remove dentures or bridges, and suction secretions).

B. Preoxygenate with FIO_2 100% by mask for 5–6 minutes (less, if time does not permit).

C. While preparing for ET intubation, if patient is not breathing spontaneously, go to basic cardiac life support/advanced cardiac life support (BCLS/ACLS) protocol:
   1) Appropriately place patient in supine position (using C/spine precautions, when indicated).
   2) Position patient's head properly (chin lift, with head tilt or jaw thrust, as indicated).
   3) Insert oropharyngeal or nasopharyngeal airway, if needed.
   4) Manually ventilate with Ambu bag-valve mask device.
   5) Cricoid pressure should be applied by an assistant (to reduce risks of GI regurgitation and aspiration to better visualize larynx for easier intubation).

4. Assemble equipment and ensure its readiness.
   A. Arrange for suction source and appropriate suction tips.
   B. Assemble appropriately sized laryngoscope blades.
      1) Miller/straight blade
      2) MacIntosh/curved blade
   C. Provide appropriately sized ETTs.
      1) Sizes 6–9 mm inside diameter fit adults. Men usually take 8–9 mm. Women usually take 7–8 mm. Also useful to have 6–7 mm ETTs available, in case needed.
   D. Inflate, then deflate ETT balloon cuff to confirm patency.
   E. Ensure that laryngoscope assembles correctly and that its light source is working. (Helpful to have backup laryngoscope light bulb as well.)

5. Start IV line with 18 gauge catheter to infuse normal saline or lactated Ringer's solutions. Start a separate IV line to administer medications.

6. Prepare and label all drugs that are likely to be needed.

7. Monitor patient, if at all possible, using cardiac monitor, pulse oximetry, and BP measurement via automatic cuff or arterial line.

8. Have crash cart and personnel ready that are BCLS/ACLS prepared.

EQUIPMENT SELECTION

1. Oropharyngeal and nasopharyngeal airways in range of sizes.
2. Oxygen source and backup.
3. Ambu bag–valve-mask ventilation device, with oxygen attachment port and various sizes of masks.
4. Suction source; rigid/tonsil tip (Yankauer) suction tip; and soft tracheal suction catheters.
5. Laryngoscope with both straight (Miller) and curved (MacIntosh) blades in a variety of sizes; extra laryngoscope light bulbs.
6. Water-soluble, viscous Xylocaine (2%) to lubricate ETT and its stylet.
7. Two 10-mL syringes to inflate ETT balloon cuff.
8. Forceps (i.e., Magill type) to direct ETT tip, or to remove foreign bodies or other obstructing matter.
9. Tape and skin adhesive solution (i.e., Mastisol or equivalent) to secure the ETT and prevent its dislodgement. Also have available cloth twill tape (umbilical tape), IV tubing, and/or Velcro straps as alternate means to tie down ETT in patients with beards or facial dressings.

PHARMACOLOGIC AGENTS

1. No drugs are needed to intubate an unconscious patient orotracheally. Promptly use laryngoscope with cricoid pressure, intubate, and ventilate.
2. Rapid-sequence/crash intubation is used to intubate conscious patients. This increasingly common technique can reduce the risk of GI regurgitation and aspiration when intubating orotracheally. The procedure is to simultaneously (in rapid sequence) give IV sedative hypnotic and short-acting, rapid-onset muscle relaxant, with or without a narcotic analgesic. Typical choices include:
    A. Thiopental 2–5 mg/kg IV.
        1) Patients with cardiovascular compromise may benefit from a smaller initial dose (25–50 mg IV, q1–2 min, prn).
    B. Etomidate 0.2–0.3 mg/kg IV is preferable to thiopental for patients with cardiovascular compromise.
        1) Etomidate causes less cardiovascular and respiratory depression than do barbiturate hypnotics.
        2) Given IV over 30–60 seconds. Onset of action: 1 minute. Duration of effect: 3–5 minutes.
    C. Succinylcholine 1.0–1.5 mg/kg IV.
    D. Additional agents are optional and may be given before those just listed.
        1) For analgesia: Fentanyl 25–50 μg IV (may repeat once after 1 minute, prn), or morphine sulfate
        2) For severe reactive airways disease, or for increased intracranial pressure (ICP): Lidocaine 1 mg/kg IV
        3) To reduce likelihood of fasciculations caused by succinylcholine: Pancuronium or vecuronium 1 mg IV
    E. Rapid-sequence/crash intubation requires excellent technical skills.
3. An alternative option is to intubate an awake patient by utilizing a drug trio of a topical anesthetic, an analgesic, and mild sedation. This useful approach permits the patient to remain awake, retain intact airway reflexes, and breathe spontaneously. Examples of drug choices include:
    A. Xylocaine (10%) oral spray can anesthetize the tongue and posterior pharynx effectively.
        1) In addition, further topicalization is required to anesthetize the larynx and subglottic region.
    B. Fentanyl and morphine sulfate are often used for analgesia.
    C. Sedation can be obtained with thiopental or a benzodiazepine (such as Versed/midazolam).
    D. Awake intubation requires excellent technical skills.
4. To review ABG interpretation and medical ventilation, refer to the references listed following this section.

PRECAUTIONS

1. Endotracheal intubation is a life-saving procedure that nonetheless can be risky in and of itself. Moreover, the pharmacologic agents used with ET intubation are both life-saving and potentially deadly (if used incorrectly or inappropriately).
2. To reiterate, endotracheal intubation should *only* be done by those medical providers who are properly trained in the procedure and who are familiar with the pharmacologic agents (such as skeletal muscle relaxants and IV

anesthetics) that may be needed. *This brief review is no substitute for special-ized training or procedural skill.*

3. Continuous observation and monitoring are needed for any patient receiving drugs used with intubation. Conscious sedation flow sheets may be appropri-ate to monitor and record a patient's reactions to these drugs. Such effects may have adverse neurologic, hemodynamic, and metabolic consequences.

4. Laryngoscopy and intubation may stimulate the autonomic nervous system to such a degree that adverse effects can result:
   A. Hemodynamic instability, further compromising patients with CVA, in-creased intracranial pressure (ICP), or cardiovascular (CV) disease.

5. Mechanical ventilation may in and of itself cause complications.
   A. Positive-pressure ventilation can lead to reduced venous return to the heart, producing decreased cardiac output and subsequent hypotension.
   B. Barotrauma may result, such as a consequence of a paralyzed patient being given a very large tidal volume. (This can be especially worrisome in asthmatics who must be intubated.)

6. Other
   A. Subcutaneous emphysema, pneumomediastinum, pneumothorax, or pleural effusion may be caused by intubation and/or mechanical ventila-tion.

TECHNIQUE

1. Depending upon how quickly a patient's condition deteriorates, give psycho-logical preparation by briefly informing conscious patient of need for ET intubation and what to expect. Limit teaching to simple, focused explana-tions:
   A. Need to intubate to help patient breathe better
   B. What to expect, immediately and once connected to ventilator
   C. Need to comply once intubation drugs wear off
   D. How to summon help.

2. The following are important aspects for the ACNP to be aware of to assist with the intubation process.
   A. Correctly positioning a patient's head and neck is an important aspect of successful technique. Place the patient in the "sniffing position" with the patient's neck flexed and head slightly extended. Place folded towels under the occiput to elevate it a few inches above the bed, thereby flexing the neck properly. When upward traction is pulled on the laryngoscope handle, the head will then be extended effectively. This correctly aligns the oral, pharyngeal, and laryngeal axes for easier ETT insertion.
   B. Apply cricoid cartilage pressure (Sellick maneuver) until ETT proper placement is verified. This occludes the esophagus (helping prevent GI regurgitation and aspiration) and helps bring the larynx into view (for easier intubation). Ideally an assistant can apply the cricoid cartilage pressure throughout the ETT placement.
   C. Placing the laryngoscope in your left hand, open the patient's mouth with your gloved right hand and insert the blade into the right side of the patient's mouth. Sweep the patient's tongue leftward as you advance the blade midline to the base of the tongue.
      1) If a curved/MacIntosh blade is used, insert its tip into the patient's valecula.

     2) If a straight/Miller laryngoscope blade is used, position its tip below the patient's epiglottis.

D. Lift the handle up and forward at a 45-degree angle to expose vocal cords. (Aim as though pulling away from you toward the junction of the ceiling with the wall.) Avoid putting pressure on the patient's lips and teeth. Don't use the teeth as a fulcrum and don't pinch the tongue between the blade and the patient's teeth. Keeping your left wrist stiff and lifting from the arm and shoulder eases the technique for you while helping prevent dental damage to the patient.

E. Insert the lubricated ETT through patient's right side of mouth using your right hand, and keep advancing the tip through the vocal cords while directly visualizing them. A lubricated curved stylet inserted into the ETT can help direct the tip of the tube to the glottic opening. This is especially useful for larynxes located very anteriorly. Bend or coil the proximal end of the stylet to prevent the distal end from extending beyond the ETT and damaging tissue.

F. Remove the stylet once the proximal end of the ETT balloon cuff reaches the vocal cords (when the cuff just disappears from sight). Then advance the ETT 1–3 cm further into the trachea. Inflate the balloon cuff with just enough air to prevent leaks with positive-pressure ventilation (usually 20 mm Hg in a low-pressure cuff). Correctly placed, the ETT will usually rest near the 23-cm mark at front incisors in average-sized men, and near the 21-cm mark in average-sized women. This positions the ETT tip 3–4 cm above the carina, allowing adequate ventilation of both lungs.

G. Clinically check for correct ETT placement. Observe for equal bilateral chest expansion and auscultate for equal bilateral breath sounds during ventilation. Right main-stem bronchus intubation often occurs when the ETT has been advanced too far. (By contrast, left main-stem bronchus intubation seldom occurs.) This can be detected by auscultating decreased breath sounds on the left. (If not corrected, the nonventilated lung can collapse.) Auscultate the epigastrium for loud, gurgling sounds with ventilation. If heard, it means that the ETT is in the esophagus, not the trachea, and must immediately be removed and repositioned.

     1) Additional means may be used to help verify correct ETT placement, but are not considered as reliable by themselves.

       a. Rising pulse oximetry (due to rising arterial oxygen saturation).

       b. Rising capnography. This monitor of end-tidal CO_2 attaches to the proximal end of an ETT and registers a color change or infrared reading when exposed to CO_2.

H. The ETT is then taped to the skin over the patient's maxilla, as this part of the face does not move. For patients in whom taping would be inadequate (i.e., with facial dressings or beards), properly secure the ETT in position with cloth twill tape (umbilical tape), Velcro straps, or IV tubing. Loop these over the patient's ears once the straps are brought around the neck.

I. Promptly order CXR to confirm proper ETT tip placement at several cm above the carina (T2 level). (Recall that flexing or extending a patient's head can advance or withdraw the ETT a distance of 2–5 cm, respectively.)

FOLLOW-UP

1. Periodically check the balloon cuff pressure with a manometer. Low-pressure cuffs require pressure below 15–20 mm Hg (just above the point when an audible leak occurs). Pressures in excess of 20–30 mm Hg can lead to potentially grave complications (i.e., mucosal ischemia, pressure necrosis, tracheoesophageal fistula, tracheal stenosis).
2. Once intubated, a patient can no longer protect his or her airway and is completely dependent upon medical caregivers to provide:
   A. Patency of ETT and airway
   B. A means for the patient to call for help
   C. Vigilant infection control
   D. Effective cough/pulmonary toilet/suction of secretions
   E. Humidified inspired air
   F. Measures to prevent aspiration around ETT:
      1) Elevate HOB ≥30 degrees.
      2) Consider NG tube insertion.

Review Questions

2.46 Miss KD is a 19-year-old barbiturate overdose patient brought to the ER by her distraught family. Gastric lavage and activated charcoal are quickly prepared to begin treating her. Meanwhile, Miss KD's respiratory status is declining rapidly and she is becoming progressively more altered in her mental status. She begins retching with dry heaves. Preparations are made for her immediate intubation. These measures include all, EXCEPT:
   A. Prepare airway by clearing foreign material, then preoxygenating patient.
   B. Assemble equipment and ensure its readiness.
   C. Give psychological preparation to the patient and her family by describing in detail what to expect.
   D. Have crash cart and personnel ready that are BCLS/ACLS prepared.
2.47 Indications for ET intubation include all, EXCEPT:
   A. It provides patent airway for patients with airway obstruction risk.
   B. It is the only means to improve hypercarbia.
   C. It facilitates mechanical ventilation in patients with ARF.
   D. It protects bronchial tree from GI contents aspiration in obtunded patients.
2.48 Mrs. LR is a 54-year-old woman in acute COPD exacerbation, unresponsive to ER therapy. She is admitted to the acute care unit with increasing work of breathing and gradually decreasing sensorium. The decision is made to intubate her and place her on mechanical ventilation. Your collaborating physician asks you to help assist by giving informed consent explanations to the patient and her concerned daughter who is present. As you briefly describe the possible risks associated with this procedure, you recall that any of these are possible, EXCEPT:
   A. Pleural effusion, which may be due to intubation and/or ventilation
   B. Barotrauma, which may result from mechanical ventilation

C. Decreased venous return to the heart due to mechanical ventilation and PEEP, leading to increased cardiac output

D. Pneumothorax, which may be caused by intubation and/or mechanical ventilation

2.49 The curved laryngoscope blade (MacIntosh type) is used:

A. By insertion of its tip into the patient's valecula

B. By positioning its tip sufficiently below the patient's epiglottis

C. More easily by those who are left handed

D. Because the straight laryngoscope blade (Miller type) is harder to use

2.50 Mr. DW is a 28-year-old firefighter hospitalized for acute smoke inhalation and progressive dyspnea, unresponsive to aggressive therapy. He is diagnosed with early ARDS and the decision is made to intubate him. In your institution, qualified ACNPs may be called upon to intubate, in collaboration with their attending physicians. Upon initially attempting to intubate Mr. DW, you are unable to visualize his vocal cords. You decide to use these means to facilitate his successful intubation (circle all that apply):

A. Reposition patient's head to ensure the neck is extended and the head is slightly flexed.

B. Lift the laryngoscope handle up and forward at a 75-degree angle to expose vocal cords.

C. Assign an assistant to apply cricoid cartilage pressure (Sellick maneuver) until proper ETT placement is verified.

D. Reposition patient's head to ensure the neck is flexed and the head is slightly extended.

Answers and Rationales

2.46 **C** All of these are suitable preparations for immediate intubation EXCEPT answer C. Detailed explanations are inappropriate in an emergent situation with the patient's condition rapidly deteriorating. If time permits, limit teaching to simple, focused explanations.

2.47 **B** All of these are appropriate indications for ETT intubation EXCEPT answer B. While intubation and mechanical ventilation can improve hypercarbia more precisely and effectively than can other methods, they are not the only means to do so.

2.48 **C** All of these are possible risks associated with ET intubation EXCEPT answer C. One of the possible complications from mechanical ventilation and PEEP can be decreased venous return to the heart, leading to *decreased* cardiac output—*not* increased.

2.49 **A** The curved laryngoscope blade (MacIntosh type) is used by insertion of its tip into the patient's valecula. The straight laryngoscope blade (Miller type) is positioned with its tip below the patient's epiglottis. Either blade type may be used by right- or left-handed operators. It is up to operator preference and the requirements of an individual patient's anatomy as to which type is preferable in a given situation.

2.50 **C, D** Proper positioning of the patient's head and neck (into the "sniffing position") is important for successful intubation. This involves positioning the patient's head to ensure the *neck is flexed* and the *head* *is slightly extended—not* vice versa. Correct technique also involves lifting the laryngoscope handle up and forward at a 45-degree angle to expose vocal cords—*not* 75 degrees. Another useful technique is to have an assistant apply cricoid cartilage pressure (Sellick maneuver) throughout the procedure, until proper ETT placement is verified.

References

Anup, A.B. (1996). *Arterial Blood Gas Analysis Made Easy*. Valhalla, NY: Author, pp. 11–93.

Adjuncts for airway control, ventilation, and oxygenation. (1994). In R.O. Cummins (ed.). *Textbook of Advanced Cardiac Life Support*. Dallas: American Heart Association, pp. 1–17.

Danzl, D.F. (1996). Advanced airway support. In J.E. Tintinalli, R.L. Krome, & E. Ruiz (eds.). *Emergency Medicine: A Comprehensive Study Guide* (4th ed.). New York: McGraw-Hill, pp. 39–49.

Freeland, M.J. (1996). Procedure: Endotracheal intubation. In R.E. Rakel (ed.). *Saunders Manual of Medical Practice*. Philadelphia: W.B. Saunders Co., pp. 148–150.

Ingenito, E.P., & J.M. Drazen. (1994). Mechanical ventilatory support. In K.J. Isselbacher, E. Braunwald, J.D. Wilson, et al. (eds.). *Harrison's Principles of Internal Medicine, Vol. 2* (13th ed.). New York: McGraw-Hill, pp. 1244–1248.

Kaur, S., & Heard, S.O. (1996). Airway management and endotracheal intubation. In J.M. Rippe, R.S. Irwin, M.P. Fink, & F.B. Cerra (eds.). *Intensive Care Medicine, Vol. I.* (3rd ed.). Boston: Little, Brown & Co., pp. 1–15.

Matthay, M.A. (1995). General principles of managing the patient with respiratory insufficiency/treatment modalities. In R.B. George, R.W. Light, M.A. Matthay, & R.A. Matthay (eds.). *Chest Medicine: Essentials of Pulmonary and Critical Care Medicine* (3rd ed.). Baltimore, MD: Williams & Wilkins, pp. 568–574.

Papadakis, M.A. (1997). Acid-base disorders. In L.M. Tierney, Jr., S.J. McPhee, & M.A. Papadakis (eds.). *Current Medical Diagnosis and Treatment, 1997* (36th ed.). Stamford, CT: Appleton & Lange, pp. 815–825.

Weinberger, S.E., & J.M. Drazen. (1994). Disturbances of respiratory function. In K.J. Isselbacher, E. Braunwald, J.D. Wilson, et al. (eds.). *Harrison's Principles of Internal Medicine: Vol. 2* (13th ed.). New York: McGraw-Hill, pp. 1152–1159.

Wilson, R.F., & C. Barton. (1996). Blood gases: Pathophysiology and interpretation. In J.E. Tintinalli, R.L. Krome, & E. Ruiz (eds.). *Emergency Medicine: A Comprehensive Study Guide* (4th ed.). New York: McGraw-Hill, pp. 108–117.

Pneumothorax

DEFINITION

Pneumothorax, or air in the pleural space, can be classified as spontaneous (without trauma or obvious cause), traumatic (direct or indirect chest trauma), or iatrogenic.

ETIOLOGY/INCIDENCE

Because the pleural pressure is normally negative and lower than the alveolar pressure, if the visceral pleura is disrupted and a connection is established between the alveoli and the pleural space, air will accumulate in the pleural space. The incidence of primary pneumothorax is about 9 cases per 100,000 population per year.

TYPES OF PNEUMOTHORAX

1. Primary spontaneous pneumothorax occurs in individuals without any lung disease. Thought to occur from rupture of subpleural apical blebs in response to high negative pressures. Affects mainly tall, thin men between the ages of 20 and 40 years. Familial factors and cigarette smoking may also be important.
2. Secondary spontaneous pneumothorax occurs as a complication of pre-existing lung disease such as COPD, asthma, TB, or PCP.
3. Traumatic pneumothorax results from penetrating or nonpenetrating chest trauma.
4. Iatrogenic pneumothorax may follow procedures such as thoracentesis, pleural biopsy, subclavian line placement, or bronchoscopy

SIGNS AND SYMPTOMS

Chest pain on the affected side and dyspnea are the two prominent symptoms and usually occur during rest.

PHYSICAL FINDINGS

1. Physical examination may be unremarkable in patients with a small pneumothorax.
2. In larger pneumothoraxes, decreased chest movement may be seen.
3. Decreased fremitus.
4. Hyperresonance.
5. Diminished or absent breath sounds.
6. A marked tachycardia (>135 bpm), hypotension, and mediastinal or tracheal shift should alert the ACNP to the possibility of a tension pneumothorax. This usually occurs in the setting of penetrating trauma, lung infection, CPR, or positive-pressure mechanical ventilation. It is caused by air in the pleural space that exceeds ambient pressure throughout the respiratory cycle. A check-valve mechanism allows air to enter the pleural space on inspiration and prevents egress of air on expiration.

DIFFERENTIAL DIAGNOSIS

1. Bullous lesion
2. Myocardial infarction
3. Pulmonary embolism
4. Pneumonia

DIAGNOSTIC TESTS/FINDINGS

1. The diagnosis of pneumothorax is generally confirmed on CXR by the finding of a radiolucent area at the periphery without lung markings that is separated from the partially collapsed lung by a radiopaque pleural stripe.
2. In tension pneumothorax, CXR shows a large amount of air in the affected hemithorax and a contralateral shift of mediastinal structures.
3. Arterial blood-gas analysis reveals hypoxemia.

MANAGEMENT/TREATMENT

1. Treatment depends upon the severity of the pneumothorax and the nature of the underlying disease.
2. The patient with a new, small pneumothorax <15% should be hospitalized, placed on bed rest, and treated symptomatically for cough and chest pain. Obtain serial CXRs every 24 hours.
3. Patients with a small pneumothorax that has been stable in size for several days to weeks can be followed closely with serial CXRs on an outpatient basis. Many small pneumothoraxes resolve spontaneously.
4. Patients with larger pneumothoraxes >15% require chest tube placement. Chest tube is placed under water-sealed drainage and suction applied until the lung expands.
5. Options to prevent recurrence include intrapleural doxycycline or minocycline, insufflation of talc, laser therapy, and pleural ablation by thoracoscopy or thoracotomy.

Patient Education

1. Advise all patients who smoke to discontinue.
2. Warn patients that the risk of recurrence in spontaneous pneumothorax is 50%.
3. Avoid exposure to high altitudes, flying in unpressurized aircraft, and scuba diving.

Review Questions

2.51 Which of the following are the most common symptoms associated with a pneumothorax?
   A. Chest pain with ST-segment elevation
   B. Dyspnea and chest pain on the affected side
   C. Dyspnea and chest pain on the unaffected side due to afferent nerve pathways
   D. Chest pain with ST-segment depression
2.52 The difference between a spontaneous and tension pneumothorax is:
   A. A spontaneous pneumothorax has a known etiology.
   B. A tension pneumothorax is caused by air in the pleural space that exceeds ambient pressure throughout the respiratory cycle.
   C. A tension pneumothorax is usually caused by rupture of subpleural apical blebs, which occurs in response to high negative intrapleural pressure.
   D. A tension pneumothorax mainly occurs in tall, thin men between the ages of 20 and 40 years.
2.53 Characteristics of patients at risk for a spontaneous pneumothorax include:
   A. Female, thin, tall, cigarette smoking
   B. Female, obese, short, cigarette smoking
   C. Male, obese, short, cigarette smoking
   D. Male, thin, tall, cigarette smoking

2.54 A 52-year-old male who is in cardiogenic shock and ARDS is on mechanical ventilation 100% FIO_2 and PEEP of 10 cm. The RN at the bedside pages you stat because the SaO_2 has decreased from 94% to 70%. The patient is tachycardiac and hypotensive. Which of the following is the most likely possibility?

A. Bacterial endocarditis
B. Severe bronchospasm
C. Ventricular septal defect
D. Tension pneumothorax

2.55 The immediate treatment for this patient is:

A. IABP
B. Inotropic therapy to maintain BP
C. Rapid infusion of IV fluids
D. Immediate chest tube placement

Answers and Rationales

2.51 **B** Dyspnea and chest pain on the affected side.

2.52 **B** In a tension pneumothorax, air in the pleural space exceeds ambient pressure throughout the respiratory cycle. A mediastinal or tracheal shift can occur.

2.53 **D** Males who are thin, tall, and smoke cigarettes have a higher incidence of spontaneous pneumothorax.

2.54 **D** A patient on mechanical ventilation with PEEP is at increased risk for a pneumothorax. The rapid and dramatic decrease in SaO_2, and tachycardia and hypotension are clinical signs of a possible tension pneumothorax.

2.55 **D** Chest tube insertion is the immediate treatment for tension pneumothorax.

References

Feinsilver, S. (1997). Respiratory System. In R. Conn, W. Borer, & J. Snyder (eds.). *Current Diagnosis 9*. Philadelphia: W.B. Saunders Co., p. 337.

Sahn, S. (1997). Diseases of the pleura. In R. Bone (ed.). *Current Practice of Medicine, Vol. 1*. New York: Churchill Livingstone, pp. 8.2–8.3.

Stauffer, J. (1997). Lung: Pleural effusion. In L. Tierney, S. McPhee, & M. Papadakis (eds.). *Current Medical Diagnosis and Treatment* (36th ed.). Stamford, CT: Appleton & Lange, pp. 317–318.

CHAPTER 3

Cardiovascular Disorders

Anna Gawlinski, RN, DNSc, CS-ACNP, CCRN
Kathy McCloy, RN, MSN, CS-ACNP
Debbie Caswell, RN, MN, ANP-C, CCRN
William J. Quiñones-Baldrich, MD

Hypertension

DEFINITION

Systolic blood pressure (SBP) ≥140 mm Hg ± diastolic blood pressure (DBP) ≥90 mm Hg based on the average of two or more readings taken at each of two or more visits after the initial screen.

Ranges for classification of hypertension (HTN) are as follows:

Category	Systolic (mm Hg)	Diastolic (mm Hg)
Stage 1 (mild)	140–159	90–99
Stage 2 (moderate)	160–170	100–109
Stage 3 (severe)	180–209	110–119
Stage 4 (very severe)	>210	>120

From JNC, 1993.

ETIOLOGY/INCIDENCE

1. United States has 35 million people with HTN and 25 million borderline HTN.
2. Age: Incidence rises with age; systolic blood pressure rises with age and it also correlates with cardiovascular problems more than diastolic.
3. Sex: Males in all age groups have higher incidence.
4. Race: More common and more severe in blacks.
5. Positive family history.
6. Obesity.
7. Increased salt intake.

PATHOPHYSIOLOGY

Systemic arterial pressure is primarily determined by cardiac output and peripheral vascular resistance, which are regulated by the following mechanisms:

1. Autonomic nervous system (Baroreceptor Reflex): Baroreceptors located in the carotid sinus, aorta, and left ventricular (LV) wall sense changes in blood pressure (BP).

    If BP is too high, increased stretch of baroreceptors occurs, which stimulates vagal cholinergic neurons to decrease heart rate and vascular tone, resulting in a lowering of blood pressure.

    If BP is too low, decrease stretch of baroreceptors occurs, which results in stimulation of sympathetic adrenergic neurons, resulting in an increase in heart rate, contractility, and vasoconstriction which leads to an increase in blood pressure.

2. Intravascular fluid volume: If fluid volume is decreased, venous return decreases, which results in a reduction in cardiac output and renal blood flow. Aldosterone stimulation occurs with retention of sodium and water in the renal tubules, thus, increasing blood pressure.

    If fluid volume and blood pressure are increased, venous return is increased. This results in increased cardiac output and renal blood flow, which causes an increased glomerular filtration rate (GFR) and diuresis, which tends to normalize BP.

3. Renin-angiotensin system: When blood pressure is low there is decreased blood flow and perfusion pressure to the kidneys. This results in renin production in the juxtaglomerular cells of the kidneys. Increased renin production causes the plasma globulin substrate, angiotensin I, to be converted to angiotensin II by the angiotensin converting enzyme (ACE). Angiotensin II causes peripheral vascular vasoconstriction and increased blood pressure. When angiotensin II is present, a negative feedback system occurs to decrease renin production.

    If blood pressure is high, there is increased blood flow and perfusion pressure to the kidneys. Renin production by the juxtaglomerular cells of the kidneys is decreased. Decreased renin causes vasodilation and decreased blood pressure.

4. Vascular autoregulation: Every organ regulates flow to protect itself from increases in blood pressure. Normal vasodilatation can be impaired by interaction between endothelial mediators such as prostacyclins, nitric oxide, endothelium-derived relaxing factor, prostaglandin, thromboxane, superoxide anion, serotonin, adenosine diphosphate, endothelium-derived relaxing factors, and endothelium-derived contracting factors.

SIGNS AND SYMPTOMS

Hypertension is a silent disease, but has deleterious effects on several organs; therefore, a thorough history is important and should include all organ systems.
    The medical history should include the following:

1. Family history of high blood pressure, premature coronary artery disease (CAD), stroke, cardiovascular disease (CVD), diabetes mellitus, and dyslipidemia

2. Patient history or symptoms of cardiovascular, cerebrovascular, or renal disease; diabetes mellitus, dyslipidemia; or gout

3. Known duration and levels of elevated blood pressure

4. History of weight gain, leisure time physical activities, and smoking or other tobacco use

5. Dietary assessment, including sodium intake, alcohol use, and intake of cholesterol and saturated fats

6. Results and side effects of previous antihypertensive therapy
7. Symptoms suggesting secondary hypertension
8. Psychosocial and environmental factors (e.g., family situation, employment status and working conditions, educational level) that may influence blood pressure control

PHYSICAL FINDINGS

Initial Physical Exam

The initial physical exam should include the following:
1. Blood pressure measurement:
    A. Two or more blood pressure measurements separated by 2 minutes with the patient either supine or standing for at least 2 minutes
    B. Verification in the contralateral arm (if values are different use the higher value)
2. Physical findings during the exam should inform the ACNP of the following:
    A. The extent of target organ disease (Table 3–1 lists the common organs affected by HTN and the manifestation of the disease)
    B. The presence of further risk factors for cardiovascular disease
    C. Causes of secondary hypertension
        Table 3–2 indicates the components of the physical exam and abnormal findings.

DIFFERENTIAL DIAGNOSIS

1. Essential HTN: Has no identifiable cause, accounts for over 90% of all cases. Onset is usually between ages 30 and 50, and there is a positive family history.
2. Secondary HTN: Has an identifiable etiology, occurs in a wide age range, is abrupt in onset and severe, with a negative family history.
    Screening techniques to differentiate between essential and secondary HTN are listed on Table 3–3.

T A B L E 3–1.   Manifestations of Target Organ Disease*

Organ System	Manifestations
Cardiac	Clinical, electrocardiographic, or radiologic evidence of coronary artery disease; left ventricular hypertrophy by echocardiography; left ventricular dysfunction or cardiac failure
Cerebrovascular	Transient ischemic attack or stroke; headache
Peripheral vascular	Absence of one or more major pulses in extremities (except for dorsalis pedis) with or without intermittent claudication; aneurysm
Renal	Serum creatinine >1.5 mg/dL; proteinuria ($\geq 1 +$); microalbuminuria
Retinopathy	Hemorrhages or exudates (white patches), with or without papilledema; vascular changes: Grade I, atherosclerotic changes with narrowing of the arteries; Grade II, AV nicking; Grade III, exudates; Grade IV, papilledema

---

* Adapted from Joint National Committee on Detection, Evaluation, and Treatment of Blood Pressure: The Fifth Report. National Heart, Lung & Blood Institute, U.S. Department of Health and Human Services, NIH Publication 93–1088, 1993, with permission.

TABLE 3–2. **Abnormal Findings on Physical Examination***

System	Finding
Vital signs	Widely variable BP readings in same arm
	Marked difference in BP readings in upper vs. lower extremities
	Tachycardia
	Bradycardia
Eyes	Arteriolar narrowing, arteriovenous nicking, hemorrhages, exudates, papilledema
Neck	Distended neck veins, carotid bruits or diminished pulsations, thyromegaly
Lungs	Crackles, wheezes
Heart	Increased size, precordial heave, clicks, murmurs, S_3 and S_4, arrhythmias
Abdomen	Abdominal aortic pulsations, aortic bruits, renal bruits, abdominal or flank masses, enlarged kidneys
Extremities	Delayed or absent femoral pulsations, diminished or absent peripheral pulses, bruits, peripheral edema
Neurologic	Focal neurologic signs, TIA, or stroke

* Adapted from Joint National Committee on Detection, Evaluation, and Treatment of Blood Pressure: The Fifth Report. National Heart, Lung & Blood Institute, U.S. Department of Health and Human Services, NIH Publication 93–1088, 1993, with permission.
BP, blood pressure; TIA, transient ischemic attack.

TABLE 3–3. **Differential Diagnosis of Secondary Hypertension***

Cause	Screening	Confirm
Coarctation	Arm and leg blood pressures, CXR	Angiography
Cushing's syndrome	Cushingoid appearance, 1 mg dexamethasone suppression test, plasma cortisol	High-dose dexamethasone suppression test
Drug induced	History of amphetamines, oral contraceptives, estrogens, corticosteroids, licorice, thyroid hormone	History Drug screening
Pheochromocytoma	History of paroxysmal HTN, headache, perspiration, palpitations or fixed diastolic >130 mm Hg, 24-hour urinary metanephrine VMA	Catecholamine levels, angiography, CT scan
Primary aldosteronism	Serum K, urine K, stimulated PRA	Aldosterone levels, venography with differential level, CT scan
Renal disease	History of congenital disease, DM, Proteinuria, Pyelonephritis, obstruction, UA, BUN, creatinine	Creatinine clearance, IVP, UTZ, biopsy
Renovascular disease	Suspect in young female or elderly patient with atherosclerosis, especially if abrupt in onset negative family history and abdominal bruit present	Digital subtraction of digital arterial angiography and differential renal vein renins, captopril test (renal perfusion)
Increased ICP	Neuro exam	Lumbar puncture, ICP

* Adapted from Joint National Committee on Detection, Evaluation, and Treatment of Blood Pressure: The Fifth Report. National Heart, Lung & Blood Institute, U.S. Department of Health and Human Services, NIH Publication 93–1088, 1993, with permission.
CXR, chest x-ray; HTN, hypertension; VMA, vanillylmandelic acid; CT, computed tomography; DM, diabetes mellitus; UA, urinalysis; BUN, blood, urea, nitrogen; IVP, intravenous pyelography; UTZ, ultrasound; ICP, intracranial pressure; PRA, plasma renin activity.

DIAGNOSTIC TESTS/FINDINGS

1. Complete blood count (CBC).
2. Urinalysis (UA) provides evidence of primary renal disease—proteinuria.
3. Serum BUN or creatinine—to evaluate extent of renal compromise.
4. Serum electrolytes (e.g., potassium [K]) is a screening test for primary aldosteronism (decreased K is found in hyperaldosteronism). Results should be known before initiating diuretic therapy.
5. Electrocardiogram (ECG)—provides baseline data regarding cardiovascular (CV) risk, ECG may show left ventricular hypertrophy (LVH), ischemic changes caused by HTN.
6. Chest x-ray (CXR)—evaluation for cardiomegaly CHF, rib notching seen with coarctation of aorta.
7. Fasting blood sugar (FBS)—CV risk.
8. Lipid profile—CV risk.

MANAGEMENT/TREATMENT

1. Nonpharmacologic: Lifestyle modifications are initial therapy in patients with mild to moderate HTN (DBP < 95) and simultaneous with drug therapy for severe HTN (stage 3 or 4). Lifestyle modifications lower blood pressure, improve lipid profile, and reduce overall cardiovascular risk.
   A. Alcohol—limit to <1 oz/day or ethanol (24 oz of beer, 8 oz of wine, or 2 oz of whiskey).
   B. Lose weight if overweight.
   C. Exercise (aerobic) 30–60 minutes five to seven times a week.
   D. Reduce sodium intake to <2 g.
   E. Stop smoking.
   F. Reduce cholesterol intake for overall health.
2. Pharmacologic: If patient has moderate HTN, or if no response to lifestyle changes after 2–3 months, pharmacologic interventions are implemented. Table 3–4 lists pharmacologic interventions for HTN treatment. The acute care nurse practitioner (ACNP) should choose a medication that is effective, affordable, treats coexisting disease when present, and has convenient dosing and favorable side effects. Recognize that it may take several months to achieve blood pressure–lowering goals.

Medication Selection for Selected Populations
(Kaplan, 1994)

Young Patient. ACE inhibitor, α-blocker, or β-blocker

Rationale. α-blocker or diuretic/captopril combination causes the least sexual dysfunction (*Arch Intern Med* 1988;148:788). ACE inhibitor does not impair exercise.

Blacks. Diuretic, calcium channel blockers (CCB), or α-blockers, ACE inhibitor (β-blockers are less effective as monotherapy)

Rationale. Blacks have increased prevalence, severity, morbidity and mortality from HTN compared to caucasians. There is a 1.3-fold increase in nonfatal stroke, a 1.8-fold increase in fatal stroke and, a 1.5-fold increase in cardiac deaths and a fivefold increase in end-stage renal disease (Gillum, 1991).

TABLE 3-4.   Pharmacologic Interventions for Hypertension*

Drug	Dosage Range (mg/day)	Adverse Effects	Reactions/Interactions
Thiazide Diuretics			
Chlorothiazide	125–500 mg	Polyuria, urinary frequency, hypokalemia, hyponatremia, hypomagnesemia, hypercalcemia, hyperuricemia, hyperglycemia, elevated serum lipids, weakness, fatigue, sexual dysfunction, photosensitivity, rash, blood dyscrasias, hepatitis, orthostatic hypotension	• Avoid use in severe renal failure, anuria; sulfonamide or thiazide sensitivity. Use cautiously in hepatic disease, diabetes mellitus, gout, lupus.
Hydrochlorothiazide	12.5–50 mg		• NSAIDs may antagonize diuretic effects.
Bendroflumethiazide	2.5–5.0 mg		• Cholestyramine and colestipol decrease absorption of thiazides.
Methylchlothiazide	2.5–5.0 mg		• Thiazides decrease effects of antidiabetics and cause increased lithium absorption; may predispose to lithium toxicity.
Trichlormethiazide	1.0–4.0 mg		
Chlorthalidone	12.5–50 mg		
Indapamide	2.5–5.0 mg		
Potassium-Sparing Diuretics			
Spironolactone	25–100 mg	Hyperkalemia, headache, rash, hyperpigmentation, drowsiness, ataxia, GI disturbances, gynecomastia (spironolactone), renal calculi (triamterene), orthostatic hypotension; give with food to minimize GI upset	• Avoid use in severe renal disease, anuria; hyperkalemia, hypersensitivity.
Triamterene	50–150 mg		• Increased lithium action (amiloride), digitalis (spironolactone).
Amiloride	5–10 mg		• Salicylates decrease diuretic effects.
			• ACE inhibitors, salt substitutes, potassium supplements ↑ risk of hyperkalemia.
β-Blockers			
Acebutolol	200–1200 mg	Bradycardia, CHF, insomnia, depression, sedation, fatigue, impotence, GI disturbances, claudication, bronchospasm, altered lipid profile, masks symptoms of hypoglycemia, reduced exercise tolerance	• Avoid use with CHF, heart block, COPD, peripheral vascular disease, diabetes mellitus, renal or hepatic impairment.
Atenolol	25–100 mg		• Antagonized by sympathomimetics.
Metoprolol	50–200 mg		• NSAIDs decrease effects of β-blockers.
Nadolol	20–240 mg		• Rifampin, phenobarbital, and nicotine can decrease serum levels of some agents.
Propanolol	40–240 mg		• Some agents: Increased β-blockade with use of cimetidine.
Propanolol (extended release)	80–240 mg		• Use cautiously with cardiodepressants.
Pindolol	10–60 mg		
Timolol	20–40 mg		

Table continues

TABLE 3–4. (Continued)

Drug	Dosage Range (mg/day)	Adverse Effects	Reactions/Interactions
α₁-Adrenergic Blockers			
Prazosin	1–20 mg	Orthostatic hypotension, first-dose syncope, tachycardia, dizziness, headache, dry mouth, GI upset, pharyngitis, rhinitis, epistaxis, red sclera, tinnitus, impotence, priapism (prazosin), incontinence, urinary frequency	• Avoid use with hypersensitivity. Use cautiously in elderly patients, or with hepatic disease.
Doxazosin	1–16 mg		• Increased hypotensive effect with use of β-blockers, nitroglycerin.
Terazosin	1–20 mg		• Decreased antihypertensive effect with use of indomethacin
ACE Inhibitors			
Captopril	6.25–150 mg	Hypotension, acute reversible renal failure, hyperkalemia, blood dyscrasias (in high doses), angioedema, cough, rash, fever, loss of taste sensation	• Contraindicated with hypersensitivity, bilateral renal artery stenosis, or stenosis in one viable kidney. Use cautiously in patients with renal insufficiency, lupus, sodium or volume depletion.
Enalapril	2.5–40 mg		• Increased antihypertensive effect with diuretics.
Lisinopril	5.0–40 mg		• Decreased effect with use of NSAIDs, antacids. Hyperkalemia may result with use of NSAIDs, potassium supplements, or potassium-sparing diuretics.
Quinipril	5.0–80 mg		
Ramipril	1.25–20 mg		
Fosinopril	10–40 mg		
Benazepril	10–40 mg		
Calcium Channel Blockers			
Diltiazem	120–360 mg	Bradycardia, heart block, CHF (verapamil, diltiazem), headache, drowsiness, GI upset, nocturia, polyuria, constipation, higher risk of tachycardia, dizziness, flushing, peripheral edema with nifedipine and other agents of the dihydropyridine class	• Contraindicated with hypersensitivity, atrioventricular conduction defects, sick sinus syndrome. Use cautiously in patients with renal or hepatic disease, or CHF.
CD	120–360 mg		• Verapamil's action decreased by rifampin, carbamazepine, phenobarbital, phenytoin.
SR	80–480 mg		• Actions of calcium channel antagonists increased by cimetidine.
Verapamil (sustained release)	120–480 mg		• Increased serum levels of digoxin, carbamazepine, prazosin, quindine, theophylline, and cyclosporine with use of calcium channel blockers.
Nifedipine (sustained release)	30–90 mg		
Amlodipine	2.5–10 mg		
Isradipine	2.5–10 mg		
Nicardipine	60–120 mg		

Table continues

TABLE **3–4.** (*Continued*)

Drug	Dosage Range (mg/day)	Adverse Effects	Reactions/Interactions
Central Sympatholytics			
Clonidine (transdermal)	0.1–0.6 mg 1 patch weekly	Rebound hypertension, orthostatic hypotension, fatigue, drowsiness, dry mouth, nausea, diarrhea, abdominal pain, constipation, bradycardia, heart block; myocarditis, fever, liver damage, hemolytic anemia (methyldopa), sexual dysfunction, Raynaud's phenomenon, rash, contact dermatitis from patch (clonidine)	• Contraindicated with hypersensitivity, acute liver disease (methyldopa). Use cautiously in recent MI, cerebrovascular disease, history of depression (clonidine).
Methyldopa	250–2000 mg		• Tricyclic agents decrease antihypertensive effect of clonidine. Alcohol use increases antihypertensive effect of clonidine.
Guanabenz	4.0–64 mg		
Guanfacine HCL	1.0–3.0 mg		• Methyldopa used concomitantly with β-adrenergic blockers can cause paradoxic hypertension. Methyldopa enhances lithium toxicity, impairs tolbutamide metabolism, can cause adverse mental effects if used with haloperidol, and potentiates effects of levodopa.
			• Use of CNS depressants can cause increased sedation (especially with guanabenz).
Peripheral Acting Adrenergic Antagonists			
Reserpine	0.05–0.25 mg	Bradycardia, GI disturbances, diarrhea, drowsiness, dizziness, visual changes, nasal congestion, sexual dysfunction, mental confusion, depression (reserpine), orthostatic hypotension, sodium and water retention (guanethidine), aching limbs, chest pain, palpitations, dyspnea on exertion, orthostatic hypotension (guanadrel)	• Avoid use in peptic ulcer disease or with ulcerative colitis (reserpine). Use carefully in renal disease, coronary disease, heart failure, cerebrovascular disease, depression, debilitated and elderly patients (reserpine), concurrent digitalis use, concurrent MAO inhibitor use, peptic ulcer disease, pheochromocytoma (guanethidine, guanadrel).
Guanadrel	10–75 mg		• Reserpine used with digitalis or quinidine may increase arrhythmias; diuretics increase antihypertensive effects; decreases effects of levodopa, ephedrine; potentiates effects of CNS depressants.
Guanethidine	10–100 mg		• MAO inhibitors antagonize effects of peripheral antagonists.

Table continues

TABLE 3–4.   (Continued)

Drug	Dosage Range (mg/day)	Adverse Effects	Reactions/Interactions
			• Hypotensive effects of guanethidine and guanadrel potentiated by other antihypertensive agents, alcohol. BP lowering effects antagonized by tricyclics, phenothiazines, haloperidol, indirect-acting sympathomimetics. *Note:* direct-acting sympathomimetics will increase hypotensive effects of guanadrel.
Direct Vasodilators Hydralazine Minoxidil	50–300 mg 2.5–80 mg	Palpitations, tachycardia, T-wave changes, angina, blood dyscrasias, rash, hypertrichosis, edema, heart failure, pulmonary hypertension, pericardial effusion (minoxidil), headache, dizziness, peripheral neuritis, muscle cramps, sodium retention, lupus-like syndrome, impotence, GI disturbance (hydralazine)	• Contraindicated in hypersensitivity, hydralazine contraindicated in coronary heart and/or valvular disease. Minoxidil contraindicated with MI, aortic aneurysm, or pheochromocytoma. Use minoxidil carefully with recent MI, renal disease. • Antihypertensive effect of hydralazine increased with quinidine, other antihypertensive agents, MAO inhibitors. • Use of minoxidil with guanethidine may potentiate orthostatic hypotension.
Loop Diuretics Bumetanide Furosemide Ethacrynic acid	0.5–5 mg 20–320 mg 25–100 mg	Electrolyte disturbances, hyperglycemia, metabolic alkalosis, hyperuricemia, dehydration, elevated blood lipids, blood dyscrasias, rash, hearing loss, photosensitivity, GI upset, GI bleeding, pancreatitis (ethacrynic acid)	• Avoid use in hypersensitivity, anuria. Do not use bumetanide in hepatic coma. Use cautiously in severe liver disease, diabetes mellitus, progressive azotemia. Avoid extremely rapid diuresis, can predispose to circulatory collapse, thromboembolic disorder. • Use of aminoglycosides or cisplatin can increase risk of ototoxicity. • Hypokalemia can increase risk of digitalis toxicity. • Indocin increases both antihypertensive and diuretic effects of loop diuretics.

Table continues

TABLE **3–4.** (*Continued*)

Drug	Dosage Range (mg/day)	Adverse Effects	Reactions/Interactions
			• Loop drugs decrease lithium excretion and may potentiate lithium toxicity. • Furosemide and ethacrynic acid can increase effect of oral anticoagulant.
Angiotensin II Receptor Antagonist Losartan	25–100 mg	Upper respiratory infection, sinusitis, nasal congestion, cough, dizziness, insomnia, diarrhea, GI upset, muscle ache, back pain, leg pain	• Avoid use with hypersensitivity. Use cautiously in patients with impaired hepatic or renal function. Use cautiously in patients with suspected volume depletion. • Hyperkalemia may result with use of sodium substitutes or vitamin K supplements.

* From Sadowski A.V., & Redeker, N.S. (1996). The hypertensive elder: A review for the primary care provider. *Nurse Pract 21*, 99–118, with permission.

NSAIDs, nonsteroidal anti-inflammatory drugs; GI, gastrointestinal; ACE, angiotensin converting enzyme; CHF, congestive heart failure; COPD, chronic obstructive pulmonary disease; MI, myocardial infarction; CNS, central nervous system; MAO, monoamine oxidase.

Elderly. Diuretic, CCB, ACE inhibitor, or α-blocker started at low dose to avoid postural hypotension. β-blockers effective but more likely to cause side effects.

Rationale. More than 60% of elderly have BP >140/90 mm Hg. Rule-out Pseudohypertension and "white coat" hypertension prior to initiating therapy. Elderly demonstrate blunted baroreceptor sensitivity and impaired cerebral autoregulation. Therefore, avoid medications associated with postural hypotension (e.g., labetolol, guanethidine). Sudden onset of HTN in elderly patients suggests the presence of atherosclerotic renovascular disease.

Diabetes Mellitus (DM). ACE inhibitor, CCB or α-blocker

Rationale. Consider more aggressive control of BP to <130/85 mm Hg as diabetic HTN carries twice the risk of CV mortality compared to nondiabetic HTN. ACE inhibitors have been shown to decrease the progression of diabetic nephropathy (Diabetes Control and Complication Trial Research Group, 1993). β-Blockers may increase insulin resistance, prolong insulin-induced hypoglycemia, and mask symptoms such as tachycardia.

Congestive Heart Failure (CHF). ACE inhibitor, diuretic, or α-blocker

Rationale. ACE inhibitors as well as combination therapy with hydralazine and isosorbide have been shown to decrease morbidity and mortality (The SOLVD Investigators, 1992; Kaplan, 1994).

Follow-up

• If BP within normal limits recheck in 2 years
• If mild HTN recheck in 1 year

T A B L E 3–5.   Lifestyle Modifications for Hypertension Control and/or Overall Cardiovascular Risk*

Lose weight if overweight

Limit alcohol intake to no more than 1 oz of ethanol per day (24 oz of beer, 8 oz of wine, or 2 oz of 100-proof whiskey)

Exercise (aerobic) regularly

Reduce sodium intake to <100 mmol/day (<2.3 gms of sodium or <6 gms of sodium chloride)

Maintain adequate dietary potassium, calcium, and magnesium intake

Stop smoking

Reduce dietary saturated fat and cholesterol intake for overall cardiovascular health

Reducing fat intake also helps reduce caloric intake—important for control of weight and type II diabetes

---

* Adapted from Joint National Committee on Detection, Evaluation, and Treatment of Blood Pressure: The Fifth Report. National Heart, Lung & Blood Institute, U.S. Department of Health and Human Services, NIH Publication 93–1088, 1993, with permission.

- If 140/100 recheck in 2 months ×3
- If 160/100 recheck in 1 month
- If 180/110 recheck in 1 week
- If >210/120 treat immediately

PATIENT EDUCATION

1. Assess patient's understanding and acceptance of diagnosis.
2. Discuss concerns and clarify misunderstandings.
3. Provide patient with written information regarding the exact numeric BP value and their target BP goal with treatment.
4. Emphasize the need to continue treatment regimen even if BP is not elevated.
5. Discuss lifestyle modifications such as diet and exercise (Table 3–5).
6. Discuss action, dose, effects, and side effects of medication regimen.

Review Questions

3.1 The most common etiology of secondary hypertension is:
   A. Drug induced
   B. Renovascular causes
   C. Stress induced
   D. Pregnancy

3.2 Mr. F. is a 55-year-old African-American man with known CAD who presents with severe headache, hypertension (180/95), and tachycardia. Which class of medications is best first-line therapy in this type of patient?
   A. β-Blocker
   B. ACE inhibitor
   C. Diuretic
   D. Combination therapy with β-blocker and diuretic

3.3 When treating HTN in the elderly patient the ACNP must be aware that drug selection is based on:
   A. The patient's age

    B. The step method, gradually introducing medications after failure at dietary and other lifestyle modifications

    C. The cost of the medication

    D. Existing medical conditions, possible drug interactions, side effects, age, and cost

3.4 A 60-year-old man was started on Lasix 40 mg QD for HTN and is seen in the acute care setting with complaint of severe muscle pain, cramping, weakness, polyuria and polydypsia. Serum electrolytes show a K level of 2.9; glucose of 280. The most likely diagnosis as the cause of HTN is:

    A. Cushing's syndrome

    B. Hyperaldosteronism

    C. Pheochromocytoma

    D. Hypokalemia due to the diuretic

3.5 The diagnosis of the above patient is made with which of the following tests:

    A. 24-hour urine for free cortisol

    B. 24-hour urine for aldosterone

    C. Renal ultrasound

    D. 24-hour serum total metanephrines

Answers and Rationales

3.1   **B**   Renovascular causes are the most common etiology of secondary hypertension.

3.2   **A**   β-Blockers should be used in the HTN patient with known CAD and tachycardia.

3.3   **D**   Medical conditions, possible drug interactions and side effects, age, and cost must be considered in the elderly to promote compliance with the medical regimen.

3.4   **B**   Primary aldosteronism may be manifested by hypertension and hypokalemia, which may first become evident during treatment with diuretics (7% have serum potassium <3.5 mEq/L).

3.5   **B**   Primary aldosteronism is diagnosed by 24-hour urine for aldosterone. Electrolytes such as urine sodium, cortisol, and serum plasma renin activity (PRA) and potassium are also helpful.

References

Aristizabal, D., & Frohlich, E.D. (1992). Hypertension due to renal arterial disease. *Heart Dis Stroke 1*, 227–234.

Coles, W.H. (1994). Hypertension and retinal vessels. *Heart Dis Stroke 3*, 304–308.

Diabetes Control and Complication Trial Research Group. (1993). *N Engl J Med 329*, 977–986.

Dustan, H.P. (1992). Prevention of Hypertension. *Heart Dis Stroke 1*, 337–339.

Frohlich, E.D. (1993). Detection, evaluation, and treatment of hypertension: JNC-5. *Heart Dis Stroke, 2* 459–460.

Glifford, R.W., & Bravo, E.L. (1993). What the primary care physician should know about pheochromocytoma. *Heart Dis Stroke 2*, 477–482.

Gillum, R.F. (1991). Cardiovascular disease in the United States: An epidemiologic overview. In E. Saunder (ed.). *Cardiovascular Diseases in Blacks*. Philadelphia: F.A. Davis Co., pp. 3–16.

Hall, W.D. (1992). Treatment of systolic hypertension. *Heart Dis Stroke 1*, 271–273.

Kaplan, N.M. (1993). Essential workup of the hypertensive patient. *Heart Dis Stroke 2*, 104–108.

Kaplan, N.M. (1994). Hypertension. In M. Freed & C. Grines (eds.). *Essentials of Cardiovascular Medicine*. Birmingham, MI: Physician's Press, pp. 2–32.

Kaplan, N.K. (1997). Systemic hypertension: Mechanisms and diagnosis. In E. Brunwald (ed.). *Heart Disease: A Textbook of Cardiovascular Medicine* (5th ed.). Philadelphia: W.B. Saunders Co., pp 807–839.

Lynn, M.N. (1996). A new antihypertensive class: The angiotensin receptor antagonist. *Nurse Pract 21*(3), 106–114.

Macklis, R.M., Mendelsohn, M.E., & Mudge, G.H. (1994). Systemic hypertension. In *Introduction to Clinical Medicine* (3rd ed.). Boston: Little, Brown & Co., pp. 192–195.

Massie, B.M. (1997). Systemic hypertension. In L.M. Tierney, S.J. McPhee, & M.A. Papadakis (eds.). *Current Medical Diagnosis & Treatment* (36th ed.). Stamford, CT: Appleton & Lange, pp. 412–431.

McKenzie, C.R., & Peterson, L.R. (1995). Hypertension. In G.A. Ewald & C.R. McKenzie (eds.). *Manual of Medical Therapeutics* (28th ed.). Boston: Little, Brown & Co.

Sadowski, A.V., & Redeker, N.S. (1996). The hypertensive elder: A review for the primary care provider. *Nurse Pract 21*, 99–118.

The Fifth Report of the Joint National Committee on Detection, Evaluation, and Treatment of High Blood Pressure (JNC V). (1993). *Arch Intern Med 153*, 186–208.

The SOLVD Investigators. (1992). Effect of enalapril on mortality and the development of heart failure in asymptomatic patients with reduced left ventricular ejection fraction. *N Engl J Med 327*, 685–691.

Wood, M.H. (1996). Current considerations in patients with coexistent diabetes and hypertension. *Nurse Pract 21*(4), 19–31.

Hypertensive Crisis

DEFINITION

1. Hypertensive crisis: Indicates the presence of hypertension that is potentially life threatening, usually defined as a diastolic blood pressure greater than 120 to 130 mm Hg (Calhoun & Oparil, 1990). The immediacy of lowering BP divides hypertensive crisis in hypertensive emergencies and urgencies (Zimmerman, 1995).

2. Hypertensive emergency: Defined as a substantial increase in blood pressure above baseline that is associated with new or progressive end-organ damage (EOD) of the neurologic, cardiovascular, and renal system (Zimmerman, 1995). The presence of acute or ongoing EOD is more important than the absolute level of BP. However, hypertensive emergency may be defined as a systolic blood pressure >220 mm Hg and a diastolic blood pressure >120 mm Hg. The goal of BP reduction needs to be individualized, but it is reasonable to attempt a 25% reduction of mean arterial pressure or reduce the diastolic pressure to 100 to 110 mm Hg over a period of minutes to hours (McKenzie & Peterson, 1995).

3. Hypertensive urgency: Defined as severe hypertension (DBP >130 mm Hg) without evidence of immediate complications (i.e., elevated BP, associated

symptoms, with no EOD). Retinal hemorrhage and papilledema are present. BP in urgent conditions can be lowered less rapidly, usually over 24 hours (Zimmerman, 1995).

ETIOLOGY/INCIDENCE

Hypertensive crisis is relatively rare and occurs in approximately 1% of hypertensive patients. Although rare, it can develop in previously normotensive patients (McKenzie & Peterson, 1995; Teplitz, 1993).

Many clinical conditions can lead to or cause an HTN crisis and the mechanisms that transform a stable HTN state into an HTN crisis are complex. Thus the pathogenesis underlying specific end-organ damage varies.

The organs at greatest danger of physiologic disturbance during a hypertensive emergency are the heart, kidney, and brain. The danger in the heart is ischemia and/or infarction with acute left ventricular insufficiency, congestive heart failure, and pulmonary edema. In the brain, the danger is risk of edema with altered level of consciousness and/or intracranial bleeding (Hoyt, 1995).

SIGNS AND SYMPTOMS

1. Depending on the degree of respiratory or CV compromise an abbreviated Hx should note:
   A. Prior Dx & Tx of HTN
   B. Prior coexisting CV, neuro, renal, and DM
   C. Known duration and level of BP
   D. Allergies
   E. Psychosocial/environmental factors contributing to BP
   F. Effectiveness of previous antihypertensive medication
   G. Diet and ETOH Hx
   H. Cardiac risk factors (Teplitz, 1993)
2. HTN emergencies may produce either widespread symptoms or the patient may be relatively asymptomatic until EOD occurs.
3. HTN urgencies usually result in elevated DBPs between 100 and 120, with minimal or no end-organ damage (Teplitz, 1993).
4. Cardiovascular
   A. With increasing pressures CV dysfunction may become apparent as orthopnea, dyspnea, anginal symptoms, and even frank pulmonary edema.
   B. Tachycardia is frequently seen with HTN emergencies and further increases oxygen demand.
   C. Cardiac output and peripheral vascular resistance may increase. Due to the increase in peripheral vascular resistance left ventricular failure may ensue, resulting in a decrease in cardiac output.
5. Neurologic
   A. Ocular fatigue, decreased visual acuity, visual blurring, occipital headaches, drowsiness, and encephalopathic changes.
   B. Transient paresthesias and CVAs tend to occur with higher pressures.

PHYSICAL FINDINGS

1. BP determination: Both arms; appropriately sized cuff; lying, sitting, standing if possible.

2. CV: Left ventricular heave, sustained apical impulse, S_4, murmurs of aortic insufficiency and mitral regurgitation, and signs of left ventricular failure.
3. Neuro: Slow or dulled responses, transient weakness or numbness, paresthesias, CVA, cerebral thrombotic or hemorrhagic events. Hypertensive encephalopathy occurs with very high blood pressures and is characterized by transient focal central nervous system (CNS) deficits, severe headache, visual disturbances, vomiting, and even convulsions, stupor, and coma (Macklis, 1994).
4. Retinal changes: Papilledema of optic disc.

DIFFERENTIAL DIAGNOSIS

Table 3–6 list the differential diagnosis for hypertensive crisis.

DIAGNOSTIC TESTS/FINDINGS

1. CBC.
2. UA provides evidence of primary renal disease—proteinuria.
3. Serum blood urea nitrogen (BUN) or creatinine—to evaluate extent of renal compromise.
4. Serum electrolytes—e.g., K is a screening test for primary aldosteronism (decreased K is found in hyperaldosteronism); also, results should be known before initiating diuretic therapy.
5. ECG—provides baseline data regarding CV risk; ECG may show LVH, ischemic changes caused by HTN.
6. CXR—evaluation for cardiomegaly CHF, rib notching seen with coarctation of aorta.
7. FBS—CV risk.
8. Lipid profile—CV risk.

TABLE 3–6.   Differential Diagnosis for Hypertensive Crisis*

Emergencies	Urgencies
Hypertensive encephalopathy	Accelerated hypertension
Acute aortic dissection	Perioperative hypertension
Acute myocardial ischemic syndromes	Severe hypertension associated
Unstable angina	with the following:
Myocardial infarction	Congestive heart failure
Acute left ventricular dysfunction	Stable angina
Acute renal insufficiency	Transient ischemic attacks
Excess catecholamine states	Renal failure from other causes
Pheochromocytoma crisis	
MAO inhibitor and tyramine interaction	
Antihypertensive withdrawal	
Acute intracranial events	
Hemorrhagic cerebrovascular accident	
Thrombotic cerebrovascular accident	
Subarachnoid hemorrhage	
Eclampsia	

* From Zimmerman, J.M. (1995). Hypertensive crises: Emergencies and urgencies. In W.C. Shoemaker, S.M. Ayres, A. Grenvik, & P.R. Holbrook (eds.). *Textbook of Critical Care* (3rd ed.). Philadelphia: W.B. Saunders Co., pp. 552–529, with permission.

MAO, monoamine oxidase.

MANAGEMENT/TREATMENT

General Principles of Treatment

Hypertensive crisis is a life-threatening event. Stabilization of blood pressure is the primary goal. Although various recommendations for the extent of BP reduction have been proposed, each case must be individualized. A reasonable goal for most HTN emergencies is to lower the mean artery pressure (MAP) by approximately 25% or to reduce diastolic BP to 100–110 mm Hg over several minutes to hours.

TABLE 3–7. Parenteral Antihypertensive Agents*

Drug	Class	Dose/Route	Onset of Action	Adverse Effects
Sodium nitroprusside (Nipride)	Arteriolar and venous vasodilator	0.3–10 μg/kg/min continuous IV infusion	Immediate	Hypotension, nausea, vomiting, muscle twitching, thiocyanate and cyanide intoxication
Nitroglycerin	Venous and arteriolar vasodilator	5–300 μg/min continuous IV infusion	1–2 minutes	Headache, tachycardia, vomiting
Diazoxide	Arteriolar vasodilator	50–100 mg IV bolus repeated, up to 150 mg, or 15–30 mg/min continuous IV infusion	1–2 minutes	Hypotension, nausea, vomiting, flushing, aggravation of angina or CHF, hyperglycemia, cerebral ischemia, fluid retention
Hydralazine hydrochloride (Apresoline)	Arteriolar vasodilator	10–20 mg IV 10–50 mg IM	10–20 minutes 20–30 minutes	Reflex tachycardia, headache, vomiting, palpitations
Phentolamine mesylate (Regitine)	α-Adrenergic blocker	5–15 mg IV	1–2 minutes	Tachycardia, flushing, dizziness, orthostatic, hypotension
Labetalol hydrochloride (Normodyne, Trandate)	α- and β-Adrenergic blocker	20–80 mg IV bolus q 10 min up to 300 mg total dose; 0.5–2.0 mg/min continuous IV infusion	5–10 minutes	Nausea, vomiting, heart block, bronchoconstriction, orthostatic hypotension
Enalapril (Vasotec)	ACE inhibitor	1.25–5 mg q 6 h IV	15 minutes	Response variable, precipitous fall in BP in high renin states
Esmolol (Brevibloc)	β-Adrenergic blocker	500 μg/kg/min for 4 minutes, then 50–300 μg/kg/min IV	1–2 minutes	Hypotension orthostatic, dizziness
Trimethaphan camsylate	Ganglionic blocker	0.5–5 mg/min continuous IV infusion	1–5 minutes	Orthostatic hypotension, blurred vision, dry mouth, tachycardia, paresis of bowel and bladder
Nicardipine hydrochloride	Calcium channel blocker	5–10 mg/hr continuous IV infusion	1–3 minutes	Tachycardia, headache, flushing

* From Zimmerman, J.M. (1995). Hypertensive crises: Emergencies and urgencies. In S.M. Ayres, A. Grenvik, P.R. Holbrook, W.C. Shoemaker (eds.). *Textbook of Critical Care* (3rd ed.). Philadelphia: W.B. Saunders Co., pp. 522–529 and Teplitz, L. (1993). Hypertensive crisis: review and update. *Crit Care Nurse* 12:20–36, with permission.

CHF, congestive heart failure; IV, intravenous; IM, intramuscular; BP, blood pressure.

TABLE 3–8. Oral Antihypertensive Agents*

Drug	Class	Dose	Onset	Adverse Effects
Nifedipine	Calcium channel blocker	10 mg PO or SL	5–10 minutes	Hypotension, tachycardia, headache, palpitations, flushing, dizziness
Clonidine	Central α-adrenergic agonist	0.1–0.2 mg PO, then 0.1 mg qh (max = 0.8 mg)	30–60 minutes	Sedation, dry mouth, orthostasis, bradycardia
Captopril	ACE inhibitor	6.25–25 mg PO	15 minutes	Hypotension

* From Zimmerman, J.M. (1995). Hypertensive crises: Emergencies and urgencies. In W.C. Shoemaker, S.M. Ayres, A. Grenvik, P.R. Holbrook (eds.). *Textbook of Critical Care* (3rd ed.). Philadelphia: W.B. Saunders Co., pp. 552–529, with permission.

Rationale. Under normal circumstances (normotensive patients) cerebral blood flow is controlled at a fixed level by autoregulation (constriction and vasodilatation) from MAP as low as 50 mm Hg and to as high as 150 mm Hg (Hoyt, 1995). In patients with chronic HTN, this autoregulatory mechanism adapts to higher pressures because of structural changes in resistance vessels that allow tolerance of elevated pressures without incurring cerebral damage. Excessive reduction of BP can compromise cerebral perfusion and precipitate ischemic events in patients with altered cerebral autoregulation (Zimmerman, 1995).

HTN emergencies require lowering of BP as quickly as possible (within minutes); immediate parenteral antihypertensive therapy is administered. Table 3–7 lists parenteral agents recommended for HTN emergencies.

HTN urgencies are treated with rapid-acting antihypertensive agents (oral or parenteral) that can reduce BP within hours. Oral medications are listed in Table 3–8. The goal of treatment is to gradually reduce blood pressure over hours to normal levels.

PATIENT EDUCATION

1. Instruct patient on diagnosis and meaning of symptoms.
2. Reassure patient that the emergent situation is being addressed and that the problem is being corrected.
3. Prepare patient for any emergent procedures necessary to treat HTN emergency/urgency.
4. Discuss the outcome of treatment and continued need for treatment and monitoring.
5. Encourage patient to ask questions and discuss fears and concerns.

Review Questions

3.6 A hypertensive crisis puts a patient at risk for:
   A. Cardiac ischemia
   B. Congestive heart failure

C. Cerebral edema
D. All of the above

3.7   Signs and symptoms of hypertensive urgency include:
A. Systolic BP >160
B. Normal diastolic pressure
C. Nonoliguric renal failure
D. Retinal hemorrhage

3.8   A patient is admitted to the intensive care unit (ICU) with severe hypertension, episodic palpitations, headache (HA), sweating, weight loss, and glucose intolerance. Pheochromocytoma is suspected. Which initial therapy for control of the blood pressure is inappropriate?
A. Nitroprusside
B. Phentolamine
C. Labetalol
D. Propranolol

3.9   A 60-year-old black man is admitted with the diastolic blood pressure of >130 mm Hg and retinal hemorrhage. The most appropriate first-line medication therapy to reduce BP is:
A. Nitroprusside
B. Phentolamine
C. Nifedipine
D. Propranolol

3.10 In patients with hypertensive emergencies, what general guidelines can be used as a target for BP reduction?
A. Decrease MAP by 25%
B. Decrease systolic BP by 25%
C. Decrease diastolic BP by 25%
D. Diastolic BP should be <90 mm Hg

Answers and Rationales

3.6   **D** All of the above are complications of hypertensive crisis.
3.7   **D** Retinal hemorrhage of papilledema and DBP >130 mm Hg are signs of HTN urgency.
3.8   **A** α-Adrenergic blockade with phentolamine is the treatment of choice for HTN due to pheochromocytoma. Nitroprusside is ineffective in lowering BP in a patient with HTN due to pheochromocytoma. β-Blockade can also be used in combination to control tachycardia and arrhythmias.
3.9   **A** Intravenous nitroprusside is appropriate first-line therapy to reduce BP in this patient.
3.10 **A** Decrease in MAP by 25% within the first 24 hours.

References

Calhoun, D.A., & Oparil, S. (1990). Treatment of hypertensive-crisis. *N Engl J Med* 323, 1177–1183.
DeVault, G.A. (1990). Hypertensive emergencies: Pathogenesis, diagnosis, therapy. *J Crit Illness 5*, 812.

Hoyt, J.W. Hypertensive emergencies. (1995). Proceedings from *Multidisciplinary Critical Care Board Review*. Anaheim, CA: Society of Critical Care Medicine, p. 317.

Kaplan, N.M. (1992). Treatment of hypertensive emergencies and urgencies. *Heart Dis Stroke 1*, 373–378.

Kaplan, N.K. (1997). Systemic hypertension: Mechanisms and diagnosis. In E. Braunwald (ed.). *Heart Disease: A Textbook of Cardiovascular Medicine* (5th ed.). Philadelphia: W.B. Saunders Co., pp. 307–339.

Macklis, R.M., Mendelsohn, M.E., & Mudge, G.H. (1994). *Introduction to Clinical Medicine* (3rd ed.). Boston: Little, Brown & Co.

McKenzie C.R., & Peterson, L.R. (1995). Hypertension. In G.A. Ewald & C.R. McKenzie (eds.). *Manual of Medical Therapeutics* (28th ed.). Boston: Little, Brown & Co.

Teplitz, L. (1993). Hypertensive crisis: Review and update. *Crit Care Nurse 12*, 20–36.

Zimmerman, J.L. (1996). Hypertensive crises: Emergencies and urgencies. In Shoemaker, W.C., Ayres, S.M., Grenvik, A, & Holbrook, P.R. (eds.). *Textbook of Critical Care* (3rd ed.). Philadelphia: W.B. Saunders Co., pp. 522–529.

Hyperlipidemia

DEFINITION

Hyperlipidemia is defined as an undesirable or abnormal plasma lipid phenotype and encompasses elevated levels of total cholesterol, low-density lipoprotein (LDL) cholesterol, and triglycerides.

ETIOLOGY/INCIDENCE

1. It is estimated that 20% of U.S. adults have high total cholesterol ($\geq$240 mg/dL) and that another 31% have borderline-high total cholesterol (200–239 mg/dL).
2. Elevated plasma levels of total cholesterol and LDL cholesterol and low plasma levels of high-density lipoprotein (HDL) cholesterol are major but modifiable risk factors for CAD.
3. In addition, triglyceride elevation may correlate with increased risk for atherosclerotic disease, although the nature of this risk is less clear. Very high plasma triglycerides are associated with pancreatitis.
4. Clinical trials: Meta-analysis of primary and secondary prevention trials from 1970 to the present suggest that for every 10% reduction in cholesterol there is an estimated 13–14% reduction in CAD mortality and an 8–10% reduction in total mortality (Gould et al., 1994; Woodhead, 1996).
5. In individuals who have had LDL intensively reduced, angiographic studies have shown a slowing of progression, and even regression of atherosclerotic lesions (Wissler & Vesselinovich, 1977; Brown et al., 1990; Panel II, 1994).

Primary Prevention

Clinical trials demonstrate that lowering serum cholesterol reduces new CAD events and CAD mortality in patients without established CAD (Grundy, 1994).

Secondary Prevention

Clinical trials demonstrate conclusively that lowering serum cholesterol reduces morbidity and mortality from CAD in patients with established CAD (Scandinavian Sinvastatin Survival Group, 1994; Grundy, 1994).

SIGNS AND SYMPTOMS

Because hyperlipidemic subjects are usually asymptomatic, routine screening of total and HDL cholesterol is necessary to detect those at risk for premature atherosclerotic disease.

PHYSICAL FINDINGS

Patients with hyperlipidemia may have the following:
1. Tendon and tuberous xanthomas.
2. Xanthelasmas.
3. Lipemia retinalis.
4. Recurrent pancreatitis.
5. Corneal arcus.
6. High uric acid levels.
7. Glucose intolerance.

DIAGNOSTIC TESTS/FINDINGS

1. Step 1: Initial classification:
   A. Serum total cholesterol and HDL cholesterol should be measured in all adults older than age 20.
   B. All samples should be drawn in a steady state (i.e., absence of active weight loss or acute illness).
   C. Table 3–9 summarizes the initial classification of cholesterol levels.
2. Step 2: Evaluate patient clinically for CAD risk factors (see Table 3–10).
3. Step 3: Use LDL cholesterol levels for treatment decisions in adults with the following:
   A. HDL cholesterol <35 mg/dL
   B. Borderline-high total cholesterol (200–239 mg/dL) when two or more risk factors for CAD are present.
   C. High total cholesterol (≥240 mg/dL) (diet or medication therapy is selected based on LDL cholesterol level and patient risk as described in Table 3–11.)
4. Step 4: Patients with established CAD should undergo lipoprotein analysis and be classified according to LDL cholesterol (Table 3–11).

T A B L E 3–9.   Initial Classification Based on Total and High-Density Lipoprotein (HDL) Cholesterol*

Total cholesterol	<200 mg/dL	Desirable blood cholesterol
	200–239 mg/dL	Borderline-high blood cholesterol
	≥240 mg/dL	High blood cholesterol
HDL cholesterol	<35 mg/dL	Low HDL cholesterol

* From Grundy, S.M. (1994). Guidelines for cholesterol management: Recommendations of the National Cholesterol Education Program's Adult Treatment Panel II. In *Heart Disease and Stroke*, *3*, 125, with permission.

TABLE 3–10. Risk Status Based on Presence of Risk Factors for Coronary Heart Disease Other than Low-Density Lipoprotein Cholesterol*,†

Positive Risk Factors
Age
    Men: ≥45 years
    Women: ≥55 years or premature menopause without estrogen replacement therapy
Family history of premature coronary heart disease (definite myocardial infarction or sudden death before 55 years of age in father or other male first-degree relative, or before 65 years of age in mother or other female first-degree relative)
Current cigarette smoking
Hypertension (≥140/90 mm Hg‡ or on antihypertensive medication)
Low HDL cholesterol (<35 mg/dL‡)
Diabetes mellitus
Negative Risk Factor§
High HDL cholesterol (≥60 mg/dL)

---

* From Grundy, S.M. (1994). Guidelines for Cholesterol Management: Recommendations of the National Cholesterol Education Program's Adult Treatment Panel II. In *Heart Disease and Stroke 3*, 125, with permission.

† High risk, defined as a net of two or more risk factors for coronary heart disease, leads to more vigorous intervention. Age (defined differently for men and for women) is treated as a risk factor because rates of coronary heart disease are higher in the elderly than in the young and in men than in women of the same age. Obesity is not listed as risk factor because it operates through other risk factors that are included (hypertension, hyperlipidemia, decreased HDL cholesterol, and diabetes mellitus), but it should be considered a target for intervention. Physical inactivity similarly is not listed as a risk factor, but it too should be considered a target for intervention, and physical activity is recommended as desirable for everyone.

‡ Confirmed by measurements on several occasions.

§ If the HDL cholesterol level is ≥60 mg/dL, subtract one risk factor (because high HDL cholesterol levels decrease risk of coronary heart disease).

HDL, high-density lipoprotein; LDL, low-density lipoprotein.

Once a Hyperlipidemia is Identified

1. Screen for the presence of secondary hyperlipidemia, including medications, alcohol abuse, diabetes mellitus, thyroid disorders, nephrotic syndrome, and obstructive jaundice.
2. Carefully review family history for genetic causes. If severe hypercholesterolemia is present, family members should be screened.
3. Assess possible contribution of lipid abnormalities to history (e.g., angina, claudication, pancreatitis) and physical examination findings (e.g., xanthomas, xanthelasma, hepatosplenomegaly).
4. Estimate risk for coronary heart disease and other atherosclerotic disease to guide intensity of further management (see Table 3–10).

TABLE 3–11. Therapy for LDL Cholesterol Levels*

Patient Category	LDL Levels (mg/dL)	
	Diet	*Drug*
Without CHD + <2 RF	≥160	≥190
Without CHD + 2 or >RF	≥130	≥160
With CHD	≥100	≥130

LDL, low-density lipoprotein; CHD, coronary heart disease; RF, risk factors.

* From Drown, D.J., & Engler, M.M. (1994). New guidelines for blood cholesterol by the National Cholesterol Education Program (NCEP). *Prog Cardiovasc Nurs 9*(1), 44, with permission.

MANAGEMENT/TREATMENT

1. General therapeutics.
   A. The ACNP should begin with diet and risk factor modification measures (exercise, weight control, smoking cessation, etc.) as first-line therapy for all patients with hypercholesterolemia.
   B. The ACNP should initiate drug therapy only after an adequate trial of dietary therapy has failed to lower LDL cholesterol levels to within desired range after 6 months.
   C. Exceptions include:
      1) Patients with established CAD and an LDL cholesterol >100 mg/dL: in these patients, medication therapy is started with target lipid levels of total serum cholesterol <160 mg/dL, LDL cholesterol <100 mg/dL, and HDL cholesterol >45 mg/dL.
      2) Patients with very high LDL levels (>220 mg/dL): Medication therapy may be initiated concurrently with Step II diet (Table 3–12).
   D. The Step I diet serves as dietary recommendations of the National Cholesterol Education Program for the general public.
   E. The more intensive fat-controlled Step II diet is designed for patients with genetic hyperlipidemia, established CAD or atherosclerotic disease, or for whom the Step I diet has proven insufficient (Table 3–12).
   F. The ACNP should refer the patient to a dietician to promote patient/family understanding of dietary restrictions with Step II diet therapy. The assistance of a registered dietician is useful in assisting the patient to understand the diet and maintaining compliance.
2. Initiate therapy with dietary and risk factor modification.
3. Goal is LDL cholesterol.
4. Follow-up:
   A. The ACNP should assess total cholesterol dietary compliance and risk factor modification strategies (exercise, weight control, smoking cessation, etc.) at 4 to 6 weeks and 3 months after beginning therapy.
   B. Total cholesterol can be followed instead of LDL to determine the effectiveness of therapy (advantages: does not require fasting or lipoprotein

TABLE 3–12. **Dietary Therapy for High Blood Cholesterol***

Nutrient†	*Step I Diet*	*Step II Diet*	Recommended Intake
Total fat			≤30% of total calories
Saturated fatty acids	8–10% of total calories	<7% of total calories	
Polyunsaturated fatty acids			Up to 10% of total calories
Monounsaturated fatty acids			Up to 15% of total calories
Carbohydrates			≥55% of total calories
Protein			Approximately 15% of total calories
Cholesterol	<300 mg/day	<200 mg/day	
Total calories			To achieve and maintain desirable weight

* Modified from Grundy, S.M. (1994). Guidelines for cholesterol management: Recommendations of the National Cholesterol Education Program's Adult Treatment Panel II. *Heart Dis Stroke 3,* 126, with permission.

† Calories from alcohol not included.

analysis, and is less expensive). Total cholesterol levels of 240, 200, and 160 mg/dL correspond to LDL cholesterol levels of 160, 130, and 100 mg/dL, respectively.

   C. Once the total cholesterol goal has been achieved, the ACNP can use lipoprotein analysis to confirm that LDL cholesterol is at an acceptable level. (Quion & Gotto, 1994).

  5. Medication Therapy

   A. Table 3–13 lists single-agent lipid medications and their dosing schedule. HMG-CoA reductase inhibitors (RIs) (also called "statins") are the most effective and best tolerated cholesterol-lowering medications and should be considered as the preferred first-line agent.

   B. Starting dose of any of the following:

    1) Lovastatin 20–40 mg qhs
    2) Pravastatin 20–40 mg qhs
    3) Simvastatin 10–20 mg qhs

   C. Patients with CAD will live longer when treated with an HMG-CoA RI. In the 4S trial there was a 34% risk reduction in major cardiac events, a 42% risk reduction in CV mortality, and a 30% reduction in all-cause mortality associated with statin treatment (The Scandinavian Simvastatin Survival Study Group, 1994). The CARE and REGRESS trials demonstrated that even patients with "normal" levels of total cholesterol and

TABLE 3–13.   **Single-Agent Lipid Medication Dosing Schedule***

	Starting Dose	Progressive Dosing	Maximal Dose
Resins			
Cholestyramine (Questran)	4 gm before main meal	4–8 gm bid before meals	8 gm tid before meals
Colestipol (Colestid)	5 gm before main meal	5–10 gm bid before meals	10 gm tid before meals
Statins			
Lovastatin (Mevacor)	10–20 mg before supper or bedtime	10–20 mg bid	40 mg bid or 80 mg before supper or bedtime
Pravastatin (Pravachol)	10–20 mg at bedtime	20–30 mg at bedtime	40 mg at bedtime
Simvastatin (Zocor)	5–10 mg before supper or bedtime	5–10 mg bid	20 mg bid or 40 mg before supper or bedtime
Others			
Niacin†	100–250 od bid after meals	500 mg bid after meals	1–2 gm bid or tid after meals
Gemfibrozil (Lipid)	600 mg qd or bid before meals		600 mg bid before meals
Fish oils‡	2 capsules tid with meals	4 capsules tid with meals	6 capsules tid with meals
Probucol (Lorelco)	250 mg bid		500 mg bid

* From Bays, H.E., Dujovne, C.A., & Lansing, A.M. (1992). Drug treatment of dyslipidemias: Practical guidelines for the primary care physician. *Heart Dis Stroke 1*, 360, with permission.

† To avoid a significantly increased risk of toxicity, the total dose of niacin should probably not exceed 4 gm/day. Doses of sustained-released preparations >1.5 gm/day have been associated with increased liver toxicity.

‡ Fish oils are generally available in lipid concentrates with 300–600 mg of eicosapentanoic acid and/or docosahexanoic acid per capsule.

LDL cholesterol benefit from treatment with an HMG-CoA RI (Sacks et al., 1991; Jukema et al., 1995).
   D. Patients who fail to achieve target lipid level (LDL <100 mg/dL with CAD) at 6 weeks to 3 months after initiation of therapy should have their dose increased or an additional agent (niacin or cholesterol-binding resin) added.
   E. Set therapeutic goals based on LDL cholesterol as described in Table 3–3 (therapeutic goals are the same as for dietary therapy).
   F. When baseline LDL cholesterol is very high (>160 mg/dL in patients with established CAD, or >190 mg/dL in patients without CAD but with multiple risk factors), it is unlikely that diet alone will be able to achieve therapeutic goals (LDL <100 mg/dL and <130 mg/dL, respectively); therefore, initial therapy with diet and medications should be considered.
6. Follow-up:
   A. Total serum cholesterol may be used instead of LDL cholesterol during the follow-up period: Total serum cholesterol of 240, 200, and 160 mg/dL correspond to LDL cholesterol of 160, 130, and 100 mg/dL, respectively.
   B. LFTs should be checked prior to initiating therapy and every 6 months for patients receiving an HMG-CoA RI.
   C. Once total cholesterol is within target range, lipoprotein analysis should be performed to confirm that LDL cholesterol is at an acceptable level.
   D. Cholesterol testing should be repeated at 4–6 weeks and 3 months after the initiation of drug therapy. More frequent laboratory testing may be needed to exclude drug toxicity.
   E. Once LDL cholesterol is at an acceptable level, total serum cholesterol should be followed every 2–3 months during the first year and every 4–6 months thereafter; lipoprotein analysis should be repeated yearly.
   F. Certain patient subsets (young adults, premenopausal females, the elderly, diabetics) warrant special considerations (Quion & Gotto, 1994).
7. Special groups
   A. Young adult males and premenopausal females: Most young adult males (age <35) and premenopausal females with LDL cholesterol levels between 160 and 220 mg/dL are at low risk of CAD in the short term. In general, drug therapy can be withheld in these groups unless extreme elevations in LDL cholesterol (>220 mg/dL) or multiple risk factors are present—especially DM and patients with a family history of premature CAD.
   B. Postmenopausal females: In the absence of contraindications such as breast cancer, postmenopausal women should benefit from estrogen replacement therapy, which has been shown to reduce the incidence of CAD and beneficially affect LDL and HDL cholesterol levels.
   C. Elderly patients: Age by itself should not preclude diet and drug therapy when hypercholesterolemia is present.
   D. Diabetics: There appears to be a synergistic effect between DM and hypercholesterolemia in the development of CAD. Therefore, initiation levels and therapeutic goals, even in the absence of CAD, should be similar to recommendations for those with established CAD (initiation level, LDL >100 mg/dL; therapeutic goal <100 mg/dL) (Quion & Gotto, 1994).
8. The ACNP should refer to cardiologist/lipid specialist for the following:
   A. Failure of diet/medications to control hyperlipidemia.

B. Uncomfortable in monitoring metabolic impact of combined medication therapy.
C. Patient with severe refractory lipid disorders or those who require complex management such as LDL apheresis therapy.

PATIENT EDUCATION

1. Instruct patient on normal and abnormal lipid levels.
2. Discuss risk associated with high lipid levels.
3. Discuss low-fat diet plan and goal of therapy.
4. If patient requires medications, stress importance that diet and risk factor modification must be an integral part of effective medication therapy.
5. Provide medication instruction regarding drug, action, dose, and side effect to report to ACNP/physician.
6. Discuss the fact that once medication therapy is initiated it is often necessary to maintain it for years or a lifetime.
7. Discuss need for follow-up and future health management.
8. Allow time for patient questions and verbalization of concerns/fears.

Review Questions

3.11 A 48-year-old male smoker with no other CAD risk factors and no known CAD would have antilipid medications started at what lipid level?
A. Cholesterol >220
B. LDL >190
C. HDL >35
D. LDL >160

3.12 A 60-year-old female patient with a history of DM is being discharged. Lipid acting drug therapy should be considered for this individual with the following:
A. HDL Cholesterol level <35
B. HDL Cholesterol level >35
C. Cholesterol level >200
D. LDL cholesterol level >100

3.13 A 50-year-old male smoker who is in the intermediate care unit following acute myocardial infarction (AMI) would
A. Have a desired lipid level of cholesterol <220
B. Have a desired lipid level of LDL <130
C. Have a desired lipid level of cholesterol <240
D. Be placed on antilipid therapy while hospitalized as secondary prevention strategy

3.14 You are discharging a patient and note that the patient has high-risk LDL cholesterol (130–159) and less than two risk factors. Your first step as the ACNP should be to:
A. Refer to a cardiologist/lipid specialist
B. Provide information on Step I diet and physical activity
C. Initiate antilipid therapy
D. Restart the lipid profile as an outpatient

3.15 Patients placed on the medication classification of "HMG-CoA RI" should have the following baseline blood work:
A. LFTs
B. Hct/Hbg
C. Thyroid
D. Electrolytes

Answers and Rationales

3.11 **B** This patient's age and smoking history are 2 CV risk factors, anti-lipid medications would be started at LDL >190 mg/dL. Diet therapy would be tried at LDL >160.

3.12 **D** There is a synergistic effect between diabetes mellitus and hypercholesterolemia in the development of CAD. Therefore, initiation of antilipid therapy and therapeutic goals, even in the absence of CAD, are similar to recommendations for those with established CAD (initiation level, LDL >100 mg/dL; therapeutic goal <100 mg/dL).

3.13 **D** This patient with known CAD will live longer treated with an HMG-CoA RI and would be placed on antilipid therapy while hospitalized as secondary prevention strategy.

3.14 **B** Provide information on Step I diet and physical activity.

3.15 **A** LFTs should be taken at baseline and every 6 months in patients on HMG-CoA RI.

References

Expert Panel on Detection, Evaluation, and Treatment of High Blood Cholesterol in Adults. (1993). Summary of the second report of the National Cholesterol Education Program (NCEP) Expert Panel on Detection, Evaluation, and Treatment of High Blood Cholesterol in Adults (Adult Treatment Panel II). *JAMA 269*, 3015–3023.

Expert Panel on Detection, Evaluation, and Treatment of High Blood Cholesterol in Adults (Adult Treatment Panel II). (1994). National Cholesterol Education Program: Second report of the Expert Panel on Detection, Evaluation and Treatment of High Blood Cholesterol in Adults (Adult Treatment Panel II). *Circulation 89*, 1329–1445.

National Institutes of Health: National Heart, Lung and Blood Institute. (1993). *New cholesterol guidelines released: Heart memo*. Fall, 1993.

National Institutes of Health: National Heart, Lung and Blood Institute. (1993). *Second Report of the Expert Panel on Detection, Evaluation, and Treatment of High Blood Cholesterol in Adults: Executive Summary*.

Bays, H.E., Dujovne, C.A., & Lansing, A.M. (1992). Drug treatment of dyslipidemias: Practical guidelines for the primary care physician. *Heart Dis Stroke 1*, 357–365.

Brown, G., Albers, J.J., Fisher, L.D., et al. (1990). Regression of coronary artery disease as a result of intensive lipid-lowering therapy in men with high levels of apolipoprotein B. *N Engl J Med 323*, 1289–1298.

Detection, evaluation and treatment of high blood cholesterol in adults. Panel II. (1994). *Circulation 89*(3), 1329–1448.

Drown, D.J., & Engler, M.M. (1994). New guidelines for blood cholesterol by the National Cholesterol Education Program (NCEP). *Prog Cardiovasc Nurs 9*(1), 43–44.

Drown, D.J. (1994). Low density cholesterol (LDC-C) and the need for pharmacologic intervention (National Cholesterol Education Program [NECP]). *Prog Cardiovasc Nurs 9*(2), 38–40.

Gould, A.L., Rousson, J.E., Santenelle, N.C., et al. (1995). Cholesterol reduction yields clinical benefits: A new look at old data. *Circulation 91*, 2279–2282.

Grundy, S.M. (1994). Guidelines for cholesterol management: Recommendations of the National Cholesterol Education Program's Adult Treatment Panel II. *Heart Dis Stroke 3*, 123–127.

Jukema, J.W., Bruschke, A.V.G., van Boven, A.J., et al. (1995). Effects of lipid lowering by pravastatin on progression and regression of coronary artery disease in symptomatic men with normal to moderately elevated serum cholesterol levels. The Regression Growth Evaluation Statin Study (REGRESS). *Circulation 91*, 2528–2540.

Quion, J.A.V., & Gotto, A.M. (1994). Dyslipidemia. In M. Freed & C. Grines (eds.). *Essentials of Cardiovascular Medicine.* Birmingham, MI: Physician's Press, pp. 34–52.

Reaven, G.M. (1993). Are triglycerides important as a risk factor for coronary disease? *Heart Dis Stroke 2*, 44–48.

Sacks, F.M., Pfeffer, M.A., Moye, L., et al. (1991). Rationale and design of a secondary prevention trial of lowering normal plasma cholesterol levels after acute myocardial infarction: The Cholesterol and Recurrent Events Trial (CARE). *Am J Cardiol 68*, 1436–1446.

Schlant, R.C. (1993). Treatment of hypercholesterolemia in patients with known coronary artery disease. *Heart Dis Stroke 2*, 373–376.

The Scandinavian Simvastatin Survival Study Group. (1994). Randomized trial of cholesterol lowering in 4,444 patients with coronary heart disease. The Scandinavian Simvastatin Survival Study (4S). *Lancet 344*, 1383–1389.

Wissler, R.W., & Vesselinovich, D. (1977). Regression of atherosclerosis in experimental animals and man. *Mod Concepts Cardiovasc Dis 46*, 27.

Woodhead, G.A. (1996). The management of cholesterol in coronary heart disease risk reduction. *Nurse Pract 45*.

Angina Pectoris

DEFINITION

1. Angina pectoris is a common complaint of patients with CAD. It is the subjective report of chest discomfort associated with ischemia. It is typically described as a feeling of discomfort in the chest, is usually substernal, and lasts approximately 5–10 minutes. It may radiate to the arms, neck, mandible, back, or epigastrium. The quality of discomfort is often described as "pressure" or "squeezing" rather than sharp pain.
2. Angina is by definition transient and reversible.
3. It may be classified into one of several clinical syndromes that impact prognosis and therapy. These include chronic stable angina (fixed or variable threshold), new-onset angina, or unstable angina (progressive, rest, or postinfarct angina).
4. While angina often accompanies ischemia, some patients may experience ischemia without angina (silent ischemia).

ETIOLOGY/INCIDENCE

1. CAD remains the leading cause of mortality in the United States. It is estimated that 7.2 million individuals have prevalent CAD. Almost 1 million

Americans die from CAD-related events every year, and significant morbidity (myocardial ischemia, left ventricular dysfunction, arrhythmias, and hospitalization) occurs in many others.
2. Clinical manifestations of CAD include angina pectoris, myocardial infarction, heart failure, and sudden death.

PATHOPHYSIOLOGY

1. Angina is caused by transient myocardial ischemia caused by an imbalance between myocardial oxygen requirements (MvO_2) and oxygen supply.
2. Angina is due to either atherosclerotic (>90%) or nonatherosclerotic CAD (e.g., spasm, coronary artery anomalies).

SIGNS AND SYMPTOMS

Evaluation and Diagnosis of CAD

1. The evaluation of chest pain is a critical step in the care of patients with CAD. It is an important and common diagnostic challenge faced by the ACNP. Many conditions produce chest pains that may mimic myocardial ischemia including gastrointestinal, musculoskeletal, pulmonary, neurologic, psychiatric, and other cardiac disorders; CAD may be overdiagnosed in these cases.
2. CAD may be underdiagnosed when it manifests with atypical symptoms (dyspnea, nausea, vomiting, diaphoresis, and fatigue).
3. CV risk factors should be assessed (age, gender, family history, diabetes, smoking, hypercholesterolemia, hypertension, postmenopausal status).
4. It is important for the ACNP to detect signs of diseases that may contribute to or accompany atherosclerotic heart disease (e.g., diabetes mellitus [retinopathy or neuropathy], xanthelasma, tendinous xanthomas, hypertension, myxedema, or peripheral vascular disease).
5. Evaluation should include a R/O of diseases that may produce other forms of chest pain such as aortic stenosis or regurgitation, hypertrophic cardiomyopathy, and mitral valve prolapse.
6. Symptom characteristics, the presence of CAD risk factors, and ECG findings should be combined to estimate a patient's likelihood of having angina due to CAD.

PHYSICAL FINDINGS

Often physical signs are found during an attack of angina:
1. Dyspnea and diaphoresis.
2. New-onset S_4 frequently occurs because of decreased compliance of the ischemic ventricle.
3. Arrhythmias may be present, which may or may not be the cause of the angina.
4. Presence of a heart murmur may indicate valvular causes of angina: mitral valve prolapse, aortic stenosis, mitral stenosis, or idiopathic hypertrophic subaortic stenosis.
5. A significant elevation in systolic and diastolic blood pressure may occur during an angina attack, but hypotension may also occur with ischemia due to decreased cardiac output (CO).

DIFFERENTIAL DIAGNOSIS

1. Musculoskeletal: Costochondritis pain is often sharp in quality and usually persists for 1 or more hours, and is often worse at the end of the day and relieved by positional changes or heat; localized (point) tenderness may be present on physical exam.
2. Gastrointestinal: Pain due to peptic ulcer disease, esophageal reflux, esophageal spasm, cholecystitis, cholelithiasis, and pancreatitis. Gastrointestinal (GI) pain is not related to exertion, but may be related to anxiety; often related to meals; may last up to several hours; often relieved by bowel movement, antacid, and/or positional change. GI pain may be relieved by nitroglycerin (NTG) or calcium channel blockers (e.g., esophageal spasm). GI pain may precipitate anginal pain. The patient may have both GI disease and angina.
3. Pulmonary: Pain due to pulmonary embolism, pleurisy, pneumothorax, pneumonia with pleuritis, pulmonary hypertension.
4. Cardiovascular: Pain due to myocardial infarction, pericarditis, dissecting aortic aneurysm.
5. Infectious: Pain from herpes zoster.
6. Psychological: Anxiety-induced pain (Macklis, 1994).

DIAGNOSTIC TESTS/FINDINGS

1. Nitroglycerin test: Relief of chest pain or discomfort by the administration of NTG is strongly suggestive of angina pectoris but not diagnostic.
2. ECG: The ECG may show transient ischemic changes such as T-wave inversion or ST-segment depression or elevation during episodes of chest discomfort. ECG during ischemia: Horizontal or down-sloping ST-segment depression and/or T-wave inversion. Ischemia-free periods may show nonspecific ST-segment and T-wave changes, Q waves, and/or intraventricular conduction delay (IVCD), but ECG is often normal.
3. LV function studies (e.g., echo, left ventriculogram): During ischemia may show regional wall motion abnormalities and/or elevations in end-diastolic pressure. May be normal during ischemia-free periods or show persistent wall motion abnormalities due to infarction, stunned, or hibernating myocardium.

MANAGEMENT/TREATMENT

1. The therapeutic focus in patients with coronary disease is to address the symptoms *and* the underlying atherosclerosis disease process and improve the long-term patient outcome.
2. Patients with CAD and angina should be treated with therapies that have demonstrated effectiveness in altering the natural history of atherosclerosis, decrease cardiac events, and improve survival.
3. The ACNP in consultation with the physician should approach these goals of treatment in a stepwise fashion.

Risk Stratification (UCLA Practice Guidelines, 1995; Pepine, 1994)

1. All patients with known or suspected CAD, regardless of whether they present with chronic stable angina or unstable angina that has stabilized on

medical therapy, should undergo evaluation to estimate the likelihood of adverse outcome (risk stratification).

2. This process is necessary because subjective complaints of angina do not accurately reflect the true anatomic and functional severity of the atherosclerotic disease process.

3. Exercise or pharmacologic stress testing should be done as part of the inpatient or outpatient evaluation of low-risk patients with chest pain or unstable angina. Physiologic stress testing has prognostic value in chest pain and unstable angina to predict death and MI.

4. Choosing the initial stress testing modality should be based on an evaluation of the patient's resting ECG, the physical ability to perform exercise, and the imaging modality that is the most readily available.

5. The ACNP should consult with the physician regarding the results of stress testing, since false-positives and negatives may occur. Patient risk is based on the clinical presentation, risk factors, and stress testing results and not just a simple normal/abnormal reading of the stress test. History is important in decision making in these patients.

6. The ACNP should refer all patients to a cardiologist with a "high-risk" stress test result. Patients with unstable angina not responsive to medical therapy are usually referred for coronary angiography and revascularization.

7. The ACNP should refer patients with lifestyle-limiting symptoms that persist despite appropriate medical therapy. Coronary angiography and revascularization are reserved for these patients.

8. Randomized trials have begun to define the relative roles of percutaneous transluminal coronary angioplast (PTCA) versus medical therapy for patients with single-vessel CAD, and PTCA versus coronary artery bypass grafting (CABG) for patients with multivessel CAD.

CHRONIC STABLE ANGINA (Pepine, 1994)

Can be fixed threshold or variable threshold.

1. Fixed-threshold angina
   A. Angina can usually be predicted or reproduced whenever a fixed level of activity (often quantified by the heart rate–blood pressure product) is exceeded and typically relieved within a few minutes by rest or NTG.
   B. Myocardial ischemia is due to the presence of relatively fixed coronary atherosclerotic narrowing, which limits myocardial oxygen delivery during periods of increased oxygen demand.

2. Variable-threshold angina
   A. Angina may occur at different levels of activity (rate–pressure product), and may vary dramatically from day to day and even hour to hour.
   B. Cold, meals, smoking, emotion and anxiety can precipitate ischemia.
   C. Myocardial ischemia is due to the presence of an atherosclerotic coronary narrowing as well as transient increases in coronary vascular tone, resulting in both fixed and dynamic obstruction.

CHRONIC STABLE ANGINA (Pepine, 1994; UCLA Practice Guidelines, 1995)

1. Therapy
   A. Identify and control precipitating factors: pulmonary embolism (PE), GI bleed, sepsis, hyperthyroidism, hypoxemia, anemia, etc.
   B. Modify risk factors: hypertension control, weight reduction, smoking cessation, treatment of hyperlipidemias

C. Modify activity pattern: Instruct patient to avoid excessive fatigue, take rest periods, modify early morning activities due to an increased tendency for angina to occur in the A.M. (e.g., make bed slowly), minimize exposure to extremes of temperature, eat several smaller meals rather than a few large meals, avoid anxiety-provoking situations, and prophylaxis against activities known to precipitate angina with nitrates, and an extra dose of a short acting β-blocker).

D. Also, consider an individualized exercise prescription based on results of a symptom-limited exercise test. An aerobic exercise program consisting of moderate intensity activity 30–60 minutes five to seven times a week should be prescribed.

E. Perform a stress test off antianginal medications to confirm the diagnosis of ischemic heart disease and to risk stratify.

F. Cardiac catheterization and coronary angiography are indicated for high-risk test results.

2. Initiate stepped-care drug therapy (Fig. 3–1 outlines the management of chronic stable angina)

A. Aspirin: 160 mg/day or 325 mg/day (shown to decrease the incidence of death and nonfatal MI).

B. Nitrates are important first-line agents for the treatment of angina (Oates & Wood, 1987).

1) Sublingual NTG or inhaled spray to treat episodes or as prophylaxis against activities known to precipitate angina. If angina occurs more than three or four times per week, longer acting nitrates (transdermal or oral) should be prescribed.

2) A 10- to 12-hour nitrate-free interval is needed to minimize nitrate tolerance, which is caused by a depletion of intravascular sulfhydryl groups necessary to convert nitrates to nitric oxide (active agent). Table 3–14 lists doses and action of commonly used nitrate preparations.

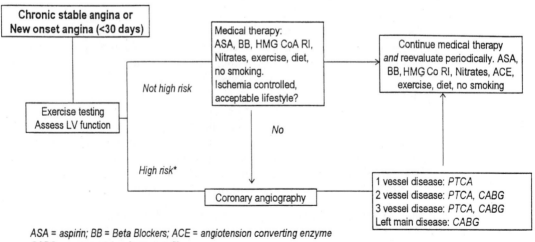

ASA = aspirin; BB = Beta Blockers; ACE = angiotension converting enzyme
CABG = coronary artery bypass grafting;:
LV = left ventricular; PTCA = percutaneous transluminal coronary angioplasty

FIGURE 3–1. Evaluation and management of chronic stable angina or new-onset angina. (Adapted from Gersh, B.J., Braunwald, E., & Rutherford, J.D. [1997]. Stable angina pectoris. In E. Braunwald [ed.]. *Heart Disease: A Textbook of Cardiovascular Medicine* [5th ed.]. Philadelphia: W.B. Saunders Co., pp. 1290–1316, with permission.)

TABLE 3–14. **Doses and Action of Commonly Used Nitrate Preparations***

Preparation	Dose	Onset	Duration
Sublingual nitroglycerin	0.3–0.6 mg	2–5 min	10–30 min
Aerosol nitroglycerin	0.4 mg	2–5 min	10–30 min
Sublingual/chewable isosorbide dinitrate	2.5–10.0 mg	10–30 min	1–2 hr
Oral isosorbide dinitrate	5–40 mg	30–60 min	4–6 hr
Oral isosorbide mononitrate	10–20 mg	30–60 min	6–8 hr
Oral sustained-release nitroglycerin	2.5–9.0 mg	30–60 min	2–8 hr
2% nitroglycerin ointment	0.5–2.0 in.	20–60 min	3–8 hr
Transdermal nitroglycerin patches	5–15 mg	>60 min	12–14 hr†

* From Winters, K.L., & Eisenberg, P.R. (1995). Angina pectoris. In: G.A. Ewald & C.R. McKenzie (eds.). *Manual of Medical Therapeutics: The Washington Manual* (28th ed.). Boston: Little, Brown & Co., pp. 85–93, with permission.
† Recommended maximum duration of application.

    C. β-Adrenergic antagonists are considered first-line agents in symptom management of stable angina. They reduce the frequency of episodes of angina and increase the exercise threshold for angina (Winters & Eisenberg, 1995).

        1) In general, β-blockers are prescribed if an arrhythmia, tachycardia, or hypertension is present. Table 3–15 lists doses and action of selected β-adrenergic antagonists.

    D. Cholesterol-lowering medications: Initiation of an HMG-CoA RI in patients with documented CAD results in a reduction in myocardial infarction, unstable angina, need for revascularization, and all-cause mortality compared to patients treated with diet alone. This is true regardless of whether the patient has undergone CABG, PTCA, or is being treated medically.

        1) These benefits are seen early such that patients should be started on therapy prior to or at the time of hospital discharge. Patients with CAD and an LDL cholesterol >100 mg/dL should be started on medication to lower cholesterol.

TABLE 3–15. **Doses and Actions of Selected β-Adrenergic Antagonists***

Agent	Oral Dose	Half-Life	Actions
β_1-selective			
Atenolol†,‡	50–100 mg qd	6–9 hr	β_1
Metoprolol†,‡	50–100 mg bid	3–4 hr	β_1
Acebutolol	200–600 mg bid	3–4 hr	β_1, ISA
Nonselective			
Propranolol†,‡	20–80 mg qid	4–6 hr	β_1, β_2
Propranolol-LA†	80–160 mg qd	10 hr	β_1, β_2
Nadolol†	40–160 mg qd	20–24 hr	β_1, β_2
Timolol‡	10–20 mg bid	3–4 hr	β_1, β_2
Pindolol	5–20 mg tid	3–4 hr	β_1, β_2, ISA
Labetalol	100–600 mg bid	6–8 hr	α, β_1, β_2

* From Winters, K.L., & Eisenberg, P.R. (1995). Angina pectoris. In G.A. Ewald & C.R. McKenzie (eds.). *Manual of Medical Therapeutics: The Washington Manual* (28th ed.). Boston: Little, Brown & Co., pp. 85–93, with permission.
† FDA-approved for treatment of angina.
‡ FDA-approved for treatment of MI.
ISA, intrinsic sympathomimetic activity; LA, long acting; FDA, Food and Drug Administration.

     2) The target lipid levels in patients with coronary artery disease is a total serum cholesterol <160 mg/dL, LDL cholesterol <100 mg/dL, and HDL cholesterol >45 mg/dL. HMG-CoA RI are the most effective and best-tolerated cholesterol-lowering medication and should be considered as the preferred first-line agent.

     3) Starting doses of common HMG-CoA RIs are:
       a. Lovastatin 20–40 mg qhs
       b. Pravastatin 20–40 mg qhs
       c. Simvastatin 10–20 mg qhs

E. Patients who fail to achieve target lipid levels (LDL <100 mg/dL) at 6 weeks to 3 months after initiation of therapy should have their dose increased or an additional agent (niacin or cholesterol-binding resin) added.

F. ACE inhibitors: These agents are not antianginal but have potent vascular and cardiac protective effects. Patients with coronary artery disease after myocardial infarction have improved survival and less heart failure when treated with ACE inhibitors. The risk of myocardial infarction or unstable angina, even the need for revascularization, is reduced with ACE inhibitor use. Patients with LV dysfunction should be started and maintained on an ACE inhibitor. In a patient with CAD and hypertension, ACE inhibitors are an excellent first-line agent. ACE inhibitors may also benefit patients with CAD by reversing endothelial dysfunction and lowering the risk of atherosclerosis progression.

G. Calcium channel blocker (CCB).
     1) In patients with angina there is a increased risk of coronary events with CCB as compared to angina control with β-blockers.
     2) These agents decrease chest pain but do not decrease the risk of a cardiac event or improve outcome. They should not be prescribed.
     3) In patients with CAD and hypertension these agents should be reserved for patients who are intolerant of or fail to have their blood pressure controlled with β-blockers, ACE inhibitors, diuretics, α-blockers, and their combination.
     4) CCBs should be considered for palliative use only in patients who have failed to respond to all other therapy. In patients with CAD following myocardial infarction, the risk of a subsequent cardiac event and mortality is not reduced and is in fact increased with CCB.
     5) In patients with CAD there may be an increased risk of myocardial infarction. In patients following angioplasty there is an increased risk of adverse events with CCB compared to placebo.

H. When ischemic control or lifestyle is unacceptable to the patient the ACNP should consult with the collaborating physician for possible referral for coronary angiography and revascularization.

Unstable Angina

DEFINITION

1. Unstable angina is a clinical syndrome characterized by angina of new onset; angina at rest or with minimal exertion; or a crescendo pattern of angina with episodes of increasing frequency, severity, or duration.

2. In the spectrum of CAD, unstable angina falls between stable angina and myocardial infarction.
3. Although the pathophysiology is heterogeneous, in most patients the transition from stable to unstable angina indicates abrupt progression of coronary stenosis due to rupture or fissuring of atherosclerotic plaques, resulting in thrombus formation, increased platelet reactivity, and increased coronary vasomotor tone (Fuster et al., 1992).
4. In a small subset of patients, unstable ischemic symptoms can be precipitated by conditions that increase cardiac demand (such as severe anemia, hyperthyroidism, hypertension, hypoxia, or heart failure) (Winters & Eisenberg, 1995).

MANAGEMENT/TREATMENT (Braunwald et al., 1990; Ewald & McKenzie, 1995; Pepine, 1994)

The goals of treatment are to aggressively relieve ischemic symptoms with antianginal drugs (using IV preparations when necessary), inhibit thrombosis in high-risk patients, and prevent progression of atherosclerosis.
1. Figure 3–2 outlines the management of unstable angina.
2. Management includes hospitalization in a monitored setting; bed rest; sedation; and correction of precipitating conditions such as hypertension, anemia, and hypoxemia.
3. Treatment of ischemia: In general, IV nitroglycerin is preferred to oral or cutaneous preparations because of the ability to rapidly achieve predictable blood levels of the drug.
   A. NTG 100 mg/250 mL @ 20 μg/min by continuous infusion titrated up to 100 μg/min until relief of chest pain or limiting side effects (hypotension with SBP <90 mm Hg).
   B. Topical, oral, or buccal nitrates are acceptable for patients without ongoing chest pain.
4. Anticoagulants and antiplatelets—IV heparin decreases the incidence of MI in patients with unstable angina (Theroux et al., 1988; Telford et al., 1981).
   A. Heparin 80 U/kg IV bolus; start @ 1000 U/hr and titrate to maintain a partial thromboplastin time (aPTT) between 1.5 to 2.5 times control.
   B. Aspirin (acetylsalicylic acid [ASA]) has been shown to reduce both mortality and the occurrence of nonfatal infarction in patients with unstable angina when administered either in low (160 mg qd) or high (325 mg q6h) dosages (Lewis et al., 1983; Cairns et al., 1985).
5. The combination of heparin and aspirin has not been shown to provide a greater reduction in the risk of MI but has been associated with increased bleeding complications (Theroux et al., 1988). To avoid reactivation of unstable angina, aspirin should be started before the discontinuation of heparin.
6. Patients in whom PTCA is contemplated should be treated with aspirin, but this may be associated with more bleeding complications in patients referred for CABG.
7. Patients should receive a β-adrenergic antagonist when not contraindicated. β-Blockers reduce the risk of progression to AMI and improve survival in patients with acute coronary insufficiency. The target resting heart rate for between blockade is 50–60 bpm.

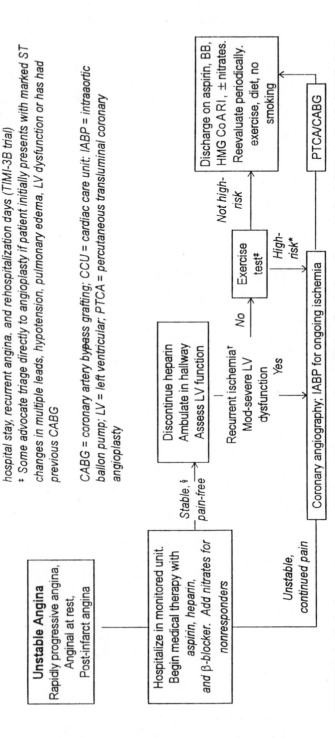

FIGURE 3-2. Evaluation and management of unstable angina. (Adapted from Gersh, B.J., Brunwald, E. & Rutherford, J.D. [1997]. Stable angina pectoris. In E. Braunwald [ed.]. *Heart Disease: A Textbook of Cardiovascular Medicine* [5th ed.]. Philadelphia: W.B. Saunders Co., pp. 1290–1316, with permission.)

8. Metoprolol
    A. 5-mg increments by slow (over 1–2 minutes) IV administration.
    B. Repeated every 5 minutes for a total initial dose of 15 mg.
    C. Followed in 1–2 hours by 25–50 mg PO q6h.
    D. If a very conservative regimen is desired, initial doses can be reduced to 1–2 mg.
9. Propranolol
    A. 0.5- to 1.0-mg IV dose
    B. Followed in 1–2 hours by 40–80 mg PO q6–8 h.
10. Esmolol
    A. Starting maintenance dose of 0.1 mg/kg/min IV.
    B. Titration in increments of 0.05 mg/kg/min every 10–15 minutes as tolerated by blood pressure until the desired therapeutic response has been obtained, limiting symptoms develop, or a dose of 0.20 mg/kg/min is reached.
    C. Optional loading dose of 0.5 mg/kg may be given by slow IV administration (2–5 minutes) for more rapid onset of action.
11. Atenolol
    A. 5-mg IV dose
    B. Followed 5 minutes later by a second 5-mg IV dose and then 50–100 mg PO qd initiated 1–2 hours after the IV dose.
12. Narcotic analgesics such as morphine sulphate (MS) are reserved for treatment of patients with pain that is refractory to aggressive medical therapy.
    A. MS 2–5 mg IV, may repeat every 5–30 minutes.
13. Intra-aortic balloon pump (IABP) counterpulsation is indicated in patients with ischemic symptoms that are refractory to medical therapy. Because this procedure is associated with a 10–15% risk of significant vascular complications, it should only be used to stabilize the patient's condition before CABG or PTCA.

Review Questions

3.16 A 75-year-old man awaiting CABG has persistent angina with ECG changes despite use of IV NTG @ 100 μg/min, 50% face mask SaO$_2$ 97%, BP 95/60, HR 62. The best course of action would be:
    A. Increase NTG infusions to 150 μg/min
    B. Intubate and institute control mechanical ventilation
    C. Add dopamine 5 μg/kg/min to increase BP
    D. Call collaborating physician to consider IABP counterpulsation therapy

3.17 Which of the following medications should this patient be receiving?
    A. ASA and heparin
    B. NTG and NTP
    C. Dopamine @ low dose 5 μg/kg/min
    D. Lasix and potassium

3.18 Which of the following are diagnostic imaging techniques that can be used to stress patients who cannot take a standard stress test because of physical limitations?
    A. CT scan
    B. PET scan

C. Dobutamine echo

D. Esophageal echo

3.19 Unstable angina is characterized by all of the following but one. Which one does not characterize unstable angina?

A. Increasing frequency of chest pain

B. Chest pain at rest

C. Elevation of ST segments

D. Increasing severity of symptoms

3.20 Research to date shows beneficial effects of all but one of the following treatments for unstable angina.

A. ASA

B. β-Blockers

C. Heparin

D. CCB

Answers and Rationales

3.16 **D** Intra-aortic balloon counterpulsation is indicated in patients with ischemic symptoms that are refractory to medical therapy.

3.17 **A** ASA and heparin inhibit thrombosis in high-risk patients.

3.18 **C** Dobutamine echo.

3.19 **C** ECG during ischemia: horizontal or down-sloping ST-segment depression and/or T-wave depression.

3.20 **D** CCB should be considered for palliative use only in patients who have failed to respond to all other therapy. In patients with CAD following myocardial infarction, the risk of a subsequent cardiac event and mortality is not reduced and is in fact increased with CCB.

References

Braunwald, E., Jones, R.H., Mark, D.B., et al. (1994). Diagnosing and managing unstable angina. *Circulation 90*(1), 613–622.

Braunwald, E., Mark, D.B., Jones, R.H., et al. (1994). *Unstable Angina: Diagnosis and Management.* Clinical Practice Guideline No. 10 (amended) AHCPR Publication No. 94-0602. Rockville, MD: Agency for Health Care Policy and Research and the National Heart, Lung, and Blood Institute, Public Health Service, U.S. Department of Health and Human Services.

Cairns, J.A., Gent, M., & Singer, J., et al. (1985). Aspirin, sulfinpyrazone, or both in unstable angina: Results of a Canadian multicenter trial. *N Engl J Med 313*, 1369–1375.

Douglas, P.S., & Ginsburg, G.S. (1996). The evaluation of chest pain in women. *N Engl J Med 334*(20), 1311–1315.

Fuster, V., Badimon, L., Badimon J.J., & Chesebro J.H. (1992). The pathogenesis of coronary artery disease and the acute coronary syndromes, *N Engl J Med 326*, 242–250, 310–318.

Gersh, B.J., Braunwald, E., & Rutherford, J.D. (1997). Stable angina pectoris. In E. Braunwald (ed.). *Heart Disease: A Textbook of Cardiovascular Medicine* (5th ed.). Philadelphia: W.B. Saunders Co., pp. 1290–1316.

Lewis, H.D.J., Davis, J.W., & Archibald, D.G., et al. (1983). Protective effects of aspirin against acute myocardial infarction and death in men with unstable angina: Results of a Veterans Administration Cooperative Study. *N Engl J Med 309*, 396–403.

Macklis, R.M., Mendelsohn, M.E., & Mudge, G.H. (eds.). (1994). Cardiovascular diseases. *Introduction to Clinical Medicine* (3rd ed.). Boston: Little, Brown & Co., pp. 177–207.

Massie, B.M., & Amidon, T.A. (1997). Angina pectoris. In L.M. Tierney, Jr., S.J. McPhee, & M.A. Papadakis (eds.). *Current Medical Diagnosis & Treatment* (36th ed.). Stamford, CT: Appleton & Lange, pp. 347–357.

Oates, J.A., & Wood, A.J.J. (1987). Nitrate therapy in stable angina pectoris. *N Engl J Med 316*, 1635–1642.

Pepine, C.J. (1994). Angina pectoris. In M. Freed & C. Grines (eds.). *Essentials of Cardiovascular Medicine*. Birmingham, MI: Physician's Press, pp. 54–86.

Telford, A.M., & Wilson, C. (1981). Trial of heparin versus atenolol in prevention of myocardial infarction in intermediate coronary syndrome. *Lancet 1*, 1225–1228.

Theroux, P., Ouimet, H., McCans, J., et al. (1988). Aspirin, heparin or both to treat acute unstable angina. *N Engl J Med 319*, 1105–1111.

UCLA Practice Guidelines Committee. (1995). *Practice Guidelines for Chest Pain and Unstable Angina*. Regents of the University of California. Division of Cardiology.

Winters, K.L., & Eisenberg, P.R. (1995). Angina pectoris. In G.A. Ewald & C.R. McKenzie (eds.). *Manual of Medical Therapeutics: The Washington Manual* (28th ed.). Boston: Little, Brown & Co., pp. 85–93.

Acute Myocardial Infarction

DEFINITION

AMI is defined as necrosis to myocardial tissue that results from cessation of blood flow to a portion of the myocardium. Progressive myocardial necrosis begins in the subendocardium and spreads to the epicardium.

ETIOLOGY/INCIDENCE

The mechanism of AMI is a ruptured atherosclerotic plaque that occurs in a moderate (<70%) stenosis. Collagen fibers are exposed, which activates platelets, initiates the coagulation cascade, and results in acute coronary occlusion. Without reperfusion therapy, progressive myocardial necrosis, ventricular dysfunction, arrhythmias, and in some cases death may ensue.

Types of Infarcts: Q-Wave Versus Non–Q-Wave MI

1. Q-wave: Q-waves on the ECG occurs with complete thrombotic coronary occlusion, which occurs in 80% of AMI patients and usually results in transmural myocardial necrosis.
2. Non–Q-wave: A non–Q-wave (previously called "subendocardial") MI occurs in patients who have well-developed collateral flow or who spontaneously reperfuse.
   A. This type of infarct results in a smaller infarction, better preservation of LV function, and lower in-hospital mortality.
   B. Non–Q-wave infarctions are "incomplete" (i.e., residual viable myocardium supplied by a diseased coronary artery), reinfarction rates are higher than those observed with Q-wave MI; by 1 year, mortality rates are similar.

C. Aggressive diagnostic and therapeutic evaluation is necessary in non–Q-wave MI (Grines, 1994).

SIGNS AND SYMPTOMS

Chest pain occurs with myocardial cellular ischemia (an imbalance between oxygen supply and demand) while local metabolic changes occur.

Myocardial Infarction Pain

1. Location: Substernal, can radiate to one or both arms (primarily left), to the neck, jaw, teeth, and back
2. Quality: Squeezing, crushing, pressure, heaviness, dull, aching, deep, strangling, tightness
3. Intensity: Can be mild to excruciating
4. Duration: >15–30 minutes; if pain was intermittent it is important to determine when pain become constant.
5. Precipitating trigger: What precipitated pain or what precipitated pain to become constant
6. Relieved by morphine (nitroglycerin may decrease pain by increasing collateral flow)
7. Nonverbal clues to assess for pain: Clenched fist over chest, facial expression of apprehension, pain or grimaces, degree of eye contact, ineffectiveness of narcotics, decreased movement in bed due to fear of pain.

Atypical MI Presentations

1. Atypical presentations such as fatigue, weakness, dyspnea, and heart failure are common in elderly and diabetics.
    A. Up to 20% of infarcts may be "silent," or unrecognized by the health care provider or patient.
2. The sensation of pain may be masked in the elderly, diabetic, or hypertensive patient due to peripheral neuropathy or altered sensorium.
3. Women describe pain more vaguely than men; they also present with more atypical symptoms then men, such as weakness and fatigue.

OBJECTIVE

Chest pain is not always the hallmark symptom of a cardiac problem. The following are other objective findings, some of which may be the presenting symptom instead of chest pain.
1. Dyspnea—The ACNP needs to R/O possible AMI with any elderly patient presenting with a chief complaint of dyspnea, regardless of a history of pulmonary or cardiac congestion. Some patients may have decreased pain sensation due to peripheral neuropathy (as in diabetes).
2. Nausea, vomiting (commonly seen with inferior infarctions).
3. Decreased level of consciousness.
4. Temperature elevation.
5. Blood pressure lability (either increased or decreased).
6. Heart sounds:
    A. Softer S_1 and S_2 heart sounds
    B. Newly developed S_4 heart sounds or becomes louder with pain

    C. S_3 heart sound indicates ventricular failure

    D. Transient pericardial friction rub or systolic murmur

7. Lung sounds—crackles in lung bases (Baldwin, 1995).

DIAGNOSTIC TESTS/FINDINGS (From Grines, 1994)

Electrocardiogram

1. The first ECG may be nondiagnostic (in approximately 44% of patients) and show nonspecific ST-segment and T-wave changes or only hyperacute T waves.
2. The ACNP must repeat the ECG in 20–30 minutes to assess for ST-segment elevation and consideration of thrombolytic/reperfusion therapy.

Guidelines for Reperfusion Therapy

1. ECG changes consistent with AMI: ST-segment elevation ≥1 mm in two or more contiguous leads (anterior, inferior, lateral) confirms the diagnosis.
    A. A pseudoinfarction pattern may be seen in patients with LV hypertrophy, Wolff-Parkinson-White syndrome, and pericarditis.
2. A new left bundle branch block (LBBB) should be treated as an MI if there is a strong clinical suspicion.
3. If the ECG does not show ST-segment elevation or is uninterpretable, the ACNP should consider use of posterior chest leads, which may detect a posterior MI due to circumflex occlusion.
4. For paced rhythms, the ACNP should consult with the cardiologist to temporarily reprogram pacemaker to a lower rate; this allows the intrinsic rhythm to be observed (*note:* in some patients, pacemaker-induced repolarization abnormalities may persist).
5. Table 3–16 shows ECG changes associated with different MIs, and the location of the coronary artery lesion.

Enzymes

1. AMI treatment should be initiated immediately, without waiting for enzyme elevation.
2. The ACNP should obtain creatine phosphokinase (CPK) total and CK-MB q6–8h times 3; at least 3 negative values are required to rule out MI.
3. Creatine kinase–MB band levels usually rise by 8–10 hours and return to normal within 48 hours.
4. Myocardial assays such as troponin I and T allow for more rapid diagnosis of AMI. Clinical studies have demonstrated improved time-dependent sensitivity and improved specificity for troponin I and T compared to CK-MB (Apple et al., 1995; Adams et al., 1993). Patients with acute MI have an earlier rise in troponin I and T than CK-MB (Mair et al., 1995; Katus et al., 1991). Using troponin I by 7 hours after symptom onset there is a 95% detection of patients who are shown to have an MI.
5. Lactate dehydrogenase isoenzyme 1 (LDH-1) exceeds LDH-2 at 3–5 days. Obtain daily times 3 if patient presents more than 24 hours after suspected MI.

TABLE 3–16.   Myocardial Infarction and Coronary Artery Lesion*

Type	Affected Artery	Affected Area	ECG Findings
Anterior infarction	Left coronary artery or branches	Anterior portion, left ventricle Two thirds of ventricular septum Bundle of His, right and left branches	V_3–V_4: Q waves V_2–V_6: R-wave progression missing
Anteroseptal infarction	Left coronary artery Left anterior descending artery	Anterior wall, left ventricle Intraventricular septum	V_1–V_4: Q waves R wave, poor progression
Inferior infarction	Right coronary artery Dominant left circumflex artery	Inferior or diaphragmatic left ventricular wall AV node Sinus node	II, III, aVF: New or deeper Q waves, ST-segment elevation, or T wave inverted
Posterior infarction	Right coronary artery Circumflex artery	Posterior left ventricle	V_1–V_2: Reciprocal changes; ST-segment depression; R waves tall, symmetric and reversed poles
Right ventricular infarction	Distal right coronary artery	Right ventricle Left ventricle inferior wall	II, III, aVF, V_3R, and V_4R: ST-segment elevation, Q waves
Lateral infarction	Circumflex artery Left anterior descending artery	Lateral wall, left ventricle	I, aVL, V_5, V_6: New or deeper Q waves, ST-segment elevation

* Adapted from Baldwin, K.M., Garza, C.S., Martin, R.N., et al. (1995). Acute myocardial infarction. In *Davis's Manual of Critical Care Therapeutics*. Philadelphia: F.A. Davis Co., pp. 87–92, with permission.
ECG, electrocardiographic; AV, atrioventricular.

6. A technetium pyrophosphate scan may be useful if LDH levels are equivocal or the patient presents more than 3 days after suspected MI.

Echocardiogram

1. In patients with continued chest pain and nondiagnostic ECGs the ACNP should consult with the cardiologist and consider ordering an echocardiogram.
2. Regional hypokinesis may indicate critical ischemia or infarction, which may be old or new. Myocardial thinning suggests old infarction.
3. Nondiagnostic ECG and absence of regional or global LV dysfunction on a high-quality echo (i.e., visualizes all endocardial surfaces) places the patient at very low probability of infarction.

Emergency Cardiac Catheterization (Grines, 1994)

1. The ACNP should refer patients with cardiac risk factors who have continued chest pain and abnormal but nondiagnostic ECGs (e.g., ST-segment depression, T-wave inversion) for emergent cardiac catheterization.
2. Regional LV hypokinesis and thrombotic coronary occlusion confirm the diagnosis of MI.
3. PTCA can provide immediate coronary artery reperfusion.
4. A stent can aid in stabilizing the artery and decrease early reocclusion.

MANAGEMENT/TREATMENT (Grines, 1994)

Management of the critically ill MI patient is primarily done by the physician. The ACNP consults with the collaborating physician throughout the treatment of this patient.

Therapeutic management is divided into interventions for the following phases:
1. Acute-phase treatment
   A. Reperfusion therapy
   B. Medical therapy (research-based interventions)
2. Postacute phase

Acute Phase: Reperfusion Therapy

The ACNP needs to be familiar with the rationale for reperfusion therapy as well as the specific institutional protocols and procedures for reperfusion therapy. The following information will aid the ACNP in this process.
1. If AMI patients with ST-segment elevation or LBBB are treated with reperfusion therapy within 12 hours, there is a reduction in mortality.
2. Thrombolytic therapy is clearly beneficial to many MI patients; several limitations exist including acute patient eligibility (only 25–35% of infarcts treated in the United States).
3. Emergent PTCA and stenting is used in many institutions for reperfusion therapy.
4. Advantages to PTCA include high infarct vessel patency rates (>95%), low rates of recurrent ischemia and reinfarction, avoidance of intracranial bleeding, shortened length of hospital stay, and ability to treat thrombolytic-ineligible patients.
5. PTCA may be the treatment of choice for some; if PTCA is not readily available, the ACNP needs to reassess patients for thrombolytic therapy or consider transferring to an institution with cardiac catheterization and PTCA facilities.
6. Table 3–17 lists AMI treatment based on ECG and chest pain duration.

Thrombolytics for Reperfusion Therapy

The ACNP needs to be familiar with institutional protocols for medications used for reperfusion therapy. Table 3–18 delineates various thrombolytic regimens, dosages, and important clinical information for the ACNP when ordering these agents.

Primary PTCA for Reperfusion Therapy

1. Studies suggest more rapid and more complete recovery of wall motion with primary PTCA, less post-MI ischemia, shorter hospitalization, and less need for further revascularization procedures.
2. Mortality is significantly reduced in acute MI patients, especially those at high risk (anterior MI, sinus tachycardia [HR >100], and elderly age [>70]), with primary angioplasty compared to thrombolytic agents.
3. Primary PTCA improves survival from 20% (medical therapy alone) to 50% in cardiogenic shock.

TABLE 3–17.   Reperfusion Based on ECG and Chest Pain Duration*

Condition	Treatment			Comments
	Lytic	Medical (No Lytic)	Acute Cath, Direct PTCA	
ST elevation or LBBB	X		X	• Mortality reduction if treated with lytics in setting of bundle branch block (24% vs. 19%, $p < .01$), anterior ST elevation (17% vs. 13%, $p < .00001$), or inferior ST elevation (8.4% vs. 7.5%, $p < .08$) treated within 24 hr (greatest benefit observed if treated within 12 hr (*Lancet* 1994; 343:311).
Chest pain duration (ST elevation or LBBB)				• If lytics are administered within 6 hr, mortality reduction is 24%. If treated within 1 hr, mortality reduction approaches 50%; MI may actually be aborted in some.
<6 hr	X		X	
6–12 hr, ongoing pain	X		X	• 17–27% mortality reduction with lytics, regardless of pain status (*Lancet* 1993;342:767; *Lancet* 1993;342:759)
6–12 hr, no pain	X	X	X	• Reperfusion therapy is generally reserved for large infarcts (anterior MI or ST elevation in five or more leads). • If small infarct or patient has increased risk of bleeding (elderly, hypertensive, etc.), medical therapy may be appropriate.
12–24 hr, ongoing pain			X	• Ongoing pain suggests viable myocardium (intermittent opening and closing of artery or well-developed collaterals). • Reperfusion rates with lytics are inversely proportional to time delay. In contrast, PTCA reperfusion rates are independent of time (*Circulation* 1987;76:142).
12–24 hr, no pain		X		• No proven benefit of lytics (*Lancet* 1993;342:767; *Lancet* 1993;342:759)
>24 hr		X		• No proven benefit but limited data available.
ECG†				
ST-segment depression		X	X	• Patients who infarct with ST depression have mortality rates of 10–18% (*J Am Coll Cardiol* 1990;16:223), a higher prevalence of multivessel disease, and lower ejection fractions than infarcts without ST elevation (*J Am Coll Cardiol* 1991;17:45A) • A trend toward increased mortality was observed among patients treated with thrombolytics; therefore, lytics are generally avoided in this setting (*Lancet* 1994;343:311)
Ischemic T-waves only		X		• Low risk; no benefit from lytics (*Lancet* 1986; 1:349). Consider echo to screen for regional hypokinesis and cath if a strong clinical suspicion exists.
Normal ECG		X		• If repeated ECGs are entirely normal, the probability of MI is low (*Am J Cardiol* 1991; 68:171)

* Adapted from Grines, C.L. (1994). Myocardial Infarction. In M. Freed & C. Grines (eds.). *Essentials of Cardiovascular Medicine*. Birmingham, MI: Physicians' Press, p. 90, with permission.

† If initial ECG does not show ST elevation or LBBB, it should be repeated in 30 minutes.

ECG, electrocardiogram; Cath, catheterization; PTCA, percutaneous transluminal coronary angioplasty; LBBB, left bundle branch block; MI, myocardial infarction.

TABLE 3–18.   Thrombolytic Regimens*

Thrombolytic Agent	Dosage/Heparin	Acute Patency	Systemic Lysis	Comments
Streptokinase (SK)	1.5 million U IV over 30–60 min Heparin: No	50%	Yes	• Least expensive and least likely to cause intracranial bleeding (*Lancet* 1990;27:121; Lancet 1992;339:753; *N Engl J Med* 1992;327:1; *N Engl J Med* 1993; 329:673). • Drug of choice for the elderly (age >75 years) and patients with severe hypertension (*Lancet* 1993;342:1523). • IV heparin is not necessary for reduction in mortality or reinfarction (*N Engl J Med* 1993; 329:673); subcutaneous heparin is of questionable benefit (*Lancet* 1990;27:121; *Lancet* 1992;339: 753; *N Engl J Med* 1992;327:1).
Urokinase (UK)	1.5 million U IV bolus and 1.5 million U IV over 1 hr Heparin: Unknown	70%	Yes	• Expensive. • No proven advantage over SK. • IV heparin is commonly used acutely, but no data on benefit.
Anistreplase (anisoylated plasminogen streptokinase activator complex [APSAC])	30 U IV bolus over 3–5 min Heparin: No	70%	Yes	• Expensive. • No proven benefit over SK (*Lancet* 1992;339:753). • Avoid if culture-proven streptococcal infection within the past several months or prior SK/APSAC allergy or use in the past 1–2 years. • Bolus dosing facilitates prehospital administration. • IV heparin is not necessary to maintain patency or improve clinical outcome (*J Am Coll Cardiol* 1994;23:11).
Tissue plasminogen activator (t-PA)	100 mg maximum: • 15 mg bolus *and* • 0.75 mg/kg over 30 min *and* • 0.5 mg/kg over next 60 min Heparin: Yes	80%	No	• Expensive. • Highest risk of intracranial bleed (*Lancet* 1990;27:121; *Lancet* 1992;339:753; *N Engl J Med* 1992;327:1; *N Engl J Med* 1993; 329:673). • Slight mortality advantage over SK if accelerated dosing regimen and IV heparin are used, and patients are treated early (<4 hr) (*N Engl J Med* 1993;329:673). • Acute IV heparin is *essential* to maintain coronary patency and should be continued for 3–7 days.

* Adapted from Grines, C.L. (1994). Myocardial Infarction. In M. Freed & C. Grines (eds.). *Essentials of Cardiovascular Medicine*. Birmingham, MI: Physicians' Press, pp. 99–101, with permission.

† Pharmacy cost at William Beaumont Hospital.

4. The use of Reopro should be considered as an adjunct to direct angioplasty. Reopro inhibits platelet aggregation by preventing the binding of fibrinogen, von Willebrand factor, and other adhesive molecules to the GPIIa/IIIb receptor. In the EPIC and CAPTURE trials the acute complication, mortality, and reintervention rates were significantly reduced.

5. Direct coronary stenting should be considered to increase the initial success rate and decrease subsequent restenosis.

6. If primary PTCA is used the ACNP should be familiar with the inclusion criteria based on chest pain duration, ECG, comorbid conditions, as well as thrombolytic exclusion due to bleeding risk. These patients may benefit from primary PTCA for reperfusion.

7. The ACNP needs to recognize AMI patients in cardiogenic shock so immediate cardiology referral is made and proper treatment is initiated in collaboration with the cardiologist (see "Shock").

Other Interventions for Therapeutic Management of AMI

In consultation with the physician, the ACNP should initiate additional therapy that is research based and has been found to impact AMI mortality and morbidity (therapies # 1 through 5, below). The following section on adjunct AMI therapy in acute and post acute phase is compiled from the following references: UCLA AMI Practice Guidelines (1997); Altman & Braunwald (1997); Hennekens et al. (1996); and Grines (1994).

1. Aspirin
   A. Dose
      1) 160–324 mg chewed acutely then PO daily
      2) Contraindications: active bleeding
   B. Evidence from clinical trials
      1) Acute therapy: enhanced patency and reduced reocclusion after lysis, reduced reinfarction, stroke, and death (ISIS-2, 1988)
2. Anticoagulants
   A. Dose
      1) IV heparin: Bolus 100 U/kg followed by an infusion of 1000–1300 U/hr (adjust to achieve aPTT 2–2.5 × normal) (*Note:* dosage and use may change based on thrombolytic agent used; see Table 3–18.)
   B. Indications
      1) IV heparin when tissue plasminogen activator (t-PA) is used, and for patients who present with anterior MI, low cardiac output, atrial fibrillation (AFIB), or LV thrombus; Low-dose subcutaneous (SQ) heparin in all others, during periods of immobilization
   C. Evidence from clinical trials
      1) The use of IV heparin is probably necessary for 1% mortality benefit of accelerated t-PA over streptokinase (SK) (GUSTO, 1993). After t-PA, IV heparin should be given for 5–7 days to reduce reocclusion rates.
      2) Routine heparin is probably not necessary after SK or anisoylated plasminogen streptokinase activator complex (APSAC), since it did not reduce rates of reinfarction or death; a significant increase in bleeding complications was observed, however (GISSI-2, 1990; ISIS-3, 1992; GUSTO, 1993).
3. β-Blockers
   A. Dose

     1) Metoprolol 5 mg IV q2min × 3, followed in 15 minutes by 50 mg PO bid × 2, and then 100 mg PO bid if tolerated, *or*

     2) Atenolol 5 to 10 mg IV followed by 100 mg PO qd

  B. Indications

     1) All MI patients except those with hypotension, bradycardia, severe heart failure, or a history of bronchospasm

  C. Evidence from clinical trials

     1) Acute β-blockade has been shown to limit infarct size and reduce mortality by 13% (Yusufet et al., 1985), to significantly reduce ventricular fibrillation and cardiac rupture (Norris et al., 1984), and to reduce reinfarction and intracranial hemorrhage after lytics (Roberts et al., 1991).

4. ACE Inhibitor

  A. Dose

     1) Captopril (initial dose: 6.25, titrate to 50 mg PO bid–tid as tolerated)

     2) Lisinopril (10 mg PO qd), ramipril (2.5–5 mg PO bid) and others probably as effective; start low-dose within few days of MI, titrate, continue indefinitely

  B. Indications

     1) Symptomatic heart failure, asymptomatic patients following MI with ejection fractions <40%

  C. Evidence from clinical trials

     1) Reduced short- and long-term mortality in asymptomatic patients following MI with ejection fraction <40% (Pfeffer et al., 1992; ISIS-4 and GISSI-3, unpublished data).

     2) Reduced rates of recurrent MI, progression to heart failure, and need for rehospitalization (Pfeffer et al., 1992).

5. Nitroglycerin

  A. Dose

     1) NTG 100/250 mL D_5W @ 10–20 μg/min IV, increase by 5–10, μ/min q5min till relief of chest pain or SBP <90.

     2) Avoid if hypotensive, RV infarct.

     3) Tolerance (lack of efficacy) may occur after 1 day of continuous therapy

  B. Indications

     1) Ischemic chest pain/AMI

  C. Evidence from clinical trials

     1) IV nitroglycerin may decrease infarct size and mortality for patients treated within 4 hours of anterior MI (Yusuf et al., 1988).

6. Morphine

  A. Dose

     1) 2–5 mg IV q5–30min for pain.

     2) Avoid if chronic lung disease (increased risk of respiratory depression).

     3) Morphine effects may be reversed with naloxone (0.4–2.0 mg IV).

  B. Indications

     1) In addition to its analgesic properties, morphine dilates peripheral venous and arterial beds, thereby reducing both preload and afterload.

  C. Evidence from clinical trials

     1) No studies proving efficacy

7. Oxygen
    A. Dose
        1) Start @ 2–4 L/min by nasal cannula.
    B. Indications
        1) Pulse oximetry should be used to determine need for oxygen therapy if SaO_2 <97%.
    C. Evidence from clinical trials
        1) Given by convention but no clear data support its routine use
        2) May increase vascular resistance
8. Lidocaine (not considered for every AMI patient, see indications)
    A. Dose
        1) Loading dose (IV bolus 1 mg/kg followed by 0.5 mg/kg bolus 10 minutes later); infusion rate 1–4 mg/min; reduce dose for the elderly and patients with CHF
    B. Indications
        1) Sustained or recurrent, hemodynamically significant nonsustained VT
        2) Toxic signs: Confusion, drowsiness, respiratory depression, perioral numbness, seizures
    C. Evidence from clinical trials
        1) Prophylactic lidocaine is not recommended—38% increase in mortality, primarily due to asystole (Yusuf et al., 1990).

Postacute Phase: Therapeutic Management

1. Aspirin
    A. Dose
        1) 160–324 mg PO daily
        2) Contraindications: Active bleeding
    B. Evidence from clinical trials
        1) Long-term aspirin therapy following MI: Significant reduction in mortality and reinfarction (Antiplatelet Trailists' Collaboration, 1988).
2. Chronic β-blocker
    A. Dose
        1) Propranolol 60 mg tid–qid
        2) Timolol 20 mg qd
        3) Start acutely and continue at least 2 years
    B. Indications
        1) All MI patients unless low-risk subset. Patients with good LV function—without angina, arrhythmia, or ischemia during functional testing—have an excellent survival, making the benefit of secondary prevention with long-term β-blockade controversial (i.e., side effects may outweight benefits).
        2) Contraindications: Symptomatic bradycardia, heart block, asthma, COPD.
    C. Evidence from clinical trials
        1) Long-term β-blockade reduces the rate of reinfarction and death (primarily sudden death) up to 6 years after MI (*JAMA* 1982;347:1707; *N Engl J Med* 1981;304:801).
        2) No data available as to whether β-blockade is beneficial in MI patients who have undergone PTCA or CABG. Generally, if the patient

is revascularized, asymptomatic, and does not have exercise-induced ischemia, β-blockers are withheld.

    3) No difference between nonselective and selective agents, although β-blockers without intrinsic sympathomimetic activity (ISA) appear to be more effective than those with ISA (Yusuf et al., 1985).

3. Chronic Warfarin
   A. Dose
      1) Start Coumadin loading dose of 10 mg PO hs; Goal—INR 2.5–4.5
   B. Indications
      1) Patients with LV thrombus or chronic risk of thromboembolic complications (AFIB, low cardiac output, prolonged immobilization)
      2) Contraindications: Active bleeding
   C. Evidence from clinical trials
      1) Long-term anticoagulation (without aspirin) has been shown to reduce the rate of recurrent MI and death (*N Engl J Med* 1990;323: 147; *Lancet* 1970;1:203).
      2) Compared to aspirin alone, warfarin failed to show a reduction in reclusion (Meijer et al., 1993) or mortality (EPSIM, 1982).
      3) Additional studies comparing warfarin and aspirin, alone or in combination, are ongoing.

4. ACE Inhibitors
   A. Dose
      1) Captopril 50 mg PO bid–tid as tolerated
      2) Continue indefinitely
   B. Evidence from clinical trials
      1) Reduced rates of recurrent MI progression to heart failure, and need for rehospitalization (Pfeffer et al., 1992)

5. NTG SL: The ACNP should ensure that at the time of discharge every MI patient is given NTG sublingually (SL)
   A. Dose
      1) NTG 1/150 grain SL prn chest pain.
      2) The ACNP needs to ensure that the patient knows what to do if chest pain reoccurs at home and how to use NTG.
      3) Oral/topical nitrates are not routinely recommended.
   B. Indications
      1) Chest pain
   C. Evidence from clinical trials
      1) Oral nitrates given at day 1 after MI did not alter mortality at 1 month (ISIS-4 and GISSI-3, unpublished data).

6. Antiarrhythmic
   A. Indications
      1) Not recommended unless sustained ventricular tachycardia (VT) >48 hours after MI
   B. Evidence from clinical trials
      1) Suppression of chronic premature ventricular contractions (PVCs) following acute MI with encainide or trend for increased mortality with moricizin (CASTII, 1992).
      2) Amiodarone may be beneficial in patients ineligible for β-blockers (Ceremuzynski et al., 1992) and for those with complex ectopy (Bukart et al., 1990).
      3) Implantable defibrillator trials in progress.

7. HMG-CoA RI
    A. Indications
        1) Recommended for all AMI patients
    B. Evidence from clinical trials
        1) In patients with CAD use of HMG-CoA RI lowers the risk of recurrent events, need for revascularization, and mortality.
        2) In the 4S trail there was a 34% risk reduction in major cardiac events, a 42% risk reduction in cardiovascular mortality, and a 30% reduction in all-cases mortality associated with stain treatment. The CARE and REGRESS trials demonstrated that even patients with "normal" levels of total cholesterol and LDL cholesterol benefit from treatment with HMG-CoA RI.
        3) Patients should be educated that these medications are for the treatment of atherosclerosis, not because the patient has failed dietary treatment.

Nonpharmacologic Interventions

1. Exercise
    A. Patients should receive specific instructions for a daily aerobic exercise program. Exercise increases HDL, reduces the risk of MI, and improves survival in patients with CAD.
    B. Either a home-based program or supervised cardiac rehabilitation is recommended.
    C. Evidence from clinical trials
        1) A summary of 22 randomized trials of exercise following MI (4554 patients) showed a trend toward a reduction in cardiovascular death, sudden death, and reinfarction (O'Connor et al., 1989). Many of these trials included several interventions for risk factor reduction besides exercise; conclusive evidence of the independent contribution of exercise is lacking.
        2) Refer to AHCPR Guidelines (1994) for benefits of cardiac rehabilitation.
2. Smoking Cessation
    A. Patients should be offered intensive smoking cessation intervention during hospitalization that includes counseling on relapse prevention.
    B. Patients should review a relapse prevention manual and be given written information about outpatient behavior modification programs and option of nicotine replacement therapy.
    C. Evidence from clinical trials
        1) Patients who continue to smoke after they present with unstable angina have 5.4-fold increase in the risk of death from all causes compared to patients who stop smoking.
3. Low-Cholesterol Diet
    A. Patients and family members should receive counseling on the National Cholesterol Education Program Step II diet.
    B. Information on outpatient dietary modification programs should be provided.
    C. Evidence from clinical trials
        1) Although dietary intervention alone has not been shown to be beneficial, there may still be benefit when diet is used in combination with exercise and cholesterol-lowering education in patients with CAD.

PATIENT EDUCATION

1. Instruct the patient about the diagnosis of AMI and healing process that occurs.
2. Discuss reasons for reperfusion therapy and effect on progression of necrosis.
3. Identify cardiac risk factors that can be modified for secondary prevention of CAD.
   A. Control of HTN, DM
   B. Smoking cessation
   C. Low-fat diet
   D. Home exercise program
   E. Stress management
   F. Compliance with medication regimen
4. Discuss the need for exercise stress testing prior to initiating home exercise program.
5. Consider referral to cardiac rehabilitation program to enhance compliance with risk factor modification.
6. Discuss medications and their role in prevention or progression of atherosclerotic disease and impact on AMI outcome.
7. Instruct the patient on what to do if chest pain reoccurs, the importance of not delaying, and on the use of NTG.

Review Questions

3.21 ST-segment elevation and deep, wide Q waves in leads II, III, and aVF are a sign of which of the following:
   A. Acute inferior MI
   B. Old inferior MI
   C. Anterior wall ischemia
   D. Subendocardial ischemia without necrosis

3.22 A posterior wall MI is diagnosed by:
   A. Tall R waves in V_5 and V_6
   B. Deep side Q waves in the anterior leads
   C. ST-segment elevation in V_1 and V_2
   D. Tall R waves in V_1 and V_2

3.23 A 65-year-old man was brought to the emergency room (ER) with 8/10 pressure like substernal chest pain of 2 hours duration. The ECG showed ST-segment elevation in V_1–V_3. What would be the ACNP's first step?
   A. Call the cardiologist immediately.
   B. Assess patient eligibility for thrombolytic/reperfusion therapy.
   C. Administer sublingual NTG for chest pain.
   D. Repeat the ECG to ensure these are not transient changes.

3.24 Immediate medical therapy for this patient that has been shown to benefit mortality and morbidity includes:
   A. NTG to relieve chest pain
   B. Oxygen by nasal cannula
   C. ASA, β-blockers, ACE, and heparin
   D. Lidocaine prophylactically

3.25 This patient developed an S_3, increasing shortness of breath (SOB), respirations and SaO_2 decreased to 92%. The most likely cause is:
A. CHF
B. Arrhythmias
C. Pericarditis
D. HTN crisis

Answers and Rationales

3.21 **A** ST-segment elevation in leads II, III, and aVF is a sign of an acute inferior wall MI.

3.22 **D** Tall R waves in leads V_1 and V_2 may represent a posterior wall infarct, although there are other causes of tall R waves in V_1 and V_2.

3.23 **B** The ACNP should quickly assess the patient's Hx for eligibility for thrombolytic therapy (indications and contraindications) then call and consult with the cardiologist.

3.24 **C** ASA, β-blockers, ACE, and heparin have been shown to decrease mortality and morbidity in the AMI patient.

3.25 **A** These are signs of CHF, which is a complication of AMI.

References

Adams, J.E., 3rd, Bodor, G.S., Davilla-Roman, V.G., et al. (1993). Cardiac troponin I. A marker with high specificity for cardiac injury. *Circulation 88*, 101–106.

Antiplatelet Trialists' Collaboration. (1988). Secondary prevention of vascular disease by prolonged antiplatelet treatment. *Br Med J 296*, 320–331.

Antman, E., & Braunwald, E. (1997). Acute myocardial infarction. In E. Brunwald (ed.). *Heart Disease: A Textbook of Cardiovascular Medicine* (5th ed.). Philadelphia: W.B. Saunders Co., pp. 1185–1288.

Apple, F.S., Voss, E., Lund, L., et al. (1995). Cardiac troponin, CK-MB and myoglobin for the early detection of acute myocardial infarction and monitoring of reperfusion following thrombolytic therapy. *Clin Chim Acta 237*, 59–66.

Baldwin, K.M., Garza, C.S., Martin, R.N., et al. (1995). Acute myocardial infarction. In *Davis's Manual of Critical Care Therapeutics*. Philadelphia: F.A. Davis Co., pp. 72–92.

Burkart, F., Pfister, M., Kiowski, W., et al. (1990). Effect of antiarrhythmic therapy on mortality in survivors of myocardial infarction with asymptomatic complex ventricular arrhythmias: Basel Antiarrhythmic Study of Infarct Survival (BASIS). *J Am Coll Cardiol 16*, 1711–1718.

Ceremuzynski, L., Kleczar, E., Krzeminska-Pakula, M., et al. (1992). Effect of amiodarone on mortality after myocardial infarction: A double-blind, placebo-controlled, pilot study. *J Am Coll Cardiol 20*, 1056–1062.

Clinical Guidelines Committee. (1996). *Acute Myocardial Infarction*. Regents of the University of California: UCLA Division of Cardiology.

Grines, C.L. (1994). Myocardial infarction. In M. Freed & C. Grines (eds.). *Essentials of Cardiovascular Medicine*. Birmingham, MI: Physician's Press, pp. 99–122.

Hennekens, C.H., Albert, C.M., Godfried, S.L., et al. (1996). Adjunctive drug therapy of acute myocardial infarction—evidence from clinical trials. *N Engl J Med 335*, 1660–1667.

ISIS-3 (Third International Study of Infarct Survival) Collaborative Group. (1992). ISIS-

3: A randomized comparison of streptokinase vs tissue plasminogen activator vs anistreplase and of aspirin plus heparin vs aspirin alone among 41,299 cases of suspected acute myocardial infarction. *Lancet 339*, 753–770.

Mair, J., Morandell, D., Genser, N., et al. (1995). Equivalent early sensitivities of myoglobin, creatine kinase MB mass, creatine kinase isoform ratios, and cardiac troponins I and T for acute myocardial infarction. *Clin Chem 41*, 1266–1272.

Mair, J., Wagner, I., Jakob, G., et al. (1994). Different time courses of cardiac contractile proteins after acute myocardial infarction. *Clin Chim Acta 231*, 47–60.

Massie, B.M., & Amidon, T.A. (1997). Acute myocardial infarction. In L.M. Tierney, Jr., S.J. McPhee, & M.A. Papadakis (eds.). *Current Medical Diagnosis & Treatment* (36th ed.). Stamford, CT: Appleton & Lange, pp. 357–369.

Meijer, A., Verheugt, F.W.A., Werter, C.J.P.J., et al. (1993). Aspirin versus Coumadin in the prevention of reocclusion and recurrent ischemia after successful thrombolysis: A prospective placebo-controlled angiographic study. Results of the APRICOT Study. *Circulation 87*, 1524–1530.

Norris, R.M., Barnaby, P.F., Brown, M.A., et al. (1984). Prevention of ventricular fibrillation during acute myocardial infarction by intravenous propranolol. *Lancet 2*, 883.

O'Connor, G.T., Burning, J.E., et al. (1989). An overview of randomized trials of rehabilitation with exercise after myocardial infarction. *Circulation 80*, 234–244.

Pfeffer, M.A., Braunwald, E., Moye, L.A., et al., on behalf of the SAVE Investigators. (1992). Effect of captopril on mortality and morbidity in patients with left ventricular dysfunction after myocardial infarction. *N Engl J Med 327*, 669–677.

Roberts, R., Rogers, W.J., Mueller, H.S., et al. for the TIMI Investigators. (1991). Immediate versus deferred beta-blockade following thrombolytic therapy in patients with acute myocardial infarction. Results of the Thrombolysis in Myocardial Infarction (TIMI) II-B Study. *Circulation 83*, 422–437.

Roux, S., Christeller, S., & Ludin, E. (1992). Effects of aspirin on coronary reocclusion and recurrent ischemia after thrombolysis: A meta-analysis. *J Am Coll Cardiol 19*, 671–677.

The Cardiac Arrhythmia Suppression Trial II Investigators. (1992). Effect of the antiarrhythmic agent moricizine on survival after myocardial infarction. *N Engl J Med 327*, 227–233.

The E.P.S.I.M. Research Group. (1982). A controlled comparison of aspirin and oral anticoagulants in prevention of death after myocardial infarction. *N Engl J Med 307*, 701–708.

The GUSTO Investigators. (1993). An international randomized trial comparing four thrombolytic strategies for acute myocardial infarction. *N Engl J Med 329*, 673–682.

The International Study Group. (1990). In-hospital mortality and clinical course of 20 891 patients with suspected acute myocardial infarction randomized between alteplase and streptokinase with or without heparin. *Lancet 336*, 71–75.

Yusuf, S., Collins, R., MacMahon, S., & Peto, R. (1988). Effect of intravenous nitrates on mortality in acute myocardial infarction: An overview of the randomized trials. *Lancet 1*, 1088–1092.

Yusuf, S., Peto, R., Lewis, J., et al. (1985). Beta blockade during and after myocardial infarction: An overview of the randomized trials. *Prog Cardiovasc Dis 27*(5), 335–371.

Yusuf, S., Sleight, P., Held, P., & McMahon, S. (1990). Routine medical management of acute myocardial infarction. Lessons from overviews of recent randomized controlled trials. *Circulation 82*, II-117–II-134.

Wenger, N.K., Froelicher, E.S., Smith, L.K., et al. (1995). *Cardiac Rehabilitation*. Clinical Practice Guideline No. 17. Rockville, MD: U.S. Department of Health and Human Services, Public Health Service, Agency for Health Care Policy and Research and the National Heart, Lung, and Blood Institute. AHCPR Publication No. 96-0672.

Winters, K.J., & Eisenberg, P.R. (1995). Myocardial infarction. In G.A. Ewald & C.R. McKenzie (eds.). *Manual of Medical Therapeutics: The Washington Manual* (28th ed.). Boston: Little, Brown & Co., pp 94–113.

Heart Failure

DEFINITION

1. Heart failure (HF) is defined as a pathophysiologic disturbance in which an abnormality in cardiac function leads to an inability of the heart to pump blood at a rate commensurate with metabolic requirements. This results in a clinical syndrome or condition characterized by (1) signs and symptoms of intravascular and interstitial volume overload, including shortness of breath, rales, edema; or (2) manifestations of inadequate tissue perfusion, such as fatigue or poor exercise tolerance. The term "heart failure" will be used in preference to the commonly used "congestive heart failure" because many patients with heart failure do not manifest pulmonary or systemic congestion (Konstam, 1994).
2. Patients with advanced HF are commonly categorized by LV dysfunction (ejection fraction [EF] <40%) and functional limitation using the New York Heart Association (NYHA) Functional Classification.
3. Table 3–19 lists the NYHA Functional Classification for patients with HF.

ETIOLOGY/INCIDENCE

1. Approximately 2 million Americans suffer from the effects of HF each year.
2. 400,000 new cases are diagnosed each year.
3. HF accounts for approximately 250,000 deaths annually, with a 10% 1-year mortality rate and a 50% mortality rate at 5 years.

TABLE 3–19.   New York Heart Association Functional Classification for Patients with Heart Failure*

Functional Class I
Patients with cardiac disease but without resulting limitations of physical activity. Ordinary activity does not cause undue fatigue, palpitation, dyspnea, or anginal pain.
Functional Class II
Patients with cardiac disease resulting in slight limitations of physical activity. They are comfortable at rest. Ordinary physical activity results in fatigue, dyspnea, palpitations, or angina pectoris.
Functional Class III
Patients with cardiac disease resulting in marked limitation of physical activity. They are comfortable at rest. Less than ordinary physical activity causes fatigue, palpitation, dyspnea, or anginal pain.
Functional Class IV
Patients with cardiac disease resulting in inability to carry on any physical activity without discomfort. Symptoms of cardiac insufficiency or of the anginal syndrome may be present even at rest. If any physical activity is undertaken, discomfort is increased.

---

* Adapted from Goldman, L., Hashimoto, B., Cook, E.F., & Loscalzo, A. (1981). Comparative reproducibility and validity of systems for assessing cardiovascular functional class. Advantages of a new specific activity scale. *Circulation 64,* 1227, with permission.

TABLE 3–20. **Causes of Heart Failure**

Common Causes	Less Common Causes
CAD, with myocardial ischemia potentially the most reversible cause of HF	Congenital heart disease
HTN	Infiltrative cardiomyopathy: amyloid, sarcoid, restrictive
Idiopathic dilated cardiomyopathy	Hemochromatosis
Valvular heart disease	Thyroid disease
Drugs: alcohol, cocaine, methamphetamine	Pheochromocytoma
	Chronic renal disease
	Viral and HIV cardiomyopathy

CAD, coronary artery disease; HF, heart failure; HTN, hypertension; HIV, human immunodeficiency virus.

4. This syndrome accounts for 1.8 million office and 1.5 million hospital visits per year.
5. HF is the leading diagnosis among adults discharged from community hospitals.
6. More than $10 billion in resources each year go into the treatment of patients with HF (Konstam, 1994).
7. Table 3–20 lists causes of HF.

PATHOPHYSIOLOGY

1. HF is a clinical syndrome that describes the systemic response to inadequate pump function or myocardial failure. The circulation mounts a series of interrelated compensatory mechanisms designed to meet the metabolic demands of the body, maintain cardiac output, and maintain an adequate tissue perfusion (Fig. 3–3).
2. HF can result from volume or pressure overload, impaired myocardial functioning, myocardial filling disorders of the heart, or increased metabolic demands of the body.
3. Hypertrophy is then associated with depressed myocardial functioning and loss of the ability to develop adequate contractile tension. Ventricular dilation occurs as pump function declines.
4. Activation of the sympathetic nervous system (SNS) and the renin-angiotensin-aldosterone system (RAAS) occurs in response to decreased cardiac output and leads to augmented peripheral vascular resistance and a maldistribution of peripheral blood flow. Systemic and pulmonary congestion ensue.
5. A chronic derangement of the circulation occurs as neurohormonal compensatory mechanisms, activated to restore arterial blood pressure and adequate tissue perfusion, are overwhelmed.
6. The majority of patients with HF have moderate to severe LV systolic dysfunction. Systolic dysfunction, or impaired myocardial contractility, commonly occurs from a sustained overload with severe ventricular hypertrophy or from loss of myocardium, either segmental (i.e., CAD) or diffuse with focal loss of myocardium, fibrosis, and resultant secondary hypertrophy as in cardiomyopathy.
7. Diastolic dysfunction occurs in approximately 40% of patients with chronic HF. Diastolic dysfunction is impaired early diastolic relaxation, increased stiffness of the ventricular wall, or both (Braunwald, 1997). Diastolic dys-

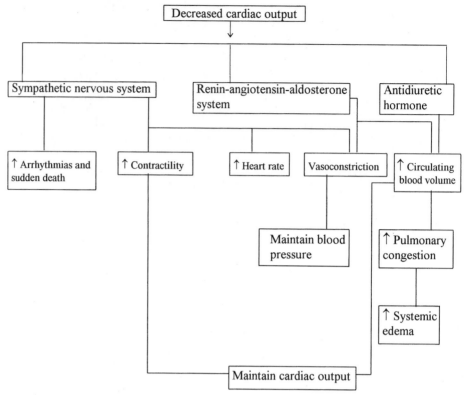

FIGURE 3–3. Neurohormonal mechanisms associated with heart failure. (Adapted from Cheitlin, M., Sokolow, M., & McIlroy, M. [1993]. *Clinical Cardiology* [6th ed.]. Norwalk, CT: Appelton & Lange, p. 321, with permission.)

function is present when the ventricles can no longer fill adequately at normal pressure to maintain normal stroke volume.

8. Diastolic dysfunction commonly occurs secondary to chronic hypertension, coronary artery disease, hypertrophic cardiomyopathy, valvular disease, chronic renal failure, diabetes, idiopathic cardiomyopathy, and restrictive or constrictive states.

SIGNS AND SYMPTOMS

1. A thorough detailed history of the patient presenting with HF should include symptoms suggestive of volume overload and/or low cardiac output:
   A. Dyspnea on exertion (DOE) (often the earliest symptom)*
   B. Orthopnea*
   C. Paroxysmal nocturnal dyspnea*
   D. Lower extremity edema
   E. Fatigue/decreased exercise tolerance
   F. Unexplained confusion, altered mental status, or fatigue in an elderly patient
   G. Abdominal symptoms associated with ascites and/or hepatic engorgement, such as early satiety, nausea, and vomiting

* The most common presenting signs of HF (Konstam, 1994).

2. History should also include previous MI, CAD, angina or equivalent, poorly controlled hypertension, or other heart disease, diabetes, renal, pulmonary, thyroid, or gastrointestinal disease.
3. A social history should include tobacco use, alcohol consumption, and recreational drug use.

PHYSICAL FINDINGS

1. Neurologic: Anxiety, restlessness, lethargy, altered mental status (i.e., confusion in the elderly)
2. Cardiovascular: Cardiomegaly; lateral displacement of the apical impulse with LV heave; S_3, S_4 gallop; murmur of mitral regurgitation (MR); tachycardia; elevated jugular venous pressure (JVP); hypotension
3. Pulmonary: Tachypnea, crackles, wheezes, cough, pulmonary edema
4. GI: Abdominal distention and/or increased abdominal girth, ascites, hepatomegaly, positive hepatojugular reflex.
5. Integument: Cold, clammy skin; pallor or cyanosis, edema-dependent, sacral, or ascites.
6. Table 3–21 lists physical findings suggestive of right- and left-sided HF.

DIFFERENTIAL DIAGNOSIS

1. Pneumonia
2. Chronic obstructive pulmonary disease
3. Bronchial asthma
4. Pulmonary embolism
5. Renal or liver dysfunction with edema

DIAGNOSTIC TESTS/FINDINGS

1. Hemodynamic monitoring with a pulmonary artery (PA) catheter may be warranted in the patient with symptomatic HF.
2. Table 3–22 lists diagnostic tests commonly used in the management of HF.

MANAGEMENT/TREATMENT

1. The goals of therapy for the patient with HF focus on improving myocardial function by enhancing contractility, decreasing preload and afterload, reg-

TABLE **3–21. Physical Findings Suggestive of Right- and Left-Sided Heart Failure**

Right-Sided Failure	Left-Sided Failure
Predominantly systemic congestion	Predominantly pulmonary congestion
Elevated systemic venous pressure	Pulmonary venous congestion
Neck vein distention	Dyspnea*
Hepatomegaly	Orthopnea*
Ascites	Paroxysmal nocturnal dyspnea*
Peripheral edema	Wheeze, cough, hemoptysis
Weight gain	Cardiomegaly
Tricuspid regurgitation	MR

* Most common presenting signs of heart failure.
MR, mitral regurgitation.

TABLE 3–22.   Diagnostic Tests Used in the Management of Heart Failure*

Test	Finding	Suspected
ECG	Acute ST-T wave changes	Myocardial ischemia
	Atrial fibrillation, other tachyarrhythmia	Thyroid disease or heart failure due to rapid ventricular rate
	Bradyarrhythmias	HF due to low HR
	Previous MI	HF due to reduced LV performance
	Low voltage	Pericardial effusion
	Left ventricular hypertrophy	Diastolic dysfunction
CBC	Anemia	HF due to or aggravated by decreased oxygen-carrying capacity
Electrolytes, BUN, Cr.	Elevated serum Cr.	Volume overload due to renal failure
		Low cardiac output
Cholesterol	Hyperlipidemia	Risk for CAD
UA	Proteinuria	Nephrotic syndrome
	Red blood cells or cellular casts	Glomerulonephritis
Serum albumin	Decreased	Increased extravascular volume due to hypoalbuminemia
Additional labs	HIV	HIV cardiomyopathy
	Serum iron, serum ferritin	Diabetic or liver disease
T_4 and TSH (obtain only if atrial fibrillation, evidence of thyroid disease, or patient >65)	Abnormal T_4 or TSH	HF due to or aggravated by hypo/hyperthyroidism
CXR	Cardiomegaly, pulmonary edema, congestive heart failure	
Echocardiography	Identify potential secondary cause HF/cardiomyopathy, evaluate degree of valvular regurgitation, estimate extent of RV involvement, determine degree of LV dilatation, evaluate for presence of LV thrombus, estimate LVEF	
Exercise treadmill test, sestamibi, PET, cardiac catheterization	If at risk for/suspect CAD, i.e., presence of angina, MI, risk factors	
CPX	Quantitate functional capacity, assess prognosis, guide exercise prescription	

* Adapted from Konstam, M., Dracup, K., Baker, D., et al. (1994). Heart failure: Evaluation and care of patients with left ventricular systolic dysfunction. Clinical practice guideline no. 11. AHCPR Publication No. 94-0612. Rockville, MD: Agency for Health Policy and Research, Public Health Service, U.S. Department of Health and Human Services, with permission.

ECG, electrocardiogram; MI, myocardial infarction; HR, heart rate; HF, heart failure; LV, left ventricular; CBC, complete blood count; BUN, blood urea nitrogen; Cr., creatinine; UA, urinalysis; CAD, coronary artery disease; HIV, human immunodeficiency virus; T_4, thyroxine; TSH, thyroid-stimulating hormone; CXR, chest x-ray; RV, right ventricular; LVEF, left ventricular ejection fraction; PET, positron emission tomography; CPX, cardiopulmonary exercise testing.

ulating heart rate, identifying and treating precipitating factors, and identifying underlying pathologic mechanisms. The ACNP consults with the collaborating physician regarding pharmacologic, nonpharmacologic, and mechanical methods of treating HF in order to attain successful patient outcomes such as reduction in mortality, alleviation of symptoms, and improvement in functional capacity.

2. The ACNP in consultation with the collaborating physician should consider hospitalization for initial management or during follow-up for:
   A. Hypoxia: SaO_2 <90%
   B. Pulmonary edema
   C. Anasarca
   D. Symptomatic hypotension: SBP <80–90 with significant volume excess
   E. CHF refractory to outpatient management
   F. Severe complicating medical illness (i.e., pneumonia)
   G. Clinical or ECG evidence of acute myocardial ischemia
   H. Inadequate social support (may contribute to decreased compliance) (Konstam, 1994)

3. In the acute and critical care setting, management of patients with HF is directed by the physician and requires close collaboration by the ACNP with the physician and the multidisciplinary team.

4. The ACNP will consult with the collaborating physician whether the patient's condition warrants hemodynamic monitoring to guide therapy. The principle of hemodynamically guided therapy is to define each individual patient's optimal filling pressures, cardiac index (CI), and systemic vascular resistance (SVR) using short-acting intravenous medications and then match and maintain those hemodynamic goals using oral vasodilators and diuretics (Fonarow, 1994; Stevenson, 1996).

5. Hemodynamically guided targets for the treatment of HF in the acute setting are (UCLA Clinical Practice Guidelines, 1994):
   A. Pulmonary capillary wedge pressure (PCWP): ≤15 mm Hg
   B. SVR: 800–1200 dynes/sec/cm^{-5}
   C. Right atrial pressure (RAP): <8 mm Hg
   D. CI: 2.5–4.5 L/min/m^2
   E. SBP: >80 mm Hg

6. The goals of pharmacologic management are aimed at minimizing neurohormonal sequelae associated with HF. Table 3–23 describes medications commonly used for HF management.

7. Afterload reduction is considered a mainstay of management for HF in the acute-care setting to improve CI and decrease LV filling pressures. Initially, vasodilators and diuretics are administered to rapidly optimize the patient's hemodynamic status.

8. Vasodilators decrease systemic resistance and are associated with improvement in mitral regurgitation, which is believed to improve forward stroke volume (SV) (Stevenson, 1996).

9. Afterload reduction is rapidly and efficiently attained with the intravenous vasodilator nitroprusside (NTP). NTP is initiated at 20 μg/min and rapidly titrated to the following hemodynamic goals: SBP ≥85 mm Hg, CI ≥2.5 L/min/m^2, and SVR 800–1200 dynes/sec/cm^{-5}. The maximum dosage of NTP is 300 μg/min.

10. Intravenous diuretics are given every few hours in conjunction with the vasodilator. Intravenous diuretics dispose of excess fluid volume that accu-

TABLE 3–23.   Medications Commonly Used in the Treatment of Heart Failure*

Class	Drug	Dosage	Mechanism of Action
Vasodilators	Sodium nitroprusside	20–300 μg/min IV drip	Dilates arterial smooth muscle
	Nitroglycerin	20–300 μg/min IV drip	Dilates arterial and venous smooth muscle
	Captopril (ACE inhibitor)	6.25–100 mg PO q8h	Inhibits angiotensin I conversion to angiotensin II resulting in vasodilatation
	Enalapril (ACE inhibitor)	2.5–20 mg PO bid	Inhibits angiotensin I conversion to angiotensin II resulting in vasodilatation
	Lisinopril (ACE inhibitor)	2.5–20 mg PO bid	Inhibits angiotensin I conversion to angiotensin II resulting in vasodilatation
	Prazosin	1–10 mg PO q6–8h	Arterial and venous smooth muscle dilation
	Hydralazine	25–100 mg PO q6h	Arterial smooth muscle dilation
	Isosorbide dinitrate	10–100 mg PO q6–8h	Venous smooth muscle dilation
Diuretics	Loop diuretic:		Induce diuresis of sodium and water
	Furosemide	20–240 mg PO/IV bid	
	Bumex	10 mg PO/IV qd	
	Thiazide diuretic:		Induce diuresis of sodium and water
	Hydrochlorothiazide	25–50 mg PO qd	
	Thiazide related:		Induce diuresis of sodium and water
	Metalazone	2.5–10 mg PO qd	
	Potassium sparing:		Induce diuresis of sodium and water
	Spironolactone	25–100 mg PO bid	
	Amiloride	5–10 mg PO qd	
Inotropes	Dobutamine	2.5 μg/kg/min titrate to maximum 20 μg/kg/min	Synthetic catecholamine, β_1; β_2-, α_1-adrenoreceptor stimulating qualities.
	Dopamine	Renal dose: 2–3 μg/kg/min	Synthetic catecholamine, β_1-, β_2-, α_1-adrenoreceptor stimulating qualities.
	Milrinone	50 μg/kg bolus followed by 0.375–0.75 μg/kg/min infusion	Phosphodiesterase inhibitor → intracellular cAMP → enhanced cardiac contractility and peripheral vasodilation.
	Digoxin	0.125–0.25 mg PO qd	Inhibits sodium pump → increases intracellular Na concentration → promotes calcium influx into myocardial cell → increased contractility. Inhibits impulse conduction at SA and AV node.

Table continues

TABLE 3-23. (Continued)

Class	Drug	Dosage	Mechanism of Action
Anticoagulant	Warfarin	2–20 mg PO qd	Inhibits synthesis of vitamin K–dependent clotting factors.
Antiarrhythmic	Amiodarone	Suggested loading dose: 600 mg/day PO for 2 wk 400 mg/day PO for 2 wk Maintenance dose: 200 mg PO qd	Lengthens effective refractory period by prolonging the action potential duration in all cardiac tissue. Noncompetitively blocks α- and β-adrenergic receptors. Some coronary and peripheral vasodilator effects.
HMG-CoA reductase inhibitor	Statins: Lovastatin Pravastatin Simvistatin Fluvastatin Atorvastatin	20–80 mg PO qd 10–40 mg PO qd 10–40 mg PO qd 10–40 mg PO qd 10–40 mg PO qd	Inhibit HMG-CoA reductase, the enzyme that catalyzes the rate-limiting step in cholesterol synthesis.

* Adapted from Konstam, M., Dracup, K., Baker, D., et al. (1994). Heart failure: Evaluation and care of patients with left ventricular systolic dysfunction. Clinical practice guideline No. 11. AHCPR Publication No. 94-0612. Rockville, MD: Agency for Health Policy and Research, Public Health Service, U.S. Department of Health and Human Services, with permission.

IV, intravenous; ACE, angiotensin converting enzyme; PO, orally; cAMP, cyclic adenosine monophosphate; SA, sinoatrial; AV, atrioventricular.

mulates in response to the maladaptive volume-retention reflexes activated in HF (Stevenson, 1996). The ACNP should consult with the collaborating physician to determine dosages of diuretics. The dosage of diuretic will vary with each individual patient in order to attain a PCWP of 15–18 mm Hg and to resolve signs of systemic congestion. In addition, the ACNP may consult with the collaborating physician regarding use of low-dose dopamine (2–3 μg/kg/min) to enhance renal perfusion and efforts at diuresis.

11. Intravenous NTG may also be used in this setting to reduce filling pressures. NTG (100 mg/250 D$_5$W) is initiated at 20 μg/min and titrated to a PCWP of 15–18 mm Hg and a SBP $\geq$85 mm Hg.

12. For low-CI states (CI <2.0 L/min/m^2) the ACNP in consultation with the collaborating physician should consider addition of an inotropic agent such as dobutamine. Dobutamine (500 mg/250 mL D$_5$W) can be titrated to doses of 5–20 μg/kg/min in order to increase CI to 2.5–4.5 L/min/m^2 (UCLA Clinical Practice Guidelines, 1994).

13. For patients who fail to respond to high doses of dobutamine or develop a tolerance to the agent due to down-regulation of β-receptors, addition of a phosphodiesterase inhibitor, such as milrinone, should be considered.

14. Once hemodynamic targets have been attained and maintained for a minimum of 4 hours, the ACNP in consultation with the collaborating physician initiates weaning of the intravenous vasodilator(s) while oral drugs are substituted to achieve the same hemodynamic goals.

15. ACE inhibitors are the cornerstone of management of LV dysfunction. Multiple clinical trials have demonstrated reduced mortality with the use of

ACE inhibitors in the setting of HF (Cohn, 1991; Pfefer, 1992; The SOLVD Investigators, 1992).

16. Isosorbide dinitrate is frequently added to the medication regimen in order to maintain a PCWP of 15–18 mm Hg. Isosorbide dinitrate is started at 10 mg and increased every 2–8 hours in 10 mg increments to keep SBP >85 or a maximum of 80 mg PO tid.

17. Digoxin is indicated in patients with symptomatic HF. Digoxin has been shown to reduce symptoms and improve functional capacity in HF. However, digoxin has not been shown to improve survival in HF (Garg et al., 1997). For patients who remain symptomatic on ACE inhibitors, give digoxin 0.125–0.25 mg PO qd. Digoxin levels should be monitored every 2–3 months.

18. Patients with HF are at increased risk for ventricular arrhythmias and sudden death. Management of ventricular arrhythmias remains problematic, as no antiarrhythmic therapy to date has been shown to reduce the risk of sudden death in HF patients. Patients with history of syncope, cardiac arrest, nonsustained ventricular ectopy, or sustained ventricular arrhythmias are at risk for sudden death and should be referred to a cardiologist/arrhythmia specialist for 24-hour Holter monitoring, possible electrophysiology study, and possible implantable cardioverter defibrillator (ICD) placement.

19. Amiodarone may be used in patients with sustained ventricular arrhythmias and in patients with atrial fibrillation. Amiodarone is started at 600 mg/day for 2 weeks then decreased to a maintenance dose of 200 mg/day. All patients receiving amiodarone therapy must have baseline thyroid, liver, and pulmonary functions tests prior to the initiation of therapy with amiodarone. (See also "Arrhythmias" for management of ventricular arrhythmias.)

20. The ACNP must closely follow the patient's fluid and electrolyte status, as activation of the neuroendocrine systems, renal dysfunction, and diuretic therapy may predispose the patient to electrolyte imbalance. Serum electrolytes must be monitored frequently with aggressive diuresis to maintain the following levels: serum potassium, 4.4–5.0 mEq/dL; serum magnesium, >1.8 mEq/dL; and serum sodium, 134–145 mg/dL.

21. Anticoagulation with warfarin, maintaining an INR of 2.0–3.0, is indicated in HF patients with any one of the following conditions: atrial fibrillation, LV thrombus on echocardiogram or ventriculography, previous history or symptoms consistent with embolization, and prosthetic heart valves (INR 2.5–3.5). (See also "Arrhythmias" for specific management of anticoagulation with warfarin.)

22. HMG-CoA RIs should be used in patients with underlying CAD. These agents have proven more effective than other cholesterol-lowering agents in lowering plasma concentrations of LDL and total cholesterol. (See "Coronary Artery Disease" for specific management of hyperlipidemia.) Table 3–23 includes specific HMG-CoA RIs and appropriate doses.

23. Management of patients with HF refractory to pharmacologic management is directed by the cardiologist. The ACNP, in consultation with the collaborating physician, should refer patients who develop symptomatic hypotension that does not respond to inotropic therapy for consideration for mechanical assist devices, such as the IABP, and left and/or right ventricular assist device. These devices provide a mechanical means of augmenting cardiac function and in some cases are used as a bridge to cardiac trans-

plantation for patients with end-stage HF. The patient with ischemic cardiomyopathy who develops angina that does not readily resolve with pharmacologic management should also be considered for early intervention with IABP.

24. Cardiac transplantation is now an accepted therapeutic option for end-stage HF when medical and surgical management have failed. (See "Cardiac Transplantation".)

25. Nonpharmacologic therapy consists of dietary and fluid restrictions that will augment pharmacologic management. In the acute setting, the ACNP may tailor these general guidelines to the degree of HF evident.
    A. Salt restriction is limited to a maximum of 2 gm/day
    B. A fluid restriction, usually a maximum 2 L/day, is strictly adhered to; however, with severe volume overload (anasarca) or hyponatremia, a 1000- to 1500-ml restriction may be appropriate until the patient's condition has stabilized.
    C. Daily weights should be obtained during hospitalization and following discharge.
    D. All patients should receive instruction to decrease the amount of saturated fats to <30% of total calories (in the absence of cardiac cachexia) and abstain from alcohol ingestion.
    E. Upon discharge, exercise training—walking a minimum of 4 days per week, increasing gradually until able to walk for 20–30 minutes (approximately 2 miles) without symptoms—is advised.

PATIENT EDUCATION

The ACNP will educate the patient and family regarding the following (Dracup, 1996):

1. General counseling
    A. Explanation of HF and reason for symptoms
    B. Cause or probable cause of heart failure
    C. Expected symptoms
    D. Symptoms of worsening HF
    E. What to do if symptoms worsen
    F. Self-monitoring with daily weights
    G. Explanation of treatment plan
    H. Role of family members or other care givers in treatment plan
    I. Availability and value of qualified local support groups
    J. Clarification of patient and family responsibilities
    K. Smoking cessation
2. Dietary recommendations
    A. Sodium restriction
    B. Avoidance of excessive fluid intake
    C. Fluid restriction
    D. Alcohol restriction/abstinence
3. Activity recommendations
    A. Recreational, leisure, and work activity
    B. Exercise
    C. Sexual difficulties and coping strategies
4. Medications
    A. Benefits for quality of life
    B. Dosage

C. Adverse events and what to do if they occur
D. Coping mechanisms for complicated therapeutic regimens
E. Availability of lower cost medications or financial assistance
5. Prognosis
   A. Life expectancy
   B. Advance directives
   C. Advice for family members in the event of sudden death

Review Questions

3.26 A 76-year-old woman with a history of DM, HTN, is admitted to the coronary care unit (CCU) with shortness of breath. She also has vague complaints of weakness and fatigue for 1 month and has noted a 5-lb weight gain over the past 4 days despite loss of appetite. Her vital signs are as follows: BP 168/90, HR 110 bpm, respiratory rate (RR) 24 breaths/min, SaO_2 90%. The admission CXR shows cardiomegaly, interstitial edema in the lung fields. What would be an appropriate therapy for this patient?
   A. Dobutamine
   B. Furosemide
   C. Antibiotics
   D. Metroprolol

3.27 A PA catheter is inserted in the above patient. Initial hemodynamic readings are as follows:
   PAP: 50/26 mm Hg
   PCWP: 24 mm Hg with v wave
   RAP: 10 mm Hg
   CI: 2.1 L/min/m^2
   SVR: 1500 dynes/sec/cm^{-5}
   $S\overline{v}O_2$:   59%
   UO: 30 mL/hr
   What would be the next appropriate pharmacologic agent to use for this patient?
   A. Nitroglycerin
   B. Morphine sulfate
   C. Milrinone
   D. Nitroprusside

3.28 After 12 hours of intravenous nitroprusside (titrated to 200 μg/kg/min) and diuretics the patient's hemodynamics are as follows:
   PAP: 38/18 mm Hg
   PCWP: 16 mm Hg with v wave
   RAP: 8 mm Hg
   CI: 3.5 L/min/m^2
   SVR: 856 dynes/sec/cm^{-5}
   $S\overline{v}O_2$:   63%
   UO: 100 mL/hr
   What would be the recommended pharmacologic agent(s) to administer next?
   A. Dobutamine 5 μg/kg/min
   B. Wean NTP to off to maintain SVR 800–1000

C. No further medications are necessary
D. Enalapril 5 mg PO, wean NTP to maintain SVR 800–1000 mg, continue intravenous furosemide prn to maintain PCWP 15–18 mm Hg

3.29 The principle pharmacologic agents used in the management of HF, once hemodynamically guided therapy is achieved, consists of what medications?
A. Diuretics
B. ACE inhibitors
C. Digoxin
D. All of the above

3.30 Which of the following electrolytes must be closely monitored in advanced HF patients because pharmacologic therapy (i.e., diuresis) may lead to ventricular arrhythmias?
A. Hypokalemia, hyponatremia
B. Hyperkalemia, hypermagnesemia
C. Hypokalemia, hypomagnesemia
D. Hypernatremia, hyperkalemia

Answers and Rationales

3.26 **B** Furosemide. The patient's vital signs and physical exam are consistent with volume overload. A diuretic is indicated initially.
3.27 **D** Nitroprusside. Physical exam and hemodynamic data indicate a low cardiac output with an elevated SVR. The agent of choice is intravenous NTP to achieve rapid afterload reduction.
3.28 **D** Transition to oral vasodilators is indicated with optimization of hemodynamics. ACE inhibitors are the vasodilators of choice. Continued monitoring of volume status is warranted and IV lasix may be indicated for increased filling pressures.
3.29 **D** Numerous clinical trials have demonstrated mortality benefit in patients treated with ACE inhibitors. Diuretics, digoxin, and ACE inhibitors in combination are considered the cornerstone of HF management.
3.30 **C** Hypokalemia (serum potassium <3.5 mEq/dL) and hypomagnesemia (serum magnesium <1.8 mEq/dL) are common electrolyte imbalances that occur with diuretic therapy. Frequent monitoring of both serum potassium and magnesium is indicated in advanced heart failure patients, as hypokalemia and hypomagnesemia may lead to life-threatening ventricular arrhythmias.

References

Cohn, J.N., et al. (1991). A comparison of enalapril with hydralazine-isosorbide dinitrate in the treatment of chronic congestive heart failure. *N Engl J Med 325*, 303–310.
Dracup, K. (1996). Heart failure secondary to left ventricular systolic dysfunction: Therapeutic advances and treatment recommendations. *Nurse Pract 21*(19), 56–68.
Garg, R., Gorlin, R., Smith, T., & Yusef, S. (1997). The effect of digoxin on mortality and morbidity in patients with heart failure: The digitalis investigation group. *N Engl J Med 336*(9), 525–533.

Goldman, L., Hashimoto, B., Cook, E.F., & Loscalzo, A. (1981). Comparative reproducibility and validity of systems for assessing cardiovascular functional class: Advantages of a new specific activity scale. *Circulation 64*, 1227.

Konstam, M., Dracup, K., Baker, D., et al. (1994). Heart failure: Evaluation and care of patients with left ventricular systolic dysfunction. Clinical practice guideline no. 11. AHCPR Publication No. 94–0612. Rockville, MD: Agency for Health Policy and Research, Public Health Service, U.S. Department of Health and Human Services.

Kuho, S.H. (1994). Vasodilator therapy in heart failure. *J Heart Lung Transplant 13*(5), 122–125.

Miller, M.M. (1994). Current trends in the primary care management of chronic congestive heart failure. *Nurse Pract 19*(5), 64–70.

Pfefer, M.A., et al. (1992). Effect of captopril on mortality and morbidity in patients with left ventricular dysfunction after myocardial infarction: Results of the survival and ventricular enlargement trial. *N Engl J Med 327*(10), 669–677.

Smith, T.W., Kelly, R.A., Stevenson, L.W., & Braunwald, E. (1997). Management of heart failure. In E. Braunwald (ed.). *Heart Disease: A Textbook of Cardiovascular Medicine* (5th ed.). Philadelphia: W.B. Saunders Co., pp. 492–514.

Stevenson, W.G., et al. (1995). Improving survival in patients with advanced heart failure: A study of 737 consecutive patients. *J Am Coll Cardiol 26*, 1400–1417.

The SOLVD Investigators. (1992). Effect of enalapril on mortality and the development of heart failure in asymptomatic patients with reduced left ventricular ejection fractions. *N Engl J Med 327*, 685–691.

UCLA Division of Cardiology. (1994). UCLA Heart Failure Practice Guidelines.

Young, J.B. (1994). Asymptomatic left ventricular dysfunction: To treat or not to treat? *J Heart Lung Transplant 13*(5), 135–140.

Valvular Heart Disease

DEFINITION

1. The heart moves blood throughout the body via the vascular system. Within the heart, unidirectional blood flow is maintained by the valves. Diseases affecting or damaging the cardiac valves impair the heart's ability to maintain an effective cardiac output.
2. There are four cardiac valves. The semilunar valves, located in the ventricular outflow tracts, are the aortic and pulmonic valves. The atrioventricular (AV) valves, located between the atria and the ventricles, are the mitral and tricuspid valves.
3. This section will outline the major valvular abnormalities: aortic regurgitation (AR), aortic stenosis (AS), mitral regurgitation (MR), and mitral stenosis (MS). In addition, infective endocarditis (IE) will be discussed.

PATHOPHYSIOLOGY

1. The pathophysiologic consequence of valvular lesions is loss of unidirectional blood flow. Valvular disorders are characterized into two functional types, regurgitation and stenosis.
2. Regurgitation (also referred to as insufficiency) is blood flowing backwards across the valve. Effective forward blood flow may eventually diminish, while blood volumes and pressures behind the valve increase. Figures 3–4, 3–5, 3–6, 3–7 outline the pathophysiology for acute and chronic AR and MR, respectively.

Acute aortic regurgitation

↓

Increased left ventricular diastolic pressure

↓

Increased left atrial pressure

↓

Increased pulmonary vascular pressure

FIGURE 3–4. Acute aortic regurgitation. (From Shackenbach, L.H. [1987]. Physiologic dynamics of acquired valvular heart disease. *J Cardiovasc Nurs 1* [3], 1–17. Copyright 1987, Aspen Publishing Inc, with permission.)

3. Stenosis is a narrowing of the valve and impedance of forward blood flow. Effective forward flow requires greater pressure to open the valve and move the blood volume. Eventually, forward blood flow diminishes and blood volume and pressures behind the valve increase. Figure 3–8 and 3–9 outline the pathophysiology for AS and MS, respectively.
4. The major etiologies of valve degeneration include rheumatic heart disease, myxomatous degeneration, endocarditis, calcification, and chordal rupture. Other causes include papillary muscle dysfunction associated with CAD, AMI, or arrhythmias.

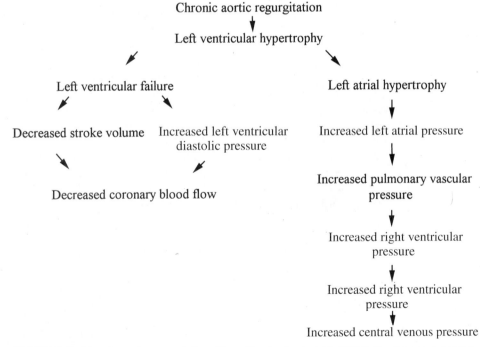

FIGURE 3–5. Chronic aortic regurgitation. (From Shackenbach, L.H. [1987]. Physiologic dynamics of acquired valvular heart disease. *J Cardiovasc Nurs 1* [3], 1–17. Copyright 1987, Aspen Publishing Inc, with permission.)

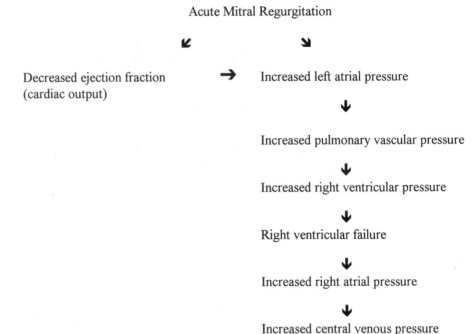

FIGURE 3–6. Acute mitral regurgitation. (From Shackenbach, L.H. [1987]. Physiologic dynamics of acquired valvular heart disease. *J Cardiovasc Nurs 1* [3], 1–17. Copyright 1987, Aspen Publishing Inc, with permission.)

SIGNS AND SYMPTOMS

1. Presenting signs and symptoms of valvular heart disease are affected by many variables including the specific heart valve involved.
2. When patients with valve disease are symptomatic, common complaints include fatigue, poor exercise tolerance, difficulty lying flat, and signs of left- or right-sided heart failure. Chest pain and dizziness may also be reported. However, the ACNP must recognize that many patients may remain asymptomatic indefinitely, depending upon the valvular abnormality.
3. Signs of HF may also be present in patients with advanced disease including jugular venous distention, pulmonary rales, peripheral coldness, hepatic congestion, peripheral edema, ascites, and muscle wasting.
4. Examination of the heart reveals characteristic pathologic changes depending upon the valve affected. Refer to each valvular abnormality for physical findings and treatment recommendations.

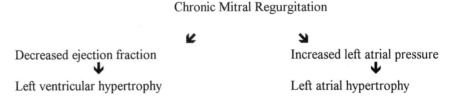

FIGURE 3–7. Chronic mitral regurgitation. (From Shackenbach, L.H. [1987]. Physiologic dynamics of acquired valvular heart disease. *J Cardiovasc Nurs 1*[3], 1–17. Copyright 1987, Aspen Publishing Inc, with permission.)

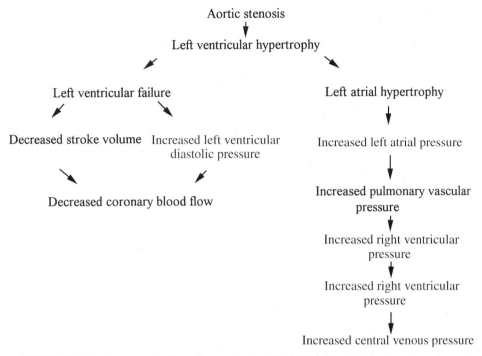

FIGURE 3–8. Aortic stenosis. (From Shackenbach, L.H. [1987]. Physiologic dynamics of acquired valvular heart disease. *J Cardiovasc Nurs 1*[3], 1–17. Copyright 1987, Aspen Publishing Inc, with permission.)

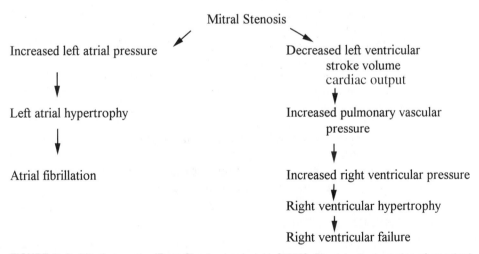

FIGURE 3–9. Mitral stenosis. (From Shackenbach, L.H. [1987]. Physiologic dynamics of acquired valvular heart disease. *J Cardiovasc Nurs 1*[3], 1–17. Copyright 1987, Aspen Publishing Inc, with permission.)

AORTIC STENOSIS (AS)

ETIOLOGY/INCIDENCE

1. AS can be classified as either acquired (more common) or rheumatic.
2. Acquired AS may be caused by idiopathic fibrosis and calcification as an individual ages. In degenerative (senile) calcific AS, the cusps are immobilized by deposits of calcium along their flexion lines at their bases that eventually prevent the cusps from opening normally during systole. This form of AS appears to be due to years of normal mechanical stress on the valve and is the most frequent cause of AS requiring aortic valve repair. Diabetes and hypercholesterolemia are risk factors for degenerative AS (Braunwald, 1997).
3. Atherosclerotic changes of the aorta or aortic valve may also lead to AS. This form of AS occurs most frequently in patients with severe hypercholesterolemia.
4. Congenital AS is a common cause of AS. The lesions are unicuspid and bicuspid valves or malformed tricuspid valves, and calcification precipitates symptoms (Shackenbach, 1996).
5. Rheumatic endocarditis is a rare cause of AS.

SIGNS AND SYMPTOMS

1. The natural history of AS is well defined. Adults with AS remain asymptomatic during a long latent period in which there is gradual obstruction and an increase in pressure load on the myocardium. Symptoms do not usually commence until the sixth decade of life.
2. The classic triad of symptoms of AS are angina pectoris, syncope, and dyspnea. The prognosis of symptomatic AS is poor when left untreated (relief of obstruction). The onset from the time of symptoms to the time of death is approximately 2 years in patients with heart failure, 3 years in those with angina, and 5 years in those with syncope (Braunwald, 1997).
3. Dyspnea is the most common initial complaint. Dyspnea is usually noted on exertion and is due to LV failure.
4. Angina results from the combination of increased oxygen demand and reduction of oxygen delivery by the excessive compression of coronary vessels (Braunwald, 1997).
5. Syncope is most commonly due to reduced cerebral perfusion that occurs during exertion when arterial pressure declines consequent to systemic vasodilatation in the presence of a fixed cardiac output (Braunwald, 1997).
6. Symptoms of low cardiac output (i.e., fatigue, peripheral cyanosis) usually are not present until late in the course of AS.

PHYSICAL FINDINGS

1. Arterial pulse: Rises slowly, small, and sustained; systolic and pulse pressures reduced in advanced stages; pulsus alternans in presence of LV dysfunction.
2. Carotid pulse: Delayed upstroke and decreased volume; palpation of apex and carotid arteries reveals distinct lag in carotid pulsation.
3. Jugular venous pulse: Prominent a waves; v waves may be present with pulmonary HTN, RV failure, and tricuspid regurgitation.

4. Palpation: Suprasternal thrill, best appreciated with patient leaning forward in full expiration, noted best at second intercostal space may radiate to carotids/suprasternal notch; point of maximal impulse (PMI) displaced laterally and inferiorly with LV failure; presystolic distention of the LV (prominent precordial a wave palpable and visible).

5. Auscultation: S_1 normal or soft; S_2 may be single (calcification or immobile leaflets render A_2 soft or absent); S_4 prominent; harsh, rasping, mid to late peaking systolic murmur best heard at the base, often radiating to the carotids and apex of the heart; associated with a systolic thrill; augmented by squatting or lying flat, reduced intensity with Valsalva strain.

DIAGNOSTIC TESTS/FINDINGS

1. ECG: Left ventricular hypertrophy most common ECG finding, found in 85% of patients with severe AS (Braunwald, 1997); left atrial enlargement may be present. Atrial fibrillation, a late sign, may occur in approximately <10% of cases.

2. CXR: Cardiomegaly (when LV failure present); poststenotic dilatation of the ascending aorta common; calcification of aortic valve may be present.

3. Echocardiography/Doppler echocardiography/transesophageal echocardiography (TEE): Estimate valve area, gradient, regurgitant flow, assess LV wall thickness.

4. Cardiac catheterization: Estimate valve area, gradient, and presence of regurgitant flow; assess LV function, and the presence or absence of associated valvular disease and coronary artery disease.

MANAGEMENT/TREATMENT

1. Patients with asymptomatic mild AS should receive noninvasive assessment of the severity of obstruction with Doppler echocardiography at a minimum of every 2 years.

2. Patients with severe asymptomatic AS should be followed every 6–12 months including clinical examination, ECG, and echocardiogram.

3. Asymptomatic patients should be instructed to report any symptoms that may be related to AS.

4. Endocarditis prophylaxis is indicated for all patients with AS (Table 3–24).

5. Medical therapy may be indicated for patients with AS. The ACNP may be required to treat symptoms associated with HF in the patient with AS.

TABLE **3-24.** **Antibiotic Prophylaxis for Dental, Oral, Respiratory Tract, or Esophageal Procedures**

Procedure	Antibiotic	Dose (Adults)
Prophylactic regimen for dental, oral, respiratory tract, or esophageal procedures	For most patients standard general prophylaxis: oral amoxicillin For amoxicillin/penicillin allergy: clindamycin, or azythromycin, or cephalexin	2.0 gm PO 1 hr before the procedure Clindamycin 600 mg or azythromycin 500 mg 1 hr prior to procedure; cephalexin 2.0 gm 1 hr prior to procedure

* Adapted from Dajani, A.S., Bisno, A.L., Chung, K.J., et al. (1997). Prevention of bacterial endocarditis. Recommendations by the American Heart Association. *JAMA 277*(22), 1794–1801. Copyright 1990, American Medical Association, with permission.

PO, orally.

The ACNP should consult with the collaborating physician regarding judicious use of diuretics and vasodilators, which may lead to hypotension and subsequent inability to maintain an adequate SV. (See also "Heart Failure.")

6. Atrial fibrillation may be present in severe AS. (Management of atrial fibrillation is outlined in "Arrhythmias.") The presence of atrial fibrillation should prompt the ACNP and collaborating physician to search for evidence of mitral valve disease.

7. Invasive and/or surgical intervention is usually reserved for symptomatic patients and hemodynamic evidence of severe obstruction.

8. Valve replacement is the surgical treatment of choice in adults with symptomatic AS and is associated with improvements in LV function.

9. Timing of aortic valve replacement (AVR) remains a critical decision in the treatment of patients with AS. General indications for AVR include:
   A. Peak systolic gradient ≥50 mm Hg
   B. Valve area ≤0.75 cm^2 (mild: 1.2–2.0 cm^2, moderate: 0.75–1.2 cm^2, severe: <0.75 cm^2)
   C. Ventricular enlargement (systolic transverse axis dimension ≥5.5 cm or cardiothoracic ratio ≥0.55)

10. The operative risk in patients without LV failure ranges from 2–8%. Risk factors for higher operative mortality include NYHA class, impairment of LV function, advanced age, and the presence of associated aortic regurgitation (Braunwald, 1997).

11. The 5-year actuarial survival rate is 85% with AVR.

12. In patients with AS and CAD, AVR and myocardial revascularization should be performed together.

13. Percutaneous aortic valvuloplasty (PTAV) is a therapeutic option for patients who are considered poor candidates for AVR (i.e., elderly with heart failure).

14. Mortality with PTAV is approximately 3–7% with restenosis rates of up to 50% of patients at 6 months.

15. PTAV may be recommended in nonsurgical candidates including patients in cardiogenic shock due to critical AS, patients with critical AS who require an urgent noncardiac operation, as a "bridge" to AVR in patients with severe heart failure who are at extremely high operative risk, and in pregnant women with critical AS (Braunwald, 1997).

16. Approximately 5% of patients undergo operative valvuloplasty, commissurotomy, and reconstruction of the aortic annulus; however, these procedures have not proven comparable to AVR (Baumgartner, 1994).

AORTIC REGURGITATION (AR)

ETIOLOGY/INCIDENCE

1. AR may be caused by primary disease of the aortic valve leaflets or the wall of the aortic root or both (Braunwald, 1997).

2. Primary disease of the aortic valve may be caused by rheumatic fever, infective endocarditis, trauma, and a congenital bicuspid valve.

3. AR is also noted in patients with Marfan's syndrome, Ehlers-Danlos syndrome, myxomatous proliferation of the aortic valve, and other related diseases of connective tissue.

4. Marked dilatation of the aorta leading to AR results from a variety of disease

states such as annuloaortic ectasia, syphilitic aortitis, ankylosing spondylitis, giant cell arteritis, and systemic HTN.

5. Patients with chronic severe AR may remain asymptomatic as the LV gradually undergoes enlargement. With the deterioration of LV function and presence of symptoms, survival rates decrease to approximately 75% at 5 years from onset of symptoms.

SIGNS AND SYMPTOMS

1. As previously stated, many patients with AR remain asymptomatic. Symptoms usually present in the fourth and fifth decades of life.
2. Exertional dyspnea, orthopnea, and paroxysmal nocturnal dyspnea are the predominant complaints.
3. Sensation of forceful heartbeat is often reported, especially in the supine position. May be accompanied by thoracic pain.
4. Angina may be present, especially nocturnal angina with diaphoresis.
5. Tachycardia, may be associated with palpitations, head pounding.
6. Symptoms of overt LV failure may be present in late stages. (See also "Heart Failure.")

PHYSICAL FINDINGS

1. Arterial pulse: *Corrigan's* pulse characterized by abrupt distention and quick collapse, readily visible in the carotid arteries; *bisferious* pulse (characterized by two systolic peaks) may be present; wide pulse pressure, systolic arterial pressure is elevated and diastolic pressure is abnormally low.
2. Palpation: Apical impulse diffuse, hyperdynamic, and displaced laterally and inferiorly; systolic retraction may be present over suprasternal region; rapid ventricular filling wave often palpable at apex; systolic thrill often palpable at base or suprasternal notch and carotid arteries.
3. Auscultation:
   A. Chronic AR: S_1 is soft or absent; S_2 may be absent or single; S_3 gallop correlates with increased LV end-diastolic pressure; high-frequency, blowing early-peaking, diastolic decrescendo murmur best heard with the diaphragm of the stethoscope with patient sitting leaning forward and in deep fixed expiration; severity of murmur correlates with duration of the murmur rather than intensity.
   B. Acute AR: Mid to late diastolic apical rumble; *Austin-Flint* murmur heard in mid-diastole, caused by turbulent antegrade flow across the mitral orifice that may be narrowed by the rapidly rising LV diastolic pressure caused by the severe AR (Braunwald, 1997); murmurs of AR augmented by any measures that increase arterial pressure such as vasopressors, squatting, or isovolumetric exercises; reduced by amyl nitrate, Valsalva strain that reduces arterial pressure.
4. Head-bobbing with each heartbeat may be visible with chronic severe AR.
5. Patients with acute AR often present gravely ill, with tachycardia, severe peripheral vasoconstriction, and pulmonary congestion and edema.

DIAGNOSTIC TESTS/FINDINGS

1. ECG:
   A. Chronic AR: Left axis deviation, left ventricular diastolic volume overload pattern; characterized by an increase in initial forces (Q waves in leads I, aVL, V_3 to V_6) and small r in V_1.

    B. Acute AR: LV hypertrophy may be present; nonspecific ST-T–wave changes may be present.

2. CXR: Cardiomegaly may be present with LV dilatation (less likely with acute AR); severe aneurysmal dilatation of the ascending aorta may be present in aortic root disease (i.e., Marfan's syndrome); pulmonary vascular congestion may be present with acute AR.

3. Echocardiography: Increased motion of the septum and posterior wall (left ventricular end-diastolic diameter and extent of systolic shortening are both augmented); identify and quantify AR (i.e., thickening of valve cusps, prolapse of the valve, flail leaflet, vegetations, dilatation of the aortic root).

4. Cardiac catheterization: Quantify degree of AR, aortography, assessment of LV function, and assessment of coexisting CAD.

MANAGEMENT/TREATMENT

1. The ACNP in consultation with the collaborating physician will manage patients with AR.
2. All patients with AR require endocarditis prophylaxis (Table 3–24).
3. Asymptomatic patients with mild to moderate AR:
   A. Annual echocardiogram to evaluate AR, LV function
   B. Consider digoxin if LV dilatation present.
4. Symptomatic patients with preserved LV function:
   A. Diuretics to relieve volume overload.
   B. Afterload reduction with vasodilator.
   C. Frequent follow-up (q3–6mo) to evaluate progression of symptoms, echocardiogram to evaluate AR/LV function.
   D. Systolic HTN may increase regurgitation, treat medically to maintain SBP <140 mm Hg, avoid use of β-blockers due to negative inotropic effects. (See "Hypertension.")
   E. Atrial rhythms and bradyarrhythmias tolerated poorly and require prompt treatment. (See "Arrhythmias" for management of these rhythms)
5. Symptomatic patients with severe chronic AR and/or evidence of impaired LV contractile function warrant referral to the cardiac surgeon for AVR. The ACNP consults with the collaborating physician regarding management of symptoms of HF due to AR. (See "Heart Failure.")
6. The operative mortality in patients without LV failure ranges from 3–8%. A late mortality of approximately 5–10% per year is noted in patients with preoperative marked cardiac enlargement and prolonged LV dysfunction.
7. Patients presenting with acute AR require immediate consultation with the collaborating physician and the cardiac surgeon for emergent evaluation and consideration for emergent AVR. The use of vasodilators (nitroprusside) and/or positive inotropes (i.e., dobutamine, dopamine) may be indicated to stabilize the patient prior to surgical intervention.

MITRAL STENOSIS (MS)

ETIOLOGY/INCIDENCE

1. The predominant cause of MS is rheumatic fever (Braunwald, 1997). Approximately 25% of patients with rheumatic fever have pure MS; approxi-

mately 40% have combined MS and mitral regurgitation (MR). The majority of patients with rheumatic MS are female.

2. Pathophysiologic findings of MS include fibrous thickening of the valve leaflets, fusion of the commissures, thickening and shortening of the chordae tendinae, and leaflet calcification as a result of acute and recurrent inflammation.
3. Other causes of MS include malignant carcinoid, systemic lupus erythematosus, and rheumatoid arthritis. Calcification of the mitral annulus is a less frequent cause of MS (as compared to MR).

SIGNS AND SYMPTOMS

1. The clinical presentation of MS depends in large part on the severity of the reduced valve area. Normal cross-sectional area of the mitral valve orifice is 4–6 cm^2. If the valve area is reduced to <2 cm^2, a significant pressure gradient develops between the left atrium and the left ventricle during diastole. Hemodynamic grades of MS are:
   A. Minimal: >2.5 cm^2
   B. Mild: 1.4–2.5 cm^2
   C. Moderate: 1.0–1.4 cm^2
   D. Severe: <1.0 cm^2
2. The predominant presenting complaint with MS is dyspnea. Reduced exertional capacity is also frequently reported.
3. Later manifestations of MS include increased fatigue and signs and symptoms of pulmonary congestion (i.e., orthopnea, paroxysmal dyspnea [PND]).
4. Patients with advanced MS may present with signs of pulmonary HTN and right-sided heart failure (i.e., peripheral edema, hepatomegaly, ascites).
5. Hemoptysis and chest pain may also be reported.

PHYSICAL FINDINGS

1. General: Pinkish purple, ruddy cheeks, "mitral facies," secondary to low cardiac output, systemic vasoconstriction with severe MS.
2. Arterial pulse: Usually normal.
3. Jugular venous pulse: Prominent a wave (sinus rhythm), prominent v wave (atrial fibrillation).
4. Palpation: RV lift may be present at left parasternal region; palpable tapping S_1, diastolic thrill when patient in left lateral recumbent position.
5. Auscultation: Accentuated S_1 that decreases with increased severity of MS, opening snap (OS) best heard at the apex with diaphragm of stethoscope following A_2; A_2-OS interval correlates to the severity of narrowing of the valve; low-pitched early to mid-diastolic rumble best heard at apex with the bell of stethoscope, may radiate to axilla or left sternal area, presystolic accentuation may be present in patients with severe MS; duration of diastolic murmur correlates with severity of MS. Diastolic murmur and OS reduced during inspiration, augmented during expiration; diastolic murmur reduced during Valsalva strain, augmented during sudden squatting, coughing, isovolumetric exercise, amyl nitrate.
6. GI: Ascites, hepatomegaly (late findings).
7. Peripheral edema may be present.

DIAGNOSTIC TESTS/FINDINGS

1. ECG: Left atrial (LA) enlargement, RV hypertrophy when pulmonary HTN present, atrial fibrillation may be present due to the chronic increase in LA pressure.
2. CXR: Left atrial enlargement, pulmonary vascular redistribution, interstitial edema, Kerly's B lines may be present due to edema and distention of the pulmonary lymphatics; RV enlargement and prominence of pulmonary arteries with pulmonary HTN.
3. Echocardiography: Major diagnostic tool; assess for thickened mitral leaflets, abnormal fusion of mitral commissures with restricted separation during diastole, left atrial enlargement, intra-atrial thrombus; assess mitral valve area, assess degree of pulmonary HTN.
4. Cardiac catheterization: Assess valve area, associated MR, pulmonary HTN, and presence of CAD.

MANAGEMENT/TREATMENT

1. The ACNP in consultation with the collaborating physician will manage patients with MS.
2. Endocarditis prophylaxis is indicated in all patients with MS (Table 3–24).
3. Diuretics may be indicated for relief of vascular congestion, fluid overload. (See "Heart Failure.")
4. When MS is accompanied by atrial fibrillation, the goal of therapy is to slow the ventricular rate and convert to sinus rhythm. Digoxin, β-blockers are recommended. Cardioversion may be indicated if pharmacologic therapy fails. Anticoagulation with warfarin is recommended to reduce the risk of thromboembolism. (See "Arrhythmias" for management of atrial fibrillation.)
5. Mitral valve replacement (MVR) is indicated for patients with moderate to severe MS (mitral valve area <1.0 cm^2/m^2 body surface area [BSA]) (Braunwald, 1997). Symptomatic patients with moderate to severe MS warrant referral to the cardiac surgeon for MVR by the collaborating physician. The operative mortality rate for MVR is 1–4%.
6. PTMV can be an effective means of increasing mitral valve area in selected patients who are considered unsuitable for surgery (i.e., elderly with associated severe ischemic heart disease, MS complicated by pulmonary, renal, or neoplastic disease). The risk of death from PTMV is approximately 1% and the restenosis rate is approximately 4% at 1 year.

MITRAL REGURGITATION (MR)

ETIOLOGY/INCIDENCE

1. Abnormalities in the structural components of the mitral valve may lead to MR.
2. The etiologies of MR include rheumatic heart disease, mitral valve prolapse, ischemic heart disease with papillary muscle dysfunction, LV dilation of any cause, mitral annular calcification, hypertrophic cardiomyopathy, infective endocarditis, mitral valve prolapse, and congenital abnormalities.

SIGNS AND SYMPTOMS

1. Early manifestations of MR include dyspnea and reduced exertional capacity.
2. Late or chronic manifestations of MR include increasing fatigue, orthopnea, and PND secondary to low cardiac output.
3. Acute presentation: Pulmonary edema.
4. Angina pectoris is rare unless coexisting CAD is present.

PHYSICAL FINDINGS

1. Carotid arterial pulse: Sharp upstroke with normal or reduced volume (with HF).
2. Palpation: PMI is brisk, hyperdynamic, displaced to the left; LV filling wave may be palpable in early diastole (LV lift).
3. Auscultation: Diminished S_1; wide splitting of S_2; S_3 due to increased early filling due to the augmented LV volume load; high-pitched, blowing, constant, holosystolic murmur best heard at the apex, may radiate to axilla and left infrascapular area, commences immediately after S_1, radiation to aortic area with posterior leaflet involvement, may become accentuated during acute myocardial ischemia if papillary muscle dysfunction present. Valsalva strain and appropriate medical therapy (diuretics, vasodilators) reduce the intensity of the murmur; isometric exercise augments the murmur of MR.

DIAGNOSTIC TESTS/FINDINGS

1. ECG: Left atrial enlargement, atrial fibrillation, LVH and RVH may be present.
2. CXR: Left atrial and left ventricular enlargement; calcification of the mitral annulus may be present; interstitial edema with Kerly's B lines may be present in acute MR.
3. Echocardiography: Identify structural cause of MR, grade severity of MR, assessment of LV function; Doppler ultrasound facilitates detection of MR by identifying turbulent flow within left atrium during systole.
4. Cardiac catheterization: Evaluate presence of CAD, grade severity of MR, assess LV function.

MANAGEMENT/TREATMENT

1. The ACNP in consultation with the collaborating physician will manage patients with MR.
2. Endocarditis prophylaxis is indicated in all patients with MR (Table 3–24).
3. Medical therapy centers around reducing pulmonary venous congestion and augmenting forward CO in place of regurgitation into LA. Medical management of MR includes all measures used in the treatment of HF. (See "Heart Failure" for specific management guidelines.)
   A. Diuretics to reduce volume overload
   B. Vasodilators to reduce systemic vascular resistance and LV afterload
4. Symptomatic patients with moderate to severe MR warrant referral to the cardiac surgeon for mitral valve repair or mitral valve replacement (MVR) by the collaborating physician. Operative mortality rates with mitral valve

repair is approximately 2% and 2–7% in patients with pure MR, New York Heart Association Functional Class II or III.

INFECTIVE ENDOCARDITIS (IE)

DEFINITION

1. Bacterial or fungal infection of the endocardial surface of the heart, including the valves.
2. IE is classified according to underlying anatomy (i.e., native valve, prosthetic valve) and infecting organism.

ETIOLOGY/INCIDENCE

1. Approximately 70% of patients presenting with IE (who do not use intravenous drugs) have evidence of underlying valvular abnormalities.
2. The major causes of native valve endocarditis include mitral valve prolapse, no underlying disease, degenerative lesions of the mitral and aortic valves, congenital heart disease, and rheumatic heart disease.
3. Prosthetic valve endocarditis accounts for 5–15% of cases of IE. Aortic valve prosthesis is more often affected than mitral. Endocarditis occurs within the first postoperative year in 1–2% of patients.

PATHOPHYSIOLOGY

1. Infection occurs most commonly when transient bacteria present in the bloodstream localize in sterile vegetations usually in areas of high pressure. The manifestations of infection result directly from vegetations on the valve and from circulating immune complexes. Complications arise from valve decompensation, embolization of vegetations, and extension of infection into nearby tissue.

SIGNS AND SYMPTOMS

1. Nonspecific symptoms: Malaise, fatigue, night sweats, anorexia, weight loss.
2. Fever is present in almost all patients with IE. Fever is usually low grade (<39°C). Elderly patients, patients with renal failure, CHF, or those previously treated with antibiotics may be afebrile.
3. CV: Cardiac murmur is common; a new cardiac murmur may arise or a change in an existing murmur may occur; IE must be investigated in any patient with heart murmur and fever; signs of congestive heart failure.
4. Respiratory: Pulmonary emboli may be present in IV drug users with tricuspid involvement.
5. Peripheral physical findings:
   A. *Janeway lesions*: Small, nontender, peripheral hemorrhages with slight nodular character; petichiae—on conjunctivae, palate, buccal mucossa, and upper extremities
   B. *Osler's nodes*: Small tender nodules, usually on finger or toe pads, persist for hours or days
   C. *Roth's spots*: Oval, retinal hemorrhages with a pale center.
6. Musculoskeletal: Arthritis, arthralgia.
7. Neurological: Headache, cerebral emboli, mycotic aneurysms.

DIAGNOSTIC TESTS/FINDINGS

1. Blood cultures: Positive blood cultures constitute definitive diagnosis.
2. Other laboratory findings may include normochromic normocytic anemia, elevated sedimentation rate, proteinuria, microscopic hematuria, and positive rheumatoid factor.
3. Echocardiography: Transthoracic and transesophageal echocardiography (TEE) may demonstrate vegetations and/or intracardiac abscess.

MANAGEMENT/TREATMENT

1. The ACNP must consult with the collaborating physician and infectious disease specialist regarding the appropriate antibiotic regimen for the patient with IE.
2. Obtain blood cultures. Treat with antibiotics until organisms isolated. (See "Infection" for suggested antibiotic regimens.) Karchmer (1997) provides a comprehensive review of causative organisms and appropriate therapy for IE.
3. Organisms that are commonly found to cause IE on native valves (in non-IV drug abusers) include streptococci (50–70%), enterococci (10%), and staphylococci (25%) (Karchmer, 1997).
4. Organisms commonly found to cause IE on prosthetic valves include staphylococci (40–50%), fungi, gram-negative aerobic organisms (20%), streptococci and enterococci (5–10%), and diptheroids (5–10%) (Karchmer, 1997).
5. Prolonged high-dose antibiotic therapy and/or valve replacement may be indicated for patients with evidence of severe valve dysfunction, persistent positive blood cultures despite antibiotic therapy, fever persisting for >1 week of therapy, severe congestive heart failure, recurrent emboli despite treatment, and evidence of myocardial or valve ring abscess.
6. The most important aspect of therapy is *prevention* of IE by administering antibiotics prior to procedures that may result in bacteremia in susceptible individuals. Procedures/circumstances warranting IE prophylaxis include (but are not limited to) (Dajani, 1997):
   A. Dental manipulations known to induce gingival bleeding or mucosal bleeding, including professional cleaning
   B. Tonsillectomy and/or adenoidectomy
   C. Surgical operations that involve intestinal or respiratory mucosa
   D. Rigid bronchoscopy and surgery of the upper respiratory tract
   E. Sclerotherapy for esophageal varices
   F. Esophageal dilatation
   G. Urethral catheterization if urinary tract infection is present
   H. Urinary tract surgery if urinary tract infection is present
   I. Genitourinary procedures including indwelling bladder catheter, cystoscopy, prostatectomy
   J. Prostatic surgery
   K. Gastrointestinal surgery, including cholycystectomy
   L. Previous endocarditis
   M. Incision and drainage of infected tissue
   N. Vaginal delivery complicated by infection
7. Table 3–24 outlines antibiotic prophylaxis for dental, oral, respiratory tract or esophageal procedures as recommended by the American Heart Association. For antibiotic prophylaxis for additional procedures refer to Dajani, et al, 1997.

PATIENT EDUCATION

1. Educate patient and family regarding disease condition.
2. Educate patient and family regarding endocarditis prophylaxis.
3. Educate patient and family regarding signs and symptoms of worsening condition to report to ACNP/collaborating physician.
4. Educate patient and family regarding activity limitations during acute periods.
5. For patients with HF secondary to valve disease, provide teaching regarding medications, fluid limitations, and sodium restriction. (See "Heart Failure.")
6. Educate patient and family regarding follow-up appointment prior to discharge.

Review Questions

3.31 The classic triad of symptoms associated with aortic stenosis includes:
   A. Chest pain, orthopnea, fatigue
   B. Chest pain, dyspnea, syncope
   C. Shortness of breath, headache, palpitations
   D. Dyspnea, fatigue, syncope

3.32 A 40-year-old man with a congenital bicuspid aortic valve is planning to have dental work after discharge from the hospital. As the ACNP you inform the patient that prophylactic antibiotic therapy is indicated. The patient is allergic to Penicillin (PCN). What antibiotic regimen would the ACNP order for this patient?
   A. Clindamycin 600 mg PO 1 hour prior to the procedure
   B. Amoxicillin 2 gm PO 1 hour before the procedure
   C. No antibiotic prohylaxis is recommended
   D. None of the above

3.33 An 80-year-old woman with a history of rheumatic heart disease is in the hospital for treatment of new-onset atrial fibrillation with rapid ventricular rate. On cardiac auscultation you hear a diastolic murmur, decrescendo in nature, with presystolic accentuation and an opening snap. Which of the following is the most likely etiology of this murmur?
   A. Mitral stenosis
   B. Aortic stenosis
   C. Mitral regurgitation
   D. Aortic regurgitation

3.34 Which of the following is a FALSE statement regarding mitral stenosis?
   A. The relationship between the timing of the A_2 and the OS relates inversely to the severity of the mitral stenosis.
   B. The OS precedes the systolic low-pitched rumbling murmur.
   C. The duration of the diastolic murmur of mitral stenosis is a guide to the severity of mitral narrowing.
   D. The primary etiology of mitral stenosis is rheumatic heart disease.

3.35 Marfan's syndrome is associated with which one of the following valvular diseases?

A. Mitral stenosis
B. Aortic stenosis
C. Aortic regurgitation
D. Mitral regurgitation

Answers and Rationales

3.31   **B**   The classic triad of symptoms associated with aortic stenosis is chest pain, dyspnea, and syncope.

3.32   **A**   Antibiotic prophylaxis is recommended by the American Heart Association in this setting. As the patient is PCN allergic, clindamycin is recommended.

3.33   **A**   See Question 3.34.

3.34   **B**   MS is characterized by a diastolic low-pitched rumbling murmur preceded by an OS. Presystolic accentuation of the murmur occurs in severe mitral stenosis.

3.35   **C**   Marfan's syndrome is associated with aortic regurgitation.

References

Baumgartner, W.A., Owens, S.G., Caneron, D.E., & Reitz, B.A. (eds.). (1994). *The Johns Hopkins Manual of Cardiac Surgical Care*. St. Louis: Mosby-Year Book Inc.

Braunwald, E. (1997). Valvular heart disease. In E. Braunwald (ed.). *Heart Disease: A Textbook of Cardiovascular Medicine* (5th ed.). Philadelphia: W.B. Saunders Co., pp. 1007–1076.

Dajani, A.S., et al. (1997). Prevention of bacterial endocarditis: Recommendations by the American Heart Association. *JAMA 227*(22) 1794–1801.

Karchmer, A.W. (1997). Infective endocarditis. In E. Braunwald (ed.). *Heart Disease: A Textbook of Cardiovascular Medicine* (5th ed.). Philadelphia: W.B. Saunders Co., pp. 1077–1104.

Shackenbach, L.H. (1996). Patients with valvular disease. In J.M. Clochesy, C. Breu, S. Cardin, et al. (eds.). *Critical Care Nursing* (2nd ed.). Philadelphia: W.B. Saunders Co., pp. 428–457.

Shackenbach, L.H. (1987). Physiologic dynamics of acquired valvular heart disease. *J Cardiovasc Nurs 1*(3), 1–17.

Arrhythmias

DEFINITION

1. The term "arrhythmia," meaning imperfection in a regularly recurring motion, refers to all cardiac rhythms other than normal sinus rhythm (Wagner, 1994).

2. This section will provide an overview of arrhythmias that are encountered in the acute-care setting and may be life threatening. These include symptomatic bradycardia/complete heart block (CHB), ventricular fibrillation (VF), VT, asystole, atrial fibrillation (AF), and wide complex tachycardia (SVT vs. VT).

ETIOLOGY/INCIDENCE

1. An initial tachyarrhythmia is associated with 80–90% of all nontraumatic cases of cardiac arrest in adults (Cummins, 1994).
2. Ventricular arrhythmias are common in patients with HF and account for sudden death in approximately 50% of this patient population.
3. The incidence of atrial fibrillation in the U.S. population is approximately 2.2 million cases. Advancing age, diabetes, heart failure, valvular disease, hypertension, and myocardial infarction predict the occurrence of AF within a population (Blackshear et al. 1996).

DIAGNOSTIC TESTS/FINDINGS

1. For all arrhythmias discussed an immediate 12-lead ECG and assessment of the patient is warranted to diagnose and document the arrhythmia, and to determine if ischemia and/or infarction are possible etiologies of the arrhythmia.
2. Holter monitoring may detect suspected arrhythmias in the acute-care and outpatient settings.
3. An echocardiogram may be indicated, for example, to rule out the possibility of intra-atrial thrombi or to assess LV function.
4. Electrophysiology studies (EPS) are indicated for the diagnosis of VT and SVT, to test drug efficacy, to stimulate an arrhythmia, and to evaluate the need for an implantable antitachycardia device.

SYMPTOMATIC BRADYCARDIA/COMPLETE HEART BLOCK

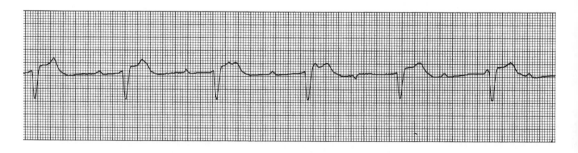

SIGNS AND SYMPTOMS/PHYSICAL FINDINGS

1. Serious signs and symptoms associated with symptomatic bradycardia/complete heart block (CHB) are related to the slow ventricular rate.
   A. Signs: Hypotension, shock, pulmonary congestion, heart failure, AMI
   B. Symptoms: Chest pain, shortness of breath, decreased level of consciousness

ECG Characteristics

1. Bradycardia
   A. P wave: 40–60/min; vector and duration unchanged
   B. QRS: 40–60/p min; vector and duration unchanged; regular.
   C. PR: 1:1

2. CHB
   A. P wave: 60–100/min; vector unchanged; vector and duration unchanged if an escape junctional rhythm is present, typically 40–60/min; vector may be changed and duration will be lengthened if an escape idioventricular rhythm is present at <40/min, if no escape rhythm, ventricular asystole results
   B. PR: No relationship; no P waves are conducted

MANAGEMENT/TREATMENT

1. *Treatment of symptomatic bradycardia/CHB requires immediate consultation with the collaborating physician.*
2. Atropine 0.5–1.0 mg IVP, may repeat to maximum dose of 3 mg IVP.
3. Isoproteronol (2 mg/250 mL D_5W) 2–20 μg/kg/min.
4. Epinepherine (2 mg/250 mL D_5W) 2–10 μg/min.
5. Dopamine (400 mg/250 mL D_5W) 5–20 μg/kg/min.
6. Temporary transcutaneous pacing: Initial settings—rate, 80–100/min; MA, start at 40 MA and increase until ventricular capture is established.
7. Temporary transvenous pacing: Initial settings—rate, 80–100/min; MA, Set at 1.5–3 times the threshold established for ventricular capture.

VENTRICULAR FIBRILLATION (VF)

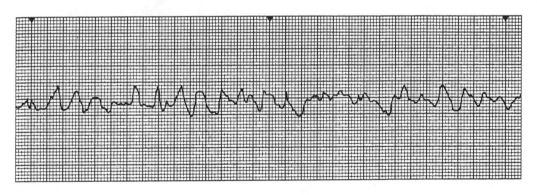

SIGNS AND SYMPTOMS/PHYSICAL FINDINGS

1. Cardiac arrest
2. Pulseless
3. Apneic

ECG Characteristics

1. P waves: None
2. QRS: None
3. Chaotic undulations, may be obvious or fine and difficult to see

MANAGEMENT/TREATMENT

1. *Treatment of VF requires immediate activation of the ACLS protocol for VF and immediate notification of the collaborating physician.*

2. Assess airway, breathing, circulation (ABC) per ACLS protocol.
3. Perform cardiopulmonary resuscitation (CPR) until defibrillator available.
4. Defibrillate up to three times (200, 300, and 360 J). Assess rhythm after each defibrillation.
5. If defibrillation is unsuccessful, continue CPR.
6. Intubate, establish IV access.
7. Medication sequence with defibrillation. Defibrillate per ACLS protocol after each dose:
   A. Epinephrine: 1 mg IVP, may repeat q3–5 min.
   B. Lidocaine: 1.0–1.5 mg/kg IVP. May repeat in 3–5 minutes to maximum dose of 3 mg/kg. A single dose of 1.5 mg/kg in cardiac arrest is acceptable.
   C. Bretylium: 5 mg/kg IVP. Repeat in 5 minutes at 10 mg/kg.
   D. Magnesium sulfate: 1–2 gm IV with torsades de pointes or suspected hypomagnesemic state or refractory VF.
   E. Procainamide: 30 mg/min in refractory VF (maximum total 17 mg/kg).
8. Assess electrolytes, acid-base balance.

VENTRICULAR TACHYCARDIA (VT)

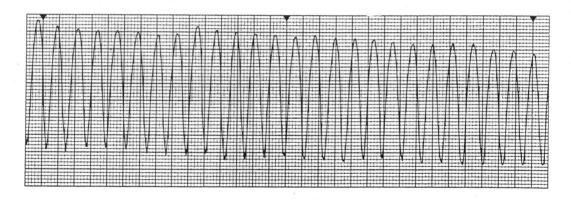

SIGNS AND SYMPTOMS/PHYSICAL FINDINGS

1. Serious signs and symptoms related to ventricular arrhythmias include:
   A. Signs: Hypotension, shock, pulmonary congestion, congestive heart failure, AMI
   B. Symptoms: Chest pain, shortness of breath, decreased level of consciousness

ECG Characteristics

1. Ventricular tachycardia
   A. P waves: 60–100/min if SR is present, may not be present
   B. QRS: 100–250/min; vector may change; duration >0.16 second; slightly irregular
2. Accelerated ventricular tachycardia
   A. QRS: 60–100/min
   B. Idioventricular rhythm: 20–60/min
3. See Table 3–25 for distinguishing SVT with bundle branch block or aberrant conduction from VT

TABLE 3–25. Distinguishing SVT with Bundle Branch Block or Aberrant Conduction from VT*

V_1 or MCL_1		V_6 or MCL_6	
Ventricular			
Monophasic R		Biphasic rS with R:S ratio <1.0	†
Taller left peak		Monophasic Q	
Biphasic RS		Notched QS	
Biphasic qR		Biphasic qR	
Any one of the following in V_1 or V_2:		Intrinsicoid deflection ≥70 ms	
(a) R >30 ms			
(b) Slurred or notched S descent			
(c) QRS onset to S nadir >60 ms			
Supraventricular with Bundle Branch Block or Aberration			
Bimodal rR′ or Triphasic rsR′		Triphasic qRs with R:S ratio >1.0	†
All of the following in V_1 and V_2:		Intrinsicoid deflection ≤50 ms	
(a) R ≤30 ms or no R			
(b) Straight S descent			
(c) QRS onset to S nadir ≤60 ms			
And, no Q in V_4			
Unhelpful QRS Morphologies			
Slurred or notched taller right peak		Monophasic R	
		Taller left or right peak	
		Biphasic Rs with R:S ratio >1.0	

* Adapted from Drew, B.J. (1991). Bedside electrocardiographic monitoring: State of the art for the 1990's. *Heart Lung, 20*(6), 610–623, with permission.
† Applies only to tachycardias with a positive waveform in V_1.
SVT, supraventricular tachycardia; VT, ventricular tachycardia.

MANAGEMENT/TREATMENT

1. *Treatment of VT requires immediate activation of the ACLS protocol for VT and immediate notification of the collaborating physician.*
2. For VT *without* a pulse, see "Ventricular Fibrillation."
3. For symptomatic VT (see Signs and Symptoms/Physical Findings) prompt direct current (DC) cardioversion at 100, 200, or 360 J (per ACLS protocol). Follow with medication sequence as outlined in 5.
4. For hemodynamically stable VT follow the medication sequence below.
5. Medication sequence for VT:

A. Lidocaine: 1–1.5 mg/kg IVP; may repeat to a maximum of 300 mg; follow with IV drip (lidocaine 2 gm/250 mL D_5W) 2–4 mg/min

B. Procainamide: 20–30 mg/min; follow with IV drip (procainamide 2 gm/250 mL D_5W) 2–4 mg/min

C. Bretylium: 0.5–0.75 mg/kg IV; follow with IV drip (bretylium 2 gm/250 mL D_5W) 2–4 mg/min

D. Amiodarone (for VT refractory to other agents): Initial rapid loading dose 150 mg IV (15 mg/mL over the first 10 minutes), followed by 900 mg IV over the next 6 hours (1 mg/min), then maintenance dose of 0.5 mg/min IV drip. Oral amiodarone dosing: 600 mg PO qd for 2 weeks, then 400 mg PO qd for 2 weeks, followed by a maintenance dose of 200 mg PO qd. Baseline thyroid function tests, liver function tests, and pulmonary function tests are obtained for patients on amiodarone.

6. Assess electrolyte, acid-base status.
7. Assess for underlying cause (i.e. myocardial ischemia).
8. For refractory VT consider EPS, ablation, ICD, orthotopic heart transplantation.

ASYSTOLE

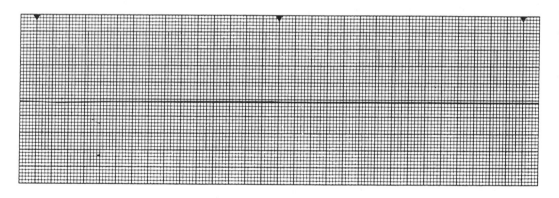

SIGNS AND SYMPTOMS/PHYSICAL FINDINGS

1. Cardiac arrest

ECG Characteristics

1. P waves: None
2. QRS: None

MANAGEMENT/TREATMENT

1. *Treatment of asystole requires immediate activation of the ACLS protocol for asystole and immediate notification of the collaborating physician.*
2. Check rhythm in two different leads to differentiate asystole from fine VF.
3. Assess airway, breathing, circulation (ABC) per ACLS protocol. Patient will be unresponsive, apneic, and pulseless.
4. Perform CPR.
5. Epinephrine 1 mg q3–5min.
6. Atropine 0.5–1.0 mg IVP.

7. Temporary transcutaneous pacing: Initial settings—rate, 80–100/min; MA, start at 40 MA and increase until ventricular capture is established.
8. Temporary transvenous pacing: Initial settings—rate, 80–100/min; MA, Set at 1.5–3 times the threshold established for ventricular capture.
9. If no response to resuscitation efforts, in consultation with the collaborating physician consider termination of efforts.

ATRIAL FIBRILLATION (AF)

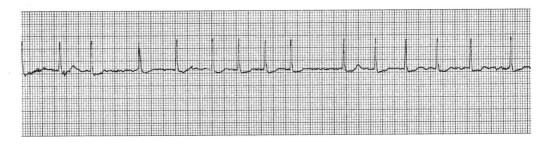

SIGNS AND SYMPTOMS/PHYSICAL FINDINGS

1. May be asymptomatic.
2. Signs and symptoms of hemodynamic compromise associated with atrial fibrillation include: hypotension, shortness of breath, congestive heart failure.

ECG Characteristics

1. P waves: Discrete atrial activity replaced by chaotic depolarization 300–750/min; baseline constantly affected; may distort ST segment and T waves
2. QRS: Up to 200/min; vector and duration unchanged; typically irregular, suspect complete block if ventricular rate is regular

MANAGEMENT/TREATMENT

1. *Treatment of AF requires immediate consultation with the collaborating physician.*
2. Identify potential contributing factors (i.e., pulmonary infection, hyperthyroidism, PE, hypersympathetic state associated with acute ETOH ingestion, underlying heart disease).
3. DC cardioversion is mandatory with rapid ventricular rate and hemodynamic compromise.
4. Continuous ECG monitoring recommended.

AF <48 HOURS

1. Pharmacologic control of ventricular rate, consider digoxin, β-blocker, diltiazem, or verapamil (see below for dosages).
2. Cardioversion *may* be attempted *without* prior anticoagulation.
3. Consider antithrombotic therapy: Initiate heparin drip to maintain activated partial thromboplastin time (aPTT) 50–80 seconds (see "Unstable Angina" for specific dosing regimen for heparin); add warfarin (see Table 3–26).
4. Observe for pharmacologic conversion to SR.

TABLE 3–26. **General Recommendations for Antithrombotic Therapy with Warfarin for AF**

1. A recommended guideline for initiating warfarin therapy is to give 5 mg/day for 5 days, checking PT with INR daily until it is in the therapeutic range; then check PT/INR weekly for up to 2 weeks. Intervals between subsequent PT/INR determinations should be based upon ACNP/collaborating physician's judgment of the patient's reliability and response to warfarin. Intervals of 1–4 weeks are usually acceptable. Maintenance doses initially range from 4–5 mg/day, yet may range from 1–20 mg/day (Gersh & Opie, 1995).
2. Adjust warfarin to maintain an INR of 2.0–3.0 (Hirsh et al. 1995).
3. In patients *without* clinical or echocardiographic evidence of risk factors* administer either warfarin (INR 2.0–3.0) or aspirin 325 mg/day. If risk factors emerge, change treatment from aspirin to warfarin; may occur in 10–15% of cases.
4. Warfarin may be discontinued after 3 weeks in patients who have successfully converted to sinus rhythm. Discontinuation of warfarin in the setting of sinus rhythm will be determined by the collaborating physician.
5. Use of warfarin may be discontinued approximately 5 days prior to a major procedure or continued at a decreased dose for a minor procedure. Early hospital admission for heparin administration during warfarin cessation may be warranted in high-risk patients (i.e., mechanical valve prosthesis, severe mitral stenosis, left ventricular dysfunction in the setting of AF).

* Risk factors: Previous TIA or stroke, hypertension, heart failure, diabetes, clinical coronary artery disease, mitral stenosis, prosthetic heart valves, or thyrotoxicosis (Laupacis et al. 1995).

AF, atrial fibrillation; PT, prothrombin time; INR, international normalized ratio; ACNP, acute-care nurse practitioners; TIA, transient ischemic attack.

AF >48 HOURS

1. Pharmacologic rate control and anticoagulation during hospitalization, continue medications at home for at least 3 weeks: elective cardioversion as outpatient or may rehospitalize.
2. Antithrombotic therapy indicated: Initiate heparin drip to maintain aPTT 1.5–2.0 times control (see "Unstable Angina" for specific dosing regimen for heparin); add warfarin (see Table 3–26).
3. Requires at least 3 weeks of anticoagulation with warfarin *prior to and following* elective chemical or electrical cardioversion to minimize systemic embolization (see Table 3–26).

AF PRECIPITATED BY AN ACUTE ILLNESS

1. Control ventricular rate as below; SR will return in most patients spontaneously with resolution of underlying precipitating event.

Pharmacologic Therapy/Chemical Cardioversion

1. Acute therapy: Rate control with digoxin, β-blocker, diltiazem, verapamil
   A. Digoxin: 0.5 mg IVP followed by 0.25 mg IVP q4–6h × 2
   B. Metroprolol: 5 mg IVP q5min up to 15 mg total; propranolol: 0.5–1.0 mg q5min up to 5 mg total
   C. Diltiazem: 20 mg over 2 minutes followed by 20 mg 20 minutes after the initial dose; follow with a 5-, 10-, or 15-mg/hr continuous IV infusion
   D. Verapamil: 5–10 mg slow IVP q30 min
2. Elective chemical conversion (Di Marco, 1994).
   A. Class 1A (procainamide, quinidine)
   B. Propafenone, sotolol (Class III), and amiodarone (Class III) may be successful in 50% of Class IA failures.

C. If AF is <48 hours, conversion rates are 70–90% for Class 1A agents.

D. If AF is >48 hours, conversion rates are 20–30% for all agents.

3. Elective electrical conversion (Di Marco, 1994).

A. Elective cardioversion is usually attempted (100, 200, 360 J) after a trial of chemical cardioversion.

B. If no response, consider IV procainamide (500–750 mg; rate not to exceed 30–50 μg/min) and reattempt electrical cardioversion using 360 J.

AF WITHOUT OVERT CARDIAC DISEASE

1. Control ventricular rate. (See above for specific medications and dosages.)

2. If <48 hours electrical or pharmacologic cardioversion.

3. If duration unknown anticoagulate for 3–4 weeks prior to electrical or pharmacologic cardioversion (see Table 3–26).

AF WITH SIGNIFICANT HEART OR VALVULAR DISEASE

1. Anticoagulate per above (see Table 3–26).

2. Treat underlying disease.

3. Control ventricular rate: β-blockers, diltiazem, amiodarone.

4. Digoxin alone often ineffective.

5. Amiodarone exhibits minimal proarrhythmic effects. Oral amiodarone dosing: 600 mg PO qd for 2 weeks, then 400 mg PO qd for 2 weeks, followed by a maintenance dose of 200 mg PO qd. Obtain baseline thyroid function tests, liver function tests, and pulmonary function tests for all patients starting amiodarone.

6. Avoid Class IA agents (quinidine, procainamide) due to increased proarrhythmic effects and negative inotropic effects in patients with significant myocardial dysfunction.

7. Ensure continued antithrombotic therapy with chronic AF (see Table 3–25).

8. When maintenance of SR and/or control of ventricular rate unsuccessful, consultation with the collaborating physician may be warranted regarding catheter ablation, surgical modification of AV conduction.

SUPRAVENTRICULAR TACHYCARDIAS (SVT)

AV Nodal Re-entrant Tachycardia (see p. 224)

SIGNS AND SYMPTOMS/PHYSICAL FINDINGS

1. While the rapid tachycardia is uncomfortable, it is usually benign because it tends to occur in young people without heart disease, and thus it is well-tolerated.

2. If not tolerated, symptoms such as palpitations, SOB, chest pain, hypotension, and CHF can occur.

ECG Characteristics

1. Rapid, regular tachycardia

2. Rate ranges from 150–250 bpm, usually 180–250 bpm

3. Onset and termination abrupt (i.e., paroxysmal)

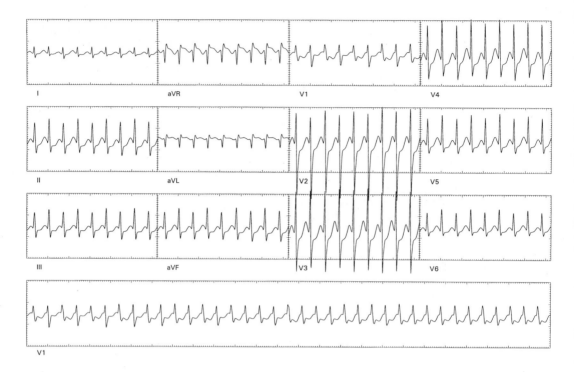

4. QRS normal and narrow (<0.12 second) unless there is aberrancy, which is rare
5. PR sequence:
   A. Common form: P waves are buried within the QRS or just barely visible at the J point which may look like part of the QRS rather than a retrograde P wave.
   B. P waves follow the QRS with an RP interval of 0.12 second or longer.
6. P wave polarity: Negative in the inferior leads (II, III, aVF).
7. Comments: Accounts for 60–70% of supraventricular tachycardia (SVT). Often initiated by premature atrial contraction (PAC). Re-entry in AV node (AVN) with antegrade conduction down slow, α-AVN pathway and retrograde conduction up fast, β-AVN pathway.
8. Table 3–25 outlines characteristics that distinguish SVT with bundle branch block or aberrant conduction from VT.

MANAGEMENT/TREATMENT

1. Immediate: AV nodal re-entrant tachycardia (AVNRT) is usually easily terminated with vagal maneuvers (carotid sinus massage) or drugs that block impulses at the AV node such as adenosine or verapamil. AVNRT can be readily terminated with pacing or DC cardioversion as well; however, these more uncomfortable procedures are rarely necessary.
2. Long-term: If a patient's lifestyle is hindered by frequent recurrences of AVNRT and the patient prefers not to take antiarrhythmic drugs, one of the dual pathways can be rendered incapable of transmitting impulses by radiofrequency (RF) ablation. RF ablation is done with the patient awake in the cardiac electrophysiology laboratory. Skill must be applied to prevent

both pathways from being damaged by the RF waves, which can cause complete AV block and require insertion of a permanent pacemaker.

AV Re-entrant Tachycardia (Orthodromic SVT)/WPW Syndrome (see p. 226, top)

SIGNS AND SYMPTOMS/PHYSICAL FINDINGS

1. Having an accessory pathway is not a problem in itself; problems arise only when the patient develops an SVT or atrial fibrillation with rapid ventricular conduction.
2. Hearts are usually normal, but can be associated with Ebstein's anomaly, cardiomyopathy, and mitral valve prolapse.
3. Symptoms such as palpitations, syncope, SOB, chest pain, hypotension, and CHF can occur.

ECG Characteristics

1. Short PR interval of ≤0.12 seconds, because ventricular depolarization begins earlier, taking up part of the PR segment.
2. Regular rhythm, rate 150–250 bpm.
3. Slurred initial deflection of the QRS complex (called delta wave) that may be negative or positive depending upon where the pathway is located, and which lead is recorded. The delta wave can vary between being absent (no pre-excitation) to being extremely wide (maximal pre-excitation). The wider the delta wave, the shorter the PR interval.
4. ST-segment and T-wave changes are common.
5. Comments: Wolff-Parkinson-White syndrome, concealed bypass tracts. SVT often initiated by PAC. Terminates suddenly with carotid sinus massage (see p. 226, bottom). In patients with manifest WPW, AF can conduct extremely rapidly, resulting in aberrant conduction and an irregular wide complex tachycardia that resembles VT and may degenerate into VF.

MANAGEMENT/TREATMENT

1. About 75% or more have paroxysmal SVTs, which can be divided into two main types: (1) re-entrant atrioventricular tachycardias, subdivided into "orthodromic" or "antidromic" tachycardia, and (2) atrial tachyarrhythmias (PAT, flutter, or fibrillation) with antegrade conduction over the accessory pathway (pre-excitation).
2. Orthodromic and antidromic tachycardias can be treated with any pharmacologic or vagal maneuver that can change the refractory period of either the AV node or accessory pathway, disrupting the re-entrant circuit, and terminating the tachycardia. The patient can be taught vagal maneuvers such as Valsalva, carotid sinus massage, squatting, gag reflex, immersion of face in ice water, etc. Adenosine or verapamil IV are the drugs of choice for terminating the arrhythmia, and β-blockers, digitalis, verapamil, pronestyl, quinidine, flecainide, and encainide can be used to prevent further SVTs.
3. Atrial flutter or fibrillation with rapid ventricular rate and hemodynamic deterioration should be DC cardioverted. If it is not an emergency, Pronestyl IV can be given. Drugs that block the normal AV nodal pathway should be avoided so as not to cause more impulses to travel to the ventricles over the accessory pathway.

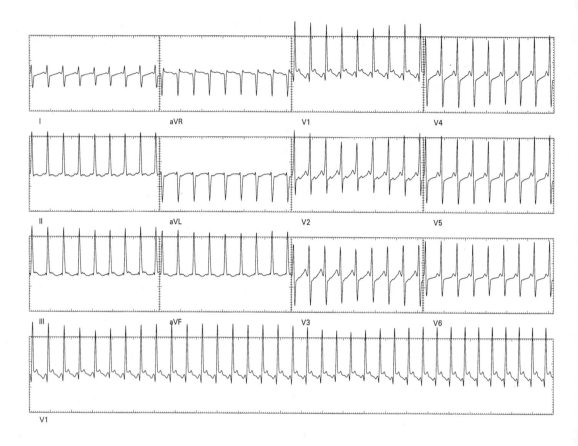

25mm/s
10mm/mV (Limb)
10mm/mV (Chest)
100Hz

Vent. rate(BPM) 105
PR interval(ms) 73
QRS duration(ms) 122

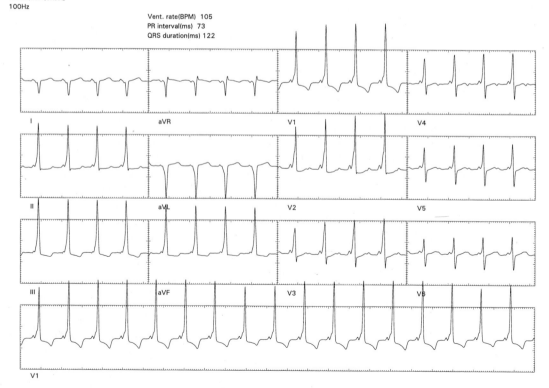

4. If the SVTs are frequent and the patient cannot tolerate antiarrhythmic medications, nonsurgical ablation can permanently interrupt the pathway. Open heart surgery can also be performed, and the pathway can be surgically interrupted.

Review Questions

3.36 A 72-year-old woman presents to the emergency room S/P syncopal episode. The monitor shows CHB. The patient's BP is 90/60. What is the most appropriate action the ACNP should take?
   A. Synchronized cardioversion at 50 J
   B. Dopamine 5 μg/kg/min
   C. Atropine 0.5 mg
   D. Transcutaneous pacing

3.37 Which of the following is the treatment for stable VT?
   A. Administer lidocaine 0.5 mg/kg IV, followed by a 2-mg/min drip
   B. Administer lidocaine 1 mg/kg IV bolus, followed by a 2-mg/min drip
   C. Administer lidocaine 2 mg/kg IV bolus, followed by a 2-mg/min drip
   D. Administer lidocaine 1 μg/kg IV bolus, followed by a 2-μg/min drip

3.38 The ACNP is called by the nurse to evaluate a patient with a wide complex tachycardia. The patient's vital signs are stable. The ACNP orders a 12-lead ECG. The ACNP confirms the diagnosis of VT. Which of the following is NOT a true statement regarding the ECG identification of VT?
   A. The presence of AV dissociation favors the diagnosis of VT
   B. Concordant pattern of R waves in all precordial leads
   C. QRS with R R' pattern in V1 with left R wave taller than right R wave
   D. QRS with RBBB pattern in V_6 with QRS <0.14 second

3.39 What is the appropriate action to take with the patient in Question 3.38 if BP decreases to 88/50 and chest pain occurs?
   A. Prepare for immediate DC cardioversion
   B. Adenosine 6 mg IVP, followed by 12 mg IVP if no response
   C. Lidocaine 1 mg/kg IV bolus, followed by a 2-mg/min drip
   D. Verapamil 5 mg IVP

3.40 The ACNP is called to evaluate a 76-year-old man 3 days postoperative for a hemicolectomy. The patient's heart rhythm is a narrow complex tachycardia at a rate of 140 bpm. The patient's blood pressure is 110/70 mm/Hg. The patient is mildly diaphoretic but has no other complaints. The ACNP determines the patient is in SVT. What is the first line of action the ACNP should take?
   A. DC cardioversion at 50 J
   B. Call the collaborating physician, order adenosine 6 mg IVP
   C. Verapamil 5 mg IVP, repeat in 5 minutes if no response
   D. Synchronized cardioversion at 50 J

Answers and Rationales

3.36   **C**   Atropine is the drug of choice for complete heart block. The ACNP should also prepare for transcutaneous pacing in the event of continued hemodynamic compromise.

3.37   **B**   Lidocaine 1 mg/kg IV bolus is the recommended first-line pharmacologic therapy for VT according to the American Heart Association's
Advanced Cardiac Life Support Guidelines. This dose is followed by
a 2-mg/min drip.

3.38   **D**   12 Lead ECG criteria favoring VT includes the presence of AV dissociation, concordant pattern of R waves in all precordial leads, and
QRS with R R' pattern in V1 with left R wave taller than right R
wave.

3.39   **A**   Unstable VT – Treatment is immediate DC cardioversion

3.40   **B**   Adenosine 6 mg IVP is the first-line therapy for hemodynamically
stable SVT, according to the American Heart Association's Advanced
Cardiac Life Support Guidelines. The ACNP should also consult with
the collaborating physician in this setting.

References

Blackshear, J.L., Kopecky, S.L., Litin, S.C., et al. (1996). Management of atrial fibrillation in adults: Prevention of thromboembolism and symptomatic treatment. *Mayo
Clin Proc 71*, 150–160.

Brugada, P., Brugada, J., Mont, L., et al. (1991). A new approach to the differential
diagnosis of a regular tachycardia with a wide QRS complex. *Circulation 83*(5),
1649–1659.

Chou, T., & Knilans, T.K. (1996). *Electrocardiography in Clinical Practice: Adult and
Pediatric* (4th ed.). Philadelphia: W.B. Saunders Co.

Cummins, R.O. (1994). *Textbook of Advanced Cardiac Life Support.* Dallas: American
Heart Association.

Drew, B.J. (1991). Bedside electrocardiographic monitoring: State of the art for the
1990's. *Heart and Lung 20*(6), 610–623.

Di Marco, J.P. (1994). Cardiac arrhythmias and conduction disturbances. In M. Freed &
C. Grines (eds.). *Essentials of Cardiovascular Medicine: Abridged Pocket Edition.*
Birmingham, MI, Physicians' Press, pp. 63–76.

Gersh, B.J., & Opie, L.H. (1995). Antithrombotic agents: Platelet inhibitors, anticoagulants, and fibrinolytics. In L.H. Opie (ed.). *Drugs for the Heart.* Philadelphia, W.B.
Saunders Co., pp. 248–287.

Golzari, H., Cebul, R.D., & Bahler, R.C. (1996). Atrial fibrillation: Restoration and maintenance of sinus rhythm and indications for anticoagulation therapy. *Ann Intern
Med 125*(4), 311–323.

Harvey, M.A. (1992). Study guide to core curriculum for critical care nursing (2nd ed.)
Philadelphia, W.B. Saunders Co.

Hirsch, J., Dalen, J., Deykin, D., et al. (1995). Oral anticoagulants: Mechanism of action,
clinical effectiveness, and optimal therapeutic range. *Chest 108*(4), 231S–246S.

Laupacis, A., Albers, G., Dalen, J., et al. (1995). Antithrombotic therapy in atrial fibrillation. *Chest 108*(4), 352S–359S.

Stevenson, W. (1995). Mechanisms and management of arrhythmias in heart failure.
Curr Opin Cardiol 10, 274–281.

Pericarditis

DEFINITION

Pericarditis is characterized by inflammation of the visceral and parietal pericardium, which may be fibrinous, serous, hemorrhagic, or purulent in nature.

Pericarditis can lead to pericardial effusion or progress to chronic constrictive pericarditis or cardiac tamponade.

ETIOLOGY/INCIDENCE

1. Viral infections are the most common cause of acute pericarditis and are probably responsible for the majority of cases classified as idiopathic. Other etiologies include:
   A. Myocardial infarction
   B. Uremia
   C. Infectious (bacterial, tuberculosis)
   D. Collagen vascular disease
   E. Radiation therapy
   F. Malignancy
   G. Blunt chest trauma
   H. Postoperatively after cardiac surgery.
2. The majority of episodes are self-limiting and resolve completely within 2–6 weeks.
3. The major early complication is cardiac tamponade (15%). Other complications include chronic constrictive pericarditis (<10%), recurrent severe chest pain (25%), and arrhythmias such as PAC's and SVT (Freed & Band, 1994).

SIGNS AND SYMPTOMS

1. The acute presentation includes chest pain, a pericardial friction rub, and serial ECG changes.
2. Pericardial chest pain includes the following characteristics:
   A. Quality: Sharp
   B. Location: Retrosternal
   C. Radiation: To shoulders, trapezius ridge, and neck
   D. Aggravating factors: Deep breathing (can be mistaken for pleuritis)
   E. Alleviating factors: Positioning (such as sitting up and leaning forward)
3. Pericarditis pain can mimic other conditions such as an acute abdominal process, aortic dissection, or myocardial infarction.
4. The pain of myocardial ischemia differs from pericardial pain by the following:
   A. Duration (ischemic pain lasts minutes to hours rather than hours to days)
   B. Quality (ischemic pain is pressure or burning rather than sharp and pleuritic)
   C. No relationship to deep inspiration, flat supine position, or leaning forward
5. Other signs and symptoms include dyspnea, fever, malaise, myalgias, and those specific to any underlying systemic diseases.

PHYSICAL FINDINGS (Freed & Band, 1994)

1. Pericarditis may initially present an arrhythmia such as SVT. It can also present as cardiac tamponade.
2. The single pathognomonic finding of acute pericarditis is the classic three-

component friction rub. Three rapidly consecutive sounds are produced by cardiac movement during atrial systole, ventricular systole (most common), and ventricular diastole (least common). A three-component friction rub is present in only 50% of cases. The friction rub is heard best at the lower left sternal border and less often at the apex. It may be missed on auscultation due to its intermittent nature. The sounds have a high-pitched squeaking or crunching quality, likened to a wet shoe leather sound.

3. ECG abnormalities occur in 90% of cases. Diffuse concave ST-segment elevation and PR-segment depression are early ECG changes of pericarditis. ST-segment elevation differs from myocardial infarction in that it is diffuse and the elevation is without reciprocal ST-segment depression or pathologic Q waves. The T wave remains upright until elevated ST segments descend to the isoelectric line. This finding contrasts to the T waves of myocardial infarction, which usually become inverted while the ST segment is still elevated.

4. In addition to chest pain, pericardial friction rub, and ECG changes, pericarditis is also characterized by the presence of a pericardial effusion. The speed of accumulation and the volume of accumulation determine the hemodynamic significance. Because the pericardium stretches, large effusions (>100 mL) that develop slowly may produce no hemodynamic effects. Smaller effusions that appear rapidly can lead to tamponade. Dyspnea and cough are common, especially with tamponade.

5. An increase in JVP is an early sign of a hemodynamically significant effusion. Hemodynamic monitoring can reveal an RA pressure tracing with a blunted Y but sharp X descent. Muffled heart tones and loss of friction rub may also be present. The presence of pulsus paradoxus (inspiratory fall in systolic BP >10 mm Hg) indicates impending hemodynamic compromise and should be considered a cardiac emergency (see "Cardiac Tamponade").

DIAGNOSTIC TESTS/FINDINGS

1. Depending on the suspected etiology, the diagnosis of pericarditis may require one or more of the following tests:
   A. Tuberculin skin test, blood cultures (infective endocarditis)
   B. Viral titers and cultures
   C. Human immunodeficiency virus (HIV) test
   D. Fungal serology
   E. Antistreptolysin O (ASO) titers (rheumatic fever)
   F. Cold agglutinins (mycoplasma)
   G. Heterophile antibody (mononucleosis)
   H. Thyroid function test (hypothyroidism)
   I. BUN/creatinine (uremia)
   J. Antinuclear antibodies (ANA), rheumatoid factor, and sedimentation rate (lupus, rheumatoid arthritis)
2. If pericarditis is accompanied by myocarditis, cardiac isoenzymes may be increased. Therefore, cardiac enzymes cannot be used conclusively to distinguish pericarditis from myocardial infarction.
3. Indications for pericardiocentesis and pericardial biopsy include suspected purulent pericarditis, tamponade, or the need for a surgical procedure (e.g., pericardial stripping).

MANAGEMENT/TREATMENT (Freed & Band, 1994;
Lorell & Braunwald, 1997)

1. For pericardial chest pain:
   A. Aspirin (650 mg PO q3–4h) *or*
   B. Indomethacin (25–50 mg PO q6h) results in relief of pain in most patients.
2. Morphine (2–15 mg IM/IV q4–6h) or meperidine (25–50 mg PO/IM/IV q3–4h) may be used to supplement PO pain relief medications.
3. If pain persists beyond 48–72 hours or is extremely severe, the ACNP should consult with the physician.
   The physician may consider use of steroids.
   A. Prednisone 60–80 mg/day in divided doses. In general, high-dose therapy is required for 5–7 days followed by tapering doses of anti-inflammatory agents.
4. Anticoagulation is not recommended due to risk of pericardial bleed. If anticoagulation is necessary for coexistent medical conditions (e.g., prosthetic valve), the ACNP should consult the physician first. IV heparin should be used rather than warfarin; protamine sulfate should be used to reverse heparin's effects when abrupt clinical deterioration occurs in association with an increasing effusion.
5. Table 3–27 lists specific treatments of pericarditis based on etiology.

PATIENT EDUCATION

1. Instruct patient on meaning of symptoms and diagnosis
2. Reassure patient that the pain is being addressed and that the problem is being corrected.
3. Prepare patient for any procedures/tests.
4. Discuss the outcome of treatment and continued need for monitoring and necessary treatment.
5. Encourage patient to ask questions and discuss fears and concerns.

Review Questions

3.41 The classic ECG change in acute pericarditis is:
   A. concordant ST-segment elevation in most leads except aVR and V_1
   B. PR-segment elevation
   C. Decrease in QRS voltage
   D. PR-segment depression and concave upward ST-segment elevation

3.42 A 50-year-old S/P AMI patient is day 3 postinfarct. The nurse pages the ACNP to report that the patient has a new episode of chest pain, rated 4/10, described as sharp and increases with inspiration. The patient also has a temperature of 37.9°C. The most likely reason for the chest pain is:
   A. Extension of the infarction
   B. Papillary muscle dysfunction
   C. Pericarditis
   D. Myocarditis

TABLE 3–27.   Treatment of Pericarditis Based on Etiology*

Etiology	Therapy
Aortic dissection	• Surgical correction.
Collagen vascular	
SLE (Lupus)	• Nonsteroidal anti-inflammatory drugs
Rheumatoid arthritis	• Corticosteroids for severe disease.
	• Immunosuppressive therapy for steroid-resistant cases.
Drug-induced	• Eliminate inciting agent.
	• Steroids may hasten recovery.
Idiopathic	• Rest and nonsteroidal anti-inflammatory drugs; steroids should be avoided.
Infectious	
Bacterial	• *Streptococcus pneumococcus*: Penicillin G ($200–250 \times 10^3$ U/kg/day IV divided into six doses) for at least 10–14 days Pericardial and blood isolates must be sent for susceptibility testing.
	• *Staphylococcus aureus*: Vancomycin (15 mg/kg IV to produce peak of 25–40 μg/mL and trough of 5–10 μg/mL) or nafcillin (200 mg/kg/day IV divided into six doses if susceptible) for at least 14–21 days.
Fungal	• Amphotericin B (0.3–0.7 mg/kg/day IV over 4–6 hr up to minimum of 1 gm) $\pm$ 5-flucytosine (up to 100–150 mg/kg/day in three or four divided doses).
TB	• Combination therapy with isoniazid (300 mg/day), rifampin (600 mg/day), pyrazinamide (PZA) (25 mg/kg/day), and corticosteroids (prednisone 1 mg/kg/day).
Viral	• Rest, nonsteroidal anti-inflammatory drugs, and close observation.
	• Corticosteroids should be avoided.
Infiltrative/metabolic	• Directed against the primary disease.
Malignant	• Terminally ill patient: Pericardiocentesis as needed. Secondary interventions include balloon pericardiostomy, sclerotherapy, or surgery through subxyphoid route for palliative "partial window."
	• Recurrent, symptomatic effusions when long-term prognosis is good: Radiation therapy for sensitive tumor types; otherwise, complete pericardiectomy. Intrapericardial sclerotherapy falling out of favor.
Post-MI	• Symptomatic therapy including rest, aspirin, analgesics, and close monitoring.
Postpericardiotomy	• Routine therapy with aspirin, nonsteroidal anti-inflammatory drugs.
	• If no response within 48 hr, steroids are administered.
Radiation	• None recommended if asymptomatic.
	• Steroids for severe intractable pain.
	• Extensive pericardiectomy for large recurrent effusions, severe effusive-constrictive, or constrictive pericarditis in those with good prognoses. Operative mortality ~20%.
Uremic	• Dialysis (intensify regimen if already on).
	• Surgical drainage for nonresponders or recurrences.

* Adapted from Freed, M., & Band, J.D. (1994). Pericardial disease. In M. Freed & C. Grines (eds.). *Essentials of Cardiovascular Medicine.* Birmingham, MI: Physicians' Press, pp. 419–422, with permission.
SLE, systemic lupus erythematosis; TB, tuberculosis; PZA, pyrazinamide; MI, myocardial infarction.

3.43 Your first step would be to:
   A. Consult with the physician
   B. Start indocin 25 mg PO q6h
   C. Give NTG 1/150 SL
   D. Obtain an ECG

3.44 In pericarditis cardiac isoenzymes are:
   A. Always elevated
   B. Always normal
   C. May be increased if pericarditis is accompanied by myocarditis
   D. May be increased if pericarditis is accompanied by pericardial effusion

3.45 If Indocin does not control the pain of pericarditis, the ACNP may consider supplemental therapy with:
   A. NTG IV drip
   B. Motrin
   C. Heparin
   D. Morphine

Answers and Rationales

3.41 **D** PR-segment depression and concave upward ST-segment elevation are early ECG changes of pericarditis.

3.42 **C** Pericarditis commonly presents itself with sharp chest pain that increases with inspiration and may be associated with fever.

3.43 **D** An ECG can document changes associated with pericarditis and is an important diagnostic test to R/O other causes of chest pain.

3.44 **C** Cardiac enzymes cannot be used to conclusively to distinguish pericardial from a myocardial infarction because they may be elevated if there is a concomitant myocarditis.

3.45 **D** Morphine 2–4 mg IV can be beneficial to control pain and decrease the workload of the heart by decreasing venous return.

References

Freed, M. & Band, J.D. (1994). Pericardial Disease. In M. Freed & C. Grines (eds.). *Essentials of Cardiovascular Medicine*. Birmingham, MI: Physician's Press, pp. 417–422.

Lorell, B.H., & Braunwald, E. (1997). Acute pericarditis. In E. Braunwald (ed.). *Heart Disease: A Textbook of Cardiovascular Medicine* (5th ed.). Philadelphia: W.B. Saunders Co., pp. 1487–1491.

Porembka, D.T. (1995). Pericarditis and endocarditis. In *Multidisciplinary Critical Care Board Review Course*. Anaheim, CA: Society of Critical Care Medicine, pp. 219–242.

Cardiac Tamponade

DEFINITION

Cardiac tamponade is a hemodynamic syndrome caused by compression of the heart due to increased fluid in the pericardial space that is under increased pressure. The fluid may be bloody, serosanguineous, serous, or purulent. In rare cases air in the pericardial space may produce a similar syndrome. The hemodynamic abnormalities in cardiac tamponade are reversed if fluid is removed to normalize pressure in the pericardial space.

ETIOLOGY/INCIDENCE

1. Traumatic causes of cardiac tamponade
   A. Cardiac perforation from any catheter placed within the heart
   B. Penetrating chest wounds
   C. Blunt trauma to the anterior chest wall
2. Medical causes of cardiac tamponade
   A. Various neoplastic syndromes resulting in pericardial effusion
   B. Clogged mediastinal or chest tubes following cardiac surgery
3. Infection
   A. Inflammation/pericarditis
4. Ruptured aortic aneurysm with bleeding into the pericardial cavity
5. AMI
6. Chronic renal failure (Baldwin et al., 1995; Hancock, 1994).

PATHOPHYSIOLOGY

Normally, the parietal pericardium directly contacts the heart and has a restraining effect when one or more chambers of the heart undergo acute enlargement. However, when the volume of pericardial fluid is increased to >100 mL, the parietal pericardium in not in contact with the heart, and a uniform pressure level is exerted throughout the pericardial space. The pressure exists equally on all chambers of the heart.

The pressure within a pericardial effusion is related to the volume of fluid, and rate of accumulation. In most cases of moderate or severe tamponade there is at least 500 mL of fluid (often the volume is >1000 mL). The pericardium has little capacity to stretch during a short period of time but a great capacity to stretch over a longer period. Cardiac tamponade may occur with as little as 200 mL of fluid when that amount of effusion develops over a few minutes, as in hemopericardium caused by trauma. Effusion as large as 2000 mL may develop with no rise in intrapericardiac pressure when this amount develops over months or years, as in cases of myxedema (Hancock, 1994).

SIGNS AND SYMPTOMS

The speed of air, blood, or fluid accumulation determines the degree of decline in cardiac function and the signs and symptoms observed.

Chronic Tamponade

The slower the accumulation, the longer the increased pressure that can be tolerated and the larger the amount of fluid that can be accommodated. Several hundred milliliters of accumulation may be tolerated before signs and symptoms occur. Symptoms include SOB, weight loss, and anorexia.

Acute Tamponade

A rapid increase of 50–100 mL or more can lead to hypotension, which indicates there is limited cardiac reserve and is a cardiac emergency.

Classic symptoms of cardiac tamponade include Beck's triad:

1. Systemic hypotension
2. Muffled heart sounds
3. Jugular venous distention

PHYSICAL FINDINGS

Subjective

1. Midthoracic chest pain
2. Dyspnea and shortness of breath

Objective

1. Evidence of precordial trauma or history of predisposing medical condition
2. Decreased urine output
3. Cough
4. Weak, tachycardic pulse
5. Cool, pale, diaphoretic skin
6. Pulsus paradoxus >10–15 mm Hg during inspiration (Mechanism: Inspiration-induced expansion of right heart volume and bowing of the intraventriculum into the LV causes impaired left ventricular filling and decreased cardiac output.)

   With slow development of tamponade, the pericardium has a chance to dilate slowly; 1000–2500 mL of fluid may be present. This leads to signs and symptoms that resemble right-sided heart failure and include:

1. Tachycardia
2. Edema
3. Hepatic engorgement
4. Positive hepatojugular reflex
5. Jugular venous distention

   With fast development of tamponade, the signs and symptoms resemble cardiogenic shock and include:

1. Agitation and confusion.
2. Decreased CO.
3. Distended neck veins.
4. Hypotension.
5. Faint heart sounds.
6. Cool clammy skin.
7. Electrical alternans (alternating large and small QRS complexes or altered direction of complexes). Alternans of all components of the ECG complex (P, QRS, T) can also occur which is pathognomonic for cardiac tamponade (Baldwin, 1995).

DIFFERENTIAL DIAGNOSIS

1. Tension pneumothorax
2. Right ventricular myocardial infarction
3. Right ventricular failure
4. Cardiogenic shock

DIAGNOSTIC TESTS/FINDINGS

Combined clinical and hemodynamic assessment (right heart catheterization and/or echocardiogram) are essential for the diagnosis of tamponade.

1. Echocardiogram: An echo-free space may be observed, indicating fluid accumulation in the pericardial sac.
2. Hemodynamic monitoring: Equalization of the following pressures: Intrapericardiac, mean RA, RV diastolic, pulmonary capillary wedge, and LV diastolic. Compared to constrictive pericarditis, there is a pronounced pulsus paradoxus, a lack of "dip and plateau" in the ventricular pressure tracing, decreased or absent Y descent in the right atrial waveform, and the absence of Kussmaul's sign (inspiratory rise in right atrial pressure).
3. ECG abnormalities such as ST-T wave changes and/or electrical alternans may occur, but this is a nonspecific finding. Low voltage complexes in the precordial leads of an ECG, post-AMI recurrent arrhythmias, and pulseless electrical activity may also be seen in tamponade.
4. Lab tests: If an infectious process is suspected, culture and sensitivity of pericardial fluid is warranted.
5. Radiographic tests including CT scan, carbon dioxide angiography, and CXR may show enlargement of the cardiac silhouette with fluid accumulation.

MANAGEMENT/TREATMENT

If hemodynamic instability is present the ACNP should immediately consult with the collaborating physician and obtain an immediate cardiology referral for management of this patient. The ACNP should initiate treatments outlined below for hemodynamic instability while waiting for physician consultation. The ACNP may also assist in procedures discussed in the management of this patient based on standardized procedures and competencies.

In consultation with the physician the ACNP orders the following to support cardiac function:

1. *Intravascular volume expansion* with 300–500 mL of normal saline over 30–60 minutes and parenteral inotropes may be used to temporarily support hemodynamics while preparing for pericardiocentesis.
2. *Inotropic agents* such as dopamine, dobutamine, or isoproterenol which increases cardiac contractility. CO is increased by improving stroke volume, and decreasing systemic vascular resistance. Heart rate also increases.
3. *Oxygen* increases oxygen content of the lungs. Helps to deliver adequate amounts of oxygen to the cells.
4. *Pericardiocentesis*: The ACNP may assist with evacuation of the tamponade with pericardiocentesis—removal of as little as 20–50 mL of fluid may improve CO. A pericardial catheter may be inserted, connected by gravity to a drainage bag or to a low-suction drainage container for a longer time period (hours or days).
5. *Surgical Intervention: The ACNP may consult with the collaborating physician and refer the patient to the CT surgeon if surgical intervention is necessary.*
   A. Prepare patient for a pericardial window (an opening into the pericardium that allows for fluid drainage into the pleural space).
   B. Prepare patient for thoracotomy to identify and repair the source of bleeding.

C. Subxyphoid pericardiotomy as a palliative procedure for those with poor prognoses—reaccumulation of fluid is common.
D. Complete pericardiectomy when long-term survival can be expected, especially for patients with effusive-constrictive pericarditis or loculated effusions.

PATIENT EDUCATION

1. Instruct patient on meaning of symptoms and diagnosis.
2. Reassure patient that the emergent situation is being addressed and that the problem is being corrected.
3. Prepare patient for any emergent procedures necessary to treat tamponade.
4. Discuss the outcome of treatment and continued need for monitoring and necessary treatment.
5. Encourage patient to ask questions and discuss fears and concerns.

Review Questions

3.46 The ECG change that is observed in tamponade is:
   A. Concordant ST-segment elevation in most V leads
   B. PR-segment elevation
   C. Electrical alternans
   D. T waves become negative in inferior leads (II, III, aVF)

3.47 The echocardiographic finding in patients with cardiac tamponade is:
   A. An echo-free space between the pericardium and epicardium
   B. Decrease in systolic wall motion
   C. Decrease in ventricular dimensions
   D. All of the above

3.48 A 60-year-old female day 5 S/P AMI, whose clinical course was complicated by CHB, required a transvenous pacemaker. She was doing well during the day shift with a BP at 110/70 and pulse 85 ventricular paced. During the night shift her BP decreased from 110 to 90 systolic, urine output diminished, she became progressively agitated, her skin was pale cool and clammy. Which of the following is the most likely cause of her change in symptoms?
   A. Pulmonary embolism
   B. Aortic aneurysm
   C. Pericarditis
   D. Cardiac tamponade

3.49 Which of the following would be appropriate treatment for this patient?
   A. Normal saline 500 mL wide open
   B. Dopamine (400 mL/250 mL) titrate to SBP >100
   C. Immediate consult with a cardiologist
   D. All of the above

3.50 A 56-year-old man has adenocarcinoma of the lung and was treated with chemotherapy and radiation. He is admitted for increasing SOB. His physical exam reveals signs of right-sided heart failure. Other findings include muffled heart sounds and electrical alternans on the ECG. Which of the following is the most likely diagnosis?

A. Aortic aneurysm
B. Cardiac tamponade
C. Pericarditis
D. Pulmonary embolism

Answers and Rationales

3.46   **C**   Electrical alternans can occur due to fluid around the pericardium, which can decrease transmission of electrical voltage from the myocardium.

3.47   **D**   Although the classic sign of cardiac tamponade is an echo-free space, all of the above can be found on the echocardiogram in a patient with cardiac tamponade.

3.48   **D**   The patient's symptoms indicate there is a decrease in cardiac function. Transvenous pacemakers can perforate the ventricle and lead to cardiac tamponade.

3.49   **D**   All of the above are necessary for this patient to maintain cardiac function and to emergently treat the tamponade with pericardial centeses.

3.50   **B**   Pericardial effusion can result from radiation therapy to the chest. As the effusion increases, symptoms of cardiac tamponade can occur. The patient's signs and symptoms indicate impaired cardiac function most probably due to cardiac tamponade.

References

Baldwin, K.M., Garza, C.S., Martin, R.N., et al. (1995). *Davis's Manual of Critical Care Therapeutics.* Philadelphia: F.A. Davis Co.

Freed, M., & Band, J.D. (1994). Pericardial Disease. In M. Freed & C. Grines (eds.). *Essentials of Cardiovascular Medicine.* Birmingham, MI: Physician's Press, p. 422.

Hancock, E.W. (1994). Cardiac tamponade. *Heart Dis Stroke 3*, 155–158.

Lorell, B.H., & Braunwald, E. (1997). Pericardial effusion with cardiac compression: Cardiac tamponade. In E. Braunwald (ed.). *Heart Disease: A Textbook of Cardiovascular Medicine* (5th ed.). Philadelphia: W.B. Saunders Co., pp. 1942–1997.

Shock

DEFINITION

1. Shock is a syndrome in which tissue oxygen delivery is inadequate to meet metabolic demands and maintain proper end-organ function.
2. Manifestations of shock include, hypotension, oliguria, mental status changes, lactic acidosis and those of the underlying disorder (e.g., hematemesis in upper GI bleed, urticaria and wheezing in anaphylaxis).
3. The clinical course of shock may be complicated by multiple organ dysfunction syndrome (MODS) characterized by disseminated intravascular coagulation (DIC), adult respiratory distress syndrome (ARDS), mesenteric ischemia, myocardial ischemia/dysfunction, hepatic/renal failure, and cerebral anoxia.

4. The prognosis of shock is dependent on the type and severity of shock, the time from symptom onset until initiation of treatment, presence of comorbidities, and the development of complications.
5. With early treatment, septic and cardiogenic shock are associated with mortality rates in excess of 50%; if left untreated, shock is uniformly fatal (Freed, 1996).

CLASSIFICATION OF SHOCK (Baldwin et al., 1995)

1. *Hypovolemic:* Characterized by loss of circulating fluid volume, either blood or plasma (usually a minimum of 15–25% loss).
2. *Cardiogenic:* Inability of the left ventricle to pump blood forward to meet metabolic tissue oxygen demands.
3. *Distributive or vasogenic shock:* An abnormality in the vascular system that produces a maldistribution of blood volume. Distributive shock includes the following three types:
   A. *Neurogenic:* Generalized vasodilation and loss of vasomotor tone resulting in a massive increase in the vascular capacity, pooling of blood in the periphery, and decreased venous return to the heart.
   B. *Anaphylactic:* Result of an antigen-antibody reaction in which histamine or histamine-like substances are released; a histamine-induced dilation of the venous and arterial system plus a loss of fluid and protein into the tissue spaces from leaking capillaries results in decreased venous return to the heart and pooling of blood in the periphery.
   C. *Septic:* A generalized infection of the blood, usually by gram-negative bacteria, which results in fever, cellular dysfunction, marked vasodilation, peripheral pooling of blood, and decreased SVR.

ETIOLOGY/PATHOPHYSIOLOGY (Baldwin et al., 1995; Rice, 1997)

1. Hypovolemic Shock
   A. Decreased fluid volume due to internal/external losses.
      1) External fluid losses due to conditions such as hemorrhage, severe vomiting, severe diarrhea, dehydration.
      2) Internal fluid losses such as third spacing due to conditions such as ileus, intestinal obstruction, and burns
   B. Pathophysiologic events of hypovolemic shock are described in Figure 3–10.
2. Cardiogenic Shock
   A. Ineffective forward flow due to left ventricular dysfunction caused by conditions such as myocardial infarction, heart failure, cardiomyopathy, acute arrhythmias, acute pericardial tamponade, severe heart valve dysfunction, massive pulmonary embolism, tension pneumothorax.
   B. Pathophysiologic events of cardiogenic shock are described in Figure 3–11
3. Distributive Shock: Alteration in distribution of circulating volume; decreased vascular resistance, increased vascular capacitance from:
   A. Neurogenic causes such as spinal cord injuries, anesthetic paralysis, reflex vasodilation.

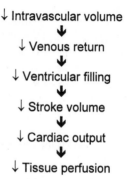

↓ Intravascular volume
↓
↓ Venous return
↓
↓ Ventricular filling
↓
↓ Stroke volume
↓
↓ Cardiac output
↓
↓ Tissue perfusion

(↓, decreased)

FIGURE 3–10. Pathophysiology of hypovolemic shock. (From Rice, V. [1997]. *Shock: A Clinical Syndrome*. California: American Association of Critical-Care Nurses, with permission.)

    1) Pathophysiologic events of neurogenic shock are described in Figure 3–12

B. Anaphylactic causes such as adverse drug reactions, pollen hypersensitivity, hypersensitivity to insect stings, hypersensitivity to foreign proteins in serum.

    1) Pathophysiologic events of anaphylactic shock are described in Figure 3–13

C. Septic causes such as gram-negative bacteria endotoxins (most common causative factor), gram-positive bacteria (toxic shock), fungi, viruses, rickettsiae.

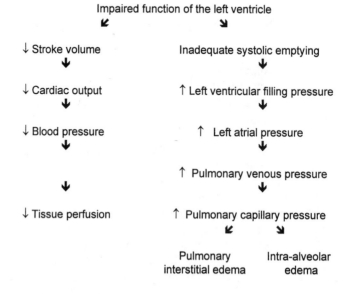

Impaired function of the left ventricle

↓ Stroke volume	Inadequate systolic emptying
↓ Cardiac output	↑ Left ventricular filling pressure
↓ Blood pressure	↑ Left atrial pressure
	↑ Pulmonary venous pressure
↓ Tissue perfusion	↑ Pulmonary capillary pressure

Pulmonary interstitial edema   Intra-alveolar edema

(↑, increased; ↓, decreased)

FIGURE 3–11. Pathophysiology of cardiogenic shock. (From Rice, V. [1997]. *Shock: A Clinical Syndrome*. California: American Association of Critical-Care Nurses, with permission.)

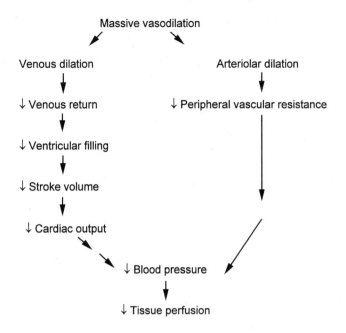

(↓, decreased)

FIGURE 3–12. Pathophysiology of neurogenic shock. (From Rice, V. [1997]. *Shock: A Clinical Syndrome.* California: American Association of Critical-Care Nurses, with permission.)

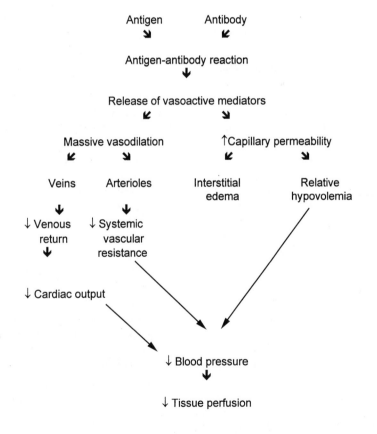

(↑, increased; ↓, decreased)

FIGURE 3–13. Pathophysiology of anaphylactic shock. (From Rice, V. [1997]. *Shock: A Clinical Syndrome.* California: American Association of Critical-Care Nurses, with permission.)

TABLE 3–28. Characteristics of the Systemic Inflammatory Response
Syndrome (SIRS)*

Definitions:
  A widespread systemic inflammatory response
  An abnormal host response characterized by generalized activation of the inflamma-
    tory reaction
Causes:
  Burns
  Pancreatitis
  Local tissue necrosis
  Trauma
  Infection
  Radiation
  Any cause of intense local inflammation
Clinical presentation (two or more of the following):
  Temperature >38°C or <36°C
  Heart rate >90 bpm
  Respiratory rate >20/min or arterial carbon dioxide tension <32 mm Hg
  White blood cell count >12,000/mm^3 or <4000/mm^3 or a 10% increase in immature
    neutrophils (bands) on the white blood cell differential count

---

* From American College of Chest Physicians/Society of Critical Care Medicine Consensus Conference Committee. (1992) Definitions for sepsis and organ failure and guidelines for the use of innovative therapies in sepsis. *Chest 101*(6):1644–1655, with permission.

    1) Characteristics of systemic inflammatory response syndrome (SIRS)
       are described in Table 3–28

SIGNS AND SYMPTOMS

As the patient progresses through the shock states (early, intermediate and
late) different signs and symptoms are observed. The following description of
the signs and symptoms associated with the various stages of shock is taken
from Baldwin et al. (1995).
1. Early stage of shock—referred to as "nonprogressive" or "compensated"
   shock
   A. This stage of shock can be reversed
   B. There is a temporary decrease in CO and BP, which stimulates the sym-
      pathetic nervous system responses and renin-angiotensin-aldosterone
      responses to compensate and prevent further deterioration.
   C. If shock does not become severe enough to enter the progressive phase
      there is normalization of the CO and arterial blood pressure.
   D. Compensatory mechanisms are activated to maintain vital signs when
      there is a 10% loss of circulating volume.
2. Intermediate stage of shock—referred to as "progressive" shock
   A. There is circulatory deterioration due to the inability for compensatory
      mechanics to maintain adequate hemodynamics. Reduced blood flow to
      the myocardium results in cellular dysfunction from insufficient oxygen
      and nutrients causing further deterioration of cardiac function.
   B. The heart normally has great reserves and can pump 300–400% more
      blood than needed; however, if cardiogenic shock continues, the myocar-
      dium will eventually fail.
   C. Clotting in the small vessels results from ischemic cellular wastes caus-
      ing agglutination and sluggish blood flow in the microvasculature and
      decreased flow of oxygen and nutrients to the cells.

    D. Increased capillary permeability results from capillary hypoxia and decreased nutrients.

    E. Decreased blood flow to the intestine increases endotoxin's formation, released by gram-negative bacteria, and absorption. Endotoxin plays an important role in septic shock.

    F. This cellular deterioration results in diminished active transport of sodium and potassium through the cell membrane resulting in increased intracellular sodium and cellular swelling.

    G. Depressed mitochondrial function increases adenosine triphosphate production by anaerobic metabolism, causing excess lactic acid production and acidosis.

    H. Release of hydrolases from the lysosomes, causing further cellular deterioration.

    I. Depressed cellular metabolism of nutrients.

    J. Areas of necrosis develop within organs (especially in the liver, lungs, and heart) and MODS occurs.

3. Late stage of shock—referred to as "irreversible" shock

    A. Pancreatic release of myocardial depressant factor causes progressive myocardial depression. Cardiac deterioration is the most significant factor in progression.

    B. Increased capillary permeability leads to movement of fluids into tissues (third spacing of fluid).

    C. Shock becomes irreversible at a cellular level when the cells are depleted of high-energy phosphate compounds.

    D. Although improvement may be noted for a brief time tissue damage is extensive and may not be reversed by therapy.

    E. When MODS is not responsive to therapy death may ensue.

PHYSICAL FINDINGS (Baldwin et al., 1995)

Subjective

1. The amount of subjective data that can be obtained will vary with the stage and type of shock.

2. Patients may be restless, anxious, or confused and not able to adequately describe what is happening to them in the early stage of shock. They often express a feeling of impending doom without being able to pinpoint the cause of the feeling.

3. Patients may describe a mechanism of injury that initiated the shock or factors that placed the patient at risk for the development of shock.

Objective

1. Neurologic

    A. Level of consciousness ranges from inability to concentrate, restlessness, agitation, anxiety, and/or confusion to bizarre behavior, lethargy, and/or apathy, to unconsciousness and unresponsiveness as shock progresses.

    B. Pupils progress from normal and reactive to dilated and reactive and, eventually, to dilated with sluggish reaction.

2. Respiratory

    A. Tachypnea: Initially rapid deep breathing that progresses to rapid, shallow breathing in the intermediate stage. In late-stage shock, rapid, shallow breathing with an irregular pattern.

    B. SaO_2 decreases as hypoxia from physiologic shunting occurs.

    C. Lung sounds are initially clear, but may progress to crackles as shock progresses and ARDS ensues.

  3. Cardiovascular:

    A. Pulse: Initial tachycardia from sympathetic stimulation may be seen progressing to tachycardia with arrhythmias and weak rapid, thready peripheral pulse as shock worsens. In late-stage shock, an extremely slow and weak or absent pulse may be noted.

    B. Blood pressure varies with the stage. Initially systolic blood pressure is maintained or rises and diastolic blood pressure rises. This may result in decreased pulse pressure. Systolic blood pressure drops as shock progresses; diastolic rises as a result of vasoconstriction causing a narrowing pulse pressure. Further progression results in frank hypotension with a widening pulse pressure. If shock is untreated, cardiovascular collapse results.

    C. Orthostatic symptoms: Initially no symptoms are present. Lightheadedness when sitting occurs in the intermediate stage and progresses to hemodynamic instability with position change in the late stage.

    D. Edema progressing to anasarca can be seen in late-stage shock as fluid leaks into the tissues.

  4. Gastrointestinal

    A. Bowel sounds become hypoactive as blood is shunted to other organs and progress to absent bowel sounds (paralytic ileus).

    B. Gastrointestinal bleeding from stress ulcer formation occurs in intermediate and late shock.

  5. Renal

    A. Decreasing urine output: Urine output is slightly decreased but within normal limits in early shock progressing to oliguria of <20 mL/hr in the intermediate stage. Anuria and renal failure are seen in the late stage as renal function deteriorates.

    B. Thirst: Occurs in the early stage of shock, becomes markedly increased in the intermediate stage, and severe in late shock (if the patient is alert and oriented enough to report it).

  6. Musculoskeletal

    A. Generalized muscle weakness and wasting occurs as blood is shunted to vital organs. Muscle aches may occur as lactic acid production increases in ischemic muscles.

  7. Integumentary

    A. Skin is warm and flushed in the early stage of septic shock. In all other types, blood is shunted to the vital organs in the early stages, so skin becomes cool and pale. As all types progress, skin becomes cold and clammy, cyanosis may be seen, there is decreased capillary refill, and edema from fluid shifts is seen. Late-stage skin changes result in cold, mottled, ashen, or cyanotic skin.

  8. Temperature changes

    A. Changes in core temperature: Core temperature is normal, but decreases with exposure to cold in all types of shock except septic. In sepsis, temperature may increase or decrease.

DIFFERENTIAL DIAGNOSIS

1. Hemodynamics and physical findings aid in differentiating the type of shock.
2. Hemodynamic profiles for the various types of shock are listed in Table 3–29

TABLE 3–29.   **Hemodynamic Profiles for the Major Types of Shock***

Parameters	Hypovolemic Shock	Cardiogenic Shock	Neurogenic Shock	Anaphylactic Shock	Septic Shock
Right atrial pressure	↓	↑	↓	↓	↓
Pulmonary artery occlusion pressure	↓	↑	↓	↓	↓
Cardiac output/index	↓	↓	↓	↓	N↑
Arterial blood pressure	↓	↓	↓	↓	↓
Pulmonary artery pressure	N↑↓	↑	N↓	N↓	N↓↑

* From Rice, V. (1997). *Shock: A Clinical Syndrome*. California: American Association of Critical-Care Nurses, with permission.

N, normal; ↑, increased; ↓, decreased.

DIAGNOSTIC TESTS/FINDINGS

1. Hemodynamic monitoring with a pulmonary artery catheter to aid in the diagnosis and management of shock. See Table 3–29 for specific hemodynamics with each type of shock.
2. Continuous mixed venous oxygenation monitoring to assess adequacy of tissue oxygenation and aid in determining type of shock may be indicated. $S\bar{v}O_2$ is usually low in hypovolemic and cardiogenic shock. $S\bar{v}O_2$ is abnormally increased in septic shock.
3. Pulse oximetry and transcutaneous oxygen monitoring to evaluate arterial oxygen saturation.
4. Chest x-ray is vital in the work-up of pulmonary, cardiovascular, and system problems.
5. ECG to assess for myocardial ischemia/injury.
6. Cardiac catheterization/angiography to evaluate coronary anatomy.
7. Noninvasive cardiology studies (e.g., ECG, echocardiogram, or multiple gaited acquisitions scan) to evaluate ejection fraction and wall motion.
8. Peritoneal lavage and/or exploratory surgery may be indicated to assess for intra-abdominal bleed in hypovolemic shock.
9. Gastrointestinal endoscopy may be indicated to evaluate stress ulcers/gastritis.
10. CT scan, magnetic resonance imaging (MRI) or spinal x-rays may be indicated (e.g., evaluate for spinal cord injury in neurogenic shock).

Laboratory Tests

The ACNP consults with the collaborating physician to determine appropriate laboratory tests. These may include:
1. Hematocrit and hemoglobin
2. White blood cell (WBC) count and differential
3. Arterial blood gases (ABGs)
4. Serum lactate
5. Serum electrolytes chemistries

6. Urinalysis
7. Cardiac enzymes
8. Blood culture
9. Culture and sensitivity

MANAGEMENT/TREATMENT (Baldwin et al., 1995; Rice, 1997)

A multidisciplinary approach is necessary for the management of these critically ill patients. The physician will determine the treatment plan and referrals. The ACNP will consult with the collaborating physician and multidisciplinary team members throughout the treatment of these critically ill patients.

1. For all forms of shock the ACNP will:
   A. Assess hemodynamic parameters to evaluate the cardiovascular response to treatment.
   B. Assess blood pressure to determine the cardiovascular response to treatment
   C. Assess urinary output via catheter to evaluate renal function
   D. Assess cardiac rhythm for tachycardia and life-threatening ventricular arrhythmias (ventricular tachycardia and/orfibrillation)
   E. Maintain a patent airway and adequate ventilation, and use supplemental oxygen to ensure that sufficient oxygen is delivered to the lungs
   F. Provide enteral nutrition or parenteral nutritional support to prevent a negative nitrogen balance (Baldwin et al., 1995)
2. Goals of therapy for all forms of shock are:
   A. Mental status: Alert and oriented
   B. SaO_2 >90%
   C. MAP >60 mm Hg
   D. CI >2.2 L/min/m^2
   E. Urine output >30 mL/hr
   F. Clearing of metabolic lactic/ketoacidosis with pH 7.3–7.5
   G. Temperature >35° and <38°C
3. For hypovolemic shock:
   A. Apply pressure to control external hemorrhage.
   B. Apply medical antishock trousers (controversial) to assist with major organ perfusion.
   C. Prepare patient for exploratory surgery to ascertain the extent of injury and repair damage.
   D. In extreme emergencies, untyped and uncrossmatched blood (0-negative) or type-specific, uncrossmatched blood may be given.
   E. Replace calcium if large amount of packed red blood cells (RBCs) are administered.
4. For cardiogenic shock:
   A. Maintain adequate CO and arterial BP with inotropes and vasodilators.
   B. Decrease preload and afterload, which maintains adequate CO/CI.
   C. Maintain adequate tissue oxygenation ($S\bar{v}O_2$ 60–80%).
   D. Monitor mechanical assistive devices—intra-aortic balloon pump, external counterpulsation device, ventricular assist device—to assess left ventricular function.
   E. Prepare patient for surgery—coronary artery bypass graft—to reperfuse the infarcted part of the left ventricle.

5. For distributive shock:
    A. Neurogenic-minimizing spinal cord trauma by proper stabilization of the trauma patient.
    B. Ascertain cause—if pain, treat with analgesics; if anxiety and stress, identify and alleviate stressor.
    C. Anaphylactic—identify and remove causative antigen.
        1) Epinephrine: 1:10,000 solution, administered 0.3 mL SQ q5–25 min or IV 0.5–1.0 mg 5 min
        2) Benedryl: 25–50 μ-mg IV
        3) Aminophylline: IV 5 to 6 mg-bolus followed by drip at 0.6–1.0 mg/kg/min
    D. Septic (See "Septic Shock" in Chapter 11 for more detailed treatment.)

Pharmacologic Therapy (Baldwin et al., 1995; Rice, 1997)

1. Volume expanders to replace lost intravascular volume and blood components. Examples include:
    A. Crystalloids: Should be used in the early phases of fluid replacement for hypovolemic, neurogenic, and septic shock. Ringer's solution, and normal saline solution commonly used.
    B. Colloids: Such as albumin and plasma substitutes (dextran, hetastarch) may be used in hypovolemic, cardiogenic, and septic shock but are not recommended for trauma.
    C. Blood or blood products: Packed RBCs, whole blood autotransfusion, and synthetic blood products may be used in severe hemorrhage with hypovolemic shock.
2. Sodium bicarbonate to reverse the metabolic acidosis that occurs as shock progresses.
3. Inotropic agents to increase cardiac function by improving myocardial contractility and increasing CO/CI and arterial blood pressure; and organ perfusion in hypovolemic, cardiogenic, and septic shock. Examples include:
    • Dopamine (Intropin)
    • Norepinephrine (Levophed)
    • Dobutamine (Dobutrex)
    • Epinephrine
4. Vasodilators to decrease afterload, SVR, and preload. These may also dilate the coronary arteries to improve myocardial oxygen supply in hypovolemic and cardiogenic shock. Reverses vasoconstriction and improves tissue perfusion in septic shock. Examples included:
    • Nitroglycerin (Tridil)
    • Nitroprusside (Nipride)
5. Diuretics to increase urine excretion by affecting water and electrolyte absorption within the glomerulus in hypovolemic shock. Examples include:
    • Furosemide (Lasix)
    • Bumetanide (Bumex)
    • Torsemide (Demadex)
6. Reperfusion therapy with emergent CABG, which has been shown to decrease mortality by restoring circulation to the ischemic portion of the left ventricle. Other types of reperfusion may be administered depending on the CA lesions involved, the physician, and overall patient condition. (see "Acute Myocardial Infarction.") Examples include:

- Coronary artery bypass
- PTCA/stent
- Tissue plasminogen activator (Activase)
- Streptokinase (Streptase)

7. Antihistamines to block the action of histamine, thus reversing broncho-constriction, hypotension, and vasodilation in anaphylactic shock. Examples include:
   - Epinephrine (Adrenalin)
   - Diphenhydramine (Benadryl)
8. Steroids to stabilize capillary walls, thus decreasing fluid shifts out of the vasculature in anaphylactic shock.
9. Bronchodilator to relieve bronchoconstriction in anaphylactic shock and is longer acting than epinephrine. An example is aminophylline (theophylline).
10. Vagolytics to counteract the bradycardic effects of the vagus nerve on the heart, thus producing increased heart rate in neurogenic shock. An example is atropine sulfate.
11. Antibiotics to treat infection from gram-positive and gram-negative aerobic and anaerobic bacteria in septic shock. Examples include:

- An aminoglycoside, such as gentamicin (Garamycin) or tobramycin (Nebcin), for gram-negative bacteria
- A third-generation cephalosporin, such as cefotaxime (Claforan) or ceftazidime (Fortaz), for both gram-negative and gram-positive bacteria
- A penicillin agent, such as nafcillin (Nafcil, Unipen) or piperacillin (Pipracil), for gram-positive bacteria
- Chloramphenicol (Chloromycetin) or clindamycin (Cleocin) for anaerobic bacteria
- Amphotericin B or fluconazole (Diflucan) for fungi

   A. Before the source is identified, at least a two-drug combination should be given.
   B. When the source is identified, therapy may be tailored to the causative organism.

Other Therapies for Septic Shock

Several drugs are thought to interrupt the septic process and are being used experimentally to treat septic shock. Below is how these drugs are thought to work. (See "Septic Shock" in Chapter 11 for further details.)
1. Naloxone: Interacts with the endogenous opiate system
2. Monoclonal antibodies: Interact with endotoxin or tumor necrosis factor
3. Nonsteroidal anti-inflammatory drugs: Inhibit prostaglandin formation
4. Allopurinol: Inhibits production of toxic oxygen free radicals
5. Human endotoxin antiserum: Causes production of antibodies to endotoxin
6. Prostacyclin and prostaglandin E_2 (PGE_2) analogs: Cause vasodilation and increased peripheral tissue perfusion

Referrals

1. The ACNP should consult with the collaborating physician to determine appropriate referrals.

2. Besides referrals to specialists, the ACNP considers referrals to multidisciplinary team members such as respiratory therapist, physical therapist, clinical nurse specialist, social worker, and chaplain.

PATIENT EDUCATION

Due to acuity of the patient's illness, education in the acute period is often given to the family; as the patient improves, information is given to the patient.
1. Explain the disease process and treatment.
2. Discuss the severity of illness and treatment options with the patient (if appropriate) and family.
3. Clarify patient wishes regarding resuscitation orders and end-of-life issues.
4. Implementation of weekly family conferences may be helpful in providing information regarding the complexity of the disease/treatment, providing support, answering questions, and addressing end-of-life issues based on the patient's request and prognosis.

Review Questions

3.51 Shock associated with high preload is most likely to be:
   A. Neurogenic
   B. Cardiogenic
   C. Hypovolemia
   D. Septic

3.52 Drugs that dilate arterioles include:
   A. Phentolamine and nitroprusside
   B. Dopamine and dobutamine
   C. Amrinone and epinephrine
   D. Nitroglycerin and high-dose dopamine

3.53 The pathophysiology of anaphylaxis includes:
   A. A late, delayed reaction to an antigen-antibody reaction
   B. Bronchodilation in response to histamine
   C. Widespread vasoconstriction
   D. Hypovolemia from increased capillary permeability

3.54 Medications that can be administered to reverse the pathophysiologic changes that develop in anaphylactic shock include:
   A. Epinephrine and aminophylline
   B. Morphine and furosemide
   C. Epinephrine and isoproterenol
   D. Aminophylline and gentamicin

3.55 A 50-year-old woman is admitted postoperatively for repair of a hip fracture and splenectomy after a motor vehicle accidence. Three hours postoperatively her level of consciousness (LOC) is decreased. VS are BP of 82/56, P 120, RR 28, UO 20 mL/hr. Her skin is cool and clammy. No C/O SOB, lung sounds clear. Temp 36.5°C. WBCs 9000.
   Based on the above information, what condition appears to be developing?
   A. LV failure
   B. Neurogenic shock

C. Septic shock

D. Hypovolemic shock

Answers and Rationales

3.51   **B**   Cardiogenic shock is associated with high preloads.

3.52   **A**   Phentolamine and nitroprusside dilate arterioles.

3.53   **D**   Patients with anaphylaxis develop shock because of increased capillary permeability, which leads to leakage of fluid out of the intravascular space and results in intravascular volume depletion and vasodilation decreasing left ventricular preload.

3.54   **A**   Epinephrine: 10,000 dilution 3–5 ml should be injected IV slowly in 1-mg increments for anaphylactic shock. If bronchospasm is present, aminophylline will provide relief.

3.55   **D**   The most probable cause is hypovolemic shock.

References

Antman, E.M. (1997). Cardiogenic shock. In E. Braunwald (ed.). *Heart Disease: A Textbook of Cardiovascular Medicine* (5th ed.). Philadelphia: W.B. Saunders Co., pp. 1725–1727.

Baldwin, K.M., Garza, C.S., Martin, R.N., et al. (1995). Shock. In *Davis's Manual of Critical Care Therapeutics*. Philadelphia: F.A. Davis Co., pp. 153–178.

Freed, M. (1994). Shock. In M. Freed & C. Grines (eds.). *Essentials of Cardiovascular Medicine*. Birmingham, MI: Physician's Press, pp. 217–251.

Kollef, M., & Goodenberger, D. (1995). Shock. In G.A. Ewald & C.R. McKenzie (eds.). *Manual of Medical Therapeutics: The Washington Manual* (28th ed.). Boston: Little, Brown & Co., pp. 190–194.

Rice, V. (1997). *Shock: A Clinical Syndrome*. CA: American Association of Critical-Care Nurses.

Tierney, L.M., Jr., & Messina, L.M. (1997). Shock. In Tierney, L.M., Jr., S.J. McPhee, & M.A. Papadakis (eds.). *Current Medical Diagnosis & Treatment* (36th ed.). Stamford, CT: Appleton & Lange, pp. 459–462.

Cardiac Transplantation

DEFINITION

1. Orthotopic heart transplantation (OHT) involves retaining a large portion of the right and left atrium in a recipient and implanting a donor heart in the atrium, together with direct end-to-end anastamoses of the aorta and the pulmonary artery. The procedure, initially described in 1960 by Lower and Shumway, involves a median sternotomy incision and the use of cardiopulmonary bypass.

2. Once considered an experimental therapy, cardiac transplantation is now considered the treatment of choice for end-stage heart failure refractory to medical and surgical intervention.

ETIOLOGY/INCIDENCE

1. Currently more than 30,297 orthotopic heart transplant surgeries have been performed as reported from 257 centers worldwide (Hosenpud et al., 1995).
2. Heart transplant recipients have an in-hospital mortality rate of <5%, a 1-year survival rate approaching 85%, and survival rates of 75–80% at 5 years (Mudge, 1993).
3. Improved surgical technique and immunosuppressive therapies contribute to the success of OHT. Success, however, has resulted in a critical donor shortage, which further demonstrates the importance of appropriate donor selection and timing for OHT.
4. Donor supply remains at about 2000 annually, while each year approximately 40,000 persons under the age of 65 die from conditions for which heart transplant may be indicated.

PHYSIOLOGY

Physiology of the donor heart:
1. The donor heart is denervated at the time of transplant.
2. The vena cava and the sinus node of the recipient remain intact with OHT, accounting for the two p waves often visualized on the ECG of the transplant recipient. Only the sinus node of the donor heart will conduct through to the ventricles and stimulate synchronized atrioventricular contraction.
3. The transplanted heart has a blunted response to exercise secondary to the denervated heart's reliance on circulating catecholamines to respond to increased demand. Cardiopulmonary exercise testing (CPX) in heart transplant patients demonstrates a maximal exercise tolerance and anaerobic threshold approximately 70% predicted of normal for gender and age (Kobashigawa & Stevenson, 1993).
4. Reinnervation of the recipient heart may occur within 1 year after transplantation; however, maximum exercise responses remain depressed.
5. Cardiac medications that are not effective on the denervated heart are listed in Table 3–30.

SIGNS AND SYMPTOMS/PHYSICAL FINDINGS

1. OHT is the treatment of choice for end-stage heart failure. (See "Heart Failure" for the specific signs and symptoms of HF.)
2. Table 3–31 lists indications for cardiac transplantation.

TABLE **3–30.** **Medications that Are Not Effective on the Donor Heart**

Medication	Comment
Digoxin	Little effect on the SA node Not likely to achieve rate control in atrial fibrillation May have positive inotropic effect
Atropine	Parasympathetic effects will not increase heart rate
Nifedipine, hydralazine	No reflex tachycardia

SA, sinoatrial.

TABLE 3–31. Indications for Cardiac Transplantation*

Accepted Indications	Possible Indications
1. Peak Vo_2 <10 mL/kg/min	1. Peak Vo_2 <14 mL/kg/min
2. Severe ischemia limiting daily activities and not treatable by other medical or surgical treatments	2. Unstable ischemia not treatable by other medical or surgical therapy
3. Recurrent symptomatic dysrhythmias that are refractory to all therapy	3. Unstable fluid balance or renal function in patients who are compliant with sodium and fluid restriction and diuretics

* Adapted from Mudge, G.H., Goldstein, S., Addonizio, L.J., et al. (1993). Task force 3: Recipient guidelines/prioritization. *J Am Coll Cardiol* 22(1), 21–30, with permission.

MANAGEMENT/TREATMENT

Perioperative Care of the Heart Transplant Patient

1. Care of the cardiac transplant patient is very complex, thus the ACNP will work closely with the collaborating physician and the multidisciplinary transplant team.
2. Perioperative care of the OHT patient primarily focuses on immunosuppression, treatment of RV dysfunction, bradycardia, and acute renal failure (ARF).

IMMUNOSUPRESSION

1. Immunosupression to prevent allograft rejection begins at the time of the transplant procedure and continues throughout the life of the recipient. Cardiac allograft rejection is discussed below with "Long-Term Care of the Heart Transplant Patient."
2. Immunosuppressive therapy usually consists of triple-drug therapy: Cyclosporine (CSA), corticosteroids, and azathioprine. Table 3–32 outlines suggested starting doses for CSA, corticosteroids, and azathioprine.
3. Target CSA levels in the perioperative period are 250–350 ng/mL (monoclonal method). Prophylactic cytolytic therapy with monoclonal or polyclonal antilymphocyte agents (i.e., OKT3, a murine monoclonal antibody directed to the pan T cell CD3 antigen) may be utilized in the immediate postoperative period as "induction therapy" to enhance immunosuppression and promote tolerance of the donor heart; however, this practice has not demonstrated improved benefit in cardiac transplant recipients (Kobashigawa & Stevenson, 1993).

RV DYSFUNCTION

1. Cardiac transplant recipients with preoperative pulmonary hypertension are at risk for the development of RV failure at the time of transplantation. RV failure requires urgent intervention by the ACNP, the collaborating physician, and the transplant team.
2. Elevated pulmonary vascular resistance (PVR) refractory to treatment is a contraindication to cardiac transplantation: PA systolic pressure ≥50–60 mm Hg, PVR ≥240 dynes/sec/cm^{-5}, or a transpulmonary gradient (mean PA pressure − PCWP) >15 mm Hg.

TABLE 3–32.   Suggested Dosing for CSA, Corticosteroids, and Azathioprine*

	Cyclosporine	Methyl-prednisolone	Prednisone	Azathio-prine	OKT3
Preoperative	2 mg/kg/day	None	None	2 mg/kg/day PO	None
Intraoperative	None	500 mg IV	None	None	None
Immediate postoperative	Start at 2–4 mg/kg PO bid titrating to CSA level 200–300 ng/mL	125 mg IV q 12 h for three doses	After methylprednisolone, start at 1 mg/kg/day in divided doses, gradually tapered over 2 weeks to 10 mg PO bid	2 mg/kg/day to maintain WBC >4000/μL	For patients at high risk for renal failure (creatinine level >3 mg/dL) give OKT3, 5 mg IVP qd for 4–6 days with CSA therapy initiated 2–4 days after surgery when renal function has stabilized
Long-term therapy	Titrate CSA level to 300–500 ng/mL	None	Target for 0.1 mg/kg/day by 3–4 mo after surgery; selected patients are weaned off prednisone after 6 mo	2 mg/kg/day to maintain WBC >4000/μL	No routine long-term use

* From Kobashigiwa, J.K., & Stevenson, L.W. (1993). Postoperative treatment of heart transplant patients. *J Crit Illness* 8(5), 610–611, with permission.
CSA, cyclosporine; IVP, intravenous push; WBC, white blood cell count.

3. Treatment is necessary if RV failure/dysfunction develops secondary to pre-existing pulmonary hypertension or inadequate preservation of the RV (which may occur intraoperatively). The ACNP in consultation with the collaborating physician may initiate and titrate the following medications to treat RV failure/dysfunction: Intravenous PGE_1 (0.01–0.5 μg/kg/min), intravenous nitroglycerin (2 to 200 μg/min), isoproteronol (2–20 μg/min), or dobutamine (5–20 μg/kg/min) to decrease PVR and unload the RV while maintaining or augmenting adequate BP and CO.

BRADYCARDIA

1. Bradycardia may occur secondary to sinus node dysfunction, either primary or secondary to preoperative use of negative chronotropic agents such as amiodarone. Terbutaline (2.5–5.0 mg PO tid) may be successfully used to treat bradycardia.
2. Permanent pacemaker therapy may be indicated in patients refractory to medical therapy.

ACUTE RENAL FAILURE

1. Oliguria may be present within the first 24–48 hours following transplant secondary to cardiopulmonary bypass and CSA. Aggressive use of diuretics is necessary to maintain urine output 50 mL/hr. ARF in this setting usually resolves within 72 hours.
2. For patients with pre-existing renal insufficiency (serum creatinine >3.0 mg/dL), the monoclonal antibody OKT3 may be used in place of CSA for

approximately 5 days to avoid early renal dysfunction secondary to the use of CSA.

LONG-TERM CARE OF THE HEART TRANSPLANT PATIENT

General considerations of long-term management for the ACNP to consider include:
1. Medication regimen:
   A. The ACNP consults with the collaborating physician and the multidisciplinary transplant team regarding the medication regimen for long-term care.
   B. Medications for the OHT patient are extensive and include (but not limited to):
      1) Immunosuppressive agents:
         Cyclosporine (CSA), prednisone, azathioprine
      2) Antibiotic prohylaxis:
         chlortrimazole troches, trimethoprime-sulfamethoxazole
      3) Miscellaneous:
         Diuretics, antihypertensive medication, H_2 blockers, cholesterol-lowering agent, iron supplement, vitamin C, magnesium supplement
   C. Triple-drug immunosuppression is usually maintained for long-term care. Target therapeutic serum CSA levels are 200–300 ng/dL (monoclonal method).
   D. Table 3–33 lists the medications, dosages, and major side effects of the immunosuppressive agents.
2. Major long-term problems:
   A. The major long-term problems facing cardiac transplant recipients include allograft rejection, infection, and transplant coronary artery disease (TCAD).
   B. Table 3–34 summarizes additional long-term complications encountered by cardiac transplant recipients.

Rejection

1. Cardiac allograft rejection is the natural response of the host to foreign alloantigen that, left untreated, ultimately leads to allograft destruction (Miller et al., 1993).
2. Rejection can be classified as either cell mediated (mild, moderate, severe), or antibody mediated, often referred to as humoral or vascular rejection, which is less common than cell mediated.
3. Rejection after cardiac transplantation is believed to be primarily a cell-mediated process in which the recipient T lymphocytes recognize donor tissue as foreign, become activated, proliferate, and ultimately destroy the donor organ (Gross et al., 1996).
4. Humoral rejection is characterized by the presence of antibodies that have specificity for donor HLA class antigens, generally located on the vascular endothelium, although non-HLA antigens may also be a target for antibody-mediated injury (Kobashigawa, 1995). Hyperacute rejection (humoral)

TABLE 3–33. **Major Side Effects of the Immunosuppressive Agents***

Drug	Side Effect
Cyclosporine	Hypertension
	Renal dysfunction
	Hyperkalemia
	Hypomagnesemia
	Hyperuricemia
	Hepatic dysfunction
	Seizures
	Tremors
	Paresthesias
	Anxiety
	Insomnia
	Rhinorrhea
	Gingival hyperplasia
	Hypertrichosis
	Hirsutism
Corticosteroids	Cataracts
	Osteoporosis
	Peptic ulcers
	Obesity
	Cushingoid habitus
	Labile emotions
	Easy bruisability
	Diabetes exacerbation
	Corticosteroid myopathy
	Insomnia
	Sodium retention
	Hyperlipidemia
	Avascular bone necrosis
	Growth retardation in children
Azathioprine	Leukopenia
	Thrombocytopenia
	Macrocytic anemia
	Pancreatitis
	Cholestatic jaundice
	Interstitial pneumonitis

* From Kobashigiwa, J.K., & Stevenson, L.W. (1993). Postoperative treatment of heart transplant patients. *J Crit Illness* 611, *8*(5), with permission.

causes immediate cardiac dysfunction due to preformed antibodies, usually the result of previous exposure to human antigens.

5. The mean number of rejection episodes per patient at 1 year following transplant is 1.3 ± 0.7; 37% of patients are rejection free at 1 year (Miller, 1993).

6. Cardiac allograft rejection remains one of the major causes of mortality within the first postoperative year following OHT, accounting for 17% of all deaths in this time period.

7. The majority of rejection episodes occur within the first 6 months following transplantation and are asymptomatic (Miller, 1993).

8. Major risk factors for the development of rejection include female gender (recipient or donor), HLA mismatching, and hearts from female and younger donors (Kobashigawa et al., 1993). The multiparous female heart transplant recipient appears to be at high risk for antibody-mediated rejection because of possible sensitization that may have occurred at the time of pregnancy (Miller et al., 1993).

TABLE 3–34.   Long-Term Complications Associated with Heart Transplantation

Complication	Incidence	Cause	Treatment
Nephrotoxicity		CSA postoperative Pre-existing renal insufficiency	Hemodialysis OKT3/hemodialysis to delay initiation of CSA Careful reduction of CSA dosage
HTN	50–90% of patients S/P OHT Develops within weeks to months independent of nephrotoxicity Secondary to CSA in 80% of patients Diastolic most common	Not influenced by usual demographics (age, sex, race, body weight) Relationship to CSA • Increased vascular smooth muscle tone • Production of potent vasoconstrictor endothelium • Decreased production of vasodilator prostacyclin • CSA nephrotoxicity Corticosteroids Increased sympathetic tone	Calcium channel agonist and ACE inhibitors most effective β-Blockade successful despite denervated heart dependent on circulating catecholamines Diuretics for expanded volume states Careful reduction of CSA Dietary measures Weight reduction Exercise program Immunoconversion from CSA to azathioprine or FK 506 Steroid tapering See also "Hypertension"
Hyperlipidemia	60–80% of patients S/P OHT Primary increase in LDL, tryglycerides Occurs within 6–8 mo S/P OHT	Genetic predisposition CSA Corticosteroids	HMG-CoA reductase inhibitors Gemfibrizil—monotherapy or combined Resin-binding agents bind with CSA monitor CSA levels
Malignancy	1–2% risk of malignancy per year	Clinical characteristics differ with immunosuppression therapy	
Squamous cell	40% of patients at 1 year	Azathioprine-based immunosuppression	↓CSA dose ↓azathioprine dose Frequent endomyocardial biopsy
Transplant lympho- proliferative disease	2% of patients at 1 year	CSA-based immunosuppression	High-dose acyclovir for Ebstein-Barr virus Chemotherapy for aggressive lymphoma
Osteoporosis	10% vertebral compression fractures Avascular necrosis may lead to surgical joint replacement	Chronic corticosteroid therapy	Steroid withdrawal or reduction Oral calcium Calcitonin Testosterone/estrogen Vitamin D
GI	Biliary tract disease most common Pancreatitis 2–18% of patients PUD	CSA effect on bile metabolism Pre-existing pancreatic disease Use of azathioprine	Prophylactic use of H_2 blockers
Noncardiac surgery	10–15% usually for intra-abdominal disorders	Minimize risk for complications: • Adequate volume to prevent hypotension • Hemodynamic monitoring not essential • Preop stress dose of corticosteroids • May need IV CSA	

CSA, cyclosporine; OHT, orthotopic heart transplantation; GI, gastrointestinal; TCAD, transplant coronary artery disease; PUD, peptic ulcer disease.

SIGNS AND SYMPTOMS

1. Vast majority of patients are asymptomatic.
2. Atrial arrhythmias—usually atrial fibrillation, atrial flutter (late sign).
3. Fever, malaise, orthopnea, shortness of breath.
4. Approximately 10% of rejection episodes produce obvious hemodynamic compromise.

DIFFERENTIAL DIAGNOSIS

1. Infection

DIAGNOSTIC TESTS/FINDINGS

1. Endomyocardial biopsy is considered the "gold standard" for diagnosing rejection. Table 3–35 outlines the standardized cardiac biopsy grading as established by the International Society of Heart and Lung Transplantation.
2. Echocardiography: Determine LV dimensions, volumes, and function; Doppler studies (isovolumetric relaxation time, pressure half-time).

MANAGEMENT/TREATMENT

All forms of suspected rejection require immediate consultation/referral with the transplant cardiologist.
1. Mild rejection
   A. No treatment
   B. Follow-up with frequent endomyocardial biopsy, as 18–33% of patients progress to a more significant form of rejection
2. Moderate to severe rejection
   A. Increase immunosuppressive therapy.
   B. Asymptomatic: Oral prednisone bolus and taper; or IV methylprednisolone for 3 days followed by an oral prednisone taper. Table 3–36 outlines specific treatment regimens and dosages for rejection.

TABLE **3–35.   Standardized Endomyocardial Biopsy Grading (ISHLT Scale)***

Grade	New Nomenclature	Old Nomenclature
0	No rejection	No rejection
1	A. Focal (perivascular or interstitial) infiltrate without necrosis B. Diffuse by sparse infiltrate without necrosis	"Mild rejection"
2	One focus only with aggressive infiltration and/or myocyte damage	"Focal" moderate rejection
3	A. Multifocal aggressive infiltrates and/or myocyte damage B. Diffuse inflammatory process with necrosis	A. "Low" moderate rejection B. "Borderline" severe rejection
4	Diffuse, aggressive polymorphous process with necrosis, with or without any of the following: Infiltrates, edema, hemorrhage, vasculitis	"Severe acute" rejection

* Adapted from Miller, L.W., Schlant, R.C., Kobashigawa, J., et al. (1993). Task force 5: Complications. *J Am Coll Cardiol 22*(1), 41–54, with permission.
ISHLT, International Society of Heart and Lung Transplantation

T A B L E 3–36. UCLA Cardiac Transplant Program Rejection Therapy*

Level of Rejection	Cyclosporine	Azathioprine	Prednisone	Methyl-prednisolone	OKT3
None (maintenance)	Titrate to whole blood monoclonal level of 200–300 ng/mL	2 mg/kg/day to maintain WBC >4000 μL	Target for 0.1 mg/kg/day by 3 to 4 mo after transplantation	None	None
Mild	Increase dose to aim for higher therapeutic blood level	Same as maintenance	Same as maintenance	None	None
Focal moderate, moderate without hemodynamic compromise	Same as maintenance	Same as maintenance	Prednisone 100 mg/day for 3 days, then decrease daily to 80, 60, 40 mg, then decrease daily by 2 mg until 20 mg/day is achieved (all doses to be given in split daily dose)	None	None
Moderate with hemodynamic compromise	Same as maintenance	Same as maintenance	After methylprednisolone is given, 100 mg/day for 3 days then decrease to 80, 60, 40 mg, then decrease daily by 2 mg until 20 mg/day is achieved (all doses to be given in split daily dose)	1 gm/day IV for 3 days	5 mg IVP for 10–14 day course

* From Kobashigiwa, J.K., & Stevenson, L.W. (1993). Managing complications in heart transplant patients. *J Crit Illness* 8(6), 682–683, with permission.
WBC, white blood cell count; IVP, intravenous push.

    C. Symptomatic or treatment failure with second course of steroids: OKT3 5 mg IVP for 10–14 days in addition to steroid bolus and taper (requires hospital admission).
3. Recurrent persistent rejection
    A. Low-dose methotrexate, mycophenalate mofetil, FK506, photophoresis, or total lymphoid irradiation
4. Humoral rejection
    A. Corticosteroids are the mainstay of treatment of antibody-mediated rejection. Traditional methods of treating rejection and plasmapheresis, although utilized, have not yet proven effective for humoral rejection.

Infection

1. Infectious complications are common following cardiac transplantation, with 0.5 episodes per patient within the first year.
2. Infection is associated with significant morbidity and mortality.
3. Referral and/or consultation is mandated with transplant cardiologist and infectious disease specialist.

SIGNS AND SYMPTOMS

1. Aggressive evaluation of the signs and symptoms of infection is warranted in the OHT patient, such as fever and elevated white blood cell count.

2. Low-grade fever may be significant, as immunosuppressive agents may blunt the febrile response to infection.
3. Additional signs and symptoms include malaise and SOB.

DIAGNOSTIC TESTS/FINDINGS

1. Culture and sensitivity: Blood, urine, sputum, and any suspect areas.
2. Complete blood count (CBC) with differential.
3. CXR: If abnormal respiratory signs and symptoms are present consider bronchoscopy with lavage and transbronchial biopsy. If GI symptoms are present consider endoscopy, especially when CMV suspected.
4. Lumbar puncture and/or CT scan of the head may be indicated if neurologic signs and symptoms are present to rule out brain abscess or other CNS abnormality.

MANAGEMENT/TREATMENT

1. Treat identified or suspected pathogen (i.e., triple-antibiotic therapy until positive blood culture identified). (See "Infection" Chapter 11.)
2. Types of infections common in the OHT patient include:
   A. Bacterial
      1) *Staphylococcus aureus* (wound, early postoperative)
   B. Opportunistic pathogens (later, several weeks postoperative)
      1) Viral: Cytomegalovirus (CMV)
      2) Fungi: *Candida, aspergillus*
      3) Parasites: *Pneumocystis, Toxoplasma*
3. Prophylactic treatment for opportunistic infections includes:
   A. CMV: Gancyclovir
   B. *Candida*: Chlortrimazole troches, 2 tabs PO bid
   C. *Pneumocystis*: Trimethoprim-sulfamethoxyzole (Bactrim), 1 tab PO bid, 2 days/wk
4. The regular use of vaccines remains controversial and generally not advised until 6 months following transplantation.
5. Antibiotic prophylaxis is recommended for dental, upper respiratory, and GI-GU procedures which may cause transient bacteremia; however, infective endocarditis is rare.

Transplant Coronary Artery Disease

1. TCAD is an accelerated form of coronary artery disease that occurs in heart transplant recipients and has become a major factor limiting long-term survival following OHT and is the leading cause of death after the first post-transplant year (Miller, 1993).
2. Approximately 10% of transplant recipients will develop TCAD at 1 year, increasing to 40% at 3 years.
3. Denervation of the donor heart, which occurs with heart transplantation, generally prevents any sensation of angina-like pain to signal the development of TCAD.
4. TCAD is considered to be immunologically mediated, although exact mechanisms are not well understood. TCAD is diffuse and progressive, affecting the microvasculature of the donor heart.

DIAGNOSTIC TESTS/FINDINGS

1. TCAD is commonly detected via coronary angiography. The unique angiographic hallmark of this disease is diffuse, concentric, longitudinal, and rapid pruning and obliteration of distal branch vessels (Miller, 1993).
2. Intravascular ultrasound (IVUS) is used to evaluate both actual lumen diameter and the appearance and thickness of the intima and media of the vessel. Intimal hyperplasia is a common manifestation of TCAD that correlates with concomitant angiographically significant CAD.

MANAGEMENT/TREATMENT

1. Management of transplant recipients with TCAD is determined by the transplant cardiologist. The ACNP will work closely with the collaborating physician.
2. PTCA, when indicated, initially may prove successful, yet is associated with restenosis rates of up to 50%, rendering it a palliative therapy.
3. Preventive measures that may reduce the incidence of TCAD include modification of known risk factors, reduced intake of cholesterol and saturated fats, HMG-CoA RIs, smoking cessation, regular exercise, and the use of an antiplatelet agent, such as low-dose aspirin.
4. Retransplantation remains the only definitive treatment for TCAD. Overall survival for a second OHT is less than with the primary recipient.

PATIENT EDUCATION

1. Educate patients and families preoperatively and postoperatively regarding the importance of the rigorous medication regimen and follow-up care after OHT.
2. Educate patients and families regarding expected side effects of the various medications and the effect they may have on body image and psychosocial adjustment.
3. Educate patients and families about the signs and symptoms of rejection and infectious complications. Emphasize prompt reporting of the symptoms to the health care team to facilitate early intervention. Emphasize taking medications exactly as prescribed and adhering to follow-up visits, as feelings of well-being may dissuade patients from taking immunosuppressive drugs, leading to rejection.
4. Discuss with patient and family the benefits of cardiac rehabilitation postoperatively, when necessary, to improve exercise tolerance and a sense of well-being.

Review Questions

3.56 Which of the following is the most likely medication the ACNP must consider in addition to cyclosporine and azathioprine as part of the triple-drug immunosuppressive therapy for the cardiac transplant recipient?
   A. Bactrim
   B. Corticosteroids
   C. Chlortrimazole troche
   D. Enalapril

3.57 A 38-year-old man 6 months S/P OHT is admitted to the ER with shortness of breath for 1 week, malaise, and palpitations. His wife states he
has not been following his medication regimen for the past 3 weeks as he
was feeling so good after transplant that he thought he did not need to
take his medications. On physical exam the ACNP notes JVP approxi-
mately 10 cm H_2O, bibasilar rales, and the presence of an S_3 on cardiac
auscultation. The patient's vital signs are as follows:
Temp: 38.4°C
BP: 90/60
HR: 120/bpm
RR: 26 breaths/min
SaO_2: 91%
What would be the likely diagnosis for this patient?
A. Infection
B. Rejection
C. Acute myocardial infarction
D. Pneumonia

3.58 On admission to the CCU the ACNP finds the patient's heart rate has
dropped to 60 bpm. The patient complains of lightheadedness. What
would be the most appropriate intervention for this patient?
A. Atropine 1 mg IVP, prepare for temporary pacemaker insertion
B. Dobutamine 5 μg/kg/min IV drip and titrate to HR >100
C. Isoproterenol drip, prepare for temporary pacemaker insertion
D. None of the above

3.59 The cardiac transplant patient presents to the ER with new-onset atrial
fibrillation. Which of the following is the most appropriate?
A. Procainamide 500 mg IVPB over 30 minutes followed by a procainamide drip at 2 mg/min
B. Know specific signs and symptoms of allograft rejection and obtain
immediate consultation with transplant cardiologist.
C. Digoxin 0.5 mg IVP, followed by 0.25 mg IVP in 2 hours
D. DC cardioversion immediately to prevent thrombus formation associated with atrial fibrillation

3.60 Which of the following is a definitive diagnostic test for cardiac allograft
rejection?
A. Cyclosporine level (serum)
B. Echocardiography
C. Endomyocardial biopsy
D. Immune complex T-cell morphology

Answers and Rationales

3.56   **C**   Traditional triple-drug immunosuppressive therapy includes cyclosporine, azathioprine, and corticosteroids. Some variation may exist
among institutions and with patient presentation.

3.57   **B**   The patient's history suggests that the likely cause of his symptoms
is rejection secondary to omission of immunosuppressive agents from
his medication regimen. Symptoms of volume overload are suggestive of decreased LV function.

3.58   **C**   Isoproterenol is the first-line drug the ACNP should consider when treating symptomatic bradycardia in the OHT patient. Due to denervation of the heart there will be no response to atropine in the cardiac transplant recipient. Preparation for temporary pacing is also recommended in this setting in the event the patient's heart rate does not increase in response to isoproterenol.

3.59   **B**   The ACNP must recognize atrial fibrillation as an arrhythmia associated with rejection in the cardiac transplant patient. Immediate consultation with the transplant cardiologist is indicated to rule out rejection and to treat the presenting arrhythmia.

3.60   **C**   Endomyocardial biopsy is considered the gold standard for diagnosing rejection in the heart transplant recipient.

References

Baumgartner, W.A., Owens, S.G., Cameron, D.E., & Reitz B.A. (eds.). (1994). *The Johns Hopkins Manual of Cardiac Surgical Care.* St. Louis: Mosby-Year Book Inc.

Gross, S., Coleman, B., Flavell, C., & Salamandara, J. (1996). Patients undergoing cardiothoracic surgery and transplants. In J.M., Clochesy, C. Breu, S. Cardin, et al. (eds.). *Critical Care Nursing* (2nd ed.). Philadelphia: W.B. Saunders Co., pp. 458–512.

Hosenpud, J.D., et al. (1995). The Registry of the International Society for Heart and Lung Transplantation: Twelfth official report—1995. *J Heart Lung Transplant 14,* 805–815.

Kobashigawa, J.A., Kirklin, J.K., Naftel, D.C., et al., & The Transplant Cardiologist's Database Research Group (1993). Pre-transplant risk factors for acute rejection after heart transplantation: A multiinstitutional study. *J Heart Lung Transplant 12,* 355–366.

Kobashigawa, J.A., Murphy F.L., Stevenson, L.W., et al. (1990). Low dose lovastatin safely lowers cholesterol after cardiac transplantation. *Circulation 82*(Suppl. IV), IV-281–IV-283.

Kobashigawa, J.A., & Stevenson, L.W. (1993). Postoperative treatment of heart transplant patients. *J Crit Illness 8*(5), 607–615.

Kobashigawa, J.A., & Stevenson, L.W. (1993). Managing complications in heart transplant patients. *J Crit Illness 8*(6), 678–689.

Miller, L.W., Schlant, R.C., Kobashigawa, J., et al. (1993). Task force 5: Complications. *J Am Coll Cardiol 22*(1), 41–54.

Mudge, G.H., Goldstein, S., Addonizio, L.J., et al. (1993). Task force 3: Recipient guidelines/prioritization. *J Am Coll Cardiol 22*(1), 21–31.

Perloff, M.G., & Reitz, B.A. (1997). Heart and heart-lung transplantation. In E. Braunwald (ed.). *Heart Disease: A Textbook of Cardiovascular Medicine* (5th ed.). Philadelphia: W.B. Saunders Co., pp. 515–533.

Post-Cardiac Surgery: CABG

DEFINITION

1. Surgical revascularization in the form of CABG remains in the forefront of treatment for CAD.

2. The rationale for performing surgical revascularization or aortocoronary bypass grafting is to restore adequate blood flow or blood supply and to provide nutritional support to myocardial tissue.

3. A harvested vessel or conduit is anastomosed between the aortic root and a point distal to the obstructing coronary lesion or stenosis (Gross et al., 1996).
4. The saphenous vein and the internal mammary artery (IMA) are the most commonly used conduits for myocardial revascularization. The patency rate for saphenous vein grafts at 1 year is 90% falling to 50–60% at 10 years. The IMA is the conduit of choice for the left anterior descending coronary artery and demonstrates excellent long-term patency rates of about 80% at 10 years.

ETIOLOGY/INCIDENCE

1. Approximately 355,000 CABG operations are performed annually in the United States (AHA, 1991).
2. Variation exists in reports of operative mortality. Data from the Coronary Artery Surgery Study (CASS) (1983) cites annual mortality rates in patients with single-, double-, and triple-artery bypass at 0.7, 1.4, and 1.0% respectively.
3. Increased survival is one of the most significant benefits of CABG, with approximately 90% of patients alive at 5 years and 80% surviving 10 years.
4. In addition to mortality benefits, CABG is associated with affecting positive outcomes for patients including relief of angina, improvement in functional status, and decreased need for pharmacologic therapy.
5. CABG surgery consumes more health care resources than any other single treatment or procedure.

SIGNS AND SYMPTOMS

1. Table 3–37 provides indications for CABG.
2. See also "Chest Pain and Unstable Angina, Myocardial Infarction," and "Valvular Heart Disease."

T A B L E **3–37.   Indications for Coronary Artery Bypass Grafting (CABG)***

Chronic stable angina refractory to medical therapy
Significant left main coronary occlusion (>50%)
Triple-vessel coronary disease
  Left ventricular dysfunction
  Proximal left anterior descending disease (as part of two-vessel disease)
Unstable angina pectoris
Acute myocardial infarction
  Emergent
  Delayed
Intractable ventricular irritability
Left ventricular failure
  Congestive heart failure
  Cardiogenic shock
Percutaneous transluminal coronary angioplasty failure

---

* From Gross, S., Coleman, B., Flavell, C., & Salamandara, J. (1996). Patients undergoing cardiothoracic surgery and transplants. In J.M. Clochesy, C. Breu, S. Cardin, et al. (eds.). *Critical Care Nursing* (2 ed.). Philadelphia: W.B. Saunders Co., pp. 458–512, with permission.

TABLE 3–38.   **Physical Exam Findings in High-Risk Patients***

Physical Exam	Abnormal Finding	Comment
Chest	Prior radical mastectomy	Contraindicate use of IMA
	Rales	May indicate pulmonary edema
Cardiovascular	Murmur of AR	AR may worsen during
	S_3, S_4	cardiopulmonary bypass because of a jet from aortic cannulation; LV dilatation may ensue; IABP contraindicated
Abdomen	Abdominal aortic aneurysm	May contraindicate use of IABP
Extremities	Peripheral arterial insufficiency	May complicate use of IABP
	Extensive venous variscosities in lower extremities	Insufficient venous conduits available for harvesting; consider arm veins/arteries, LIMA
		Increased risk of lower extremity cellulitis
Neurologic	Carotid bruits	Increase of perioperative CVA
	Preoperative neurologic deficits	Neurologic status may deteriorate postoperatively due to compromised cerebral perfusion

* Adapted from Antman, E.M. (1997). Medical management of the patient undergoing cardiac surgery. In E. Braunwald (ed.). *Heart Disease: A Textbook of Cardiovascular Medicine* (5th ed.). Philadelphia: W.B. Saunders Co., pp. 1715–1740, with permission.

IMA, internal mammary artery; AR, aortic regurgitation; LV, left ventricular; IABP, intra-aortic balloon pump; LIMA, left internal mammary artery; CVA, cerebrovascular accident.

PHYSICAL FINDINGS

1. A complete physical examination is necessary preoperatively in the patient undergoing CABG.
2. The ACNP must be aware of physical findings to report to the collaborating physician that may indicate a high-risk patient and may require further evaluation (Table 3–38).
3. See "Angina Pectoris and Unstable Angina," "Acute Myocardial Infarction" for physical findings of conditions that may require cardiac surgery.

DIFFERENTIAL DIAGNOSIS

1. CABG is a treatment for CAD. (See also "Angina Pectoris and Unstable Angina" for differential diagnosis specific to this condition.)

DIAGNOSTIC TESTS/FINDINGS

1. Preoperative serum laboratory tests necessary prior to cardiac surgery include:
   A. CBC, coagulation screen (PT, PTT), serum electrolytes, BUN, creatinine, and routine urine analysis (RUA). Liver function tests are often obtained for baseline information.
   B. Type and crossmatch for blood transfusion is required for all patients undergoing CABG.
   C. A history of hepatitis or thyroid disorder should initiate the determination of the patient's antibody and antigen status and thyroid function, respectively.
2. A 12-lead ECG and a CXR are essential baseline studies preoperatively.

3. Echocardiography is also useful to evaluate cardiac structure and function.
4. Cardiac catheterization is necessary to demonstrate coronary anatomy and ventricular function, to record intracardiac pressures, and to measure oxygen saturation.
5. Other diagnostic tests performed prior to cardiac surgery may include chest CT, MRI, and radionuclide scanning.
6. Carotid duplex scanning may be completed prior to cardiac surgery to evaluate for carotid artery stenosis.

MANAGEMENT/TREATMENT—POSTOPERATIVE

1. On admission to the ICU the ACNP recovering the cardiac surgery patient during the immediate postoperative period should address the following issues and hemodynamic parameters (Baumgartner, 1994).
   A. Rapid initial assessment: BP, HR and rhythm, auscultate heart and lungs, assess peripheral pulses, ensure that epicardial pacing wires are connected to the pulse generator, and test for capture.
   B. Consult with surgeon regarding intraoperative course, postoperative treatment plan.
   C. Consult with anesthesiologist regarding intraoperative course, postoperative treatment plan.
   D. Complete initial assessment:
      1) Review admission CXR
      2) Assess respiratory status: ABG, ventilation parameters
      3) Review and evaluate rhythm and 12-lead ECG
      4) Assess hemodynamic status and initiate appropriate interventions
      5) Assess chest tube output: Assess patency early to prevent cardiac tamponade
2. The ACNP in consultation with the cardiac surgeon and multidisciplinary team will be required to manage common postoperative conditions encountered in the cardiac surgery patient. These include fluid, electrolyte, and acid-base abnormalities; respiratory management; hypertension; perioperative MI; low output syndrome and shock states; cardiac tamponade; arrhythmias; hemostatic disturbances; and infection (Antmann, 1997).

COMMON POSTOPERATIVE CONDITIONS

Fluid, Electrolyte, and Acid-Base Balance

1. After extracorporeal circulation there is an increase in extracellular fluid and exchangeable total sodium and a decrease in exchangeable potassium.
2. Limit free water to 1 L/day for the first 48 hours postoperatively; IV fluid is D_5 W; sodium replacement varies with volume status.
3. Maintain serum potassium 4.5 ± 5.5 mEq/L; serum potassium will fluctuate dramatically necessitating frequent monitoring, especially in diabetics. Maintain serum magnesium at 2.0 mEq/L. Frequent monitoring of potassium and magnesium is necessary as abnormalities may predispose to arrhythmias.
4. Serum glucose levels are frequently elevated due to IV fluid and surgically induced increases in cortisol and catecholamines. Insulin may be required.
5. Mild metabolic acidosis or alkalosis may be present for the first 24 hours postoperatively, especially with rewarming. Usually does not require correction unless renal dysfunction is present or ensuing.

6. Serum total calcium, phosphorus, may be depressed for 24–48 hours postoperatively secondary to hemodilution; are usually self-correcting.

Respiratory Management

Abnormalities of respiratory function may occur after cardiac surgery secondary to the effects of anesthesia, cardiopulmonary bypass, and sternotomy. These include alveolar dysfunction secondary to right-to-left intrapulmonary shunting, decreased central respiratory drive secondary to general anesthesia (pharmacologic effects) and mechanical derangements to thoracic function, decreased respiratory muscle function secondary to pain, and exacerbation of underlying pulmonary disease (Antmann, 1997).

1. Most patients will require 6–8 hours of ventilatory support.
2. Intermittent mandatory ventilation (IMV) is ventilatory mode of choice; frequent ABGs for the first 12 hours postoperatively.
3. Criteria for successful weaning from ventilatory support include (Antmann, 1997):
   - VC >10–15 cc/kg body weight
   - FEV_1 >10 cc/kg body weight
   - PIP > −20 to −30 cm H_2O
   - Resting minute ventilation <10 L
   - Spontaneous respiratory rate under 25 on IMV of 6 while resting comfortably, alert, and no apparent work of breathing
   - A-a gradient on 100% FIO_2 <300–500 torr
   - Arterial PO_2 >80 torr in the absence of intracardiac right-to-left shunting when the FIO_2 ≤0.5%.
   - Shunt fraction (Q_s/Q_t) <10–20%
   - Dead space tidal volume (V_D/V_T) <0.55–0.66
4. Early extubation, <6 hours postoperative, is possible when low-dose synthetic narcotics and inhaled anesthetics are used, muscle relaxants are reversed, total CPB time <100 minutes, the patient is hemodynamically stable and mentally alert, and VC is ≥10 cc/kg.
5. Positive end-expiratory pressure (PEEP) is used with caution in patients with pre-existing chronic obstructive pulmonary disease (COPD) (due to barotrauma and air trapping). PEEP may not be tolerated with hypovolemia and inadequate preload.
6. Additional factors that may influence the decision not to extubate include decreased level of consciousness; hemodynamic instability; recurrent sustained malignant ventricular arrhythmias; postoperative bleeding that may require reoperation; ineffective cough; hemoglobin <10 gm/dL; and significant atelectasis, lobar consolidation, or pleural effusion.
7. *Urgent and complex respiratory problems (i.e., pulmonary edema, diaphragmatic failure, COPD) require immediate consultation with the cardiac surgeon and multidisciplinary team* (See "Pulmonary Diseases.")

Hypertension

1. Postoperative HTN is defined as an SBP >140 mm Hg (Antmann, 1977).
2. About 40–60% of patients will manifest postoperative hypertension, which is more common in patients with a preoperative history of HTN, preoperative maintenance therapy with β-blockers, and well-preserved LV function.

3. Adverse consequences of elevated SBP in the postoperative period include increased risk of postoperative bleeding, suture line disruption, aortic dissection, elevated LV afterload with reduction of LV output, injury to aorto-coronary bypass grafts, and postoperative stroke.
4. Rapid-acting, titratable intravenous agents with a short half-life are the agents of choice for acute postoperative HTN, such as sodium nitroprusside, esmolol, nitroglycerin, and labetolol.
5. Transition to oral antihypertensive agents is determined on an individual basis.
6. See "Hypertension/Hypertensive Emergencies" for specific drug dosages and further information in the management of hypertension.

Low Cardiac Output Syndrome/Shock States

1. Low cardiac output syndrome (LCOS) is a multifaceted syndrome of inadequate tissue perfusion, clinically defined as a CI less than 2.0 L/min/m^2 (Baumgartner, 1994).
2. LCOS is associated with a high incidence of cardiac death and postoperative complications (i.e., respiratory failure, neurologic sequelae, and renal failure).
3. The sequence of hemodynamic changes occurring with LCOS are diagrammed as follows:

$$\uparrow PCWP \rightarrow \downarrow SV \text{ and } \uparrow HR \rightarrow \downarrow CI \text{ and } \downarrow SV \rightarrow \downarrow BP$$

Increased PCWP may be an early sign; correlate $\downarrow$ CI with $\downarrow$ S$\overline{v}O_2$
4. See also "Shock" for the specific management for LCOS.

Myocardial Ischemia

1. The incidence of myocardial ischemia in the postoperative surgery patient varies dramatically depending on the patient, anesthetic techniques, and experience of the operating team. Myocardial ischemia occurs in approximately 3–15% of patients.
2. The highest incidence of myocardial ischemia occurs in the first 6 hours after bypass.
3. The etiology of myocardial ischemia in the postoperative period may be related to mechanical factors (graft occlusion), myocardial hypoperfusion (hypotension), increased myocardial oxygen demand (tachycardia, elevated afterload), vasospasm, and inadequate intraoperative myocardial protection.
4. See "Angina Pectoris and Unstable Angina," "Acute Myocardial Infarction" for management of myocardial ischemia.

Arrhythmias

1. The electrophysiologic mechanisms underlying arrhythmias in the postoperative cardiac surgery patient are poorly understood, yet are believed to be due to a combination of effects, including circulating catecholamines, alteration in autonomic nervous system tone, transient electrolyte imbalances, myocardial ischemia or infarction, and mechanical irritation of the heart (Antman, 1977; Ommen et al., 1997).

ATRIAL FIBRILLATION

1. AF occurs in at least 20–30% of CABG patients and 50% of valve replacement patients with the greatest incidence at the second or third postoperative day.
2. β-Blockers have been used as a prophylaxis against atrial arrhythmias in the postoperative period. Patients receiving β-blockers preoperatively should continue to receive them postoperatively (if possible), as patients whose β-blocker therapy is discontinued postoperatively have a higher incidence of postoperative atrial tachyarrhythmias (Ommen et al., 1997).
3. Initial treatment, if hemodynamically stable and LV function is preserved, is to slow the ventricular rate pharmacologically. Agents include β-blockers (metroprolol, esmolol) and calcium channel blockers (verapamil, diltiazem). Digoxin can be used; however, desired rate control is less with high levels of circulating catecholamines.
4. DC cardioversion is the treatment of choice when hemodynamic compromise is present.
5. For specific treatment guidelines and medication dosages in the treatment of AF, see "Arrhythmias."
6. Prompt anticoagulation should be strongly considered if the arrhythmia persists for 24 hours or more (Ommen et al., 1997). See also "Arrhythmias" for use of warfarin and "Acute Myocardial Infarction" for use of heparin.

PAROXYSMAL SUPRAVENTRICULAR TACHYCARDIA

1. Paroxysmal supraventricular tachycardia (PSVT) occurs less frequently than AF. PSVT may be responsive to vagal maneuvers or pharmacologic therapy.
2. Adenosine is the drug of choice for treating PSVT. May also be terminated with burst atrial pacing.
3. For management of other arrhythmias such as ventricular arrhythmias, bradyarrhythmias, and heart block(s), see "Arrhythmias."

Hematologic Disturbances

1. CBP causes derangements of the hemostatic system due to exposure of the blood to artificial surfaces, hemodilution, and the effects of heparin.
2. Platelet dysfunction is the most significant abnormality that occurs following CPB, although diminution of coagulation factors also occurs.
3. Most obvious evidence of bleeding is assessed by measuring chest tube drainage. Acceptable rate of bleeding is <100 mL/hr. Excessive bleeding, defined as 500 mL/hr for 1 hour, more than 300 mL/hr for 3 hours, or 200–300 mL/hr for 5 hours, requires return to the operating room for control of bleeding (Antman, 1997). Consider correctable extenuating circumstances (i.e., uncontrolled HTN, failure to achieve normothermia, or an abnormal coagulation status that is being corrected).
4. Frequent measurements of the coagulation profile (i.e., platelets, ACT, PT, PTT) are indicated.
5. Consider platelet transfusion for platelet count <100,000 mm^3 in the presence of bleeding and fresh frozen plasma to correct an elevated PT.
6. Other management strategies for bleeding include desmopressin (DDAVP) to increase plasma levels of von Willebrand factor; empirical administration

of protamine sulfate to counteract heparin, which may be liberated from the patient's fat stores with rewarming.

7. The ACNP must be alert to sudden cessation of bleeding from chest tubes as clotted blood may cause fluid to drain into mediastinal and/or pleural spaces. Serial CXRs may be indicated in the setting of bleeding.

8. *Bleeding episodes require immediate consultation with the attending physician or surgeon, as return to the operating room may be required to control bleeding.*

Pericarditis/Pericardiotomy Syndrome

1. The postpericardiotomy syndrome (PPS) is a common complication after cardiac surgery occurring in 10–15% of patients.

2. It is characterized by fever, anterior chest pain that is worsened with inspiration and lying supine, and a two- or three-component pericardial friction rub. PPS is usually self-limiting, although it is noted in some cases to cause cardiac tamponade. The etiology of PPS is unclear.

3. See "Pericarditis and Cardiac Tamponade" for management of pericarditis and cardiac tamponade.

Infection

1. Fever is the most common sign of postoperative infection; however, it may be present for up to 6 days postoperatively in the normally convalescing patient.

2. For temperature ≥38.5°C culture and sensitivity of blood (peripheral and line), urine, sputum, and wound(s) are indicated. Empiric antibiotic therapy is indicated.

3. Infections of the leg wound usually present with fever, induration, pain, erythema, local warmth, and drainage from the suture line.

4. Diagnostic tests of wound aspiration and Gram-stain guide therapy.

5. Infectious agents of the leg wound are usually *Staphylococcus, Streptococcus*, and gram-negative bacilli.

6. If a fungal infection is identified, topical antifungal agents should be administered in addition to oral antibiotic therapy.

7. Mediastinitis and sternal osteomyelitis are the most serious complications of a sternotomy.

8. **Mediastinitis requires immediate consultation with the collaborating physician/surgeon for aggressive treatment with appropriate antibiotic therapy and surgical exploration/correction.**

9. Mediastinitis occurs in approximately 2% of patients undergoing median sternotomy and is present within 2 weeks of surgery (Antman, 1997).

10. Presenting signs and symptoms of mediastinitis include persistent fever >101°F beyond the fourth postoperative day, leukocytosis, bacteremia, erythema at the sternal incision, and purulent discharge from the sternal wound. Wound erythema, abnormal sternal tenderness or instability, and/or mediastinal widening may not be apparent early in the development of mediastinitis.

11. Fifty percent caused by *Staphylococcus aureus* and 40% caused by gram-negative bacilli. The organism may be resistant to antibiotic prophylaxis especially if gram-negative bacillus or a β-lactamase–producing *S. aureus*.

12. Viral infections after cardiac surgery are usually the result of transfusion therapy; primarily result in hepatitis C.
13. For treatment of infective endocarditis, see "Valvular Heart Disease."

Neurologic Complications

1. Neurologic problems may occur after cardiac surgery, especially in the elderly, and include short-term memory loss, lack of concentration, and psychological problems such as depression.
2. Cerebral vascular accident (CVA) occurs in 1–5% of patients, and as high as 10% in patients over 65 years of age.
3. Risk factors for CVA or transient ischemic attack (TIA) include preoperative carotid bruit, previous CVA or TIA, postoperative atrial fibrillation, prolonged CPB >2 hours, and preoperative LV mural thrombus.
4. For treatment of CVA, see Chapter 4.

PATIENT EDUCATION

1. Assess the patient and family response to illness and the forthcoming procedure. Assess the patient's expectations of the procedure and the postoperative convalescence. Plan preoperative teaching to include this information.
2. Provide information on the patient's progress to the family and/or significant others on a daily basis postoperatively to meet their needs for information and reduction of anxiety.
3. Establish realistic and specific goals with the patient to facilitate healing and adaptation during the immediate postoperative period and during the phases of recovery and rehabilitation.
4. Discuss the usual postoperative course, medications, activity, and wound care in anticipation of discharge from the hospital.
5. Determine frequency of follow-up appointments with patient and family.

Review Questions

3.61 Which of the following is a relative contraindication to CABG?
   A. Unstable angina
   B. AMI with cardiogenic shock
   C. AMI without evidence of cardiogenic shock
   D. Multiple vessel stenosis

3.62 A 66-year-old man is brought to the SICU immediately following CABG × 5. His initial hemodynamic measurements are:
   BP: 172/88
   HR: 126/bpm
   PAP: 20/10
   PCWP: 8
   RAP: 5
   LAP: 8
   CI: 2.2
   SVR: 2300
   The nurse reports 500 mL output from the mediastinal chest tube and

250 mL from the pleural chest tube in the last hour. What is the first intervention the ACNP should consider?
A. Order 6 units of fresh frozen plasma (FFP)
B. Call the attending surgeon and prepare to take the patient back to the OR
C. Check with the nurse in 1 hour
D. Order NTP to decrease the SBP

3.63 A 77-year-old man is 3 days S/P AVR, CABG × 2. He calls his nurse as he feels palpitations. The monitor shows atrial fibrillation with a ventricular rate of 130/min. The patient's blood pressure is 110/76. What is the most appropriate intervention?
A. Digoxin 0.5 mg IVP
B. Overdrive pacing
C. DC cardioversion
D. Adenosine 6 mg IVP

3.64 A 72-year-old woman is 4 days post-CABG × 4. She has been transferred to the step-down unit. She continues to complain of substernal chest pressure when lying supine. On cardiac auscultation you note a three-component pericardial friction rub. What is the most likely cause of the patient's discomfort?
A. Incisional pain
B. Postpericardiotomy syndrome
C. Angina
D. Pulmonary embolism

3.65 What is the most appropriate medication to give the patient in Question 3.64?
A. Nonsteroidal anti-inflammatory drugs (NSAID's)
B. Morphine sulfate
C. Acetaminophen
D. Digoxin

Answers and Rationales

3.61 **B** Patients with AMI and cardiogenic shock have an increase in mortality associated with CABG surgery and should be stabilized prior to surgery.
3.62 **B** Bleeding from the chest tube(s) ≥500 mL/hr constitutes rationale to return to the OR to investigate the cause of the excessive chest tube drainage. The attending surgeon should be notified immediately by the ACNP.
3.63 **A** Digoxin is indicated to slow the patient's ventricular rate and to convert the atrial fibrillation to sinus rhythm. This patient is in atrial fibrillation with stable hemodynamics. Pharmacologic therapy is indicated. The loading dose of digoxin is commonly followed by 0.25 mg in 2 hours times two doses.
3.64 **B** The patient's pain is positional and on cardiac exam a friction rub is present which suggests postpericardiotomy syndrome.
3.65 **A** Nonsteroidal anti-inflammatory medications are indicated in patients with postpericardiotomy syndrome in order to reduce inflammation and relieve discomfort.

References

Antman, E.M. (1997). Medical management of the patient undergoing cardiac surgery. In E. Braunwald (ed.). *Heart Disease: A Textbook of Cardiovascular Medicine* (5th ed.). Philadelphia: W.B. Saunders Co., pp. 1715–1740.

Baumgartner, W.A., Owens, S.G., Cameron, D.E., & Reitz, B.A. (eds.). (1994). *The Johns Hopkins Manual of Cardiac Surgical Care*. St. Louis: Mosby-Year Book, Inc.

CASS Principal Investigators and their Associates. (1983). Coronary artery surgery study (CASS): A randomized trial of coronary artery bypass surgery. Survival data. *Circulation 68*(5), 939–950.

Edmond, M., et al. (1994). Long-term survival of medically treated patients in the coronary artery surgery study (CASS) registry. *Circulation 90*(6), 2645–2657.

Evans, S.A. (1993). The economics of cardiac surgery. *AACN Clin Issues Crit Care Nursing 4*(2), 340–347.

Foster, E.D., Fisher, L.D., Kurser, G.C., & Meyers, W.O. (1984). Comparison of operative mortality and morbidity for initial and repeat coronary artery bypass grafting: The coronary artery surgery study (CASS) registry experience. *Ann Thorac Surg 38*, 563–570.

Gross, S., Coleman, B., Flavell, C., & Salamandara, J. (1996). Patients undergoing cardiothoracic surgery and transplants. In J.M. Clochesy, C. Breu, S. Cardin, et al. (eds.). *Critical Care Nursing* (2nd ed.) Philadelphia: W.B. Saunders Co., pp. 458–512.

Kirklin, J.W., Atkins, C.W., Blackstone, E.H., et al. (1991). Guidelines and indications for coronary artery bypass graft surgery: ACC/AHA task force report. *J Am Coll Cardiol 17*, 543–589.

Ommen, S.R., Odell, J.A., & Stanton, M.S. (1997). Atrial arrhythmias after cardiothoracic surgery. *N Engl J Med 336*(20), 1429–1434.

Abdominal Aortic Aneurysm

DEFINITION

Local irreversible dilatation, outpouching, or swelling of the arterial wall at 150% of the normal aortic diameter. This greater than normal vessel configuration results in alteration in blood flow and a tendency toward rupture or thrombosis.

ETIOLOGY/INCIDENCE

1. Risk factors for AAA include:
   A. Increasing age
   B. Male gender (male/female ratio for deaths between ages 60 and 64 is 11:1; between ages 85 and 90, 3:1)
   C. Family history of aneurysms
   D. Smoking history
   E. Hypertension
   F. Peripheral vascular disease
   G. Coronary artery disease
   H. Chronic obstructive pulmonary disease
   I. Presence of other aneurysms (popliteal aneurysms associated with 35% AAA occurrence rate; femoral aneurysms with 66%)
2. Risk of rupture increases with size of aneurysm (few aneurysms <4 cm will

rupture and 3 to 6% of aneurysms >4 cm in diameter will rupture annually), hypertension, and chronic obstructive pulmonary disease.

3. In the United States, AAAs are 15th leading cause of death. Approximately 0.8% of male deaths and 0.3% of female deaths attributed to AAA in persons over age 65.

4. Overall mortality rate after rupture is 90%, although if patient reaches hospital alive the mortality rate is 50%. Operative mortality rate for emergency repair is 50% versus 5% for elective repair.

5. Natural history of most aneurysms is one of gradual enlargement with growth rates estimated to average an increase of 10% of the current diameter per year.

6. There is an estimated tenfold increase in risk in patients with a first-degree relative with an AAA.

7. Highly significant correlation between emergency admission and sudden death from ruptured aneurysm in autumn and winter has been demonstrated with temperature-induced changes in BP as the contributing factor.

PATHOPHYSIOLOGY

The true cause of abdominal aortic aneurysms (AAAs) is unknown, however, most AAAs represent a degenerative process often attributed to atherosclerosis due to the age factor and other atherosclerotic changes often found. Normal aortic tunica media consists of elastin, which provides compliance, and collagen fibers with smooth muscle cell matrix, which provides strength in the normal aorta. In experimental models digestion of elastin leads to aortic dilatation. Histologically, AAAs reveal fragmentation of the elastin layers, decreased elastin content with the aneurysm ultimately left with a thin tunica media and only a few elastin layers remaining. Atherosclerosis in the intima is typical but the medial degenerative process for aneurysm is quite different from the typical intimal-medial thickening that occurs with occlusive atherosclerotic process. Thrombus is progressively overlaid on the intimal surface of the aneurysm.

Types of Aneurysms

1. True aneurysms
   A. Fusiform is uniform spindle-shaped dilatation of the entire circumference of a segment of an artery, and is the most common shape of an AAA representing about 75% of cases.
   B. Saccular is an outpouching of one side of the aortic wall; it is uncommon in the abdominal aorta but usually found proximal to the origin of the renal arteries.
   C. Dissecting aneurysm has a cavity that is formed by the blood that has been forced between the arterial wall layers.
2. False aneurysm is one in which the attenuation does not involve any of the layers of the aortic wall but is usually a pulsating encapsulated hematoma in communication with the lumen of the ruptured vessel.

SIGNS AND SYMPTOMS

1. Most AAAs are asymptomatic, even very large aneurysms, and are found incidentally.

2. Vague abdominal pain is the most common complaint, and is described as throbbing or constant.
3. Patients may report an awareness of pulsation in the abdomen that they notice while lying down or sitting quietly.
4. Back pain unassociated with movement may be present, usually described as dull, aching, continuous. Back pain complaint in majority of patients with ruptured AAA.
5. Constipation may develop; in patients with contained rupture approximately 20% of patients develop constipation.
6. Patients may report impaired or painful orgasms due to changes in sympathetic trunk due to aneurysmal periarteritis.
7. Testicular pain has been indicated as marker for impending AAA rupture especially in men over 50 years of age who have evidence of atherosclerosis.
8. Testicular edema or scrotal ecchymosis may be clues to presence of leaking AAA.
9. Weight loss, early satiety, and nausea may occur and are most likely due to intestinal compression.
10. The triad of shock, pulsatile mass, and abdominal or back pain is highly suggestive of rupture, although shock may be absent or minimal depending on degree of blood loss.

PHYSICAL FINDINGS

1. Pulsating mass is commonly felt in the abdomen (at or above the umbilicus) which pushes examiners hands apart rather than anteriorly (aneurysm must be at least 4.5 cm to be palpable). Size estimation overinflated 20% by this method. Drawback of palpation is aneurysms are felt only laterally while anterior posterior size may actually be much greater than lateral.
2. Bruit may be heard over aneurysm.
3. Lower extremity examination may reveal femoral and/or popliteal aneurysms.
4. Ruptured aneurysms may present with vital sign changes associated with hypovolemia, shock, ecchymosis in flank, severe pain in abdomen or back of sudden onset (triad of symptoms suggestive of rupture).

DIFFERENTIAL DIAGNOSIS

1. Urinary tract infection
2. Renal obstruction
3. Ruptured disc
4. Diverticulitis
5. Pancreatitis
6. UGI hemorrhage
7. Abdominal neoplasm
8. Peptic ulcer perforation

DIAGNOSTIC TESTS/FINDINGS

1. Laboratory values are of limited diagnostic value in diagnosis of unruptured AAA. Lab values that are typically drawn preoperatively include CBC, electrolytes, BUN and creatinine, fasting blood sugar, liver function tests, coagulation profile, and urinalysis. No labs are indicated for the routine patient

presenting with AAA; this should be a clinical decision made on individual basis.

2. If patient presents with rupture, blood sample for type and crossmatch should be drawn along with minimal preoperative studies such as hematocrit, electrolytes, BUN, and creatinine.

3. Ultrasound screening is the least expensive and most frequently used examination for initial confirmation of physical finding and for follow-up. Size measurements are more accurate in the anteroposterior than lateral dimension. This test should not be used for suspected rupture.

4. CT scan is more accurate and provides a more precise interpretation of the size and location of the aneurysm, although it is more expensive than ultrasound and involves radiation exposure.

5. MRI/MRA appear comparable to CT scanning, although it is less commonly available, much more expensive, and may be more difficult to obtain.

6. Arteriography is not an accurate technique to determine the presence or size of AAAs due to the presence of thrombus contained in the aneurysm which diminishes the size of the lumen visible with the contrast.

MANAGEMENT/TREATMENT

1. All abdominal aortic aneurysms require referral to vascular surgeon.

2. Suspected rupture of aneurysm is a surgical emergency requiring emergent vascular consult. Stabilize patient and prepare for surgery.

3. Nonruptured aneurysms of <5 cm in low-risk patients may be followed up by ultrasound or CT scan at 6-month intervals. This decision to operate should be made by surgeon and patient.

4. Hypertension should be carefully controlled in those patients in whom a watch-and-wait approach is appropriate.

PATIENT EDUCATION

1. Teach nature, onset, and course of disease including risk of rupture.

2. Inform patient that routine follow-up will be necessary with either repeat ultrasound or CT scans to determine course of aneurysm progression.

3. Inform patient that if he should experience sudden, severe pain in the back or abdomen (signs of rupture) he should call 911 or go immediately to the emergency room.

4. If surgery is indicated, teach patient, family about surgical procedure, postoperative expectations, and recovery period.

5. If patient situation is such that surgery is indicated but risk of surgery is greatly increased, provide patient and family information regarding outcomes and expectations, and assist them in making a decision regarding future treatment.

6. Teach patient about any medication that may be indicated including purpose, dosage, frequency, side effects, and signs of toxicity.

Review Questions

3.66 The pathophysiologic cause of aortic aneurysm includes:
    A. Degeneration due to atherosclerosis
    B. Degeneration due to age

    C. Fragmentation of the elastin layers
    D. All of the above

3.67 The most common symptoms of a patient with aortic aneurysm is:
    A. Abdominal pain
    B. Claudication
    C. No symptoms, most are asymptomatic
    D. Constipation

3.68 During physical examination of a 65-year-old man, you notice a pulsation in the abdomen. Palpation of the aorta reveals a lateral displacement of your hands revealing about a 6-cm aorta. The patient denies postprandial pain, diarrhea, back pain, impotence, or hematuria. The therapeutic intervention that should be done is:
    A. Emergent consult with vascular surgeon
    B. Ultrasound
    C. Angiogram
    D. Kidneys, ureters, and bladder (KUB)

3.69 A 72-year-old man presents to the emergency department with complaints of severe back pain that was sudden in onset; states he has a history of 20-lb weight loss over the last year; has abdominal cramping and diarrhea after eating; and denies blood in stool or urine, diabetes mellitus, or renal failure. PMH is positive for CABG × about 2 years ago, a 40-pack-year smoking history, and hypertension × 10 years for which he takes propranolol. Vital signs are HR 88, BP 110/62, respirations 12, and temperature 97.6°F. During physical examination you would most likely find:
    A. Positive psoas and obturator sign
    B. Tenderness with rigidity and guarding in the right lower quadrant indicative of ruptured diverticulum, especially given the history of weight loss
    C. Pulsatile abdominal mass
    D. Physical examination will probably be essentially negative; however, HBsAg will probably be positive, given history of coronary artery bypass graft surgery which, further questioning reveals, required 5 U of blood to be given

3.70 The diagnostic test that should be ordered immediately is:
    A. CT scan of the abdomen and chest
    B. KUB, upright and decubitus view looking for free air
    C. Angiogram
    D. MRA

Answers and Rationales

3.66   **D**   The etiology of aortic aneurysms is unknown; however, most aneurysms have a degenerative component attributable to age and atherosclerosis. In addition, there is histologic evidence that a weakening of the elastin in the medial layer of the aorta is present in aortic aneurysms. This weakening is different than the process that occurs in the intimal layer from the atherosclerotic process

3.67   **C**   Most patients are asymptomatic and the aneurysm is discovered incidentally. Some patients will have a vague abdominal discomfort that they describe as throbbing. They may also be aware of a pulsating sensation in the abdomen that they notice while lying down. If the patient complains of back pain, suspect rupture.

3.68   **B**   Ultrasound screening is the least expensive, most readily available test for diagnosis of aortic aneurysm in the nonemergent patient. CT scan is the more accurate test; however, it may be cost prohibitive for many patients and does involve radiation exposure. Ultrasound is never indicated if rupture of the aneurysm is suspected.

3.69   **C**   The history of sudden onset of severe back pain should always raise ruptured aneurysm as part of the differential diagnosis. There are also many risk factors in his history that would lead to the suspicion of aortic aneurysm or chronic mesenteric ischemia including weight loss, postprandial pain, smoking history, coronary artery disease, and hypertension. It is important to note that this patient may not have vital sign changes such as tachycardia due to β-blockade for treatment of hypertension.

3.70   **A**   The patient is stable enough to warrant definitive diagnostics. After confirmation with CT scan, aortic aneurysm resection would be treatment. Stat consult with vascular surgeon is mandatory and should be obtained as soon as rupture is suspected.

References

Cronenwett, J., & Sampson, L. (1996). Aneurysms of the abdominal aorta and ileac arteries. In R. Dean, J. Yao, & D. Brewster (eds.). *Current Diagnosis and Treatment in Vascular Surgery.* Norwalk, CT: Appleton & Lange, pp. 220–238.

Dalsin, M., & Sawchuk, A. (1988). Surgery of the aorta. In V. Fahey (ed.). *Vascular Nursing.* Philadelphia: W.B. Saunders Co, pp. 185–222.

Power, T. (1996). Aortic dissection. In R. Rakel (ed.). *Saunders Manual of Medical Practice.* Philadelphia: W.B. Saunders Co, pp. 262–264.

Tierney, L. (1996). Diseases of the aorta. In L. Tiernery, S. McPhee, & M. Papakadis (eds.). *Current Medical Diagnosis and Treatment.* Stamford, CT: Appleton & Lange, pp. 403–433.

Deep Vein Thrombosis

DEFINITION

Single or multiple blood clots in the deep veins of the extremities and/or pelvis. Thrombosis is usually accompanied by inflammation of the vessel wall.

ETIOLOGY/INCIDENCE

1. Risk factors include:
   A. Previous history of thrombosis is greatest risk factor for deep vein thrombosis (DVT).
   B. Pregnancy.
   C. Estrogen therapy (i.e., hormone replacement therapy or birth control pills usually with ≥ 50 μg of estrogen).

D. Malignancy, especially adenocarcinoma of lung, breast, and viscera.

E. Polycythemia.

F. Advancing age (increases dramatically after age 40 and triples with each additional 20 years).

G. Obesity and immobility. Obesity will increase risk two fold.

H. Heart disease.

I. Trauma.

2. Approximately 2 million cases per year in United States; 35% of hospitalized patients develop DVT.

3. Venous thrombus, should it become detached, flows to inferior vena cava, right side of heart and into pulmonary arteries where it can lodge and occlude pulmonary flow.

4. Use of central venous catheters for access, monitoring, nutrition, and drug administration increases risk of DVT in upper body sites. Emboli from these sources deposit in pulmonary circulation.

PATHOPHYSIOLOGY

1. Virchow's triad, factors that create an environment that promotes thrombus formation, are hypercoagulability, stasis, and endothelial damage. Hypercoagulability is caused by an increased procoagulant activity that can be from increases in platelet adhesiveness and count; changes in coagulation and/or fibrinolytic factors; deficiencies of antithrombin III, protein S, or protein C; or presence of anticardiolipin antibodies. Hypercoagulability is common in postoperative or posttrauma patients due to initiation of stress response. Stasis refers to decrease or interference of blood flow in venous system. Forward flow is almost entirely dependent on action of voluntary muscles in extremities and on functional one-way valves. Stasis allows prolonged contact of activated platelets with the vessel wall, theoretically allowing thrombus formation. Endothelial damage can occur from trauma, infection, venipuncture, myocardial infarction, or chemical agents (chemotherapeutic, contrast, or blood pressor agents), or as a result of excess venous dilation.

2. Venous thrombosis usually begins in valve pockets where areas of maximum stasis occur or at sites of venous injury. Most thrombi begin as platelet aggregates in the valve pockets. Typically, these are rapidly lysed with no sequelae. However, activation of the coagulation cascade due to release of tissue factor such as may occur following surgery or trauma results in increased thrombus formation that may overwhelm the ability of the local fibrinolytic activity to dissolve the thrombus, especially in states of venous stasis.

3. Principal site of venous thrombosis is soleal sinus. Thrombus typically extends into major deep calf veins, posterior tibial veins, and peroneal veins. Other common sites include other deep veins such as iliac, femoral, popliteal, and vena cava.

4. Thrombus, after formation, continues to propagate, developing a tail of fibrin mixed with white blood cells and red blood cells. It is this tail that breaks off and embolizes, most often to the pulmonary arteries.

SIGNS AND SYMPTOMS

1. Presenting signs and symptoms will vary depending on location of affected vein, size of thrombus, and presence of collateral vessels. Many DVTs are

asymptomatic. About 80% of deep vein thrombosis will remain confined to the calf and usually undergo spontaneous lysis or recanalization. The remainder will propagate, with approximately 10–20% manifesting with pulmonary embolism.
2. Pain may be present, and made worse by standing or walking; it improves with rest or elevation. Pain may be present in about 50% of patients.
3. Swelling of affected extremity, especially sudden increase in circumference of calf or thigh.
4. Patients with pulmonary embolus may be asymptomatic or present with varying degrees of dyspnea, tachypnea, or chest pain.

PHYSICAL FINDINGS

1. Low-grade fever may be the first clinical sign.
2. Swelling of affected extremity above or below knee is verified by measuring and comparing extremity circumference. Edema is usually distal to thrombus and is unilateral.
3. May have tenderness to palpation along course of thrombus if sufficient inflammatory action.
4. Homans' sign (pain in calf upon dorsiflexion) may be present in approximately 20% of patients with DVT.
5. May have tenderness on anteroposterior but not lateral compression of calf (Bancroft's sign). Present in less than one half of patients.
6. Inflation of blood pressure cuff around calf to 80 mm Hg produces prompt calf pain (Lowenberg's sign). Present in less that one half of patients.

DIFFERENTIAL DIAGNOSIS

1. Cellulitis
2. Ruptured synovial cyst (Baker's cyst)
3. Lymphedema
4. Muscle strain or rupture
5. Extrinsic compression of vein by tumor or enlarged lymph nodes
6. Postphlebitic syndrome

DIAGNOSTIC TESTS/FINDINGS

1. Ultrasonography: Diagnosis of DVT is made by failure of deep veins to compress under gentle pressure from probe of transducer.
2. Impedance plethysmography: Diagnosis of DVT by impairment of venous drainage from lower extremity resulting in abnormal test. Not useful for identifying calf DVT.
3. Ascending contrast venography: Gold standard for diagnosis of DVT. Should be used only when it is imperative to obtain definitive diagnosis due to disadvantages (risk of sensitivity, is uncomfortable, may cause renal insufficiency or congestive heart failure, is costly). DVT is diagnosed by presence of filling defects in deep veins on more than one view.

MANAGEMENT/TREATMENT

The best treatment is prevention! Extensive deep vein thrombosis and/or suspected pulmonary embolus requires immediate medical referral.

1. Patients with DVT of calf may be managed conservatively as outpatients. All others must be admitted.
2. Heparin therapy with bolus of 5000 to 10,000-U intravenous bolus and infusion to keep aPTT 1.5–2.5 times control.
3. Monitor platelet count for signs of heparin-induced thrombocytopenia. Discontinue heparin immediately if platelet count decreases. Low-molecular-weight heparin may be utilized in this situation.
4. Warfarin 10 mg daily on days 1 and 2, then at estimated daily maintenance dose.
5. Stop heparin therapy days 5–7 when INR is 2.0–3.0.
6. Warfarin at dose titrated to keep INR between 2.0 and 3.0 for 3 months.
7. Extremity should be elevated as much as possible.
8. Warm compresses may be applied.
9. Tylenol or NSAIDs may be given as needed for pain.
10. Antiembolism stockings should be worn after acute episode, and applied prior to arising.

PATIENT EDUCATION

1. Cause, onset, and course of DVT should be explained, and risk factors should be reviewed.
2. Medication teaching should include:
   A. Check warfarin for size, consistent manufacturer.
   B. Take at same time every day.
   C. Report all new medications to their doctor, avoid aspirin.
   D. Side effects such as easy bruisability may be present.
   E. Any unusual bleeding should be reported.
   F. Need to have regular INR testing.
3. Avoid food high in vitamin K such as organ meats, green tea, green leafy vegetables such as broccoli, brussel sprouts, cauliflower, chickpeas, kale, spinach, and turnip greens.
4. Avoid any contact sports, and prolonged sitting, or standing.
5. Teach how to apply antiembolism stockings and importance of wearing.

Review Questions

3.71 Virchow's triad includes:
   A. Hypercoagulability, vasoconstriction, hypotension
   B. Hypercoagulability, hypervolemia, hypertension
   C. Pain, swelling, fever
   D. Hypercoagulability, stasis, endothelial damage

3.72 A 23-year-old woman presents with complaints of leg swelling ×2 days. She states she awoke with slight pain and heaviness in her left leg. History that would be important to elicit would be:
   A. Medication history including birth control pills
   B. Past history of thrombosis, phlebitis
   C. Recent surgery, trauma
   D. All of the above

3.73 Physical examination and history leads you to suspect deep vein thrombosis. Your next step would be:

A. Contrast venography
B. Duplex ultrasound
C. Lab tests to include PT, PTT, platelet count, CBC
D. Angiogram

3.74 Isolated DVT was diagnosed on this patient. You decide to treat as outpatient. The most important item of patient education is:
A. Importance of taking anticoagulants as prescribed, at same time of day.
B. Diet teaching to avoid foods high in vitamin K
C. To avoid prolonged sitting or standing
D. All of the above.

3.75 A 24-year-old woman is admitted following exploratory surgery for bleeding S/P motor vehicle accident. She has also been diagnosed with a pelvic fracture, and femur fracture of her left leg. You know that trauma and surgery can increase the release of tissue factor, which activates the coagulation cascade. What should be ordered to prophylax against the usual sequelae of this activation?
A. Phytonadione 10 mg SQ qd
B. CBC and platelet count 6 h for 24 hours then 9–12 hours for 24 hours then qd if stable
C. Heparin 500 U SQ q12h
D. 8 U of platelets to be transfused for platelet count <60,000

Answers and Rationales

3.71 **D** Hypercoagulability, stasis, and endothelial damage (also known as Virchow's triad) act either singly or in combination, and create an environment that promotes formation of thombus.

3.72 **D** Pharmaceutical estrogen, such as in birth control pills or hormone replacement therapy (≥50 μg), increases risk of DVT. History of thrombosis associated with higher risk of future thrombus; phlebitis will increase risk due to platelet aggregation from inflammation of vessels. Surgery and trauma cause hypercoagulability due to elicitation of stress response and coagulation cascade.

3.73 **B** Venous duplex assists in the diagnosis of DVT by showing failure of veins to compress under gentle pressure from probe of transducer. This test is noninvasive, inexpensive, and involves minimal to no risk to patient. The gold standard for diagnosis is contrast plethysmography.

3.74 **D** Patients who are managed conservatively as outpatient must receive thorough teaching and follow-up. Taking medication at the same time each day ensures steady state in blood level; ingesting foods that are high in vitamin K will decrease anticoagulation effects decreasing INR; prolonged sitting or standing will increase stasis and provide environment conducive to thrombus formation.

3.75 **C** Surgery and trauma along with venous stasis from bed rest are risk factors for deep vein thrombosis. Prevention of thrombus is always preferred over intervention once thrombus has occurred. Heparin along with TED hose or sequential compression stockings are indicated in high-risk patients as part of deep vein thrombosis prophylaxis.

References

Caswell, D. (1993). Thromboembolic phenomena. *Crit Care Nursing Clin North Am* 5(3), 489–497.

Comerota, A. (1996). Treatment of acute deep vein thrombosis. In A. Callow & C. Ernst (eds.). *Vascular Surgery: Theory and Practice*. Stamford, CT: Appleton & Lange, pp. 1463–1476.

Comerota, A. & Stewart, G. (1995). Current concepts in the etiology of postoperative deep vein thrombosis. In A. Callow & C. Ernst (eds.). *Vascular Surgery: Theory and Practice*. Stamford, CT: Appleton & Lange, pp. 1453–1462.

Adams, J., & Silver, D. Deep venous thrombosis and pulmonary embolism. In R. Dean, J. Yao, & D. Brewster (eds.). *Current Diagnosis and Treatment in Vascular Surgery*. Norwalk, CT: Appleton & Lange, pp. 375–390.

Eftychiou, V. (1996). Clinical diagnosis and management of the patient with deep venous thromboembolism and acute pulmonary embolism. *Nurse Pract* 21(3), 50–61.

Fahey, V. (1988). Venous thromboembolism. In V. Fahey (ed.). *Vascular Nursing*. Philadelphia: W.B. Saunders Co., pp. 341–370.

LaCroix, L., & Leclerc, J. (1996). Prophylaxis of venous thromboembolism. In A. Callow & C. Ernst (eds.). *Vascular Surgery: Theory and Practice*. Stamford, CT: Appleton & Lange, pp. 1477–1490.

Tanaka, D. (1996). Deep venous thrombosis. In R. Rakel (ed.). *Saunders Manual of Medical Practice*. Philadelphia: W.B. Saunders, Co., pp. 283–285.

Arterial Occlusive Disease

DEFINITION

Arterial occlusive disease is a group of diseases that result in occlusion of the branches of the aorta, medium, and small size arteries. Atherosclerotic disease is the most common cause.

ETIOLOGY/INCIDENCE

1. Arterial occlusive disease is most commonly caused by atherosclerosis. Other causes include:
   A. Immune arteritis including periarteritis nodosa; temporal arteritis, Takayasu's arteritis
   B. Thromboangiitis obliterans (Buerger's disease)
   C. Raynaud's disease
   D. Fibromuscular dysplasia
2. Most commonly involves vessels of lower extremities.
3. Incidence is related to age, at age 60, 9% of men and 4% of women have evidence on treadmill testing of arterial occlusive disease.
4. Three independent risk factors are smoking, hypertension, and hypercholesterolemia. Predisposing factors include genetic predisposition, diabetes mellitus, low high-density lipoproteins, male gender, sedentary lifestyle, and stress.
5. Ten percent of patients with arterial occlusive disease have high-grade carotid artery stenosis.

6. Coronary artery disease is commonly found in combination with arterial occlusive disease. Estimated that 20% of patients with arterial occlusive disease have severe, surgically correctable CAD. Cardiovascular disease is the leading cause of death following peripheral vascular procedures.
7. Arterial occlusive disease may be the best marker for patients with renal artery stenosis.
8. Atherosclerosis is more common and occurs earlier in diabetics than in non-diabetic patients. Persons with type II diabetes are at particularly high risk of developing lower extremity arterial occlusive disease. Arterial occlusive disease in diabetics is associated with a much worse prognosis.

PATHOPHYSIOLOGY

1. Exact cause of atherosclerotic disease is not known. It may occur as follows:
   A. Response to repair of arterial wall from ongoing intimal injury causing release of growth factors that induce smooth muscle cell migration and proliferation.
   B. Infiltration of lipids into arterial wall result from high serum lipid levels which results in proliferation of smooth muscle cells and increased deposition of lipids between cells resulting in atherosclerotic plaque formation.
   C. Predominance of lesions at points of vessel origin or branches suggests that hemodynamics plays role in determining location of lesions.
2. Early atherosclerotic lesions appear as fatty streaks composed of cells containing cholesterol. Progression of lesion results in smooth muscle proliferation within the intima. Invasion of the intima by blood-borne monocytes, and lipids which allows connective tissue matrix to continue to accumulate. Result of this process is either occlusion of flow from proliferation and development of occlusive plaque and/or development of ulcerations in lining of artery that can embolize or cause platelet aggregation.

SIGNS AND SYMPTOMS

1. Most common presenting symptom is that of intermittent claudication. Typically described as pain (may be aching, tiredness, numbness, weakness, or cramping) that begins after walking a determined distance; pain is relieved by 1–5 minutes of rest with the extremity in the vertical position. Pain returns after walking same distance after rest. Superficial femoral artery occlusion presents with calf pain while iliac artery occlusion presents with thigh or buttock pain.
2. Coldness of feet is early symptom with numbness or paresthesias developing later in course of disease. Cold feet alone not usually associated with occlusive disease.
3. Symptoms may fluctuate over time due to development of collateral circulation and development of new lesions.
4. Claudication pain may be masked in diabetic patients by coexisting peripheral neuropathy.
5. Rest pain occurs with advanced disease. Usually involves toes of affected extremity. Nocturnal leg cramps not associated with occlusive disease. May have necrotic areas on toes at this stage.
6. Nonhealing ulcer may be presenting symptom. Healing is impaired due to extremity ischemia from decreased blood flow. Ulcer due to arterial insufficiency will be painful, "punched out," gray base, no bleeding (Table 3–39).

TABLE 3–39.   Physical Findings of Ulcers of the Lower Extremities*

	Chronic Venous Insufficiency	Arterial Insufficiency	Trophic Ulcer
Location	Distally, above medial malleolus	Toes, lateral malleolus, pressure points	Pressure points, areas of decreased sensation, demonstrable neuropathy
Skin around ulcer	Pigmented, sometimes fibrotic	Shiny, atrophic skin	Callused, demonstrable neuropathy
Pain	Not severe, relieved with elevation	Severe, relieved by dependency	None, ulcer may go unnoticed
Associated gangrene	Absent	May be present	Usually absent
Bleeding from ulcer	Venous ooze	Little or none	May be brick red
Associated signs	Edema, pigmentation, possible cyanosis if foot is dependent	Decreased pulses, pallor on elevation, dependent rubor	Decreased sensation, absent ankle reflexes

* From Pousti, T.J., Wilson, S.E., & Williams, P.A. (1994). Clinical examination of the vascular patient. In F.J. Veith, et al. (eds.). *Vascular Surgery: Principles and Practice.* New York: McGraw-Hill, with permission.

7. Impotence may be the presenting symptom.
8. If patient presents with symptoms that were of abrupt onset, digit or upper extremity involvement, or in person <40 years of age, etiology other than atherosclerotic disease is suggested. Patients with acute arterial ischemia must be referred for vascular surgical consult immediately.

PHYSICAL FINDINGS

1. Trophic changes present on involved extremity such as alopecia; dry, scaly skin; thick, brittle nails. Atrophy of skin and subcutaneous tissue produces shiny, scaly, skeletonized foot.
2. Diminished or absent pulses in lower extremity. Pulses may be normal in large-vessel disease without complete occlusion and thus may not interfere with blood flow at rest. Absent dorsalis pedis pulse occurs in approximately 10% of population with no evidence of arterial occlusive disease.
3. Careful inspection between toes may reveal unsuspected ischemic ulcers. Ischemic ulcers are present with chronic ischemic arterial occlusive disease and is characteristically on distal portion of foot or over a pressure point. Ulcer is typically painful unless it occurs in diabetic patients.
4. Pallor of arterial insufficiency is evident with elevation of extremity. Lowering legs results in delayed return of color (>10 seconds) with development of dependent rubor after several minutes of dependency in advanced ischemia (Buerger's test).
5. Patients with advanced disease may have very red-appearing toes that refill very rapidly after compression; this may be mistaken for hyperemia but is due to chronic dilation of vascular bed (dependent rubor).
6. Arterial bruits may be heard over femoral artery suggesting lesion capable of producing turbulent flow.
7. Always assess cardiovascular system for other involvement.

DIFFERENTIAL DIAGNOSIS

1. Arthritis
2. Spinal stenosis (produces pseudoclaudication)
3. Herniated lumbar disc
4. Peripheral neuropathy
5. Venous stasis disease

DIAGNOSTIC TESTS/FINDINGS

1. Ankle/brachial index (ABI) noninvasively assesses lower extremity flow by determining ratio of ankle to brachial systolic blood pressure measure by Doppler device (ABI = A/B). Normal value 1.0. Mild claudication occurs at 0.80; moderate to severe claudication at 0.4–0.8; rest pain at <0.4. Arterial wall incompressibility is an important limitation with this study, occurring in 5–10% of diabetic patients.
2. A 20% decrease in ABI after exercise indicates disease and is useful if symptoms suggest arterial occlusive disease and ABI is normal.
3. Plethysmography is useful for patients who have falsely elevated ankle pressures or who have disease confined to distal arterial beds. This measures blood pressure by use of a photoelectric cell with a light-emitting diode that is taped to the end of the digit and a photosensor transduces changes in dermal arterial flow. With inflation of toe cuff followed by slow deflation, plethysmographic waveforms reappear when the systolic toe pressure is reached.
4. Air plethysmography can be used to record segmental limb blood pressure and provide waveform analysis of volume changes with arterial pulse. This technique is an indirect measure of blood flow, and changes in the waveform amplitude provide an index of local tissue perfusion. This provides information regarding the location and severity of peripheral occlusive disease. The precise anatomic location, or high-grade versus total occlusion of an artery, cannot be determined by this method.
5. Duplex scanning should be used to address specific queries concerning disease such as stenosis, occlusion, or aneurysm; to measure vessel diameter or to determine length of vessel occlusion. This technique is useful to evaluate specific diseased arterial segments or assess patency of previous arterial grafts.
6. Angiography is the gold standard for the diagnosis of anatomic disease; this is used when considering an interventional procedure. Angiography should not be used as part of the initial assessment.
7. CBC and coagulation profile should be drawn to assess for hypercoagulable state, polycythemia.
8. BUN and creatinine should be sent to assess renal function.
9. Carotid duplex should be ordered for any patient with carotid bruit, signs of carotid insufficiency, TIAs.
10. Electrocardiogram should be done as baseline and to rule out or determine extent of cardiovascular disease.

MANAGEMENT/TREATMENT

1. *Limb threatening ischemia evidenced by rest pain, ischemic ulcers, or gangrene should be referred immediately to vascular surgeon for surgical intervention.*

2. Patients with smoking history without limb-threatening ischemia should be referred for smoking cessation counseling. Cessation of smoking is of utmost importance in reducing morbidity from arterial occlusive disease.
3. Implementing a regular walking program for 30 min/day is important in development of collateral circulation and to assist in making muscles more efficient is their utilization of energy. Patient should not stop at onset of pain but continue walking until pain becomes severe, rest, and then continue walking. Patients who do not have advanced disease may avoid surgical intervention with regular walking program.
4. Weight loss is encouraged.
5. Control of diabetes, hypertension, hyperlipidemia. Hyperlipidemia may need cholesterol-lowering agent, diet counseling.
6. Pentoxifylline 400 mg tid may improve blood flow in some instances.
7. Aspirin 1 tab od may be given to decrease risk of stroke, myocardial infarction.
8. Foot care should be made a priority.
   A. Feet should be inspected and washed daily with thorough drying between toes.
   B. Apply lanolin-based moisturizer daily,
   C. Keep nails trimmed; if thickened nails, may need podiatrist referral.
   D. Wear comfortable, well-fitting shoes.
   E. Do not walk barefoot.
9. Assist patient in determining point at which quality of life is impaired by arterial occlusive lesion and surgical intervention is option.
10. Vascular surgeon consult may be helpful in determining follow-up program and expected disease progression.

PATIENT EDUCATION

1. Educate patient regarding nature, course, and onset of disease.
2. Reassure patient that claudication pain is not harmful, and that it is not dangerous to continue walking beyond point of pain.
3. Educate patient about reasons to stop smoking. Remind patient of dangers of secondhand smoke.
4. Teach patient risk factor modification such as control of hypertension, hyperlipidemia.
5. Teach patient importance of regular exercise program on outcome of illness.
6. Teach patient foot care as above.
7. Inform patient of danger signs, such as development of rest pain, ulcer, gangrene, sore that will not heal.
8. Teach medication purpose, dosage, frequency, side effects, and signs of toxicity.

Review Questions

3.76 The major risk factors for development of arterial insufficiency include:
   A. Smoking, hypertension, hypercholesterolemia
   B. Smoking, COPD, hypercoagulability
   C. Smoking, deep vein thrombosis, diabetes
   D. Hypertension, age, diet

3.77 A 50-year-old man patient presents with complaints of pain after walking about one block. He states he can then rest a few minutes and walk the same distance again. Denies edema or pain awakening him at night. He has a 50-pack-year smoking history. Physical examination reveals that dorsalis pedis or posterior tibial pulses are not palpable bilaterally. ABIs are 1.0 on the right and 0.98 on the left. Based on this information you would:

A. Order an angiogram with run-off
B. Order exercise ABI
C. Order photoplethysmography
D. Instruct him on a walking program to promote collateral circulation

3.78 A patient with arterial occlusive disease has ABI results of 0.5 on the right and 0.7 on the left. You know that this result indicates:

A. Normal ABI on left, low on right
B. Moderate to severe peripheral vascular disease
C. Severe disease on left associated with rest pain
D. Bilateral, severe arterial insufficiency and surgical consult is necessary

3.79 Esther, a 69-year-old woman patient with a history of type II diabetes mellitus, coronary artery disease, and hypertension presents to clinic with complaints of pain in her right calf that occurs after walking. Physical examination shows absent distal pulses in right lower extremity, 1+ in left, trophic changes are evident bilaterally. She denies rest pain. Vascular laboratory studies reveal ABIs of 0.56 on the right and 0.79 on the left. The most appropriate therapeutic intervention for this patient would be:

A. Femoral popliteal bypass using lesser saphenous vein
B. Trental 400 mg tid
C. Balloon angioplasty
D. A strict program of daily walking.

3.80 An 82-year-old man presents to the emergency department with complaints of severe pain in his left foot. Patient's family states his pain has been present for some time but has become severe in the last few days. While patient is lying on examination table you note that left leg is somewhat pale in appearance; however, the patient is unable to remain supine for long periods of time due to severe pain in his foot that he states is relieved by hanging foot down. You note that foot becomes deep red with dependency. Further examination reveals absent pulses, ischemic ulcer is present on second toe and plantar surface beneath great toe. The appropriate treatment plan for this patient would be:

A. Treatment plan cannot be made until diagnostic studies are completed as you do not know patients degree of disease
B. Trental 400 mg PO tid
C. Strict walking program
D. Stat consult with vascular surgeon

Answers and Rationales

3.76 **A** Smoking, hypertension, and hypercholesterolemia are the three independent risk factors for atherosclerotic arterial occlusive disease.

Other factors such as diabetes, family history, obesity, and stress are all predisposing factors but have not been shown to be independent risk factors.

3.77 **B** In some patients with arterial occlusive disease that produces claudication, ankle, brachial indices may be normal or near normal. In this situation, exercise ABIs are indicated. This is due to the ability of the circulatory system to meet the requirements of regular activity; however, exercise places extra stress on the system and the vessels are not able to supply adequate amounts of oxygen to the exercising muscles, thus producing claudication pain. Exercise ABIs, in this situation, are helpful in diagnosing degree of disease.

3.78 **B** Mild claudication occurs with ABI <0.8, moderate to severe disease between 0.4 and 0.8, and rest pain is typical at ≤0.4.

3.79 **D** Walking a little beyond onset of claudication pain enables the muscles to become more efficient in their extraction and utilization of energy. It may also help build collateral circulation. A strict walking program of at least 30 min/day has been shown to be very effective in preventing progression of disabling arterial occlusive disease.

3.80 **D** This patient has critical ischemia and needs revascularization procedure to prevent limb loss. The surgeon will most likely order an angiogram and depending on the site, type, and number of occlusions will decide upon the appropriate revascularization procedure.

References

Benjamin, M., & Dean, R. (1995). Examination of the patient with vascular disease. In R. Dean, J. Yao, & D. Brewster (eds.). *Current Diagnosis and Treatment in Vascular Surgery.* Norwalk, CT: Appleton & Lange, pp. 1–4.

Esses, G. & Brandyk, D. Noninvasive studies of vascular disease. In R. Dean, J. Yao, & D. Brewster (eds.). *Current Diagnosis and Treatment in Vascular Surgery.* Norwalk, CT: Appleton & Lange, pp. 5–12.

Fahey, V. (1988). *Vascular Nursing.* Philadelphia: W.B. Saunders Co., pp. 286–287.

Goerdt, C. (1996). Peripheral arterial disease. In R.E. Rakel (ed.). *Saunders Manual of Medical Practice.* Philadelphia: W.B. Saunders Co.

Rutherford, R. (1996). The vascular consultation. In R. Rutherford (ed.). *The Surgical Approach to Vascular Problems.* Philadelphia: W.B. Saunders Co., pp. 1–9.

Chronic Venous Insufficiency

DEFINITION

Venous insufficiency is defined as impaired return of blood in the deep venous system due to incompetent valves allowing reflux, leads to varicose veins.

ETIOLOGY/INCIDENCE

1. Risk factors associated with increased risk of varicose vein occurrence include:
    A. Family history of varicose veins, associated with development of disease in 70–80% of first-degree relatives.

    B. Age 50 years or over, peak incidence in sixth decade of life

    C. Female sex especially in early years with female/male ratio 6:1; sixth decade of life ratio decrease to 2:1.

    D. Multiparity (two or more pregnancies)

    E. Oral contraceptive use

    F. Occupation requiring standing >6 hr/day

    G. Obesity

2. Exact incidence of varicose veins hard to define due to variety of definitions used.
3. Most common in Europe and the United States.
4. Estimated 24 million adults in the United States affected by varicose veins.
5. Approximately 50% of population over age 40 have some form of varicosity or telangiectasia.
6. Between 10 and 20% of adults have significant varicose veins.
7. About 2 million people in the United States suffer from some venous ulceration as a result of chronic venous insufficiency.
8. Hidden costs associated with venous insufficiency are estimated to be between $775 million and $1 billion dollars annually.

PATHOPHYSIOLOGY

1. Arterial flow is generated by high pressure via cardiac contraction. Venous flow, however, is relatively low pressure with blood being propelled primarily by external contraction of the muscle pumps of the calf and foot, which continuously push against the force of gravity. Orderly venous flow out of the leg can only occur if the valvular system is competent. Valves prevent reversal of flow in the venous system to protect the lower extremities from the deleterious effects of continuously elevated hydrostatic pressure.
2. Valve dysfunction, due to a number of factors, is the primary cause of varicosities and venous insufficiency. Most cases are a result of deep vein thrombosis which, in most instances, resorbs, leaving scarred, unclosable valve leaflets. Valvular destruction or venous dilation leads to bidirectional venous flow resulting in venous outflow. The venous system is intricately connected; therefore, hypertension is distributed through many outlets, resulting in a cascade of breakdown of valves and loss of one-way flow. The result is development of dilated, tortuous veins, venules. The net effect of this valvular dysfunction is that the weight of the venous blood column from the right atrium is transmitted the full length of the veins so that very high venous pressure is exerted at the ankle level (hydrostatic pressure).

SIGNS AND SYMPTOMS

Severity of symptoms caused by varicose veins not correlated with number and size of varicosities.

1. Dull, aching heaviness exacerbated by periods of standing is most common complaint.
2. Leg cramps, may be worse at night.
3. Complaints of fatigue, heaviness in legs that is alleviated by rest and elevation.
4. Patient may complain of pain associated with walking, described as bursting or tight heavy sensation which does not go away with rest. This venous claudication is a result of increased arterial flow associated with exercise.

Normally, the pressure from arterial flow is matched by venous outflow through the collateral vessels without development of high venous pressures. In venous disease, these collateral channels are not sufficient to handle the severalfold increase in arterial flow generated by exercise. The pain is the result of the tense engorgement of the venous channels in the leg.

5. Edema of affected leg due to increased hydrostatic forces allowing fluid to pool in tissues in dependent areas.

6. Ulcer may be present. Venous stasis ulcers are typically in the gaiter area (lower third of leg to just below medial malleolus), most commonly on the medial malleolus, are larger and shallower with a moist granulating base (see Table 3–39). Venous stasis ulcers are almost always surrounded by stasis dermatitis. Pain may be present if ulcer develops. Pain of venous stasis ulcer is mild and is relieved by elevation of the extremity. Venous ulcers will occur in 67–90% of patients with venous insufficiency. A recurrence rate of 76% has been reported.

PHYSICAL FINDINGS

1. Edema of lower extremities may be present. Edema may be from venous disease, lymphatic disease, cardiac or orthostatic edema, or fat (see Table 3–40).

2. Brown staining of skin in gaiter area begins in the early stages with progressive staining and fibrosis of the tissue. This is due to the breakdown of extravasated red cells with hemosiderin deposition which causes the characteristic pigmentation. This process along with increased fibrin in the interstitial fluid leads to inflammation and fibrosis in the subcutaneous tissues.

3. Skin over affected area becomes hairless and dry due to decreased transport of oxygen and nutrients through obstructed capillary beds to the subcutaneous tissues.

TABLE 3–40.   Differential Diagnosis of Chronic Leg Swelling*

Clinical Feature	Venous	Lymphatic	Cardiac Orthostatic	"Lipedema"
Consistency of swelling	Brawny	Spongy	Pitting	Noncompressible (fat)
Relief by elevation	Complete	Mild	Complete	Minimal
Distribution of swelling	Maximal in ankles and legs, feet spared	Diffuse, greatest distally	Diffuse, greatest distally	Maximal in ankles and legs, feet spared
Associated skin changes	Atrophic and pigmented, subcutaneous fibrosis	Hypertrophied, lichenified skin	Shiny, mild pigmentation, no trophic changes	None
Pain	Heavy ache, tight or bursting	None or heavy ache	Little or none	Dull ache, cutaneous sensitivity
Bilaterality	Occasionally, but usually unequal	Occasionally, but usually unequal	Always, but may be unequal	Always

* From Rutherford, B. (1995). The vascular consultation. In R. Rutherford (ed.). *The Surgical Approach to Vascular Problems.* Philadelphia: W.B. Saunders Co., with permission.

4. Scaly, itchy dermatitis most commonly begins in the early phases. Dermatitis may be made worse by patient's attempts at "treating dry skin" with lotions causing blistering and worsening of dermatitis.
5. Varicosities of varying degrees most likely will be noted.
6. Progressive disease will present with the following:
   A. Stasis dermatitis is due to chronic inflammation in the subcutaneous tissues causing the skin to become atrophic and break down. Dermatitis from venous disease will have a gaiter appearance, sparing the feet. Stasis dermatitis will have a scaly presentation, much like eczema.
   B. Brawny edema will present, giving the leg an inverted champagne bottle appearance. Progression of chronic changes converts skin and subcutaneous tissue of lower leg from a diffusely edematous state to a pigmented, atrophic, tightly scarred zone, which when viewed in contrast to the proximal edema leads to description as champagne bottle leg. This process is restricted to the gaiter area, sparing the foot.
   C. Ulceration occurs in the distal third of the leg, usually above the medial malleolus (see Table 3–39).

DIFFERENTIAL DIAGNOSIS

1. Peripheral neuritis
2. Arterial insufficiency
3. Osteoarthritis
4. Edema due to CHF
5. Lymphedema

DIAGNOSTIC TESTS/FINDINGS

Vascular Laboratory

1. Doppler ultrasound to assess patency and valvular competence in the deep veins. Insufficiency is diagnosed by reversal of flow. Duplex B-mode Doppler allows imaging of superficial and deep vessels.
2. Photoplethysmography allows assessment of degree of venous insufficiency and can separate superficial venous reflux from deep venous valvular insufficiency but does not add anything to Duplex exam combined with physical examination.
3. ABI will quantitate degree of arterial insufficiency and should be done if diagnosis of coexisting arterial disease is suspected.
4. If surgery is to be done, magnetic resonance phlebography and contrast phlebography may be required.

MANAGEMENT/TREATMENT

1. Graded compression stockings to improve venous return by exerting greater pressures at the foot and ankle level than at the calf. Pressure ordered should be 40 mm Hg at the ankle.
2. Patients with severe swelling should be placed on bed rest with legs elevated above the level of the heart.
3. Diuretics may be indicated to assist in fluid removal (i.e., furosemide 20–40 mg PO qd)
4. If ulcer is present, culture may be done if ulcer appears purulent, infected.

5. Unna's boot is used for venous stasis ulcers, changed 3–14 days, depending on exudate. Unna's boot should not be used on infected ulcer. Unna's boot works on moist healing theory, which provides environmental protection while preventing release of wound moisture. This results in enhanced autolytic deAAbridement and greater collagen production than dry wounds and prevents dry crust from forming, which impedes epithelization. A moist wound allows wounds to epithelialize at twice the rate feasible in dry atmosphere.
6. If cellulitis is present:
   A. Treat with antibiotics stable in the presence of β-lactamase (i.e., cefazolin 500 mg bid).
   B. Wet to wet dressing changes to ulcer tid with normal saline.
   C. Wrap leg with elastic bandage.
7. Surgical consult for patients with intractable venous disease when conservative measures have failed.

PATIENT EDUCATION

1. Teach patient nature and course, expected outcome of disease.
2. Instruct patient on proper use of compression stockings including need to apply stocking prior to arising in the morning, proper application, care of stocking.
3. Avoid long periods of standing or sitting with feet in dependent position.
4. Elevate legs while sitting.
5. Wound care for dressing changes if applicable.
6. Follow-up for Unna's boot changes.
7. Medications purpose, dosage, side effects, toxicity if medication is to be prescribed.

Review Questions

3.81 The cause of venous insufficiency is:
   A. Valvular incompetence in the veins of the lower extremities
   B. Atherosclerosis
   C. Deposition of fibrin and hemosiderin on the subcutaneous tissues which breaks down, autolyzing the collagen leaving fibrotic scar tissue in the gaiter area
   D. Varicose veins

3.82 A 72-year-old woman presents with severe swelling of both lower extremities. She denies dyspnea, orthopnea, history of heart disease. Upon examination you find physical signs of venous insufficiency as well as an ulcer on the medial aspect of left leg just above the medial malleolus. Redness and induration, as well as some purulent appearing drainage, are noted around ulceration extending up the leg. The most appropriate treatment plan for this patient is:
   A. Unna's boot application with changes every 3–7 days
   B. Graded compression stockings
   C. Admit to hospital for leg elevation, IV antibiotics, and dressing changes
   D. None of the above

3.83 Antibiotic choice that would be appropriate for this patient include:
  A. Ampicillin 250–500 mg tid
  B. Cephazolin 500 mg bid
  C. Gentamycin 60–80 mg IV q6h
  D. Pentoxifylline 400 mg tid

3.84 Upon discharge, this patient is to be followed by home care nurses for dressing changes. The most important points for patient education include:
  A. Avoid long periods of sitting, standing
  B. Elevate legs above level of heart while lying down
  C. Symptoms that should be reported
  D. All of the above

3.85 A 67-year-old woman is seen in clinic complaining of bursting pain in her left calf associated with walking. States she recently began a walking exercise program to try to prevent further varicose veins from forming. She states that this pain occurs after walking variable distance, takes about an hour to go away, and that she must elevate her legs to obtain relief from the pain. Physical examination reveals 2+ edema of lower extremities, pulses 2+ at posterior tibial bilaterally. Few varicose veins are noted in dependent position but are not evident in recumbent position. Ankle brachial index is 0.96 on right and 1.0 on left. Your treatment plan, based on your diagnosis, includes which of the following?
  A. Angiogram of lower extremities to determine runoff, refer to vascular surgeon for possible lower extremity revascularization procedure
  B. Continue to walk past occurrence of pain to assist in enhancing muscle efficiency
  C. Graded compression stockings with 40 mm Hg pressure at ankle, elevate legs while sitting
  D. Unna's boot with changes every 7 days until pain goes away

---

Answers and Rationales

3.81 **A** Valves in the venous system act to prevent reversal of flow, thereby protecting the venous system from increased pressure. Scarred, incompetent valves allow bidirectional, inefficient venous outflow. The net effect of this is that the weight of the venous blood column from the right atrium is transmitted the full length of the venous system, dramatically increasing the hydrostatic pressure in the ankles and lower legs.

3.82 **C** Venous ulcers will only heal if edema is alleviated; therefore, leg elevation is essential to the healing process. Physical examination points to cellulitis with probable infection in the ulcer. Admitting the patient to ensure leg elevation, and for intravenous antibiotics, is definitely indicated in this situation. Moist dressing changes rather than Unna's boot is indicated for wound care.

3.83 **B** A broad-spectrum antibiotic stable in the presence of β-lactamase is always the treatment of choice in skin infections until culture results are returned.

3.84   **D** Patient education for venous insufficiency is an essential part of treatment and prevention. Most of the preventative and treatment measures for alleviating the symptoms of venous insufficiency rely on the patient recognizing the problem and how to treat, as well as how to avoid them.

3.85   **C** Based on the patient's history and physical examination this patient has venous insufficiency. The pain she describes does not have the typical claudication pattern associated with arterial insufficiency but does fit the pattern of venous claudication. The evidence of swelling, varicose veins, palpable pulses, and relatively normal ABIs also points to venous insufficiency as the etiology of her discomfort. If unsure about coexisting arterial occlusive disease, exercise ABIs may be indicated. However, based on the evidence presented, graded compression stockings and leg elevation is the treatment of choice.

References

Barr, D. (1996). The Unna's Boot as a Treatment for Venous Ulcers. *Nurse Pract 21*, 55–77.

Beaglehole, R. (1986). Incidence and risk factors: Epidemiology of varicose veins. *World J Surg 10*, 898.

dePalma, R., Bergan, J. (1996). Chronic venous insufficiency. In R. Dean, J. Yao, & D. Brewster (eds.). *Current Diagnosis and Treatment in Vascular Surgery.* Norwalk, CT: Appleton & Lange, pp. 365–374..

Fahey, V. (1988). Venous thromboembolism. In V. Fahey (ed.). *Vascular Nursing.* Philadelphia: W.B. Saunders Co., pp. 341–370.

Korstanjo, M. (1995). Venous stasis ulcers. *Dermatol Surg, 21*, 635–640.

Marston, W., & Johnson, G. (1996). Varicose veins and superficial thrombophlebitis. In R. Dean, J. Yao, & D. Brewster (eds.). *Current Diagnosis and Treatment in Vascular Surgery.* Norwalk, CT: Appleton & Lange, pp. 351–364.

Nehler, M., Moneta, G., Kim, Y., & Porter, J. (1995). Nonoperative therapy for patients with chronic venous insufficiency. In A. Callow & C. Ernst (eds.). *Vascular Surgery: Theory and Practice.* Stamford, CT: Appleton & Lange, pp. 1533–1546.

Nicolaides, A. (1995). Hemodynamic evaluation of chronic venous insufficiency. In A. Callow & C. Ernst (eds.). *Vascular Surgery: Theory and Practice.* Stamford, CT: Appleton & Lange, pp. 1515–1526.

Rutherford, B. (1995). The vascular consultation. In R. Rutherford (ed.). *The Surgical Approach to Vascular Problems.* Philadelphia: W.B. Saunders Co., pp. 1–9.

Trachtenbarg, D. (1996). Stasis ulcer. In R. Rakel (ed.). *Saunders Manual of Medical Practice.* Philadelphia: W.B. Saunders, Co., pp. 987–988

van Bemmelen, P. (1995). Venous duplex evaluation of chronic venous insufficiency. In A. Callow & C. Ernst (eds.). *Vascular Surgery: Theory and Practice.* Stamford, CT: Appleton & Lange, pp. 1527–1532.

CHAPTER 4

Neurologic Disorders

Megan M. Keiser, RN, MS, CS, ANP-C, CNRN

Headaches

DEFINITION

The most common neurologic complaint is headache, with a wide variety of neurologic as well as nonneurologic etiologies. Simply defined, a headache is the subjective sensation of pain involving the scalp, cranium, or cerebrum with or without associated symptoms. Three types of headache syndromes will be discussed here: tension headache, migraine headache, and cluster headache.

ETIOLOGY/INCIDENCE

Recent studies indicate that 93% of the population across various cultures have suffered from headache over the last 12 months. Approximately 42 million patients visit their primary care physician annually for headache. The majority of common headaches are benign. In more complicated patients who do not respond to traditional conservative therapy, referral to a physician specializing in headache management is necessary. Of these patients, only 10% of headaches were found to be caused by an organic disorder, while 90% were due to other causes including vascular, tension, and idiopathic.

Migraine headaches are the most common type of vascular headache and occur in about 6% of men and 18% of women. These statistics may be artificially low, as less than 5% of migraine sufferers consult health care providers. Migraines most often occur in the third decade of life and in lower socioeconomic groups. Migraine has also been associated with increased prevalence of depression and anxiety disorders (i.e., panic attacks). Cluster headaches are most common in adolescent and adult males (four times more than women).

PATHOPHYSIOLOGY

Although theories do exist, much is not yet understood about the pathophysiology of pain due to its subjective nature. In general, the perception of pain is thought to depend on many interacting elements of the nervous system including the somatosensory system and neurotransmitters. A painful stimulus is received and awareness of pain occurs at the thalamus. Pain-producing substances such as bradykinin, histamine, serotonin, and acetylcholine are released at the synapses closest to the stimulus. Substance P (an excitatory neu-ropeptide) is then released by nociceptors, which are free nerve endings that are located under the epidermis and deep within the tissue and respond to direct mechanical, thermal, and chemical stimuli. Substance P promotes the transmission of pain impulses. The release of endogenous opioid peptides (en-kephalins, β-endorphins, and dynorphin) from the amygdala, hypothalamus, midbrain, medulla, and dorsal horns results in analgesia. When the amount of endogenous pain-producing substances exceeds the amount of endogenous analgesia, a painful sensation results.

Depending on its classification, headache pain is suspected to be caused by the interplay between muscles, nerves, and vascular structures, which stim-ulates the release of pain-producing substances. Although headache pain is almost always self-limiting, exogenous analgesia is often utilized to reduce or eliminate symptoms.

HISTORY

The most important part of assessing a patient with a headache in the acute care setting is obtaining a detailed and accurate history from the patient and, when necessary, the significant others. This history must include the following information:

1. Specific information about their headache:
   A. Intensity on 0–10 scale
   B. Onset and duration
   C. Frequency
   D. Exact location
   E. Quality (throbbing, dull, constant, etc.)
   F. Does anything make it worse or better?
   G. Precipitators
   H. Associated symptoms (photophobia, diplopia, nausea, tinnitis, dizzi-ness, etc.)
   I. Aura
   J. Is this the worst headache of your life?
   K. Are you able to continue your normal activities?
2. Family history of headaches or migraines
3. Medical history: Recent head or neck trauma, lumbar puncture, illness (sinusitis, flu, infection), birth injury, nervous system disorders, visual problems, dental problems
4. Social history: Recent inebriation, substance abuse (alcohol, tobacco, drugs)
5. Environmental exposures: Carbon monoxide, lead, high altitudes, extreme cold
6. Occupation: Video display terminal (computer), excess reading, excess noise, bright light, number hours worked, off shifts, co-workers complain of headaches
7. Medications: Cimetidine, vasodilators, oral contraceptives, recently discon-tinued analgesic, any allergies
8. Diet: Caffeine, chocolate, MSG, recent ingestion of mushrooms, food aller-gies
9. Sleep habits

10. Psychological: Recent and long-term stressors, mechanisms to handle stressful situations

Tension Headache

Most patients who present with tension headache describe their pain as dull, constant pressure that is bilateral and diffuse in frontal and occipital regions. The pain has an episodic, gradual onset (no aura), and variable duration. They usually have a history of some benign causative factor such as stress, noise, or exhaustion.

Migraine Headache

Patients who present with migraine will usually have a positive family history as well as a personal history of headaches that may date back to childhood. Patients also commonly report diet choices that precipitate attacks (caffeine, chocolate, wine, cheese), and an episodic, recurrent pattern to attacks usually preceded by 30–40 minutes of prodrome (aura) that may consist of visual disturbances, dizziness, etc. They describe their pain as severe with a peak 1 hour after onset. The pain begins unilaterally but becomes more diffuse with a duration of 4–6 hours. The attacks can occur at any time of day (most often in the morning) but do not awaken the patient. They may have associated symptoms that include one or more of the following: Photophobia, nausea, vomiting, diarrhea, constipation, chills, tremor, diaphoresis, fatigue, and nasal congestion.

Cluster Headache

Patients who present with cluster headaches often have no family history of headache or migraine. Episodes of severe unilateral periorbital pain occur daily for several weeks, usually occurring at night awakening the patient and lasting <2 hours. The pain is often accompanied by one or more of the following: Ipsilateral nasal congestion, rhinorrhea, lacrimation, redness of the eye, and Horner's syndrome (a unilateral, small pupil that reacts to light and demonstrates accommodation; ptosis of the eyelid). Remission occurs for weeks or months before another bout of closely spaced attacks occurs.

PHYSICAL FINDINGS

Most often, a patient who presents with a chief complaint of headache (labeled as tension, migraine, or cluster) will have a completely normal physical exam as detailed below.

1. General appearance: Anxious, may show discomfort.
2. Vital signs: Usually within normal range.
3. Skin: Pallor, diaphoresis with severe headache.
4. Head: Ears, nose, throat normal.
5. Eyes: Normal funduscopic exam, patient may be photophobic.
6. Neurologic: Normal—any focal abnormality requires referral to or consultation with a physician.

TABLE 4-1. Serious Signs and Symptoms in the Patient with Headache Indicate Need for Urgent/Emergent Consultation and Work-Up

The patient complains of the "worst headache of my life"
New-onset headache in patient over 45 years of age
Changing or worsening headache
Abnormal neurologic exam:
    Motor, sensory, reflex, or gait disturbance
    Cranial nerve deficit
    Altered level of consciousness
    Progressive vision or speech disturbance
    Meningismus: Neck pain, nuchal rigidity
    Papilledema
Abnormal vital signs: Fever >101.5°F, malignant hypertension
Tenderness or pulsation of temporal arteries

Nevertheless, the practitioner must also have knowledge of what signs may indicate a more severe condition (see Table 4-1).

DIFFERENTIAL DIAGNOSES

1. New-onset headache
   A. Ocular disorders (acute angle closure glaucoma): Narrow anterior chamber, decreased visual acuity, dilated pupils, eye pain, ocular hypertension
   B. Infectious causes (sinusitis, meningitis, encephalitis, dental caries/abscess, otitis, temporal arteritis): To differentiate the source of the infection, assess for fever, nuchal rigidity, positive Kernig's sign, Brudzinsky's sign, petechiae with meningococcemia, tooth pain, sinus tenderness
   C. CNS mass lesion (hemorrhage, abscess, tumor): Altered mental status, papilledema, any focal neurologic deficits
   D. Minor head trauma (postconcussive syndrome, skull fracture, cerebral contusion): History is diagnostic, no further signs are present unless central nervous system (CNS) mass lesion has been produced (see above); patient may complain of decreased memory, attention span, and ability to concentrate
   E. Metabolic causes (hyponatremia, uremia, hypoglycemia, carbon monoxide poisoning, hypercapnia as with chronic obstructive pulmonary disease (COPD) and sleep apnea): Often have confusing presentation and are diagnosed only through laboratory data
   F. Benign causes: "Hangover" reaction, caffeine withdrawal, eyestrain
   G. Subarachnoid hemorrhage: One of the most common reasons for a patient with the chief complaint of headache to be admitted to the hospital (see Table 4-2).
2. Recurrent Headache
   A. Cervical spondylosis: Associated neck pain, radicular symptoms
   B. Pseudotumor cerebri: Typical patient is overweight female with a history of oral contraceptive use; most common associated symptom is papilledema
   C. Tic douloureux: Associated facial pain in the distribution of the affected branch of the trigeminal nerve (cranial nerve [CN] V) with trigger points precipitated by chewing, talking, brushing teeth, or drinking cold liquid
   D. CNS mass lesion: Same as above

TABLE 4-2. Summary of Subarachnoid Hemorrhage

Etiology	Craniocerebral trauma Cerebral aneurysm rupture Cerebral arteriovenous malformation Clotting abnormalities
Signs and Symptoms	"Worst headache of my life" with sudden onset, no precipitating factors, no relief with OTC analgesia. Altered consciousness Mental status changes Stiff neck Nausea and vomiting Photophobia Seizures Cranial nerve abnormalities Motor or sensory deficits
Diagnosis	If you suspect an SAH, the first test to obtain is a CT scan of the brain; If negative, a lumbar puncture must be obtained to look for the presence of blood. Routine serum blood work includes CBC, BUN, creatinine, glucose, electrolytes, PT, aPTT. Upon diagnosis of SAH and in the absence of cranial trauma, a cerebral angiogram is required to ascertain the source of the bleeding.

Treatment	The goals of treatment are to prevent rebleed and prevent secondary complications (most commonly hydrocephalus and cerebral vasospasm).
	"Triple H therapy" to prevent vasospasm:
	  Hypertension to SBP = 150
	  Hemodilution to hematocrit 31–33
	  Hypervolemia which aids in maintaining blood pressure and hematocrit in desired ranges
	Routine medications include:
	  Colace 100 mg PO bid
	  Codeine 30–60 mg SQ q4h prn
	  Nimodipine (Nimotop) 60 mg PO q4h × 21 days
	  Phenobarbital 30–60 mg PO/SQ q6h prn sedation
	  Dilantin 100 mg PO tid (although the use of anticonvulsants as seizure prophylaxis is controversial)
	SAH precautions include:
	  Dimly lit, quiet, private room
	  No stress, limited visitors
	  Complete bed rest
	  Avoid Valsalva maneuver—straining to have bowel movement, coughing, etc.

OTC, over-the-counter; SAH, subarachnoid hemorrhage; CT, computed tomography; CBC, complete blood count; BUN, blood urea nitrogen; PT, prothrombin time; PTT, partial thromboplastin time; SBP, systolic blood pressure.

DIAGNOSTIC TESTS/FINDINGS

1. Thorough history and physical exam are paramount in determining the nature of the headache as well as any potentially life-threatening etiologies. In most cases, this is sufficient and no further work-up is necessary.
2. Blood tests are indicated when patients do not respond to traditional therapy or their history and physical indicate a more complex process; these may include electrolytes, thyroid panel, complete blood count (CBC), urinalysis, serology, arterial blood gases (ABG) if hypoxia or hypercarbia are suspected

3. Radiologic exam is necessary under rare circumstances, which include an unclear clinical picture following history, physical, and laboratory studies or if the patient has any focal neurologic deficit. A computed tomography (CT) scan or magnetic resonance imaging (MRI) scan may be utilized with the MRI being the test of choice for a suspected mass lesion. Skull films may be ordered in the case of mild head trauma or the palpation of a suspected fracture. Angiography is indicated only if the CT scan shows sub-

---

TABLE 4-3.   Management of Common Headache Syndromes*

Headache Syndrome	Pharmacologic Management	Nonpharmacologic Management
Tension	Acetaminophen Aspirin NSAIDs	Supportive care to monitor stress levels and coping mechanisms. Lifestyle modification (i.e., weight loss, cessation of substance abuse, nutritional diet) has shown to decrease episodes in frequent headache sufferers. Follow-up in 2 weeks to monitor progress. Consultation with a physician if conservative treatment fails or clinical depression is suspected.
Migraine	*Acute attack* (must be taken at onset of symptoms or aura to be effective) Sumatriptan (Imitrex) 6 mg SQ, may repeat in 1 hour prn—no more than two doses/day Cafergot (ergotomine maleate 1 mg + caffeine 100 mg) 1–2 tablets, may repeat 1 tablet q30min up to 6 tablets (if attack includes nausea/vomiting Cafergot suppositories, ergotomine tartrate inhalers [0.36 mg per puff], and ergotomine SL 2-mg tablets are available) Dihydroergotamine mesylate (DHE 45) 0.5–1 mg IV or 1–2 mg SQ/IM, repeat q1h prn to max of 3 mg Midrin (a combination drug containing isometheptene mucate 65 mg, dichloralphenazone 100 mg, acetaminophen 325 mg) 2 tabs PO, may repeat q1h until relief, max of 5 tabs/day *Prophylaxis* (should be considered if patients have attacks more than two or three times per month) Aspirin 650–1950 mg/day Propranolol (Inderol) 80–240 mg/day Imipramine (Tofranil) 10–150 mg/day Ergonovine maleate 0.6–2 mg/day Cyproheptadine (Periactin) 12–20 mg/day Clonidine (Catapres) 0.2–0.6 mg/day Methysergide (Sansert) 4–8 mg/day Verapamil (Calan) 80–160 mg/day	Diet counseling—see table on food to avoid. Lifestyle modification (i.e., weight loss, smoking cessation, nutritional diet) has shown to decrease episodes in frequent migraine sufferers. During attacks, patient should stay in a dark, quiet environment and rest. Warm baths may help patient to relax. Follow-up at regular intervals to assess effectiveness of treatment (initially q2wk × 2 months, then every month for 6 months, and prn if treatment successful). Consultation with physician if patient does not respond to traditional management or condition worsens.

Table continues

TABLE **4-3.** (*Continued*)

Headache Syndrome	Pharmacologic Management	Nonpharmacologic Management
Cluster	*Acute attack* Sumatriptan (Imitrex) 6 mg SQ (see above) Dihydroergotamine mesylate (DHE 45) 1–2 mg SQ/IM (see above) Ergotamine tartrate aerosol (0.36 mg/puff)—up to 6 puffs/attack 100% oxygen inhalation (7 L/min for 15 minutes) Butorphanol tartrate nasal spray (Stadol NS) 10 mg/mL—one spray in one nostril, repeat q3–4h *Prophylaxis* Ergotomine tartrate Suppository 0.5–1 mg qhs or bid Orally 2 mg/day Subcutaneous 0.25 mg tid 5 days a week Propranolol (Inderal) 80–240 mg/day Amitriptyline (Elavil) 10–150 mg/day Cyproheptadine (Periactin) 12–20 mg/day Methysergide (Sansert) 4–6 mg/day Verapamil (Calan) 240–480 mg/day Lithium carbonate (Eskalith) 150–600 mg/day Prednisone 20–40 mg qd–qod × 2 weeks followed by gradual withdrawal	Lifestyle modification and supportive care are of limited benefit for these patients, as there are few known precipitating factors for a bout of attacks. During a bout, some patients report that alcohol, stress, glare, or ingestion of certain foods will precipitate an attack but this is highly individual—patients are certainly advised to avoid anything that they feel worsens their condition. Follow-up at regular intervals during treatment; spacing of visits will vary depending on the patient's pattern of remissions and bouts.

* In the management of all headaches, narcotic or addictive medications should be avoided, as these patients have a tendency to overmedicate due to the duration of symptoms.
NSAIDs, nonsteroidal anti-inflammatory drugs.

arachnoid hemorrhage and/or the MRI is suspicious for an aneurysm or arteriovenous malformation (AVM).

4. Electroencephalography (EEG) may be performed if the patient has a history suspicious for seizures. A position emission tomogram (PET) or single-photon emission computed tomography (SPECT) scan may follow an abnormal EEG to determine the etiology of the seizures.

5. For the patient who presents with the clinical picture of migraine, administration of ergotamine during an attack with relief of pain may be considered diagnostic in the presence of a normal physical exam.

MANAGEMENT/TREATMENT

Variable depending on type of headache syndrome (see Table 4–3).

PATIENT EDUCATION

1. Medication: Purpose, dose, side effects, and toxicity. Stress difference in treatment of acute attacks versus prophylaxis for patients with migraine and cluster headaches. May need to educate in technique for suppository insertion, use of inhalers, and subcutaneous injection if necessary.

2. Environment: Should be restful and relaxing during and between attacks. Teach methods to moderate and cope with stressful situations.

3. Diet: Stress importance of balanced diet for all patients. Migraine patients must avoid all trigger foods (see Table 4–4). Cluster headache patients must avoid any food that precipitates an attack during a bout.

TABLE 4-4.   Dietary Restrictions for Patients with Migraines

Must Avoid	Should Avoid
1. Foods containing nitrites, nitrates, amines, tyramine, and monosodium glutamate	Although less common, many fruits and vegetables have also been implicated:
2. Pickled, preserved, and marinated foods	1. Apples
3. Processed or salted meat and fish	2. Apricots
4. Strong and aged cheese	3. Avocados
5. Chocolate	4. Beans high in starch (e.g., lima, pole, pinto, garbanzo, navy, Italian)
6. Nuts and seeds	5. Carob
7. Fresh baked products with yeast	6. Cherries
8. High-sodium soup or sauce (e.g., bouillon, soy sauce, canned soup)	7. Figs
9. Alcohol (especially red wine and beer)	8. Lentils
10. Coffee, tea, cola with caffeine	9. Olives
	10. Onions
	11. Papaya
	12. Passion fruit
	13. Peaches
	14. Pears
	15. Raisins
	16. Snow peas and pea pods
	17. Red plums
	18. Sauerkraut

4. Instruct patient to keep a diary that includes date, time, and duration of attack; precipitating factors (stress, recent food ingestion, etc.); self-treatment and effectiveness. Instruct the patient to bring diary to all follow-up visits.
5. Disease course and expected outcome: There is no known cure for tension, migraine, or cluster headache syndromes. All can be treated and controlled in most cases. Patterns of attacks vary with each patient.
6. Prevention: Centers around environment in all cases and can include the use of medication in migraine and cluster headache syndromes. Avoidance of precipitating factors is also necessary as is diet modification for all migraine patients and some patients with cluster headaches.

Review Questions

4.1 A 25-year-old black male comes into the emergency room (ER) complaining of a headache and blurred vision for 2 hours. Upon obtaining a recent history, the patient states that he was hit in the head with a "fly ball" at a baseball game earlier that evening. He reports that he was unconscious for 30 seconds and then confused for several minutes. He denies any further symptoms and his neurologic exam is normal. What is the first diagnostic test to perform on this patient?
   A. Serum alcohol level
   B. Skull x-ray
   C. CT scan of the brain
   D. EEG

4.2 The following is/are the most important piece(s) of history needed to differentiate tension headaches from migraine headaches:

A. Intensity of pain
B. Quality of pain
C. Pattern of attacks (onset, location, and duration of pain; recurrence)
D. Family history

4.3 Which of the following is the current drug of choice for an acute migraine headache?
A. Cafergot (ergotamine tartrate + caffeine)
B. Amitriptyline (Elavil)
C. Propranolol (Inderol)
D. Acetaminophen (Tylenol)

4.4 A 17-year-old white male presents to clinic with episodes of severe left periorbital pain that awaken him every night and last approximately 2 hours. He denies a history of this problem in himself or any member of his family. On exam, he has marked erythema of the left eye with excessive tearing and postnasal drip. His neurologic exam is normal. The most likely diagnosis for this patient is:
A. Migraine headaches
B. Cluster headaches
C. Recurrent tension headaches
D. Conjunctivitis

4.5 For the above patient, what would your treatment plan consist of?
A. Lifestyle modification (diet, exercise, stress reduction)
B. Sumatriptan 6 mg SQ at onset of attack; education on the subcutaneous route of medication administration
C. Ophthalmologic exam to rule out ocular pathology
D. Both B and C

Answers and Rationales

4.1 **C** Brain CT scan must be performed as soon as possible to rule out a cerebral hemorrhage. Blurred vision is considered a focal sign and when coupled with loss of consciousness may indicate a more severe brain injury. Skull films are not necessary, as bones can be visualized on CT scan. Blood work and EEG may be done later if indicated.

4.2 **C** Intensity and quality of pain are purely subjective and difficult to assess, although they are important. The pattern of the attack (onset, duration, location of pain, recurrence) is what characterizes headache syndromes. Family history is generally only positive in migraine sufferers.

4.3 **A** Cafergot is the current drug of choice for migraine headache patients and can also be given as plain ergotamine tartrate as a suppository or inhalation for patients with associated nausea, making it versatile for most patients. Propranolol and amitriptyline may be used prophylactically as necessary.

4.4 **B** The location, quality, timing, duration of attacks, and associated signs as well as the patient's age and gender strongly suggest cluster headaches.

4.5 **D** Since this is the patient's first bout, an ophthalmologic exam should be performed to rule out ocular pathology, but need not supersede treatment with sumatriptan. Obviously, the patient would require education on subcutaneous injection technique.

References

Adams, R.D., & Victor, M. (1993). *Principles of Neurology* (5th ed.). New York: McGraw-Hill.

Aminoff, M.J. (1996). Nervous System. In L.M. Tierney, S.J. McPhee, & M.A. Papadakis (eds.). *Current Medical Diagnosis and Treatment.* Stamford, CT: Appleton & Lange.

Hackett, G. (1994). Management of migraine. *Practitioner 238*(2), 130–136.

Hickey, J.V. (1997). Headaches. In J.V. Hickey (ed.). *The Clinical Practice of Neurological and Neurosurgical Nursing* (4th ed.). Philadelphia: Lippincott-Raven.

Marks, D.R., & Rapoport, A.M. (1992). Cluster headache syndrome: Ways to abort or ward off attacks. *Postgrad Med 91*(3), 96–104.

Marshall, S.B., Marshall, L.F., Vos, H.R., & Chesnut, R.M. (1990). *Neuroscience Critical Care: Pathophysiology and Management.* Philadelphia: W.B. Saunders Co.

Perkins, A.T., & Ondo, W. (1995). When to worry about a headache: Head pain as a clue to intracranial disease. *Postgrad Med 98*(2), 197–208.

Reddy, M.J. (1996). Headache. In R.E. Rakel (ed.). *Saunders Manual of Medical Practice.* Philadelphia: W.B. Saunders Co.

Robbins, L.D. (1994). *Management of Headache and Headache Medications.* New York: Springer-Verlag.

Springhouse Corporation. (1996). *Nurse Practitioner's Drug Handbook.* Philadelphia: Springhouse Corporation.

Stevens, M.B. (1996). Migraine headache. In R.E. Rakel (ed.). *Saunders Manual of Medical Practice.* Philadelphia: W.B. Saunders Co.

Trachtenbarg, D.E. (1994). Tension headaches: Relieving pain without creating dependence. *Postgrad Med 95*(6), 44–56.

Weiss, J. (1993). Assessment and management of the client with headaches. *Nurse Pract 18*(4), 44–57.

Seizure Disorders (Epilepsy)

DEFINITION

A seizure is defined by Callahan (1994) as "an abnormal paroxysmal electrical discharge in the cerebral cortex." Epilepsy is defined as recurrent seizures. It is not a disease but a symptom of a central nervous system disorder.

The types of seizure disorders have been classified according to the International Classification of Epileptic Seizures below:
1. Partial seizures (seizures with focal onset)
   A. Simple partial (no impairment of consciousness)
      1)With motor signs
      2)With somatosensory or special-sensory symptoms
      3)With autonomic symptoms or signs
      4)With disturbance of higher cerebral functions
   B. Complex partial (consciousness impaired)
      1)With automatisms
      2)Without automatisms
   C. Partial seizures with secondary generalization

2. Primary generalized seizures
   A. Generalized tonic-clonic
   B. Absence/atypical absence
   C. Myoclonic
   D. Atonic
   E. Clonic
3. Unclassified epileptic seizures

ETIOLOGY/INCIDENCE

Idiopathic epilepsy (no identifiable etiology) is the diagnosis in 40-70% of patients with seizures. However, seizures can also be caused by a wide variety of potentially reversible systemic or central nervous system disorders including:
1. Systemic
   A. Drug or alcohol use/abuse/withdrawal
   B. Metabolic disorders (hypocalcemia, hypoglycemia, pyridoxine deficiency, phenylketonuria (PKU) in newborns and infants, renal failure, diabetes, hyponatremia, endocrine disorders caused by pregnancy and menstruation)
2. Cerebral
   A. Birth injury
   B. CNS infection: meningitis, encephalitis, abscess
   C. Sobarachnoid hemorrhage (SAH), cerebrovascular accident (CVA), AVM, cerebral vasospasm
   D. Cerebral trauma with or without hemorrhage
   E. Brain tumors
3. Posttraumatic (following mechanical trauma or cerebral infection)
   A. Usually occur 6–24 months after trauma
   B. May follow mild or severe trauma
   C. Considered a symptom of postconcussive syndrome

In the United States, the risk of a person experiencing at least one seizure in their life is 4% by age 20 and jumps to almost 10% by age 80. The risk of developing epilepsy by age 80 is 3.5%. The incidence of a first unprovoked seizure is approximately 59 per 100,000 persons per year and the incidence of epilepsy is 42 per 100,000 persons. These rates do not exclude febrile seizures, which occur at an incidence of 100 per 100,000 infants in the first 12 months of life and drive up the overall incidence.

Primary idiopathic epilepsy most commonly begins between ages 2 and 5. There is no age that correlates with secondary seizures except that risk and incidence increases with age.

The proportion of incidence by seizure type is reported by So (1995) as 35% complex partial, 23% generalized tonic-clonic, 14% simple partial, 8% other generalized, 7% partial unknown, 6% absence, 3% myoclonic, and 3% unclassified.

PATHOPHYSIOLOGY

The exact pathophysiology of seizures is unknown, but several theories exist. Idiopathic epilepsy is thought to result from an unknown biochemical imbalance possibly involving an excess of excitatory and/or a deficiency of inhibitory neurotransmitters. Secondary seizures due to cerebral and posttraumatic etiologies are thought to be due to the irritative effect that blood, infectious by-products, and toxins have on brain tissue. Space-occupying lesions may stimulate seizures by causing local tissue irritation usually resulting in a focal seizure pattern.

HISTORY

An accurate history of symptoms as well as a complete description of the alleged seizure (usually from a witness and not the patient) is critical in labeling or ruling out a seizure disorder. Do not use the term "seizure" when interviewing the patient/witness. Instead use terms such as "episode" or "event." The following information must be elicited.

1. History of:
   A. Birth injury
   B. Febrile or childhood seizures
   C. Cerebral trauma or lesion
   D. Immediate family member with epilepsy
   E. Drug or alcohol use/abuse
   F. Metabolic disorders (PKU, diabetes mellitus [DM], other endocrine)
   G. Psychiatric illness
2. Description of event (patient and witness)
   A. Any aura? (visual, auditory, olfactory, verbal, sensory)
   B. Any precipitating event? What was the patient doing when the episode occurred? (playing video games, using computer, watching TV, listening to loud music, smelling a particular odor)
   C. When do they usually take place? (during sleep, times of stress, menstruation, fatigue)
   D. Signs and symptoms at onset?
   E. Progression of signs and symptoms?
   F. Duration of episode?
   G. If consciousness impaired, how long until fully conscious?
3. Medication History
   A. Aminophylline, theophylline, lidocaine: Toxic levels can cause generalized seizures.
   B. Meperidine, penicillin, cimetidine: Excessive doses can cause generalized seizures.
   C. Contrast agents used for radiology procedures may cause generalized seizures as a manifestation of allergy.
   D. Phenothiazines, tricyclic antidepressants, alprostadil, amphetamines: Can trigger seizures in patients with pre-existing epilepsy.
   E. Isoniazide, vincristine may lower seizure threshold.
4. How do these episodes affect activities of daily living?

The actual signs and symptoms of seizures differ based on the seizure classification. However, the symptoms may vary between individuals although they have seizures within the same classification.

1. Generalized tonic-clonic: Preceded by aura; a cry or scream usually follows with subsequent loss of consciousness; tonic-clonic muscle contractions ensue accompanied by cyanosis, dyspnea/apnea, tongue biting, frothing, incontinence; a variable period of stupor or sleep follows the clinical seizure. Most are idiopathic.

2. Absence: Sudden, brief arrest of consciousness with loss of awareness and motor activity; usually last only 2–10 seconds; often go unnoticed by patient and witnesses; can occur several times a day. Most are idiopathic.

3. Atonic: Otherwise known as a drop attack because the patient simply goes completely limp and falls to the ground without warning or loss of consciousness; most common in patients with congenital birth defects or birth injury leading to mental retardation.

4. Simple partial: Usually consists of a clonic spasm or tremor in one extremity; may spread to adjacent areas (jacksonian march); usually localized but can progress to generalized seizure. Most common seizure type that occurs in response to a cerebral lesion.

5. Complex partial: Impaired consciousness, automatisms, hallucinations (visual, auditory, olfactory), bizarre behavior are typical; may last seconds to a few minutes and are not recalled by patient; rarely progress to generalized seizure. Often caused by a benign lesion (area of infarct or hypometabolism) in the temporal lobe.

PHYSICAL FINDINGS

The findings of the physical exam for patients with idiopathic seizures are usually normal. The presence of focal signs on neurologic exam is cause for concern and further diagnostic exams must be performed.

1. General appearance: Anxious.
2. Vital signs: Normal between episodes.
3. Skin: Bruises can be a sign of a convulsion or drop attack.
4. Head, eyes, ears, nose, and throat (HEENT): Head trauma common with drop attacks; tongue biting common with generalized seizure.
5. Neurologic: Usually normal between episodes.

DIFFERENTIAL DIAGNOSIS

The possible causes for seizures must be included as differential diagnoses (see list under "Etiology"). There are also differential diagnoses that should be considered after cerebral and systemic disorders have been ruled out prior to making the diagnosis of idiopathic epilepsy.

1. Cardiac syncope secondary to dysrhythmia, valvular heart disease, vasovagal attack, orthostatic hypotension.
2. Sleep disorders: Narcolepsy, cataplexy, night terrors, somnambulism.
3. Psychiatric disorders: Panic or rage attacks, psychogenic seizures.
4. Conditions that can cause sudden behavior change: Transient ischemic attacks (TIAs), migraine, breath-holding in children.

DIAGNOSTIC TESTS/FINDINGS

1. Thorough history and physical.
2. Blood tests: CBC, electrolytes, calcium, magnesium, phosphorus, serum glucose, renal and liver functions, urinalysis, drug screen, alcohol level, anticonvulsant levels (particularly important for emergency room patients who are "found down" in order to rule out pre-existing seizure disorder, and for patients with pre-existing epilepsy).

3. Radiologic exams: Any patient with an initial seizure must have an MRI to rule out cerebral lesions (unless they present with the suspicion of head trauma in which case a CT scan is more appropriate to rapidly diagnose a cerebral hemorrhage); other tests may be performed when clinically indicated including cerebral angiogram, lumbar puncture, PET/SPECT scan.
4. EEG: Necessary to diagnose seizure classification as baseline; may perform 24-hour EEG via Holter monitor to quantify episodes as well as capture an actual episode; also utilized in conjunction with video monitoring as a screening test for epilepsy surgery as well as postoperatively to determine surgical success.

MANAGEMENT TREATMENT

1. Medication: Regimens differ based on seizure classification. The goal is single-drug therapy, but a combination of medications is often necessary to bring seizures under control. Drug levels must be maintained within the therapeutic range (usually at the high end) to be effective (see Table 4–5).
2. Appropriate referral of epileptics for surgical evaluation and/or consultation with a neurologist regarding medical management.
3. Surgery: Excision/evacuation of any space-occupying lesion that is the etiology for the seizures. Also, several institutions have initiated a protocol for epilepsy surgery that includes preoperative evaluation via neuropsychological testing, inpatient 24-hour video EEG monitoring with sphenoidal electrodes or (when indicated) surgically placed subdural grids or strips of electrodes. If a lesion that is a amenable to surgery is determined to be the focus of the seizures, the patient undergoes Wada's test, which consists of a cerebral angiogram and instillation of a cerebral anesthetic with simultaneous EEG and neuropsychometric testing to determine hemispheric dominance. The most common procedures are temporal lobectomy for complex partial epilepsy and a corpus callosotomy for atonic epilepsy.
4. Psychotherapy for psychogenic seizures or for patients who exhibit depression as a result of or in conjunction with their diagnosis.
5. Regular follow-up varies depending on the type of seizure and the prescribed management. Patients with idiopathic epilepsy should be followed initially every 2–4 weeks until a therapeutic drug level and seizure control are obtained. Thereafter, patients are usually seen every 3–6 months based on compliance.

PATIENT EDUCATION

1. Medications: Purpose, dose, side effects, toxicity, importance of compliance with regimen, necessary blood tests. Instruct patient not to consume alcohol while taking anticonvulsants. Patients should also be given a list of drugs that may precipitate seizures or lower seizure threshold.
2. Environment: Avoid stimuli that are known to precipitate seizures; necessary safety precautions (no climbing ladders, no swimming alone, no driving, etc.); patients with atonic and frequent tonic-clonic seizures should wear helmets.
3. Management of seizure: Instruct patient and significant other about preventing injury during and after seizures (nothing in the mouth, do not attempt to restrain, turn head to side). Advise the patient to wear a Medic Alert bracelet to identify themselves as an epileptic. Instruct patient to keep

TABLE 4–5. **Pharmacologic Management for Seizure Disorders***

Seizure Type	Medications	Usual Daily Dosage	Therapeutic Level
Generalized tonic-clonic	*Drugs of choice*		6–12 µg/mL
	Carbamazepine (Tegretol)	800–1600 mg	
	Phenytoin (Dilantin)	300–400 mg	10–20 µg/mL
	Alternates/adjuncts		
	Phenobarbital (Luminal)	90–150 mg	15–35 µg/mL
	Primidone (Mysoline)	750–1250 mg	6–12 µg/mL
	Lamotrigine (Lamictal)	100–500 mg	Not established
Absence	*Drugs of choice*		
	Ethosuximide (Zarontin)	750–1250 mg	40–100 µg/mL
	Valproate (Depakene)	1000–3000 mg	50–120 µg/mL
	Alternates/adjuncts		
	Clonazepam (Klonopin)	1.5–20 mg	20–80 µg/mL
	Lamotrigine (Lamictal)	100–500 mg	Not established
Atonic or myoclonic	*Drug of choice*		
	Valproate (Depakene)	1–3 gm	50–120 µg/mL
	Alternates/adjuncts		
	Clonazepam (Klonopin)	1.5–20 mg	20–80 µg/mL
	Felbamate (Felbatol)	1200–3600 mg	Not established
Simple partial	*Drugs of choice*		
	Carbamazepine (Tegretol)	800–1600 mg	6–12 µg/mL
	Phenytoin (Dilantin)	300–400 mg	10–20 µg/mL
	Lamotrigine (Lamictal)	100–500 mg	Not established
	Phenobarbital (Luminal)	90–150 mg	15–35 µ g/mL
	Alternates/adjuncts		
	Primidone (Mysoline)	750–1250 mg	6–12 µg/mL
	Clonazepam (Klonopin)	1.5–20 mg	20–80 µg/mL
	Gabapentin (Neurontin)	900–2400 mg	Not established
	Felbamate (Felbatol)	1200–3600 mg	Not established
Complex partial	*Drugs of choice*		
	Phenytoin (Dilantin)	300–400 mg	10–20 µg/mL
	Carbamazepine (Tegretol)	800–1600 mg	6–12 µg/mL
	Lamotrigine (Lamictal)	100–500 mg	Not established
	Gabapentin (Neurontin)	1800–3600 mg	Not established
	Alternates/adjuncts		
	Phenobarbital (Luminal)	90–150 mg	15–35 µg/mL
	Primidone (Mysoline)	750–1500 mg	6–12 µg/mL
	Valproate (Depakene)	1000–6000 mg	50–120 µg/mL
	Clonazepam (Klonopin)	1.5–20 mg	20–80 µg/mL
	Felbamate (Felbatol)	1200–3600 mg	Not established

* All anticonvulsant medications must be tapered up and down while carefully monitoring drug levels and other pertinent diagnostic tests (laboratory and radiologic) to avoid serious side effects. Patients should be maintained on the lowest effective dose.

a diary of seizure activity. Patient must also report any illness accompanied by fever or vomiting, as this could lead to increased seizure activity.

4. Disease course: Explain that most epileptics must be maintained on medication for life in order to control seizures (although some patients with childhood-onset seizures may outgrow them). The advances in surgical treatment may offer future hope to some epileptics who are not currently surgical candidates.

5. Legal issues: Explain that licensed health care providers must report any diagnosis with an associated lapse of consciousness to the local health department who in turn notifies the agency responsible for granting drivers'

licenses. Their license will be revoked. The period that a patient must be seizure-free in order to regain their license varies from state to state.

6. Support groups are available for the patient and family.

STATUS EPILEPTICUS

This disorder is marked by continuous seizure activity and should be suspected any time a patient has two or more consecutive seizures without return to baseline. It is a life-threatening condition especially when it begins as or progresses to generalized tonic-clonic status epilepticus accompanied by respiratory distress.

The causes of status epilepticus in a patient with pre-existing epilepsy include abrupt withdrawal of anticonvulsants, inability to keep medications down in times of illness, menstruation, excessive fatigue or stress, and febrile illness. Other causes in epileptics as well as the general population include cerebral infection, hypoxic/metabolic encephalopathy, chronic alcoholism with acute withdrawal, drug overdose/withdrawal, hypoglycemia, hypocalcemia, and acute head trauma.

Status epilepticus, regardless of the cause, must be treated as a medical emergency. The condition will most often persist until pharmacologic intervention takes place. The drugs of choice are diazepam (Valium) 5–20 mg slow IV push (IVP) at 1–2 mg/min (maximum of 100 mg/24 hr) or lorazepam (Ativan) 4–8 mg slow IVP at 1–2 mg/min (maximum of 80 mg/24 hr). Either drug may be repeated every 5–10 minutes until the seizures subside. At that time, the etiology can be determined and treated per the previous treatment plan.

Review Questions

4.6 A 15-year-old male presents to the ER following a generalized tonic-clonic seizure at school. The patient has no significant medical history or known history of trauma. The first diagnostic test to be done is:
A. CT scan of the brain
B. Blood chemistry: Electrolytes, blood urea nitrogen (BUN), creatinine, calcium, magnesium, glucose, drug screen
C. Urine: Urinalysis (UA), toxicology
D. EEG

4.7 The above patient has another seizure while being admitted to the emergency department and has not yet regained consciousness following the first seizure. The first intervention would be to:
A. Insert a bite block
B. Intubate
C. Establish IV access and give Valium 5 mg slow IVP
D. Restrain the patient

4.8 A 17-year-old female is a patient on the orthopedic surgery floor S/P surgical reduction of a tibia/fibula fracture. She has a known history of complex partial epilepsy since early childhood. Since her menarche at age 12, she has been having generalized tonic-clonic seizures during her period. She sustained her current trauma during one of these severe seizures. You contact her neurologist and ask if you may:

A. Instruct the patient to increase her Tegretol during her menses.
B. Add a second anticonvulsant during her menses.
C. Put the patient on an oral contraceptive that will maintain her hormone levels constantly.
D. Add phenobarbital to her regimen to control generalized seizures.

4.9 A 40-year-old black male is admitted to the detoxification unit at your facility for alcohol withdrawal. Forty-eight hours after admission, you are called to see the patient because he has had a generalized tonic-clonic seizure. Your evaluation of the patient, who is now awake and cooperative, suggests alcohol withdrawal as the etiology. Your treatment plan includes:
A. Blood chemistry: Electrolytes, alcohol level, toxicology screen
B. Phenobarbital titrated to therapeutic level
C. Head CT scan if seizures do not cease within 5–7 days
D. Both A and C

4.10 Patient education for patients with idiopathic epilepsy must include:
A. Medications
B. Avoidance of precipitants to seizures
C. Safety issues (no climbing, driving, swimming alone, etc.)
D. All of the above

Answers and Rationales

4.6 **B** This would be a logical first choice, since electrolyte imbalances and drugs are common causes of seizure in patients with no history of epilepsy. If the patient exhibited objective signs of head trauma (bleeding, ecchymosis, pupil abnormality), then a CT scan of the brain would be indicated. EEG comes much later and often only if the etiology has been difficult to diagnose.

4.7 **C** The nurse practitioner should assume that the patient is in status epilepticus if he has two or more seizures without regaining consciousness. The first intervention is to administer IVP Valium. *Never* restrain or place anything in the mouth of a convulsing patient. The patient will require intubation only if they become apneic, cannot protect their airway after the seizure stops, or you are unable to break the seizure pattern and must paralyze the patient.

4.8 **C** The reason that many female epilepsy patients have increases in seizure severity and/or frequency is postulated to be due to hormonal fluctuation. Most patients do very well on a steady-dose oral contraceptive (28-day cycle, no placebos). Increasing or adding medications during menses is not effective because the medication levels are not changing with their menses—if they are in a therapeutic range, they will stay therapeutic and still have seizures.

4.9 **D** If your history and physical exam yield no risk factors for brain cancer, no history of trauma, and no focal deficits, this patient likely has had an alcohol withdrawal seizure. This type of seizure is frequently accompanied by electrolyte imbalances. The labs should be sent and the patient should be watched closely and placed on seizure precautions. If the seizures continue for more than 5 days and/or the patient has neurologic deterioration, the patient deserves a head CT scan to rule out a structural lesion. Medication is not necessary at this time as patients with true alcohol withdrawal seizures are only at minimal risk for developing status epilepticus.

4.10 **D** Patients with idiopathic epilepsy must receive comprehensive patient and family education. These are just three of the elements that must be included.

References

Adams, R.D., & Victor, M. (1993). *Principles of Neurology* (5th ed.). New York: McGraw-Hill.

Callahan, M. (1994). Seizures and epilepsy. In E. Barker (ed.). *Neuroscience Nursing*. St. Louis: Mosby-Year Book, Inc.

Hickey, J.V. (1997). Seizures and Epilepsy. In J.V. Hickey (ed.). *The Clinical Practice of Neurological and Neurosurgical Nursing* (4th ed.). Philadelphia: Lippincott-Raven.

Kupecz, D. (1995). New drugs for the treatment of epilepsy. *Nurse Pract 20*(5), 83–85.

Massey, A.D. (1996). Seizure disorder. In R.E. Rakel (ed.). *Saunders Manual of Medical Practice*. Philadelphia: W.B. Saunders Co.

Parks, B.L., et al. (1994). Drug therapy for epilepsy. *Am Fam Physician 50*(3), 639–648.

So, E.L. (1995). Classifications and epidemiological considerations of epileptic seizures and epilepsy. *Neuroimaging Clin North Am 5*(4), 513–526.

Springhouse Corporation. (1996). *Nurse Practitioner's Drug Handbook*. Philadelphia: Springhouse Corporation.

Wyler, A.R. (1993). Modern management of epilepsy: Recommended medical and surgical options. *Postgrad Med 94*(3), 97–108.

Hydrocephalus

DEFINITION

Hydrocephalus is a disturbance in the flow or absorption of cerebrospinal fluid (CSF) causing progressive ventricular dilatation.

CLASSIFICATION

There are two types of hydrocephalus:

1. Communicating hydrocephalus: A condition in which CSF cannot be properly reabsorbed due to insufficient or nonfunctional arachnoid villi. This type of hydrocephalus may be caused by a subarachnoid hemorrhage that causes the villi to become clogged. Another type of communicating hydrocephalus seen in older adults is **normal-pressure hydrocephalus** which presents with ventricular enlargement and compression of cerebral tissue, but normal CSF pressure on lumbar puncture (LP).
2. Noncommunicating hydrocephalus: A condition in which CSF in the ventricles does not circulate properly within or into the subarachnoid space. An example would be congenital hydrocephalus due to obstruction of the aqueduct of Sylvius during gestation leading to stenosis or incomplete development. This type of hydrocephalus may also be caused by an intracranial lesion (blood clot, tumor, cyst), or central nervous system infection (meningitis, encephalitis).

ETIOLOGY/INCIDENCE

No data on actual incidence of hydrocephalus are available, as hydrocephalus is most commonly seen as a result of another neurologic disease. It is known that noncommunicating hydrocephalus is most common in infants (congenital hydrocephalus) and is diagnosed during their first 3 months of life. It is also known that normal-pressure hydrocephalus is most common in patients in their sixth and seventh decades of life.

PATHOPHYSIOLOGY

Hydrocephalus is due to a mechanical obstruction of CSF outflow or absorption or an overproduction of CSF. Specific pathologic processes have been identified with each cause:

1. Obstruction of outflow: Space-occupying lesions, scar tissue formation following CNS infection or cranial surgery
2. Obstruction of absorption: SAH (arachnoid villi are obstructed by plugs of vibrin and clotted blood), CNS infection (macrophages plug arachnoid villi)
3. Overproduction of CSF: Choroid plexus papilloma (very rare benign neoplasm—its excision cures the hydrocephalus)

Also, various pathophysiologic processes have been linked to the development of normal-pressure hydrocephalus including:

1. Clogging of the arachnoid villi with blood following SAH
2. Scarring of the basal cistern following accidental or surgical head trauma
3. Fibrotic changes and plugging of the arachnoid villi following CNS infection
4. Presence of thrombi in the superior saggital sinus

HISTORY

The symptoms of hydrocephalus are characteristic but variable depending on the type of hydrocephalus present. In patients with recurrent hydrocephalus, it is important to know their typical pattern of symptoms as they tend to repeat. In new-onset hydrocephalus, the patient will likely present with signs and symptoms of an underlying disease process as well as those of hydrocephalus. Whether new-onset or recurrent, the symptoms usually consist of some combination of the following:

1. Headache
2. Visual changes: Diplopia
3. Impaired balance
4. Lethargy, irritability
5. Photophobia
6. Generalized weakness

The classic presentation of normal-pressure hydrocephalus is a triad of urinary incontinence, mental status changes, and gait disturbance. Often, these symptoms are attributed to the normal aging process and thus overlooked by the patient, family, and practitioner.

For the patient with recurrent hydrocephalus, information regarding the history of the hydrocephalus must also be obtained:

1. At what age was this diagnosed?
2. What was the underlying diagnosis?
3. What was done to correct the hydrocephalus?
4. How many surgical shunt procedures have been performed? Dates?
5. What is the current anatomic location of the shunt?
6. Have you had any other recent illnesses/injury?
    A. Febrile illness
    B. Nausea, vomiting
    C. Head, neck, chest, abdominal trauma

PHYSICAL FINDINGS

1. General appearance: Anxious, irritable, lethargic, shielding eyes from light
2. Vital signs: Usually normal
3. Head: Note tenderness over shunt site
4. Neck: Note tenderness over shunt tube site
5. Chest/abdomen: Note tenderness over shunt site
6. Neurologic: Unable to look up when extraocular movements (EOMs) are tested (setting sun eyes), uncoordination, decreased level of consciousness with increased intracranial pressure, gait abnormalities

DIFFERENTIAL DIAGNOSIS

1. New-Onset Hydrocephalus
    A. Cerebral lesion (tumor, cyst, abscess)
    B. Cerebral hemorrhage
    C. Head trauma
    D. Meningitis/encephalitis
    E. Choroid plexus papilloma
    F. Congenital hydrocephalus
    G. Alzheimer's disease (secondary to brain atrophy)
    H. Normal-pressure hydrocephalus
2. Recurrent hydrocephalus
    A. Shunt malfunction (obstruction or disconnection most common)
    B. Shunt infection

DIAGNOSTIC TESTS/FINDINGS

Select appropriate tests dependent on whether new-onset or recurrent hydrocephalus is suspected based on history and exam.

1. Suspect new-onset hydrocephalus:
    A. CT scan to diagnose dilated ventricles
    B. MRI to look for mass lesion not seen on CT scan that may be the cause of hydrocephalus
    C. LP (after increased intracranial pressure [ICP] ruled out) to determine opening pressure and to perform CSF analysis; will see increased protein, white blood cells (WBCs) and decreased glucose in CSF with CNS infection (culture necessary to determine offending organism)
    D. Rule out any source of infection, no matter how slight, prior to performing any shunt procedure, whether or not patient has any signs or symptoms

of infection (CBC, blood cultures, chest x-ray [CXR], UA, and culture and sensitivity [C&S])
2. Suspect recurrent hydrocephalus in patient with shunt:
   A. CT scan to diagnose dilated ventricles
   B. Chest/abdominal x-rays to look at shunt connections
   C. Shunt tap to determine if shunt is functioning
   D. Rule out any source of infection, no matter how slight, prior to performing any shunt procedure, whether or not patient has any signs or symptoms of infection (CBC, blood cultures, CXR, UA, C&S)

MANAGEMENT/TREATMENT

Appropriately determine and develop a treatment plan for the underlying cause of new-onset hydrocephalus (see sections "Cerebrovascular Accident," "Brain Tumors," "Central Nervous System infections," "Craniocerebral Trauma"). In conjunction, determine the appropriate treatment for the hydrocephalus.

1. Once the diagnosis of hydrocephalus has been confirmed, refer to/consult with a neurosurgeon for shunting procedure or necessary procedure to treat underlying cause.
2. Ventriculostomy: For immediate relief of increased ICP and in patients who have any infectious process rendering a shunt procedure impossible.
3. Shunt procedure: Surgical placement of the appropriate design and desired pressure flow control shunt into the right ventricle space (most shunt systems consist of a pressure-sensitive pump, a reservoir for CSF sampling, and a one-way valve to prevent backflow); a tube then is dropped subcutaneously from the head to the neck and into either the peritoneal cavity (ventriculoperitoneal [VP] shunt) or the right atrium (ventriculoatrial [VA] shunt). *Note:* VA shunts are usually reserved for patients who have excessive scar tissue in their peritoneal cavity or have some other contraindication to VP shunting.
4. Routine IV antibiotics while ventriculostomy is in place as well as pre-/intra-/postoperatively for shunt procedures to prevent devastating CNS infection and/or shunt malfunction. Best choice is a third-generation cephalosporin (ceftriaxone 50 mg/kg q12h or cefotaxime/ceftizoxime 50 mg/kg q6h). May also send CSF cultures during external ventricular drainage and following shunt procedures, although this practice is considered controversial.
5. Follow-up: 2-week postoperative visit for any suture/staple removal, evaluate incisions and shunt function based on signs and symptoms; follow-up annually and prn thereafter (also as needed to treat any underlying illness as cause for hydrocephalus).

PATIENT EDUCATION

1. Medications (usually restricted to those needed for postoperative pain management and antibiotics): Dosage, purpose, side effects, toxicity
2. Incisional care (head, neck, and abdomen/chest): Keep clean and dry; note any redness, swelling, drainage and report to health care provider.
3. Disease course and expected outcomes: Educate regarding underlying cause of hydrocephalus; explain that the hydrocephalus itself is treatable with shunt procedure; educate on signs and symptoms of recurrent hydrocepha-

lus and that shunt revisions may be necessary; educate on signs and symptoms of shunt infection and necessary interventions.

Review Questions

4.11 A 65-year-old white male presents to your urgent care center complaining of difficulty keeping his balance when walking. He states that this has been getting worse over the past few months. He denies any other complaints and says that he is otherwise healthy. On review of systems, you also discover a history of urinary incontinence and memory difficulty. The most likely diagnosis for this patient is:
A. Normal-pressure hydrocephalus
B. Meningitis
C. Parkinson's disease
D. Multiple sclerosis

4.12 The "gold standard" and most cost-effective diagnostic test for hydrocephalus is:
A. CT scan of the brain
B. Lumbar puncture
C. EEG
D. MRI of the brain

4.13 A patient presents with signs and symptoms of increased intracranial pressure including decreased level of consciousness, pupil irregularity, cranial nerve palsy. Your CT scan shows acute hydrocephalus and the absence of any space-occupying brain lesion. Your initial intervention would be to:
A. Consult with a neurosurgeon and schedule the patient for a shunt procedure.
B. Give the patient IV mannitol to reduce the swelling in his brain.
C. Consult with a neurosurgeon and place a ventriculostomy to drain fluid from the ventricles.
D. Elevate the head of the bed 30 degrees.

4.14 A 21-year-old white male presents to the ER with complaints of headache, visual disturbance, fatigue, and impaired gait. He has a history of congenital hydrocephalus with a ventriculoperitoneal shunt placed at age 18 months and a shunt revision at age 15 years. On exam, the patient has a fever of 102°F. He also has "setting sun" eyes but otherwise has a normal exam. Your initial diagnosis is recurrent hydrocephalus secondary to:
A. Shunt infection
B. Shunt obstruction
C. Shunt disconnection
D. Brain lesion

4.15 The treatment measure(s) for the patient in Question 4.14 would be to:
A. Consult with a neurosurgeon and schedule a shunt revision.
B. Tap the shunt and send CSF for laboratory analysis.
C. Consult with a neurosurgeon to externalize the shunt and empirically treat patient with ceftizoxime 50 mg/kg intravenous piggyback (VPB) every 6 hours.
D. Perform an MRI of the brain.

Answers and Rationales

4.11   **A**   This patient has an insidious onset of the classic triad of symptoms for normal-pressure hydrocephalus.

4.12   **A**   Dilated ventricles show up clearly on a head CT scan. A lumbar puncture should never be performed when increased intracranial pressure is suspected or the pressure gradient change may cause brain stem herniation. An MRI is not necessary unless a brain lesion is suspected and is unclear on CT scan. An EEG is almost never required.

4.13   **C**   A ventriculostomy is the fastest way to reduce this patient's intracranial pressure and some advanced practice nurses have been trained to perform this procedure in consultation with a neurosurgeon. Mannitol is not indicated at this time as the fluid is not in the brain tissue. The patient will likely require a shunt procedure when he is stabilized. Elevating the head of the bed will not hurt the patient, but will also not help.

4.14   **A**   The clinical picture points to a shunt infection due to the severely elevated temperature. He likely also has mild hydrocephalus, as by-products from the infectious process often clog the shunt—given this fact, a shunt obstruction may be a secondary diagnosis.

4.15   **C**   The shunt should be externalized by a neurosurgeon so that infected CSF does not continue to circulate around this patients brain. Also, this patient should be empirically treated with a third-generation cephalosporin while his CSF results are pending. While B is correct, it is diagnostic and the question asks for treatment. "A" is incorrect, as you must eradicate the infection before placing or revising a shunt. Although a CT scan would likely be performed to view the ventricles, an MRI is not indicated at this time.

References

Adams, R.D., & Victor, M. (1993). *Principles of Neurology* (5th ed.). New York: McGraw-Hill.

Aminoff, M.J. (1996). Nervous system. In L.M. Tierney, S.J. McPhee, & M.A. Papadakis (eds.). *Current Medical Diagnosis and Treatment.* Stamford, CT: Appleton & Lange.

Barker, E. (1994). Cranial surgery. In E. Barker (ed.). *Neuroscience Nursing.* St. Louis: Mosby-Year Book, Inc.

Hickey, J.V. (1997). Intracranial pressure: Theory and management of increased intracranial pressure. In J.V. Hickey (ed.). *The Clinical Practice of Neurological and Neurosurgical Nursing* (4th ed.). Philadelphia: Lippincott-Raven.

Marshall, S.B., Marshall, L.F., Vos, H.R., & Chesnut, R.M. (1990). *Neuroscience Critical Care: Pathophysiology and Patient Management.* Philadelphia: W.B. Saunders Co.

Brain Tumors

DEFINITION

Cancer of the brain is a devastating disease with serious implications for patient, family, and health care provider. Tumors in the brain are often difficult to diagnose and treat until well into their destructive course. These tumors reveal themselves slowly, with malingering symptoms that are often over-looked, misdiagnosed, or ignored. The care and treatment of these patients is complex and dictated not only by tumor type but also by tumor position within the brain.

CLASSIFICATION

Brain tumors are most commonly classified by cell type, location, and malig-nancy. Table 4–6 discusses some of the more common tumor types and their characteristics.

ETIOLOGY/INCIDENCE

Approximately 40,000 primary brain tumors (a rate of 17 per 100,000 popula-tion) and 20,000 secondary brain tumors are diagnosed each year. The annual death rate, from the American Cancer Society, resulting from brain cancer is 8 deaths per 100,000 population.
Risk factors:

A. Higher incidence in male and whites.
B. Primary tumors seen more frequently in those 40–60 years old.
C. Nearly 20% of cancer affects the brain, but only 2% originates in the brain.
D. About 75% of brain tumors occur supratentorially.
E. The majority of brain tumors are glioma (45%); only 15% are metastatic.
F. The most common primary carcinomas that metastasize to the brain are lung, breast, gastrointestinal tract, and genitourinary tract.

PATHOPHYSIOLOGY

The pathophysiology of brain tumors is similar to all cancerous tumors. It in-volves the proliferation of abnormal cells, which leads to the formation of a tumor, which causes the death or destruction of normal cells and/or structures. The rate of cell proliferation, the site of invasion, and the prognosis vary by cell type.

HISTORY

Patients with brain tumors often have no symptoms or subtle symptoms that may not justify the performance of CT or MRI of the brain. Common complaints can be focal or nonfocal. The nonfocal symptoms include:

1. Headache (rarely the presenting symptom)
2. Nausea, vomiting
3. Difficulty with cognition (poor attention, diminished judgment/insight, emo-tional lability)
4. Memory disturbance
5. Speech disturbance
6. Auditory disturbance
7. Dizziness
8. Seizures

The exception to this rule is the pituitary adenoma. Although the pituitary gland is considered a part of the endocrine system, the diagnosis of a pituitary

TABLE 4–6.   **Tumor Types and Characteristics**

Tumor	Clinical Features	Treatment and Prognosis
Glioblastoma multiforme	Presents commonly with nonspecific complaints and increased intracranial pressure. As it grows, focal deficits develop.	Course is rapidly progressive, with poor prognosis. Total surgical removal is usually not possible, and response to radiation therapy is poor.
Astrocytoma	A glioma that presents similar to glioblastoma multiforme but course more protracted, often over several years. Cerebellar astrocytoma, especially in children, may have a more benign course.	Prognosis is variable. By the time of diagnosis, total excision is usually impossible; tumor often is not radiosensitive. In cerebellar astrocytoma, total surgical removal is often possible.
Medulloblastoma	A glioma seen most frequently in children. Generally arises from roof of fourth ventricle and leads to increased intracranial pressure accompanied by brain stem and cerebellar signs. May seed subarachnoid space.	Treatment consists of surgery combined with radiation therapy and chemotherapy.
Ependymoma	Glioma arising from the ependyma of a ventricle, especially the fourth ventricle; leads early to signs of increased intracranial pressure. Arises also from central canal of spinal cord.	Tumor is not radiosensitive and is best treated surgically if possible.
Oligodendroglioma	Slow-growing glioma. Usually arises in cerebral hemisphere in adults. Calcification may be visible on skull x-ray.	Treatment is surgical, which is usually successful.
Brain stem glioma	Presents during childhood with cranial nerve palsies and then with long-tract signs in the limbs. Signs of increased intracranial pressure occur late.	Tumor is inoperable; treatment is by irradiation and shunt for increased intracranial pressure.
Cerebellar hemangioblastoma	Presents with disequilibrium, ataxia of trunk or limbs, and signs of increased intracranial pressure. Sometimes familial. May be associated with retinal and spinal vascular lesions, polycythemia, and hypernephromas.	Treatment is surgical.
Pineal tumor	Presents with increased intracranial pressure, sometimes associated with impaired upward gaze (Parinaud's syndrome) and other deficits indicative of midbrain lesion.	Ventricular decompression by shunting is followed by surgical approach to tumor; irradiation is indicated if tumor is malignant. Prognosis depends on histopathologic findings and extent of tumor.
Craniopharyngioma	Originates from remnants of Rathke's pouch above the sella, depressing the optic chiasm. May present at any age but usually in childhood, with endocrine dysfunction and bitemporal field deficits.	Treatment is surgical, but total removal may not be possible.

Table continues

TABLE 4-6. *(Continued)*

Tumor	Clinical Features	Treatment and Prognosis
Acoustic neuroma	Ipsilateral hearing loss is most common initial symptom. Subsequent symptoms may include tinnitis, headache, vertigo, facial weakness or numbness, and long-tract signs. (May be familial and bilateral when related to neurofibromatosis.) Most sensitive screening tests are MRI and brain stem auditory evoked potential.	Treatment is excision by translabyrinthine surgery, craniectomy, or a combined approach. Outcome is usually good.
Meningioma	Originates from the dura mater or arachnoid; compresses rather than invades adjacent neural structures. Increasingly common with advancing age. Tumor size varies greatly. Symptoms vary with tumor site (e.g., unilateral exophthalmos [sphenoidal ridge]; anosmia and optic nerve compression [olfactory groove]). Tumor is usually benign and readily detected by CT scanning; may lead to calcification and bone erosion visible on plain x-rays of skull.	Treatment is surgical. Tumor may recur if removal is incomplete. Patients may receive radiation if removal is incomplete to decrease risk of recurrence.
Primary cerebral lymphoma	Associated with AIDS and other immunodeficient states. Presentation may be with focal deficits or with disturbances of cognition and consciousness. May be indistinguishable from cerebral toxoplasmosis.	Treatment is by whole-brain irradiation; chemotherapy may have an adjunctive role. Prognosis depends upon CD4 count at diagnosis.

* Adapted from Aminoff, M.J. (1996). Nervous system. In L.M. Tierney, S.J. McPhee, & M.A. Papadakis (eds.). *Current Medical Diagnosis and Treatment.* Stamford, CT: Appleton & Lange, with permission.)
MRI, magnetic resonance imaging; CT, computed tomography; AIDS, acquired immunodeficiency syndrome.

adenoma may be made by an endocrinologist, a neurologist, or a neurosurgeon. This is usually determined by the presenting symptom that necessitates referral to one of these specialists. These symptoms are summarized in Table 4–7.

PHYSICAL FINDINGS

Focal neurologic findings must always be worked-up. Unfortunately, most brain tumors do not produce focal findings until they are well advanced. These focal findings will vary depending on the location of the tumor and may include the following clinical picture.

1. General appearance: Normal
2. Vital signs: Normal
3. Eyes: Diminished visual acuity, papilledema, pupil abnormality, impaired extraocular movements, hemianopia

TABLE 4-7. **Signs and Symptoms of Pituitary Adenomas**

General	Prolactin-Secreting Adenoma	ACTH-Secreting Adenoma	Growth Hormone–Secreting Adenoma
Diminished visual acuity	Galactorrhea	Cushing's syndrome	Giantism before puberty or epiphyseal closure
Bitemporal hemianopia	Amenorrhea	Moon facies	Acromegaly after puberty or epiphyseal closure
Paresis of extraocular muscles	Infertility	Buffalo hump	Enlarged jaw, nose, tongue, hands, feet
Headache	Loss of pubic hair	Abdominal striae	Thickened facial features
	Impotence	Pendulous abdomen	Enlarged heart and pulmonary disease
	Increased serum prolactin levels	Ecchymoses	Diabetes mellitus
		Hypertension	Serum growth hormone levels >10 ng/mL
		Muscle weakness	
		Osteoporosis	
		Increased cortisol levels	
		Adrenal hyperplasia	

4. Neurologic: Weakness, hemiparesis, sensory disturbance, impaired gait, aphasia, agraphia

If the patient has more advanced disease, they may present to the clinic or ER with signs and symptoms of increased intracranial pressure including the above as well as altered level of consciousness, seizures, headache, hemiplegia, cranial nerve palsy, altered vital signs (Cushing's triad), and impaired brain stem reflexes (cough, gag, corneal).

The patient with a pituitary adenoma frequently presents with physical findings that are not initially considered neurologic in origin. For a summary of these findings, see Table 4–7.

DIFFERENTIAL DIAGNOSIS

1. Migraine headaches
2. Epilepsy
3. Cerebrovascular accident
4. Cerebral abscess
5. Cerebral hemorrhage
6. Endocrine disorders (in the case of a pituitary adenoma)

DIAGNOSTIC TESTS/FINDINGS

1. Brain CT scan or MRI: A CT scan will reveal many lesions but enhancement with contrast medium may be necessary. An MRI will reveal lesions more clearly and may assist to diagnose the type of lesion.
2. Skull radiographs: Only ordered for known tumors that are very close to the surface of the brain in order to determine if there is any bone involvement or erosion.
3. EEG: In a patient who presents with seizure, an EEG may be ordered; slow waves are characteristic of space-occupying lesion.
4. Angiogram: Determine vascularity of tumor.
5. Stereotactic brain biopsy: To determine tumor type.
6. Metastatic work-up: Chest x-ray, bone scan, mammogram, prostate exam, chest/abdominal/pelvic CT if indicated.

TABLE 4–8.   Endocrine Studies for Pituitary Adenomas

Hormone	Normal Level
Prolactin	Premenopausal women: 2.2–19.2 mEq/L Postmenopausal women: 1.0–12.8 mEq/L Men: 1.9–11.7 mEq/L
Growth hormone	Women: 0–30 ng/mL Men: 0–8 ng/mL
Cortisol	6 A.M. to 8 A.M.: 10–25 gm/L 4 P.M. to 6 P.M.: <10 gm/L
17-Ketosteroids (urine)	Women: 6–15 mg/24 hours Men: 8–20 mg/24 hours
17-Hydrocorticosteroids (urine)	4–12 mg/24 hours

7. The endocrine work-up for pituitary adenoma includes serum and urine levels of several hormones (see Table 4–8).

MANAGEMENT/TREATMENT

See chart on tumor classification—treatment varies depending on tumor type.

1. Referral to neurosurgeon and neuro-oncologist for long-term management.
2. Surgery: Craniotomy for tumor excision; the transphenoidal approach is often utilized for pituitary microadenoma excision.
3. Radiation therapy.
4. Chemotherapy (see Chapter 9 for chemotherapy guidelines): Agents that are commonly used to treat brain tumors are carmustine (BCNU), lomustine (CCNU), cisplatin (Platinol), procarbazine hydrochloride, and etoposide (VePesid). Selection of an agent, dosage, and route will vary greatly dependent on tumor type and should always be managed by a qualified neuro-oncologist.
5. Medical management of increased intracranial pressure due to tumor-related cerebral edema.
   A. Minimize activities that increase ICP (coughing, suctioning, Valsalva, seizures, stress, fever).
   B. Cerebrospinal fluid drainage.
   C. Blood pressure control to maintain cerebral perfusion pressure.
6. Medications
   A. Osmotic diuretics: Mannitol (Osmitrol) 12.5 gm as a 15–20% solution IV over 3–5 minutes for signs and symptoms of increased ICP and/or severe cerebral edema on CT scan.
   B. Corticosteroids: Dexamethasone (Decadron) initial dose 10 mg IV/PO, then 4–6 mg IV/PO q6h; must taper patient off of Decadron if they are on regular dosing for >72 hours. Routine taper is to reduce the dose by 1 mg/day or every other day as tolerated until discontinued—slower tapering is required for patients who have been on corticosteroids for a lengthy period or who do not tolerate rapid taper. Also, the prescription of corticosteroids requires concurrent prescription of an H_2 blocker to prevent gastric ulcers; the drugs of choice include ranitidine (Zantac) 150 mg PO bid, cimetidine (Tagamet) 200 mg PO bid, and famotidine (Pepcid) 20 mg PO bid.

   C. Barbiturates (reduce cerebral metabolism): On rare occasions, the use of barbiturates is required to allow time for the brain to recover from surgery or increased ICP. Pentobarbital (Nembutal) is the drug of choice and is given 1–3 mg/kg/hr IV infusion after an initial loading dose (usually 5–34 mg/kg) sufficient to produce burst suppression of the EEG.

   D. Anticonvulsants: The administration of anticonvulsants is controversial even in the presence of a seizure as the presenting symptom of a brain tumor. Many neurosurgeons feel that controlling/treating cerebral edema is sufficient in preventing seizures. In the patient with recurrent seizures due to tumor location and/or edema, the anticonvulsant of choice is phenytoin (Dilantin) 1 gm IV/PO loading dose and then 300 mg/day in divided doses.

7. Support groups for patient and family

PATIENT EDUCATION

1. Disease course and expected outcome: Varies depending on tumor type.
2. Medications: Purpose, dose, side effects, and toxicity. Give patients specific information on their current steroid dose and the need to taper off of steroids slowly only when directed to do so.
3. Signs and symptoms of increased ICP.
4. Necessary follow-up.

Review Questions

4.16 The presenting symptom(s) of a brain tumor:
   A. Is usually only headache
   B. May be indicative of increased intracranial pressure
   C. May be focal or nonfocal
   D. Both B and C

4.17 Which test is the most diagnostic for a brain tumor?
   A. MRI of the brain
   B. CT scan of the brain
   C. Tumor biopsy
   D. EEG

4.18 Mary is a 22-year-old white female with a history of headache, amenorrhea, and weight gain without a change in eating habits. Her physical exam reveals a blood pressure of 144/90, moon facies, buffalo hump, and abdominal striae. Her pregnancy test is negative. You suspect that Mary may have:
   A. Hypothyroidism
   B. A pituitary adenoma
   C. Multiple sclerosis
   D. Hysterical pregnancy

4.19 Given the differential diagnosis in Question 4.13, which of the following diagnostic tests would be appropriate?
   A. MRI of the brain
   B. Serum cortisol level
   C. Serum prolactin level
   D. All of the above

4.20 A patient presents to the ER following a witnessed generalized tonic-clonic seizure with confusion, an enlarged right pupil, and paresis of the left extremities. A stat CT scan of the brain reveals a large mass in the right temporal lobe with massive cerebral edema. After paging the neurosurgeon stat, your first intervention would be to:
A. Administer mannitol 12.5 gm IVPB
B. Administer dilantin 1 gm slow IVP
C. Send the patient for a stat MRI of the brain
D. Schedule a stereotactic biopsy of the lesion

Answers and Rationales

4.16 **D** Headache is an early symptom in only one third of patients with a brain tumor. The signs and symptoms are usually vague, focal or nonfocal, and represent increased intracranial pressure.

4.17 **C** The gold standard for the diagnosis of brain tumor is a tissue biopsy, either open or stereotactically. This will diagnoses tumor type on which treatment will be based.

4.18 **B** Given the history and physical exam, the most likely diagnosis is pituitary adenoma. Obviously, hypothyroidism needs to be ruled out as part of the work-up.

4.19 **D** The patient's symptoms are classic for a pituitary adenoma but an MRI is necessary to determine its presence. Also, a serum cortisol level is necessary to determine the tumor's secretory ability. A prolactin level should also be done, as this patient is amennorrheic.

4.20 **A** The most important issue at this time is to treat the cerebral edema with mannitol. Dilantin may be indicated later if the patient has intractable seizures. An MRI and stereotactic biopsy must be postponed until after the patient has been evaluated and stabilized.

References

Adams, R.D., & Victor, M. (1993). *Principles of Neurology* (5th ed.). New York: McGraw-Hill.

Aminoff, M.J. (1996). Nervous System. In L.M. Tierney, S.J. McPhee, & M.A. Papadakis (eds.). *Current Medical Diagnosis and Treatment*. Stamford, CT: Appleton & Lange.

Barker, E., Perrin Ross, A., & Bohan, E. (1994). Recognition and treatment of brain tumors. In E. Barker (ed.). *Neuroscience Nursing*. St. Louis: Mosby-Year Book, Inc.

Bronstein, K.S. (1995). Epidemiology and classification of brain tumors. *Neurooncology* 7(1), 79–89.

Chang, L., Miller, B.L., & McIntyre, H.B. (1994). Critical care in neurologic disease. In F.S. Bongard & D.Y. Sue (eds.). *Current Critical Care Diagnosis and Treatment*. Norwalk, CT: Appleton & Lange.

Hickey, J.V. & Armstrong, T. (1997). Brain tumors. In J.V. Hickey (ed.). *The Clinical Practice of Neurological and Neurosurgical Nursing* (4th ed.). Philadelphia: Lippincott-Raven.

Marshall, S.B., Marshall, L.F., Vos, H.R., & Chesnut, R.M. (1990). *Neuroscience Critical Care: Pathophysiology and Management*. Philadelphia: W.B. Saunders Co.

Newton, H.B. (1994). Primary brain tumors: Review of etiology, diagnosis, and treatment. *Am Fam Physician 49*(4), 787–797.

Springhouse Corporation. (1996). *Nurse Practitioner's Drug Handbook*. Philadelphia: Springhouse Corporation.

Central Nervous System Infections

DEFINITION

Infections of the CNS often become acute, life-threatening conditions. Prompt diagnosis and treatment are essential to the prevention of significant morbidity and mortality. The two most common infections are encephalitis (inflammation of the brain) and meningitis (an inflammation of the pia mater and arachnoid membranes that cover the spinal cord). A cerebral abscess is an infected space-occupying lesion in the brain most often due to a primary infection elsewhere in the body.

ETIOLOGY/INCIDENCE

The etiology of these infections is related to the microbe that causes the infection. These microbes may be viral (enteroviruses, adenoviruses, mumps virus, Epstein-Barr, herpes simplex), fungal—most commonly in the immunocompromised (*Candida albicans, Coccidioides immitis*, crytococci, *Mycobacterium tuberculosis*, syphilis), and bacterial (*Streptococcus pneumoniae, Haemophilus influenzae, Neisseria meningitidis*). Encephalitis is most commonly caused by an arbovirus, most of which are from the Bunyaviridae, Flaviviridae, or Togaviridae families. Most arboviruses that cause encephalitis occur as epidemics. Mononucleosis and vaccinations for measles, mumps, and rubella have also been linked to encephalitis.

Cerebral abscesses are caused by primary infections that extend into the cerebral tissue. Approximately one half of cerebral abscess are caused by a primary infection in or near the brain. Some of the more common infections are otitis media, mastoid infection, and sinusitis. Although uncommon, cerebral abscesses may also occur as a complication of intracranial or oral surgery and cerebral trauma. Abscesses that are carried to the brain from other infectious sites in the body are sometimes called metastatic cerebral abscesses. Their sources include lung infection/abscess, empyema, skin infection, bacterial endocarditis, bronchiectasis, and congenital heart or lung disease.

Infections of the CNS occur in all age groups. Meningitis tends to be more common in children than adults, and the reverse is true for encephalitis. These diseases have no preference based on sex or ethnic origin. The incidence of acute encephalitis is approximately 15 cases per 100,000 population. The incidence of meningitis varies by infectious agent. The most common is tuberculosis (TB) meningitis, averaging approximately 10 million cases annually worldwide.

PATHOPHYSIOLOGY

Meningitis is primarily caused by the normal flora of the nasopharynx. Often an upper respiratory infection will cause these organisms to become blood borne. These organisms are able to overcome the host defenses and cause a widespread inflammatory response involving the pia, arachnoid, CSF, and ventricles. This does not usually involve brain tissue. A purulent exudate is rapidly formed and circulated throughout the CSF. This process is what leads to the symptoms and may occasionally cause hydrocephalus due to clogging and obstruction of the choroid plexus and arachnoid villi with the purulent exudate.

The herpes simplex virus type 1 (HSV-1) is the most common cause of sporadic, focal encephalitis in the United States. The majority of cases of encephalitis worldwide are caused by mosquito bites, which inoculate the offending organism into the host's body. This leads to a mild or severe nonsuppurant inflammation with varying degrees of tissue destruction depending on the organism. After the virus gains entry, it invades the polymorphonuclear leukocytes and mononuclear cells, which congest and swell. This results in vasculitic lesions, myelin destruction, widespread nerve cell degeneration, necrosis, and/or hemorrhage.

A cerebral abscess forms when the brain tissue (usually within the white matter) is inoculated with a pathogen from a primary infection elsewhere in the body. The infected tissue goes through a series of changes beginning with edematous, congested tissue with a preponderance of polymorphonuclear leukocytes. Over the next 10–14 days the lesion becomes a mass of liquified necrotic tissue that encapsulates with a wall of connective tissue of variable thickness.

HISTORY

Patients with CNS infections usually have no long-term complaints. Encephalitis patients may be too sick at the time of presentation to give a history. Their symptoms usually come on rapidly weeks after the primary infection. The primary infection is usually reported as "the flu" including headache, nausea, and vomiting.

Meningitis patients often report a sudden onset of symptoms within the past few hours including headache, photophobia, fever, and nuchal rigidity. Patients with a fungal meningitis must be assessed for a history of human immunodeficiency virus (HIV) and other causes of immunocompromise. If the patient has a past history of splenectomy, sickle cell anemia, pneumonia, sinusitis, alcoholism, or head trauma the etiology may be pneumococcal. A history of HIV or immunosuppressive therapy should be worked-up for a fungal origin. If the patient has had a known exposure to a patient with meningococcal meningitis, this is likely the offending organism due to the contagious nature of this pathogen. In such a case, all close contacts must be isolated and treated.

Patients with cerebral abscess go through two stages of symptoms. The first stage takes place at the time of initial formation of the abscess during which time the patient may complain of headache, chills; fever, malaise, confusion, drowsiness, and speech disorders. It should be noted that some patients may be completely asymptomatic during this initial phase and that any symptoms may subside in response to antibiotic treatment for a suspected systemic infection. The second stage symptoms are due to the expanding cerebral mass. These patients often present with the vague signs and symptoms of a brain tumor including recurrent headache that increases in severity, confusion, drowsiness, and stupor. They may also continue to have the aforementioned flu-like symptoms.

All patients with an infection of the CNS must be asked questions that could assist the practitioner in identifying the infectious agent and/or an immunocompromised state. These questions include:

1. Any recent travel?
2. Any recent illness or exposure to illnesses?
3. Positive purified protein derivative (PPD) skin test?
4. History of cold sores (HSV-1)?
5. Complete past medical and surgical history.

PHYSICAL FINDINGS

Meningitis

1. General appearance: Toxic
2. Vital signs: Fever, tachycardia, hypotension
3. Skin: Petechial hemorrhage and ecchymosis of skin and mucous membranes (most common with meningococcal meningitis)
4. Eyes: Photophobia, ocular palsy
5. Ear, nose, and throat (ENT): Deafness and vertigo (CN VIII)
6. Musculoskeletal: Joint pain, Kernig's sign, Brudzinsky's sign, nuchal rigidity
7. Neurologic: Headache, decreased level of consciousness, seizures, unilateral or bilateral sensory loss

Encephalitis

1. General appearance: Anxious, lethargic
2. Vital signs: Unstable with diffuse CNS infection, fever
3. Eyes: Nystagmus, ocular paralysis
4. Abdominal: Nausea, vomiting
5. Musculoskeletal: Nuchal rigidity
6. Neurologic: Severe headache, ataxia, dysphasia, hemiparesis, stupor progressing to coma, confusion, olfactory or gustatory hallucinations, seizures

Cerebral Abscess

1. General appearance: Ill, lethargic
2. Vital signs: Fever, unstable if severe increased ICP present
3. Neurologic: Speech and visual disturbance, hemiparesis, seizures, severe headache, stupor progressing to coma

DIFFERENTIAL DIAGNOSIS

1. Subarachnoid hemorrhage
2. Epidural abscess
3. Epilepsy

THERAPEUTIC MANAGEMENT

Diagnostic

1. Blood studies: CBC, electrolytes, liver/renal panel (prior to starting antibiotics), cultures (positive in 50% meningitis cases), serology to diagnose certain types of viral encephalitis.

TABLE 4–9. Cerebrospinal Fluid Findings with Central Nervous System Infection

Lumbar Puncture Data	Aseptic Meningitis	Bacterial Meningitis	Viral Encephalitis
Cultures	No growth	Growth	No growth
Gram's stain	Negative	Positive in 70–90% of cases	Negative
Latex agglutinin	Negative	Available for *S. pneumoniae, H. influenzae, N. meningitidis*	Negative
WBC	<1000, mostly mononuclear lymphocytes	>1000; <10,000/mm^3, mostly polymorphonuclear cells	Elevated with increased lymphocytes
Protein	Normal to slightly elevated	Increased; 100–500 mg/dL	Elevated
Glucose	Normal to slightly decreased	Decreased; <40 mg/dL	Normal to low
Opening Pressure	Increased	Increased	Moderate to high
Color	Clear to cloudy	Turbid cloudy	Clear to bloody

2. Brain CT scan: Must be done to rule out space-occupying lesion or cerebral edema prior to performing lumbar puncture. CT scan is the test of choice when a cerebral abscess is suspected.
3. Lumbar puncture with CSF analysis (see Table 4–9). The lumbar puncture is rarely performed on a patient with a cerebral abscess because increased ICP is often present. If an LP is indicated, the results usually show an elevated WBC count from a few to thousands with lymphocytes being the predominant cell, elevated protein, normal glucose, and an elevated CSF opening pressure.
4. If a cerebral abscess is identified on CT scan, identification of the primary infection may help to identify the pathogen. Chest, skull, and sinus radiographs or chest CT scan may be necessary to identify the primary infection.
5. Urine, sputum, and nasopharynx cultures may be indicated to identify any sources of infection.

MANAGEMENT/TREATMENT

1. Referral to or consultation with neurologist, neurosurgeon, and infectious disease specialist is necessary to formulate treatment plan.
2. Medications:
   A. Antibiotics must be started immediately in suspected cases of meningitis or encephalitis. Empiric treatment with cefotaxime (200 mg/kg/day IV) is presumptive treatment; ampicillin (200 mg/kg/day IV) is added in newborns, adults over age 50, and the immunocompromised. Antibiotics may need to be administered intrathecally if no improvement on antibiotics within 24 hours.
   B. Antiviral therapy for HSV-1 encephalitis must be started before the patient progresses to coma or the mortality rate is 70–80%. If treatment with acyclovir (Zovirax) is begun prior to coma, the mortality rate remains 28%, with a high rate of variable morbidity in those that survive.

C. The antibiotics of choice for a cerebral abscess are penicillin G 20 million U with chloramphenicol 4–6 gm daily in divided doses.

D. In cases where increased ICP is suspected due to cerebral edema resulting from any infectious process, mannitol and/or corticosteroids may be required (see recommendations in "Brain Tumor," section).

E. Analgesia: Nonsteroidal antiinflammatory drugs are effective.

F. Antipyretics: Acetaminophen as needed for fever >101°F.

G. Anticonvulsants (usually dilantin 300 mg/day) if seizures are present.

H. IV hydration.

3. Respiratory support: Mechanical ventilation as needed.

4. Surgery: In the case of a cerebral abscess, if initial antibiotic treatment is ineffective surgical excision of the abscess will be necessary. The goal is to perform a craniotomy and excise the abscess and the entire membrane. If the membrane cannot be removed, then the abscess is drained and the sac is injected with antimicrobial agents. Future drainage of the sac may be necessary.

5. Ventriculostomy to reduce ICP and/or to treat hydrocephalus.

6. Support and counseling for patient and family.

PATIENT EDUCATION

1. Disease course and expected outcome: Instruct patient and family in severity of illness and need for intensive care management. Explain the potential complications and that morbidity is high. Mortality is dependent on the organism involved.

2. Medications: Explain the necessary medications and their route, dose, side effects, toxicity.

3. Procedures: Explain all procedures prior to performing and state rationale; obtain informed consent from patient or family as needed.

Review Questions

4.21 The most appropriate diagnostic testing sequence for a patient with suspected CNS infection is:
   A. Lumbar puncture, MRI, blood work
   B. Lumbar puncture, CT scan, blood work
   C. CT scan, lumbar puncture, blood work
   D. Blood work, lumbar puncture, CT scan

4.22 A 22-year-old white male presents to the ER lethargic, complaining of a severe headache and nausea. His history is significant for the flu 2 weeks ago. On exam, the patient has a fever of 102°F, nuchal rigidity, and mild difficulty with word-finding. The most likely diagnosis for this patient is:
   A. Meningitis
   B. Encephalitis
   C. Cerebral abscess
   D. Brain tumor

4.23 A 37-year-old black female is admitted to the infectious disease service with a diagnosis of lung abscess. She is being treated with IV antibiotics and begins to improve. On hospital day 3, she becomes confused and ex-

hibits right hemiparesis. You order a CT scan of the brain because you
suspect:
A. A right-sided meningioma
B. A left-sided meningioma
C. A right-sided cerebral abscess
D. A left-sided cerebral abscess

4.24 In performing a lumbar puncture on a patient with a normal brain CT
scan and suspected meningitis with a known exposure to a patient with
meningococcal meningitis, you would expect to find:
A. Positive Gram's stain
B. Elevated protein
C. Decreased glucose
D. All of the above

4.25 For the patient in Question 4.24, the most common symptoms are:
A. Headache, fever, photophobia, nuchal rigidity, petechial hemorrhage
and echymosis of the skin and mucous membranes
B. Headache, fever, malaise, nausea, vomiting, nuchal rigidity
C. Headache, fever, hemiparesis, stupor
D. Headache, fever, seizures, pupillary abnormality

Answers and Rationales

4.21   **C**   A CT scan must *always* precede a lumbar puncture in a patient presenting with the signs and symptoms of CNS infection. The lumbar
puncture can be performed before, during, or after the blood work.

4.22   **A**   This patient has a classic picture for viral encephalitis. A patient
with meningitis would have more meningeal irritation and a patient
with a cerebral abscess would likely have further focal abnormality
(weakness, pupillary dysfunction, etc.)

4.23   **D**   A cerebral abscess would be suspected, as the patient has the known
risk factor of a lung abscess as well as new neurologic symptoms.
The abscess would likely be on the left side of the brain given the
patient's right hemiparesis.

4.24   **D**   All of the above would be true for a patient with bacterial meningitis,
which would be the most likely case for this patient, given the contagious nature of meningococcal meningitis.

4.25   **A**   These are the symptoms most specific for meningococcal meningitis.
Those listed in B are more specific to encephalitis, while C and D
are more often related to cerebral abscess.

References

Adams, R.D., & Victor, M. (1993). *Principles of Neurology* (5th ed.). New York: McGraw-
Hill.

Cammermeyer, M., & Appledorn, C. (1996). *Core Curriculum for Neuroscience Nursing*
(3rd ed. Update). Chicago: American Association of Neuroscience Nurses.

Hickey, J.V. (1997). Selected infections of the nervous system. In J.V. Hickey (ed.). *The
Clinical Practice of Neurological and Neurosurgical Nursing* (4th ed.). Philadelphia:
Lippincott-Raven.

Marshall, S.B., Marshall, L.F., Vos, H.R., & Chesnut, R.M. (1990). *Neuroscience Critical Care: Pathophysiology and Management*. Philadelphia: W.B. Saunders Co.

Maxson, S., & Jacobs, R.F. (1993). Viral meningitis: Tips to rapidly diagnose treatable causes. *Postgrad Med 93*(8), 153–164.

Metcalf, J. (1994). Neurologic infections. In E. Barker (ed.). *Neuroscience Nursing*. St. Louis: Mosby-Year Book, Inc.

Morganlander, J.C. (1994). Lumbar puncture and CSF examination: Answers to three commonly asked questions. *Postgrad Med 95*(8), 125–131.

Schissel D. (1996). Meningitis. In R.E. Rakel (ed.). *Saunders Manual of Medical Practice*. Philadelphia: W.B. Saunders Co.

Springhouse Corporation. (1996). *Nurse Practitioner's Drug Handbook*. Philadelphia: Springhouse Corporation.

Transient Ischemic Attacks

DEFINITION

A TIA is an episode of sudden, brief, variable neurologic deficits caused by focal cerebral ischemia. A TIA usually lasts 5–15 minutes followed by full recovery of neurologic function within 24 hours. The majority last less than 1 hour. Reversible ischemic neurologic deficit (RIND) is defined as a neurologic deficit, similar to a TIA, lasting >24 hours with complete recovery of function, usually within 48 hours. Many patients have recurrent attacks, which may be indicative of an impending stroke. Discovering the cause and providing appropriate treatment for a TIA/RIND may prevent a more serious event.

ETIOLOGY/INCIDENCE

The causes for TIAs mimic those for stroke, as a TIA is considered a ministroke. These can be subdivided into the following groups:

1. Vascular diseases
   A. Carotid stenosis
   B. Extracranial atherosclerosis
   C. Arteritis
   D. Thromboembolic events
2. Hematologic disorders
   A. Hypercoagulability
   B. Polycythemia
3. Cerebrovascular insufficiency
   A. Diminished cardiac output
   B. Subclavian steal syndrome (decreased blood supply to the subclavian artery)
   C. Mechanical obstruction of one of the major blood vessels in the neck

A valid estimate of the incidence of TIAs is not available because many attacks go unreported due to the usually subtle nature of the symptoms. It is known that, following a stroke, many patients or their significant others report that the patient has suffered one or more episodes likely to have been TIAs preceding their stroke.

Risk factors include:

1. Age >50
2. Male
3. Black
4. Smoking tobacco
5. Hypertension
6. Diabetes
7. Obesity
8. Lack of exercise
9. High-fat diet

PATHOPHYSIOLOGY

There are two common pathophysiologic processes by which TIAs are classified. They are differentiated based on the cerebral blood supply affected by one or more etiologic mechanisms.

1. Vertebrobasilar TIA: Results from inadequate blood flow from vertebral arteries; most often secondary to a partially obstructed subclavian artery, which supplies the vertebrobasilar system.
2. Carotid TIA: Results from inadequate blood flow from the carotid artery; most often secondary to carotid stenosis.

HISTORY

A patient who presents complaining of symptoms consistent with TIA must be adequately interviewed in an attempt to determine the extent of their illness and risk for stroke. The following answers must be elicited:

1. Specific information about attack:
   A. When was your first attack?
   B. How often do these attacks occur?
   C. How long do they last?
   D. What are your exact symptoms? May need to prompt patient and localize the symptoms to specific area of body.
2. Medical history
   A. Postural hypotension
   B. Arrhythmias—atrial fibrillation, heart block
   C. Hypertension
   D. Atherosclerosis
   E. Diabetes mellitus non–insulin-dependent diabetes mellitus ([NIDDM] and insulin-dependent diabetes mellitus IDDM)
   F. Hyperlipoproteinemia
   G. Smoking
   H. Recent surgery—particularly involving cardiac bypass
3. Family history
   A. TIAs
   B. Stroke
   C. Atherosclerosis
4. Diet and exercise history

The majority of patients who present with TIA will have a history for cerebrovascular disease and one or more risk factc medical history. The classic symptoms during an attack assist to differentiate between the two pathophysiologic classificati

1. Vertebrobasilar TIA: Dizziness, diplopia, dark/blurred vision, visua. deficits, ptosis, dysarthria (difficulty articulating words), dysphagia (difficulty swallowing), perioral paresthesias, general weakness, acute confusion, and occipital headache that may precede other symptoms and persist for a few days following the attack
2. Carotid TIA: Transient unilateral blindness/neglect, altered level of consciousness, numbness of tongue, contralateral sensory or motor deficits, aphasia, dysarthria, dyslexia, diffuse ipsilateral headache following attacks, focal seizures

PHYSICAL FINDINGS

Most often, by the time a patient has arrived at a clinic or emergency room following a TIA, their objective signs have resolved. The patient's report is all the practitioner has to rely upon. Nevertheless, the practitioner must perform a complete exam to detect subtle residual deficits and detect risk factors for stroke.

1. General appearance: Normal, perhaps mild anxiety
2. Vital signs: Possible hypertension, postural hypotension, irregular heart rate on palpation and auscultation
3. Eyes: Funduscopic exam may show atherosclerotic changes (such as retinal emboli); possible orbital bruit; may see visual field deficit for 24 hours after attack of which patient is not aware
4. Neck: Possible carotid and/or supraclavicular bruit
5. Peripheral pulses: May be diminished or absent
6. Neurologic: Usually normal between attacks; may see slightly hyperactive deep tendon reflexes for 24 hours after attack

DIFFERENTIAL DIAGNOSES

1. Migraine with atypical aura
2. Focal seizure disorder
3. Cerebral mass lesion
4. Cerebrovascular abnormality (aneurysm, AVM)
5. Cerebrovascular accident (CVA, stroke)
6. Temporal arteritis
7. Ocular disorders (in the absence of generalized symptoms)

Most differential diagnoses are ruled in or out during the routine diagnostic work-up for TIA.

DIAGNOSTIC TESTS/FINDINGS

1. Thorough history and physical exam is necessary but not sufficient.
2. Blood tests including CBC, platelets, prothrombin time (PT), partial thromboplastin time (PTT), sedimentation rate, electrolytes, serum glucose, cal-

334 , lipid profile, thyroid panel. Antinuclear antibodies (ANA), serology, d toxicology screen if indicated.

Radiologic exams.

A. Head CT scan should be performed, as 10–20% of patients with TIA will have evidence of cerebral infarction in the territory of the brain consistent with their symptoms.

B. MRI is more sensitive for infarcts that are <1 cm as well as being preferred for patients with vertebrobasilar TIAs or when the vascular territory cannot be clearly identified based on symptoms.

C. Ultrasound vascular evaluation such as carotid duplex study is indicated for carotid territory symptoms, while transcranial Doppler study is a useful screening test for patients with vertebrobasilar or brain stem symptoms.

D. Magnetic resonance angiography (MRA) is an alternative to ultrasound studies and can be performed during a noncontrast MRI. The advantage is that both intracranial and extracranial vessels can be examined.

4. Other diagnostic tests as indicated including:

A. Echocardiogram and Holter monitoring to rule out a cardiac source of microemboli. A transesophageal echocardiogram (TEE) may be helpful in identifying clots in the atria that may have showered emboli into the cerebral blood flow.

B. Cerebral angiography should be performed in patients with carotid stenosis on duplex study in preparation for carotid endarterectomy as well as those who continue to have an unclear diagnosis following less invasive studies. Emergent angiography must be performed if carotid or vertebral artery dissection is suspected—in these patients, the symptoms consistent with TIA usually do not clear completely.

C. EEG to rule out focal seizures as a diagnosis or a symptom of cerebral ischemia.

D. If no clear etiology has been found, more detailed coagulation studies may be indicated. Also, a lumbar puncture may be performed for signs of meningeal inflammation (*Note:* A lumbar puncture must *never* be performed until increased intracranial pressure and cerebral mass lesion have been ruled out by CT scan or MRI.)

MANAGEMENT/TREATMENT

1. Medications: For patients with long-term history of TIAs, enteric coated aspirin 325 mg daily is the drug of choice if the etiology is not amenable to surgery. For patients with cardiac emboli as the etiology, heparinization followed by warfarin is indicated possibly in combination with aspirin or dipyridamole (Persantine) 100 mg PO bid. Warfarin is the treatment for arterial dissection, which usually heals spontaneously in 3–6 months, at which time patients are switched to aspirin. Ticlopidine (Ticlid) 250 mg bid with meals is available for patients with recurrent TIAs on aspirin or those who do not tolerate aspirin. Patients on Ticlid must be monitored for diarrhea and leukopenia (biweekly CBC).

2. Referral to or consultation with a physician following diagnostic work-up if patient is a surgical candidate, does not respond to medical management options, or presents an unclear clinical picture.

3. Surgery: Carotid endarterectomy is indicated for patients with demonstrated 70–90% carotid stenosis if they do not present excessive surgical

risk due to their age or medical history. If surgery is deemed too great a risk, patients are managed on medications as above.

4. Follow-up in 2 weeks (or sooner if pathology is found) to review results of diagnostic work-up and begin appropriate treatment. Continue follow-up every 2 weeks to determine effectiveness of therapy until patient has been free from TIAs for 6 months. Then, follow-up as needed for re-evaluation and routine labs.

PATIENT EDUCATION

1. Medication: Purpose, dosage, side effects, toxicity, importance of compliance with regimen, necessary laboratory evaluation. Advise patient to inform practitioner if any other medications are taken, as they may interfere with the action of their anticoagulants. Also, make certain that patients inform other health care providers, including dentists, that they are taking anticoagulants. Wearing a Medic Alert bracelet should be encouraged.
2. Disease course and expected outcome: Once diagnosed, TIAs can be treated medically or surgically as indicated. However, patients must be informed that even with treatment, 30–60% of patients with TIAs will suffer a stroke within 7–10 years. Education on the warning signs of stroke as well as to seek treatment immediately must be performed.
3. Prevention: As most patients with TIAs have one or more risk factors that are preventable, education in the reduction or modification of risk factors is important.
   A. Low-fat diet
   B. Regular exercise
   C. Weight loss
   D. Controlling hypertension
   E. Controlling diabetes
   F. Smoking cessation
   G. Moderate alcohol intake

Review Questions

4.26 Determining a medical versus surgical treatment plan for TIAs (in the absence of significant surgical risk factors) will depend on the results of which test?
   A. Carotid duplex study
   B. MRI of the brain
   C. Echocardiogram
   D. Cerebral angiography

4.27 Patients on Ticlid must be monitored closely for:
   A. Dehydration
   B. Leukopenia
   C. Signs and symptoms of stroke
   D. All of the above

4.28 Mrs. R, a 70-year-old woman, presents to urgent care with a 3-month history of episodes during which she describes dysphasia, diplopia, dizziness, and tingling in her right arm. These episodes have occurred five

times over the past 3 months and they last 5–15 minutes. Mrs. R has a past medical history significant for smoking (one PPD × 50 years) and hypertension. Her physical exam reveals a patient in no acute distress, weight 200 lbs, height 62 inches, blood pressure 156/80, otherwise normal. Given this clinical picture, the most likely cause for Mrs. R's episodes is:
A. Transient ischemic attacks
B. Simple partial seizures
C. Cerebral neoplasm
D. Multiple sclerosis

4.29 For the above patient, what diagnostic test(s) would you order to work-up Mrs. R related to your suspected diagnosis?
A. An MRI of the brain
B. Transcranial Doppler
C. Carotid Doppler
D. A and B

4.30 The therapeutic management plan for Mrs. R would include all of the following EXCEPT:
A. Aspirin 325 mg PO qd
B. Referral to a surgeon for possible carotid endarterectomy
C. Smoking cessation
D. Weight loss

Answers and Rationales

4.26   **A**   A carotid duplex study showing severe carotid stenosis would be an indication for surgery. Echocardiogram and cerebral angiography are suggested as surgical preparation. An MRI is not necessary.

4.27   **D**   Ticlid is a drug given to patients with TIAs. Patients on Ticlid must be observed for dehydration secondary to diarrhea and leukopenia. All patients should have a biweekly CBC. Also, all patients should be watched for a worsening of their condition, which can lead to a stroke.

4.28   **A**   Given Mrs. R's clinical picture and her risk factors, TIA would be the most likely diagnosis at this time.

4.29   **D**   Mrs. R's symptoms are most clearly indicative of a vertebrobasilar TIA. The best tests for her evaluation are transcranial Doppler and MRI. A carotid Doppler is best for patients with symptoms pointing to the carotid territory.

4.30   **B**   Mrs. R has not been proven to have carotid occlusion sufficient to warrant a surgical evaluation. She may very well, at her age, have some degree of occlusion. However, her symptoms do not indicate a carotid source for her TIAs. All of the other interventions would be appropriate given her diagnosis and risk factors.

References

Adams, R.D., and Victor, M. (1993). *Principles of Neurology* (5th ed.). New York: McGraw-Hill.

Aminoff, M.J. (1996). Nervous system. In L.M. Tierney, S.J. McPhee, M.A. Papadakis (eds.). *Current: Medical Diagnosis and Treatment*. Stamford, CT: Appleton & Lange.

Chaturvedi, S., & Hachonski, V. (1994). Transient ischemic attacks: Rethinking concepts in management. *Postgrad Med 96*(5), 42–54.

Springhouse Corporation. (1996). *Nurse Practitioner's Drug Handbook.* Philadelphia: Springhouse Corporation.

Whitney, F. (1994). Stroke. In E. Barker (ed.). *Neuroscience Nursing.* St. Louis: Mosby-Year Book, Inc.

Wityk, R.J. (1996). Transient ischemic attack. In R.E. Rakel (ed.). *Saunders Manual of Medical Practice.* Philadelphia: W.B. Saunders Co.

Cerebrovascular Accident (Stroke)

DEFINITION

The National Survey of Stroke in the United States defines stroke:
A clinical syndrome consisting of a constellation of neurological findings, sudden or rapid in onset, which persists for more than 24 hours, and whose vascular origins are limited to: (a) thrombotic or embolic occlusion of a cerebral artery resulting in infarction, or (b) spontaneous rupture of a vessel resulting in intracerebral or subarachnoid hemorrhage. This definition excludes occlusion or rupture due to traumatic, neoplastic, or infectious process which produce vascular pathology (Naradzay & Gaasch, 1996).

ETIOLOGY/INCIDENCE

There are two main etiologies for stroke—embolic and hemorrhagic. Each of these mechanisms has other causes linked to them.

1. Thromboembolic: Atherosclerosis, microemboli from surgery, fat emboli from long bone fracture, air emboli from posterior fossa surgery, coagulopathy, microemboli from atrial fibrillation
2. Hemorrhagic: Hypertension, cocaine use, anticoagulation, aneurysm, AVM
   Stroke is the third leading cause of death in the United States with an annual incidence of 1–2 per 1000. Approximately 500,000 new strokes occur in the United States each year. The risk factors are the same as those previously stated for TIAs.

PATHOPHYSIOLOGY

The pathophysiology of stroke is relatively simple. In the case of a thromboembolic stroke, a thrombus or embolus lodges in a major vessel that supplies blood to the brain and arrests blood supply to the brain. In the case of a hemorrhagic stroke, a major vessel ruptures due to a variety of reasons. In the case of an aneurysm or AVM, there is a pre-existing weakness in the vessel and it either leaks (leading to subarachnoid hemorrhage [SAH]) or it ruptures (leading to an intracerebral hemorrhage [ICH]). Cocaine-related strokes are due to an erosion of the vessel from the cocaine leading to vessel wall weakness and rupture. "Hypertensive bleeds" are strokes caused by uncontrolled hypertension leading to vessel rupture as the pressure in the cerebral arteries exceeds their capacity.

In both cases, the brain tissue supplied by the affected vessel becomes ischemic and will die within 3–5 minutes. In some cases, damage to this area may be minimized if the cerebral circulation has collateral avenues to deliver blood to the area supplied by the affected vessel.

HISTORY

With the advent of new therapies for stroke, the history has become increasingly important. As in the case of recombinant tissue plasminogen activator (rt-PA) for myocardial infarction, rt-PA for stroke has a "window of opportunity" during which time the drug must be given. It is important to pinpoint the exact onset of symptoms and what they consisted of; this becomes difficult because often the symptoms begin slowly or are mistaken for a TIA and when they do not clear, the patient seeks medical attention. Too often, by the time the patient gets to the hospital, it is too late to utilize rt-PA. Please see Table 4–11 for current inclusion and exclusion criteria for the use of rt-PA.

In general, the history will be different for each stroke patient, but they may report one or more of the following over the past 24 hours:

1. Confusion
2. Unilateral weakness
3. Unilateral numbness or tingling
4. Speech difficulty
5. Swallowing difficulty
6. Visual disturbance

By the time they get to the hospital, the patient may be unable to give a history due to decreased level of consciousness and/or aphasia. The family may be the only source of information. Be certain to obtain a medical and surgical history including whether or not the patient has the following:

1. Hypertension
2. Diabetes
3. Smoking
4. Recent surgery
5. Recent trauma
6. TIAs
7. Cardiovascular disease
8. Dysrhythmias

PHYSICAL FINDINGS

1. General appearance: Lethargic to stupor/coma
2. Vital signs: Possible hypertension, tachycardia, respiratory pattern abnormalities
3. Skin: Check for pressure points/sores depending on duration of time between stroke and presentation at hospital
4. Neurologic: Pupillary abnormality, hemiplegia, hemiparesis, facial droop, aphasia, seizures, coma, nystagmus, meningeal signs. These focal findings will vary based on the vessel involved. Table 4–10 summarizes the findings for four commonly affected vessels.

DIFFERENTIAL DIAGNOSES

1. Cerebral aneurysm rupture
2. Arteriovenous malformation
3. Hydrocephalus

TABLE 4–10. Clinical Characteristics Following CVA

Vessel	Clinical Characteristics Follow
Carotid artery	Contralateral motor and/or sensory loss (fleeting blindness); possible spatial (right brain); possible speech deficit (
Anterior cerebral artery	Confusion; personality changes; incontinence motor and/or sensory loss; leg more involved than arm, difficulty with eye movement (tracking)
Middle cerebral artery	Contralateral motor and/or sensory loss; contralateral motor loss in lower face; arm involved more than leg; ipsilateral visual field loss; possible communication deficit (left brain); possible spatial perceptual deficit (right brain)
Posterior cerebral artery	Contralateral sensory loss, ipsilateral visual field deficit; possible communication deficit (left brain); possible spatial perceptual deficit; graying of vision

CVA, cerebrovascular accident.

4. Craniocerebral trauma
5. Cerebral lesion: Tumor, abscess

DIAGNOSTIC TESTS/FINDINGS

1. Brain CT scan: First test to be done, as a hemorrhagic stroke must be ruled out in order to administer anticoagulants or rt-PA.
2. Blood tests: CBC, electrolytes, liver/renal profiles, clotting studies, lipid panel.
3. Angiogram: Any patient with a hemorrhagic stroke evidenced by SAH must have an angiogram to rule in/out aneurysm or AVM.
4. Other tests as part of work-up same as for TIA and include carotid duplex, MRA, echocardiogram, EEG, lumbar puncture as needed.

MANAGEMENT/TREATMENT

Preventive therapies were discussed in the section of TIA. This discussion will focus on treating the patient following a stroke.

1. Referral to or consultation with neurosurgeon and/or neurologist to determine treatment plan; early rehabilitation referrals
2. Medication:
   A. Intravenous rt-PA 0.9 mg/kg (maximum of 90 mg) with 10% of dose given as a bolus followed by an infusion lasting 60 minutes—given for thrombotic stroke only in order to dissolve clot; rt-PA must be given within 3 hours of the onset of ischemic stroke symptoms. The inclusion and exclusion criteria are listed in Table 4–11. Patients receiving rt-PA must be closely monitored for any bleeding complication, and if any complication is suspected the infusion must cease immediately. Procedures that may cause minor bleeding should be postponed when possible until after the infusion is completed—indwelling urinary catheter for at least 30 minutes, nasogastric tube for at least 24 hours, central venous and arterial punctures for as long as possible (weighing the risk vs. benefit of performing such procedures).

TABLE 4–11. Inclusion and Exclusion Criteria for rt-PA in Thromboembolic Stroke

Inclusion Criteria	Exclusion Criteria
Patient arrives in emergency room within 3 hours of symptom onset	Current use of anticoagulants or a PT >15 seconds
CT scan of brain confirms the absence of hemorrhage	Use of heparin in the previous 48 hours and a prolonged PTT
Qualified medical exam verifies signs and symptoms consistent with ischemic stroke	A platelet count <100,000/mm^3
	Another stroke of serious head injury in the previous 3 months
Persons who have been on aspirin are eligible if they do not have any exclusion criteria	Major surgery within the preceding 14 days
	Pretreatment SBP >185 mm Hg or DBP >110 mm Hg
	Neurologic signs that are improving rapidly
	Isolated mild neurologic deficits
	Prior intracranial hemorrhage ·
	Blood glucose <50 mg/dL or >400 mg/dL
	Seizure at the onset of stroke
	Gastrointestinal or urinary bleeding within the preceding 21 days
	Recent myocardial infarction

rt-PA, recombinant tissue plasminogen activator; PT, prothrombin time; CT, computed tomography; PTT, partial thromboplastin time; SBP, systolic blood pressure; DBP, diastolic blood pressure.

B. Anticoagulation: Heparin 5000-U bolus followed by 1000 U/hr until PTT is in desired range (institutional policy varies as to the optimum PT/PTT value). Warfarin sodium (Coumadin) is generally started as soon as the patient is at the desired PT or PTT at a maintenance dose of 2–10 mg/day. The duration of anticoagulation therapy varies considerably and ranges from 90 days to lifetime.

C. Anticonvulsants: Controversial; some physicians use prophylactically if the stroke involves the temporal lobe; others use only if seizures present as a complication of the stroke; the medication should be selected based on the seizure type.

D. Nimodipine (Nimotop) 30 mg PO q6h for 4 weeks may reduce the deficit produced by cerebral ischemia.

E. Vasopressors as needed to maintain cerebral perfusion pressure.

F. Supportive/comfort: Analgesia, antipyresis, sedation.

3. Surgery

A. Aneurysm clipping if indicated

B. AVM—interventional neuroradiologic procedures common

1) Placement of coils so AVM clots off

2) Instillation of glue during angiogram: No flow through AVM

3) May still require surgical excision

C. Evacuation of ICH if necessary

4. Intensive care management

A. Management of increased ICP (as previously outlined)

B. Respiratory support: Mechanical ventilation as needed

C. Cardiovascular support

D. Nutritional support: Early enteral or parenteral feeding

E. Early rehabilitation: Physical, occupational, and speech therapy

5. Support and counseling for patient and family

PATIENT EDUCATION

1. Disease course and expected outcome: Explain severity of illness and need for extensive rehabilitation; explain likelihood of residual deficit.
2. Counsel on end-of-life decisions for those patients with no likelihood of recovery: Durable power of attorney, resuscitation status, etc.
3. Explain all treatments, procedures, and medications to patient and family; obtain informed consent when necessary.
4. Prevention: Patients and family members must be instructed in how to prevent another stroke. This education must include lifestyle and diet modification as outlined in the section on TIA.

Review Questions

4.31 Mr. Smith is a 67-year-old black male brought to the hospital by his wife, who stated that he fell down 20 minutes ago and has been unable to speak or move his right side since then. Mr. Smith has no significant past medical history. On exam, Mr. Smith is conscious, very anxious, his speech is garbled and unintelligible, he has a left facial droop, and he is completely right hemiplegic. The most likely etiology for his symptoms is:
   A. Cerebrovascular accident
   B. Traumatic brain injury
   C. Brain tumor
   D. Alzheimer's disease

4.32 Given Mr. Smith's clinical picture, which of the following would be the first diagnostic test that must be performed?
   A. CT scan of the brain
   B. MRI of the brain
   C. Cerebral angiogram
   D. EEG

4.33 Following the performance of necessary blood tests and in the absence of cerebral hemorrhage, the best initial therapy for Mr. Smith would be:
   A. Administration of heparin 5000-U bolus
   B. Administration of rt-PA bolus
   C. Intubation and mechanical ventilation
   D. Intravenous fluids and direct observation

4.34 In a patient with a hemorrhagic CVA, which test must be performed to determine the possible cause:
   A. Cerebral angiogram
   B. CT scan
   C. MRI
   D. EEG

4.35 The goal(s) of therapy following CVA include:
   A. Minimize complications
   B. Minimize disability
   C. Prevent further strokes
   D. All of the above

Answers and Rationales

4.31 **A** Mr. Smith has all of the classic symptoms of a stroke or CVA. Although he did have a fall that could lead a practitioner to suspect traumatic brain injury, rarely does a patient maintain consciousness following an injury severe enough to cause Mr. Smith's symptoms.

4.32 **A** Given the suspicion of a stroke, the first test to perform would be a CT scan to determine the presence or absence of hemorrhage.

4.33 **B** Administration of rt-PA is the treatment most appropriate in a patient who has had a recent onset of CVA symptoms. Prior to giving rt-PA, a hemorrhagic stroke must be ruled out—rt-PA is exclusively for dissolving clots that give rise to thromboembolic stroke. The PT/PTT should also be checked, as rt-PA is a potent anticoagulant and a baseline must be established. Heparin would be the next choice if Mr. Smith met any exclusion criteria for rt-PA.

4.34 **A** Many hemorrhagic strokes are caused by AVM or aneurysm that may require surgical treatment. An angiogram is the most appropriate test to reveal the presence of these lesions.

4.35 **D** Treatment of patients following CVA is geared toward maximizing their quality of life by minimizing their deficits. Prompt recognition and management is necessary to achieve these goals.

References

Aminoff, M.J. (1996). Nervous system. In L.M. Tierney, S.J. McPhee, & M.A. Papadakis (eds.). *Current Medical Diagnosis and Treatment.* Stamford, CT: Appleton & Lange.

Cammermeyer, M., & Appeldorn, C. (1996). *Core Curriculum for Neuroscience Nursing* (3rd edition update). Chicago: American Association of Neuroscience Nurses.

Hickey, J.V. (1997). Stroke and other cerebrovascular diseases. In J.V. Hickey (ed.). *The Clinical Practice of Neurological and Neurosurgical Nursing* (4th ed.). Philadelphia: Lippincott-Raven.

Marshall, S.B., Marshall, L.F., Vos, H.R., & Chesnut, R.M. (1990). *Neuroscience Critical Care: Pathophysiology and Management.* Philadelphia: W.B. Saunders Co.

Naradzay, J.F.X., & Gaasch, W.R. (1996). Acute stroke. *Emerg Med Clin North Am 14*(1), 197–216.

Pryse-Phillips, W., & Yegappan, M.C. (1994). Management of acute stroke: Ways to minimize damage and maximize recovery. *Postgrad Med 96*(5), 75–82.

Smucker, W.D. (1995). Systematic approach to diagnosis and initial management of stroke. *Am Fam Physician 52*(1), 225–234.

Springhouse Corporation. (1996). *Nurse Practitioner's Drug Handbook.* Philadelphia: Springhouse Corporation.

Whitney, F. (1994). Stroke. In E. Barker (ed.). *Neuroscience Nursing.* St. Louis: Mosby-Year Book, Inc.

Craniocerebral Trauma

DEFINITION

Simply defined, craniocerebral trauma is any injury to the scalp, cranium, or brain due to several etiologic mechanisms of injury. The resulting injuries are classified according to the areas involved as follows:

1. Scalp
   A. Laceration
   B. Burn
   C. Avulsion
   D. Abrasion
2. Cranium
   A. Linear fracture
   B. Basilar fracture
   C. Comminuted fracture
   D. Depressed fracture
   E. Compound fracture
3. Brain
   A. Contusion
   B. Concussion
   C. Dural tear
   D. Hemorrhage
      1) Subarachnoid
      2) Subdural
      3) Epidural
      4) Intracerebral

ETIOLOGY/INCIDENCE

The mechanisms of head injury are numerous, as outlined below.

1. Direct trauma which includes:
   A. The head striking a stationary object (deceleration injury)
   B. A moving object striking the stationary head (acceleration injury)
   C. A lateral blow rotating the brain about the saggital axis (rotational injury)
2. Indirect trauma which includes:
   A. Blast injury such as an explosion
   B. Hyperextension or hyperflexion causing shearing and tensile strains
   C. Falls that transmit force from spinal column to brain
3. Penetrating trauma which includes:
   A. Missile (gunshot wounds, shrapnel, etc.)
   B. Stabbing
   C. Impalement

The incidence of head trauma is vastly underreported because many minor injuries are nonconsequential. The number of reported injuries each year numbers in the hundred thousands. The number of male victims is at least twice as high as female victims and 70% of all fatal accidents involve head injury. The most common causes of head injury are vehicular accidents, sports-related injuries, acts of violence, and falls. Many injuries are directly linked to the ingestion of alcohol or drugs immediately preceding the injury.

PATHOPHYSIOLOGY

The pathophysiology of brain injury is complicated and directly related to the severity of injury, which in turn determines prognosis. When any area of the body receives a forcible injury or trauma, swelling is likely to occur. The main problem with a brain tissue injury is that the cranium is a rigid vault and cannot expand to accommodate brain tissue swelling. The Monroe-Kellie doctrine states that when one of the contents of the skull (those being blood, brain, and CSF) increases, another must decrease in order to compensate and maintain normal intracranial pressure. The brain attempts to perform compensatory strategies until all blood and CSF contents have been minimized as much as possible. If, at this time, the brain tissue continues to swell, the brain will herniate towards the path of least resistance, which is down through the foramen magnum causing compression of the brain stem and death of the patient.

HISTORY

The history of a patient with head trauma must include all of the circumstances of the accident or injury:

1. Exact time and place of injury?
2. How did injury occur?
3. Any loss of consciousness?
4. Any seizures?
5. Cardiopulmonary arrest?
6. Posttraumatic amnesia?

The symptoms of specific injuries vary. Some common symptoms with all head trauma include headache, mental status changes, visual changes, and weakness (usually unilateral). Many patients with head trauma are not able to communicate due to impaired consciousness or speech difficulty. Bystander reports are very important in determining the mechanism of injury and likely intracranial pathology.

PHYSICAL FINDINGS

The physical complaints and exam vary based on the type in injury. Table 4–12 summarizes some key findings.

When a patient presents with head trauma, all other body systems must be assessed for traumatic injury. Particularly common in vehicular accidents is associated musculoskeletal injury (long bone and/or rib fracture, neck sprain or fracture), cardiothoracic injury (cardiac contusion, pneumothorax, etc.) and abdominal injury (vital organ laceration or contusion).

Physical Findings Consistent with Brain Death

1. Completely unresponsive to all stimuli (including deep pain).
2. Permanent apnea.
3. No cephalic or brain stem reflexes.
4. Absence of hypothermia or drug intoxicator that would explain above findings.
5. In rare cases (medicolegal issues) an angiogram may be done to demonstrate an absence of cerebral blood flow or an EEG to demonstrate absence of electrical brain activity.

DIFFERENTIAL DIAGNOSIS

In the case of head trauma, the diagnosis is often clear. The differentials come into play when determining the pathology. In addition to the diagnoses listed

TABLE 4–12.   Physical Findings Following Craniocerebral Trauma

Injury	Physical Findings
Concussion	Headache, fatigue, dizziness, loss of balance, diplopia, photophobia, memory and attention disturbances, irritability, personality changes
Cerebral contusion	Altered LOC, dysphasia, hemiparesis, flexor posturing, focal/generalized seizures, pupil alterations
Brain stem contusion (range from mild to severe)	Absent response to stimuli, fever >102.5°F, tachycardia, tachypneic, perspiration, pupil changes, absent brain stem reflexes (doll's eyes), Battle's sign (bruising behind ear), vomiting, hiccups, otorrhea, flaccid bilateral paresis, cranial nerve deficits
Intracranial hematoma—subdural, epidural intracerebral	Signs and symptoms of increased intracranial pressure: Early—deterioration in LOC, changes in pupil size/shape/light response, mono/hemiparesis, sensory deficit, cranial nerve palsy, headache, seizure Later—continued decreased LOC progressing to stupor/coma, pupillary changes (dilation and nonreaction to light), vomiting, headache, hemiplegia, decortication or decerebration, respiratory irregularities, impaired brain stem reflexes
Subarachnoid hemorrhage	Headache, nuchal rigidity, photophobia, altered LOC
Linear skull fracture	Headache, obvious tissue trauma (edema, laceration, erythema, ecchymosis)
Comminuted skull fracture	Same as linear fracture and often associated with cerebral contusion because bone splinters and causes local brain tissue injury
Depressed skull fracture	Same as linear fracture and may feel "step-off" over fracture site when skull is palpated; usually associated with severe scalp bruising and laceration; degree of neurologic symptoms (increased ICP) dependent on amount of brain involved
Basilar skull fracture	Same as linear fracture; fracture extends to anterior, middle, or posterior fossa; frequently results in dural tear and CSF leak; unique findings include subconjunctival hemorrhage, periorbital ecchymosis, epistaxis, anosmia, visual defect, rhinorrhea, Battle's sign
Penetrating trauma	Look for entry and exit wound; brain extruding from wound poor prognostic sign; examine wound for dirt, debris; signs and symptoms related to sudden, severe rise in ICP; usually have associated scalp, cranium, and brain tissue pathology that may include any or all of the preceding injuries

LOC, loss of consciousness; ICP, intracranial pressure; CSF, cerebrospinal fluid

under classifications of head trauma, other potentially serious sequelae of head trauma must be ruled out, including:

1. Vascular injuries: Traumatic aneurysm, carotid cavernous fistula, thrombus formation and vascular occlusion, vertebral artery thrombosis
2. Cranial nerve injury:
   A. CN I: Most common, associated with anterior fossa fracture
   B. CN II: Associated with frontal lobe injury or blow
   C. CN III, IV, VI: Associated with sphenoid or cavernous sinus injury
   D. CN V: Superior orbital or basilar fracture
   E. CN VII, VIII: Parietotemporal injury near petrous ridge

F. CN IX, X, XI: Foramen magnum fractures
G. CN XII: Very rare

In the case of a patient who was "found down" and has no obvious sign of recent head trauma (absence of local scalp injury), other differential diagnoses must be considered including:

1. Seizure
2. Cerebrovascular accident
3. Drug overdose
4. Space-occupying brain lesion other than traumatic hemorrhage
5. Subacute or chronic subdural hematoma (most often in elderly or alcoholic patients up to several weeks following trauma)

DIAGNOSTIC TESTS/FINDINGS

In a patient admitted with obvious head trauma, the diagnosis is based on exam and the following diagnostic work-up.

1. Brain CT scan: Indicated in all cases of head trauma in which focal deficits are present or when reports indicate loss of consciousness or seizure. Clearly indicates the presence of blood. Bone windows are useful in determining the presence of skull fracture, particularly those that are not clear on skull x-ray.
2. Skull x-rays: When fracture suspected in absence of need for CT scan.
3. Cervical spine films: Up to 20% of head injuries have associated injury to the cervical spine; must visualize down to C7 to rule out fracture or subluxation; DO NOT remove cervical collar until C-spine cleared by radiologist.
4. Laboratory: Blood toxicology/alcohol screen, blood urea nitrogen (BUN) creatinine, electrolytes, serum osmolarity, CBC, coagulation panel.
5. Transcranial Doppler: Demonstrates vasospasm associated with trauma.
6. Cerebral angiography: If posttraumatic vascular anomalies suspected.

MANAGEMENT/TREATMENT

1. Referral to or consultation with neurosurgeon or trauma surgeon.
2. Medications to reduce ICP and maintain cerebral perfusion pressure (CPP) >70 mm Hg:
    A. Osmotic diuretics: Mannitol (Osmitrol) 25 gm (125 mL of 20% solution) IV over 10 minutes q4h prn for signs and symptoms of increased ICP and/or severe cerebral edema on CT scan (maintain serum osmolarity 300–310 mOsm/L). Frequently, the use of mannitol is dependent on the ICP reading with doses being given for ICP >15–20 mm Hg. The maximum daily dose is 25 gm and mannitol may not be given if the serum osmolarity is >310.
    B. Barbiturates (reduce cerebral metabolism): On rare occasions, the use of barbiturates is required to allow time for the brain to recover from surgery or increased ICP. Pentobarbital (Nembutal) is the drug of choice and is given 1–3 mg/kg/hr IV infusion after an initial loading dose (usually 5–34 mg/kg) sufficient to produce burst suppression of the EEG. An alternative to the use of pentobarbital is propofol (Diprivan) 3–6 mg/kg/hr. This drug causes burst slowing on the EEG and

rarely causes burst suppression. This drug is being used more often because it is short acting, so patients can be clinically evaluated more rapidly after it is discontinued.

C. Anticonvulsants: The administration of anticonvulsants is controversial even in the presence of an initial posttraumatic seizure. If utilized, the drug of choice is phenytoin (Dilantin) 1 gm IV loading dose and then 300 mg/day in divided doses. Dilantin has been found to be effective in preventing early (within the first 2 weeks) posttraumatic seizures but should not be used for long-term prophylaxis. Often times it will be discontinued after 10–14 days if the patient has not had any seizure activity.

D. Vasopressors: To maintain blood pressure (BP) at a range sufficient to keep CPP (CPP = MAP − ICP) at least 70 mm Hg, the drug of choice is a dobutamine drip of 3–20 μg/kg/min titrated to keep CPP >70. A second-line drug is a phenylephrine drip at 40–200 μg/min titrated to keep CPP >70. The choice between these two drugs is often made based on hemodynamic readings, with dobutamine being used if the cardiac index is less than 3.0 L/min/m^2 and phenylephrine being used if the CVP or pulmonary artery wedge pressure (PAWP) acceptable but the CPP is low. If the CPP, central venous pressure (CVP), and PAWP are low, albumin 5% 250 mL IV is given over 20 minutes and may be repeated in 30 minutes at a volume not to exceed 500 mL over 2 hours.

E. Paralytics: The use of paralytics in the management of patients with craniocerebral trauma is restricted for those patients who require maximum ventilatory support. The use of paralytics to control an agitated patient is discouraged. However, if the agitation is refractory to sedation and makes routine management difficult, it may be indicated. The drugs that may be used are pancuronium bromide (Pavulon) 0.1 mg/kg IV initially with repeat 0.01 mg/kg q 30–60 mins prn and vecuronium bromide (Norcuron) 0.3 mg/kg initially with repeat 0.015 mg/kg q 12–15 mins. It is extremely important to place patients on around-the-clock dosing of sedatives and analgesics while paralyzed.

F. Stress ulcer prophylaxis: The drugs of choice include ranitidine (Zantac) 150 mg PO bid, cimetidine (Tagamet) 200 mg PO bid, and famotidine (Pepcid) 20 mg PO bid.

G. Sedation: For use in patients who are paralyzed, agitated, or anxious. The current drug of choice is midazolam (Versed) 2 mg IV q2h prn. Care must be taken in the extubated patient, as Versed may cause mild respiratory depression.

H. Analgesia: The drug of choice in head trauma patients is morphine sulfate 2 mg IV q2h prn. Care must be taken in extubated patients, as morphine may cause profound respiratory depression.

I. Antipyretic: Acetaminophen (Tylenol) 650 mg PR for temperature 100°F. Lower fevers must be aggressively treated in head trauma patients, as the cerebral metabolic rate rises dramatically for each degree above normal body temperature. Cooling blankets should be utilized if the patient does not respond to acetaminophen after 30 minutes. If shivering is caused by cooling measures and the patient is intubated, norcuron 0.1 mg/kg may be used and repeated at 0.05–0.1 mg/kg/hr prn.

J. Intravenous fluids: Volume replacement with colloids or blood.

K. Antibiotics: Broad spectrum for dirty wounds or prophylaxis in presence of internal ICP monitor; best choice is a third-generation cephalosporin (ceftriaxone 50 mg/kg q12h or cefotaxime/ceftizoxime 50 mg/kg q6h.

3. Hemodynamic monitoring: Arterial lines and pulmonary artery catheters are utilized in the majority of patients following head injury. Blood pressure must be aggressively maintained in the high normal range, as studies have shown that even a brief episode of hypotension significantly increases mortality. A jugular bulb catheter may be placed in order to measure the oxygenation of the blood as it leaves the brain. This information tells the practitioner how well oxygenated the brain is, with the normal value being 65–74.

4. Fluid management: Following head trauma, the patient's fluids and electrolytes must be managed carefully. Although much disagreement exists, the majority of the research indicates that the solution of choice for the maintenance IV is D_5NS or $D_{5.45}NS$ with 20 mEq of KCl per liter. The total fluid rate (including IV, total parenteral nutrition [TPN], enteral nutrition) should be 1.5 mL/kg/hr. A replacement IV of NS (if Na <145) or $D_{0.45}NS$ (is Na >146) is recommended. Fluid replacement is determined by the patient's hemodynamic status. The current recommendation is to monitor intake and output every 4 hours with fluid replaced over 2 hours only if CVP <10 or PAWP <14.

5. Surgical:
   A. Craniotomy/craniectomy in order to:
      1) Remove hematoma
      2) Débride open wounds
      3) Elevate skull fractures
      4) Perform temporal lobectomy in presence of refractory increased ICP (done as a last resort)
   B. Ventriculostomy to monitor ICP and drain CSF as needed: Considered by most as secondary to the use of medications to reduce ICP; frequently used in patients who have hemorrhaged into their ventricles.
   C. Intraparenchymal fiberoptic catheter or microtransducer to monitor ICP: Considered a basic monitoring appliance for patients with significant head trauma, as the ICP will frequently rise before signs and symptoms become evident.

6. Respiratory: Mechanical ventilation as needed; tape from ETT should not cross jugular area. Continuous pulse oximetry and arterial blood gases at least every 4 hours are necessary, as recent studies show that even a brief episode of hypoxemia significantly increases mortality. Tracheostomy may be necessary for long-term ventilatory support. The use of hyperventilation as a strategy to reduce ICP is no longer accepted, as recent studies show that this practice causes significant cerebral ischemia. The P_{CO_2} that is currently desired is 30–35 mm Hg. Premedicating patients with lidocaine 2% 75 mg IV/ETT 3–5 minutes prior to suctioning has been shown to decrease the ICP spikes that are common with this procedure.

7. Nutrition: Early TPN, PPN, or enteral nutrition, jejunostomy tube may be necessary.

8. Positioning: Head of bed up 30 degrees and neutral head position to promote venous return of cerebral blood flow.

9. Rehabilitation: Early initiation of physical therapy, occupational therapy, speech therapy, neuropsychometric testing; transfer to rehabilitation facility as soon as possible.

10. Follow-up for mild head injury: Evaluate in 2 weeks to confirm resolution of symptoms; no repeat x-ray is necessary for simple skull fracture. Follow-up for moderate to severe head injury is dependent on the treatment and subsequent rehabilitation required.

PATIENT EDUCATION

1. Medications: Dose, rationale, route, side effects, toxicity.
2. Procedures: Explain all tests and procedures prior to performing, obtain informed consent when necessary.
3. Disease course and expected outcome: Highly variable depending on severity of injury; be certain to be honest with family members especially when explaining prognosis and brain death.
4. Discharge planning: Begin as soon as survivability established; explain care needs and placement issues to patient and family; discuss expected length of rehabilitation.
5. Education and support: Refer to support groups and provide educational materials on injury, facilities, etc.

Review Questions

4.36 The Monroe-Kellie doctrine states that:
   A. The skull is a rigid compartment.
   B. When one of the contents of the skull (brain, CSF, or blood) increases in volume . . . another must decrease in volume.
   C. The brain always maintains a normal ICP.
   D. The brain can compensate for any increase in ICP.

4.37 Billy is a 17-year-old white male who was brought by ambulance after being involved in a fight on his way to school this morning. Witnesses stated that he was hit in the head with a baseball bat and lost consciousness for 2 minutes. Afterwards, he complained of a headache and blurred vision, but went to school. While in school Billy had a generalized tonic-clonic seizure and was brought to the hospital. Currently, Billy is extremely agitated, noncommunicative, and has a left hemiparesis. There is clear fluid dripping from his right ear. The first test to order on Billy is:
   A. A CT scan of the brain
   B. An MRI of the brain
   C. A microscopic analysis of the fluid coming from his ear
   D. An EEG

4.38 It is discovered that Billy has a right frontotemporal cerebral contusion and a basilar skull fracture. There is significant cerebral edema and Billy's level of consciousness is deteriorating. Your next intervention would be to:
   A. Administer Versed 5 mg IV
   B. Call the neurosurgeon and set up for insertion of an ICP monitor
   C. Administer mannitol 12.5 gm IV
   D. Administer dilantin 1 gm IV

4.39 Mrs. Baker is a 70-year-old black female who presents to the ER with complaints of diplopia, dizziness, memory difficulty, and headache for the past 10 days. During the history she tells you that she fell 3 weeks ago and hit her head on a step. She has a large bruise over her left eye. What is your most likely differential diagnosis:
   A. Brain tumor
   B. Traumatic brain injury
   C. Alzheimer's disease
   D. Senility

4.40 Given the above differential diagnosis, what would be the first diagnostic test you would order?
   A. Neuropsychometric testing to determine the severity of Mrs. Baker's cognitive dysfunction
   B. An MRI of the brain to look for a brain mass or plaques
   C. A CT scan of the brain to look for hemorrhage
   D. A toxicology screen

Answers and Rationales

4.36 **B** The doctrine states that unless this happens, ICP will rise continually until one of the contents decreases or herniation takes place.

4.37 **A** The first and most important test is the CT scan of the brain to rule out hemorrhage that requires surgical evacuation.

4.38 **C** Although this patient will require an ICP monitor, he needs an immediate dose of mannitol in an attempt to reduce his cerebral edema. Considering the findings of the CT scan and his deteriorating status, this intervention will provide the maximum benefit at this time. Versed is not indicated, as his level of consciousness is deteriorating.

4.39 **B** Given the fact that Mrs. Baker's symptoms were acute in onset and subsequent to her fall as well as the fact that no symptoms preceded the fall, the most likely diagnosis would be a traumatic brain injury. A woman of this age can develop a subdural hematoma and have relatively few symptoms initially. Over a period of days to weeks, the hematoma becomes subacute and then chronic and the patient will begin to note symptoms.

4.40 **C** With the above information in mind, the first diagnostic test should be a CT scan and if a subacute or chronic subdural hematoma is present, it will likely require surgical evacuation (this depends on the size and the degree of shift present).

References

American Association of Neurological Surgeons, Joint Section on Neurotrauma and Critical Care. (1995). *Guidelines for the Management of Severe Head Injury.* New York: The Brain Trauma Foundation.

Cammermeyer, M., & Appeldorn, C. (1996). *Core Curriculum for Neuroscience Nursing,* (3rd ed. Update). Chicago: American Association of Neuroscience Nurses.

Doberstein, C., Rodts, G.E., & McBride, D.Q. (1994). Neurosurgical critical care. In F.S. Bongard & D.Y. Sue (eds.). *Current Critical Care Diagnosis and Treatment.* Norwalk, CT: Appleton & Lange.

Hickey, J.V., & Cook, H. (1997). Craniocerebral injuries. In J.V. Hickey (ed.). *The Clinical Practice of Neurological and Neurosurgical Nursing* (4th ed.). Philadelphia: Lippincott-Raven.

Marshall, S.B., Marshall, L.F., Vos, H.R., & Chesnut, R.M. (1990). *Neuroscience Critical Care: Pathophysiology and Management.* Philadelphia: W.B. Saunders Co.

Springhouse Corporation. (1996). *Nurse Practitioner's Drug Handbook.* Philadelphia: Springhouse Corporation.

Walleck, C., & Mooney, K. (1994). Neurotrauma: Head injury. In E. Barker (ed.). *Neuroscience Nursing.* St. Louis: Mosby-Year Book, Inc.

Spinal Cord Injury

DEFINITION

Spinal cord injury is any injury to the spinal cord resulting from trauma. Injuries are classified by the area of the spine involved as follows:
1. Vertebral injury
    A. Simple fracture
    B. Compression fracture: Wedge, hyperflexion injury
    C. Comminuted fracture: Burst fracture with bone fragments
    D. Tear drop fracture: Small fragment from anterior edge breaks off
    E. Dislocation: One vertebra overrides the other
    F. Subluxation: Dislocation of one vertebra over another
    G. Fracture-dislocation
2. Spinal cord injury
    A. Concussion: Temporary loss of function 24–48 hours
    B. Contusion: Bruising of cord; possible necrosis
    C. Laceration: Permanent residual deficits
    D. Transection
    E. Hemorrhage
    F. Damage to blood vessels supplying cord

ETIOLOGY/INCIDENCE

The most common causes of spinal cord injury include vehicular accidents, diving accidents, falls, sports injuries, and gunshot wounds. The mechanisms of injury include flexion, extension, rotation, and compression. All are related to an excessive force being applied to the spine causing bone and tissue injury. In an incomplete injury, the spinal cord is injured but not transected or necrotic. In a complete injury, the spinal cord is either transected or has become necrotic due to prolonged ischemia.

Approximately 12,000 new spinal cord injuries occur each year. Of these, 4000 die before reaching the hospital. The ratio of males to females is 4:1. The peak age group affected is 20–24 years in males and 25–29 years in females.

PATHOPHYSIOLOGY

Spinal cord injury results from compression, contusion or transection of the spinal cord. In an unstable bony injury, if alignment is maintained, the spinal cord may be spared. Once injured, the spinal cord becomes edematous and may be further injured by the presence of bone fragments or other foreign bodies. A period of spinal shock begins. If no intervention is taken, the process of spinal cord necrosis begins. This is a rapid process related to vascular disruption, biochemical alteration (vasoactive amines which collect in wound tissue causing vasospasm), and neuronal effects which may lead to demyelination and liquification of spinal cord in severe disruption.

HISTORY

A thorough history of the accident is necessary to determine the probable pathology and treatment plan. Questions should include:

1. Exact time and place of accident?
2. Circumstances of injury?
3. Onset of symptoms immediately?
4. Any associated multisystem trauma?
5. Current symptoms?

The signs and symptoms will vary depending on the severity and location of injury. Refer to Table 4–13 for a detailed description.

PHYSICAL FINDINGS

Table 4–13 arranges the physical findings by the type of injury or syndrome.
   The single common finding with all types of traumatic spinal cord injury is pain with local tissue swelling at the site of injury.
   When assessing the physical findings of a patient with suspected spinal cord injury, neurologic localization is essential. Identifying the level of pre-

T A B L E 4–13.   Spinal Cord Injuries

Injury	Physical Findings
Anterior cord syndrome	Paralysis below level of injury; loss of pain and temperature sensations below level of injury; preservation of sensations of touch, motion, position, and vibration
Central cord syndrome	Motor weakness greater in upper than lower extremities; arm paralysis with lower motor neuron lesions; varying degrees of sensory deficits; varying severity of bladder/bowel dysfunction
Posterior cord syndrome	Intact motor function; loss of sense of touch, position, and vibration; dissociation between patient's perception of own ability and actual motor ability due to sensory loss
Brown-Séquard syndrome	Ipsilateral motor paralysis below level of injury; ipsilateral loss of position and vibration sense below level of injury; contralateral loss of pain and temperature sensation
Horner's syndrome	Ipsilateral findings—smaller pupil, eyeball sinks, eyelid droops, absence of facial sweating
Cauda equina syndrome	Ipsilateral dysesthesia and weakness of the lower extremity; because the cauda equina is the bundle of lumbar, sacral, and coccygeal peripheral nerve roots, recovery from cauda eguina injuries is possible as peripheral nerves are able to regenerate
Complete spinal cord transection	Below level of injury—flaccid, total paralysis of all skeletal muscles; loss of all spinal reflexes (deep tendon and superficial); loss of pain, proprioception, touch, temperature and pressure sensations; absence of somatic and visceral sensations; Above level of injury—hyperesthesia

TABLE 4–14. Levels of Spinal Cord Innervation

Level	Innervation
C5	Elbow flexors (biceps, brachialis)
C6	Wrist extensors (extensor carpi radialus longus and brevis)
C7	Elbow extensors (triceps)
C8	Finger flexors (flexor digitorum profundus) to the middle finger
T1	Small finger abductors (abductor digiti minimi)
L2	Hip flexors (iliopsoas)
L3	Knee extensors (quadriceps)
L4	Ankle dorsiflexors (tibialis anterior)
L5	Long toe extensors (extensor hallucis longus)
S1	Ankle plantarflexors (gastrocnemius soleus)

served function is done based on the affected muscle groups and whether or not the reflexes are present. Table 4–14 summarizes the different levels of spinal cord innervation.

Also necessary is identifying the patient's intact sensory level using a standard dermatome (see Fig. 4–1).

DIFFERENTIAL DIAGNOSIS

The diagnosis of a patient with a history of trauma to the spine and focal findings as above is usually unmistakable. The difficulty arises when attempting to determine the syndrome and/or fracture type as described above. Other possible diagnoses that should be considered, but are usually quickly ruled out based on radiographic tests, are ruptured intravertebral disc (herniated nucleus pulposus) and cauda equina syndrome.

DIAGNOSTIC TESTS/FINDINGS

1. Spine x-rays: Narrow to area of suspected injury (cervical, thoracic, lumbosacral).
2. CT scan of the spine: May be ordered but usually will not show clear pathology outside of bony structures; adjunct to plain x-ray for patient with fracture or subluxation.
3. MRI of spine: Clearly shows bone, spinal cord, nerve roots. May combine with MRA to evaluate spinal blood supply; most useful in patients with neurologic evidence of spinal cord injury in absence of fracture.
4. Laboratory: CBC, electrolytes, BUN, creatinine, toxicology/alcohol screen.
5. Somatosensory evoked potentials may determine completeness of spinal cord injury; useful in patients who are unable to cooperate with exam due to altered mental status.

MANAGEMENT/TREATMENT

1. At the scene: Immediate immobilization; maintain airway, breathing, and circulation.
2. Medications:
   A. Methylprednisolone 30 mg/kg load over 15 minutes within 8 hours of injury followed by 5.4 mg/kg/hr to begin 45 minutes after load and continue for 23 hours; must prophylax for stress ulcer while infusing this steroid—ranitidine (Zantac) 50 mg IV q12h

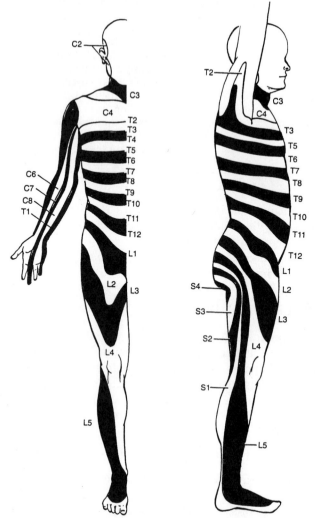

FIGURE 4–1. Cutaneous distribution of the spinal nerves (dermatomes). (From Conn, P.M. [1995]. *Neuroscience in Medicine.* Philadelphia: J.B. Lippincott, with permission.)

   B. Analgesia: Morphine 10 mg IM q4h prn

   C. Vasopressors: Titrate dopamine drip 1–10 μg/kg/min

3. Referral to or consultation with a neurosurgeon or orthopedic surgeon.
4. Surgery: Spinal stabilization with bony fusion and/or instrumentation—indicated for unstable fractures and/or in elderly patients. The procedure varies depending on type of fracture. Débridement of open wounds may also be required.
5. Nonsurgical immobilization (indicated for stable fractures): Immobilization of cervical fractures may be accomplished with a halo device or a cervical collar depending on the type of fracture. Immobilization of thoracic and lumbar fractures may be accomplished using a body cast or with a wide variety of commercial body jackets/vests that are available. The use of halos and body casts is also indicated for patients who may not be compliant with a device that can be removed.
6. Respiratory management: Mechanical ventilation as needed; chest physical therapy, quad coughing.

7. Nutrition: Early TPN, Peripheral Parenteral Nutrition (PPN), or enteral nutrition.
8. Prophylaxis against common complications:
   A. Deep vein thrombosis, pulmonary embolism
      1) Antiembolic hose
      2) Sequential compression devices
      3) Heparin 5000 U SQ bid
   B. Gastrointestinal (ulcer, paralytic ileus)
      1) Antacids around the clock
      2) Nasogastric decompression
      3) Ranitidine (Zantac) 150 mg PO bid or 50 mg IV q12h
   C. Pressure sores
      1) Kinetic therapy beds
      2) Frequent position change
   D. Pneumonia
      1) Assisted coughing
      2) Ventilatory support as needed
      3) Chest x-ray when indicated: Routine daily chest x-ray rarely performed any more

PATIENT EDUCATION

1. Medications: Dose, rationale, route, side effects, toxicity.
2. Procedures: Explain all tests and procedures prior to performing; obtain informed consent when necessary.
3. Disease course and expected outcome: Highly variable depending on severity of injury; be certain to be honest with family members especially when explaining prognosis.
4. Discharge planning: Explain care needs to patient and family; discuss expected length of rehabilitation.
5. Education and support: Refer to support groups and provide educational materials on injury, facilities, etc.

Review Questions

4.41 Sam is a 22-year-old construction worker who is brought to the trauma center following a 20-foot fall. He is fully conscious and complaining of severe lower back pain. On exam, he has no movement, sensation, or reflexes in his lower extremities. The first diagnostic test to be performed would be:
   A. A CT scan of the spine
   B. Vertebral x-rays
   C. An MRI of the spine
   D. Somatosensory evoked potentials
4.42 You immediately suspect that Sam has a spinal cord injury. In addition to immobilization, the first treatment measure for a patient with suspected spinal cord injury is:
   A. Analgesia
   B. Mechanical ventilation

C. Methylprednisolone IV bolus

D. Kinetic therapy

4.43 Sam has been moved to the acute care unit and has a confirmed burst fracture of L2. He is a complete paraplegic. He is awake and alert with stable vital signs. Of the following, which therapies would be appropriate for Sam?

A. Sequential compression device

B. Assisted coughing

C. Morphine 2–5 mg IV

D. All of the above

4.44 Bonnie is a 30-year-old woman who was out swimming in the lake when she dove off of the dock. Her husband saw her float to the top of the water 60 seconds later and pulled her out of the water. She was not breathing and received immediate cardiopulmonary resuscitation. An ambulance transported her to the emergency room. Bonnie remains unconscious and on exam has no respiratory effort, no response to deep pain, and no deep tendon reflexes. She is placed on a ventilator. Your primary concern is that Bonnie:

A. May have sustained a spinal cord injury

B. May have has a seizure

C. May have has a traumatic brain injury

D. May be suffering from drug or alcohol intoxication

4.45 Which of the following is true regarding the administration of methylprednisolone for acute spinal cord injury?

A. It must be started within 8 hours of injury.

B. A loading dose followed by a continuous infusion must be completed within 24 hours.

C. Prophylaxis against stress ulcers must be given during the infusion.

D. All of the above.

Answers and Rationales

4.41 **B** Vertebral x-rays may reveal a fracture that requires surgical stabilization or a bone fragment that must be emergently removed. In many cases, x-rays may be followed by CT or MRI to determine the amount of bony impingement of the spinal cord before surgery.

4.42 **C** Methylprednisolone must be given within 8 hours of injury. It is effective in minimizing secondary injury to the spinal cord by reducing the edema within the cord. Analgesia is also necessary but can be given after the methylprednisolone. Kinetic therapy beds and mechanical ventilation are routinely used only for patients with a cervical fracture and/or multiple trauma.

4.43 **A** Given Sam's current status, prophylaxis against deep venous thrombosis (DVT) would be appropriate utilizing sequential compression devices. Sam is stable, awake and alert, and able to cooperate with care. Appropriate analgesia at this time would be morphine IM or codeine SQ. He does not require assisted coughing, as this is usually reserved for quadraplegics.

4.44   **A**   Given the history and exam, a spinal cord injury is quite possible and should be assumed until proven otherwise.

4.45   **D**   All of these statements are true.

References

Cammermeyer, M., & Appeldorn, C. (1996). *Core Curriculum for Neuroscience Nursing* (3rd ed. update). Chicago: American Association of Neuroscience Nurses.

Doberstein, C., Rodts, G.E., & McBride, D.Q. (1994). Neurosurgical critical care. In F.S. Bongard & D.Y. Sue (eds.). *Current Critical Care Diagnosis and Treatment.* Norwalk, CT: Appleton & Lange.

Fehlings, M.G., & Louw, D. (1996). Initial stabilization and medical management of acute spinal cord injury. *Am Fam Physician 54*(1), 155–162.

Hickey, J.V., Cook, H. (1997). Vertebral and spinal cord injuries. In J.V. Hickey (ed.). *The Clinical Practice of Neurological and Neurosurgical Nursing* (4th ed.). Philadelphia: Lippincott-Raven.

Marshall, S.B., Marshall, L.F., Vos, H.R., & Chesnut, R.M. (1990). *Neuroscience Critical Care: Pathophysiology and Management.* Philadelphia: W.B. Saunders Co.

Springhouse Corporation. (1996). *Nurse Practitioner's Drug Handbook.* Philadelphia: Springhouse Corporation.

Walleck, C. (1994). Neurotrauma: Spinal cord injury. In E. Barker (ed.). *Neuroscience Nursing.* St. Louis: Mosby-Year Book, Inc.

Multiple Sclerosis

DEFINITION

Multiple sclerosis (MS) is a chronic, progressive, demyelinating disease of the CNS characterized by periods of remission and exacerbation. It is the most common neurologic disease afflicting young adults.

ETIOLOGY/INCIDENCE

The exact etiology remains unknown, although several theories have been proposed including:

1. Abnormality of immune regulation
2. Chronic infection of the CNS
3. Environmental factors encountered in childhood
4. Genetic predisposition

MS is becoming increasingly prevalent in the United States and Europe possibly due to increased longevity and better epidemiologic data collection. It is most prevalent among people living in northern climates, urban areas, in high socioeconomic groups, and in Caucasians (over 90% of patients in the United States are Caucasian). The overall prevalence in the United States averages 50 cases per 100,000. The risk increases incrementally (based on the closeness of the relation) if a family member is afflicted. The total number of cases in the United States today is approaching 350,000. The mean age at onset is 30 years and MS affects women three times as often as men.

PATHOPHYSIOLOGY

The principal findings in MS are multiple plaques in the brain and spinal cord. These plaques are characterized by demyelination of nerve fibers, gliosis, and inflammatory cells. The plaques range in size from 1–4 cm and are more prevalent in the white matter as well as in the periventricular regions of the brain stem (90% of patients), the optic nerves and chiasm, cerebellum, cerebrum, and cervical spinal cord.

These demyelinated plaques slow the speed and conduction of nerve impulses, which gives rise to the symptoms. The pathogenesis involved in the exacerbation and remission is not understood, but it has been postulated that this pattern is controlled to some degree by the immune response.

HISTORY

The family history and symptomatology are important to differentiate MS from other neurodegenerative disorders.

1. Family history of MS?
2. Symptoms:
    A. Visual disturbances (diplopia, nystagmus)
    B. Emotional lability
    C. Bowel, bladder, sexual dysfunction
    D. Impaired coordination
    E. Extremity weakness, numbness, aching
    F. Speech changes (slurring, stuttering)
    G. Dizziness, vertigo
3. Does anything aggravate symptoms?
    A. Heat
    B. Exercise
    C. Stress

PHYSICAL FINDINGS

The symptoms may be vague and may precede recognizable signs for many months or years—do not rule out diagnosis based on a normal exam. The following represent signs found during an exacerbation or in patients with longstanding symptoms and often are the presenting factors for which the patient has sought care.

1. General appearance: Normal to depressed; may have speech slurring
2. Eyes: Decreased visual acuity, nystagmus, pale optic discs, internuclear ophthalmoplegia
3. Skin: May see evidence of trauma from falls, burns, or pressure sores due to sensory deficit
4. Neurologic: Intention tremor, asymmetric weakness more common in lower extremities, atypical sensory loss—patchy, unable to correlate to a dermatome, impaired vibratory sensation and position sense, hyperreflexia with or without Babinski's sign, spastic gait, ataxia
5. Psychologic: Depression, mild dementia

DIFFERENTIAL DIAGNOSIS

Differential diagnoses vary depending on the symptomatology and duration of disease. Problems arise in diagnosing MS during the initial exacerbation and due to the fact that patients may present with progressive myelopathy or an uncommon pattern to their symptoms. Disorders that must be ruled out include:

1. Brain and spinal cord tumors
2. Neurosyphilis
3. Myasthenia gravis
4. Friedreich's ataxia
5. Conversion reaction
6. Chiari malformation
7. Collagen vascular disease (i.e., systemic lupus erythematosis)
8. HIV encephalopathy
9. Vitamin B_{12} deficiency

DIAGNOSTIC TESTS/FINDINGS

Kaufman (1996) wrote the following cautionary statement to clinicians:

> MS is diagnosed only when physiologically consistent symptoms and signs and laboratory tests converge to suggest involvement of white matter projections from multiple areas within the CNS. Signs and symptoms fluctuate with time. No other pathology can exist to explain the complaints and findings. The diagnosis is not secure without appropriate positive laboratory findings
>
> Many findings within the diagnostic exam are characteristic of MS and others serve to rule out other etiologies for the clinical findings.

1. Thorough history and physical exam.
2. Blood tests: Not indicated.
3. Radiologic tests: MRI scan much preferred to CT scan; may show plaques in the form of high-intensity areas involving brain and spinal cord on T2-weighting. Any enhancing areas are suggestive of acute inflammation. Possibility of false-positive and false-negative reading. Serial MRI is recommended to monitor progression of disease.
4. Lumbar puncture: Cerebrospinal fluid findings are most diagnostic; shows increased protein, lymphocytes, IgG, myelin basic protein; presence of oligoclonal bands; should always be preceded by MRI to rule out possibility of increased intracranial pressure.
5. Evoked potentials (visual, auditory, somatosensory): All will show prolonged impulse conduction with MS.
6. Urodynamic studies if indicated: Show abnormalities consistent with neurogenic bladder.
7. Psychological evaluation if conversion reaction or depression are suspected.

MANAGEMENT/TREATMENT

1. The nurse practitioner will consult with a neurologist as well as other members of the health care team (physical therapist, occupational therapist etc.) to discuss the treatment plan, especially for patients refractory to standard management.
2. Medications and therapies: Multidisciplinary approach.
   A. Symptomatic treatment
      1) Fatigue: Amantadine (Symmetrel) 100 mg PO bid, assess for depression

   2) Depression: Amitriptyline (Elavil) 25 mg bid–tid and counseling
   3) Spasticity: Baclofen (Lioresal) 5–20 mg PO tid and physical therapy
   4) Bladder spasms: Anticholinergics, timed voiding
   5) Urinary retention: Intermittent catheterization
   6) Constipation: Fiber, fluids, softeners, laxatives
   7) Neuralgia: Carbamazepine (Tegretol) initially 100 mg PO bid up to
      600–1400 mg/day usually combined with a tricyclic antidepressant
   8) Chronic aching: Antidepressants, phenothiazines
   9) Postural tremor: Propranolol (Inderal) 10–40 mg PO tid–qid
   B. Disease-specific
   1) Exacerbation: Methylprednisolone (Solu-Medrol) 0.5–1 gm IV daily
      for 3–7 days to speed recovery, followed by a prednisone taper of 60
      mg daily for 3 days and then decreasing the dose by increments of
      10 mg daily until discontinued; an alternative is adrenocorticotropic
      hormone (ACTH) 25–60 U IM or IV over 8 hours daily and tapered
      gradually over a 2 to 4-week period.
   2) Relapsing remitting: Interferon beta-1b (Betaseron) 8 million IU (0.25
      mg) SQ qod results in fewer relapses and MRI lesions. The new inter-
      feron beta-1a (Avonex) 3–9 million IU SQ three times weekly for 6
      months has been recently released.
   3) Progressive: Monthly IV boluses of cyclophosphamide (Cytoxan) and
      methylprednisolone (Solu-Medrol) in younger patients; low-dose aza-
      thioprine sodium (Imuran) 50–100 mg PO daily and methotrexate
      7.5–15 mg/wk have stabilized disease progression in some patients.
3. Physical therapy: For restoration of strength and maintenance of function,
   can be done in pool for patients with advanced disease or exacerbation.
4. Occupational therapy: Energy conservation while performing activities of
   daily living, adaptive devices.
5. Follow-up regularly depending on the patient's patterns of exacerbation and
   remission or disease progression; at least every 3–6 months and as needed.
6. Emergent and inpatient care of patients with multiple sclerosis is rarely
   necessary and is usually related to severe exacerbation.

PATIENT EDUCATION

1. Medications: Purpose, dosage, side effects, toxicity, necessary blood test
   monitoring. Advise patient to report any side effects as well as decreased
   effectiveness of regimen.
2. Diet: Stress importance of good nutrition and adequate hydration.
3. Activity: Stress importance of adequate rest and the need for regular exercise and physical and occupational therapy.
4. Environment: Avoid overheating, overexerting, and unnecessary stress all
   of which may exacerbate disease.
5. Elimination: Empty bladder every 2 hours to avoid retention or incontinence; teach self-catheterization if necessary; teach prevention of and proper
   treatment for constipation.
6. Disease course and expected outcome: Explain that MS is chronic and can
   be progressive—there is no cure and no way to prevent the disease. In some
   patients, the disease progresses to complete disability and may be fatal due
   to complications of immobility (pneumonia, aspiration, etc.). Explain that
   in most cases, symptoms can be controlled medically and patients live out
   their normal lifespan.

7. Encourage attendance at local support groups and the joining of national associations. Also encourage to wear a Medic Alert bracelet.

Review Questions

4.46 The exacerbations and remissions of multiple sclerosis are thought to be related to all of the following except:
A. The immune response
B. Cold climate
C. Stress
D. Exercise

4.47 The management plan for multiple sclerosis includes:
A. Symptomatic management with medication
B. Surgery to remove the plaques
C. Physical therapy
D. A and C

4.48 Jane is a 30-year-old white female who presents to the neurology clinic with a 2-year history of progressive visual disturbance, emotional lability, impaired coordination, extremity weakness and aching, and dizziness. She says that she notices the symptoms more on very warm days and just after going to the gym. Given Jane's history, the most likely diagnosis is:
A. Multiple sclerosis
B. Myasthenia gravis
C. Brain tumor
D. Exhaustion

4.49 Due to your suspected diagnosis, which of the following diagnostic tests would most rapidly confirm your suspicion?
A. Tensilon challenge test
B. An MRI of the brain
C. A lumbar puncture with CSF analysis
D. Evoked potentials

4.50 Three months later, Jane presents in the ER with an acute exacerbation of her disease. She has profound lower extremity weakness and is unable to perform her activities of daily living or ambulate unassisted. She is very depressed about her condition. Which of the following therapies would be indicated for Jane in her current condition?
A. Admit to the hospital
B. Administer methylprednisolone 250 mg IV q6h for 3–5 days
C. Order a psychological evaluation
D. All of the above

Answers and Rationales

4.46 **B** The symptoms of multiple sclerosis are aggravated by heat, exercise, and stress and are related to the immune response. Cold has not been shown to cause exacerbations.

4.47 **D** There is no cure for multiple sclerosis. The symptoms are managed medically with medications, physical and occupational therapy, counseling, and follow-up. Patient education is crucial. There is no surgical procedure to remove the plaques, as they are diffusely present throughout the central nervous system.

4.48　**A**　Jane's clinical picture is classic for the onset of multiple sclerosis.

4.49　**C**　Jane has the early symptoms of multiple sclerosis. Although there is no way to definitively diagnose this disease, the CSF often will show changes such as increased protein. An MRI and evoked potentials do not usually show changes until later in the disease progression. A tensilon challenge test is indicated when myasthenia gravis is suspected.

4.50　**D**　Jane is unable to function and is depressed. She requires a more thorough evaluation and acute management. All of these interventions would be appropriate.

References

Adams, R.D., & Victor, M. (1993). *Principles of Neurology* (5th ed.). New York: McGraw-Hill.

Donohoe, K. (1994). Autoimmune disorders. In E. Barker (ed.). *Neuroscience Nursing*. St. Louis: Mosby-Year Book, Inc.

Hickey, J.V., & Cook, H. (1997). Selected degenerative diseases of the nervous system. In J.V. Hickey (ed.). *The Clinical Practice of Neurological and Neurosurgical Nursing* (4th ed.). Philadelphia: Lippincott-Raven.

Kaufman, M.D. (1996). Multiple sclerosis. In R.E. Rakel (ed.). *Saunders Manual of Medical Practice.* Philadelphia: W.B. Saunders Co.

Springhouse Corporation. (1996). *Nurse Practitioner's Drug Handbook.* Philadelphia: Springhouse Corporation.

van Oosten, B.W., et al. (1995). Multiple sclerosis therapy: A practical guide. *Drugs* 49(2), 200–212.

Williams, R., Rigby, A.S., Airey, M., et al. (1995). Multiple sclerosis: Its epidemiological, genetic, and health care impact. *J Epidemiol Commun Health 49,* 563–569.

Myasthenia Gravis

DEFINITION

Myasthenia gravis (MG) is a progressive autoimmune disorder of the nervous system that causes sporadic weakness of the skeletal or voluntary muscles predominantly in the face, lips, tongue, neck, and throat. It can, however, manifest as weakness in any muscle group.

ETIOLOGY/INCIDENCE

Adult MG is a chronic autoimmune disease. It is thought to be due to T cells and various antibodies attacking and impairing or destroying the nicotinic acetylcholine receptors at the motor end-plate. A tumor of the thymus gland has been found in up to 10% of patients with MG, although this has not been definitely identified as a risk factor or etiology. Juvenile MG is also autoimmune with an earlier onset. Congenital MG is not autoimmune related, but is caused by many other neuromuscular defects.

MG is an uncommon disease with a wide variety of published prevalence rates ranging from 0.5–14.2 per 100,000 (Phillips, 1994). It is known that the prevalence has risen steadily since the 1950s, when data collection began. This is due to an increased lifespan of MG patients secondary to improving treatment. The National Myasthenia Gravis Foundation estimates that there are at least 100,000 patients in the United States with MG and another 25,000 yet undiagnosed. The incidence is highest in women ages 18–25 and in men ages 50–60 with a 3:2 predominance in women. No other demographic pattern exists.

PATHOPHYSIOLOGY

MG is caused by a deficiency in the amount of normal, active acetylcholine receptors at the postsynaptic membrane of the neuromuscular junction. The amount of acetylcholine at the neuromuscular junction is normal; however, there is a reduced number of normal acetylcholine receptors on which they are able to bind. The patient's body produces antibodies against the acetylcholine receptors and these cause the destruction of the receptors via a process of T-cell–mediated immunity. This is theorized to occur after sensitization in the thymus to a protein that appears similar to the acetylcholine receptor.

HISTORY

1. Family history present in 10–20%
2. Symptoms:
   A. Voluntary muscle weakness exacerbated by continuous use, warmer climate, stress
   B. Increased fatigue
   C. Diplopia
   D. Dysphagia
   E. Difficulty/weakness chewing
   F. Difficulty swallowing/choking
   G. Fluid regurgitation through nose when drinking
   H. Progressive hypophonia

PHYSICAL FINDINGS

Clinical findings are often vague, making early diagnosis difficult. Commonly, MG patients are diagnosed only after complications ranging from falls to aspiration pneumonia. The signs and symptoms that should point the practitioner in the direction of MG are related to ocular and oral weaknesses.
1. General appearance: May be emaciated due to difficulty eating
2. Vital signs: Usually normal, may see orthostatic hypotension with dehydration
3. Skin: Poor turgor due to decreased fluid intake, possibly dehydration
4. Eyes: Diminished visual acuity, visual field deficit, ptosis, strabismus
5. Mouth: Excess salivation (due to inability to swallow), possibly drooling in severe cases, diminished tongue strength
6. Neurologic: Generalized muscle weakness occurs in descending pattern with the muscles innervated by cranial nerves becoming weak most commonly (order or involvement is ocular, bulbar, neck, proximal extremity, and distal extremity)

T A B L E 4-15.   Myasthenic Versus Cholinergic Crisis

	Myasthenic Crisis	Cholinergic Crisis
Cause	No apparent cause An infection is a common precipitating event	Precipitated by the toxic effects of cholinesterase inhibitors; a problem of over medication
Presentation	The patient's usual myasthenic symptoms but more intense Swallowing and respiratory difficulty may be severe	Abdominal cramping and diarrhea Generalized weakness Excessive pulmonary secretions Impaired respiratory function
Diagnosis	By exam Improved muscle strength when Tensilon is injected IV	By exam No improvement or deterioration in muscle strength when Tensilon is injected
Management	Ventilatory support for vital capacity of <1000 (use as guideline for elective intubation) Plasma phoresis or IVIG Temporary withholding of cholinesterase inhibitors Resume cholinesterase inhibitors in 2–3 days if patient shows responsiveness to them—the best dosage and combination of drugs must be determined	Same as for myasthenic crisis except that plasma phoresis usually not indicated

IVIG, intravenous immunoglobulin.

Patients with myasthenia gravis can go into a crisis state. Two such states exist: myasthenic crisis and cholinergic crisis. These two conditions are summarized in Table 4–15.

DIFFERENTIAL DIAGNOSIS

1. Eaton-Lambert syndrome
2. Amyotrophic lateral sclerosis (Lou Gehrig's disease)
3. Space-occupying brain lesion (tumor, hemorrhage)
4. Muscular dystrophy

DIAGNOSTIC TESTS/FINDINGS

A single test is insufficient to diagnose MG or to rule out other differential diagnoses. Three tests are required for diagnosis. If they do not confirm MG, other studies would be required (such as MRI, LP, blood tests) to determine the cause of symptoms.

1. Acetylcholine antibody assay: Elevated up to 95% of the time in MG patients (less in patients exhibiting ocular only symptoms)
2. Tensilon (edrophonium) challenge test: Patients are given IV Tensilon; the test is positive for the diagnosis of MG if muscle strength improves; false-negatives have been reported with ocular MG.

3. Electromyography (EMG): A nerve stimulation test showing sp⌐ stimulation and muscle contraction; muscle response time is slo⌐ MG

MANAGEMENT/TREATMENT

1. Medications:
   A. Acetylcholinesterase inhibitors: Dosage must be individualized depending on response and tolerance of adverse side effects.
      1) Pyridostigmine (Mestinon) 30–120 mg q4h while awake
      2) Pyridostigmine 180 mg timed-released tablets are available for patients to take every night at bedtime if they suffer from nocturnal weakness or weakness on arising.
      3) Neostigmine bromide (Prostigmin) initially 15–30 mg PO tid (range is 15–375 mg daily).
   B. Immunosupressants
      1) Prednisone 10–25 mg daily, increase by 10 mg daily until improvement is noted and maintain dose until maximum improvement is noted; then taper slowly to lowest possible dose to maintain desired effect.
      2) Azathioprine (Imuran) is a second-line choice after prednisone or if prednisone cannot be used; gradually increase dose to 150–200 mg/day. Onset of improvement is gradual, often taking up to 12 months; after 12–24 months of improvement, the drug can be gradually tapered and discontinued.
      3) Cyclophosphamide (Cytoxan) is rarely used any more due to toxicity.
   C. Adjunct medications for side effects
      1) Atropine 0.4 mg PO bid: Diarrhea/salivation from acetylcholinesterase inhibitors
      2) Potassium chloride, calcium carbonate, vitamin D supplement: Decreased levels from steroids
      3) Antacids: Nausea, vomiting from immunosuppressants
2. Consultation with neurologist regarding treatment plan and for patients who are refractory to traditional therapy; ACNP in consultation with neurologist would refer to surgeon for thymectomy if indicated.
3. Plasmaphoresis and plasma exchange to cleanse the body of these abnormal acetylcholine receptor antibodies; only gives short-term improvement and must be performed regularly; especially useful in acute myasthenic crisis, which is manifested by severe motor weakness and respiratory muscle involvement. The procedure takes 3–5 hours and treatment usually consists of a course of five treatments over a 2-week period.
4. Intravenous immunoglobulin (IVIG) is indicated for short-term treatment of a serious relapse of myasthenia. Improvement occurs within 4–5 days.
5. Thymectomy has become common and leads to improvement in almost all MG patients, although improvement is not as pronounced in patients with ocular MG.
6. Diet: High protein, high fiber, sources of potassium and calcium, restrict calories only if excessive weight gain in prednisone.
7. Follow-up every 2 weeks for first 3 months after diagnosis to determine responsiveness to treatment and reinforce treatment.

•UCATION

ns: Purpose, dosage, side effects, toxicity; necessary blood monitor-
:ertain drugs (e.g., potassium with prednisone, CBC with other
ippressants). Certain medications may exacerbate myasthenic
:akness. They include pancuronium, vecuronium, quinine, quini-
ainamide, gentamicin, kanamycin, neomycin, streptomycin, clin-
lindomycin, trimethadione, morphine, chloroquine, β-blockers,
1annel blockers, and d-penicillamine. Myasthenics should always
ir physician prior to beginning any new medication, as several
otner medications may intensify muscle weakness.

2. Diet: As above.
3. Activity: Exertion may exacerbate symptoms.
4. Environment: Warm temperatures may exacerbate symptoms.
5. Disease course and expected outcome: Explain that MG is a chronic disease for which there is no cure; it is characterized by periods of exacerbation and remission; there is no way to prevent its occurrence; most patients can be controlled on medication and live out their full expected lifespan.
6. Instruct patient that they should wear a Medic Alert bracelet.

Review Questions

4.51 The following diagnostic tests may assist in the diagnosis of MG:
   A. Acetylcholine antibody assay
   B. Tensilon challenge test
   C. EMG
   D. All of the above

4.52 The procedure that cleanses the body of acetylcholine receptor antibodies and gives short-term improvement for MG patients is called:
   A. Thymectomy
   B. Plasmapheresis
   C. Dialysis
   D. Immunosuppression

4.53 Mary is a 20-year-old student who presents to the ER with sudden onset of severe muscle weakness, drooling, and respiratory difficulty. She has a history of myasthenia gravis. You administer Tensilon and Mary shows no improvement in muscle strength. You suspect that Mary is experiencing:
   A. Myasthenic crisis
   B. Cholinergic crisis
   C. Pneumonia
   D. Pulmonary embolism

4.54 Assuming your above diagnosis is correct, what other symptoms would you assess Mary for?
   A. Diarrhea, abdominal cramping
   B. Diplopia
   C. Difficulty swallowing
   D. Headache

4.55 As previously stated, Mary is having respiratory difficulty. Which of the following facts would indicate that elective intubation is advisable?

A. Respiratory rate of 32
B. Excessive respiratory secretions
C. Vital capacity of <1000
D. Inability to manage oral secretions

Answers and Rationales

4.51 **D** All of the tests listed may assist in making the diagnosis of MG. If the diagnosis is still unclear, further tests must be performed to determine the cause of the patient's symptoms.

4.52 **B** Plasmapheresis is the test described and must be performed regularly. Thymectomy is a surgical procedure that has led to improvement in most MG patients. Immunosuppressants may be used orally or intravenously on a regular basis. Dialysis is not effective in cleansing the blood of the receptor antibodies responsible for MG.

4.53 **B** Given Mary's history, symptoms, and no response to Tensilon, a cholinergic crisis is likely.

4.54 **A** Diarrhea and abdominal cramping are additional symptoms to cholinesterase inhibitor toxicity. The other signs mentioned are those of myasthenia gravis and are frequently not present due to the excess of medication on board.

4.55 **C** All of these facts indicate respiratory difficulty, but elective intubation is indicated for a vital capacity <1000.

References

Adams, R.D., & Victor, M. (1993). *Principles of Neurology* (5th ed.). New York: McGraw-Hill.

Donohoe, K. (1994). Autoimmune disorders. In E. Barker (ed.). *Neuroscience Nursing.* St. Louis: Mosby-Year Book, Inc.

Hart, J.J. (1996). Myasthenia gravis. In R.E. Rakel (ed.). *Saunders Manual of Medical Practice.* Philadelphia: W.B. Saunders Co.

Hickey, J.V., & Cook, H. (1997). Selected degenerative diseases of the nervous system. In J.V. Hickey (ed.). *The Clinical Practice of Neurological and Neurosurgical Nursing* (4th ed.). Philadelphia: Lippincott-Raven.

Juhn, M.S. (1993). Myasthenia gravis: Diagnostic method and control measures for a chronic disease. *Postgrad Med 94*(5), 161–174.

Phillips, L.H. (1994). The epidemiology of myasthenia gravis. *Neurol Clin North Am 12*(2), 263–271.

Springhouse Corporation. (1996). *Nurse Practitioner's Drug Handbook.* Philadelphia: Springhouse Corporation.

Guillain-Barré Syndrome (Acute Idiopathic Polyneuropathy)

DEFINITION

Guillain-Barré syndrome (GBS) is an acute form of polyneuritis thought to be due to an autoimmune process within the peripheral nervous system. GBS is characterized by rapidly progressive, symmetric motor weakness and can be fatal if the diaphragm becomes involved or due to the complications of immobility.

CLASSIFICATIONS

There are three different classifications of GBS according to symptomatology. They are, in order of incidence:

1. Ascending GBS: Weakness and paresthesia/dysasthesia begins in legs and ascends to trunk, arms, and cranial nerves; respiratory distress in 50% of patients; most common presentation (a less common pure motor type of ascending GBS also exists, although usually milder and without dysasthesia).
2. Descending GBS: Weakness and paresthesia/dysasthesia begins in the areas innervated by the cranial nerves and descends to the trunk and extremities; rapid respiratory involvement in most patients.
3. Miller-Fisher variant GBS: Ataxia, ophthalmoplegia, areflexia, no sensory symptoms, respiratory difficulty uncommon.

ETIOLOGY/INCIDENCE

GBS is currently the most common cause of acute nontraumatic paralysis in the United States, as polio has been virtually eliminated. The published annual incidence rates vary from 0.4 to 1.7 per 100,000. GBS is thought to be slightly more common in women. There are two peak age groups—young adults and adults from 50–80 years old. GBS seems to occur most often during the "cold and flu" season (fall, winter) but this fact has not been proven demographically.

Etiology

The exact cause of GBS is not known. It is thought to be due to demyelination of the peripheral nerves through a cell-mediated autoimmune reaction. Precipitating factors are thought to play a major role in the development of this condition:

1. Infection: 60–70% of patients with GBS report a recent respiratory or gastrointestinal infection that may be viral or bacterial; viral infections include cytomegalovirus (CMV), Epstein-Barr virus (EBV), HSV, herpes zaster virus (HZV), influenza A, measles, mumps, rubella, adenovirus, enteric cytopathic human orphan (ECHO), coxsackie, hepatitis B virus (HBV), HIV; bacterial infections include *Mycoplasma, H. pylori, Borrelia burgdoferi.*
2. Surgery: 5–10% of patients with GBS report recent surgery and/or the use of spinal/epidural anesthesia.
3. Vaccination: A small percent age of GBS patients report having received vaccines within 8 weeks prior to the onset of GBS symptoms (antirabies, swine influenza, oral polio).

PATHOPHYSIOLOGY

GBS is an acute, acquired, inflammatory disease involving demyelination of peripheral nerve fibers with sparing of the axons. The term "acute inflamma-

tory demyelinating polyneuropathy" (AIDP) is also used to identif
inflammation that results in myelin destruction is thought to be
autoimmune reaction following a recent systemic or localized infec
by certain viral or bacterial organisms. GBS patients have areas of fc
tion by T-cell lymphocytes and macrophages in a segmental pattern throughout
cranial nerve, autonomic, motor, and sensory pathways. These macrophages
attack and progressively destroy the myelin, which slows and eventually blocks
the conduction of nerve impulses to muscles, resulting in motor weakness, paralysis, and sensory disturbance and loss. IgM antibodies selective against myelin have been found in the serum of GBS patients.

History

1. Any recent illness? Surgery? Vaccination?
2. Any recent trauma to spine or peripheral nerves?
3. Any family history of nervous system disorders (MS, MG, chronic inflamma-
   tory demyelinating polyneuropathy [CIDP])?
4. Symptoms:
   A. Weakness: Where/when did it begin?
   B. Sensory changes: Where/when did it begin?
   C. Pain (neuralgia) lower extremities, flank, back
   D. Difficulty swallowing, talking
   E. Difficulty breathing
   F. Impaired balance
   G. Visual changes
   H. Acute/subacute, progression of symptoms

PHYSICAL FINDINGS

1. General appearance: May be in respiratory distress, anxious
2. Vital signs: Orthostatic hypotension, tachycardia, irregular heart beat, tachypnea
3. Skin: Diaphoresis
4. Cardiovascular: Dysrhythmia, hemodynamic instability
5. Respiratory: Tachypnea, may hear adventitious sounds due to aspiration
6. Genitourinary: Bladder distention due to urinary retention
7. Abdomen: Diminished bowel sounds, abdominal distention
8. Neurologic: Pupillary abnormality, cranial nerve dysfunction, generalized
   motor weakness or paralysis, sensory abnormalities, areflexia or hyporeflexia

DIFFERENTIAL DIAGNOSIS

1. Poliomyelitis: Purely motor with areflexia
2. Myasthenia gravis: No sensory or reflex involvement
3. Botulism: Associated bradycardia
4. Tick paralysis: No sensory loss

DIAGNOSTIC TESTS/FINDINGS

1. Lumbar puncture with CSF studies: Increased protein, few or no cells, normal opening pressure
2. Nerve conduction studies: Demyelination evidenced by reduction in the amplitude of the muscle action potential with distal nerve stimulation

MANAGEMENT/TREATMENT

1. Consultation with neurologist, physiatrist, and necessary surgeons to implement management plan
2. Medical: Hospitalization mandatory!
   A. Respiratory support: Hourly assessment of vital capacity; intubation and mechanical ventilation may be necessary (indicated for vital capacity <1000); tracheostomy for long-term ventilatory support.
   B. Cardiovascular support: Electrocardiograph (ECG), arterial line, may require hemodynamic monitoring with pulmonary artery (PA) catheter, temporary pacing for complete heart block or symptomatic bradycardia, adequate hydration and volume expansion.
   C. Nutrition: Early TPN; PEG tube if necessary to prevent aspiration.
   D. Plasmaphoresis may reduce duration and severity of symptoms; must be started 7–14 days after onset of the disease to be effective; 3–4 treatments 1–2 days apart is customary with a second course of treatment for those patients who deteriorate after the first round.
   E. Pain management with nonsteroidal anti-inflammatory drugs (NSAIDs), antidepressants (Elavil), or narcotic analgesia.
   F. Adjunctive therapies to prevent complications (nosocomial infections, aspiration, pneumonia, pulmonary embolus, gastrointestinal (GI) bleed, cardiac failure, respiratory failure, joint contractures, pressure sores) are necessary: physiotherapy to chest and extremities, specialty beds, antiembolic hose, routine urine/sputum cultures, etc.
3. Early rehabilitation
   A. Physical therapy, occupational therapy
   B. Speech therapy for treatment and swallowing evaluation
4. Psychosocial support and counseling
5. Discharge planning: Over 80% of patients require inpatient rehabilitation for short stay or several months; 10% of patients have severe residual disability that may require placement in a long-term care facility.
6. Follow-up dependent on disposition and condition.

PATIENT EDUCATION

1. Medications: Dosage, frequency, purpose, side effects, toxicity.
2. Diet: Explain why patient may not have oral food and fluids; importance of adequate nutrition and hydration during acute and rehabilitation phases of treatment through any available route.
3. Diagnostic and treatment procedures: Full explanation must precede procedure as well as obtaining informed consent when necessary.
4. Discharge planning: Explain that patients will likely not go straight home from hospital but will go to a rehabilitation program; telling the patient and family this early will assist them in selecting a suitable location for postacute care.

5. Disease course and expected outcome: Explain that GBS is likely secondary to a preceding viral or bacterial illness that probably could not have been prevented; explain that 90% of patients recover fully without residual symptoms but that this may take several months; explain that 10% of patients will have severe disability and that 3% may go on to have recurrent episodes of acute neuropathy or develop CIDP.

Review Questions

4.56 All of the following are true about the CSF of a patient with GBS except:
   A. Elevated protein
   B. Decreased glucose
   C. Few or no cells
   D. Normal opening pressure

4.57 One characteristic that differentiates GBS from other similar neurologic illnesses is:
   A. Motor weakness or paralysis
   B. Sensory disturbance
   C. Neuralgia
   D. Diminished bowel sounds

4.58 Bob is a 23-year-old white male who is brought to the ER by his roommate, complaining of profound weakness in all four extremities, back pain, and lower extremity "pins and needles." His only medical history is about of bronchitis 2 weeks ago. On exam, Bob's muscle strength ranges from 2–3 in all muscle groups. He is diaphoretic, tachypneic, tachycardiac, and mildly hypotensive at 88/50. The most likely diagnosis is:
   A. Spinal cord injury
   B. Multiple sclerosis
   C. Guillain-Barré syndrome
   D. Septicemia

4.59 Bob begins to have difficulty breathing. His respirations are shallow with the use of abdominal muscles at a rate of 40 per minute. His vital capacity is 900. The most appropriate intervention at this time would be to:
   A. Intubate and place on a ventilator
   B. Order an albuterol breathing treatment
   C. Try to calm Bob down, he is just hyperventilating
   D. Order an aminophylline drip

4.60 Bob is being admitted to the neurointensive care unit (ICU). All of the following would be included in his admitting orders EXCEPT:
   A. Arterial line to continuously monitor
   B. Schedule for plasma phoresis in A.M.
   C. Morphine sulfate 2 mg IV q2h prn
   D. Elavil 25 mg PO qid

Answers and Rationales

4.56   **B**   The CSF of a GBS patient shows elevated protein, few or no cells, and normal opening pressure.

4.57   **C**   The complaint of neuralgia in the flank, back, and lower extremities is very common with GBS and helps to differentiate it from other neurologic illnesses. This pain may be severe and must be adequately treated, especially in the patient who is unable to communicate. Controlling the pain may require narcotic analgesia and/or Elavil.

4.58   **C**   Bob's history and presentation are classic for GBS. His neuralgia, weakness, and recent history of upper respiratory infection should clue the practitioner in to this diagnosis.

4.59   **A**   With GBS, the patient's respiratory status often declines rapidly and it takes several days for them to improve. The practitioner should intubate electively now due to the fact that Bob's vital capacity is <1000 and he is in obvious distress.

5.60   **B**   Steroids have not been found to be helpful in the treatment of GBS. Plasma phoresis may reduce the duration and severity of symptoms but should not commence until 7–14 days after onset. Morphine is acceptable to control Bob's acute pain and Elavil is known to be effective treatment for neuralgia. An arterial line is mandatory to monitor Bob's blood pressure and ABGs. A PA catheter may also be necessary if Bob's hemodynamic status deteriorates.

References

Adams, R.D., & Victor, M. (1993). *Principles of Neurology* (5th ed.). New York: McGraw-Hill.

Dematteis, J.A. (1996). Guillain-Barre syndrome: A team approach to diagnosis and treatment. *Am Fam Physician 54*(1), 197–200.

Donohoe, K. (1994). Autoimmune disorders. In E. Barker (ed.). *Neuroscience Nursing.* St. Louis: Mosby-Year Book, Inc.

Harjai, K.J. (1996). Guillain-Barre syndrome. In R.E. Rakel (ed.). *Saunders Manual of Medical Practice.* Philadelphia: W.B. Saunders Co.

Hickey, J.V., & Cook, H. (1997). Selected degenerative diseases of the nervous system. In J.V. Hickey (ed.). *The Clinical Practice of Neurological and Neurosurgical Nursing* (4th ed.). Philadelphia: Lippincott-Raven.

Marshall, S.B., Marshall, L.F., Vos, H.R., & Chesnut, R.M. (1990). *Neuroscience Critical Care: Pathophysiology and Management.* Philadelphia: W.B. Saunders Co.

Sheth, R.D., Riggs, J.E., Hobbs, G.R., & Gutman, L. (1996). Age and Guillain-Barre syndrome severity. *Muscle Nerve 19*, 375–377.

Springhouse Corporation. (1996). *Nurse Practitioner's Drug Handbook.* Philadelphia: Springhouse Corporation.

Parkinson's Disease (Paralysis Agitans)

DEFINITION

Parkinson's disease (PD) is a chronic, slowly progressive, degenerative condition resulting in impaired voluntary movement and loss of control of the autonomic nervous system. The course of PD may span more than 10 years and usually results in death due to complications such as aspiration or other infection. The disease progression is described by the Hoehn-Yahr staging scale and is based on the severity of symptoms and disability as follows:

Stage 0: No signs of disease
Stage I: Unilateral disease
Stage II: Bilateral or midline involvement
Stage III: Stage II plus impaired balance
Stage IV: Severe disability, unable to walk
Stage V: Wheelchair-bound, bedridden

ETIOLOGY/INCIDENCE

Although PD is considered idiopathic, there may be some etiologic correlation
between parkinsonism and encephalitis, head trauma, cerebral ischemia, long-
term use of certain drugs (primarily phenothiazines and reserpine), and exposure to certain toxins. Quite often, parkinsonian symptoms from a reversible
cause are misdiagnosed as PD.

It is estimated that as many as 1 million Americans suffer from PD and as
the number of persons over 60 years of age increases, so too does the incidence of
PD. This disease strikes approximately 1 in 100 persons over the age of 60.
Over 40,000 new cases are diagnosed each year in the United States. It effects
men slightly more often than women. The mean age at onset is between 58
and 62 years.

PATHOPHYSIOLOGY

Parkinson's disease is an idiopathic condition resulting from a degeneration
and depigmentation of the substantia nigra, which leads to a deficiency of the
inhibitory neurotransmitter dopamine. This loss of dopamine is thought to account for many of the hypotonic motor symptoms experienced.

HISTORY

An accurate history from the patient is critical in differentiating Parkinson's
disease from potentially reversible parkinsonian symptoms.

1. Medical history
   A. Head trauma
   B. Stroke
   C. Encephalitis
   D. Current medications
2. Specific symptoms
   A. Gait/posture disturbance: Stooped position and poor balance leading to
      falls; shuffling gait
   B. Slowing or difficulty initiating movements (bradykinesia)
   C. Stiffness (cogwheel rigidity)
   D. Resting tremor of hands: Exaggerated by anxiety, absent during sleep,
      decreased during purposeful movement; an action tremor may be present
      in some cases, usually only in advanced disease
   E. Muscle cramps and aching
   F. Constipation
   G. Urinary frequency and stress incontinence
   H. Speech difficulty: Slurring, hypophonic
   I. Dementia: Progressive memory difficulty, recent occurs first followed by
      distant

3. Nonspecific complaints from patient and family leading to discovery of symptoms
   A. Falling frequently
   B. Difficulty grooming, dressing, feeding
   C. Walking slower
   D. Never smiles
   E. Dizziness
   F. Generalized aches
   G. Arms shake when patient becomes angry, sad
   H. Speaks very softly
   I. Excessive sweating
   J. Difficulty swallowing
   K. Can't read their writing, it's so small (micrographia)
4. Onset/progression of symptoms
   A. At what age did first symptom appear?
   B. Insidious onset is typical with progression over years.

PHYSICAL FINDINGS

Use of the mnemonic TRAP will assist the practitioner to cover all areas of exam: *T*remor, *R*igidity, *A*kinesia, and *P*ostural hypotension.

1. General appearance: Masked facies; hypophonic, slow, monotonous speech; palilalia (involuntary sentence repetition) and echolalia in advanced disease; patient sits immobile on examining table and is slow to respond to commands (bradykinesia).
2. Vital signs: Orthostatic hypotension.
3. Skin: Seborrheic dermatitis, greasy face, excess perspiration.
4. Eyes: Decreased eyeblink, impairment of upward gaze and convergence, positive glabellar reflex (uncontrollable blinking when tap on forehead) or Myerson's sign (uncontrollable blinking when tap on bridge of nose).
5. Mouth: Drooling.
6. Abdomen: Diminished bowel sounds, possible fecal mass if constipated.
7. Musculoskeletal system: Digital impedance, rigidity of extremities, either jerky ("cogwheel") or smooth ("lead pipe"); pill rolling tremor with thumb and index finger unilateral or bilateral; in advanced disease, will see tremor spread to other extremities, lips, tongue, jaw, etc. Rigidity and tremor are usually presenting signs.
8. Neurologic: Gait disturbance with decreased balance, lack of arm swing, small and shuffling steps, inability to turn torso without turning rest of body (en bloc).
9. Psychological: Dementia, depression, anxiety.

The early signs of PD are blepharoclonus, Myerson's sign, digital impedance, and lack of arm swing. These may be the only abnormalities in the exam in a patient presenting with PD.

DIFFERENTIAL DIAGNOSIS

1. Parkinsonism with the following associated syndromes can be differentiated from idiopathic Parkinson's disease:
   A. With ocular dysmotility can indicate progressive supranuclear palsy
   B. With cerebellar signs and symptoms can indicate olivopontocerebellar degeneration

C. With autonomic insufficiency can indicate Shy-Drager syndrome (multiple system atrophy)
2. Secondary parkinsonism must be considered, especially in younger patients: Parkinsonian symptoms due to head trauma, hyperparathyroidism, encephalitis, toxins and occupational exposures (carbon tetrachloride, carbon monoxide, cyanide, methanol), drugs (Compazine, Reglan, Haldol, reserpine, lithium)
3. Essential tremor: Differentiated from Parkinson tremor as it is a kinetic, not resting, tremor of the hands and head in the absence of bradykinesia and rigidity
4. Depression: Main manifestation is psychomotor slowing with most other parkinsonian features absent
5. Normal pressure hydrocephalus

DIAGNOSTIC TESTS/FINDINGS

Clinical presentation is virtually diagnostic, as there are no definitive tests. Further diagnostic tests are performed to rule out other possible causes for parkinsonian symptoms.

1. Blood tests: CBC, toxicology screen, urinalysis, specific chemistry—all performed to rule out other causes for symptoms.
2. Radiologic tests: CT scan or MRI to rule out hydrocephalus, ischemia, infarct, focal lesion if history of head trauma; usually normal or show mild atrophy consistent with age; advanced cases of PD may show increased cortical atrophy and ventricular dilatation.
3. Lumbar puncture: Perform if CNS infection is suspected; usually normal.
4. EEG: may see generalized slowing, but usually normal.
5. Psychological assessment: Rule out depression as cause or effect of parkinsonism.

MANAGEMENT/TREATMENT

Treatment is aimed at controlling or reducing symptoms; no treatment has been shown to definitively slow the progression.

1. Medications: Many have disturbing side effects that can become severe and symptoms may become refractory to medication, either of which necessitates a "drug holiday" for 3–7 days and then restarting medication at the lowest effective dose. The following medications have proven to reduce the symptoms of PD:
   A. Dopaminergics to reduce rigidity, bradykinesia
      1) Levodopa-carbidopa (Sinemet): Dosing varies widely in strength and frequency; pills come as Sinemet 10/100, 25/100, and 25/250 with the first number indicating the dose in milligrams of carbidopa and the second number being the dose in milligrams of levodopa. The maximum daily dose is 200 mg of carbidopa and 2000 mg of levodopa.
      2) Amantidine (Symmetrel): 100 mg PO bid or tid; useful for patients who have a decreased response to or are on maximum doses of Sinemet.
   B. Anticholinergics to reduce tremor, rigidity
      1) Trihexyphenidyl (Artane): 1 mg PO on day 1, 2 mg PO on day 2, then increase 2 mg every 3–5 days until a total of 6–10 mg is given daily usually divided tid with meals

> 2) Benztropine mesylate (Cogentin): Initially 0.5–1 mg daily, increased 0.5 mg every 5–6 days to maximum of 6 mg daily divided bid or tid
>
> C. Dopamine agonists to control motor fluctuations
>> 1) Bromocriptine (Parlodel): Initial dose of 1.25 mg PO bid with meals; may increase every 14–28 days up to 100 mg daily until maximal therapeutic response is achieved
>> 2) Pergolide mesylate (Permax): Approved only as an adjunct to the use of levodopa-carbidopa; initially 0.05 mg PO daily for the first 2 days with increases of 0.1–0.15 mg every third day over the next 12 days, then increase by 0.25 mg every third day until optimum response occurs; mean therapeutic dose is 3 mg usually in divided doses tid.
>
> D. MAO-B inhibitor for newly diagnosed PD patients and for motor fluctuation
>> 1) Selegiline hydrochloride (Eldepryl): Used in order to make reductions in the dose of Sinemet possible; given as 10 mg daily taken as 5 mg at breakfast and at lunch; after 2–3 days of therapy, begin gradual decrease of Sinemet dosage.

2. Referral to or consultation with a physician to determine treatment options. Referral to a neurosurgeon if surgery is an option.
3. Surgical procedures: The ACNP will likely not see Parkinson's disease (as the primary diagnosis) in the inpatient setting unless the patient has a surgical procedure.
   A. Thalamotomy: Reduces tremor
   B. Pallidotomy: Reduces tremor, rigidity, bradykinesia
   C. Fetal cell transplant: Highly controversial and investigational; involves transplanting cells from the substantia nigra of an aborted fetus into the brain of a patient with PD
4. Exercise: Regular program to improve range of motion and muscle strength; referral to a physical therapist to help design program.
5. Diet: A reduction in protein intake has been shown to reduce symptoms in some patients.
6. Psychotherapy necessary in 15–25% of patients.
7. Follow-up every month until treatment plan has become effective, then every 3–6 months and prn.

PATIENT EDUCATION

1. Medications: Purpose, dosage, side effect: take levodopa before meals to improve efficacy unless it produces nausea, do not crush Sinemet. Explain "drug holidays" and when they may be necessary. Inform patient as to which side effects should be reported to health care provider. Instruct patient that they cannot take Demerol while on Sinemet, as it can produce a potentially fatal cardiac arrest.
2. Treatment plan: Medical, surgical, exercise, diet
3. Disease course and expected outcome: explain the chronic and progressive nature of PD and that there is no way to prevent its occurrence and no cure. Explain that symptoms may be fairly controlled on medication but that eventually the patient will be disabled.
4. Complications: instruct on methods to reduce complications such as falls, aspiration, infection, depression.
5. Encourage participation in local support groups and national associations.

Review Questions

4.61 The classic symptoms on Parkinson's disease include all of the following EXCEPT:
A. Shuffling gait
B. Intention tremor
C. Bradykinesia
D. Cogwheel rigidity

4.62 The first-line drug for the treatment of Parkinson's disease is:
A. Levodopa-carbidopa (Sinemet)
B. Amantidine (Symmetrel)
C. Bromocriptine (Parlodel)
D. Benztropine (Cogentin)

4.63 Mr. Crosby is a 67-year-old white male who presents to the clinic with his wife. He has no complaints. However, his wife describes that he has been clumsy and falling all the time despite walking very slowly, speaking so softly that she cannot hear him, and always looks sad. She also says that he acts depressed because he has stopped doing his normal activities (such as golf, bowling, walks). The possible diagnosis/diagnoses for this patient is:
A. Brain tumor
B. Clinical depression
C. Parkinson's disease
D. All of the above

4.64 Mr. Crosby refuses treatment at his first clinic visit, but comes back in 2 months late complaining that his symptoms are worsening. The most disturbing symptom for him is a severe bilateral hand tremor. Following a thorough diagnostic work-up, no structural lesion or depression is found. The drug(s) of choice for this patient to control his symptoms is/are:
A. Sinemet
B. Sinemet and Cogentin
C. Symmetrel
D. Sinemet and Symmetrel

4.65 Mr. Crosby is not improving as much as he would like. All he wants is for his symptoms to be reduced. What other treatment option would be the most appropriate to discuss with him at this time?
A. Thalamotomy
B. Fetal cell transplant
C. Pallidotomy
D. Adding Eldepryl to his medication regimen

Answers and Rationales

4.61 **B** The classic symptoms of Parkinson's disease include cogwheel rigidity, bradykinesia, flat affect, shuffling gait, lack of arm swing, and *resting* tremor (not intention tremor).

4.62 **A** The drug of choice for PD is Sinemet. The others listed as choices may be added if the patient's condition warrants.

4.63   **B**   This patient exhibits the classic picture of early Parkinson's disease, although all of the other choices must be ruled out as differentials.

4.64   **B**   The patient has a tremor which is best treated with Cogentin as well as bradykinesia which is best treated with Sinemet. Most patients with PD require more than one drug to control all of their symptoms. Treatment should focus on the most bothersome symptoms for each patient.

4.65   **C**   A pallidotomy would be an acceptable procedure as Mr. Crosby has both tremor and bradykinesia. Thalamotomy has been shown to reduce tremor but does little for bradykinesia. Fetal cell transplant is a last resort. The addition of Eldepryl would not be inappropriate, but may not give the patient as dramatic an improvement as the surgery.

References

Adams, R.D., & Victor, M. (1993). *Principles of Neurology* (5th ed.). New York: McGraw-Hill.

Ahlskog, J.E. (1994). Treatment of Parkinson's disease: From theory to practice. *Postgrad Med 95*(5), 52–69.

Bunting, L., & Fitzsimmons, B. (1994). Degenerative disorders. In E. Barker (ed.). *Neuroscience Nursing.* St. Louis: Mosby-Year Book, Inc.

Fitzsimmons, B., & Bunting, L.K. (1993). Parkinson's disease: Quality of life issues. *Nur Clin North Am 28*(4), 807–818.

Hickey, J.V., & Cook, H. (1997). Selected degenerative diseases of the nervous system. In J.V. Hickey (ed.). *The Clinical Practice of Neurological and Neurosurgical Nursing* (4th ed.). Philadelphia: Lippincott-Raven.

Slevin, J.T. (1996). Parkinson's disease. In R.E. Rakel (ed.). *Saunders Manual of Medical Practice.* Philadelphia: W.B. Saunders Co.

Springhouse Corporation. (1996). *Nurse Practitioner's Drug Handbook.* Philadelphia: Springhouse Corporation.

Alzheimer's Disease

DEFINITION

Alzheimer's disease (AD) is the most common cause of dementia. Although this disorder is associated with deficits in memory and personality, motor and sensory deficits also occur. This disease is chronic and incurable. The signs and symptoms develop progressively over a period of years.

ETIOLOGY/INCIDENCE

Although the exact etiology is unknown, several theories have been proposed. First, genetic predisposition in the form of an autosomal dominant trait is thought to play a role, as immediate relatives have a four times greater chance of developing Alzheimer's disease. Second, the "abnormal protein theory" blames the disease on accumulations of plaques containing an abnormal protein (42–amino acid piece of β-amyloid precursor protein) in the brain of Alzheimer's patients. Third, the "slow virus theory" suggests that a virus (with an incubation period of several years) enters the brain in old age as the blood-brain barrier deteriorates. The fact that aluminum deposits have been found in the brain of patients with AD has been disproven as an etiology of AD.

No one theory has any more proof than the others. The only risk factors presently accepted in Alzheimer's disease are advanced age, female gender, small head size, family history of dementia, and family history of Down's syndrome. Some studies have linked a history of head trauma to be a risk factor for AD due to the fact that head trauma causes increased amyloid production and decreased intracellular synaptic connections, both of which increase the risk of AD.

It is estimated that over 4 million persons in North America now suffer from Alzheimer's disease and it has become the fourth leading cause of death. The actual incidence increases with age (8–10% of persons over 65 and up to 50% of persons over 85). Alzheimer's disease tends to affect women more often than men and the onset of symptoms is typically in the sixth decade. Low educational level is associated with fewer synaptic connections between neurons and has been proposed as an explanation for the earlier and more frequent occurrence of AD among those with little education. It has also been calculated that the health care cost Alzheimer's disease is over $45 billion every year.

PATHOPHYSIOLOGY

Although the exact mechanism is unknown, many abnormalities have been found in the brains of Alzheimer's patients on postmortem exam. Gross exam reveals an atrophic brain with loss of almost 30% of normal brain weight. Atrophy, as evidenced by enlarged sulci and atrophic gyri, is most prevalent in the anterior frontal and temporoparietal areas. Microscopic pathologic brain changes include:

1. Neurofibrillary tangles: Twisted clumps of protein with a predominance in the hippocampus and cerebral cortex
2. Neuritic plaques: Clusters of dying neurons, more prevalent in the hippocampus; the core of these plaques is made up of β-amyloid (starch-like protein)
3. Neurotransmitter deficiency: Especially acetylcholine and norepinephrine; caused by degeneration of the cortex, hippocampus, and hypothalamus
4. Cerebrovascular abnormalities: Diminished oxygen metabolism and blood flow; thickening of capillaries that make up the blood-brain barrier resulting in impaired cerebral perfusion

HISTORY

When soliciting the history of a patient with Alzheimer's disease, it is necessary to interview the patient as well as significant others separately. The description of symptoms, their time of onset, and progression helps the clinician to determine the stage of the disease. Three stages of Alzheimer's disease have been described and each has progressively worsening signs and symptoms (Table 4–16).

Also important in gathering the history is to determine whether the patient has any immediate family members with a history of dementia. It is also necessary to gather data that may rule out treatable causes of dementia using the mnemonic DEMENTIA (Fig. 4–2).

The National Institute of Neurological and Communicative Diseases and

TABLE 4–16. Stages of Alzheimer's Disease*

Stage	Duration	Signs and Symptoms
I	1–3 years	Defective new learning, impaired remote recall, topographic disorientation, poor construction, poor word list generation, anomia, apathy, irritability, depression, normal motor system
II	2–10 years	Increasing impairment of recent and remote recall, poor construction, spatial disorientation, fluent aphasia, acalculia, ideomotor apraxia, indifference, apathy
III	8–12 years	Severely deteriorated intellectual functioning, limb rigidity, flexion posture, urinary and fecal incontinence

* From Cummings, J.L., & Benson, D.F. (1992). *Dementia: A Clinical Approach.* Stoneham, MA: Butterworth, with permission.

Stroke-Alzheimer's Disease and Related Disorders Association (NINCDC-ARNDA) has published criteria for definite, probable and possible AD. These criteria are summarized as follows (McKhann et al. 1984):

1. Definite AD: Clinical criteria for probable AD as well as histopathologic evidence of AD (autopsy of biopsy).
2. Probable AD: Dementia established by clinical exam, documented by mental status questionnaire, and confirmed by neuropsychometric testing; deficits in two or more areas of cognition; progressive worsening of memory and other cognitive functions; no disturbance of consciousness; onset between ages 40 and 90; absence of systemic disorders or other brain diseases capable of producing a dementia syndrome.
3. Possible AD: Presence of a systemic disorder or other brain disease capable of producing dementia but not thought to be the sole cause of the dementia; gradual progressive decline in a single intellectual function in the absence of any other identifiable cause.
4. Unlikely AD: Sudden onset, focal neurologic signs, seizures or gait disturbance early in the course of the illness

PHYSICAL FINDINGS

1. General appearance: Apathy, indifference, depression, fear, anxiety, irritability

D = drug reactions/interactions
E = emotional disorders
M = metabolic/endocrine disorders
E = eye and ear disorders
N = nutritional loss
T = tumors
I = infection
A = arteriosclerosis

FIGURE 4–2. Mnemonic for the differential diagnoses for dementia. (From Gwyther, L.P. [1985]. *Alzheimer's Disease: A Manual for Nursing Home Staff.* Washington, DC: Alzheimer's Disease Association and American Health Care Association, with permission. Courtesy of M. Elliott, M.D.)

2. Vital signs: Normal
3. Neurologic: Limb rigidity, flexion posture, apraxia, anomia, poor construction, topographic disorientation, gait disturbance, impaired memory/judgment

DIFFERENTIAL DIAGNOSIS

It is imperative to rule out treatable causes of dementia during the diagnostic process. These include:

1. Medication-induced dementia: Antihypertensives, sedatives, antidepressants, neuroleptics
2. Dementia due to metabolic abnormality: Malnutrition, dehydration, alcohol toxicity, thyroid abnormality, electrolyte imbalance
3. Depression
4. Infection: May see confusion in any febrile elderly patient, but dementia is very prevalent in tertiary syphilis
5. Normal-pressure hydrocephalus
6. Space-occupying brain lesion: Tumor, abscess, hemorrhage (particularly chronic subdural hematoma)
7. Hypoxia
8. Sensory deficits: Can produce confusion (i.e., conditions causing decreased auditory or visual acuity)
9. Vitamin B_{12} deficiency

DIAGNOSTIC TESTS/FINDINGS

1. Blood tests: CBC, electrolytes, BUN, creatinine, toxicology screen, thyroid panel, folate, B_{12}, fluorescent treponemal antibody absorption test (FTA-ABS), albumin, glucose.
2. Urinalysis.
3. Lumbar puncture with CSF analysis to rule out treatable causes of dementia such as neurosyphillis, encephalitis, etc.
4. Brain imaging: CT scan will show ventricular dilatation and sulci enlargement consistent with brain atrophy in stage III and late stage II. MRI may be necessary to rule out brain tumor.
5. EEG Will show diffuse slowing in stage II, worsening in stage III.
6. PET/SPECT scanning: Will see decreased uptake of glucose in temporoparietal region; keep in mind that this test is expensive and not widely available.
7. Neuropsychometric testing: To determine the extent of intellectual dysfunction; done as a baseline to determine the rate of disease progression.
8. Brain biopsy: Definitive diagnosis can only be made if the expected pathologic changes are present in a tissue sample.

MANAGEMENT/TREATMENT

1. Frequently, the ACNP will see AD patients only when their condition exposes them to injury (such as falls, burns, exposure). ACNPs often collaborate with a neurologist to make the diagnosis following which the NP is qualified to manage the patient medically as well as to educate the patient (the two mainstays of treatment).
2. Medication to increase availability of acetylcholine (acetylcholinesterase inhibitors): Tacrine hydrochloride (Cognex) initially 10 mg qid may be increased by 10 mg qid every 6 weeks if tolerated to a maximum of 40 mg

qid. Cognex is approved for mild to moderate Alzheimer's disease; weekly monitoring of LFTs is required, as 50% of patients will develop a transient increase in their LFTs, usually in the mild range.

3. Treatment of behavioral manifestations.
   A. Agitation
      1) Haloperidol (Haldol) 0.5–3 mg/day
      2) Thioridazine (Mellaril) 10–75 mg/day
      3) Trazodone (Desyrel) 150–400 mg/day
      4) Buspirone (BuSpar) 15–30 mg/day
      5) Thioridazine (Mellaril) 20–200 mg/day
      6) Propranolol 80–240 mg/day
      7) Carbamazepine (Tegretol) 800–1200 mg/day
   B. Delusions
      1) Haloperidol (Haldol) 0.5–3 mg/day
      2) Thioridazine (Mellaril) 10–75 mg/day
   C. Depression
      1) Nortriptyline (Pamelor) 20–75 mg/day
      2) Sertraline (Zoloft) 50–200 mg/day
      3) Fluoxetine (Prozac) 5–40 mg/day
   D. Apathy
      1) Tacrine (Cognex) 80–160 mg/day
      2) Methylphenidate (Ritalin) 5–60 mg/day
   E. Anxiety
      1) Oxazepam (Serax) 20–60 mg/day
      2) Lorazepam (Ativan) 0.5–6 mg/day
   F. Insomnia
      1) Temazepam (Restoril) 15–30 mg qhs prn
      2) Thioridazine (Mellaril) 10–75 mg/day
      3) Trazodone (Desyrel) 150–400 mg/day
      4) Chloral hydrate (Noctec) 500–1000 mg qhs prn
4. Diet: Maintain adequate nutrition and hydration; may require meal supplements, thick liquids, soft foods, tube feedings and/or someone to feed them in late disease.
5. Refer for counseling and strategies to improve functioning for as long as possible.

PATIENT EDUCATION

Patient and caregiver education is the mainstay of treatment for patients with AD. The education regarding the routine that is necessary to minimize the difficulties that both patient and caregiver face must begin at the time of diagnosis.

1. Nonpharmacologic strategies to manage symptoms of AD:
   A. Simple communication
   B. Identify and eliminate precipitants of agitation and aggression
   C. Maintaining nutrition and hydration
   D. Minimizing the use of medication
   E. Maintain a calm and routine environment
   F. Maximize the safety of the patient's environment
   G. Provide sheltered freedom where wandering and pacing can occur without danger or obstruction
2. Medication: Dosage, purpose, side effects, toxicity; instruct family members

and/or caregivers to give prn medications only when necessary to avoid the patient becoming dependent.
3. Diet: Need for supervision and assistance; explain that patient may need to be reminded to eat; educate in enteral feedings if this becomes necessary.
4. Activity: Explain need for supervision to prevent patient from wandering
5. Support services: Adult day care, caregiver support groups, Alzheimer's Association (800-272-3900)
6. Legal issues: Recommend that the patient begin getting their affairs in order prior to a decline in cognitive functioning (power of attorney, living will/advanced directive, etc.). Inform patient that the some states require that patients with AD be reported and evaluated for continuing driving priviledges.
7. Disease course and expected outcome: Explain the progressive nature of this fatal disease and that there is no cure; explain that the progression can last from 2 to 12 years before debilitation and death occur.

Review Questions

4.66 The early symptoms of AD include:
A. Confusion
B. Memory difficulty
C. Irritability
D. Both B and C

4.67 Of the utmost importance in the work-up of dementia is:
A. Ruling out treatable causes for the symptoms
B. Referring the patient for psychiatric care
C. Counseling the patient that they probably have Alzheimer's
D. Warning the family that the patient will get worse

4.68 The definitive diagnostic test in Alzheimer's disease is:
A. CT scan of the brain
B. MRI of the brain
C. Brain biopsy
D. EEG

4.69 An unidentified elderly white female presents to the emergency room escorted by police after being found wandering in the street. She is acutely confused and agitated with repeated attempts to strike emergency personnel. She is uncooperative with the exam, but her vital signs are normal and she appears to have no focal abnormalities, although she insists that it is 1952. With nothing further to go on, your list of differential diagnoses includes:
A. Acute psychotic episode
B. Alzheimer's disease
C. Craniocerebral trauma
D. All of the above

4.70 Two hours later, the patient's daughter arrives at the ER and informs you that the patient was diagnosed with AD 5 years ago. She says that her mother has received no treatment, as she has no insurance. Given this information and the current condition of the patient, your treatment plan would include:

A. Referral to the Alzheimer's Association to assist her with funding for treatment
B. Cognex 10 mg PO qid
C. Haldol 1 mg PO tid
D. Both A and C

Answers and Rationales

4.66   **D**   Early symptoms of AD include defective new learning, impaired remote recall, topographic disorientation, poor concentration, anomia, apathy, depression, irritability and poor word list generation. True confusion is not present until late stage II or stage III.

4.67   **A**   Remember that this question deals with the work-up of suspected dementia during which time treatable causes must be ruled out. The other choices deal with a treatment plan once AD is diagnosed.

4.68   **C**   Although a brain biopsy is the only definitive diagnostic test, most patients do not have this performed until post-mortem. The CT scan, MRI, and EEG are used to assist in the diagnosis in the absence of a brain biopsy.

4.69   **D**   This patient is elderly and the most likely diagnosis is Alzheimer's disease. However, since there is no definitive test for AD, you must include psychosis and trauma as well as multiple other possibilities on your list of differential diagnoses until you perform diagnostic tests to rule them out.

4.70   **D**   Patients with AD and their families/caregivers must receive all treatment options and information on the many resources available to them. Referral to the Alzheimer's Association can achieve this goal. The fact that this patient has been diagnosed with AD as well as her severe dementia indicates that Cognex is not appropriate. Haldol would be an appropriate method of controlling her agitation and making her routine care easier to accomplish.

References

Adams, R.D., & Victor, M. (1993). *Principles of Neurology* (5th ed.). New York: McGraw-Hill.

Bunting, L., & Fitzsimmons, B. (1994). Degenerative disorders. In E. Barker (ed.). *Neuroscience Nursing*. St. Louis: Mosby-Year Book, Inc.

Cummings, J.L., & Benson, D.F. (1992). *Dementia: A Clinical Approach*. Stoneham, MA: Butterworth.

Evans, M.J. (1995). *Neurologic and Neurosurgical Nursing*. Springhouse, PA: Springhouse Corporation.

Gwyther, L.P. (1985). *Alzheimer's Disease: A Manual for Nursing Home Staff*. Washington, DC: Alzheimer's Disease Association and American Health Care Association.

Hickey, J.V., & Cook, H. (1997). Selected degenerative diseases of the nervous system. In J.V. Hickey (ed.). *The Clinical Practice of Neurological and Neurosurgical Nursing* (4th ed.). Philadelphia: Lippincott-Raven.

McKhann, G., Drachman, D., Folstein, M., et al. (1984). Clinical diagnosis of Alzheimer's disease: Report of the NINCDS-ADRDA Work Group, Department of Health and Human Services Task Force on Alzheimer's Disease. *Neurology 34*, 939–944.

Moss, R.J. (1996). Alzheimer's disease. In R.E. Rakel (ed.). *Saunders Manual of Medical Practice*. Philadelphia: W.B. Saunders Co.

CHAPTER 5

Musculoskeletal and Connective Tissue Disorders

Eileen Simpson, RN, MSN, ANP, GNP, PNP
Dorothy Anderle Johnson, RN, DNSc, FNP.

Bursitis

DEFINITION

The inflammation of a bursae sac. Bursitis may be acute or chronic in nature. Bursae are structures lined with synovial membranes that secrete and absorb liquid. The bursae provides a lubricating mechanism between structures such as bones, ligaments, tendons, muscles and skin. Most bursitis occurs in the shoulder, but other common forms exist.

ETIOLOGY/INCIDENCE

1. Trauma (especially those involved in occupations such as carpet layers and plumbers)
2. Acute or chronic infection
3. Inflammatory arthritis
4. Gout
5. Rheumatoid arthritis
6. Tuberculosis (rare)
7. Gonorrhea

SIGNS AND SYMPTOMS

1. Pain, localized bursal swelling, frequently accompanied by cellulitis.
2. Systemic signs of infection are common
3. Regional lymphadenopathy
4. Limited range of motion of affected joint
5. Acute bursitis: Pain, localized tenderness, limitation of motion
6. Chronic bursitis: May follow previous attacks of bursitis or repeated trauma, pain, swelling, tenderness, muscle weakness
7. Septic bursitis:

A. Pain with flexion of affected joint
B. Local skin abrasion, lacerations or draining sinuses
C. Cellulitis

PHYSICAL FINDINGS

1. Smooth surface at affected joint
2. Erythema
3. Edema
4. Tenderness to palpation and movement
5. Passive range of motion (ROM) limited due to pain
6. Regional lymphadenopathy

DIFFERENTIAL DIAGNOSIS

1. Septic joint
2. Joint effusion
3. Arthritic conditions
4. Periarticular tendons or muscle tears
5. Osteomyelitis
6. Tuberculosis (TB)
7. Cellulitis
8. Gout/pseudogout
9. Gonorrhea

DIAGNOSTIC TESTS/FINDINGS

1. Joint aspiration (done by an experienced acute care nurse practitioner [ACNP] or a physician); send for:
   A. Cell count and differential
   B. Crystals
   C. Glucose
   D. Total protein
   E. Gram's stain and culture: Most common organisms include *Staphylococcus saureus* and streptococci.
2. X-ray to demonstrate calcific deposits and tendons.
3. Complete blood count (CBC) and white blood cell count (WBC) may be elevated, indicating systemic infection.
4. Sedimentation rate may be elevated, indicating infection.
5. Blood cultures may be indicated in immunocompromised patients or in patients where the Gram's stain of joint aspirate reveals gram-negative or gram-positive cocci.

MANAGEMENT/TREATMENT

1. Rest.
2. Traumatic bursitis will often resolve spontaneously if the area of inflammation is immobilized.
3. Splint area where feasible.
4. Elimination of precipitating trauma.
5. Protection of area from future trauma.
6. Ice for 24 hours.

7. Injection therapy using combination of corticosteroids and local anesthesia usually done by an experienced ACNP or referred to a physician.
8. Burrow's solution soaks.
9. Antibiotics for secondary infection (see below).
10. Physical therapy.
11. Medications:
    A. Motrin (ibuprofen): Used as an analgesic for mild to moderate pain and inflammation suppression, 300–800 mg PO three to four times a day take with food. Reevaluate for continued need for medication in 10 days.
    B. Naprosyn (naproxen): Used as an analgesic for mild to moderate pain and inflammation 500 mg, PO as an initial dose then 250 mg q6–8h. Take with food.
    C. Toradol (ketorolac): Used for short-term management of moderate pain. Use not to exceed 5 days total; PO dose 20 mg initially then 10 mg q4–6h; IM 60 mg initially then 30 mg q6h.
    D. Indocin: Used in the management of inflammatory disorders; PO dose 25–50 mg two to four times per day or 75-mg extended-release capsule once or twice daily (not to exceed 200 mg or 150 mg of SR/day).
12. Antibiotics:
    A. Dicloxacillin: Antibiotic that is effective against *S. aureus* and *S. epidermidis*; PO dose 125–250 mg q6h (up to 6 g m/day) for 10 days.
    B. Augmentin (amoxicillin/clavulanate): Antibiotic that is effective against streptococci, pneumococci, enterococci, *Haemophilus influenzae*, *Escherichia coli*, *Proteus mirabilis*, *Neisseria menigitidis*, *N. gonorrhoeae*, *Shigella*, *Salmonella*, *Moraxella catarrhalis*; PO dose 250–500 mg amoxicillin with 125 mg clavulanate q8h for 10 days.
    C. Keflex/Ancef: Antibiotic effective against many gram-positive cocci including staphlococci and streptococci; PO dose 250–500 mg q6h for 10 days. AncefIV 250 mg–1.5 gm q6–8h for 10 days.
    D. Ciprofloxacin: Antibiotic effective against many gram-positive and gram-positive pathogens; PO dose 500–750 mg q12h for 10 days; IV dose 400 mg q12h for 10 days.
    E. Clindamycin: Antibiotic effective against most gram-positive aerobic cocci and has good activity against some anaerobic bacteria; PO dose 150–300 mg q6h for 10 days; IV dose 300–600 mg q6–8hr, for 10 days.
    F. Nafcillin: Antibiotic effective against most gram-positive aerobic cocci; PO dose 250–100 mg q4–6h for 10 days (oral nafcillin is irradically absorbed from the gastrointestinal [GI] tract); IV 500–2000 mg q4–6h for 10 days.
    G. Unasyn: Effective against β-lactamase enzymes; IM, IV doses 1.5–3 gm q6–8h for 10 days.
13. Systemic corticosteroids:
    A. Prednisone: Used systemically and locally for inflammation. Prednisone PO, 15–30 mg/day for 3 days.

For chronic bursitis, the ACNP may need to consult an orthopedic surgeon, as both the bursa and underlying bone may need to be excised surgically.

PATIENT EDUCATION

1. Explain the importance of resting the affected area.
2. Instruct patient how to maintain splint used to immobilize affected extremity.

3. Instruct patient how to perform pendulum exercises (for shoulder bursitis).
4. Instruct patient on preventative measures such as the fact that early active movement inhibits development of limiting adhesions.
5. Instruct patient on the use of knee pads for those involved in prolonged kneeling activities.

Low Back Pain

DEFINITION

Low back pain affects the area between the lower rib cage and gluteal folds and often radiates into the thighs; 1% of patients with acute low back pain have sciatica, which is defined as pain in the distribution of a lumbar nerve root, often accompanied by neurosensory and motor deficits.

Low back musculoligamentous strain usually presents after a specific episode of bending, twisting, or lifting. There may be tearing of muscle fibers or distal ligamentous attachments of the paraspinal muscles usually at the iliac crest or lower lumbar/upper sacral region.

ETIOLOGY/INCIDENCE

1. The number one cause of restricted activity in people under 45 years old and the third common cause of restricted activity in people between 45 and 65 years old.
2. About 6.5 million people in the United States are bedridden because of back pain.
3. About $6 billion dollars a year is spent in this country on evaluation and treatment of low back pain.
4. Low back pain is the most common etiology for workers' compensation.
5. Low back pain is second only to headache among the leading causes of pain.
6. Total national cost to care for those afflicted with low back pain is estimated at $20 billion a year.
7. Men and women are equally affected by low back pain. In addition, injuries to the low back usually occur in the third and fourth decades of life.
8. Those who work in occupations that are exposed to constant vibration, repetitive lifting in the forward bent and twisted positions suffer more from low back pain.
9. Those with a history of obesity and poor muscle tone have an increased incidence of low back pain. The combination of excessive weight and poor abdominal muscle tone displaces a person's center of gravity forward, resulting in increased lumbar lordosis and thereby causing the patient to assume a mechanically disadvantageous position, which places stress on the low back.
10. Other causes:
    A. Paravertebral muscle sprain
    B. Disc degeneration/protrusion/extrusion
    C. Poor posture
    D. Trauma

SIGNS AND SYMPTOMS

A precipitating injury is identified in only 40% of patients who complain of back pain.

1. Pain radiating across the low back often radiating to the buttock and upper thigh posteriorly.
2. Antalgic gait: Twisted to one side and bent forward.
3. Inability to walk tip toe: Inability to tip toe suggests S1 nerve root compression.
4. Inability to heel walk: Inability to heel walk indicates poor dorsiflexion and is a quick screen for L5 nerve root compression.
5. Asymmetry of the lower back and limb length discrepancies: Asymmetric paravertebral muscle spasm may lead to scoliotic posture in a patient with disc herniation.
6. Limited range of lumbar motion through extension and side-to-side bending.
7. Rigidity and prominence of paraspinal muscles upon palpation.
8. Pain associated with straining or lifting weakness or paresthesia and decreased deep tendon reflexes.
9. Fever: May indicate epidural abscess or osteomyelitis. The ANCP needs to refer patients with this finding to the physician.

PHYSICAL FINDINGS

1. Standing
   A. Assess ROM: Check flexion, extension, lateral bending and rotation.
   B. Assess muscle spasm.
   C. Palpate to assess for trigger zones, myofascial nodes, sciatic nerve tenderness, and sacroiliac joint tenderness. Costovertebral angle (CVA) tenderness upon palpation may indicate kidney infection or presence of stone.
2. Sitting
   A. Hidden straight leg raising test (patient in sitting position extends leg, which stretches the sciatic nerve in an indirect manner).
   B. Motor exam of the quadriceps muscle.
   C. Reflex exam of patellar and Achilles tendons: A decrease in these reflexes may indicate injury to back in the L4–L5–S1 area.
3. Lying down
   A. Abdominal exam: Abdominal aortic anuerysm or abdominal or pelvic masses may cause back pain.
   B. Rectal exam: Decreased sphincter tone may be indicative of neurologic dysfunction, or palpation of a mass in the rectum may be indicative of a malignant process.
   C. Straight leg raising: Pain in the back with leg raises over 30 degrees is indicative of nerve root irritation.
   D. Sensory, vibratory and temperature perception exam: Decreased vibratory and sensation is indicative of a neoplasm or massive midline disc herniation.
   E. Perform exam of hip and pelvis. Pathology in these areas can be manifested as back pain.

DIFFERENTIAL DIAGNOSIS

1. Spondylolysis
2. Spondylolisthesis
3. Spinal infections
4. Circulatory disorders
5. Metastatic tumor
6. Gynecologic disorders
7. Psychogenic pain syndrome and malingering
8. Compression fractures
9. Cauda equina syndrome
10. Renal calculi
11. Abdominal aortic anuerysm
12. Metabolic disorders
13. Osteoporosis

DIAGNOSTIC TESTS/FINDINGS

1. Lumbar/sacral spine x-rays to rule out fractures, inflammation, or malignancies; plain anteroposterior (AP) lateral lumbar spine x-rays are indicated especially in patients who are over 50 years old.
2. Urinalysis to rule out presence of occult blood or infection.
3. CBC with differential and a sedimentation rate (increased sedimentation rate may be indicative of cancer, high WBC may indicate infection).
4. Serum CA (increased level may indicate malignancy).
5. Serum alkaline phosphatase (increased level may indicate malignancy).
6. Magnetic resonance imaging (MRI) scan to rule out pathology in the muscle and tissue fibers.
7. Computed tomography (CT) scan to rule out bony abnormalities.
8. Myelography may be indicated in some cases.

MANAGEMENT/TREATMENT

1. Bed rest for 48 hours.
2. Sleep on a firm mattress, so that the patient's weight is evenly distributed.
3. Ice applied to area for the first 24 hours to decrease inflammatory response and edema, decrease muscle spasms, and increase patient's pain threshold.
4. Moist heat applied to area after the first 24 hours and to continue for 5 days—moist heat provides better penetration.
5. Massage.
6. Reduction diet if patient is overweight.
7. Medications:
   A. Motrin (ibuprofen): Used as an analgesic for mild to moderate pain and inflammation suppression, 300–800 mg PO three to four times a day, take with food. Re-evaluate for continued need for medication in 10 days.
   B. Naprosyn (naproxen): Used as an analgesic for mild to moderate pain and inflammation suppression, 500 mg PO as an initial dose then 250 mg q6–8h. Take with food. Use cautiously in patients with a history of gastritis or GI bleeding.
   C. Toradol (ketorolac): Used for short-term management of moderate pain. Not to exceed 5 days total; PO dose 20 mg initially then 10 mg q4–6h;

IM 60 mg initially then 30 mg q6h. Use with caution in patients with chronic renal insufficiency.

D. Orudis KT (ketoprofin): Used for management of mild to moderate pain, in three to four divided doses or 200 mg PO qid as extended release tablet; take medication with a full glass of water and remain in upright postion for 15–30 minutes after taking.

E. Soma (carisoprodol): Used as an adjunct to rest and physical therapy for treatment of muscle spasm; 350 mg, three to four times a day. Use with caution in patients with altered mental status.

F. Flexeril (cyclobenzaprine): Used as a skeletal muscle relaxant in combination with rest and physical therapy; 10 mg tid. Use with caution in patients with altered mental status.

G. Vicodin (hydrocodone/acetominophen): One to two tabs q4h prn pain. Used to manage moderate to severe pain. Binds to opiate receptors in the central nervous system (CNS). Use cautiously in the elderly due to its sedative effects.

H. Colace (docusate sodium): Used for prevention of constipation. Promotes incorporation of water into stool, resulting in softer fecal mass; 50–500 mg PO once daily. Administer with a full glass of water. May be administered on an empty stomach for more rapid results.

8. Admission to the acute or subacute hospital should be considered with intractible pain or unsteady gait: For pain management and physical therapy.

9. Epidural steroids to alleviate acute pain: Referral to orthopedic surgeon for treatment.

10. Surgery may be indicated in some cases: Referral to neurosurgeon is necessary.

11. Manipulative therapy (controversial).

12. Low back patient education to include:
    A. Group instruction in anatomy and causation of symptoms
    B. Ergonomic information such as proper seating, standing, and lifting techniques
    C. Simple exercise program and obstacle course simulations of home and work environments

13. Patients who fail to improve after therapeutic measures need referral for investigation of other causes.

Special Considerations for the Elderly

In geriatric patients the need to treat the whole patient exists. In essence, a broad evaluation should be done on geriatric patients, not just a focused exam on the obvious area of injury. This is due to the fact that back pain in the elderly may represent a variety of maladies including but not limited to bone fragility, pre-existing degenerative arthritis, malignancies, and other disorders.

Diagnostic and Prognostic Red Flags in Cases of Low Back Pain

Patients with these conditions may need a more in-depth work-up or the ANCP may need to refer these patient to an orthopedist or surgeon for evaluation.

1. Pain unrelieved by rest or any postural modification
2. Pain unchanged despite treatment for 2–4 weeks
3. Colicky pain or pain associated with a visceral function
4. Fever or immunosuppressed status
5. High risk for fracture (older age, osteoporosis)
6. Known or previous history of cancer
7. Associated malaise, fatigue, or weight loss
8. Possible neurologic impairment
9. Severe morning stiffness as a primary complaint
10. Bowel or bladder dysfunction
11. Unable to ambulate or to care for self
12. Compensable cause of injury
13. Out of work, disabled, or seeking disability
14. Repeated failed surgical or medical treatment for low back pain or other chronic illnesses

PATIENT EDUCATION

Instruct patient to:

1. Sleep on a firm mattress
2. Not lift loads over 5 lb for the first 2 weeks after injury
3. Perform proper body mechanics and lifting with large leg muscles
4. Perform reconditioning exercises to strengthen abdominal muscles
5. Understand purpose, dosage, side effects, and toxic effects of medication

Fractures

DEFINITION

A fracture is a break in the surface of a bone, either across its cortex or through its articular surface. Types of fractures include:

1. Open fracture: One which communicates with the outside environment
2. Simple fracture: One in which there is no communication with the outside environment
3. Impaction: Where distal bone fragment is driven into a proximal one
4. Avulsion: Where a bone is pulled off where tendon or ligament inserts
5. Greenstick: An incomplete fracture in which one side of the bone is bent
6. Compression fracture: Occurs when there is anterior wedging of the vertebral body in the anterior spinal column, usually stable in nature and rarely involving neurologic deficit
7. Intertrochanteric fracture: A fracture of the hip that occurs along a line between the greater and lesser trochanter with variable comminution

ETIOLOGY/INCIDENCE

1. Trauma (falls, gunshot wounds, motor vehicle accidents, physical abuse).
2. Metastasis of cancer (usually causes pathologic fractures).
3. History of exposure to undue or prolonged stress such as heavy lifting, repeated falls.

4. History of long-term use of steroids
5. Patients with a history of osteoporosis have a higher incidence of fractures.
6. Female have a 2:1 higher incidence of hip fractures than do males.
7. Blacks have the lowest incidence of hip fractures, while white northern Europeans have the highest.
8. People who smoke, drink alcohol, and are inactive have increased chance of having a hip fracture after suffering a fall.

SIGNS AND SYMPTOMS

The ACNP may see a variety of fractures; however, the most common fractures seen in the acute care setting will be:

1. Extremity fractures
   A. Pain
   B. Swelling
   C. Ecchymosis
   D. Inability to bear weight on the affected limb
   E. Loss of feeling or numbness in limb affected by injury
   F. Difficulty ambulating or moving the extremity
   G. Displacement or angulation of the extremity
   H. Decreased range of motion of the extremity
2. Compression fracture of the spine
   A. Usually seen in the elderly with a history of osteoporosis or those with a history of taking long-term steroids.
   B. Complaint of sudden back pain with a history of minimal trauma.
   C. Discomfort at the level of the fracture.
   D. Most fractures occur at the middle or lower level or the dorsal spine.
   E. Pain upon palpation of lumbar spine or sacrum.
   F. Limited range of motion of the spine.
3. Hip fracture
   A. Inability to ambulate.
   B. Shortening and external rotation of the injured limb.
   C. Pain (can be referred to the knee).
   D. Ecchymosis.
   E. Hip fractures most often occur in the intracapsular, intertrochanteric, and subtrochanteric area of the proximal femur.
   F. Any motion may elicit pain.
   G. Femoral neck fractures are the most commonly missed hip fractures. Many times this fracture does not show up radiographically until 5 or more days after the initial injury. Due to this fact it would be advantageous to have the patient ambulate. If the patient is unable to ambulate, the ACNP must refer the patient for a bone scan to definitely rule out the presence of fracture.
4. Pelvic fracture
   A. Pain
   B. Point tenderness of pubis and/or iliac spines, swelling and ecchymosis of medial thigh, genitals, and lumbosacrum
   C. Instability of pelvis
   D. Peripheral neuropathy
   E. Crepitus
   F. Difficulty or inability to ambulate

PHYSICAL FINDINGS

1. Deformity of affected extremity or spine.
2. Swelling of affected extremity.
3. Inability to use part affected.
4. Neurovascular and sensory compromise. These injuries need immediate reduction to improve neurovascular flow and/or surgical intervention. The ACNP should refer this patient to a surgeon or orthopedist.
5. Shortening of extremity.
6. Inability to bear weight on extremity affected.
7. Ecchymosis.
8. Crepitus at injury site.
9. Rotation of extremity affected by injury.
10. Small puncture wounds or extensive abrasions around the suspected fracture is an open fracture until proven otherwise. The ACNP needs to refer this patient to a surgeon for surgical débridement.
11. Assess for nervous or circulatory status: Check the 5 P's—pain, pulselessness, paralysis, paresthesia, and pallor.

DIFFERENTIAL DIAGNOSIS

1. Soft tissue injury.
2. Sprains.
3. Strains.
4. Muscle spasms.
5. Joint subluxation or dislocation. Hip dislocation is a medical emergency; however, it is rare in the elderly. The ACNP should refer this patient to an orthopedic surgeon.
6. Compartment syndrome.
7. Open fractures.

DIAGNOSTIC TESTS/FINDINGS

1. X-rays: Most radiographs should be taken in two planes, each at 90 degrees to the other. This usually includes AP lateral views of the joint proximal and distal to an extremity fracture, to rule out the presence of associated dislocation or subluxation. In addition, patients with suspected hip fractures need to have an AP view of the pelvis. This view allows comparison with the uninvolved side, which may be helpful in identifying nondisplaced or impacted fractures.
2. Complete neurologic exam including deep tendon reflexes (DTRs), assessment of dermatomes, assessment of sensation.
3. Labs:
   A. CBC: A baseline hemoglobin (Hgb) and hematocrit (Hct) and serial Hgb and Hct should be done to assess for the presence of bleeding. It is possible that a patient may have two to four units of occult blood loss in the event of a pelvic or hip fracture.
   B. Urinalysis (UA): To assess for the presence of blood in the urine, which would indicate associated genitourinary trauma in patients with pelvic or hip fractures.
   C. Electrolyte panel.
4. Rectal exam: To assess sphincter tone and presence of blood in stool.

5. Compression: Distraction test for stability of pelvic ring (if the illiac crest can be pressed together or pulled apart, the pelvis is unstable).
6. Electrocardiogram (ECG) in all patients over the age of 65 years.
7. Bone scans may be done in the event that an x-ray is negative and based on clinical exam, a fracture is still suspected.

MANAGEMENT/TREATMENT

1. Immobilization and reduction of injury if extremity is affected.
2. Splinting.
3. Ice.
4. Elevation if there is an injury to an extremity.
5. Care of surgical staples in the case of a patient with an open reduction internal fixation (ORIF)—staples are usually removed within 2 weeks postoperatively and Steri Strips are applied to the postoperative site.
6. Medications:
   A. Pain medications
      1) Motrin (ibuprofen): Used as an analgesic for mild to moderate pain and inflammation suppression, 300–800 mg PO three to four times/day, take with food. Re-evaluate for continued need for medication in 10 days. Use with caution in patients with a history of gastritis, GI bleeding, or chronic renal insufficiency.
      2) Vicodin (hydrocodone/acetaminophen): Used as an analgesic for moderate to severe pain suppression, one to two tablets, PO q4h. Binds to opiate receptors in the CNS. Use with caution in the elderly due to its sedative effects.
      3) Darvocet N-100 (propoxyphene/acetaminophen): Used as an analgesic for moderate to severe pain suppression, one to two tablets, PO q4h. Binds to opiate receptors in the CNS. Use with caution in the elderly due its sedative effects.
   B. Medications used for deep venous thrombosis (DVT) and pulmonary emboli (PE) prophylaxis (Coumadin will usually be prescribed for DVT prophylaxis in patients who have undergone total joint replacement. Heparin or Lovenox will be used in other instances. However, choice of DVT medications may vary depending on the surgeon's preference.)
      1) Heparin/Lovenox: Used for prophylaxis and treatment of DVT and PE. Doses:
         • Heparin 5000 U, SQ, q12hs or
         • Lovenox 30 U, SQ, q12h (Note: This medication is more expensive than heparin.)
         Use cautiously in patients with a history of bleeding disorder and those with history of gastrointestinal bleeding. Monitor partial thromboplastin time (PTT) and platelet count every 3–4 days during heparin therapy. Monitor CBC and platelet count periodically during Lovenox therapy.
      2) Coumadin (warfarin): Used for prophylaxis and treatment of DVT and PE. It interferes with hepatic synthesis of vitamin K–dependent clotting factors (II, VII, IX, and X). Use cautiously in patients with a history of ulcer or liver disease. Loading dose of 6–10 mg/day for 2–4 days then adjust daily dose by results of prothrombin time (PT) or International Normalized Ratio (INR). Therapeutic INR for patients with DVT or PE prophylaxis is 2–3. Therapeutic INR for pa-

tients who have undergone orthopedic surgeries is 1.5–2.2. Coumadin has many drug interactions; be cautious when dosing. May be used for a few weeks postoperatively then discontinued.

C. Stool softeners

1. Colace (docusate sodium): Used for prevention of constipation. Promotes incorporation of water into stool resulting in softer fecal mass; 50–500 mg PO once daily. Administer with a full glass of water. May be administered on an empty stomach for more rapid results.

7. Antiembolic stockings.
8. Abductor pillows for patients S/P hip fractures.
9. Physical and occupational therapy as indicated.
10. ORIF as indicated for patients who have suffered operable fractures. Evaluated by an orthopedic surgeon.
11. Hyperextension exercises as indicated for compression fractures of the spine.
12. Patients who have suffered a compression fracture of the spine may need to be hospitalized for pain control.
13. Pelvic fractures that do not involve the pelvic ring are considered stable. These fractures are not treated operatively, but with bedrest and protected ambulation.
14. Patients with hip fractures must be admitted and placed on best rest and maintained in a position of comfort with slight hip flexion and external rotation. Progressive ambulation with physical therapy and weight bearing per orthopedic surgeons protocol.
15. Tetanus prophylaxis.
16. Teach patient crutch training and hip precautions; usually done by physical therapist.
17. Patients discharged from acute care facility need home health physical therapy evaluation.
18. If patient is discharged on Coumadin, PT/INR need to be closely monitored.
19. Consider calcium requirements of 1000-1500 mg/day and supplement accordingly.

PATIENT EDUCATION

1. Discuss treatment plan including pain medications.
2. Discuss discharge plans with patient and family.
3. Instruct patient on the importance of follow-up with orthopedic surgeon after discharge.
4. Instruct patients who are discharged on Coumadin not to take acetylsalicylic acid (ASA) or nonsteroidal anti-inflammatory drugs (NSAIDs) and that blood tests will need to be done routinely on an outpatient basis.

Disc Herniation

DEFINITION

1. Disc herniation occurs when damage occurs to the annular fiber of the disc. The damaged disc can be defined as degenerated, protruded, extruded, and sequestered.

2. Degeneration results from tearing of circumferentially arranged laminar fibers of the anulus without bulging of the peripheral disc margin.
3. A protruded disc is caused by extensive breakdown of the anulus with bulging of the outer anular fibers and posterior longitudinal ligament which may trap a lumbar nerve root innervating the lower extremity and cause sciatica.
4. An extruded disc occurs when a portion of the nucleus pulposus ruptures through the outmost fibers of the anulus but not through the posterior longitudinal ligament.
5. A sequestered disc ruptures through both the anulus and the posterior longitudinal ligament and lies free within the spinal canal. At this stage, the disc usually causes disabling sciatica.

ETIOLOGY/INCIDENCE

1. About 95% of disc herniations occur at the L4–L5 and L5–S1 area of the spine.
2. Degenerative disc disease is one of the most common back disorders seen in any medical practice. However, the pathophysiology of degenerative disc disease remains unclear.
3. Continued axial loading stress on the spine resulting from daily bipedal weight bearing is a contributing factor to disc degeneration.
4. Repetitive percussion-type activities (e.g., construction work) and lifting weights may contribute to disc disease.
5. Those with a history of cigarette smoking have a higher incidence of disc disease, since nicotine has been shown in animal studies to impair the availability of nutrients to the discs.
6. Those with a history of cigarette smoking have a higher incidence of suffering low back pain. A smoker's cough predisposes a person to back injury, and nicotine has been shown in animal studies to impair the availability of nutrients to the discs.

PATHOGENESIS

1. Trauma
2. Enzymatic changes and changes in the metabolism of the nutrients sent to the discs
3. Dehydration of the discs
4. Obesity
5. Congenital anomalies

SIGNS AND SYMPTOMS

1. Sudden onset of low back pain (usually from the L4–L5 and L5–S1 levels) and subsequent radicular pain.
2. Dull and aching in quality or pain may be acute and crippling in severity.
3. Aggravated by exertion and lessened by rest.
4. May have weakness in lower extremities indicating major compression of affected nerve root.
5. Pain may be exacerbated by any type of Valsalva maneuver (i.e., coughing, sneezing, or laughing).
6. Paraspinal muscle spasm.
7. Pain is generally worse in the leg than in the back.

8. Morning pain that resolves in the afternoon is characteristic of discogenic pain.
9. Patients with S1 nerve root irritation may complain of numbness in the buttock, posterior thigh, calf, lateral aspect of the ankle, foot, and lateral toes.
10. Patients with L5 root compression may complain of pain radiating to the dorsum of the foot.

PHYSICAL FINDINGS

1. Standing
   A. Assess ROM: Check flexion, extension, lateral bending, and rotation.
   B. Assess muscle spasm.
   C. Palpate to assess for trigger zones, myofascial nodes, sciatic nerve tenderness, and sacroiliac joint tenderness. CVA tenderness upon palpation may indicate kidney infection or presence of stone.
2. Sitting
   A. Hidden straight leg raising test (patient is in sitting position, leg is extended, which stretches the sciatic nerve in an indirect manner; positive findings, back pain).
   B. Motor exam of the quadriceps muscle.
   C. Reflex exam of the patellar and Achilles tendons: A decrease in these reflexes may indicate injury to back in the L4–L5–S1 area.
3. Lying down
   A. Abdominal exam: Abdominal aortic aneurysm or abdominal or pelvic masses may cause back pain.
   B. Rectal exam: Decreased sphincter tone may be indicative of neurologic dysfunction, or palpation of a mass in the rectum may be indicative of a malignant process.
   C. Straight leg raising: Pain in the back with leg raises over 30 degrees is indicative of nerve root irritation.
   D. Sensory, vibratory and temperature perception exam: Decreased vibratory sensation is indicative of a neoplasm or massive midline disc herniation.
   E. Perform exam of hip and pelvis: Pathology in theses areas can be manifested as back pain.

DIFFERENTIAL DIAGNOSIS

1. Spondylolysis
2. Spondylolisthesis
3. Spinal infection
4. Circulatory disorders
5. Metastatic tumor
6. Gynecologic disorders
7. Psychogenic pain syndrome and malingering
8. Compression fractures
9. Cauda equina syndrome
10. Renal calculi
11. Abdominal aortic aneurysm
12. Metabolic disorders
13. Osteoporosis

14. Arthritis
15. Facet syndrome

DIAGNOSTIC TESTS/FINDINGS

1. Lumbar/sacral spine x-rays to rule out fractures, inflammation, or malignancies: Plain AP lateral lumbar spine x-rays are indicated especially in patients who are over 50 years old.
2. Urinalysis to rule out presence of occult blood or infection.
3. CBC with differential and sedimentation rate (increased sedimentation rate may be indicative of cancer, high WBC may indicate infection).
4. Serum CA (increased level may indicate malignancy).
5. Serum alkaline phosphatase (increased level may indicate malignancy).
6. MRI to rule out pathology in the muscle and tissue fibers.
7. CT scan to rule out bony abnormalities.
8. Myelography may be indicated in some cases.

MANAGEMENT/TREATMENT

1. Bed rest with bathroom privileges for 48 hours.
2. Sleep on firm mattress: May need a bedboard under mattress.
3. Ice applied to area for the first 24 hours to decrease inflammatory response and edema, decrease muscle spasms, and increase patient's pain threshold.
4. Moist heat applied to area after the first 24 hours to continue for 5 days; moist heat provides better penetration.
5. Massage.
6. Reduction diet if patient is overweight.
7. Medications:
   A. Motrin (ibuprofen): Used as analgesic for mild to moderate pain and inflammation suppression, 300–800 mg PO three to four times a day, take with food. Re-evaluate for continued need for medication in 10 days.
   B. Naprosyn (naproxen): Used as an analgesic for mild to moderate pain and inflammation suppresion, 500 mg, PO as an initial dose then 250 mg q6–8h. Take with food. Use cautiously in patients with a history of gastritis or GI bleeding.
   C. Toradol (ketorolac): Used for short-term management of moderate pain. Not to exceed 5 days total; PO dose 20 mg initially then 10 mg q4–6h; IM 60 mg then 30 mg q6hs. Use with caution in patients with chronic renal insufficiency.
   D. Orudis KT (ketoprofin): Used for management or mild to moderate pain, in three to four divided doses or 200 mg PO sid as extended release tablet. Take medication with a full glass of water and remain in upright position for 15–30 minutes after taking.
   E. Soma (carisoprodol): Used as an adjunct to rest and physical therapy for treatment of muscle spasm; 350 mg, three to four times a day. Use with caution in patients with altered mental status.
   F. Flexeril (cyclobenzaprine): Used as a skeletal muscle relaxant in combination with rest and physical therapy; 10 mg, tid. Use with caution in patients with altered mental status.
   G. Vicodin (hydrocodone/acetominophen): One to two tabs q4h prn pain. Used to manage moderate to severe pain. Binds to opiate receptors in the CNS. Use cautiously in the elderly due to its sedative effects.

H. Colace (docusate sodium): Used for prevention of constipation. Promotes incorporation of water into stool resulting in softer fecal mass; 50–500 mg PO sid. Administer with a full glass of water. May be administered on an empty stomach for more rapid results.

8. Admission to the acute or subacute hospital should be considered with intractable pain or unsteady gait: For pain management and physical therapy.

9. Epidural steroids to alleviate acute pain: Referral to an orthopedic physician for treatment.

10. Surgery may be indicated in some cases: Referral to a neurosurgeon is necessary.

11. Manipulative therapy (controversial).

12. Low back patient education to include:
    A. Group instruction in anatomy and causation of symptoms
    B. Ergonomic information such as proper seating, standing, and lifting techniques
    C. Simple exercise program and obstacle course simulations of home and work environments

Patients who fail to improve after therapeutic measures need referral for investigation of other causes.

Special Considerations for the Elderly

In geriatric patients, the need to treat the whole patient exists. In essence, a broad evaluation should be done on geriatric patients—not just a focused exam on the obvious area of injury. This is due to the fact that back pain in the elderly may represent a variety of maladies including but not limited to bone fragility, pre-existing degenerative arthritis, malignancies, and other disorders.

Diagnostic and Prognostic Red Flags in Cases of Low Back Pain

Patients with these conditions may need a more in-depth work-up or the ANCP may need to refer these patients to an orthopedic physician or surgeon for evaluation.

1. Pain unrelieved by rest or any postural modification
2. Pain unchanged despite treatment for 2–4 weeks
3. Colicky pain or pain associated with visceral function
4. Fever or immunosuppressed status
5. High risk for fracture (older age or osteoporosis)
6. Known or previous history of cancer
7. Associated malaise, fatigue, or weight loss
8. Possible neurologic impairment
9. Severe morning stiffness as a primary complaint
10. Bowel or bladder dysfunction
11. Unable to ambulate or care for self
12. Compensable cause of injury
13. Out of work, disabled, or seeking disability

14. Repeated failed surgical or medical treatment for low back pain or other illnesses

PATIENT EDUCATION

Instruct patient to:

1. Sleep on firm mattress
2. Not lift loads over 5 lb for the first 2 weeks after injury
3. Perform proper body mechanics and lifting with large leg muscles
4. Perform reconditioning exercises to strengthen abdominal muscles
5. Understand purpose, dosage, side effects, and toxic effects of medications

References

Brown, D.E., & Neumann, R.D. (1995). *Orthopedic Secrets.* St. Louis, C.V. Mosby Co.

Bueff, H.U., & VanDer Reis, W. (1996). Low back pain. *Prim Care 23*, 345–364.

Deglin, J.H., & Vallerand, A.H. (1997). *Davis's Drug Guide for Nurses* (5th ed.). Philadelphia: F.A. Davis Co.

Deyo, R.A., Rainville, J., & Kent, D. (1992). What can the history and physical exam tell us about low back pain. *JAMA 268*, 760–765.

Dunwoody, C.J. (1991). Pelvic fracture patient care, reflections on the past, implications for the future. *Nurs Clin North Am 26*, 65–71.

Frymoyer, J.W. (1988). Back pain and sciatica. *N Engl J Med 318*, 291–299.

Frymoyer, J.W. (1992). Predicting disability from low back pain. *Clin Orthop 279*, 101–109.

Haye, K. (1991). That old hip. *Nurs Clin North Am 26*, 43–40.

Heckman, J.D. (1991). Fractures, emergency care and complications. *Clin Symp 43*, 2–27.

Hockberger, R. (1986). The lowdown on low back pain. *Emerg Med 18*, 122–171.

Hoppenfeld, S. (1976). *Physical Examination of the Spine and Extremities.* San Mateo, CA: Appleton & Lange.

Kirkaldy-Willis, W.H. (1987). Low back pain. *Clin Symp 39*, 2–32.

Lee, Y.L., & Yip, K.M.H. (1996). The osteoporotic spine. *Clin Orthop 323*, 91–97.

Martin, R.E. (1996). Initial assessment and management of common fractures. *Prim Care 23*, 405–409.

Miller, M.D. (1990). Orthopedic trauma in the elderly. *Emerg Med Clin North Am 8*, 325–339.

Nachemson, A.L. (1992). Newest knowledge of low back pain, a critical look. *Clin Orthop 279*, 8–20.

Pedinoff, S., Pinals, R.S., Schwartsz, S.A., & Spengler, D.M. (1991). A rational workup for low-back pain. *Patient Care 25*, 43–67.

Raby N., Berman, L., & de Lacy, G. (1996). *Accident and Emergency Radiology, A Survival Guide.* Philadelphia: W.B. Saunders Co.

Richardson, J.D., Pold, H.C., & Flint, L.M. (1987). *Trauma Clinical Care and Pathophysiology.* Chicago: Year Book Medical Publishers, Inc.

Rockwood, C.A., Green, D.P., Bucholz, R.W., & Heckman, J.D. (1996). *Fractures in Adults, Vol. 2.* Philadelphia: Lippincott-Raven, pp. 1575–1613.

Shields, C.B., & Williams, P.E. (1986). Low back pain. *Am Fam Physician 33*, 173–182.

Sonzogni, J.J. (1992). Lumbosacral spine injuries part 1: Evaluation. *Emerg Med 24*, 169–188.

Sonzogni, J.J. (1992). Lumbosacral spine injuries part 2: Specific disorders. *Emerg Med 24*, 27–57.

Spoelhof, G.D., & Bristow, M. (1989). Back pain pitfalls. *Am Fam Physician 40*, 133–138.

Swezey, R.L. (1988). Low back pain in the elderly: Practical management concerns. *Geriatrics 43*, 39–44.

Tintinalli, J.E., Ruiz, E., & Krome, R.L. (1996). *Emergency Medicine, A Comprehensive Study Guide.* New York: McGraw-Hill.

Wheeler, A.H. (1995). Diagnosis and management of low back pain and sciatica. *Am Fam Physician 52*, 1333–1340.

Zuckerman, J.D., & Schon, L.C. (1990). *Comprehensive Care of Orthopaedic Injuries in the Elderly.* Baltimore: Urban & Schwarzenberg.

Review Questions

5.1 Which of the following statements is NOT considered to be characteristic of those afflicted with low back pain?

A. Affects men and women equally.

B. Affects those involved in occupations exposed to constant vibration and repetative lifting.

C. Low back pain is the number one cause of restricted activity in people under the age of 45 years.

D. Affects only those with a history of cancer.

5.2 A 55-year-old male patient presents to your office with a history of low back pain radiating to the paraspinal area of the lumbar sacral spine. The pain occurred suddenly after bending over to pick up his grandson approximately 1 hour prior to arrival. Your initial physical exam and diagnostic work-up would include:

A. Physical exam in the standing, sitting, and lying positions to include an abdominal, neurologic, and rectal exam

B. Lumbar sacral x-rays to R/O fracture/dislocation

C. Urinalysis to check for presence of blood or infection

D. CT scan and MRI

  1. A and B
  2. B and C
  3. C and D
  4. A, B, and C
  5. All of the above

5.3 An 80-year-old female S/P left femoral head fracture and subsequent total hip replacement. She also has a history of hypothyroidism and atrial fibrillation. Current medications include Synthroid, Coumadin, digoxin, Motrin, and Tagamet. She is admitted to the subacute unit under your care. Therapeutic interventions and admission orders that would be appropriate for this patient would include:

A. Hip precautions

B. Admission labs to include baseline CBC, SMA7, INR, thyroid-stimulating hormone (TSH) and digoxin level

C. Aggressive pulmonary toilet including incentive spirometry, O_2 at 2L per nasal cannula prn shortness of broath, and baseline pulse oximetry.

D. Demerol 100 mg IM q4h for pain control

1. A and B
2. B and C
3. C and D
4. A, B, and C
5. All of the above
6. None of the above

5.4 Mrs. Jones is a 60-year-old female with a complaint of severe pain and swelling of the right shoulder for 1 week. On exam she has tenderness and limited range of motion of the right shoulder. There is pain with flexion, her WBC is 16,500 mL and she has a fever of 101°F. An x-ray was done of the shoulder that reveals calcification around the tendons. You suspect which of the following?
A. Septic bursitis
B. Chronic bursitis
C. Gout
D. Rheumatic arthritis

5.5 Your initial management plan for the patient in the previous scenario would include:
A. Heat, Toradol IM
B. Physical therapy
C. Serum sedimentation rate, ciprofloxacin PO
D. Blood cultures, IV Ancef and Naprosyn

Answers and Rationales

5.1   **D** The spine is a site of metatasis of cancer. However, it is uncommon, especially in those patients who are under the age of 50 years. The people most commonly at risk for neoplastic metastasis are over the age of 50 who have had back pain for over 1 month.

5.2   **D** (A) Examining a patient in various positions will help to pinpoint **(4)** the etiology of the low back pain. An abdominal exam will help to rule out the presence of abdominal anuerysm or abdominal or pelvic masses that may cause referred pain to the low back. Rectal exam will help to assess for decreased sphincter tone or presence of mass in the rectum. A neurologic exam will help to detect the presence of neurologic deficits or the presence of cauda equina syndrome or disc herniation. (B) X-rays are indicated in low back pain where there is a history of trauma. In this case there is a history of trauma when the patient picked up his grandson. (C) A urinalysis is indicated to assess for the presence of blood, which may be a sign of infection or stone.

5.3   **D** (A) Hip precautions are necessary to prevent stress on the hip joint **(4)** thus averting possible dislocation or dislodgment of surgical hardware. (B) These specific lab test are indicated to monitor for anemia, electrolyte imbalances, toxic or subtherapeutic drug levels and hypo- or hypercoagulation. (C) Patients who are at prolonged bed rest are at risk for pneumonia and atelectasis. A patient such as this needs proper pulmonary toilet.

5.4   **A** Septic bursitis usually presents with tenderness, erythema, swelling, pain with flexion of affected joint, limited ROM, fever, and elevated WBC.

5.5   **D** (1) Blood cultures to assess for specific causative organism and septicemia. (2) Ancef, a broad-spectrum antibiotic given IV instead of PO; it is more effective in this case. (3) Naprosyn given for inflammation and pain control.

Rheumatoid Arthritis

DEFINITION

Rheumatoid arthritis (RA) is a systemic autoimmune disorder of unknown etiology. The major feature is chronic, symmetric, and erosive synovitis of peripheral joints. Proliferative and inflammatory responses in the one-cell synovial lining tissue of the joint produces an erosive tissue called pannus. Pannus contains growth factors and inflammatory cytokines. A persistent inflammatory process occurs and continues to produce cytokines, which leads to destruction of cartilage and other extra-articular structures. The major histocompatibility locus (HLA) controls immune responses, an association of HLA-DR1 and HLA-DR4 with rheumatoid arthritis may indicate a defect in T-cell function on the immune response in RA.

ETIOLOGY/INCIDENCE

1. Prevalence: 1–2% of adult population
2. Female to male ratio: 2.5:1
3. Primary cause is as yet unknown

SIGNS AND SYMPTOMS

For the diagnosis of rheumatoid arthritis, the patient must have four of seven criteria present. Criteria 1 through 4 must be present for at least 6 weeks.

1. Morning stiffness: Morning stiffness in and around the joint, lasting at least 1 hour before maximal improvement.
2. Arthritis of three or more joints: At least three areas simultaneously have had soft tissue swelling or fluid observed by a health care provider.
3. Arthritis of hand joints: At least one area swollen.
4. Symmetric arthritis: Simultaneous involvement of the same joint areas on both sides of the body.
5. Rheumatoid nodules: Subcutaneous nodules, over bony prominence, or extensor surfaces, or in juxta-articular region observed by a health care professional.
6. Serum rheumatoid factor: Demonstration of abnormal amounts of serum rheumatoid factor by any method for which the result had been positive <5% of normal control subjects.
7. Radiographic changes: Radiographic changes typical of rheumatoid arthritis on posteroanterior hand and wrist radiographs adjacent to the involved joints (osteoarthritis changes alone do not qualify).

PHYSICAL FINDINGS

There are over 100 different types of arthritis. Because diagnosis and treatment of these disorders are clinically based, a complete and thorough history and physical remain the hallmark of diagnosis and treatment. In most rheumatic disorders the target organ is the joint.

1. Initial presentation: There is an insidious development of symptoms over several weeks, pain, symmetric swelling of multiple joints, morning stiffness.
2. Musculoskeletal exam
   A. Observe the joint for the following:
      1) Deformity
      2) Immobilization
      3) Muscle spasm and shortening
      4) Bone and cartilage destruction
      5) Ligament laxity
      6) Changed tendon function (i.e., tendon rupture)
      7) Synovitis
   B. Assess for joint pain
      1) Intra-articular
         a. Pain with active and passive ROM
         b. Tender parallel to joint surface and around joint
         c. Generalized pain
      2) Extra-articular
         a. Pain more with active and specific ROM
         b. Localized usually along tendon or ligament perpendicular to joint surface
         c. Can point to pain
3. Assess for extra-articular manifestations of rheumatoid arthritis such as:
   A. Skin
      1) Rheumatoid nodules
      2) Vascular lesions (i.e., splinter hemorrhages at fingertips)
   B. Ocular
      1) Episcleritis inflammation of the episclera
      2) Scleromalacia perforans erosion through sclera into the choroid
   C. Respiratory
      1) Inflammatory circoarytenoid joint (dysphonia, laryngeal pain)
      2) Interstitial lung disease
      3) Interstitial fibrosis
   D. Cardiac
      1) Inflammatory pericarditis
      2) Rheumatoid nodules in myocardium or valves
   E. GI: Gastritis or peptic ulcer disease with NSAIDs
   F. Neurologic
      1) Myelopathies related to cervical spine instability
      2) Entrapment neuropathies
      3) Ischemic neuropathies
      4) Mononeuritis multiplex
   G. Hematologic
      1) Anemias
      2) Felty's syndrome (RA and splenomegaly and leukopenia)

DIFFERENTIAL DIAGNOSIS

1. Osteoarthritis
2. Systemic lupus erythematosus
3. Ankylosing spondylitis
4. Systemic sclerosis
5. Polyarticular gout

DIAGNOSTIC TESTS/FINDINGS

No laboratory test, histologic, or radiographic findings conclusively determine diagnosis of rheumatoid arthritis.

General Laboratory

1. Urinalysis
   A. Analysis for protein and microscopic presence of cells
   B. Toxicity related to gold or penicillamine
   C. Hematuria toxicity to gold
2. Hematology
   A. Complete blood count with differential and platelet count
   B. Anemia
      1) Of chronic disease
      2) Due to gastrointestinal bleeding
      3) Hemolysis
      4) Iron deficiency
3. Blood chemistries
   A. Serum electrolytes, liver function, renal function, and mineral metabolism
      1) Monitor effects of treatment
      2) Early toxicity reflected by liver and kidney changes
4. Serologic tests
   A. Autoantibodies: Immunogloblin that is directed against a normally occurring protein or cell component
   B. Rheumatoid factor (RF) positive
      1) First autoantibody discovered
      2) IgM antibody directed against the constant portion of IgG
      3) 80% of rheumatoid arthritis patients have a positive RF
      4) Positive rheumatoid factor associated with severe disease, erosions of bone, extra-articular manifestations, greater disability
      5) RF will change with remission of disease
5. Acute-phase reactants
   A. Measured indirectly through erythrocyte sedimentation rate (ESR)
   B. Measured directly through C-reactive protein (CRP) (Changes in CRP occur and return more quickly but take 1 day to perform.)
   C. ESR elevated
   D. C-reactive protein elevated
6. Synovial fluid analysis
   A. Plays an important role in understanding pathophysiology of the joint.
   B. Unique and valuable information about what is going on inside joints.
   C. Alters diagnosis and affects treatment.

TABLE 5–1. Synovial Fluid Analysis

	Type	Clarity	Cell Count	Disorder
Group 1	Noninflammatory	Clear	<2000 monocytes	OA, osteonecrosis
Group 2	Inflammatory	Translucent	2000–20,000 monocytes	SLE, RA, crystalline arthritis
Group 3	Infection	Translucent	2000–20,000 monocytes, polymorphonuclear (PMN)	Infection, crystalline arthritis
Group 4	Traumatic	Bloody	Red blood cells	Bleeding disorders, trauma

OA, osteoarthritis; SLE, systemic lupus erythematosus; RA, rheumatoid arthritis.

D. Perform to rule out bacterial infection in severely inflamed joint (R/O septic joint).
E. See Table 5–1 for synovial fluid analysis.

MANAGEMENT/TREATMENT

1. Medication: General guidelines for the ACNP to consider when prescribing:
   A. It is recommended that all medications except analgesics be prescribed with consultation of a rheumatologist because of the side effects and the drug interactions.
   B. Decision to use any medication is based on the risk versus benefit ratio to the patient.
   C. Use the safest drug for the greatest benefit.
   D. In order to determine efficacy of drug therapy, use of the following medications need to be given in dosages that have been proven effective in RA. These drugs need to be given for the time proven effective.
   E. Therapy may include a combination of medications with different mechanisms.
   F. Intensity of treatment reflects the type, and severity of disorder.
   G. Types, combinations, and dosage vary depending on the provider.
   H. Single-drug therapy has been disappointing. Combination drug therapy is increasing (i.e., corticosteroid, slow-acting antirheumatic, NSAIDs).
   I. Control inflammation as aggressively as possible, inflammation is reversible, the damage done is not.
2. The ACNP may prescribe the following analgesics for relief of pain:
   A. Acetaminophen (Tylenol, Panadol, Anacin-3); 1000–4000 mg/day in three to four doses; taken as prescribed usually free of side effects; contraindications include alcohol use, kidney disease, hepatitis, or other liver disease.
   B. Acetaminophen with codeine: 1200–2400 acetaminophen combined with 60–480 mg of codeine per day in two to four doses.
      Side effects include constipation, dizziness or lightheadedness, drowsiness, nausea, vomiting, and over time psychological and physical dependence.
      Contraindications include drug or alcohol abuse, asthma, and kidney or thyroid disease.

TABLE 5–2. **Nonsteroidal Anti-inflammatory Drugs (NSAIDs)**

Drug	Dosage		
Diclofenac sodium (Voltaren)	100–150 mg/day in 2 doses	NSAIDs have similar side effects, such as: Abdominal pain, GI bleeding, gastric ulcers, diarrhea, fluid retention, heartburn, rash, indigestion, ringing in ears, interstitial nephritis, worsening of hypertension, pseudoallergic reactions (wheezing, rhinitis, laryngeal edema), inhibit platelet aggregation	A significant portion of patients have increased morbidity and mortality as a result of serious reactions to NSAIDs. These adverse effects occur in the following patients: Elderly, history of ulcers, smokers, current corticosteroid use, sensitivity or allergy to aspirin, kidney (intrinsic renal dysfunction), reduced renal blood flow
Diflunisal (Dolobid)	500–1000 mg/day in 2 doses		
Etodolac (Lodine)	600–1200 mg/day in 1–4 doses		
Fenoprofen calcium (Nalfon)	1800–2400 mg/day in 3–4 doses		
Flurbiprofen (Ansaid)	200–300 mg/day in 2–3 doses		
Ibuprofen (Motrin, Advil, Nuprin)	1200–3200 mg/day in 3–4 doses		
Indomethacin (Indocin)	50–200 mg/day in 2–4 doses		
Ketoprofen (Orudis, Oruvial)	150–200 mg/day in 3–4 doses		
Meclofenamate sodium (Meclomen)	200–400 mg/day in 3–4 doses		
Nabumetone (Relafen)	500–1000 mg/day in 1–2 doses		
Naproxen (Naprosyn)	500–1500 mg/day in 2–3 doses		
Naproxen sodium (Aflaxen, Anaprox, Aleve)	500–1650 mg/day in 2 doses		
Oxaprozin (Daypro)	1200–1800 mg/day in 1 dose		
Phenylbutazone (Butazolidin)	300–2400 mg/day in 3–4 doses or q4h (long-term use not more than 400 mg/day)		
Piroxicam (Feldene)	20 mg/day in 1 dose		
Sulindac (Clinoril)	150–200 mg/day in 2 doses		
Tolmetin sodium (Tolectin)	1200–2400 mg/day in 3 doses		

TABLE 5–3. Corticosteroids

Drug	Dose	
Cortisone (Cortone Acetate)	5–150 mg/day in 1 dose	Side effects of corticosteroids include: Hypothalmic-pituitary-adrenal axis suppression, growth retardation, amenorrhea, osteoporosis, aseptic bone necrosis, myopathy, glucose intolerance, hyperlipidemia, sodium and water retention, hypertension, hypokalemic alkalosis, euphoria, depression, acne, hirsutism, impaired wound healing, striate cataracts, glaucoma, susceptibility to infection
Dexamethasone (Decadron, Hexadrol)	0.75–9 mg/day in 1 dose	
Hydrocortisone (Cortef, Hydrocortone)	20–240 mg/day in 1 dose or several doses	
Methylprednisolone (Medrol)	4–160 mg/day in 1 dose or several doses	
Prednisolone (Prelone)	5–200 mg/day Aristocort	
Prednisolone sodium (Pediapred)	5–60 mL/day in 1–3 doses	
Prednisone (Deltasone, Orasone, Predincen-M, Sterapred)	1–60 mg/day in 3–4 doses evenly throughout day	
Triamcinolone (Aristocort)	4–60 mg/day in 1 dose or several doses	

3. The ACNP will consult with the collaborating physician regarding use of NSAIDs. Table 5–2 provides common medications.
4. The ANCP should consult with the collaborating physician regarding use of corticosteroids, which are potent anti-inflammatory agents (Table 5–3). The lowest dose should be used for the shortest time.
5. Tables 5–4 and 5–5 provide a list of antirheumatologic medications and their mechanisms of action. The ACNP in consultation with the rheumatologist should consider prescribing these medications for the modification of disease progress. The ACNP should be aware that there is a delayed onset of action (3 weeks to 3 months) and that the long-term efficacy is disappointing. Only methotrexate has been continued for more than 2 years by 50% of patients.
6. Prescribe guidelines for rest.
   A. General
      1) Nighttime sleep: 8–10 hours
      2) Day rest periods: 30–60 minute periods
      3) Proper positioning and posture (i.e., firm comfortable mattress [use of egg crate], pillows for neck that will put neck in flexion)
      4) Relaxation techniques (i.e., guided imagery)
   B. Joint
      1) Activity modification to avoid overuse or prevent injury

TABLE 5-4.   Slow-Acting Antirheumatic Drugs

Drug	Dose	Side Effects	Contraindications
Gold Auranofin (oral) Injectable gold Thiomalate (Myochrysine) Aurothioglucose (Solganol)	3–9 mg/day 1 dose or 2–3 doses 10 mg in a single dose week 1, 25 mg in a single dose week 2, 25–50 mg/wk 1 dose following weeks	Adverse 30% of patients, dermatitis, stomatitis, pruritis, gray-blue discoloration of mucous membranes, proteinuria, nephrotic syndrome leukopenia, thrombocytopenia, aplastic anemia, diarrhea (oral)	Kidney disease, skin disease
Methotrexate (Rheumatrex, oral) injectable	7.5–25 mg/wk in 1 dose of 3 divided	Decreased white blood cell count (WBC), megloblastic anemia, cirrhosis, pulmonary interstitial inflammation, nausea, vomiting, diarrhea, mouth ulcers	Liver disease, alcohol abuse, immune-system deficiency, liver disease
Hydroxychloroquine sulfate (Plaquenil)	200–600 mg/day in 2 doses	Retinopathy, skin rash, dyspepsia	Retinal abnormality
Penicillamine (Cuprimine, Depen)	125–150 mg in a single dose to start, increased to not more than 1500 mg in 1–3 doses	Rash, dermatitis, proteinuria, hematuria, neutropenia, thrombocytopenia	Penicillin allergy
Sulfasalazine (Azulfidine)	2–3 mg/day in 2–4 doses	Nausea, vomiting, hemolysis, blood dyscrasias, headache, rash, may cause male infertility	Allergy to sulfa drugs or aspirin
Azathioprine (Imuran)	50–150 mg/day in 1–3 doses	Nausea, dyspepsia decreased WBC, pancreatitis	Use of allopurinol
Cyclophosphamide (Cytoxan)	50–150 mg/day PO or IV in 1 dose	Hemorrhagic inflammation of urinary bladder, nausea, oral ulcers, decreased RBC, alopecia	Use with caution in liver or kidney
Cyclosporine (Sandimmune)	200–400 mg/day in 1–2 doses	Kidney damage, hypertension, increased body hair	Use with caution with hypertension

    2) Use of orthoses/splinting to reduce swelling, rest individual joint, un-load joint (i.e., cane) as needed, reduce biomechanical stress, position joint in proper alignment

7. May refer to physical or occupational therapy for exercise prescription:
   A. Relieve stiffness, maintain joint movement, increase elasticity of muscle and periarticular tissue, maintain flexibility
   B. Range of motion exercise at least once a day in acute joint inflammation:
     1) Isometric
       a. Improve muscle tone, strength, endurance
       b. Muscle contraction with joint movement

TABLE 5-5. Mechanisms of Action and Monitoring of Antirheumatic Drugs

Drug	Mechanism of Action	Monitoring
Gold	Inhibits PMN function Inhibits T- and B-cell activity Inhibits activation of macrophages	PO: CBC, (UA), biweekly to monthly Injectable: CBC, UA prior to each injection initially, then monthly
Methotrexate	Decreases PMN chemotaxis Decreases DNA synthesis	CBC, LFTs monthly
Hydroxychloroquine	Inhibits IL-1 release (in vivo)	Funduscopic and visual field exam every 6 months
Penicillamine	Inhibits T-cell function Inhibits antigen presentation	CBC, UA biweekly initially or changing dose, then monthly
Sulfasalazine	Decreases PMN migration Decreases lymphocyte response	CBC, LFTs, monthly × 3 months then every 1-2 months
Azathioprine	Interferes with DNA synthesis Decreases lymphocyte growth	CBC, 1-2 weekly initially then 1-3 months, LFTs 1-3 months
Cyclophosphamide	Decreases circulating T and B cells	CBC, UA monthly after initial weekly tests
Cyclosporine	Blocks synthesis of IL-2	CBC, serum creatinine, blood pressure weekly, then 2-4 weeks on maintenance dose

PMN, polymorphonuclear neutrophil leukocytes; DNA, deoxyribonucleic acid; CBC, complete blood count; UA, urinalysis; LFTs, liver function tests; IL-1, interleukin-1.

      c. Maintain contraction for 5-6 seconds, exhale during contraction, inhale with relaxation, no more than two muscle groups at a time, five to ten repetitions per day

   2) Dynamic

      a. Joint motion

      b. Changes in muscle length with repetitive muscle contraction and relaxation shortening and lengthening contractions

      c. Warm-up and cool down necessary, only move joint in pain-free zone, incorporate functional movement and body positions, progressively increase resistance and repetitions, reduce if joint swelling or increased pain

  8. Prescribe treatment to decrease inflammation, function, and pain

    A. Heat application (usually patient preference): Decrease; pain swelling and increases flexibility (i.e., hot packs, paraffin wax, topical cream/gels)

    B. Cold application (usually patient preference): Decrease pain, swelling and inflammation (i.e., ice packs, ice massage, cold baths, vapocoolant spray)

    C. Splints

      1) Reduce pain and inflammation by immobilizing/supporting joint and joint structures, improves functional use

      2) Types

         a. Resting: Used day and night to reduce joint inflammation and pain

         b. Functional: Improves function, provides stability and alignment to joint

         c. Soft splints: Day and night use to decrease stiffness, pain, improve function (i.e., gloves, wraps)

D. Assistive devices
   1) Increase independence
   2) Identify the type of devices necessary to aid in daily tasks to prevent stress and pain in joints
   3) Types
      a. Elevated toilet seat, tub rails and grab bars, car swivel seat cushion, toilet tongs for hygiene
      b. Dressing sticks, long handles, combs/brushes, swivel or rocker or angles utensils, doorway ramps
9. Joint arthroplasty: The ACNP should consult with the collaborating physician to determine need for referral to the orthopedic surgeon. Factors to consider are joint pathology, pain, and function.

PATIENT EDUCATION

The ACNP needs to educate the patient about the disease process, goals of treatment, and medication regimens.

1. Medications
   A. NSAIDs (Table 5–2)
      1) Take with food, glass of milk
      2) Two or more different drugs not beneficial; may increase risk of toxicity
      3) Report dark/tarry stools
   B. Corticosteroids (Table 5–3)
      1) Take with food.
      2) Single daily dose with breakfast.
      3) Do not stop medication abruptly. Dose must be tapered gradually.
      4) Identification carried on person who is steroid user.
      5) Inform about mood swings.
      6) Educate regarding diabetes.
      7) Intra-articular injection: Ice can be applied for pain for 24 hours following injection.
   C. Slow-acting antirheumatic drugs (Table 5–4)
      1) Gold
         a. PO, take with a glass of milk/water
         b. If stomach upset occurs, take with food
      2) Methotrexate
         a. Take with food or glass of milk/water
         b. Take once a week
      3) Hydroxychloroquine
         a. Take with food or glass of milk/water
         b. Report visual changes
      4) Penicillamine: Take with food or glass of milk/water
      5) Sulfasalazine
         a. Take with food or glass of milk/water
         b. May change the color of urine to orange
      6) Azathioprine
         a. Take with food
         b. Shape of pill may cause underdosing
      7) Cyclophosphamide
         a. Take oral medication with breakfast
         b. Drink a lot of fluid all day

8) Cyclosporine
    a. Take at the same time of day every day
    b. Report edema

2. Biobehavioral treatment
  A. Cognitive behavior therapy
    1) Learning new cognitive and behavioral coping skills to reduce physical and psychological disability
    2) Sessions: 5–10 weeks, 1–2 hours per session, 10–12 individuals in class
    3) Examples of cognitive skills:
      a. Relaxation
      b. Diversion
    4) Examples of behavioral skills:
      a. Goal setting
      b. Pacing techniques
  B. Self-management/self-help programs
    1) Learning disease-related information, exercises, problem-solving skills, training in adopting new behaviors, and communication skills
    2) Sessions: 5–7 weeks, 2 hours per session
    3) Examples:
      a. Arthritis self-management class
      b. Fibromyalgia self-help class

3. Use of modalities for inflammation, pain and function
  A. Splints
  B. Orthoses
  C. Assistive devices
  D. Heat
  E. Cold

References

Arnett, F.C., Edworth, S.M., Bloch, D.A., et al. (1988). The American Rheumatism Association 1987 revised criteria for the classification of rheumatism arthritis. *Arthritis Rheum 31*, 315–324.

Golding, D.N. (1982). *A Synopsis of Rheumatic Diseases* (4th ed.). London: Wright PSG.

Katz, W.A. (1987). *Diagnosis and Management of Rheumatic Diseases* (2nd ed.). Philadelphia: J.B. Lippincott Co.

Kelly, W.N., Harris, E.D., Ruddy, S., & Sledge, C.B., (1989). *Textbook of Rheumatology.* Philadelphia: W.B. Saunders Co.

Mitchell, D.M., Spitz, P.W., Young, D.Y., et al. (1986). Survival, prognosis, and causes of death in rheumatoid arthritis. *Arthritis Rheum 29*, 706–714.

Schumacher, R.H. (ed.). (1993). *Primer on Rheumatic Disease* (10th ed.). Atlanta: Arthritis Foundation.

Wagner, S.T., Belza, B.B., & Gall, E.P. (1996). *Clinical Care in the Rheumatic Diseases.* Atlanta: American College of Rheumatology.

Review Questions

5.6   Rheumatoid arthritis is:
  A. An erosive disease
  B. A degenerative disease

C. A disease that affects mainly men
D. An inflammatory disease

5.7 J.K. has rheumatoid arthritis and has been admitted for a total knee arthroplasty. What other conditions would you expect to find in a patient with RA?
A. Poor wound healing
B. An anemia
C. Normal bone
D. Hypertension

5.8 Which medications would J.K. most likely be taking for his RA?
A. Hydroxychloroquine (Plaquenil)
B. Prednisone
C. Naproxyn
D. Methotrexate

5.9 Which medication is considered a slow-acting antirheumatic medication?
A. Hydroxychloroquine (Plaquenil)
B. Prednisone
C. Naproxyn
D. Methotrexate

5.10 Which of the following are included in the criteria in making a diagnosis of RA?
A. Morning stiffness
B. Symmetric arthritis
C. Rheumatoid nodules
D. Vasculitis

Answers and Rationales

5.6 **A,** Rheumatoid arthritis is an inflammatory erosive disease that affects
D mainly women.

5.7 **A,** Rheumatoid arthritis patients have thin skin that does not heal eas-
B ily and usually anemia of chronic disease.

5.8 **A,** Medications with different mechanisms of action are used to control
B, rheumatoid arthritis to decrease inflammation and disease progres-
C, sion.
D

5.9 **A** Hydroxychloroquine (Plaquenil) is a slow-acting antirheumatic medication.

5.10 **A,** Vasculitis may be a manifestation of rheumatoid arthritis but it is
B, not part of the diagnostic criteria.
C

Systemic Lupus Erythematosus

DEFINITION

Inflammatory multisystem disease of unknown etiology.

Characterized by the production of antibodies to components of the cell nucleus in association with a many clinical manifestations. Whether systemic lupus erythomatosus (SLE) represents a single pathologic disorder with many different symptoms or a group of related conditions remains unknown. The ACNP should be aware that SLE is a syndrome and therefore patients present with a different constellation of symptoms and in varying severity.

ETIOLOGY/INCIDENCE

1. Disease of young women
2. Peak incidence between 15 and 44 years of age
3. Increased incidence in African American, age 90 and female
4. Strong familial aggregation with a higher frequency among first-degree relatives (25–50% of monozygotic twins: 5% dizygotic twins SLE occurs concordantly)

SIGNS AND SYMPTOMS

Criteria for diagnosis of SLE includes the patient having 4 or more of the 11 criteria listed in Table 5–6 serially or simultaneously, during any interval of observation.

PHYSICAL FINDINGS

The ACNP should be aware that the patient's physical findings may increase in type and severity. The waxing and waning of symptoms is common in rheumatic disease.

1. Skin manifestations
   A. Malar rash: "Butterfly" rash across nose malar eminence sparing the nasal folds precipitated by exposure to sunlight
   B. Discoid lupus: Chronic subcutaneous lesions
   C. Subacute cutaneous lupus erythematosus (SCLE): Nonfixed, nonscarring, exacerbating, and remitting; many with SCLE have antibody to Ro (SSA)
   D. Vasculitis
   E. Alopecia
   F. Livedo reticularis
   G. Telangiectasia
2. Musculoskeletal manifestations
   A. Arthralgias and arthritis are the most common presenting conditions.
   B. Arthritis:
      1) May involve any joint but typically small joints of hands, wrists, and knees
      2) Usually symmetric
      3) Typically not erosive but joint deformities may occur (Jaccoud's arthritis)
   C. Myositis.
   D. Avascular necrosis.
   E. Myalgia
3. Renal manifestations
   A. Proteinuria
   B. Hematuria
   C. Pyuria (>5WBC/hpf) in the absence of infection

TABLE 5–6. **Criteria for Diagnosis of SLE**

Criteria	Definition
Malar rash	Fixed erythema, flat or raised, over the malar eminence, tending to spare the nasolabial folds
Discoid rash	Erythematous raised patches with adherent kerotic scaling and follicular plugging; atrophic scarring may occur in lesions
Photosensitivity	Skin rash as a result of unusual reaction to sunlight, by patient history or health care professional observation
Oral ulcers	Oral or nasopharyngeal ulceration, usually painless, observed by a health care professional
Arthritis	Nonerosive arthritis involving two or more peripheral joints characterized by tenderness, swelling, or effusion
Serositis	Pleuritis; history of pleuritic pain or rub heard by a health care provider or evidence of pleural effusion *or* Pericarditis; documented by ECG or rub or evidence of pericardial effusion
Renal disorder	Persistent proteinuria >0.5 gm/day or >3+ if quantitation not performed *or* Cellular casts; may be red cells, hemoglobin, granular, tubular, or mixed
Neurologic disorder	Seizures in the absence of offending drugs or known metabolic derangement (e.g., uremia, ketoacidosis, or electrolyte imbalance) *or* Psychosis; in the absence of offending drugs or known metabolic derangement (e.g., uremia, ketoacidosis, or electrolyte imbalance)
Hematologic disorder	Hemolytic anemia; with reticulocytosis *or* Leukopenia; <4000/mm^3 total on two or more occasions *or* Lymphopenia; <1500 mm^3 on two or more occasions *or* Thrombocytopenia; <100,000/mm^3 in the absence of offending drugs
Immunologic disorder	Positive LE cell preparation *or* Anti-DNA; antibody to native DNA in abnormal titer *or* Anti-Sm; presence of antibody to SM nuclear antigen *or* False-positive serologic test for syphilis known to be positive for at least 6 months
Antinuclear antibody	An abnormal titer of antinuclear antibody by immunofluorescence or an equivalent assay at any point in time and in the absence of drugs known to be associated with "drug-induced lupus" syndrome

* From Yan, E.M., Cohen, A.S., Fries, J.F., et al. (1982). The 1982 revised criteria for the classification of systemic lupus erythematous. Arthritis Rheum *25*, 1271–1277, with permission.
ECG, electrocardiogram; SLE, systemic lupus erythematosus.

D. Elevated creatinine
E. Abnormality on renal biopsy
4. Neuropsychiatric manifestations
   A. Headache
   B. Seizures
   C. Cerebral vascular accidents
   D. Cranial neuropathy
   E. Organic brain disorder
   F. Transverse myelitis
   G. Psychosis
   H. Mononeuritis multiplex
   I. Sensory peripherial neuropathy
5. Cardiovascular
   A. Pericarditis
   B. Pericardial effusion
   C. Contraction disturbance
   D. Libman-Sacks endocarditis
   E. Myocarditis
   F. Vasculitis
   G. Raynaud's phenomenon
6. Gastrointestinal manifestations
   A. Diffuse abdominal pain
   B. Anorexia
   C. Nausea
   D. Peritonitis
7. Pulmonary manifestations
   A. Pneumonitis
   B. Pulmonary hemorrhage
   C. Pulmonary embolism
   D. Pulmonary hypertension
   E. Pleurisy
   F. Pleural effusion
8. Hematologic manifestations
   A. Cytopenias
      1) Anemia, hemolytic anemia Coombs'-positive and Coombs'-negative
      2) Leukopenia
      3) Lymphopenia
      4) Thrombocytopenia
   B. Clotting abnormalities
      1) False-positive Venereal Disease Research Laboratories (VDRI) test for syphilis
      2) Lupus anticoagulant
      3) Anticardiolipin antibody
   C. General
      1) Fatigue
      2) Fever
      3) Loss of appetite
      4) Loss of weight

DIFFERENTIAL DIAGNOSIS

1. Rheumatoid arthritis
2. Scleroderma

3. Polymyositis
4. Mixed connective tissue disease (MCTD)

DIAGNOSTIC TESTS/FINDINGS

The ACNP should consider the criteria for diagnosis when ordering diagnostic tests.
1. Antinuclear antibody (ANA)
   A. Antinuclear antibodies not diagnostic of SLE: Titers 1/80 have less significance than those with greater titers.
   B. The ACNP may find the patterns identified with ANA tests to be helpful in making a diagnosis. These include the following:

Pattern	Disease
Rim or peripheral	SLE
Nucleolar or centromere	Systemic sclerosis
Diffuse or speckled in low titers	No underlying disorder

The ACNP should be aware that if the ANA is positive, additional testing for the related protein antigen is indicated. The ACNP may find the identification of the autoantibody to be helpful in making a diagnosis. The following autoantibodies may be reported in the results of an ANA panel.

Autoantibody	Disorder	Frequency
RF	Rheumatoid arthritis	70–80%
Anti-ds DNA	SLE	40–70%
Anti-ss DNA	Drug-induced SLE	80%
Anti-SM	SLE	20–30%
Sci-70	Diffuse scleroderma	70%
SS-A, SS-B	Primary Sjögren's syndrome	70–90%
Anti-U, RNP	MCTD	>95%

2. Complement
   A. C3 and C4 measure the complement pathways.
   B. CH50 measures of the entire complement pathway.
   C. Low levels are usually related to consumption of complement by immune complex activation of the classical pathway.
   D. Decrease in complement may preceed a flare-up of disease.
3. Renal biopsy for lupus nephritis
4. Positive direct Coombs' test for hemolytic anemia
5. Acute-phase reactants elevated
6. General hematologic tests for monitoring of medications and disease
   A. Urinalysis analysis for protein and microscopic presence of cells
   B. Lupus nephritis

MANAGEMENT/TREATMENT

The ACNP should be aware of the different treatment modalities available but should consider all of the organ systems involved in SLE before implementing.
1. Medication
   A. General guidelines for the ACNP to consider

    1) It is recommended that all medications except analgesics be prescribed with consultation of a rheumatologist because of the side effects, drug interactions, and the multisystem involvement of SLE.

    2) Medications generally prescribed for SLE patients. See "Rheumatoid Arthritis" for dose, side effects, mechanisms of action, and monitoring of these medications.

  B. NSAIDs

  C. Corticosteroids (topical, PO, and IV)

  D. Hydroxychloroquine and chloroquine (especially for skin manifestations)

  E. Methotrexate

  F. Azathioprine

  G. Cyclophosphamide

2. Prescribe guidelines for rest
  A. General
    1) Nighttime sleep: 8–10 hours
    2) Day rest periods: 30–60 minute periods
    3) Proper positioning and posture (i.e., firm comfortable mattress)
    4) Relaxation techniques (i.e., guided imagery)
  B. Joint
    1) Activity modification to avoid overuse or prevent injury
    2) Use of orthoses/splinting to reduce swelling, rest individual joint

3. Prescribe guidelines for exercise (see "Rheumatoid Arthritis")
  A. Relieve stiffness, maintain flexibility
  B. Types:
    1) Isometric
    2) Dynamic

4. Prescribe treatment to decrease inflammation and pain, and increase function; see "Rheumatoid Arthritis" for heat, cold applications, splints, and assistive devices.

5. Joint arthroplasty: The ACNP should consult with the orthopedic surgeon when the patient's joint pathology, pain and function are indictive of surgery. SLE patients usually experience total hip arthroplasty because of avascular necrosis secondary to corticosteroid use.
  A. Preoperative measures
    1) Stop aspirin and NSAIDs 1 day to 1 month before surgery according to half-life.
    2) Evaluate the need for IV corticosteroids (i.e., long-term use of corticosteroids).
      a. Prevent postoperative infection
      b. Dental check-up
      c. Urine culture (asymptomatic bacturia)
      d. Closure of any open skin wounds

6. Consultation
  A. Physical and occupational therapy for:
    1) Exercise
    2) Splints and orthoses
    3) Assistive devices
    4) Total joint precautions
  B. Rheumatologist: Any worsening of condition
  C. Social services: Sexual and marital counseling, family counseling
  D. Orthopedic surgeon: Total joint arthroplasty

PATIENT EDUCATION

The ACNP needs to educate the patient about the disease process, goals of treatment, and medication regimens.

1. Medication (see "Rheumatoid Arthritis")
    A. NSAIDs
    B. Corticosteroids (topical, PO, and IV)
    C. Hydroxychloroquine and chloroquine
    D. Methotrexate
    E. Azathioprine
    F. Cyclophosphamide
2. Family planning: The ACNP should educate the patient about the necessity of planning pregnancies because of the toxicities of the medications and the multiple system involvement of SLE.
3. Biobehavioral education
    A. Cognitive behavior therapy: See "Rheumatoid Arthritis" for cognitive-behavior therapy
    B. Self-management/self-help programs
        1) See "Rheumatoid Arthritis" for self-management
        2) Arthritis Foundation SLE self-help class
4. Education of modalities for inflammation, pain, and function
5. Education for avoiding sun exposure by using sunblock and care in using photosensitizing antibiotics

References

Golding, D.N. (1982). *A Synopsis of Rheumatic Diseases* (4th ed.). London: Wright PSG.

Katz, W.A. (1987). *Diagnosis and Management of Rheumatic Diseases* (2nd ed.). Philadelphia: J.B. Lippincott Co.

Kelly, W.N., Harris, E.D., Ruddy, S., & Sledge, C.B. (1989). *Textbook of Rheumatology*. Philadelphia: W.B. Saunders Co.

Klippel, J.H. (ed.). (1988). Systemic lupus erythematosus. *Rheum Dis Clin North Am 14*.

Schumacher, R.H. (ed.). (1993). *Primer on Rheumatic Disease* (10th ed.). Atlanta: Arthritis Foundation.

Wagner, S.T., Belza, B.B., & Gall, E.P. (1996). *Clinical Care in the Rheumatic Diseases*. Atlanta: American College of Rheumatology.

Yan, E.M., Cohen, A.S., Fries, J.F., et al. (1982). The 1982 revised criteria for the classification of systemic lupus erythematosus. *Arthritis Rheum 25*, 1271–1277.

Review Questions

5.11. Mrs. Smith presents in the emergency room with newly diagnosed SLE. Which of the following symptoms might she present with?
    A. A seizure
    B. A rash when in the sun
    C. A red rash on her nose and cheeks
    D. Pleurisy on x-ray

5.12. Which of the following diagnostic tests would be most helpful in ruling out SLE in Mrs. Smith?
   A. ANA
   B. ANA panel
   C. RF
   D. UA

5.13. Which of the following are true of SLE?
   A. It is an inflammatory disease
   B. It is a multisystem disease
   C. It is increased in men
   D. Its etiology is unknown

5.14. In monitoring SLE activity, which of the following laboratory tests would be most valuable?
   A. C3/C4
   B. VDRL
   C. RF
   D. CBC

5.15. Mrs. Smith has persistent proteinuria, hematuria, and casts. Which of the following conditions would you suspect?
   A. Lupus nephritis
   B. Diabetes
   C. Rheumatoid arthritis
   D. Osteoarthritis

Answers and Rationales

5.11   **A,** All of these symptoms are part of the criteria for diagnosis.
       B,
       C,
       D

5.12   **A,** The ANA will be positive in SLE patients and the ANA panel will
       B, indicate the antigen for specificity of disease. The UA will indicate
       D lupus nephritis.

5.13   **A,** SLE is a multisystem disease of unknown etiology, which has various
       D clinical manifestations.

5.14   **A,** C3/C4 measure complement and will be decreased with active SLE.
       D The CBC will monitor cytopenias, leukopenia, and thrombocyto-
       penia.

5.15   **A** The symptoms indicate lupus nephritis, which may be life threaten-
       ing and should be diagnosed and treated quickly.

Gout

DEFINITION

Tissue deposition of crystals of monosodium urate from supersaturated extra-cellular fluids that results in one or more clinical manifestations.

1. Gouty arthritis: Recurrent attacks of severe acute or chronic articular and periarticular inflammation

2. Tophi: Accumulation of articular, osseous, soft tissue, and cartilaginous crystalline deposits
3. Uric acid calculi
4. Gouty nephropathy: Renal impairment

ETIOLOGY/INCIDENCE

1. Adult men with a peak incidence in fifth decade
2. Most prominent cause of inflammatory arthritis in men over age 30

SIGNS AND SYMPTOMS/PHYSICAL FINDINGS

1. Acute gouty arthritis
   A. Metatarsophalangeal (MTP) joint of the first toe is involved most often; ankle, tarsal area, and knee are also frequently affected.
   B. First episode: Abrupt onset, often during the night, patient awakes with dramatic joint pain and swelling.
   C. Early attacks tend to resolve spontaneously over 3–10 days even without treatment.
   D. Subsequent attacks occur more frequently, involve more joints, and last longer.
   E. Polyarticular gout can be present in first attack.
2. Intercritical gout
   A. Intervals between attacks
   B. Usually symptom free but crystals may be found in synovial fluid
3. Chronic tophaceous gout
   A. Subcutaneous monosodium urate crystals containing tophi occur in advanced gout.
   B. More common location, of tophi include:
      1) Synovium
      2) Subchondral bone
      3) Olecranon bursa
      4) Infrapatellar and Achilles tendons
      5) Subcutaneous tissue on the extensor surface of forearms
      6) Helix of ear
      7) Heart valves
4. Gouty nephropathy
   A. Urolithiasis
   B. Proteinuria

DIFFERENTIAL DIAGNOSIS

1. Cellulitis
2. Osteoarthritis
3. Rheumatoid arthritis
4. Pseudogout

DIAGNOSTIC TESTS/FINDINGS

1. Synovial fluid contains monosodium urate crystals
2. Nodules with urate crystals

MANAGEMENT/TREATMENT

The ACNP should be aware that the early symptoms of gout may resolve in 3–5 days without treatment. The ACNP should be aware of the type of gout, the history of the number of attacks, and the duration between attacks before considering management and treatment. Some medication regimens and treatment modalities are as follows:

1. Prescribe medications after consideration of the following:
   A. Two types
      1) Treating gouty arthritis includes NSAIDs, corticosteroids, and colchicine.
      2) Treating long-term complications by decreasing uric acid levels includes probenecid, sulfinpyrazone, and allopurinol.

   Table 5–7 provides common medications for the treatment of gout.

1. Acute gout:
   A. Colchicine
   B. NSAIDs at or near maximum recommended dose (long-acting not recommended)

TABLE 5–7. **Gout Medications**

Drug	Dose	Side Effects	Contraindications
Allopurinol (Loprin, Zyloprim)	100–300 mg/day in 1 dose, reserved for urate overproducers, nephrolithiasis or other renal insufficiency	Pruritic rash, dyspepsia, diarrhea	Hyperuricemia
Probenecid (Benemid, Probalan)	0.5 gm/day initially, advanced to not more than 1 gm bid; colchicine may be needed for 6 months or more to avoid acute attacks	Rash, dyspepsia, nephrolithiasis, headache	Glomerular filtration rate (GFR) <50–60 mL/min, inability to ingest 2 L of fluids a day, past history of nephrolithiasis, inability to ingest salicylates
Colchicine	0.6–1.2 mg/day in 1–2 doses for prevention, 0.6 mg q2h (no more than 8 doses/day to stop acute attacks) IV 1. 3 mg total single dose 2. 4 mg total daily dose 3. After a full course of IV colchicine, no additional by any route 4. Adjust dose in renal and hepatic failure	Toxicity in 80% nausea, vomiting, abdominal cramping, thrombophlebitis, neuromuscular syndrome	IV 1. Combined renal and hepatic disease 2. GFR <10 mL 3. Extrahepatic biliary obstruction

       C. Corticosteroids (intrarticular injections)
2. Intercritical gout:
    A. The decision to provide prophylactic treatment depends on many issues and should be considered after a pattern of frequency has been established.
    B. Antihyperuricemic drugs:
       1) Two choices: Probenecid (uricosuric agent) and allopurinal can be used if uric acid level excreation is < 700 mg/day normal renal function
          a. Probenecid first: Does not interfer with purine or pyrimidine metabolism
          b. Allopurinol
            i. History of renal calculi
            ii. Presence of tophi
            iii. Failure of uricosuric agent
3. Prescribe a weight-reduction diet and program.
4. Prescribe a program for the elimination of alcohol ingestion.
5. Prescribe rest for the affected joint.

PATIENT EDUCATION

The ACNP needs to educate the patient about the disease process, goals of treatment, and medication regimens.
1. Medication
    A. Allopurinol
       1) Take immediately after a meal
       2) Stop taking and report first sign of a rash
       3) May experience hives, itching
       4) May experience acute attack with initial doses
    B. Probenecid
       1) Take with food or an antacid
       2) Do not take with aspirin or other salicylates
       3) Avoid alcohol
       4) May experience headache, joint pain, skin rash, dyspepsia
2. Biobehavioral programs
    A. Weight reduction
    B. Elimination of alcohol ingestion
3. Education for rest and elevation of the affected joint
4. Demonstrate the use of cold packs and prn ice massage
5. Consultation
    A. Rheumatologist: Any worsening of condition
    B. Pharmacist: Drug interactions

References

Boss, G.R., & Seegmiller, J.E. (1979). Hyperuricemia and gout: Classification, complications, and management. *N Engl J Med 300*, 1459–1468.

Fox, I.H., & Kelly, W.N. (1979). Management of gout. *JAMA 242*, 361–364.

Golding, D.N. (1982). *A Synopsis of Rheumatic Diseases* (4th ed.). London: Wright PSG.

Katz, W.A. (1987). *Diagnosis and Management of Rheumatic Diseases* (2nd ed.). Philadelphia: J.B. Lippincott Co.

Kelly, W.N., Harris, E.D., Ruddy, S., & Sledge, C.B. (1989). *Textbook of Rheumatology.* Philadelphia: W.B. Saunders Co.

Schumacher, R.H. (ed.). (1993). *Primer on Rheumatic Disease* (10th ed.) Atlanta: Arthritis Foundation.

Wagner, S.T., Belza, B.B., & Gall, E.P. (1996). *Clinical Care in the Rheumatic Diseases.* Atlanta: American College of Rheumatology.

Review Questions

5.16 Gouty nephropathy includes which of the following:
A. Urolithiasis
B. Proteinuria
C. Glucosuria
D. Polyuria

5.17 In normal synovial fluid you would expect to find which of the following?
A. Clear pale yellow, pH 7.5.
B. Clear white, pH 7.0
C. Cloudy but white, pH 7.9
D. Cloudy, yellow, pH 7.0

5.18 R.K. presents with a great toe that is red to midfoot, swollen, and tender. Which of the following treatments would be appropriate?
A. Start PO antibiotics
B. Start IV antibiotics
C. Joint fluid analysis
D. Warm foot soaks

5.19 Your education program in a patient with gout would include which of the following:
A. Weight reduction
B. Rest
C. Red wine with dinner
D. Hot packs

5.20 Gout is more prevalent in which of the following:
A. Men
B. Women
C. Young adults
D. Asians

Answers and Rationales

5.16 **A,** Kidney stones and protein in the urine are symptoms of gouty ne-
      B phropathy. Polyuria and glucosuria are associated with diabetes mellitus.

5.17 **A** This is part of the description for normal synovial fluid. The synovial fluid for gout contains monosodium urate crystals.

5.18 **C** The differential diagnosis would include a septic joint and gout. In order to make the diagnosis you would analyze the joint fluid. Treatment and management would be determined by the results.

5.19   **A,** Rest for the joint will enhance the other modalities of treatment and
       B reduce the stress of weight bearing. Decreasing weight will reduce
       the dynamic force on the joint.
5.20   **A** Gout has a higher prevalence in middle aged or older men.

Osteoarthritis

DEFINITION

Osteoarthritis is the most common joint disease, and is a degenerative monoar-
ticular disorder affecting the hands and large weight-bearing joints. It is characterized by pain, deformity, enlargement of the joints, limitation of movement,
formation of new cartilage, and new bone growth in the joint margin (osteo-
phytes).

ETIOLOGY/INCIDENCE

Osteoarthritis affects about 60 million people in the United States; it is estimated that 50% have clinical signs by 60 years of age.

SIGNS AND SYMPTOMS/PHYSICAL FINDINGS

1. General
   A. Usually local.
   B. Pain early in disease occurs after joint use, relieved with rest.
   C. Later pain occurs with minimal motion and can occur at rest.
   D. Night pain may occur at this point.
   E. Pain on passive range of motion.
   F. Crepitus with joint range of motion.
   G. Bony deformity.
   H. Stiffness <30 minutes.
   I. Absence of warmth.
2. Hands
   A. Herberden's nodes: Spurs found at distal interphalangeal (DIP) joints.
   B. Bouchard's nodes: Spurs found at the proximal interphalangeal (PIP)
      joints.
   C. Nodes develop slowly over a number of years.
   D. Gelatinous cysts may appear before the node appears.
   E. DIP joints are the most frequent sight of hand involvement. PIP joints
      are also affected. MCP joints are rarely involved.
3. Knee: Localized tenderness over the knee and pain with passive or active
   range of motion and crepitus
4. Hip
   A. Insidious onset of pain, may be followed by a limp
   B. Pain is usually localized in the groin or the inner aspect of the thigh,
      buttocks, sciatic region, or knee
   C. Loss of hip motion marked by loss of internal rotation or extension
5. Foot: First metatarsophalangeal joint aggravated by tight shoes
6. Spine
   A. Lumbar spine symptoms include local pain, stiffness, radicular pain due
      to compression of nerve roots

B. Spinal stenosis common in lumbar spine; results from degenerative spurs, disc herniation
7. A. Osteoarthritis of the glenohumeral joint is rare without trauma or some other predisposing condition.

DIFFERENTIAL DIAGNOSIS

1. Seronegative rheumatoid arthritis
2. Gout
3. Charcot's joint
4. Paget's disease

DIAGNOSTIC TESTING

The ACNP should become familiar with viewing radiographs and with the findings for identifying osteoarthritis.

1. Radiologic findings
   A. Joint space narrowing
   B. Subchondral bony sclerosis
   C. Marginal osteophyte formation
   D. Cyst formation
2. Laboratory data not helpful except in negative sense

MANAGEMENT/TREATMENT

The ACNP should be aware that the main goals of treatment are to relieve pain and improve/maintain function.

1. Prescribe medications (see "Rheumatoid Arthritis")
   A. NSAIDs
   B. Analgesics
2. Recommend a biobehavioral program: Self-management for education about the disease process
3. Prescribe guidelines for rest
   A. General
   B. Joint
4. Prescribe guidelines for exercise (see "Rheumatoid Arthritis")
   A. Isometric
   B. Dynamic
5. Prescribe treatment to increase function and decrease pain
   A. Heat application
   B. Cold application
   C. Splints
   D. Assistive devices
6. Recommend joint arthroplasty: The ACNP should consult with the orthopedic surgeon when the patient's joint pathology, pain, and function indicate the need for surgery.
7. Consultation
   A. Physical and occupational therapy for:
      1) Exercise
      2) Splints and orthoses

      3) Assistive devices

      4) Total joint precautions

  B. Rheumatologist: Any worsening of condition

  C. Social services: Sexual and marital counseling, family counseling

  D. Orthopedic surgeon: Total joint arthroplasty

PATIENT EDUCATION

The ACNP needs to educate the patient about the disease process, goals of treatment, and medication regimens.

1. Education of medication regimen, and side effects (see "Rheumatoid Arthritis").
   A. NSAIDs
   B. Analgesics
2. Discuss biobehavioral treatment.
   A. Cognitive behavior therapy
   B. Self-management/self-help programs
   C. Weight-reduction program
3. Discuss the use of modalities for inflammation, pain, and function.
4. Pre- and postoperative education.
5. Discuss the use of rest treatment modalities.
6. Discuss the benefits of the use of a daily exercise program.

References

Golding, D.N. (1982). *A Synopsis of Rheumatic Diseases* (4th ed.). London: Wright PSG.

Katz, W.A. (1987). *Diagnosis and Management of Rheumatic Diseases* (2nd ed.). Philadelphia: Lippincott Co.

Kelly, W.N., Harris, E.D., Ruddy, S., & Sledge, C.B. (1989). *Textbook of Rheumatology.* Philadelphia: W.B. Saunders Co.

Moskowitz, R.W., Howell, D.W., Goldberg, W.H., & Mankin, H.J. (1984). *Osteoarthritis: Diagnosis and Treatment.* Philadelphia: W.B. Saunders Co.

Schumacher, R.H. (ed.). (1993). *Primer on Rheumatic Disease* (10th ed.). Atlanta: Arthritis Foundation.

Wagner, S.T., Belza, B.B., & Gall, E.P. (1996). *Clinical Care in the Rheumatic Diseases.* Atlanta: American College of Rheumatology.

Review Questions

5.21 Mr. J is a 60-year-old with osteoarthritis of the knee. His symptoms most likely would include which of the following?
   A. Pain with active and passive range of motion
   B. Tender parallel to joint surface and around the joint
   C. Generalized pain
   D. Can point to the pain

5.22 When examining the hands of a patient with OA, the ACNP may find which of the following?
   A. Herberden's nodes
   B. Bouchard's nodes

C. Nodes that developed slowly over a number of years
D. Gelatinous cysts that appeared before the nodes

5.23 Which of the following would be included in patient education for OA?
A. Discuss the use of modalities for inflammation, pain, and function.
B. Discuss the use of rest treatment modalities.
C. Discuss the benefits of the use of a daily exercise program.
D. The use of daily PO corticosteroids.

5.24 Which of the following medications are useful in the treatment of OA?
A. NSAIDs
B. Analgesics
C. PO corticosteroids
D. Plaquenil

5.25 Which of the following might the ACNP refer the patient with OA to:
A. Physical therapy
B. Social services
C. Orthopedic surgeon
D. Occupational therapy

Answers and Rationales

5.21 **A, B, C**   Local pain is indicative of extra-articular joint involvement.

5.22 **A, C, D**   Bouchard's nodes are found in the PIP joints of the hands.

5.23 **A, B, C**   Corticosteroids can be injected into the joint, but are not indicated for oral use because the mechanism of action would have no effect in osteoarthritis.

5.24 **A, B**   Hydroxychloroquine (Plaquenil) is used in rheumatoid arthritis and corticosteroids can be injected into the joint, but are not indicated for oral use because their mechanisms of action would have no effect in osteoarthritis.

5.25 **A, B, C, D**   Treating osteoarthritis is a multidisciplinary team effort. All members have a contribution.

Regional Rheumatic Pain Syndromes

DEFINITION

Regional rheumatic pain syndromes are disorders that affect tendon, ligament, muscle, and bursa that are often difficult to diagnose and treat. Tendinitis is the inflammation of the peritendon tissue or synovial sheath (tenosynovitis). Bursitis is an inflammation of the bursa. The ACNP should become familiar with the examination of the extra-articular area of the joint in order to identify the disorders.

PHYSICAL FINDINGS

See Table 5–8 for common areas of tendinitis and bursitis.

TABLE 5–8.   Common Areas of Tendinitis and Bursitis

	Site	Symptom
Supraspinatus tendinitis	Anterior shoulder pain Increased in lateral deltoid area	Often with calcium deposits Often with an osteophyte at the underside of the acromion-clavicular joint Less pain with passive range of motion (ROM) Pain at 60- to 120-degree arc of motion
Bicipital tendinitis	Chronic pain in the anterior region of the shoulder Pain with supination or shoulder flexion against resistance Pain with extension of shoulder	Tender over bicipital groove
de Quervain's tendinitis	Pain in wrist around radial styloid Complication of pregnancy	Pain is increased with thumb folded across palm and wrist turned toward ulna
Lateral epicondylitis (tennis elbow)	Pain occurs with hand shaking, lifting a briefcase or other similar activities	Hallmark: Localized tenderness directly over the lateral epicondyle
Anserine bursitis	Knee pain especially with stairs	Pain at medial aspect of knee
Infrapatellar bursitis	Knee pain	Below patella swelling and tender
Calcaneal bursitis	Plantar surface of heel pain	Calcaneum pressure produces tenderness
Trochanteric bursitis	Aching over the trochanteric area and lateral thigh	Point tenderness over the trochanteric area

DIFFERENTIAL DIAGNOSIS

1. Osteoarthritis
2. Rheumatoid arthritis
3. Chronic fatigue syndrome
4. Fibromyalgia
5. Tendon tear

MANAGEMENT/TREATMENT

The ACNP should consider any other joint conditions and the general condition of the muscle when considering modalities for management and treatment.

1. Prescribe medications (see "Rheumatoid Arthritis").
   A. NSAIDs
   B. Analgesics
   C. Corticosteroids (intra-articular injections)
   D. Spray and stretch (vapocoolant spray with gentle stretching of muscle)
2. Prescribe a program of exercise.
   A. Stretching
   B. Dynamic: Strengthening, endurance, and conditioning

3. Prescribe a program of rest: Tendinitis may be rested for 2–3 days before beginning exercise.
4. Prescribe heat and cold modalities: Cold modalities may be used before and after exercise.

PATIENT EDUCATION

The ACNP should consider the patient's lifestyle and occupation to assess for repetitive motion activities or dysfunctional use of joint during activities.

1. Explain the medication regimen and side effects.
   A. Discuss the necessity of taking the medications in the prescribed dose for the maximum effect.
   B. Self-management programs.
2. Explain the objectives of a biobehavioral program: Cognitive-behavioral program.
3. Demonstrate the modalities of a rest program.
4. Explain the use of assistive devices for activities of daily living.
5. Discuss an exercise program that will be appropriate for the disorder.
6. Consultation.
   A. Physical and occupational therapy for:
      1) Exercise
      2) Splints and orthoses
      3) Assistive devices
      4) Total joint precautions
   B. Rheumatologist: Any worsening of condition

Fibromyalgia

DEFINITION

Fibromyalgia is a disorder characterized by widespread pain that has been present for at least 3 months and tender areas at 11 of 18 anatomic sites of unknown etiology. The ACNP should be aware that this is a disorder that is slow to respond to treatment.

ETIOLOGY/INCIDENCE

1. 3.4% of women
2. 0.5% of men in the United States
3. 25–45 years of age

SIGNS AND SYMPTOMS

1. Generalized widespread pain for > 3 months
2. Fatigue
3. Decreased quality of sleep
4. Irritable bowel
5. Cognitive dysfunction
6. Paresthesias

PHYSICAL FINDINGS

1. Tender points in the described anatomic sites
   A. Location of tender points:
      1) Occiput: Suboccipital muscle insertions
      2) Low cervical: Anterior aspects of the intertransverse spaces at C5–C7
      3) Trapezius: Midpoint of the upper boarder
      4) Supraspinatus: Above the scapula spine near the medial boarder
      5) Second rib: Costochondral junctions, lateral to junction upper surface
      6) Lateral epicondyle: 2 cm distal to condyle
      7) Gluteal: Upper outer quadrants of buttocks in anterior fold of muscle
      8) Greater trochanter: Posterior to trochanteric prominence
      9) Knee: Medial fat pad proximal to the knee joint
   B. Abnormal stage 3–4 sleep on electroencephalogram (EEG)
   C. Deconditioned muscle
   D. No joint swelling
   E. No weight loss or fever

DIFFERENTIAL DIAGNOSIS

1. SLE
2. Rheumatoid arthritis
3. Chronic fatigue syndrome
4. Multiple sclerosis
5. Depression
6. Psychological dysfunction

DIAGNOSTIC TESTS

1. None.
2. Tests may be performed to rule out any number of conditions.
3. Fibromyalgia is a diagnosis based on exclusion but diagnosed based on history and clinical assessment.

MANAGEMENT/TREATMENT

The ACNP should be aware that this is a difficult disorder to treat. A multidimensional approach is needed. The deconditioned musculature makes a "go-slow" approach necessary.

1. Prescribe medication.
   A. NSAIDs (see "Medication" section in "Rheumatoid Arthritis")
   B. Tricylic antidepressant in low doses to improve quality of sleep (e.g., amytriptyline [Elavil] 10–25 mg every night)
2. Prescribe an exercise program, which is an essential part of management.
   A. Stretching
   B. Dynamic: Strengthening, endurance, and conditioning
   C. Hydrotherapy program
   D. Spray and stretch (vapocoolant spray with gentle stretching of muscle)

PATIENT EDUCATION

1. Educate the patient about the reason for recommending medications, side effects, and regimen.

2. Discuss a biobehavioral program with prevention of relapse.
   A. Self-management program
   B. Cognitive-behavioral program
3. Discuss a program of rest balanced with daily activities.
4. Plan the type and amount of participation in an exercise program. Explain that this is an essential part of the management program.
5. Explain the sleep cycle and the correlation of lack of rest, sleep, and musculoskeletal pain.
6. Demonstrate and teach relaxation techniques.

References

Cailliet, R. (1988). *Soft Tissue Pain and Disability* (2nd ed.). Philadelphia: F.A. Davis Co.

Golding, D.N. (1982). *A Synopsis of Rheumatic Diseases* (4th ed.). London: Wright PSG.

Katz, W.A. (1987). *Diagnosis and Management of Rheumatic Diseases* (2nd ed.). Philadelphia: J.B. Lippincott Co.

Kelly, W.N., Harris, E.D., Ruddy, S., & Sledge, C.B. (1989). *Textbook of Rheumatology.* Philadelphia: W.B. Saunders Co.

Klippel, J.H. (ed.). (1988). Systemic lupus erythematosus. *Rheum Dis Clin North Am 14.*

Schumacher, R.H. (ed.). (1993). *Primer on Rheumatic Disease* (10th ed.). Atlanta: Arthritis Foundation.

Wagner, S.T., Belza, B.B., & Gall, E.P. (1996). *Clinical Care in the Rheumatic Diseases.* Atlanta: American College of Rheumatology.

Wolfe, F., Smythe, H.A., Yunus, M.B., et al. (1990). The American College of Rheumatology 1990 Criteria for the Classification of Fibromyalgia. Report of the Multicenter Criteria Committee. *Arthritis Rheum 33,* 160–172.

Review Questions

5.26 M.J. is 30 years old and has fibromyalgia. Which of the following symptoms might she present with?
   A. Tenderness at the suboccipital muscle insertions
   B. Tenderness at anterior aspects of the intertransverse spaces at C5–C7
   C. Denies fatigue
   D. Poor sleep

5.27 Which of the following treatment modalities would be indicated for M.J.?
   A. NSAIDs
   B. Elavil 10–25 mg every night
   C. Methotrexate
   D. Tylenol with codeine

5.28 Which of the following types of exercise would be most beneficial to M.J.?
   A. Stretching
   B. Dynamic: Strengthening, endurance, and conditioning
   C. Hydrotherapy program
   D. Weight lifting

5.29 Bicipital tendinitis is characterized by which of the following?
A. Chronic pain in the anterior region of the shoulder
B. Pain with supination or shoulder flexion against resistance
C. Pain with extension of the elbow
D. Pain with supination of the elbow

5.30 Mr. J complains of knee pain when climbing the stairs and at the medial aspect of the knee. Which type of soft tissue disorder would you suspect?
A. Anserine bursitis
B. Trochanteric bursitis
C. Infrapatellar bursitis
D. Calcaneal bursitis

Answers and Rationales

5.26 **A, B, D**   One of the major complaints along with the tender areas (two are described in the question) and poor sleep is overwhelming fatigue.

5.27 **A, B**   Amitriptyline medications help to improve the quality of sleep. NSAIDs will help with the generalized musculoskeletal pain.

5.28 **A, B, C**   Fibromyalgia patients generally have deconditioned muscles. It is recommended that tone and endurance be modified.

5.29 **A, B**   This is a shoulder disorder, not elbow. The movements described in the correct answer will cause the pain to be reproduced.

5.30 **A**   Anserine bursitis is a disorder that is often missed because of similar complaints associated with osteoarthritis.

Osteoporosis

DEFINITION

Characterized by low bone mass, deterioration of bone tissue leading to bone fragility, and increased risk of fracture.

ETIOLOGY/INCIDENCE

1. Postmenopausal estrogen-deficient women
2. Chronic corticosteroid use
3. Chronic alcohol and nicotine use
4. Calcium deficiency

SIGNS AND SYMPTOMS

1. Fractures

PHYSICAL FINDINGS

1. Back pain

DIFFERENTIAL DIAGNOSIS

1. Cushing's syndrome
2. Hyperthyroidism

3. Hypergonadism in men
4. Osteogenesis imperfecta and related disorders
5. Hyperparathyroidism
6. Osteomalacia

DIAGNOSTIC TESTS

1. Dual-energy x-ray absorptiometry bone density

MANAGEMENT/TREATMENT

1. Prescribe medication. The ACNP should be aware that vitamin D is usually obtained by sunlight and/or diet but should consider vitamin D deficiency in the elderly, as they show low levels of 1,25-dihydroxyvitamin D levels.
2. Table 5–9 list medications for the treatment of osteoporosis.
3. Prescribe an exercise program.
   A. Weight bearing
   B. Dynamic
   C. Extension exercise program, for low back (flexion exercises may be harmful)
4. Consultations.
   A. Physical and occupational therapy
      1) Exercise
      2) Environmental hazards
   B. Physician as needed
   C. Nutritionist: Diet high in calcium

TABLE 5–9. Medications for the Treatment of Osteoporosis

Drug	Dose	Side Effects	Contraindications
Calcitonin (Calcimar, Miacalcin)	50–100 IU qod IM in 1 dose Nasal spray: 200 U/day (1 puff)	Diarrhea, nausea, vomiting, stomach pain, inflammation of skin at injection site	Protein allergy
Conjugated estrogens (PMB, Premarin)	0.625 mg in various dosing patterns	Abdominal cramps, nausea, stomach bloating, breast swelling and tenderness, pedal edema, weight gain	Prior breast or uterine cancer
Etidronate (Didronel, EHDP)	400 mg/day first 2 weeks of a 12-week cycle	Bone pain, diarrhea, nausea, change in taste	
Alendronate disodium (Fosamax)	10 mg/day in 1 dose	Nausea, ulcerative esophagitis	
Calcium carbonate	1500–1800 mg/day		
Testosterone cypionate	200 mg IM every 3 weeks		
Vitamin D	400 IU/day usually achieved with sunlight/diet	Hypercalcemia	

PATIENT EDUCATION

1. Discuss medication regimens.
   A. Calcitonin
      1) Store medication in the refrigerator.
      2) Do not use if liquid has changed color.
      3) Do not use if liquid has particles.
      4) Eat a diet rich in calcium and vitamin D.
      5) Monitor and report any reaction or infection at injection site.
   B. Conjugated estrogens
      1) Eat a diet rich in calcium and vitamin D.
      2) Explain the change in general body habitus.
   C. Alendronate
      1) Take on an empty stomach.
      2) Take in an upright position and remain upright for 30 minutes.
   D. Calcium
      1) Take with food, as hypoacidity decreases absorption.
2. Discuss safety measures to prevent falls (vision, auditory, and environmental deficits).
3. Discuss lifelong diet rich in calcium.

References

Golding, D.N. (1982). *A Synopsis of Rheumatic Diseases* (4th ed.). London: Wright PSG.

Katz, W.A. (1987). *Diagnosis and Management of Rheumatic Diseases* (2nd ed.). Philadelphia: J.B. Lippincott Co.

Kelly, W.N., Harris, E.D., Ruddy, S., & Sledge, C.B. (1989). *Textbook of Rheumatology*. Philadelphia: W.B. Saunders Co.

Raisz, L.G. (1988). Local and systemic factors in the pathogenesis of osteoporosis. *N Engl J Med 318*, 818–828.

Schumacher, R.H. (ed). (1993). *Primer on Rheumatic Disease* (10th ed.). Atlanta: Arthritis Foundation.

Sewell, K.L. (1989). Modern therapeutic approaches to osteoporosis. *Rheum Clin Dis North Am 15*.

Wagner, S.T., Belza, B.B., & Gall, E.P. (1996). *Clinical Care in the Rheumatic Diseases*. Atlanta: American College of Rheumatology.

Yan, E.M., Cohen, A.S., Fries, J.F., et al. The (1982) revised criteria for the classification of systemic lupus erythematosus. *Arthritis Rheum 25*, 1271–1277.

Review Questions

5.31 Which type of exercises would you advise for your patient with osteoporosis?
   A. Weight bearing
   B. Dynamic
   C. Extension exercise program, for low back
   D. Passive range of motion

5.32 Mrs. Anderson is a 54-year old Caucasion female with osteopenia seen on plain x-ray. Which of the following would be the most useful in determining her future risk of fracture?

    A. Bone marker
    B. Dual-energy x-ray absorptiometry bone density
    C. CAT scan
    D. Ultrascan

5.33 Mr. O. age 75 fell recently and sustained wrist fracture. What other disease would you suspect?
    A. Osteoporosis
    B. Lupus
    C. Fibromyalgia
    D. Rheumatoid arthritis

5.34 A diet rich in calcium over a lifetime will decrease the risk of:
    A. Heart disease
    B. Osteoporosis
    C. Gout
    D. Rheumatoid arthritis

5.35 Which of the following medications should be considered in your treatment of osteoporosis?
    A. Calcitonin
    B. Corticosteroids
    C. Calcium
    D. Hormone replacement therapy
    E. Alendronate

Answers and Rationales

5.31 **A, B, C**   Exercises should be weight bearing to help with bone remodelling.

5.32 **B**   Dual-energy x-ray absorptiometry bone density will increase your knowledge about percentage of bone lost and risk of fracture. Calcium will aid with bone remodelling, and Tylenol will provide analgesia.

5.33 **A**   The incidence of osteoporosis in men increases with age.

5.34 **B**   A diet rich in calcium over a lifetime will decrease the risk of osteoporosis.

5.35 **A, C, D, E**   Corticosteroids can be a cause of osteoporosis. Many patients with rheumatologic disorders have steroid-induced osteoporosis.

CHAPTER 6

Renal Disorders

Mary B. Sherman, MD

Urinary Tract Infections

DEFINITION

An acute infection of one or all of the structures of the urinary tract including the urethra, bladder, ureters, and renal parenchyma.

ETIOLOGY/INCIDENCE

1. Infections of the bladder and urethra are almost always managed in the outpatient setting.
2. Asymptomatic bacteriuria increases with age and approaches a prevalence of 10% in women over the age of 70. Urinary tract infection (UTI) in men is associated with the development of urinary obstruction due to prostatic hypertrophy in men >65.
3. Bacterial carriage is also affected by:
   A. Pregnancy
   B. Frequency of intercourse
   C. Use of diaphragms
   D. Estrogen deficiency
   E. Previous history of UTI
4. Risk factors in hospitalized patients include:
   A. Indwelling catheters
   B. Recent or concurrent antibiotic use
   C. Diabetes mellitus
   D. Immunosuppression
   E. Poor urine output
   F. Recent instrumentation of urinary tract
5. Caused by:
   A. Bacteria: Primarily gram-negative rods, *Enterococcus* and *Staphylococcus aureus*
   B. Fungal: *Candida* sp.
   C. *Mycobacterium tuberculosis*

SIGNS AND SYMPTOMS

1. Acute cystitis
   A. Sudden onset of dysuria, frequency, suprapubic discomfort
   B. Cloudy, foul-smelling urine noted
   C. Increased white blood cells (WBC), red blood cells (RBCs), and bacteria on urinalysis (UA)
   D. Fever and leukocytosis usually absent
   E. *Escherichi coli* most common organism
2. Acute bacterial pyelonephritis
   A. Dysuria and frequency may be present
   B. Fever and chills may be prominent or hypothermia in elderly
   C. Flank pain, abdominal pain, nausea, and vomiting may be present
   D. Gram-negative rods predominate
   E. Leukocytosis with left shift
   F. Blood cultures may be positive
3. Fungal UTI
   A. Often asymptomatic
   B. Associated with recent antibiotic therapy or indwelling catheters
   C. Usually not invasive unless immunocompromised
   D. Occasionally associated with disseminated fungemia that requires systemic therapy
4. *Mycobacterium tuberculosis* UTI
   A. Uncommon in the United States due to milk pasteurization
   B. Usually not acute presentation
   C. Characterized by persistent pyuria with negative cultures
   D. Pulmonary involvement frequently found

PHYSICAL FINDINGS

1. Patients may be asymptomatic
2. Fever usually present in acute pyelonephritis
3. Hypotension may occur in urosepsis
4. Suprapubic tenderness to palpation in acute cystitis
5. Costovertebral angle (CVA) tenderness is not always present in pyelonephritis
6. Altered mental status may be only symptom in elderly

DIFFERENTIAL DIAGNOSIS

1. Lower tract disease
   A. Vaginitis: *Candida*, bacterial, *Trichomonas*, atrophic
   B. *Chlamydia* urethritis
   C. Herpes simplex
   D. Gonococcal urethritis
   E. Bladder tumors
2. Upper tract disease
   A. Nephrolithiasis
   B. Glomerulonephritis
   C. Malignancy
   D. Papillary necrosis

DIAGNOSTIC TESTS/FINDINGS

1. Positive urine dipstick for nitrate/leukocyte esterase.
2. Microscopic exam of unspun urine that reveals one or more bacteria on high power is correlated with presence of bacterial UTI.
3. Urine culture and sensitivity indicated if:
   A. High fever and urosepsis suspected
   B. Recurrent UTIs
   C. Recent broad-spectrum antibiotic exposure
   D. Structural urinary tract abnormalities
4. Complete blood count (CBC), lytes, blood urea nitrogen (BUN), creatinine, blood cultures if patient has high fever and appears toxic.
5. If nephrolithiasis is suspected, then kidney, ureter, bladder (KUB) may show stones but intravenous pylogram (IVP) or computed tomography (CT) urogram is more sensitive if serum creatinine is <2.0 mg/dL.
6. If obstruction is suspected, ultrasound is indicated.
7. If renal abscess is suspected, then CT scan is more sensitive.
8. A urine culture of >100,000 bacteria usually indicates significant infection unless there is a chronic catheter or bladder dysfunction in an asymptomatic patient.

MANAGEMENT/TREATMENT

1. Acute bacterial cystitis
   A. In young, healthy women, a single dose or short course of 1–3 days utilizing trimethoprim/sulfamethoxazole or a quinolone is usually adequate treatment.
   B. In cases of recurrent infection, age >55, or pregnancy, a longer course of antibiotics for 10–14 days may be necessary.
   C. Do not treat catheterized patients unless systemic illness is present.
   D. Recurrent infections may be controlled with chronic suppressive therapy with sulfa or Macrodantin.
   E. Recurrent infections may necessitate urologic evaluation of the urinary tract for structural abnormalities, especially in men who have lower susceptibility to urine infections.
2. Acute bacterial pyelonephritis
   A. May be treated as outpatient if patient is young and nontoxic with the same medications utilized for complicated cystitis.
   B. Toxic and/or elderly patients should be hospitalized and started on an aminoglycoside such as gentamicin or tobramycin with dosage adjusted for weight and renal function. A cephalosporin such as cefazolin 1 gm q8h or ceftriaxone 1 gm q24h or ciprofloxacin 400 mg q12h should be added depending on allergies. If gram-positive cocci are seen on culture or Gram's stain, then ampicillin 2 gm q6h should be added to the aminoglycoside to cover *Enterococcus*. The aminoglycoside should be discontinued if the cultures indicate sensitivity to less toxic drugs.
   C. If fever persists for >3 days, then abscess or obstruction should be suspected.
   D. Fluid resuscitation as indicated, monitor input and output (I&O).
   E. Monitor serum creatinine regularly if on aminoglycoside.
   F. PO antibiotics continued as outpatient, repeat UA culture and sensitivity (C&S)

3. Fungal UTI
   A. Remove catheter if possible.
   B. Fluconazole 100 mg PO for 7 days or amphotericin via bladder lavage may be indicated if symptomatic.
   C. Evaluate for presence of diabetes and improve control if present.
4. *Mycobacterium tuberculosis* pyelonephritis
   A. Characteristic scarring found on IVP.
   B. Urine culture for acid-fast bacilli (AFB) requires long incubation.
   C. Three- or four-drug regimen is usually utilized depending on incidence of drug resistance. Drugs include isoniazid, rifampin, pyrazinamide, and ethambutol or streptomycin.
   D. Consider human immunodeficiency virus (HIV) testing.

PATIENT EDUCATION

1. Explain the definition of cystitis and pyelonephritis and the possible causes.
2. Review the expected course of recovery.
3. Discuss treatment plan including antibiotics, hydration, and importance of compliance with drugs prescribed.
4. Inform patient of possible preventive strategies including frequent voiding, postcoital voiding, avoiding prolonged diaphragm insertion, and application of estrogen vaginal cream.
5. Discuss discharge plans with patient and family.
6. Explain importance of follow-up after discharge

Review Questions

6.1 Frequent urinary tract infections are associated with all of the following conditions EXCEPT:
   A. Diabetes mellitus
   B. Male sex
   C. Indwelling catheter
   D. Bladder dysfunction

6.2 A 20-year-old female is seen in the emergency walk-in clinic with dysuria and frequency. She is afebrile with a negative physical. Her urinalysis shows significant pyuria and bacteruria. She has never had a previous UTI and she has no allergies. The best antibiotic regimen in this case would be:
   A. Septra DS 4 tablets PO as a single dose
   B. Cipro 500 mg PO q12h for 7 days
   C. Nitrofurantoin 50 mg PO every morning for 3 months
   D. Ampicillin 250 mg PO q6h for 10 days

6.3 Which antibiotic is indicated if Grams' stain or preliminary culture shows gram-positive cocci?
   A. Ciprofloxacin
   B. Cephalexin
   C. Tetracycline
   D. Ampicillin

6.4 Elderly patients with pyelonephritis may present with which of the following signs?
   A. Mental status changes
   B. Temperature of 95.8°F
   C. Abdominal pain
   D. Leukocytosis

6.5 In hospitalized patients with pyelonephritis you should suspect an underlying abnormality including obstruction, stone, or abscess if the patient demonstrates:
   A. A urine culture with >100,000 gram-negative rods
   B. A persistent high fever for more than 3 days after initiating adequate antibiotic coverage
   C. Leukocytosis on admission
   D. Flank tenderness on admission

Answers and Rationales

6.1 **B**   The frequency of urinary tract infections is much lower among men, although it does increase in older men with prostatic hypertrophy.

6.2 **A**   The duration of the other regimens is too long. The nitrofurantoin dose is appropriate for chronic suppression. Resistance to ampicillin has increased in frequency and it may not be the best first choice.

6.3 **D**   Ampicillin is indicated in this case for coverage of *Enterococcus*.

6.4 **A, B, C, D**   Symptoms in the elderly may be very nonspecific.

6.5 **B**   The other findings would be expected in uncomplicated pyelonephritis.

References

Reller, L.B. (1995). The Patient with Urinary Tract Infection. In R.W. Schrier (ed.). *Manual of Nephrology*. Boston: Little, Brown & Co.

Kirby, R.R., Taylor, R.W., & Civetta, J.M. (1994). Nosocomial infections. In *Handbook of Critical Care*. Philadelphia: J.B. Lippincott Co.

Stamm, W.E. (1994). Urinary tract infections and pyelonephritis. In K.J. Isselbacher, et al. (eds.). *Harrison's Principles of Internal Medicine*. New York: McGraw-Hill.

Additional Recommended References

Presti, J.C. Jr., Stoller M.L., & Carroll, P.R. (1996). Urology. In L.M. Tierney, Jr., et al. (eds.). *Current Medical Diagnosis and Treatment*. Stamford, CT: Appleton & Lange.

Acute Renal Failure

DEFINITION

Acute renal failure (ARF) is defined as a sudden decline in glomerular filtration rate (GFR) often accompanied by a drop in urine output. Decreased GFR results in accumulation of nitrogenous wastes and alterations in fluid and electrolyte balance.

ETIOLOGY/INCIDENCE

1. Acute renal failure may occur in up to 5% of hospitalized patients. In the ICU, up to 30% of patients may exhibit some degree of acute renal insufficiency. In more severe forms of ARF mortality remains high.
2. Pathogenesis of ARF can be divided into three main categories.
   A. Prerenal characterized by a sudden reduction in renal perfusion as seen in:
      1) Acute trauma with severe blood loss
      2) Sepsis
      3) Cardiogenic shock
      4) Acute gastrointestinal bleeding
   B. Renal injury as seen with:
      1) Acute glomerulonephritis (GN)
      2) Acute tubular necrosis (ATN) due to toxins
      3) Acute interstitial nephritis (AIN)
   C. Postrenal disease caused by acute obstruction of urine outflow as seen in:
      1) Bilateral nephrolithiasis or unilateral in single kidney
      2) Acute trauma to ureters, bladder, or urethra
      3) Large tumors of the lower renal tract
      4) Bladder neck obstruction (i.e., prostatic hypertrophy)

SIGNS AND SYMPTOMS

1. Pre renal causes of ARF are usually apparent although third spacing of fluid may not always be obvious.
   A. Look for hypotension, orthostatic changes, tachycardia, flat neck veins, and dry mucous membranes.
   B. Nasogastric tube aspirates or stool may be positive for blood.
   C. Cardiogenic shock may be accompanied by pulmonary congestion, S_3 gallop, and poor peripheral perfusion.
   D. In acute trauma large amounts of blood can be lost in the peritoneum, retroperitoneum, and upper thigh.
   E. Hepatorenal syndrome is usually accompanied by ascites and a hard cirrhotic liver to palpation.
2. Renal causes of ARF are quite varied and presentation depends on the specific etiology. Some helpful scenarios include:
   A. Systemic lupus erythematosus (SLE) may be accompanied by facial rash, arthritis, pleuritis, and central nervous system (CNS) changes.
   B. Poststreptococcal glomerulonephritis is often preceded by acute strep throat or streptococcal skin infection.
   C. Acute interstitial nephritis may be associated with an allergic rash and fever.
   D. Acute vasculitis due to subacute bacterial endocarditis may be associated with fever, heart murmur, and splinter hemorrhages of the nail beds.
   E. Goodpasture's syndrome may present with hemoptysis.

F. Hemolytic uremic syndrome has recently been linked to acute diarrheal illness caused by *E. coli.*

G. Multiple myeloma may present with ARF along with anemia, weakness, and bone pain.

3. Postrenal cause of ARF usually present with difficulty urinating, decreased urination, and pain if the obstruction is sudden. Depending on the cause there may be severe flank pain, gross hematuria, and a distended bladder to palpation.

PHYSICAL FINDINGS

1. Patients with prerenal azotemia may exhibit dry mouth, skin tenting, flat neck veins, fever, abdominal pain with peritoneal signs, hypotension, tachycardia, frank tissue trauma, peripheral vasoconstriction, ascites, and occult blood-positive stool or nasogastric aspirate.

2. Primary renal diseases may exhibit few physical findings or there may be many varieties of presentation. Please refer to the previous section for some particular scenarios. Careful attention should be given to the pulmonary and cardiac exam, skin rashes, joint abnormalities, and any evidence for infection.

3. Postrenal ARF may present with flank pain radiating to the groin, gross hematuria, distended urinary bladder, and a large postvoid residual if the obstruction is at the prostate gland.

DIFFERENTIAL DIAGNOSIS

1. Prerenal causes of ARF
   A. Hypovolemia due to:
      1) Acute hemorrhage
      2) Excessive diuresis
      3) Gastrointestinal losses
      4) Third spacing of fluids in peritonitis, burns, pancreatitis
      5) Sepsis
   B. Cardiovascular disorders such as:
      1) Cardiogenic shock
      2) Renal emboli
      3) Dissection of the aorta
      4) Traumatic pericardial tamponade
      5) Positive-pressure ventilation
   C. Intrarenal vascular constriction caused by:
      1) Hepatic failure/hepatorenal syndrome
      2) Nonsteroidal anti-inflammatory drugs (NSAIDs) which inhibit prostaglandins
      3) Cyclosporine
      4) Angiotensin converting enzyme inhibitors (i.e., captopril)
2. Primary renal causes of ARF
   A. Ischemic: Any of the problems listed in the previous section may progress to cause ATN.
   B. Toxin-associated ATN:
      1) Aminoglycosides (i.e., gentamicin)
      2) Chemotherapy (i.e., cisplatin)
      3) Amphotericin

    4) Radiographic contrast
    5) Solvents (i.e., ethylene glycol)
    6) Myoglobinuria due to rhabdomyolysis, muscle trauma, cocaine
    7) Heavy metals (i.e., mercury)
    8) Myeloma light and heavy chain disease
  C. Glomerular and vascular diseases such as
    1) Idiopathic rapidly progressive glomerulonephritis (RPGN)
    2) Goodpasture's syndrome
    3) Malignant hypertension
    4) Microangiopathy (hemolytic uremic syndrome)
    5) Atheroembolic disease
  D. Systemic diseases such as:
    1) SLE
    2) Bacterial endocarditis
    3) Vasculitis (i.e., polyarteritis, Wegner's granulomatosis)
    4) Cancer (i.e., hypercalcemia, hyperuricemia, infiltration)
  E. Acute interstitial nephritis is most commonly associated with:
    1) Antibiotics (i.e., penicillins, sulfa)
    2) Diuretics
    3) NSAIDs
    4) Infections (i.e., *Legionella*, malaria)
3. Postrenal causes of ARF
  A. Nephrolithiasis involving both ureters or single kidney
  B. Tumor near ureteral vesicular junction, bladder, cervical or prostatic cancer
  C. Hemorrhage and clots
  D. Trauma or surgical ligation
  E. Retroperitoneal disease including fibrosis, hemorrhage, or tumor invasion
  F. Prostatic hypertrophy
  G. Neurogenic bladder
  H. Urethral stricture

DIAGNOSTIC TESTS/FINDINGS

1. Urinalysis including microscopic exam of fresh, spun urine. Red blood cell casts may be seen in acute glomerulonephritis and white blood cell casts are seen in pyelonephritis or in interstitial nephritis. Phase-contrast microscopy may reveal dysmorphic red blood cells in acute GN.
2. BUN/creatinine levels. On their own, both of these tests are insensitive measures of true GFR. BUN may increase with gastrointestinal bleeding and may be low in liver disease. Creatinine may be artificially low in advanced age or muscle wasting. Various drugs may also alter the serum creatinine level (see "Drug Management and Toxicity in Renal Disease"). Expect serum creatinine to rise at a rate of approximately 1.0 mg/dL/day in ARF unless there is muscle damage. Rhabdomyolysis is associated with a more rapid rise.
3. A 24-hour protein of >3.0 gm is associated with GN.
4. Bun/Creatinine ratio is a somewhat crude tool to differentiate prerenal azotemia from established ARF. In general the ratio should be 20:1 in prerenal azotemia and 10:1 in ARF.

5. Urinary spot chemistries may also be useful in diagnosing ARF

	Urine Sodium (mEq/L)	Urine Osmolality (mOsm/kg H$_2$O)	U/PCr (mg/dL)
Prerenal	<20	>500	>40
Acute renal failure	>40	<350	<20

6. The fractional excretion of sodium (FENA) is a further refinement of diagnostic criteria. It is calculated using the following equation where UNa is urine sodium and UCr is urine creatinine. In ARF the ratio is >1% and in prerenal azotemia the result is <1%.

$$\text{FENA} = \frac{(\text{UNa})(\text{PCr})(100)}{(\text{PNa})(\text{UCr})}$$

7. If vasculitis, glomerulonephritis, or connective tissue disease is suspected, then specialized tests such as antinuclear antibody (ANA), erythrocyte sedimentation rate (ESR), complement levels, antineutrophilic cytoplasmic antibody, and antiglomerulobasement membrane antibodies may be obtained. Ordering of these tests should be left to the discretion of the attending physician.
8. If multiple myeloma is suspected, order serum protein electrophoresis and urine for light chains (Bence Jones protein).
9. Urine and/or serum eosinophils may be present in acute interstitial nephritis.
10. Renal ultrasound is a good screening test to rule out hydronephrosis due to obstruction. If bilateral small kidneys are noted, then the renal failure is chronic rather than acute. CT scan or magnetic resonance imaging (MRI) may also identify obstruction. Retrograde urography is sometimes utilized by urologists to provide information on the ureters and lower urinary tract.
11. Renal biopsy performed by the nephrologist or radiologist with special immune stains and electron microscopy may elucidate the cause of the renal failure.

MANAGEMENT/TREATMENT

Patients with acute renal failure are generally managed by a nephrologist. Nevertheless, the acute care nurse practitioner (ACNP) may work collaboratively with the physician in managing the patient with ARF.

1. Maximize perfusion
   A. Intravenous fluids
   B. Plasma expanders (i.e., albumin)
   C. Blood transfusions
   D. Pressor agents (i.e., dopamine/dobutamine)
   E. Unloading agents (i.e., nipride/nitroglycerin) in cases of congestive heart failure (see Chapter 3 for management)
2. Stop fluid loss
   A. Assess and control bleeding sites

B. Replace gastrointestinal fluid losses and treat bacterial infections with appropriate antibiotics
C. Broad-spectrum antibiotics for sepsis
D. Excision of eschar and grafting in burn injuries
3. Eliminate renal toxins
A. Diuresis with saline plus IV loop diuretic may prevent ARF due to rhabdomyolysis or IV contrast dye.
B. Alkalinization of the urine with acetazolamide or sodium bicarbonate may help prevent intratubular precipitation of uric acid in hyperuricemia due to malignancy or rhabdomyolysis (acetazolamide 150–500 mg IV)
C. Withdraw nephrotoxic drugs (i.e., ACE inhibitors, NSAIDs, aminoglycosides).
D. Ethylene glycol (antifreeze) ingestion is treated with alkalinization, IV ethanol, and hemodialysis.
E. Remove possible allergenic drugs if acute interstitial nephritis is suspected.
4. Relieve obstruction
A. Foley catheter
B. Ureteral stents
C. Ureteroscopic stone removal
D. Lithotripsy
E. Percutaneous nephrostomy
5. Provide specific therapies for nephritis
A. Immunosuppression with steroids and/or cyclophosphamide for vasculitis, SLE us, rapidly progressive glomerulonephritis (RPGN).
B. Plasmapheresis is indicated for Goodpasture's syndrome, rapidly progressive idiopathic GN, and thrombotic thrombocytopenic purpura.
C. Steroids for acute interstitial nephritis.
6. Renal replacement therapy
A. Hemodialysis
B. Continuous arteriovenous hemofiltration (CAHF)
C. Peritoneal dialysis

PATIENT EDUCATION

1. Explain the definition of kidney failure and causes
2. Review the probable course of recovery
3. Review dietary adjustments necessary to maintain electrolyte and protein balance
4. Explain the rationale for studies and procedures to the patient and family
5. Referral to support groups as needed
6. Discuss discharge plans with patient and family
7. Explain importance of follow-up after discharge

Review Questions

6.6 All of the following conditions can cause prerenal azotemia that may lead to acute tubular necrosis EXCEPT:

    A. Acute gastrointestinal bleeding
    B. Cardiogenic shock
    C. Septic shock
    D. Bilateral nephrolithiasis

6.7 Nafcillin may cause acute renal failure by:
    A. Precipitation in the renal tubules
    B. Causing acute rhabdomyolysis
    C. Causing an allergic reaction with interstitial inflammation
    D. Causing hepatorenal syndrome

6.8 Prerenal azotemia is best identified by which of the following urinary findings?
    A. Urine osmolality <300 mOsm/kg H_2O
    B. Urine sodium >30 mEq/L
    C. Eosinophils in the urine
    D. Urine sodium <20 mEq/L

6.9 A 65-year-old Hispanic male had a nephrectomy 2 years ago for cancer. He has hypertension, an abdominal bruit, and a baseline serum creatinine of 1.7 mg/dL. He suddenly develops acute renal failure after receiving a new antihypertensive medicine. Which drug is a likely cause?
    A. Captopril
    B. Clonidine
    C. Hydrochlorothiazide
    D. Verapamil

6.10 What finding in the urinary sediment is most specific for acute glomerulonephritis?
    A. Granular casts
    B. Red blood cells
    C. Bacteria
    D. Red blood cell casts

Answers and Rationales

6.6 **D** Nephrolithiasis causes acute obstruction of urinary outflow.

6.7 **C** Nafcillin causes acute renal failure by producing acute interstitial nephritis.

6.8 **D** When renal perfusion is compromised in prerenal azotemia, the kidneys respond by retaining sodium and excreting only small amounts of sodium. When acute tubular necrosis occurs, the kidneys lose their ability to retain sodium and urinary sodium levels rise.

6.9 **A** Captopril is an angiotensin converting enzyme inhibitor (ACEI). It is known to cause acute renal failure in cases of renal artery stenosis with a single kidney. ACEIs block angiotensin and renin, which maintain renal perfusion in renal artery stenosis.

6.10 **D** Red blood cell casts are the most specific finding. The other findings are nonspecific.

References

Agmon, Y. & Mayer, B. (1993). Acute renal failure: A multifactorial syndrome. In E. Bourke, V. Mallick, & E. Pollak (eds.). *Contributions in Nephrology*. Basel: Karger.

Brivet, F.G., et al. (1996). Acute renal failure in intensive care units. *Crit Care Med* *24*(2).

Cronin, R.E. (1995). The patient with acute azotemia. In R.W. Schrier (ed.). *Manual of Nephrology*. Boston: Little, Brown & Co.

Kirby, R.R., Taylor, R.W., & Civetta, J.M. (1994). Acute renal failure. In *Handbook of Critical Care*. Philadelphia: J.B. Lippincott Co.

Additional Recommended References

Brady, H.R., & Brenner, B.M. (1994). Acute renal failure. In K.J. Isselbacher, et al. (eds.). *Harrison's Principles of Internal Medicine*. New York: McGraw-Hill.

Miller, S.B. (1992). Renal diseases. In M. Woodley & A. Whelan, *The Washington Manual*, Boston: Little, Brown & Co.

Morrison, G. (1996). Kidney. In L. Tierney, Jr., et al. (eds.). *Current Medical Diagnosis and Treatment*. Stamford, CT: Appleton & Lange.

Chronic Renal Failure

DEFINITION

The chronic, progressive loss of functioning nephrons that results in a decline in glomerular filtration, reduced excretion of metabolic toxins, and alterations in fluid and electrolyte homeostasis.

ETIOLOGY/INCIDENCE

1. Although there are multiple causes for chronic renal failure, they ultimately follow a common final pathway that leads to end-stage renal disease (ESRD). Much research has been done in the last 10 years in an effort to elucidate this process. It appears that when a critical number of nephrons are damaged, the remaining glomeruli must over compensate. The resulting hyperfiltration accelerates the damage to the remaining functional units. Because the kidney plays such a significant role in metabolic, fluid, and electrolyte homeostasis, chronic renal failure leads to derangements in multiple systems.
2. There are over 45,000 patients in the United States suffering from ESRD who require dialysis Since the initiation of Medicare coverage in 1972, the average age of the dialysis population has progressively risen. It is not unusual for patients in their 70's and 80's to be on chronic dialysis.
3. The top three causes of ESRD are:
   A. Diabetes mellitus, 34%
   B. Hypertension, 29%
   C. Glomerulonephritis, 14%

SIGNS AND SYMPTOMS

1. Fatigue and somnolence
2. Nausea and vomiting
3. Sleep disturbance
4. Severe itching of the skin
5. Hiccups

6. Chest pain (due to pericarditis)
7. Increased or decreased urination
8. Shortness of breath
9. Easy bruising
10. Numbness and cramping in the legs

PHYSICAL FINDINGS

1. Sallow complexion, bruising
2. Pale nail beds and conjunctiva (if anemia untreated)
3. Asterixis
4. Jugular venous distention
5. Pulmonary rales
6. Pericardial rub
7. Peripheral edema
8. Hypertension
9. Peripheral neuropathy
10. Occult blood in stool
11. Coma (end-stage uremia)

DIFFERENTIAL DIAGNOSIS

1. Diabetes mellitus: Type I diabetics are usually younger and have been on insulin since childhood. The incidence of ESRD is related to poor glucose control. Approximately one third of type I diabetics go on to have ESRD after 15–20 years. Type 2 diabetics also represent a growing proportion of ESRD patients.
2. Hypertension: A higher proportion of these patients are middle aged or elderly. However, young adults (especially African Americans) may suffer from accelerated hypertension and renal failure. Differentiation from primary renal diseases may be difficult at times, since they may cause secondary hypertension. In primary hypertension there is usually only mild proteinuria (<1 gm/24 hr) and red blood cells (RBCs) and RBC casts are absent.
3. In the pediatric and young adult population look for congenital and hereditary forms of renal disease such as Alport's syndrome (X-linked congenital hearing loss and renal failure) and reflux nephropathy. SLE, Henoch-Schönlein purpura, and focal sclerosing glomerulonephritis are also more common.
4. In middle-age, disease such as polycystic kidney disease (PCKD) and membranous glomerulonephritis increase in frequency.
5. In the elderly expect to find increasing frequency of chronic interstitial nephritis due to analgesic abuse, multiple myeloma, hypertensive glomerulosclerosis and obstructive uropathy due to prostatic hypertrophy.

DIAGNOSTIC TESTS/FINDINGS

1. Chest x-ray: Look for cardiomegaly, heart failure, pleural effusion.
2. Electrocardiogram (ECG) may show left ventricular hypertrophy, peaked T wave with hyperkalemia, ST elevations with pericarditis.
3. Urine will usually have a low specific gravity due to concentrating defects. The urine output may be variable.
4. Urine sediment may show granular casts and proteinuria.

5. Renal ultrasound will usually show small contracted kidneys. If the kidneys are normal or enlarged suspect acute renal failure, diabetes, amyloidosis, polycystic kidney disease, or infiltrative neoplasm. Patients with PCKD >30 should have visible cysts.
6. Chemistries will reveal:
   A. Elevated BUN/creatinine
   B. Hyperkalemia if GFR <10 mL/min unless diabetic where GFR may be significantly higher
   C. Hyperphosphatemia/hypocalcemia
   D. Metabolic acidosis with a low bicarbonate
   E. Hyperuricemia
   F. Elevated Parathyroid hormone (PTH) levels
7. CBC will reveal normochromic, normocytic anemia unless the patient is receiving erythropoietin.
8. Bleeding time may be prolonged.
9. Echocardiogram may show pericardial effusion.
10. Nerve conduction velocities will be abnormal in the peripheral nerves.
11. Electroencephalogram (EEG) may show diffuse changes and lowered seizure threshold.
12. The 24-hour creatinine clearance will give some measurement of the severity of renal failure.
13. Serologic studies such as ESR, ANA, serum protein electrophoresis, serum complement, etc., may help in defining the etiology.
14. Kidney biopsy is sometimes indicated, although it is usually not that helpful, since only scar tissue may be obtained.

MANAGEMENT/TREATMENT

Patients with chronic renal failure are managed by a nephrologist; however, the ACNP may work collaboratively with the physician in caring for these complicated patients.

1. Measures to delay progression of renal failure include:
   A. Control of hypertension to normal ranges
   B. Strict glucose control in type I diabetes
   C. Use of ACE inhibitors (i.e., captopril) in diabetic nephropathy
   D. Protein restriction: 0.6–1.0 m/kg/24 hr of high-biologic-value protein
2. Management of the metabolic consequences of chronic renal failure include:
   A. Anemia: Administration of erythropoietin to replace decreased production by failing kidneys. Iron supplementation is often required as well.
   B. Calcium/phosphorus metabolism: Calcium carbonate or calcium acetate is given with meals to maintain calcium levels and bind excess phosphorus. Phosphorus intake is also reduced and sometimes vitamin D in an active form is required.
   C. Fluid overload: Usually controlled with loop diuretics and occasionally the addition of Zaroxolyn. Thiazide diuretics are ineffective in moderate to severe renal failure.
   D. Hyperkalemia: Potassium-restricted diets (2.5–3.0 gm K^+) are prescribed. Loop diuretics also decrease K^+. In some cases potassium-binding resin (Kayexalate) is necessary to prevent hyperkalemia.
   E. Acidosis: If severe (bicarbonate levels <15 mmol/L), supplementation may be necessary.

3. Renal replacement is instituted when GFR falls to between 5 and 10 mL/ min. If patients have uremic symptoms such as nausea, pericarditis, or uncontrolled fluid overload at slightly higher GFRs, dialysis therapy is initiated sooner. Current methods of renal replacement include:
    A. Hemodialysis: Requires arteriovenous fistula or artificial graft. Center-based dialysis is more common but home dialysis still used if appropriate support setting.
    B. Peritoneal dialysis (PD): Access is via a peritoneal catheter. Continuous ambulatory peritoneal dialysis (CAPD) is the most common form of peritoneal dialysis, but machine-operated PD can also be utilized.
    C. Continuous arteriovenous hemofiltration (CAVH): Better tolerated in hemodynamically compromised patients but requires continuous heparinization. Use is generally reserved for the intensive care unit (ICU) setting.

COMPLICATIONS OF ESRD AND DIALYSIS

1. Complications due to ESRD include:
    A. Increased incidence of hyperlipidemia and cardiovascular morbidity—the most common cause of death in dialysis patients
    B. Increased susceptibility to infection
    C. Malnutrition
    D. Renal bone disease
    E. Pericarditis
    F. Peripheral neuropathy
    G. Dementia (aluminum toxicity)
    H. Anemia (usually ameliorated with erythropoietin)
2. Complications of hemodialysis include:
    A. Fluid overload between dialysis
    B. Hypotension and/or angina during dialysis
    C. Blood loss in the dialysis machine
    D. Graft dysfunction due to thrombosis, infection, or aneurysm
    E. Inadequate dialysis
    F. Air embolization
3. Complications of peritoneal dialysis include:
    A. Peritonitis
    B. Catheter obstruction
    C. Inadequate dialysis due to peritoneal fibrosis/adhesions
    D. Catheter site infections and erosions

PATIENT EDUCATION

1. Education is best managed by a multidisciplinary team including a nephrologist, dietician, social worker, and nursing staff.
2. Patients need detailed and repetitive diet information.
3. Patients and families need social service support and education to deal with the numerous financial and psychosocial problems that arise when patients suffer renal failure and require chronic dialysis.
4. Patients and families need education about support programs such as those run by the Kidney Foundation.
5. Special training is necessary for patients and families undertaking home hemodialysis and CAPD.

Review Questions

6.11 All of the following medications are useful for the control of metabolic abnormalities in chronic renal failure with the exception of:
  A. Calcium acetate
  B. Potassium phosphate
  C. Erythropoietin
  D. Kayexalate

6.12 Which disease is responsible for causing the greatest proportion of ESRD in the United States?
  A. Hypertension
  B. Systemic lupus erythematosus
  C. Wegner's granulomatosis
  D. Diabetes mellitus

6.13 All of the following measures can delay the onset of renal failure EXCEPT:
  A. Administration of erythropoietin
  B. Strict blood pressure control
  C. Strict glucose control in type I diabetics
  D. Angiotensin converting enzyme inhibitors in diabetic patients with early proteinuria

6.14 A 60-year-old black male with a long history of diabetes and proteinuria is seen in the emergency room (ER). He has been having substernal chest discomfort that is nonexertional and improves when he leans forward. His neck veins appear to be distended even when sitting. Which examination will be most helpful in reaching a diagnosis?
  A. Auscultation of the lungs
  B. Auscultation of the heart supine and in the left decubitus position
  C. Funduscopic exam
  D. Palpation of peripheral pulses

6.15 The most common cause of death in the dialysis population is:
  A. Cancer
  B. Hyperkalemia
  C. Cardiovascular disease
  D. Sepsis

Answers and Rationales

6.11 **B** Potassium phosphate would make the hyperkalemia and hyperphosphatemia found in chronic renal failure worse and could be life threatening if serum potassium was already high.

6.12 **D** Diabetes causes the most cases of ESRD in the United States, with hypertension a strong second.

6.13 **A** Erythropoietin raises the blood count and improves the well-being of patients but does not delay the progression of renal failure.

6.14 **B** This patient exhibits signs and symptoms of pericarditis. Auscultation of the heart in different positions can bring out the typical cardiac rub.

6.15 **C** Cardiovascular disease is the most common cause of death in the dialysis population.

References

Adler, S. & Feld, S. (1997). Diabetic nephropathy. In H.C. Gonick (ed.). *Current Nephrology,* Boston: C.V. Mosby Co.

Alfrey, A.C. (1995). Chronic renal disease. In R.W. Schrier (ed.). *Manual of Nephrology.* Boston: Little, Brown & Co.

Chantler, C. (1997). Kidney disease in children. In R.W. Schrier (ed.). *Diseases of the Kidney.* Boston: Little, Brown & Co.

Chronic renal failure. (1995) In R. Kirby, et al. (eds.). *Handbook of Critical Care.* Philadelphia: J.B. Lippincott Co.

Diabetes Control and Complications Trial (DCCT). (1993). *N Engl J Med 329.*

Fougue, D., et al. (1992). Controlled low protein diet in chronic renal failure: A Meta-analysis. *BMJ 304,* 216–220.

Lewis, E.J., et al. (1993). Effect of ACE inhibition on diabetic nephropathy. *N Engl J Med 329,* 1456.

Parving, H.H. (1996). Initiation and progression of diabetic nephropathy, *N Engl J Med 335,* 1682.

Drug Therapy in Renal Failure

DEFINITION

Drug therapy in patients with acute or chronic renal failure frequently requires careful adjustment and monitoring. Many drugs are metabolized and/or excreted by the kidneys. Other medications may exacerbate the renal condition or cause unintended side effects. Finally, some drugs may alter the serum levels of creatinine or urea nitrogen without actually altering true renal function.

ETIOLOGY/INCIDENCE

Injury to the kidney affects the entire chemical homeostasis of the body. The kidney plays a central role in the metabolism and excretion of many substances including many drugs. Therefore, decreased clearance of drugs is related to decreased GFR and reduced renal parenchyma. The presence of reduced renal function may not always be obvious in the clinical setting. In individuals with muscle wasting or in the elderly, measured serum creatinine may appear to remain normal in spite of a significant decline in GFR. A 24-hour creatinine clearance may be ordered. A rough estimate can be obtained using a formula:

$$\frac{(140 - \text{age})(\text{ideal body weight in kg})}{(\text{S creatinine})(72)}(100) = \text{Creatinine clearance (ml/min)}$$

In females the weight is multiplied by 0.85 to adjust for decreased muscle mass.

Clinical pharmacists and nephrologists should be consulted when prescribing medications in patients with a creatinine clearance <20 mL/min. Patients on dialysis almost always require significant adjustments in their medications.

DIFFERENTIAL DIAGNOSIS OF DRUG EFFECTS

1. Pseudorenal insufficiency: Common drugs that raise the serum creatinine without affecting true kidney function include:

A. Trimethoprim/sulfamethoxazole
B. Cimetidine
C. Methyldopa
D. Ranitidine
E. Levodopa
F. Ascorbic acid
G. Cephalosporins
H. Tetracycline
Some of these agents interfere with laboratory assays, while others alter tubular secretion of creatinine. Tetracycline causes increased catabolism and elevated BUN.
2. Acute renal failure or exacerbation of chronic renal failure:
A. Aminoglycosides (i.e., gentamicin)
B. IV contrast dye: Especially in diabetics with serum creatinine >2.0 mg/dL
C. NSAIDs (i.e., ibuprofen)
D. Diuretics: Excessive dehydration may precipitate acute tubular necrosis
E. Cisplatin
F. Amphotericin
3. Problems related to active metabolites:
A. Nitrofurantoin: Metabolites accumulate with GFR <50 mL/min and can cause peripheral neuropathy.
B. Meperidine: Normeperidine may accumulate and cause confusion and seizures.
C. Triamterene: Found in dyazide. Metabolite may accumulate and cause hyperkalemia.

MANAGEMENT OF DRUG DOSING IN RENAL FAILURE

1. Drugs that are metabolized by the liver generally do not need adjustment unless an active metabolite is excreted by the kidney.
2. Drugs that are primarily metabolized or excreted by the kidneys require careful dosing in renal failure.
3. If the patient's GFR is <20 mL/min, then drug dosing should be determined in consultation with a pharmacist and/or nephrologist.
4. When a patient's GRF is between 10 and 50 mL/min, many oral and IV medications require adjustment. You may consult the references for specific drugs. Nevertheless, in most classes of drugs there are some that require no dosage change. Some of the more common drugs that require no adjustment are:
A. Antiarrhythmics: Amiodarone, lidocaine, quinidine
B. Antibiotics: Dicloxacillin, erythromycin, metronidazole, cefoperazone, ceftriaxone, clindamycin, pentamidine
C. Anticonvulsants: Carbamazepine, phenobarbital, phenytoin, valproic acid
D. Antidepressants: Tricyclic antidepressants, fluoxetine, sertraline
E. Antihypertensives: Clonidine, calcium channel blockers, some β-blockers (i.e., labetalol, metoprolol, propranolol, timolol), minoxidil, nitroprusside, prazosin
F. Antimycobacterial: Isoniazid, pyrazinamide, rifampin
G. Cardiopulmonary: Albuterol, calcium channel blockers, lovastatin, nitrates, theophylline, warfarin
H. Gastrointestinal: Misoprostol, omeprazole, sucralfate

5. Do not overlook the possibility of drug toxicity from over-the-counter (OTC) medications. Excessive use of magnesium-containing antacids may cause high Mg$^+$ levels. Phosphorus-containing enemas can cause hyperphosphatemia. NSAIDs such as ibuprofen may adversely affect renal function.

6. Common oral antibiotics such as amoxicillin or Septra may be given in smaller doses or at longer intervals to prevent excess accumulation. Most oral cephalosporins, the quinolones, and clarithromycin require reduction in dosage.

PATIENT EDUCATION

1. Explain the relation of kidney disease to drug handling.
2. Emphasize the need for careful monitoring of their medications by the medical staff.
3. Review frequently used OTC medications and possible ill effects in kidney disease (i.e., ibuprofen, Naprosyn)
4. Provide information regarding patient Medic Alert materials.

Review Questions

6.16 A 50-year-old male has longstanding kidney failure with an elevated potassium and phosphorus. When he becomes constipated, which is the safest over-the-counter medication you would recommend?
A. Milk of magnesia
B. Potassium phosphate
C. Fleet enema
D. Dulcolax suppository

6.17 All of the drugs listed below may result in an elevated serum creatinine. Which drug causes a factitious elevation?
A. Cimetidine
B. Gentamicin
C. Amphotericin
D. Cisplatin

6.18 You are called to see an 80-year-old woman who is agitated, hallucinating, and 3 days postoperative after a hip pinning. She has been receiving pain medication around the clock with meperidine and Vistaril. Her creatinine clearance is 20 mL/min. The best course of action is to:
A. Obtain a single photon emission computed tomography (SPECT) scan to rule out Alzheimer's dementia
B. Perform a lumbar puncture to rule out meningitis
C. Stop the meperidine
D. Order a stat brain MRI to rule out an acute stroke

6.19 The following antibiotics do not require adjustment when the creatinine clearance is between 10 and 50 mL/min with the exception of:
A. Erythromycin
B. Metronidazole
C. Dicloxacillin
D. Amoxicillin

6.20 A 30-year-old woman with systemic lupus has a serum creatinine of 3.8 mg/dL and a creatinine clearance of 25 mL/min. She has urinary frequency, burning, and a UA consistent with a urinary tract infection. She is afebrile and without systemic symptoms. She can be safely be treated with:

A. Gentamicin 100 mg IM 98 h for 7 days

B. Septra DS 1 tablet 918 h for 7 days

C. Nitrofurantoin 100 mg 96 h for 10 days

D. Tetracycline 500 mg 96 h for 7 days

Answers and Rationales

6.16 **D** The other laxatives and enema may cause excessive levels of potassium, phosphorus, or magnesium in patients with renal failure.

6.17 **A** Cimetidine decreases tubular secretion of creatinine and may cause an increase in the serum creatinine without a true decline in GFR.

6.18 **C** Normeperidine tends to accumulate in the elderly and those with kidney disease. This metabolite can cause confusion, muscle spasm, and seizures.

6.19 **D** Amoxicillin requires adjustment in moderate to severe renal failure.

6.20 **B** The Septra dose is adjusted appropriately for the patient's GFR. Parenteral medication is not necessary and nephrotoxic drugs such as gentamicin should be avoided. Nitrofurantoin may cause peripheral nephropathy when the creatinine clearance is <50 mL/min. Finally, tetracycline may not cover frequent pathogens and can cause increased BUN in established renal insufficiency.

References

Aronoff, G.R., & Abel, S.R. (1995). Practical guidelines for drug dosing in patients with renal impairment. In R.W. Schrier (ed.). *Manual of Nephrology.* Boston: Little, Brown & Co.

Chronic renal failure. (1995). In R. Kirby, R.W. Taylor, & J. Civetta (eds.). *Handbook of Critical Care.* Philadelphia: J.B. Lippincott Co.

Hilbrands, L.B., et al. (1991). Cimetidine improves the reliability of creatinine as a marker of glomerular filtration. *Kidney Int 40*, 1171.

Sanford, J.P., Gilbert, D.N. & Sande, M.A. (1996). *Guide to Antimicrobial Therapy.* Dallas: Pfizer Drugs.

Schrier, R.W. (1991). *Clinical Use of Drugs in Patients with Kidney and Liver Disease.* Philadelphia: W.B. Saunders Co.

Renal Artery Stenosis

DEFINITION

The presence of a significant reduction in the lumen of one or both renal arteries that results in decreased perfusion. If the reduced perfusion causes a reflex elevation of renin and aldosterone, then hypertension is the result.

ETIOLOGY/INCIDENCE

1. In individuals 25–45 years of age fibromuscular dysplasia is the most common etiology. Females outnumber males and the condition is rare in African Americans.
2. In individuals over the age of 55, arteriosclerotic vascular disease is the predominate cause.
3. Other less frequent etiologies include polyarteritis nodosa, dissection of the artery, stenosis of a transplanted kidney at the anastomosis, and Takayasu's arteritis.
4. Renovascular hypertension is found in only 1–2% of unselected hypertensive patients. However, the incidence may approach 30% in a population of patients referred to a hypertension clinic for poorly controlled blood pressure.

SIGNS AND SYMPTOMS

1. Patients maybe entirely asymptomatic.
2. If hypertensive crisis occurs, then symptoms such as headache, altered sensorium, and chest pain may be prominent.
3. If hyperaldosteronism with hypokalemia occurs, then patients may present with muscle cramping and edema.
4. Suspect renal artery stenosis (RAS) in early-onset hypertension in young females or if hypertension suddenly appears over the age of 55.
5. Suspect RAS in the elderly when previously well-controlled hypertension becomes difficult to control without changes in compliance.

PHYSICAL FINDINGS

1. Bruit of the abdomen and/or flanks.
2. Sudden drop in blood pressure in response to single dose of captopril or other angiotensin-converting enzyme inhibitor.
3. If hypertensive crisis occurs, then look for hemorrhages and exudates on fundal exam, decreased sensorium, rales, and/or hyperreflexia.

DIFFERENTIAL DIAGNOSIS

1. Essential hypertension
2. Primary renal disease with secondary hypertension
3. Hyperaldosteronism due to adrenal lesions
4. Cushing's syndrome due to adrenal or pituitary lesions
5. Toxemia of pregnancy
6. Pheochromocytoma
7. Coarctation of the aorta

DIAGNOSTIC TESTS/FINDINGS

1. Hypokalemia may be present.
2. Elevated BUN/creatinine may be present, especially with a single kidney or bilateral RAS.
3. Intravenous pyelograms are no longer utilized because of their poor sensitivity.
4. Renal scan before and after administration of captopril 50 mg utilizing tech-

netium diethylenetetramine-pentaacetic acid (DTPA) may be a useful noninvasive screening study.

5. Arterial digital subtraction angiography generally produces a relatively high degree of sensitivity and specificity.
6. Renal arteriography has been considered the most specific and sensitive study but is the most costly.
7. Venous sampling for renin. If the ratio of stenotic to normal kidney is ≥ 1.5, then renovascular hypertension is more likely.
8. Doppler ultrasound may play a role in diagnosis in the future.
9. MRI angiogram is alternative when the serum creatinine is >2.0 mg/dL.

MANAGEMENT/TREATMENT

The ANCP works collaboratively with the physician in managing patients with renal artery stenosis.

1. Balloon angioplasty is most effective for fibromuscular hyperplasia but may also be successful in discreet arteriosclerotic lesion. Stenting may be utilized to prevent restenosis.
2. Operative renal artery repair or bypass is utilized in patients who fail angioplasty or who have arteriosclerotic ostial lesions not amenable to angioplasty. In general, renal vein renins should indicate renovascular hypertension (ratio ≥ 1.5) and the patients should have a stable cardiovascular status.
3. Medical management with the usual antihypertensive medications. ACEIs may be utilized, but care must be taken to avoid worsening of renal function due to decreased renal perfusion.

PATIENT EDUCATION

1. Explain the definition of renal artery stenosis and the causes.
2. Discuss the rationale behind the various diagnostic tests.
3. Review the treatment plan and emphasize the importance of compliance with antihypertensive medications.
4. Explain in general terms the risks and benefits of invasive therapy.

Review Questions

6.21 A 35-year-old black male with hypertension is statistically most likely to be suffering from:
   A. Pheochromocytoma
   B. Fibromuscular dysplasia of a renal artery
   C. Arteriosclerotic renovascular disease
   D. Essential hypertension

6.22 A renal transplant patient is given a new medication to control his hypertension. He suddenly develops a rising serum creatinine. Which drug is most likely to be responsible?
   A. Metoprolol
   B. Captopril

 C. Verapamil

 D. Furosemide

6.23 All the tests listed below are sensitive and specific tests to identify renal artery stenosis EXCEPT:

 A. Intravenous pyelogram

 B. Renal arteriogram

 C. Arterial digital subtraction arteriogram

 D. Nuclear renogram using DTPA and captopril

6.24 Percutaneous angioplasty is most effective for which disease entity?

 A. Arteriosclerotic disease of the renal ostium

 B. Fibromuscular dysplasia of the renal arteries

 C. Essential hypertension

 D. Hyperaldosteronism

6.25 During a physical exam the most specific finding that would suggest renal artery stenosis is:

 A. Hemorrhages on fundal exam

 B. S_4 on cardiac exam

 C. Continuous bruit over one of the flanks

 D. Reduced pulses in both legs compared to both arms

Answers and Rationales

6.21 **D** The patient is too young in general for arteriosclerotic renovascular disease; the wrong sex for fibromuscular dysplasia and unlikely to have pheochromocytoma due to its rarity.

6.22 **B** ACEIs may cause a sudden reduction in renal perfusion and acute renal failure in patients with renal artery stenosis and a single kidney.

6.23 **A** The IVP is no longer utilized as a screening test for RAS due to its inferior sensitivity compared to the other tests listed.

6.24 **B** Fibromuscular dysplasia of the renal arteries responds to angioplasty to a much greater degree than arteriosclerotic disease.

6.25 **C** Bruits of the upper abdomen or flank are more specific for RAS than the other listed physical findings. Reduced pulses in the lower extremities may be seen in arteriosclerotic peripheral vascular disease or in coarctation of the aorta.

References

Badr, K.F., & Brenner, B.M. (1994). Vascular injury to the kidney. In K.J. Isselbacher, et al. (eds.). *Harrison's Principles of Internal Medicine*, New York: McGraw-Hill.

Derks, F.H., et al. (1994). Renal artery stenosis and hypertension. *Lancet 344*, 237–239.

Massie, B.M. (1996). Systemic hypertension. In L.M. Tierney, Jr., et al. (eds.). *Current Medical Diagnosis and Treatment*, Stamford, CT: Appleton & Lange.

Smith, M.C., & Dunn, M.J. (1995). The patient with hypertension, In R.W. Schrier (ed.). *Manual of Nephrology*. Boston: Little, Brown & Co.

Strandness, D.E., Jr. (1994). Natural history of renal artery stenosis. *Am J Kidney Dis 24*, 630–635.

Renal Transplantation

DEFINITION

The implantation of a kidney into a host who is suffering from end-stage renal disease. The kidney is usually obtained from either a living, related donor or a cadaveric donor. The graft is almost always allogenic with the exception of identical twins. Control of immunologic rejection remains the greatest hurdle to success.

INCIDENCE

1. The first successful renal transplant was performed in 1956 between identical twins.
2. The majority of transplants in the United States are from cadaveric donors.
3. There is a growing shortage of available organs compared to demand.

PROCEDURE

1. The organs are harvested and preserved in special solutions that maintain viability up to 48 hours.
2. The transplant procedure itself is not complex. The vascular structures are anastomosed to the iliac vessels and the ureter is implanted in the bladder.
3. Donor organ undergoes HLA typing to match the major histocompatibility sites and blood type.
4. Kidneys are allocated via the United Network for Organ Sharing and are based on HLA typing and availability.
5. Close HLA matching is associated with improved graft survival.

CONTRAINDICATIONS

1. Human immunodeficiency virus (HIV)
2. Malignancy
3. Advanced age
4. Severe cardiac disease

COMPLICATIONS

1. Rejection
   A. Accelerated acute: Within a few days
   B. Acute: Within 6 months
   C. Chronic: >6 months
2. Thrombosis of vessels
3. Renal artery stenosis
4. Hypertension: Calcium channel blockers drugs of choice
5. Acquired infections from donor kidney
   A. Cytomegalovirus (CMV)
   B. Hepatitis C
   C. HIV
6. Increased incidence of malignancy
   A. Skin cancer
   B. Lymphoproliferative cancers
   C. Rarely cancer has been transmitted from the donor organ

7. Increased infectious disease due to immunosuppression
   A. Bacterial
   B. Viral
   C. Fungal
   D. Mycobacterial
8. Recurrent disease in grafts
   A. Focal glomerulosclerosis
   B. Membranous glomerulonephritis
   C. Dense deposit disease
   D. Antiglomerular basement disease (Goodpasture's syndrome)
   E. Diabetic nephropathy: Usually not symptomatic
9. Perirenal fluid collections due to lymph drainage or ureteral leak
10. Cyclosporine toxicity: Associated with increased hypertension (HTN), endothelial vascular changes, and increased serum creatinine
11. Steroid-induced problems: Diabetes, osteoporosis, weight gain, HTN

IMMUNOSUPPRESSION

1. Azathioprine: Used as primary drug 1962–1982, now secondary use
2. Prednisone
3. Cyclosporine: Responsible for improved 1-year survival of cadaveric transplants since introduction
4. Pulse IV steroids: Used to reverse acute rejection
5. OKT3 monoclonal antibodies: Used especially in steroid-resistant first rejection
6. Antilymphocytic globulin
7. Cessation of immunosuppressants usually causes immediate rejection

SIGNS AND SYMPTOMS OF REJECTION

1. Fever
2. Decreased urine output
3. Abdominal fullness or pain

PHYSICAL FINDINGS

1. Swelling/tenderness over allograft
2. Ascites
3. Bruit over allograft
4. Scrotal or labial edema

DIAGNOSTIC EVALUATION OF DECREASED GRAFT FUNCTION

1. BUN/creatinine
2. 24-hour urine for creatinine clearance
3. Ultrasound
4. Doppler arterial study
5. Nuclear renal scan
6. Renal biopsy
7. Angiogram

MANAGEMENT/TREATMENT OF COMPLICATIONS

Renal transplant patients are managed by a nephrologist and the transplant team. The ACNP may work collaboratively with the physician in managing the patient.

1. Pulse IV steroids. OKT3 for acute rejection episodes.
2. Appropriate antibiotics for acute infections, trimethoprim-sulfamethoxazole for *Pneumocystic* prophylaxis, ganciclovir for CMV.
3. Angioplasty may be indicated for renal artery stenosis.
4. Surgical exploration for vascular problems such as stenosis or thrombosis or for ureteral leakage.

PATIENT EDUCATION

1. Multidisciplinary team approach for counseling and ongoing management of transplant recipient, living donor, or donor's family.
2. Explain the basic technical aspects of surgery and the role of immunosuppression in maintaining graft function.
3. Review the probable course of recovery.
4. Emphasize strict adherence to drug regimen, since discontinuation can cause sudden, irreversible rejection.
5. Encourage all patients to consider organ donation designation in writing or via the Department of Motor Vehicles (DMV).

Review Questions

6.26 Which statement is true?
   A. Kidney donor availability compared to demand has improved significantly in the last 10 years.
   B. Immune matching does not improve graft survival.
   C. Immunosuppression can be stopped after 1 year without any serious consequences.
   D. Cyclosporine has significantly improved 1 year graft survival of cadaveric transplants.

6.27 The biggest barrier to kidney transplantation is:
   A. Availability of antirejection drugs
   B. Lack of donor kidneys
   C. HLA mismatching
   D. Availability of transplant surgical teams

6.28 Rejection of the donor kidney can occur:
   A. After 2 days
   B. After 6 months
   C. After 5 years
   D. All of the above

6.29 Acute rejection may present with all of the following findings except
   A. Fever
   B. Decreased urine output

    C. Decreased serum creatinine

    D. Tenderness over the transplanted kidney

6.30 Cyclosporine may cause various problems to the transplant recipient with the exception of:

    A. Overall decreased graft survival at 1 year

    B. Hypertension

    C. Increased susceptibility to infection

    D. Increased serum creatinine

Answers and Rationales

6.26 **D** Demand for kidneys increasingly outstrips availability. HLA matching improves graft survival and immunosuppression should be continued indefinitely unless life-threatening infection intervenes.

6.27 **B** There is significant mismatch between demand and supply of donor organs.

6.28 **D** Rejection can occur at any time in the course of transplantation.

6.29 **C** Serum creatinine increases because of reduced GFR.

6.30 **A** Cyclosporine causes HTN, increased serum creatinine, and increased susceptibility to infection due to immunosuppression.

References

Carpenter, C.B., & Lazarus, J.M. (1994). Dialysis and transplantation in the treatment of renal failure. In K.J. Isselbacherer, et al. (eds.). *Harrison's Principle of Internal Medicine.* New York: McGraw-Hill.

Kirby, R.R. et al. (1994). The renal allograft recipient. In *Handbook of Critical Care.* Philadelphia: J.B. Lippincott Co.

Spiegel, D.M. (1995). Renal replacement therapy: Dialysis and transplantation. In R.W. Schrier (ed.). *Manual of Nephrology.* Boston: Little, Brown & Co.

Surnayi, M.G., et al. (1994). Recent developments in renal transplantation. In Gonick, H.C. (ed.). *Current Nephrology.* Boston: Mosby-Year Book.

Additional Recommended References

McKay, D.B., et al. (1996). Clinical aspects of renal transplantation, In B.M. Brenner (ed.). *The Kidney.* Philadelphia: W.B. Saunders Co.

Murray, A.G., & Halloran, P.F. (1997). Advances in transplantation. In H.G. Gonick (ed.). *Current Nephrology.* Boston: Mosby-Year Book.

Fluid and Electrolyte Disturbances

HYPONATREMIA

DEFINITION

A decrease in the measured sodium (Na$^+$) concentration in the serum below 135 mEq/L.

Mild   125–134 mEq/L
Moderate   110–124 mEq/L
Severe   100–109 mEq/L

INCIDENCE/PATHOPHYSIOLOGY

1. Found in approximately 10–15% of hospitalized patients.
2. May be confused with pseudohyponatremia caused by:
   A. Hyperglycemia
   B. Hyperlipidemia
   C. Hyperproteinemia (i.e., multiple myeloma)
3. Characterized by volume states

Hypervolemia	Euvolemia	Hypovolemia
Congestive heart failure (CHF)	Syndrome of inappropriate antidiuretic hormone (SIADH) hypothyroidism	GI loss: Diarrhea, vomiting, NG tube
Renal failure	Drugs	Diuretic excess: Thiazide
Cirrhosis	Adrenal insufficiency	Laxative abuse third space losses
Nephrotic syndrome	Psychogenic polydipsia	Salt-losing nephropathy
Iatrogenic due to hypotonic fluids	Hypotonic fluids	Adrenal insufficiency
		Beer-drinkers' hyponatremia

4. SIADH results in excessive free water retention and excessive loss of Na^+ in the urine in spite of low serum sodium levels.
5. Drugs commonly associated with SIADH:
   A. Antihyperglycemics: Chlorpropamide, tolbutamide
   B. CNS medications: Barbiturates, carbamazepine, tricyclics
   C. Pain medications: Morphine, acetaminophen, indomethacin
   D. Antineoplastics: Cyclophosphamide, vincristine
   E. Cardiovascular drugs: Clofibrate, isoproterenol
6. Medical conditions frequently associated with SIADH:
   A. Malignancy: Especially small cell, tumors of the lung, pancreatic cancer, Hodgkin's lymphoma
   B. Pulmonary lesions: Pneumonia, tuberculosis (TB), fungal disease
   C. CNS disease: Stroke, meningitis, psychosis, malignancy, metabolic disease such as acute prophyria
7. Sudden onset of hyponatremia in <24 hours may be associated with increased intracranial pressure and a risk of herniation or hypoxic encephalopathy.
8. Too rapid a correction of hyponatremia may be associated with central pontine myelinolysis, a potentially fatal condition.

SIGNS AND SYMPTOMS

1. Lethargy
2. Disorientation/poor concentration
3. Muscle cramping
4. Nausea/loss of appetite

5. Nervousness
6. Headache

PHYSICAL FINDINGS

1. Altered mental status
2. Cheyne-Stokes respirations
3. Decreased temperature
4. Diminished reflexes
5. Seizure activity
6. Pupillary abnormalities if impending herniation

DIAGNOSTIC TESTS/FINDINGS

1. Bedside evaluation of fluid status with attention to skin turgor, jugular venous distention, cardiopulmonary exam, peripheral edema
2. Routine chemistries including BUN, creatinine, liver functions serum globulin, thyroid-stimulating hormone.
3. Serum osmolality: May be measured or calculated

$$2(Na^+ + K^+) + \frac{BUN}{2.8} + \frac{Glucose}{18} = Serum\ osmolality$$

4. Urine spot Na^+ and osmolality
   A. If hypovolemia then urine Na^+ usually <15 mEq/L and urine osmolality >400 mOsm/kg H_2O
   B. If euvolemia with significant hyponatremia and urine Na >30 mEq/L then may be due to diuretics or SIADH
5. Chest x-ray
6. CT or magnetic resonance imaging (MRI) scan of head if space-occupying lesion suspected
7. Cortrosyn stimulation test if adrenal insufficiency suspected

MANAGEMENT/TREATMENT

1. Mild to moderate hyponatremia
   A. Rapid correction should be avoided, especially if the condition is chronic and the patient has mild symptoms.
   B. Normal saline may be useful if the patient is hypovolemic or euvolemic.
   C. Removal of drugs that cause SIADH may be sufficient along with fluid restriction.
   D. If CHF and hypervolemia are present, diuresis with loop diuretics plus ACEIs along with free water restriction may control the hyponatremia.
2. Severe hyponatremia
   A. Correction with hypertonic saline should be restricted to severe, symptomatic hyponatremia.
   B. Patients should managed in the ICU setting and may require hemodynamic monitoring, especially if elderly.
   C. Rapid correction of hyponatremia, especially when chronic, has been associated with the development of central pontine myelinolysis. This condition may be fatal.

   D. Correction should proceed under the guidance of a physician.
   E. Most recent guidelines suggest that correction should be restricted to <10 mmol/L in 24 hours.
3. Chronic management
   A. Fluid restriction 500–1000 mL/24 hrs
   B. Withdrawal of possible causative drugs
   C. Replacement of thyroid hormone or cortisone if deficient
   D. Demeclocycline 300–600 mg bid: Avoid in the presence of hepatic dysfunction

PATIENT EDUCATION

1. Educate patients regarding the danger of diuretic or laxative abuse.
2. Instruct and explain rationale for fluid restriction.
3. Review probable hospital course with patient and family.
4. Discuss discharge planning with patient and family.

HYPERNATREMIA

DEFINITION

The presence of a serum sodium concentration >150 mEq/L.

INCIDENCE/PATHOPHYSIOLOGY

1. Less common than hyponatremia because of strong thirst drive, which usually prevents occurrence. Hypernatremia may be seen more frequently in the very young and the debilitated elderly who are unable to physically obtain water. Occasionally occurs due to iatrogenic error.
2. Associated with diabetes insipidus (DI).
   A. Central: Lack of antidiuretic hormone (ADH) secretion related to trauma, infection, tumor, stroke. Responds to arginine vasopressin or DDAVP nasal spray.
   B. Nephrogenic: Kidney tubules do not respond to ADH. As a result, urine volume rises, since the tubules are unable to reabsorb free water.
3. Acquired nephrogenic diabetes insipidus
   A. Associated with systemic diseases that affect renal tubules and medullary structures: Sickle cell, amyloidosis, sarcoidosis.
   B. Occurs in chronic renal disease with predominately interstitial and medullary distribution: Polycystic kidney disease, chronic pyelonephritis, analgesic nephropathy.
   C. Hypercalcemia and/or hypokalemia can induce nephrogenic DI.
   D. Several drugs may produce a syndrome of nephrogenic DI including lithium, demeclocycline, amphotericin, colchicine, propoxyphene.

SIGNS AND SYMPTOMS

1. Thirst
2. Weakness
3. Polyuria
4. Syncope

5. Fatigue
6. Lethargy

PHYSICAL FINDINGS

1. Decreased skin turgor
2. Obtundation
3. Seizures
4. Tachycardia
5. Hypotension
6. Edema present if increased total sodium stores

DIAGNOSTIC TESTS/FINDINGS

1. Chemistry panel including electrolytes, calcium.
2. Urine sodium and osmolality: If due to extrarenal fluid losses, then urine sodium usually <10 mEq/L; If primary renal, then urine sodium is >20 mEq/L.
3. Strict intake and output.
4. If patients are clinically stable, then overnight dehydration may be instituted with monitoring of urine output, serum, and urine sodium and osmolality testing.
5. Serum ADH levels if diabetes insipidus suspected.
6. Trial of DDAVP to rule out nephrogenic diabetes insipidus.

MANAGEMENT/TREATMENT

1. If hypernatremia is due to both sodium and water losses from osmotic diuresis or extrarenal losses, then hypotonic saline should be utilized.
2. If there is pure water loss with normal sodium stores due to diabetes insipidus, then free water replacement is indicated.
3. If there is increased total sodium stores due to elevated aldosterone or cortisol levels, then diuretics may be added to free water replacement.
4. Eliminate possible causative drugs.
5. Parenteral ADH or DDAVP nasal spray if diabetes insipidus is demonstrated.
6. Avoid correction of chronic hypernatremia (>24 hours) at a rapid rate to avoid brain edema. Correction should not exceed 1 mEq/L/r. Water deficit can be estimated:

$$\text{TBW (L)} = (0.6) \text{ (body weight in kg). In women multiply by } 0.5.$$

$$\text{Targeted TBW} = \frac{(\text{present serum Na}^+) \, (\text{present TBW})}{(\text{Normal serum Na}^+)}$$

$$\text{Total water deficit} = \text{Target TBW} - \text{Current TBW}$$

PATIENT EDUCATION

1. Instruct parents on proper fluid replacement for infants with acute diarrhea.
2. Instruct caregivers of elderly about proper fluid availability and proactive administration of fluids and avoidance of sedatives.
3. Review probable hospital course and therapy with patient and/or family.

HYPOKALEMIA

DEFINITION

The presence of a measured serum potassium <3.5 mEq/L.

INCIDENCE/PATHOPHYSIOLOGY

1. Represents the most common electrolyte disturbance in hospitalized patients.
2. Renal losses are most commonly due to diuretics. Nephrotoxic drugs such as gentamicin and amphotericin also cause renal K^+ wasting. Congenital or acquired renal tubular acidosis also cause, hypokalemia.
3. Extrarenal potassium loss may be related to diarrhea, laxative abuse, intestinal fistulas, ureteroenterostomies.
4. Metabolic causes include:
    A. Hyperglycemia causing osmotic diuresis.
    B. Elevated aldosterone: Adrenal tumors, real, licorice ingestion.
    C. Glucocorticoid excess either due to Cushings syndrome or steroid administration.
    D. Alkalosis due to nasogastric aspiration.
    E. Congenital causes include Bartters syndrome, Liddle's syndrome, and hypokalemic periodic paralysis.

SIGNS AND SYMPTOMS

1. Weakness
2. Paresthesias
3. Palpitations
4. Myalgias and muscle cramps
5. Depression
6. Constipation
7. Respiratory difficulty
8. Confusion

PHYSICAL FINDINGS

1. Hyporeflexia
2. Hypotension
3. Muscle weakness, muscle pain due to rhabdomyolysis
4. Ileus
5. Respiratory muscle weakness
6. Irregular heart rate

DIAGNOSTIC TESTS/FINDINGS

1. Chemistry panel
2. Creatine phosphokinase (CPK)
3. Serum pH
4. Digoxin level if currently prescribed. Can potentiate cardiac effects of low potassium.
5. ECG may show u waves, flattened T waves, ST depression, AV block, ventricular ectopy or tachycardia.

MANAGEMENT/TREATMENT

1. Intravenous replacement with KCl at a rate of $\leq$10 mEq/hr
2. Oral replacement
3. Hold diuretics if possible
4. Control extra renal losses
5. Addition of potassium retaining diuretics such as Aldactone or triamterene

PATIENT EDUCATION

1. Provide dietary information on high-potassium foods.
2. Educated patients about importance of compliance with potassium supplements when on diuretics.
3. Review the relation of constitutional symptoms to potassium deficiency with patient.
4. Explain expected course of recovery.

HYPERKALEMIA

DEFINITION

A measured serum potassium >5.0 mEq/L.

INCIDENCE/PATHOPHYSIOLOGY

1. Symptoms and cardiac effects become apparent with levels >6.5 mEq/L
2. Etiologies related to decreased renal excretion:
   A. End-stage renal disease
   B. Type IV renal tubular acidosis seen especially in diabetics
   C. Hypoaldosteronism, adrenal insufficiency
   D. Drugs such as ACEIs, heparin, NSAIDs
3. Hyperkalemia caused by redistribution:
   A. Acidosis
   B. Digitalis toxicity
   C. β-Blockers
4. Hyperkalemia due to increased K^+ load:
   A. Iatrogenic administration
   B. Tissue, cellular destruction from crush injuries, rhabdomyolysis, tumor necrosis
5. Pseudohyperkalemia:
   A. Hemolysis of RBCs during blood drawing or handling
   B. Thrombocythemia: Platelets >1 million
   C. Leukocytosis: WBCs >70,000

SIGNS AND SYMPTOMS

1. Weakness
2. Syncope
3. Paresthesias/tingling
4. Paralysis
5. Cardiac arrest

PHYSICAL FINDINGS

1. If ESRD is present, then findings could include reduced urine output, edema, elevated, jugular venous distention (JVD), cardiac rub, peripheral neuropathy.
2. Rhabdomyolysis may present with muscle tenderness.
3. Acute tissue trauma should be obvious.
4. Areflexia.
5. Irregular heart beat.
6. Asystole.

DIAGNOSTIC TESTS/FINDINGS

1. Chemistry panel including BUN, serum creatinine
2. CPK
3. Serum pH
4. ECG: Decreased p waves, peaked T waves, QRS progressively widens until it forms a sine wave appearance until asystole intervenes

MANAGEMENT/TREATMENT

1. Acute hyperkalemia >7.0 mEq/L
    A. Calcium gluconate 10 mL of 10% solution IV over 2–5 minutes temporarily reverses cardiac and neuromuscular membrane effects.
    B. D50 (25 gm) one to two ampules IV together with 10–20 U of regular insulin IV produces temporary shift of K^+ into cells.
    C. Sodium bicarbonate 7.5% ampule (44.6 mEq) given IV over 5 minutes also drives K^+ into cells. May be repeated every 15 minutes. Watch for circulatory overload due to Na^+ content and tetany due to alkalosis and hypocalcemia.
    D. Sodium polystyrene sulfonate (Kayexalate) is a cation-exchange resin that absorbs 1 mEq of K^+ for each 1.5 mEq of Na^+ it releases. Oral administration doses are 30–40 gm mixed with 70% sorbitol, which may come premixed. PO doses are given q2–4h prn. Kayexalate may also be administered without sorbitol via a retention enema. Dosage is 50–100 gm q1–4h. Kayexalate resin actually removes potassium permanently out of the system, but can cause Na^+ fluid overload.
    E. Dialysis (hemodialysis or peritoneal) is indicated for ESRD patients or those suffering from massive crush injuries.
2. Chronic hyperkalemia
    A. 2.5–3.0 gm K^+ diet
    B. Loop diuretics
    C. Withdrawal of drugs that exacerbate hyperkalemia
    D. Kayexalate PO
    E. Florinef replacement for hypoaldosteronism

PATIENT EDUCATION

1. Provide Information for kidney patients and family regarding the danger of excessive dietary potassium ingestion.
2. Review expected course of therapy for hyperkalemia.
3. Review high- and low-K^+ foods and dietary supplements.

HYPOVOLEMIA/HYPERVOLEMIA

DEFINITION

Hypovolemia is recognized when fluid loss causes a reduction in weight, blood pressure, skin turgor, and even cardiac output leading to decreased perfusion of vital organs.

Hypervolemia is manifested by weight gain, hypertension, pulmonary congestion, edema, and ascites. Cardiac output may vary.

INCIDENCE/PATHOPHYSIOLOGY

1. Total body water is calculated by multiplying the weight in kilograms by 0.6 for men or 0.5 for women. Approximately two thirds of this water is intracellular and one seventh is plasma in the vascular system.
2. Hypovolemia may be due to:
   A. Decreased intake
   B. Increased insensible loss due to fever or high external temperatures
   C. Acute or chronic hemorrhage
   D. Gastrointestinal losses from vomiting, NG aspiration, or diarrhea
   E. Renal losses especially from diuretics
   F. Third-space shifts due to peritonitis, burns, pancreatitis, sepsis
3. Hypervolemia may be due to:
   A. Iatrogenic fluid and/or sodium administration
   B. Congestive heart failure
   C. Cirrhosis
   D. Nephrotic syndrome
   E. Renal failure
4. Patients may demonstrate overall increased body fluid with edema and ascites but have decreased effective circulatory volume due to hypoproteinemia and third spacing.

SIGNS AND SYMPTOMS

1. *Hypovolemia*
   A. Weakness
   B. Light headedness
   C. Dry mouth
   D. Decreased urination
   E. Confusion
2. *Hypervolemia*
   A. Shortness of breath
   B. Chest pain
   C. Orthopnea
   D. Variable urine output
   E. Swelling of abdomen/extremities

PHYSICAL FINDINGS

1. *Hypovolemia*
   A. Orthostatic hypotension
   B. Skin tenting

    C. Decreased weight

    D. Dry oral mucosa

    E. Absent neck veins

    F. Tachycardia

    G. Oliguria

    H. Hypovolemic shock

2. *Hypervolemia*

    A. Hypertension

    B. Pedal edema

    C. Increased weight

    D. Pulmonary rales

    E. JVD

    F. Variable heart rate

    G. S_3 on cardiac exam

    H. Cardiogenic shock

DIAGNOSTIC TESTS/FINDINGS

1. Chemistry panel including BUN, creatinine; BUN elevated with hypovolemia
2. CBC to rule out anemia/blood loss
3. Orthostatic blood pressure
4. Stool for occult blood
5. Strict intake and output
6. Urine sodium and osmolality: Low Na^+ and high osmolality in prerenal azotemia
7. Hemodynamic monitoring

MANAGEMENT/TREATMENT

1. Hypovolemia

    A. Oral rehydration solution

    B. IV saline

    C. Blood transfusions if indicated

    D. Pressor agents: Dopamine, dobutamine, norepinephrine

    E. Corrective therapy for specific problems such as gastrointestinal hemorrhage, burns, sepsis, etc.

    F. Intra-aortic balloon counterpulsation for cardiogenic shock especially if surgery is anticipated

2. Hypervolemia

    A. Na^+-restricted diet

    B. Diuresis

    C. Nipride, ACEIs for unloading in congestive heart failure

    D. Low-dose dopamine, dobutamine for inotropic support of CHF

    E. Hemodialysis, peritoneal dialysis in renal failure

PATIENT EDUCATION

1. Explain the definition of decreased or increased fluid volume and the related causes.

2. Describe and explain the indicated interventions to correct the appropriate fluid problem
3. Review signs and symptoms of fluid overload with patients suffering from CHF, cirrhosis, nephrotic syndrome, etc.
4. Discuss compliance with medical regimens to avoid exacerbation of medical condition.
5. Review signs and symptoms of dehydration with patients suffering from diarrhea or using diuretics so they can avoid significant hypovolemia.

Review Questions

6.31 All the following conditions can cause true hyponatremia EXCEPT:
   A. Small cell carcinoma of the lung
   B. Hyperlipidemia
   C. Adrenal insufficiency
   D. Hypothyroidism

6.32 An 80-year-old white female is admitted to your service. She had been on hydrochlorothiazide (HCTZ) for hypertension. She has suffered from gradually increasing confusion over the last 2 weeks. On exam she is confused and mildly lethargic. Her vital signs are stable and her sodium is 116 mEq/L. All the following measures are indicated EXCEPT:
   A. Hypertonic saline given intravenously to raise the serum sodium to 140 mEq/L within 24 hours
   B. Discontinue diuretics
   C. Normal Na^+ diet
   D. 800 mL/24-hr fluid restriction

6.33 A 45-year-old African American male with non–insulin dependent diabetes is admitted for routine hernia repair. His serum creatinine is 1.9 mg/dL and his potassium level is 5.8 mmol/L. There is no evidence of hemolysis and his other labs are normal. The most likely condition associated with his hyperkalemia is:
   A. Uremia
   B. Rhabdomyolysis
   C. Type IV renal tubular acidosis
   D. Thrombocythemia

6.34 A 26-year-old white male is recovering from a head injury. He complains about frequent urination and severe thirst. His serum sodium is 148 mEq/L. His urine osmolality is low at 170 mOsm/kg. Which medication would be most likely to control this patient's symptoms?
   A. Lithium
   B. Demeclocycline
   C. Insulin
   D. Arginine vasopressin

6.35 All of the following conditions can produce increased total body fluid with reduced circulating intravascular volume with the exception of:
   A. Cirrhosis
   B. Untreated congestive heart failure
   C. Nephrotic syndrome
   D. Third-degree burns of 50% body surface

Answers and Rationales

6.31   **B**   Hyperlipidemia causes pseudohyponatremia by displacement of sodium from the serum fraction.

6.32   **A**   Chronic moderate hyponatremia does not require hypertonic saline and rapid correction may be detrimental.

6.33   **C**   This patient has type IV renal tubular acidosis with hyporenin, hypoaldosteronism which causes potassium retention out of proportion to the degree of renal insufficiency.

6.34   **D**   The patient is suffering from diabetes insipidus and requires vasopressin to allow his kidney to retain free water.

6.35   **B**   Untreated CHF is associated with increased intravascular volume

References

Kirby, R.R., et al. (eds.) (1994). Electrolyte disorders. In *Handbook of Critical Care.* Philadelphia: J.B. Lippincott Co.

Laureno, R., & Karp, B.I. (1997). Myelinolysis after correction of hyponatremia. *Ann Intern Med 126*, 57–62.

Mulloy, A. & Caruana, R.J. (1995). Hyponatremic emergencies. *Med Clin North Am 79*, 155–167.

Narins, R.G., et al. (1995). The patient with hypokalemia or hyperkalemia. In R.W. Schrier (ed.). *Manual of Nephrology.* Boston: Little, Brown & Co.

O'Shea, M.H. (1992). Fluid and electrolyte management. In M. Woodley & A. Whelan (eds.). *Washington Manual of Medical Therapeutics.* Boston: Little, Brown & Co.

Papadakis, M.A. (1996). Fluid and Electrolyte Disorders. In L.M. Tierney, Jr., et al. (eds.). *Current Medical Diagnosis and Treatment.* Stamford, CT: Appleton & Lange.

Schrier, R.W. (1995). The Patient with hyponatremia or hypernatremia. In R.W. Schrier (ed.). *Manual of Nephrology.* Boston: Little, Brown & Co.

Schrier, R.W. (1995). The edematous patient. In R.W. Schrier (ed.). *Manual of Nephrology.* Boston: Little, Brown & Co.

Kirby, R.R., et al. (eds.). (1994). Shock. *Handbook of Critical Care.* Philadelphia: J.B. Lippincott Co.

Steele, A., et al. (1997). Postoperative hyponatremia despite near-isotonic saline infusion: A phenomenon of desalination. *Ann Intern Med 126*, 20–25.

CHAPTER 7

Urology

Paula Gull, RN, MSN, CS, ANP, CCTC

Acute Bacterial Prostatitis

DEFINITION

An acute inflammation of the prostate.

ETIOLOGY

1. Usually caused by gram-negative rods, especially *Escherichia coli* and *Pseudomonas* species; less commonly by gram-positive organisms, such as *Enterococcus*.
2. Most likely routes of infection: Ascent up the urethra and reflux of infected urine into prostatic ducts.
3. Hematogenous and lymphatic routes are rare.

SIGNS AND SYMPTOMS

1. Fever
2. Irritative voiding complaints (urinary frequency, nocturia, urgency)
3. Perineal, sacral, or suprapubic pain
4. Varying degrees of obstructive symptoms as acutely inflamed prostate swells; may lead to urinary retention

PHYSICAL FINDINGS

1. High fever
2. Prostate warm and exquisitely tender on *gentle* rectal exam
3. Avoid vigorous manipulation of prostate; may result in septicemia. *Prostatic massage is contraindicated.*

DIFFERENTIAL DIAGNOSIS

1. Acute pyelonephritis: Discernible by location of pain and physical exam
2. Acute epididymitis: Discernible by location of pain and physical exam
3. Acute diverticulitis: History and urinalysis (UA) differentiate acute bacterial prostatitis from acute diverticulitis

4. Urinary retention secondary to benign or malignant prostatic enlargement: Distinguishable by initial or follow-up rectal exam, absence of pyuria/fever

DIAGNOSTIC TESTS/FINDINGS

1. Complete blood count (CBC) shows leukocytosis and a left shift
2. Urinalysis shows pyuria, bacteriuria, and varying degrees of hematuria
3. Urine cultures will reveal causative organism

MANAGEMENT/TREATMENT

1. Hospitalization with parenteral antimicrobial therapy:
   A. Empiric: Ampicillin (1 gm IV q6h) and aminoglycoside (i.e., gentamicin 1.5 mg/kg IV as initial dose, followed by 1.0 mg/kg IV q8h).
   B. Adjust antimicrobial therapy when organism sensitivities are known.
2. Acetaminophen for fever.
3. Monitor intake and output.
4. Stool softener for constipation and to reduce discomfort associated with straining to defecate.
5. *Urethral catheterization or instrumentation is contraindicated if urinary retention develops. Consult urologist for placement of percutaneous suprapubic tube.*
6. After patient is afebrile for 24–48 hours, appropriate oral antibiotics are used for 4–6 weeks to complete course of therapy. Effective oral agents include trimethoprim-sulfamethoxazole (DS 160/800 1 tab PO bid), quinolones depending upon sensitivities (ciprofloxacin 250–750 mg PO bid, or norfloxacin 400 mg PO bid).
7. Follow-up appointment within 1 week after discharge.

PATIENT EDUCATION

1. Explain the definition of acute bacterial prostatitis and possible cause.
2. Review probable course of recovery.
3. Discuss treatment plans including need for hospitalization, parenteral antibiotics, importance of tests.
4. Discuss discharge plans with patient and family.
5. Explain importance of completing PO antibiotic therapy.
6. Explain importance of follow-up after discharge.

Review Questions

7.1 The most likely route of infection in acute bacterial prostatitis is:
   A. Hematogenous
   B. Via lymphatics
   C. Via ascent up the urethra
   D. None of the above

7.2 Physical examination of a patient suspected of having prostatitis should include all of the following EXCEPT:
   A. Gentle rectal examination
   B. Vigorous prostate examination

C. Assessment for flank tenderness

D. Suprapubic palpation

7.3 You are asked to see Mr. Johnson, a 45-year-old male admitted to the medical floor. He has a temperature of 103°F, complains of urgency, frequency, and perineal pain. He states his urine is somewhat cloudy in appearance. Mr. Johnson denies any trauma to the genital area. On physical exam, Mr. Johnson appears acutely ill, flank tenderness is negative to percussion, abdominal assessment is unrevealing. Rectal exam reveals an exquisitely tender prostate. You order all the following tests EXCEPT:

A. CBC

B. UA

C. Urine culture

D. Prostate-specific antigen (PSA)

7.4 The nurse caring for Mr. Johnson calls you 6 hours later. Mr. Johnson is unable to void, and complains of further discomfort. You suspect Mr. Johnson has urinary retention as a result of acute prostatitis. You take the following course of action:

A. Order input and output (I & O) catheterization q6h prn no void

B. Perform prostatic massage

C. Consult urologist

D. None of the above

7.5 Which organism is most likely to cause acute bacterial prostatitis?

A. *Mycobacterium tuberculosis*

B. *Staphylococcus aureus*

C. *E. coli*

D. *Chlamydia*

Answers and Rationales

7.1   **C**   The most likely route of infection includes ascent up the urethra and reflux of infected urine into prostatic ducts.

7.2   **B**   Vigorous manipulation of the prostate may lead to septicemia.

7.3   **D**   PSA is not useful in the diagnosis of acute bacterial prostatitis. It is useful when considering benign prostatic hypertrophy (BPH) or prostate cancer. PSA levels may be elevated following digital rectal exam (DRE) (Bakerman, 1994).

7.4   **D**   The urologist may have to place a percutaneous suprapubic tube in order to relieve urinary retention.

7.5   **C**   Acute bacterial prostatitis is usually caused by gram-negative rods, such as *E. coli*.

References

Bakerman, S. (1994). *Bakerman's ABC's of Interpretive Laboratory data* (3rd ed.). Myrtle Beach, SC: Interpretive Laboratory Data, Inc.

Criste, G., Gray, D., & Gallow, B. (1994). Prostatitis: A review of diagnosis and management. *Nurse Pract 19*(7), 32–33, 37–38.

Goodson, J.D. (1995). Management of acute and chronic prostatitis. In A.H. Goroll, L.A. May, & A.G. Mulley, Jr. (eds.). *Primary Care Medicine Office Evaluation and*

Management of the Adult Patient (3rd ed.). Philadelphia: J.B. Lippincott Co., pp. 708–711.

Gray, M. (1992). *Genitourinary Disorders.* St. Louis, MO: Mosby-Year Book.

Kirkpatrick, M.O. (1996). Prostatitis. In R.E. Rakel (ed.). *Saunders Manual of Medical Practice.* Philadelphia: W.B. Saunders Co. pp. 554–555.

Presti, J.C. Jr., Stoller, M.L., & Carroll, P.R. (1996). Urology. In L.M. Tierney, Jr., S.J. McPhee, & M.A. Papadakis (eds.). *Current Medical Diagnosis and Treatment* (35th ed.). Stamford, CT: Appleton & Lange, pp. 822–857.

Benign Prostatic Hypertrophy

DEFINITION

Nonmalignant enlargement of the periurethral gland.

ETIOLOGY/INCIDENCE

1. Cause not completely understood. Androgen hormones are influential for cellular level changes.
2. Originates in the periurethral and transition zones of the prostate gland: Stromal and/or epithelial elements give rise to hyperplastic nodules.
3. Incidence is age-related.
4. Histologic prevalence:
   A. Approximately 20% in men aged 41–50
   B. 80% in men 80 years
5. Symptoms of prostate obstruction is also age-related
   A. At age 55, 25% of men report obstructive voiding problems.
   B. At age 75, 50% of men will complain of decrease in force and caliber of urinary stream.

SIGNS AND SYMPTOMS

1. Obstructive voiding symptoms: Decreased force and caliber of urinary stream, intermittent stream, urinary hesitancy
2. Irritative symptoms: Urinary frequency, urgency, nocturia

PHYSICAL FINDINGS

1. Focal or uniform enlargement of prostate on DRE
2. Possible distended urinary bladder consistent with urinary retention

DIFFERENTIAL DIAGNOSIS

1. Urethral stricture
2. Bladder neck contracture
3. Bladder calculi
4. Prostate cancer (seen with focal areas of induration)
5. Bladder cancer
6. Urinary tract infection (UTI)

7. Neurologic disease leading to voiding disorders
8. Prostatitis

DIAGNOSTIC TESTS/FINDINGS

1. Urinalysis to exclude associated infection, hematuria.
2. Serum BUN and creatinine to evaluate impairment of renal function due to obstructive uropathy.
3. PSA may be elevated in BPH and prostate cancer.
4. Culture expressed prostatic secretions (EPS).
5. Plain film of abdomen may reveal urinary tract calculi.
6. Intravenous urography is reserved for patients with hematuria or when upper urinary tract disease is suspected.
7. Consider ultrasound to measure postvoid residual.

MANAGEMENT/TREATMENT

1. Medical management
   A. Androgen blockade
      1) Finasteride (Proscar) (libido maintained) to reduce prostatic size and improve obstructive symptoms in mild to moderate BPH. Dose: 5 mg PO qd. Takes 3–6 months to see effect. Symptoms better in 30% of patients.
   B. α-Blockers (for moderate BPH)
      1) Terazosin (Hytrin): Selective long-acting α_1-blockade. Begin with small initial dose 0.5 mg PO at hs. Usual final dose is 5 mg. May increase to 10 mg qd. Postural hypotension with first dose or with initial increases in dose.
      2) Doxazosin (Cardura): Begin with 1 mg PO qhs, usual final dose is 5 mg, maximum is 16 mg/day.
      3) Prazosin (Minipress): 2–5 mg PO qhs.
2. Surgical management for patients with:
   A. Refractory urinary retention
   B. Recurrent urinary tract infection
   C. Recurrent or persistent hematuria
   D. Bladder calculi
   E. Renal insufficiency
3. Urology consult for surgery:
   A. Transurethral resection of prostate (TURP): Low mortality rate (0.1%), moderate morbidity rate (18%), very high likelihood of objective and subjective improvement of BPH signs/symptoms
      1) Retrograde ejaculation is a common occurrence.
   B. Laser TURP (VLAP): Less surgical risk than TURP, can be done as an outpatient procedure, has more minor morbidity, nearly as effective as TURP
   C. Transurethral incision of prostate (TUIP): For men with signs/symptoms of BPH with smaller prostate glands
      1) Antegrade ejaculation is usually maintained.
4. Other treatment methods under investigation:
   A. Microwave hyperthermia of prostatic tissue
   B. Self-retaining intraurethral stents

PATIENT EDUCATION

1. Explain the definition of BPH.
2. Discuss treatment plan including importance of tests.
3. Instruct patient that α-blockers can cause first-dose postural hypotension. Begin medication at bedtime to reduce side effect.
4. Explain importance of follow-up, especially when irritative or obstructive symptoms return.
5. *Inability to void requires emergent visit to physician or emergency room.*

Review Questions

7.6 Obstructive voiding symptoms include:
   A. Decreased force and caliber of urinary stream
   B. Intermittent stream
   C. Urinary hesitancy
   D. All of the above

7.7 Symptoms of BPH are primarily seen in men:
   A. Age 18–25
   B. Age 26–35
   C. Age 36–40
   D. Over age 50

7.8 Irritative voiding symptoms include:
   A. Urgency
   B. Urinary frequency
   C. Nocturia
   D. All of the above

7.9 Mr. Richards, age 51, has returned to the urologist's office where you are working. Your review of his medical record reveals that on his first visit with the urologist, Mr. Richards complained of nocturia $\times$ 2, urgency, decreased force of stream. The urologist noted an enlarged prostate without nodules. Urinalysis was negative for bacteria. The urologist suspects BPH and ordered urine culture, BUN, creatinine, and PSA (PSA to be done 2 weeks after patient's digital rectal exam). Urine culture was negative. BUN and creatinine within normal limits. PSA is in the upper range of normal limits. Mr. Richards asks you what other options are available for BPH besides surgery. Medical management can include:
   A. Watchful waiting
   B. Use of Proscar
   C. Use of α-blockers
   D. All of the above

7.10 Mr. Richards agrees to medical management. You will monitor Mr. Richards until his condition warrants referral back to the urologist for surgical intervention. Which of the patients below need referral to a urologist?
   A. Age 50 with nocturia 1–2 times
   B. Age 50 with decreased force of stream (FOS)
   C. Age 50 with nocturia 1–2 times, urgency, frequency, unremarkable UA, normal BUN and creatinine
   D. Age 50, recurrent UTI, refractory urinary retention, serum creatinine 2.5

Answers and Rationales

7.6   **D**   All of the above are obstructive voiding symptoms.
7.7   **D**   Symptoms of BPH are primarily seen in men over age 50.
7.8   **D**   All of the above are irritative voiding symptoms.
7.9   **D**   All of the above are used in the medical management of BPH.
7.10   **D**   Patients with recurrent UTI, refractory urinary retention, and renal insufficiency are good candidates for prostate surgery.

References

Goodson, J.D., & Barry, M.J. (1995). Management of benign prostatic hyperplasia. In A.H. Goroll, L.A. May, & A.G. Mulley, Jr. (eds.). *Primary Care Medicine Office Evaluation and Management of the Adult Patient* (3rd ed.). Philadelphia: J.B. Lippincott Co., pp. 705–708.

Gray, M. (1992). *Genitorurinary Disorders*. St. Louis, MO: Mosby-Year Book.

Hall, N.K. (1996). Benign prostatic hyperplasia. In R.E. Rakel (ed.). *Saunders Manual of Medical Practice*. Philadelphia: W.B. Saunders Co., pp. 556–557.

Presti, J.C., Jr., Stoller, M.L., & Carroll, P.R. (1996). Urology. In L.M. Tierney, Jr., S.J. MePhee, & M.A. Papadakis (eds.). *Current Medical Diagnosis and Treatment* (35th ed.). Stamford, CT: Appleton & Lange, pp. 822–857.

Steers, W., & Zorn, B. (1995). Benign prostatic hyperplasia. *Dis Month 41*(7), 441–497.

Prostate Cancer

DEFINITION

Malignant neoplasm of the prostate gland.

ETIOLOGY/INCIDENCE

1. Incidence increases with age (over age 50).
2. Third leading cause of cancer death among men in the United States.
3. Clinical incidence does not match the prevalence as noted at autopsy.
4. Clinical incidence high in North American and European countries, intermediate in South America, and low in Far East. This suggests environmental or dietary differences may be important for prostatic cancer growth.
5. Black and others with family history of prostatic cancer are at increased risk for developing prostatic cancer.
6. Most prostatic cancers are adenocarcinomas.
7. Most prostatic cancers arise in the periphery of the prostate (peripheral zone); 5–10% arise in the central and 20% arise in the transition zones of the gland.

SIGNS AND SYMPTOMS

1. Most prostatic cancers are detected in asymptomatic men.
2. Focal nodules or areas of induration within the prostate gland are found at time of DRE.

3. Obstructive voiding symptoms: Hesitancy, frequency, nocturia, decreased FOS. May be persistent in advanced cases.
4. Systemic symptoms: Weight loss, bone pain—seen in 20% of patients.
5. Large or locally extensive prostatic cancers can cause obstructive voiding symptoms.
6. Lymph node metastases can lead to lower extremity swelling.
7. Back pain or pathologic fractures from bone metastases to axial skeleton.

PHYSICAL FINDINGS

1. Focal nodules or area of induration within the prostate gland upon DRE. The posterior lobe of the prostate may be enlarged and asymmetric.
2. Tenderness when palpating spine if bony metastasis has occurred.

DIFFERENTIAL DIAGNOSIS

1. BPH
2. Prostatitis

DIAGNOSTIC TESTS/FINDINGS

1. Elevated PSA, but 20% of patients will have normal PSA (<4 ng/mL) and still have localized cancer. The level of PSA correlates with the volume and stage of disease in untreated patients with prostate cancer. Cancer confined to the prostate is associated with PSA <10 ng/mL. In more advanced disease, the PSA may be significantly elevated. A rising PSA after treatment is consistent with progressive disease.
2. Elevated BUN or creatinine with advanced prostatic cancer in patients with urinary retention or with ureteral obstruction.
3. Elevated alkaline phosphatase, hypercalcemia in patients with bony metastasis.
4. Hypoechoic lesions on transrectal ultrasound (patient should be prepped for biopsy at time of ultrasound).
5. Positive prostate needle biopsy (definitive test).
6. Positive radionuclide bone scan in patients with bony metastasis. Bone scan should be done on patients with advanced local lesions, symptoms of metastasis (e.g., bone pain) and elevations in PSA >10 ng/mL.

MANAGEMENT/TREATMENT

1. Referral to urologist for management of all stages of prostate cancer. The acute care nurse practitioner (ACNP) may be working closely with the urologist.
2. Based on age and health of the patient. With small-volume or well-differentiated cancers and an anticipated survival >10 years, referral to urologist for surgical (radical prostatectomy) and/or radiation therapy.
3. For metastatic disease, may use androgen deprivation medication or orchiectomy.
   A. Luteinizing hormone releasing hormone (LH-RH) agonists (Lupron Depot 7.5 mg IM every month)
   B. Antiandrogen (flutamide 250 mg PO q8 h)
      1) Flutamide and Lupron Depot must be started simultaneously to achieve benefit of the adjunctive therapy.

4. Follow-up bone scan.
5. Monitor for obstructive voiding symptoms: Decreased force and caliber of urinary stream, intermittent stream, urinary hesitancy.
6. Monitor blood urea nitrogen (BUN), creatinine.
7. Referral to urologist for pain management with bony metastasis.

PATIENT EDUCATION

1. Explain the definition of prostate cancer.
2. Discuss treatment plan, including importance of tests, and medications.
3. Discuss discharge plans with patient and family.
4. Explain importance of follow-up after discharge.

Review Questions

7.11 Most prostatic cancers arise in the:
   A. Peripheral zone
   B. Central zone
   C. Transition zone
   D. None of the above

7.12 Most prostatic cancers are detected in
   A. Young men, under age 40
   B. Men with a history of renal calculi
   C. Asymptomatic men
   D. None of the above

7.13 Mr. Lane is a 56-year-old black male who was treated for prostate cancer 1 year ago with radiation therapy. His last PSA was 2.6 ng/mL 6 months ago. His PSA done 1 week ago is now 5.5 ng/mL. He reports no change in urinary pattern or changes in his state of health. You discuss this patient with the urologist because you know that an elevated PSA correlates:
   A. Well with the stage of disease in the untreated patient
   B. With progressive disease after treatment
   C. With both A and C
   D. With none of the above

7.14 The urologist suspects that Mr. Lane has recurrence of his cancer. He asks you to order BUN, creatinine, serum calcium, alkaline phosphatase, transrectal ultrasound with prostate needle biopsy, and bone scan. Based on these results, the urologist will be able to discuss the disease management options for Mr. Lane. Such options include:
   A. Surgery (radical prostatectomy)
   B. Monthly Lupron Depot injections
   C. Daily oral flutamide in conjunction with monthly Lupron Depot injections
   D. All of the above

7.15 A DRE can reveal
   A. Rectal mass
   B. Focal nodules or area of induration within the prostate gland

C. A and B
D. None of the above

Answers and Rationales

7.11 **A** Most prostatic cancers arise in the periphery of the prostate.
7.12 **C** Most prostatic cancers are detected in asymptomatic men and may be found on DRE.
7.13 **B** An elevated PSA may not correlate well with the stage of disease in the untreated patient. An elevated PSA following treatment is consistent with progression of the disease; 20% of men will have a normal PSA (<4 ng/mL) and still have localized cancer.
7.14 **D** Disease management is based on the age and health of the patient. A patient with small-volume or well-differentiated cancer and an anticipated survival of >10 years should be referred to a urologist for radical prostatectomy. Patients with metastatic disease are candidates for daily oral flutamide and monthly injections of Lupron Depot IM.
7.15 **C** A DRE may reveal the presence of a rectal mass, areas of induration, or focal nodules on the prostate.

References

Goroll, A.H. (1995). Management of genitourinary cancers in men. In A.H. Goroll, L.A. May, & A.G. Mulley, Jr. (eds.). *Primary Care Medicine Office Evaluation and Management of the Adult Patient* (3rd ed.). Philadelphia: J.B. Lippincott Co., pp. 721–729.

Gray, M. (1992). *Genitourinary Disorders.* St. Louis, MO: Mosby-Year Book.

Presti, J.C. Jr., Stoller, M.L., & Carroll, P.R. (1996). Urology. In L.M. Tierney, Jr., S.J. McPhee, & M.A. Papadakis (eds.). *Current Medical Diagnosis & Treatment* (35th ed.). Stamford, CT: Appleton & Lange, pp. 822–857.

Wilt, T.J. (1996). Prostate cancer. In R.E. Rakel (ed.). *Saunders Manual of Medical Practice.* Philadelphia: W.B. Saunders Co., pp. 558–559.

Renal Calculi

DEFINITION

Polycrystalline aggregates composed of a small amount of organic matrix and varying amounts of crystalloid. There are five major types of renal calculi: (1) calcium oxalate, (2) calcium phosphate, (3) struvite, (4) uric acid, and (5) cystine.

ETIOLOGY/INCIDENCE

1. Requires saturated urine that is dependent upon pH, ionic strength, solute concentration.
2. In developing countries: Children, especially boys, are prone to bladder calculi.

3. In industrialized countries: Most calculi are seen in adults.
4. High humidity and elevated temperatures seem to contribute to the problem.
5. Incidence of symptomatic stones greatest during hot summer months.
6. Decreased fluid intake may lead to stone formation in predisposed individuals.
7. Genetic factors may contribute to formation of urinary calculi.
8. Persons with sedentary occupations have higher incidence than manual laborers.
9. Men affected more than women, 4:1.
10. Initial presentation in third or fourth decade.
11. Hypercalciuric stones: Caused by increased absorption of calcium in the small bowel, renal phosphate leak, hyperparathyroidism, renal tubular acidosis.
12. Hyperuricosuric stones: Caused by dietary excess or uric acid metabolism defect.
13. Hyperoxaluric stones: Caused by primary intestinal disorders (history of chronic diarrhea, inflammatory bowel, steatorrhea).
14. Hypocitraturic stones: Caused by chronic diarrhea, type I renal tubular acidosis, chronic hydrochlorothiazide treatment.
15. Uric acid stones: Caused by urinary pH<5.5, hyperuricemia, myeloproliferative disorders, malignancy with increased uric acid production, abrupt weight loss, uricosuric medications.
16. Struvite stones: Caused by urease-producing organisms (*Proteus, Pseudomonas, Providencia, Klebsiella, Mycoplasma, staphylococcus*)
17. Cystine stones: Caused by abnormal excretion of cystine, ornithine, lysine, and arginine.

SIGNS AND SYMPTOMS

1. Sudden and severe flank pain (may even awaken patient from sleep).
2. Nausea and vomiting may be present.
3. Patients are constantly moving, looking for position of comfort.
4. May radiate over anterior abdomen.
5. Pain may be referred to ipsilateral testis or labium as stone moves down ureter.
6. Complaints of urinary urgency and frequency if stone becomes lodged at ureterovesical junction.

PHYSICAL FINDINGS

1. Patient may not be able to sit or lie still.
2. May have positive costovertebral angle (CVA) tenderness.
3. About 10% of patients have microscopic or gross hematuria.
4. May pass stone.

DIFFERENTIAL DIAGNOSIS

1. Acute pyelonephritis
2. Obstructive uropathy
3. Acute cystitis
4. Acute epididymitis

5. Acute bacterial prostatitis
6. UTI
7. Appendicitis
8. Cholecystitis
9. Diverticulitis

DIAGNOSTIC TESTS/FINDINGS

1. May see hematuria with urinalysis.
2. Urine culture may indicate UTI.
3. Persistent urinary pH <5.0 suggests uric acid or cystine stone; persistent pH >7.5 suggests struvite stone (normal urine pH: 5.85).
4. Kidneys-ureter-bladder (KUB) film shows presence of stone(s).
5. Intravenous pyelography (IVP) shows extent of obstructive uropathy.
6. Baseline serum calcium, phosphate, electrolytes, BUN, creatinine, and uric acid.
7. 24-hour urine collection for urinary pH, calcium, uric acid, oxalate, phosphate, citrate excretion.
8. Stone analysis on recovered stones.
9. Serum PTH: May be elevated.

MANAGEMENT/TREATMENT

1. Medical management
   A. Fluid intake >2 L daily
      1) Ingest fluids with meals, 2 hours after meals, prior to going to sleep at night, and during the night (when get up to void).
   B. Hypercalciuric stone: caused by absorptive, resorptive, and renal disorders
      1) Three types of absorptive hypercalciuria: Types I, II, III
         a. Cellulose phosphate (10–15 gms in three divided doses) taken with meals to bind calcium with type I
         b. Thiazide therapy (limited long-term usefulness) with type I
         c. Decrease calcium intake by 50% (to approximately 400 mg/day) with type II
         d. Orthophosphates 0.5 gm tid to inhibit vitamin D synthesis with type III
      2) Surgical referral for resection of parathyroid adenoma in resorptive type
      3) Hydrochlorothiazide therapy for inability of renal tubule to handle calcium load in renal disorder type
   C. Hyperuricosuric stone (from dietary excess or uric acid metabolic defects)
      1) Allopurinol therapy (200–300 mg/day PO in divided doses)
      2) Purine dietary restriction (protein restriction)
   D. Hyperoxaluric stone (due to primary intestinal disorders)
      1) Increased fluid intake
      2) Decrease amount/duration of diarrhea or steatorrhea
      3) Oral calcium supplements with meals (calcium carbonate 1250 mg PO with meals)
   E. Hypocitraturic stone (secondary to type I renal tubular acidosis, chronic diarrhea, chronic hydrochlorothiazide treatment): Potassium citrate 20 mEq PO tid

F. Uric acid stone (urinary pH <5.5)
   1) Urinary alkalinization with 100–150 mEq of sodium bicarbonate PO every 24 hours in divided doses
   2) Allopurinol if hyperuricemia is present
G. Struvite stone (aka magnesium-ammonium-phosphate stone; urinary pH >7.0–7.5 and formed secondary to urease-producing organisms: *Proteus, Pseudomonas*; frequently become staghorn calculi)
   1) Referral to urologist for percutaneous nephrolithotomy
   2) Perioperative antibiotics, such as gentamicin 1.5 mg/kg IV initially, followed by gentamicin 1.0 mg/kg IV q8h
H. Cystine stone (abnormal excretion of cystine, ornithine, lysine, and arginine; cystine is insoluble in urine)
   1) Increased fluid intake
   2) Alkalinization of urine >pH 7.5 (use nitrazine pH paper to monitor effectiveness)
   3) D-Penicillamine: Initial dose 250 mg PO per day; usual dosage 2 gm/day
2. Surgical treatment
   A. *Upper tract obstruction with fever is a medical emergency*
      1) Referral to urologist for drainage by ureteral catheter or percutaneous nephrostomy
      2) Analgesics for pain such as Demerol or morphine sulfate
      3) Appropriate antibiotics (i.e., Ancef 1 gm IV q8h and gentamicin 1.5 mg/kg IV initially, followed by gentamicin 1.0 mg/kg IV q8h) (if suspect presence of *Pseudomonas*, use Fortaz 1 gm IV q8h instead of Ancef)
      4) Acetaminophen for fever
   B. Ureteral stones <6 mm in diameter
      1) May observe for 4 weeks for passage
      2) Provide appropriate pain medication
      3) If stone does not pass, refer to urologist for ureteroscopic stone extraction or extracorporeal shock wave lithotripsy (ESWL)
   C. Renal stones
      1) Refer to urologist for ESWL for stones <3 cm in diameter
      2) Larger stones are treated via percutaneous nephrolithotomy
      3) Perioperative antibiotics based on preoperative urine culture

PATIENT EDUCATION

1. Explain what renal/urinary calculi are and possible causes.
2. Review probable course of recovery.
3. Discuss treatment plan including importance of hydration, medication, and tests.
4. Discuss discharge plans with patient and family.
5. Explain importance of follow-up after discharge.

Review Questions

7.16 You are working on the urology service and have been called by the emergency room resident to see Mr. Payne. Mr. Payne is a 32-year-old male complaining of urinary urgency, frequency, and testicular pain. He reports that he has back pain over his left kidney that began suddenly, early this morning. He states the pain is severe, beginning in his back, moving over his abdomen and into his left testicle. He feels nauseated; denies any vomiting. On examination, you note he is in moderate distress, temperature 103°F, BP 150/90, pulse 100, respirations 24. Patient has positive CVA tenderness, and cannot sit still. He asks to urinate three times during your exam. Bowel sounds are present in all four quadrants. Mr Payne most likely has:

A. Abdominal colic
B. Renal calculi
C. Constipation
D. None of the above

7.17 Normal urinary pH is:
A. 5.85
B. <5.5
C. >7.0
D. None of the above

7.18 A KUB and IVP was ordered for Mr. Payne. The studies show multiple stones in the left ureter and in the renal pelvis. There is evidence of obstruction. Upper tract obstruction with fever requires which of the following courses of action?
A. Can be managed by watchful waiting and Tylenol
B. Is a medical emergency
C. Requires hospitalization and prompt referral to urologist
D. Both B and C

7.19 Medical management of renal calculi, based on stone analysis:
A. Includes fluid intake >2 L/day
B. May include calcium intake restriction to 400 mg day
C. May include protein restriction
D. All of the above

7.20 Carla James has returned to the emergency room 48 hours after her first visit in the ER. She was told 48 hours ago that she has a UTI. She stated this is her third urinary tract infection she has had in 3 months and it is not getting better. She is now complaining of right flank pain. You look for the previous (done 48 hours ago) UA and culture results. You note the following: Urinary pH 8.0. Urinary culture reveals *Proteus* >100,000/mL. Radiographic studies suggest the presence of a right staghorn calculus. These findings are consistent with:
A. Uric acid calculus
B. Cystine calculus
C. Hyperoxaluric calculus
D. Struvite calculus

Answers and Rationales

7.16 **B** Patients with renal calculi often cannot find a position of comfort. Pain radiates to the ipsilateral testis or labium as the stone moves down the ureter. If the stone becomes lodged at the ureterovesical junction, the patient will complain of urinary urgency and frequency.

7.17 **A** Normal urinary pH is 5.85.

7.18 **D** Upper urinary tract obstruction with fever is a *medical emergency*. Infection may be present behind an obstructed ureter. This requires hospitalization and referral to a urologist for drainage by ureteral catheter or percutaneous nephrostomy and appropriate antibiotic coverage.

7.19 **D** All patients who are stone-formers should increase their fluid intake in order to keep their urine dilute, and therefore reduce crystal formation. Patients who are calcium stone-formers may have to restrict their calcium intake to 400 mg/day. Patients who are hyperuricosuric stone-formers have either a dietary excess of uric acid or a uric acid metabolic defect; purine (protein) restriction may prevent further stone formation.

7.20 **D** Struvite stones are formed secondary to urease-producing organisms, such as *Proteus*. These stones frequently become staghorn calculi, causing flank pain. Urinary pH is >7.0.

References

Fang, L.S.-T. (1995). Approach to the patient with nephrolithiasis. In A.H. Goroll, L.A. May, & A.G. Mulley, Jr. (eds.). *Primary Care Medicine Office Evaluation and Management of the Adult Patient* (3rd ed.). Philadelphia: J. B. Lippincott Co. pp. 694–698.

Gray, M. (1992). *Genitourinary Disorders*. St. Louis, MO: Mosby-Year Book.

Herwig, K.R. (1996). Urinary stones; hypercalciuria. In R.E. Rakel (ed.). *Saunders Manual of Medical Practice*. Philadelphia: W.B. Saunders Co., pp. 533–534.

Presti, J.C. Jr., Stoller, M.L., & Carroll, P.R. (1996). Urology. In L.M. Tierney, Jr., S.J. McPhee, & M.A. Papadakis (eds.). *Current Medical Diagnosis & Treatment* (35th ed.). Stamford, CT: Appleton & Lange, pp. 822–857.

Bladder Cancer

DEFINITION

Malignant neoplasm of the urinary bladder.

ETIOLOGY/INCIDENCE

1. Epithelial malignancies make up 98% of primary bladder cancers
   A. Ninety percent of these malignancies are transitional cell carcinomas (TCC)
      1) Most often appears as papillary growths
      2) Higher grade lesions may be ulcerated and have a broad base attachment
      3) Has the best prognosis
2. Frequency of recurrence and progression is strongly correlated with grade: Common in poorly differentiated lesions
3. Carcinoma in situ (CIS) is often found in association with papillary bladder cancers
4. Adenocarcinomas make up 2% of all bladder cancers
5. Squamous cell cancers make up 7% of all bladder cancers

6. Second most common urologic cancer
7. Occurs more commonly in men than in women (2.7 : 1)
   A. Fourth most common cause of cancer in males after lung, colorectal, and prostate
   B. Eighth most common cause of cancer in females
8. Usually diagnosed in the sixth decade of life
9. Risk factors: Cigarette smoking, exposure to aromatic amines—industrial dyes or solvents, ingestion of large amounts of analgesics contain phenacetin

SIGNS AND SYMPTOMS

1. Eighty-five to 90% of patients have microscopic or gross hematuria.
2. May have urinary frequency and urgency (irritative voiding symptoms).
3. Most patients will not have any symptoms because of the superficial nature of the cancer.
4. Mass may be detected on bimanual exam: Usually large volume or deeply infiltrating cancer.
5. May have flank pain due to ureteral obstruction.
6. Hepatomegaly or positive supraclavicular lymphadenopathy with metastasis.
7. Lymphedema of lower extremities from metastasis to pelvic lymph nodes or as a result of locally advanced cancer.

PHYSICAL FINDINGS

1. May not have any physical finding other than hematuria (gross or microscopic, may be painless hematuria)
2. May detect mass on bimanual exam
3. Hepatomegaly or positive supraclavicular lymphadenopathy with metastasis
4. May have weight loss, abdominal or bone pain in advanced disease
5. May have lymphedema of lower extremities

DIFFERENTIAL DIAGNOSIS

1. Glomerulonephritis
2. Tubulointerstitial nephritis
3. Ruptured renal cyst (as in polycystic kidney disease)
4. UTI
5. Medullary sponge kidney
6. Urinary stone disease
7. Acute cystitis
8. Nonbacterial prostatitis
9. Renal cell carcinoma

DIAGNOSTIC TESTS/FINDINGS

1. Hematuria on urinalysis.
2. Anemia from chronic blood loss.
3. Positive urine cytology.
4. Filling defect seen on ultrasound/intravenous urography.
5. Cystoscopy with positive biopsy. "Gold standard" for diagnosis. All patients with hematuria in the absence of UTI or stone *need* cystoscopy.

6. Chest x-ray (CXR), abdominal and pelvic computed tomography (CT) scan, bone scan, serum chemistries including alkaline phosphatase are needed for staging.

MANAGEMENT/TREATMENT

1. Refer to urologist for transurethral resection of bladder tumor (TURBT)
2. Intravesical chemotherapy: Thiotepa, mitomycin, doxorubicin, bacille Calmette-Guérin (BCG) for superficial recurrent tumor
3. Radical cystectomy by urologist for invasive or high grade tumor
4. Chemotherapy for metastatic disease
5. Pyridium (200 mg PO tid × 2 days) as urinary analgesic to reduce irritative voiding symptoms *after* diagnosis and treatment

PATIENT EDUCATION

1. Explain the definition of bladder cancer.
2. Discuss treatment plan, including importance of tests, medications, and their side effects (irritative voiding symptoms, hemorrhagic cystitis with intravesical chemotherapy), stoma care.
3. Discuss discharge plans with patient and family.
4. Explain importance of follow-up after discharge.

Review Questions

7.21 Patients with bladder cancer may have all of the following EXCEPT?
   A. No signs of the disease due to its superficial nature
   B. Microscopic or gross hematuria
   C. Irritative voiding symptoms
   D. Glycosuria

7.22 Mr. Jones is a 65-year-old male who works with industrial dyes. He has been smoking 2 packs per day for 40 years. He comes to the office complaining of urinary frequency and urgency. He has noted a pink tinge to his urine. Aside from frequent headaches (approximately two to three per week), he reports he is in good health. He takes phenacetin for his headaches. Your differential diagnosis includes UTI, stone disease, bladder cancer. Risk factors for bladder cancer include:
   A. Exposure to aromatic amines
   B. Cigarette smoking
   C. Ingestion of large amounts of analgesics containing phenacetin
   D. All of the above

7.23 The bladder cancer that has the best prognosis is:
   A. Poorly differentiated lesions
   B. Squamous cell carcinoma
   C. Adenocarcinoma
   D. Transitional cell carcinoma

7.24 Mr. Jones is complaining of urgency, frequency, and nocturia × 2. He

denies any decrease in his force of stream or hesitancy. You recognize his urinary complaints as:
A. Obstructive in nature
B. A problem with urine concentration
C. Irritative in nature
D. None of the above

7.25 Cystoscopy allows the urologist to:
A. Visually inspect the bladder
B. Obtain biopsy specimens
C. Irrigate the bladder for urine cytologic studies
D. All of the above

Answers and Rationales

7.21 **D** Patients with bladder cancer may not have any symptom at all. Eighty-five percent of patients will have painless hematuria. A few patients will complain of irritative voiding symptoms. Glycosuria is not a presenting sign or symptom of bladder cancer.

7.22 **D** All of the above are risk factors for bladder cancer.

7.23 **D** Transitional cell carcinoma has the best prognosis of all the cell types. Approximately 90% of the cases are transitional cell carcinomas.

7.24 **C** Irritative voiding symptoms include urgency and frequency.

7.25 **D** Cystoscopy allows for visual inspection of the bladder, biopsy sampling, and irrigation of the bladder for urine cytologic studies.

References

Goroll, A.H. (1995). Management of genitourinary cancers in men. In A.H. Goroll, L.A. May, & A.G. Mulley, Jr. (eds.). *Primary Care Medicine Office Evaluation and Management of the Adult Patient* (3rd ed.). Philadelphia: J.B. Lippincott, Co., pp. 721–722.

Gray, M. (1992). *Genitourinary Disorders.* St. Louis, MO: Mosby-Year Book.

Hall, D.L. (1996). Bladder cancer. In R.E. Rakel (ed.). *Saunders Manual of Medical Practice.* Philadelphia: W.B. Saunders Co., pp. 563–565.

Moore, S., Newton, M., Grant, E.G., & Ketch, D.W. (1993). Treating bladder cancer: New methods, new management. *AJN 93*(5), 32–39.

Presti, J.C. Jr., Stoller, M.L., & Carroll, P.R. (1996). Urology. In L.M. Tierney, Jr., S.J. McPhee, & M.A. Papadakis (eds.). *Current Medical Diagnosis and Treatment* (35th ed.). Stamford, CT: Appleton & Lange, pp. 322–857.

Bladder (Voiding) Dysfunction

BROAD DEFINITION

The inappropriate expulsion (incontinence) or retention of urine by the lower urinary tract.

INCONTINENCE

DEFINITION

Involuntary loss of urine sufficient to cause social or hygienic problems. Urinary incontinence is a symptom of some other problem. There are four types of incontinence:

1. *Stress incontinence*: Reduced sphincter resistance, which allows urine to leak, especially when intra-abdominal pressure is increased by laughing, lifting, coughing; can also result from pelvic or prostate surgery, multiparity, weak pelvic floor.
2. *Urge incontinence*: Results from detrusor instability and subsequent bladder contraction at a time other than intentional urination (sudden urge to void).
3. *Overflow incontinence*: Bladder contractions are decreased or urethral resistance is increased, resulting in increasing bladder storage of urine, until intravesical pressure just exceeds outlet resistance, allowing leakage of urine.
4. *Functional incontinence*: Normal voiding systems but there are other physical or psychological reasons for inability to reach toilet.

ETIOLOGY/INCIDENCE

1. Common in the elderly, particularly females
   A. Afflicts 15–30% of older people living at home
   B. Afflicts one third of those in acute-care settings
   C. Afflicts one half of those in nursing homes
2. Medications and alcohol
   A. Anticholinergic agents
   B. Diuretics
   C. Narcotics
3. Fluid and caffeine intake
4. Restricted mobility
5. Stool impaction
6. Urologic surgery
7. Pelvic floor laxity
8. Depression
9. Endocrine/metabolic disorders
   A. Diabetes mellitus/insipidus
   B. Hypercalcemia
10. Delirium
11. Infection
12. Atrophic vaginitis or urethritis
13. Neurologic disease
14. Spinal cord injury

SIGNS AND SYMPTOMS

1. Complaints of frequency, nocturia, urgency
2. Presence of fever and/or delirium in elderly
3. Complaints of polyuria, polydipsia

4. Complaints of urinary leakage with coughing, laughing, straining
5. Urinalysis and urine culture may show evidence of UTI

PHYSICAL FINDINGS

1. May see fever, confusion, disorientation.
2. May see neuropathy: Skeletal muscle flaccidity of the lower extremities; Achilles deep tendon reflex and knee-jerk reflex may be present.
3. Rectal mass, fecal impaction.
4. Palpable bladder (indicates at least 400–500 mL volume).
5. Vaginal atrophy, cystocele, rectocele, pelvic mass, or uterine prolapse.

DIFFERENTIAL DIAGNOSIS

1. UTI
2. Frequency/nocturia secondary to diabetes mellitus or diabetes insipidus
3. Vesicovaginal fistula

DIAGNOSTIC TESTS/FINDINGS

1. Urinalysis and urine culture to exclude UTI
2. Limited pelvic ultrasound or I & O catheterization for postvoid residual
3. Serum BUN and creatinine to assess renal function
4. Urine for cytology (to rule out CIS causing bladder urgency)
5. Cystometry to assess bladder capacity, accommodation, sensation, voluntary control, contractility, response to medications
6. Fasting serum glucose, albumin and serum calcium, serum sodium

MANAGEMENT/TREATMENT

1. Treat any reversible cause such as UTI.
2. Improve environmental conditions (i.e., bedside commode, elevated toilet seats, urinal within reach, availability of walker or other mobility aids to facilitate toileting).
3. Decrease caffeine intake.
4. Treat fecal impaction and provide diet high in fiber, encourage exercise.
5. Review medications that may contribute to incontinence.
6. Low-dose estrogen (0.3–0.6 mg conjugated estrogen) for atrophic vaginitis or urethritis. Progestin should be added for women with intact uterus.
7. For detrusor instability, may use anticholinergic agents in the absence of obstruction (e.g., BPH, stricture) or glaucoma:
   A. Pro-Banthine 7.5–30 mg tid–qid
   B. Bentyl 10–20 mg tid
   C. Ditropan 2.5–5 mg tid–qid
   D. Tofranil 10–100 mg daily
   E. Sinequan 10–100 mg daily
8. For stress incontinence, may use α-agonist: Phenylpropanolamine hydrochloride, prolonged release.
9. Bladder retraining: Patient initially toilets every 30 minutes while awake, with gradual increase in voiding interval by resisting the urge to void.

10. Habit training: Patient has scheduled voiding times without teaching patient to resist urge to void.
11. Pelvic muscle or Kegel's exercises, for at least 6 weeks, to strengthen pelvic floor muscles. Useful in women after multiple genitourinary surgical repairs, females with stress incontinence, patients with urge incontinence, males after prostatic surgery. Weighted vaginal cones may be added to Kegel's exercise.
12. Intermittent catheterization is preferred over long-term use of indwelling catheters.
13. Absorbent pads/diapers improve mobility and self-esteem by reducing accidents.
14. Refer to urologist for surgery because of incontinence due to obstruction, stress incontinence due to sphincter deficiency, or postvoid residual >100 mL.

PATIENT EDUCATION

1. Explain definition of incontinence and possible cause.
2. Discuss treatment plan including importance of tests, medication, environmental modifications that facilitate toileting.
3. Discuss discharge plans with patient and family. Include keeping a voiding diary (record intake and output, nocturia, number of incontinent episodes, number of pads used) to assist with outpatient follow-up.
4. Explain importance of follow-up after discharge.

URINARY RETENTION

DEFINITION

Failure of the urinary bladder to empty itself during micturition.

ETIOLOGY/INCIDENCE

1. Bladder outlet obstruction
   A. Occurs primarily in men
   B. Second most common cause of incontinence in older men
2. Deficient detrusor contractility: Affects both men and women
3. Urethral stricture
4. Neurologic disease
5. Spinal cord injury
6. May be related to medication use, narcotics postoperatively, anticholinergics
7. Fecal impaction

SIGNS AND SYMPTOMS

1. Hesitancy to start urinary stream.
2. Decreased FOS.
3. Intermittent stream.
4. May have sense of incomplete emptying of bladder.
5. Nocturia, frequency, urgency.
6. Overflow incontinence with frequent urination (paradoxical incontinence).

7. Inability to void.
8. In thoracic or cervical spinal cord patients, bladder distention may lead to autonomic dysreflexia. Symptoms include elevated heart rate, elevated blood pressure, headache, diaphoresis; may result in cerebrovascular accident.

PHYSICAL FINDINGS

1. Enlarged prostate
2. Fecal impaction, rectal mass
3. Palpable bladder (indicates at least 400–500 mL volume)
4. May see overt neurologic symptoms (e.g., paralysis)
5. May see fever if develops UTI
6. Decreased anal reflex

DIFFERENTIAL DIAGNOSIS

1. BPH
2. Urinary retention secondary to spinal cord injury
3. Urinary retention secondary to medication use (anticholinergics, antihistamines, calcium channel blockers, opiates)
4. Malignant prostatic enlargement
5. Acute bacterial prostatitis
6. Urethral stricture
7. Bladder stone

DIAGNOSTIC TESTS/FINDINGS

1. Post void residual (PVR) >25% of total bladder capacity (voided volume plus residual urinary volume); a volume >50 mL is abnormal)
2. Positive urine culture
3. Elevated PSA
4. Serum BUN and creatinine to evaluate impairment of renal function
5. Urodynamics: Demonstrates low pressure or obstruction
6. Cystoscopy revealing stricture, enlarged prostate, trabeculated bladder, bladder diverticula
7. Ultrasound of prostate shows enlargement

MANAGEMENT/TREATMENT

1. *Acute urinary retention is a medical emergency and requires catheter drainage.*
2. *Autonomic dysreflexia is a medical emergency and requires immediate intervention*: Rapid assessment for noxious stimuli that precipitate such an event (full urinary bladder, digital disimpaction of feces, source of infection, [i.e., pressure sore]). *The precipitating event must be treated (catheterize urinary bladder) or discontinued (d/c disimpaction).* Sitting patient upright may temporarily lower blood pressure; antihypertensive medication is given to relieve hypertension associated with autonomic dysreflexia.
3. Review medication that can lead to urinary retention.
4. Treat UTI.
5. Treat constipation; include high-fiber diet.

6. Teach patient Credé's technique (with one or both hands, apply downward external suprapubic pressure in the direction of the urinary meatus during voiding) to enhance bladder emptying if due to flaccid bladder.
7. Intermittent or indwelling catheterization. May need to decompress bladder for several weeks and then perform voiding trial (by clamping indwelling catheter and allowing the patient to void on his own, then unclamp catheter and measure PVR).
8. If BPH is the cause of retention, may try medication.
   A. Proscar (androgen blockage) to reduce prostatic size and improve obstructive symptoms. Dose: 5 mg qd. May need to take medication for 6 months before individual response to medication can be determined.
   B. Hytrin (α-blocker). Begin with 0.5 mg PO hs. May increase to 10 mg hs.
   C. Minipres (α-blocker). Begin with 1 mg PO hs. May increase to 10 mg hs.
9. Referral to urologist for surgical management of outlet obstruction, or post-void residual >100 mL.

PATIENT EDUCATION

1. Explain definition of urinary retention and possible cause.
2. Discuss treatment plan including importance of tests, medications, Credé's technique to facilitate bladder emptying if retention is secondary to flaccid bladder, the need for catheterization.
3. Discuss that acute urinary retention, or symptoms of autonomic dysreflexia are medical emergencies and require prompt action.
4. Discuss discharge plans with patient and family.
5. Explain importance of follow-up after discharge.

Review Questions

7.26 Incontinence is:
   A. A symptom of some other problem
   B. An involuntary loss of urine such that it causes social or hygienic problems
   C. A symptom seen primarily in young adults
   D. Both A and B

7.27 Bladder outlet obstruction:
   A. May be related to medication use
   B. May result from upper or lower motor neuron lesions
   C. Occurs primarily in men
   D. All of the above

7.28 Mr. Sherwood is a 75-year-old male 2 week S/P laser TURP. He presents to the emergency room 8 hours following discontinuance of his Foley catheter. He states he is unable to void. He appears somewhat anxious and has a palpable bladder. You conclude that Mr. Sherwood is in acute urinary retention. This situation:
   A. Is a medical emergency
   B. Requires catheter drainage
   C. Both A and B
   D. None of the above

7.29 You are asked to see Mr. Jones, a 70-year-old gentleman on the surgical floor. He has recently undergone a total hip replacement. Today is postoperative day 3. The nurses note that he has been incontinent of urine, he sleeps, most of the day and, therefore, does not eat or drink much. He has a running IV of D5 1/2 NS at 75 mL/hr. He is being medicated every 5 hours with two tabs Vicodin. On physical exam, you detect a palpable bladder. You suspect he is in urinary retention. You can support your index of suspicion because:

A. A palpable bladder is indicative of a volume of 400–500 mL.
B. He has been regularly medicated with Vicodin.
C. He probably has overflow incontinence.
D. All of the above.

7.30 You are asked to see Mr. Lockwood, a 72-year-old gentleman in the nursing home. He complains of being incontinent of urine. He denies feeling ill and is embarrassed by his accidents. In evaluating his complaint of incontinence, you:

A. Would order a UA with culture and sensitivity (C & S)
B. Order a limited pelvic ultrasound for PVR
C. Perform a rectal exam
D. All of the above

Answers and Rationales

7.26 **D** Incontinence is an involuntary loss of urine such that the patient suffers social and hygienic consequences. It is a symptom that some other problem exists.

7.27 **D** The etiology of bladder outlet obstruction may be related to urethral stricture, upper and lower motor neuron lesions, deficient detrusor contractility, medication usage, or fecal impaction. Bladder outlet obstruction is seen primarily in men.

7.28 **C** Acute urinary retention is a medical emergency. The patient requires catheter drainage.

7.29 **D** Mr. Jones is most likely incontinent due to urinary retention. His palpable bladder suggests that he has a retained volume of at least 400 mL. Vicodin is likely a contributing factor in his retention, decreasing bladder contractions or increasing urethral resistance. This results in increased bladder storage. His incontinence is most likely ascribed as overflow incontinence, where intravesical pressure just exceeds outlet resistance, and thus, urine is able to leak.

7.30 **D** You would perform all of the above. Incontinence can result from a UTI, as a result of urinary retention, which can be assessed by PVR; and as a result of BPH, fecal impaction, or rectal mass.

References

Brunsell, S.C. (1996). Symptom: Urinary incontinence. In R.E. Rakel (ed.). *Saunders Manual of Medical Practice*. Philadelphia: W.B. Saunders Co., pp. 523–530.

Couillard, D.R., & Webster, G.D. (1995). Detrusor instability. *Urol Clin North Am 22*(3), 593–612.

Elbadawi, A. (1995). Pathology and pathophysiology of detrusor in incontinence. *Urol Clin North Am 22*(3), 499–512.

Goodson, J.D. (1995). Approach to incontinence and other forms of lower urinary tract dysfunction. In A.H. Goroll, L.A. May, & A.G. Mulley, Jr. (eds.). *Primary Care Medicine Office Evaluation and Management of the Adult Patient* (3rd ed.). Philadelphia: J.B. Lippincott Co., pp. 637–694.

Gray, M. (1992). *Genitourinary Disorders*. St. Louis, MO: Mosby-Year Book.

Norris, J.P., & Staskin, D.R. (1996). History, physical examination, and classification of neurogenic voiding dysfunction. *Urol Clin North Am 23*(3), 337–343.

Presti, J.C. Jr., Stoller, M.L., & Carroll, P.R. (1996). Urology. In L.M. Tierney, Jr., S.J. McPhee, & M.A. Papadakis (eds.). *Current Medical Diagnosis and Treatment* (35th ed.). Stamford, CT: Appleton & Lange, pp. 322–357.

Resnick, N.M. (1996). Geriatric incontinence. *Urol Clin North Am 23*(1), 55–74.

Yim, P.S., & Peterson, A.S. (1996). Urinary incontinence. *Postgrad Med 99*(5), 137–140, 143–144, 149–150.

CHAPTER 8

Endocrine Disorders

Deborah Hamwi, RN, MSN, NP
Dat Vo, MD

Diabetes

DEFINITION

Diabetes mellitus (DM) is a group of metabolic diseases characterized by hyperglycemia resulting from defects in insulin secretion, insulin action, or both. The vast majority of DM falls into two broad categories: type 1 and type 2. It is a chronic disease that affects approximately 16 million Americans, half of whom are undiagnosed.

ETIOLOGY/INCIDENCE

1. Type 1
   A. The cause is an absolute deficiency of insulin secretion.
   B. Certain human leukocyte antigens are strongly associated with the development of type 1 DM.
   C. Accounts for 10–15% of all cases of DM.
   D. Clinically characterized by hyperglycemia and a propensity to diabetic ketoacidosis (DKA).
   E. Most commonly develops in childhood or adolescence and is the predominant type of DM diagnosed before age 30.
   F. Among individuals with a genetic predisposition to DM, immune-mediated destruction of insulin-producing cells leads to a progressive loss of endogenous insulin.
2. Type 2
   A. Hyperglycemia results from both an impaired insulin secretory response to glucose and decreased insulin effectiveness.
   B. More than 90% of all diabetics in the United States have type 2 diabetes.
   C. Usually occurs after age 30; risk increases with age.
   D. Strong genetic predisposition.
   E. Commonly associated with lack of physical activity and obesity.
   F. The production of endogenous insulin is usually adequate to avoid ketoacidosis.
3. Impaired glucose intolerance (IGT): Describes plasma glucose concentrations outside the normal range following a glucose tolerance test but not high enough to be labeled diabetic.

SIGNS AND SYMPTOMS

1. Type 1
   A. Type 1 patients often present with symptomatic hyperglycemia or DKA.
   B. Polyuria.
   C. Polyphagia.
   D. Polydipsia.
   E. Weight loss despite normal or increased dietary intake.
   F. Rise in serum ketones, frequently followed by DKA.
   G. Weakness or fatigue.
   H. Blurred vision.
   I. Vaginal candidiasis.
   J. Peripheral neuropathy.
2. Type 2
   A. May be asymptomatic initially
   B. Polyuria
   C. Polydipsia
   D. Weakness or fatigue
   E. Blurred vision
   F. Vaginal candidiasis
   G. Peripheral neuropathy
3. Chronic complications of diabetes: Late clinical manifestations of DM include a number of pathologic changes that involve small and large blood vessels, cranial and peripheral nerves, the skin, and the eye. These lead to hypertension, renal failure, blindness, neuropathy, amputations of the lower extremities, heart disease, and cerebral vascular accidents (CVAs). The cause of these late manifestations correlates with the duration of the diabetic state. In type 1 DM, complications from end-stage renal disease are a major cause of death, whereas patients with type 2 DM are more likely to have diseases leading to, myocardial infarction (MI) and stroke as the main cause of death.
   A. Diabetic retinopathy
   B. Glaucoma
   C. Cataracts
   D. Diabetic nephropathy: most common cause of end-stage renal disease
   E. Foot ulcers and infections
   F. Diabetic neuropathy
   G. Skin and mucous membrane complications, including chronic pyogenic infections of the skin, eruptive xanthomas, candidal infections
   H. Cardiovascular disease
   I. Impotence
   J. Gastroparesis

PHYSICAL FINDINGS

1. Type 1
   A. Thin appearance
   B. Hypotension
   C. Change in level of consciousness
   D. Fruity breath odor
   E. Loss of subcutaneous fat, muscle wasting
   F. Eruptive xanthomas

2. Type 2
   A. Obese—localization of fat deposits on the abdomen, chest, neck, and face
   B. Generalized pruritis
   C. Vaginitis
   D. Hypertension

DIFFERENTIAL DIAGNOSIS

1. Hyperglycemia secondary to other causes
   A. Endocrine tumors—pheochromocytoma, somatostatinoma, Cushing's syndrome, glucagonoma
   B. Drugs—glucocorticoids, nicotinic acid, sympathomimetics, thiazide diuretics, phenytoin, pentamidine
   C. Liver disease—cirrhosis, hemochromatosis
   D. Muscle disorders—myotonic dystrophy
   E. Adipose tissue disorders—lipoatrophy, truncal obesity
   F. Insulin receptor disorders—acanthosis nigricans syndromes, leprechaunism
   G. Pancreatic disorders—pancreatitis, hemosiderosis

DIAGNOSTIC TESTS/FINDINGS

1. The diagnostic criteria for DM have been modified from those previously recommended by the National Diabetes Data Group and the World Health Organization. Three methods of diagnosing diabetes are available, and each must be confirmed on a subsquest day by any one of the three following methods:
   A. Symptoms of DM plus casual plasma glucose concentration ≥200 mg/dL. Casual is defined as any time of day without regard to time since last meal. Classic symptoms of DM include polyuria, polydipsia, and unexplained weight loss.
   B. Fasting plasma glucose ≥126 mg/dL. Fasting is defined as no caloric intake for at least 8 hours.
   C. Two-hour postload glucose (2hGP) ≥200 mg/dL during an oral glucose tolerance test (OGTT).
2. The corresponding categories when the OGTT is used are the following:
   A. 2hPG <140 mg/dL = normal glucose tolerance
   B. 2hPG ≥140 and <200 mg/dL = IGT
   C. 2hPG ≥200 mg/dL = provisional diagnosis of diabetes (the diagnosis must be confirmed as described above)
   For results to be valid, patients should not be stressed, should be free from acute illness, and should be normally active and receive at least 150–200 gm of carbohydrate daily for 3 days before the test. Adults should be given 75 gm of glucose dissolved in 300 mL of water in the morning following an overnight fast. (See Table 8–1 for the National Diabetes Data Group criteria for evaluating standard oral glucose tolerance test.)
3. Urinalysis: May show presence of glucose, ketones, and protein. Proteinuria is the first sign of diabetic nephropathy.
4. Blood urea nitrogen (BUN) and creatinine may be elevated, indicating renal involvement.
5. Urine glucose measurement can detect the occurrence of blood glucose levels above a variable renal threshold (150–300 mg/dL). Measurement of

TABLE 8–1. **National Diabetes Data Group Criteria for Evaluating Standard Oral Glucose Tolerance Test*,†**

	Normal Glucose Tolerance	Impaired Glucose Tolerance	Diabetes Mellitus
Fasting plasma glucose (mg/dL)	<115	116–139	>140
Points between 0 and 120 minutes (mg/dL)	<200	<200	200 at least once
Two hours post-glucose load (mg/dL)	<140	>140 but <200	>200

* From Karam, J. (1997). Diabetes mellitus and hypoglycemia. In L. Tierney, S. McPhee, & M. Papadakis (eds.). *Current Medical Diagnosis and Treatment* (36th ed.). Stamford, CT: Appleton & Lange, pp. 1069–1097, with permission.

† Give 75 gm of glucose dissolved in 300 mg of water after an overnight fast in subjects who have been receiving at least 150–200 gm of carbohydrate daily for 3 days before the test.

urine glucose is influenced by both glucose and water excretion; therefore, results correlate poorly with blood glucose levels.

6. Self-monitoring of blood glucose can be performed by patients at home and allows greater flexibility in management while achieving improved glycemic control. Particularly useful in brittle diabetics.

7. Fasting plasma triglycerides, total cholesterol, and high-density lipoprotein (HDL) cholesterol.

8. Electrocardiogram (ECG)—baseline.

9. Ophthalmologic referral.

10. Hemoglobin (Hb) A_{1c} to estimate plasma glucose control during the preceding 3 months. The normal level of glycosylate hemoglobin assayed in labs will vary; the average level is about 4–8%. "Excellent" glycemic control is presumed when Hb A_{1c} levels are less than 7.5%, "good" control when they are between 7.5% and 9%, and "poor" control when they are between 9.1% and 11%. (HB) A_{1c} should be at least quarterly.

11. Criteria for testing for diabetes in asymptomatic, undiagnosed individuals:
    A. Testing for diabetes should be considered in all individuals at age 45 years and above and, if normal, it should be repeated at 3-year intervals
    B. Testing should be considered at a younger age or be carried out more frequently in individuals who:
       1) Are obese (≥120% desirable body weight)
       2) Have a first-degree relative with diabetes
       3) Are members of a high-risk ethnic population (e.g., African American, Hispanic, Native American)
       4) Have delivered a baby weighing >9 lb or have been diagnosed with gestational diabetes
       5) Are hypertensive
       6) Have an HDL cholesterol level ≤35 mg/dL and/or a triglyceride level ≥250 mg/dL
       7) On previous testing, had impaired fasting glucose or IGT

MANAGEMENT/TREATMENT

1. Persistent hyperglycemia is the hallmark of all forms of diabetes. The goal is to achieve an acceptable serum glucose level, prevent acute symptoms

or complications of uncontrolled hyperglycemia, avoid hypoglycemia, and prevent or delay the progression of the chronic complications of diabetes. A fasting serum glucose level of <120 mg/dL and a Hb A_{1c} <7% are generally accepted criteria of good control.

2. The hospital admission guidelines for diabetes mellitus of the American Diabetes Association (1997) are to be used for determining when a patient requires hospitalization for reasons related to diabetes. Inpatient care may be appropriate in the following situations:
   A. Life-threatening acute metabolic complications of diabetes, such as diabetic ketoacidosis and hyperosmolar nonketotic state.
   B. Substantial and chronic poor metabolic control that necessitates close monitoring of the patient to determine the etiology of the problem, with subsequent modification of therapy. For admission, documentation should include at least one of the following:
      1) Hyperglycemia associated with volume depletion.
      2) Persistent refractory hyperglycemia associated with metabolic deterioration.
      3) Recurring fasting hyperglycemia >300 mg/dL that is refractory to outpatient therapy, or a glycosylated hemoglobin level of ≥100% above the upper limit of normal.
      4) Recurring episodes of severe hypoglycemia (i.e., <50 mg/dL) despite intervention.
      5) Metabolic instability manifested by frequent swings between hypoglycemia (<50 mg/dL) and fasting hyperglycemia (>300 mg/dL).
      6) Recurring diabetic ketoacidosis without precipitating infection or trauma.
      7) Repeated absence from school or work as a result of severe psychosocial problems that cannot be managed on an outpatient basis.
   C. Severe chronic complications of diabetes that require intensive treatment or other severe conditions unrelated to diabetes that significantly affect its control or are complicated by diabetes. Chronic cardiovascular, neurologic, renal, and other diabetic complications may progress to the stage where hospital admission is appropriate. In these situations, the needs governing admission for the complication (e.g., management of end-stage renal disease) are the primary guidelines for determining whether inpatient care is required. However, in applying such guidelines, the fact that diabetes is present must be considered and may result in patients who otherwise might be managed on an outpatient basis requiring admission.
   D. Uncontrolled or newly discovered insulin-requiring diabetes during pregnancy.
   E. Institution of insulin pump therapy or other intensive insulin regimens.
3. Dietary modification
   A. Revised American Diabetes Association (ADA) recommendations published in 1994 have replaced the calculated ADA diet formula. Medical nutrition therapy for diabetics should be individualized based on metabolic, nutritional, and lifestyle requirements.
   B. Emphasis for medical nutrition therapy in type 2 patients should be on achieving glucose, lipid, and blood pressure control.
   C. Type 1 diabetics need to eat at consistent times synchronized with the time-action of insulin. Adjust insulin for the amount of food eaten.
   D. Restriction of fat to 35% or less of the total calories.

E. Cholesterol restricted to 300 mg or less daily.

F. Percentage of carbohydrates will vary depending on the patient's eating habits and glucose and lipid goals.

G. Protein intake should be 10–20% of total calories.

H. Dietary fiber of 20–35 gm daily.

I. Sodium intake of 2400–3000 mg/day generally; for patients with hypertension, 2400 mg/day or less; and for patients with hypertension and nephropathy, 2000 mg/day.

J. Artificial sweeteners such as aspartame and saccharin are approved for consumption by all diabetics.

K. All newly diagnosed diabetics should be referred to a dietician for nutritional assessment and education.

L. To determine desirable body weight:
   1) Women: For first 5 ft, allow 100 lb; for each inch >5 ft, allow 5 lb
   2) Men: For first 5 ft, allow 106 lb; for each inch >5 ft, allow 6 lb
   3) For large frame, add 10%; for small frame, subtract 10%

M. To determine total caloric intake:
   1) To maintain weight: 15 kcal/lb or 30 kcal/kg
   2) To lose weight: 10 kcal/lb or 20 kcal/kg
   3) To gain weight: 20 kcal/lb or 40 kcal/kg
   4) For each decade over age 50, decrease total by 10%

4. Exercise
   A. Type 1 diabetes
      1) Exercise programs have not been exclusively shown to improve glycemic control in type 1 diabetes.
      2) Patients should be encouraged to exercise because of the potential to improve cardiovascular fitness and psychological well-being.
      3) Safe participation in all forms of exercise consistent with an individual's lifestyle should be a primary goal.
      4) Many variables, including fitness, duration and intensity of exercise, and time of exercise with respect to insulin administration and meals will affect the metabolic response to exercise.
      5) For these reasons, self-monitoring of blood glucose should be incorporated into the exercise program to provide the information necessary to adjust insulin or diet.
   B. Type 2 diabetes
      1) Exercise can improve glycemic control, reduce cardiac risk factors, and increase psychological well-being.
      2) Patients should have a pre-exercise evaluation to uncover previously undiagnosed hypertension, neuropathy, retinopathy, nephropathy, and silent ischemic heart disease.
      3) Patients taking oral medications or insulin should self-monitor their glycemic response to exercise.
      4) Exercise program should include aerobic exercise at 50–70% of an individual's maximum oxygen uptake, last 20–45 minutes, and be repeated at least three times a week. There should be cool-down exercises, and the overall program should be appropriate to the person's general physical condition and lifestyle.
      5) Elderly diabetic patients, especially those who are sedentary, should not be expected to undergo a dramatic change in lifestyle. Thus a simple walking program may be beneficial. For those elderly dia-

betic patients who are physically active, an initial exercise program should consist of moderate aerobic conditioning.

   C. General guidelines for all people with diabetes
     1) Use proper footwear
     2) Avoid exercise in extreme heat or cold
     3) Inspect feel daily and after exercise
     4) Avoid exercise during periods of poor metabolic control

5. Oral hypoglycemic agents (Table 8–2)
   A. Sulfonylureas
     1) The most commonly used oral antidiabetic drugs are the sulfonylureas, which are indicated for nonpregnant adults with type 2 diabetes. Work primarily by stimulating insulin production.
     2) Sulfonylureas should not be used in type 1 DM, in children, or during pregnancy or lactation. Caution is advised in patients with severe hepatic or renal disease or allergies to sulfa.
     3) Complications of these drugs include hypoglycemia, skin rash, blood dyscrasias, flushing, tachycardia, and nausea.
     4) Alcohol, chloramphenicol, methyldopa, miconazole, monoamine oxidase (MAO) inhibitors, salicylates, sulfonamides, warfarin, and phenylbutazone may potentiate hypoglycemic effects of sulfonylureas, and their use requires intensification of glucose monitoring and sulfonylureas dosage adjustment.
     5) In elderly patients, avoid chlorpropamide because of its long half-life and long duration of action. Sulfonylureas in general should be initiated at low doses.

   B. Antidiabetic agents: Biguanides and α-glucosidase inhibitors
     1) Biguanides: Metformin (Glucophage)
       a. May be used as primary or adjunctive therapy in type 2 diabetes and most secondary DM. Can be used in combination with a sulfonylurea.
       b. Metformin appears to stimulate a nonoxidative metabolism of glucose in peripheral tissues, increasing glucose utilization. Metformin does not produce hypoglycemia and may reduce triglycerides and low-density lipoprotein cholesterol while increasing HDL cholesterol.
       c. Frequent side effects include gastrointestinal symptoms, including anorexia, nausea, vomiting, and abdominal discomfort.
       d. Contraindicated in renal failure with creatinine >1.5, hepatic dysfunction.
       e. Daily dose is 1000–2500 mg two to three times daily. Generally start with 500 mg twice a day.
     2) α-Glucosidase inhibitors: Acarbose (Precose)
       a. Can be used alone or in combination with sulfonylureas or insulin.
       b. Reduces postprandial hyperglycemia by binding to α-glucosidase enzymes in the small intestine. It inhibits the digestion of complex carbohydrates in the upper jejunum so that they are digested throughout the length of the small intestine. The major effect is to decrease the postprandial rise in plasma glucose.
       c. Must be taken with the first mouthful of food ingested.
       d. Acarbose does not cause hypoglycemia; however, a patient on

T A B L E 8–2.   Oral Medications for Diabetes

Medications: Generic (Brand Name)	Formulations	Total Daily Dose	Onset of Action (hr)	Duration of Action (hr)	Comments
Sulfonylureas					
First Generation					
Acetohexamide (Dymelor, various generics)	250-, 500-mg tablets	250–1500 mg dosed once or twice daily (max: 1500 mg/day)	1	12–24	Rarely used.
Chlorpropamide (Diabinese, various generics)	100-, 250-mg tablets	100–500 mg dosed once daily (max 750 mg/day)	1	24–72	Prolonged hypoglycemia and alcohol intolerance possible.
Tolazamide (Tolinase, various generics)	100-, 250-, 500-mg tablets	100–500 mg dosed once daily (max: 500 mg/day)	4–6	12–24	Few side effects. No active metabolites. Preferred drug for elderly.
Tolbutamide (Orinase, various generics)	500-mg tablets	500–3000 mg dosed 2 or 3 times daily (max: 3000 mg/day)	1	6–12	Must be taken 2–3 times daily.
Second Generation					
Glimepride (Amaryl)	1-, 2-, 4-mg tablets	1–8 mg	1	24	
Glipizide (Glucotrol, Glucotrol XL, various generics)	5-, 10-mg tablets; 5-, 10-mg extended-release tablets	5–40 mg dosed once or twice daily (max: 20 mg/day)*	1–1.5	12–24	Few side effects. No active metabolites. Preferred drug for elderly.
Glyburide (DiaBeta, Micronase, various generics)	1.25-, 2.5-, 5-mg tablets	1.25–10 mg dosed once or twice daily (max: 10 mg/day)	2–4	12–24	Hypoglycemia possible if meals skipped.
Glyburide, micronized (Glynase Prestabs)	1.5-, 3-, 6-mg, micronized tablets	1.5–12 mg dosed once or twice daily (max: 12 mg/day)	1	24	Hypoglycemia possible if meals skipped.
Biguanides					
Metformin (Glucophage)	500-, 850-mg tablets (film-coated)	1000–2550 mg dosed 2 or 3 times daily (max: 2550 mg/day)	1	10–12	Take with meals. Start with low dose, and increase dose slowly to minimize GI intolerance. Does not cause hypoglycemia (may potentiate hypoglycemia of sulfonylureas or insulin). Lactic acidosis rare.
α-Glucosidase Inhibitors					
Acarbose (Precose)	50-mg scored tablets, 100-mg tablets	150–300 mg dosed three times daily (max: if <60kg, 150 mg/day; if >60, 300 mg/day)	0.5–1	4–6	Take with first bite of meal. Start with low dose and increase dose slowly to minimize GI intolerance. Does not cause hypoglycemia (may potentiate hypoglycemia of sulfonylureas or insulin).

Table continues

TABLE 8-2. *(Continued)*

Medications: Generic (Brand Name)	Formulations	Total Daily Dose	Onset of Action (hr)	Duration of Action (hr)	Comments
Thiazolinedione Insulin Resistance Reducer Rezulin (Troglitazone)	200-, 300-, 400-mg tablets	Starting dose of 200 mg/day; may be increased after 2–4 weeks (max: 600 mg/day)	2–3	12	Take with meals. Well tolerated. May cause hepatic disease; monitor liver function tests.

GI, gastrointestinal.

    acarbose who becomes hypoglycemic from another cause must be treated with glucagon or glucose and not sucrose.

    e. When acarbose is added to sulfonylurea therapy, the sulfonylurea can cause hypoglycemia.

    f. Most common side effects are flatulence, diarrhea, and abdominal discomfort.

    g. Daily dose is 150–300 mg three times daily. Start with a low dose and increase slowly. If the dose is increased too quickly, the gas and bloating are unacceptable.

    h. Use is contraindicated in patients with liver disease, bowel obstruction, or colitis.

  C. Rezulin (Troglitazone)

    1) Oral antihyperglycemic agent that acts primarily by decreasing insulin resistance.

    2) Used in type 2 diabetes. This includes type 2 patients on insulin.

    3) Improves target cell response to insulin.

    4) Decreases hepatic glucose output and increases insulin-dependent glucose disposal in skeletal muscle.

    5) Should be taken with meals.

    6) Use with caution in patients with hepatic disease.

    7) Can be used as monotherapy or combination therapy with sulfonylureas or insulin.

    8) May cause hepatic disease in a small number of patients; monitor liver function tests.

    9) Starting dose is 200 mg every day; may increase to maximum dose of 600 mg. The dose of sulfonylurea or insulin will need to be adjusted based on glucose lowering response.

  6. Insulin

  A. Indicated for type 1 diabetics as well as for type 2 diabetics who have evidence of severe insulin deficiency and a catabolic state on the basis of ketonuria, profound weight loss, or dehydration, or who are thin. In addition, patients who are symptomatic from hyperglycemia and have failed to respond to diet and/or sulfonylurea, metformin, or acarbose, as well as those with severe elevated triglyceride levels, should be treated with insulin.

  B. Preparations of purified porcine insulin, purified bovine insulin, semisynthetic human insulin, and biosynthetic human insulin are available.

  C. Insulin preparations are classified as rapid, short, intermediate, or long acting. The usual onset of action, time of peak of action, and duration

T A B L E 8–3.   Pharmacokinetics of Insulin after Subcutaneous Injection*

Insulin Type	Onset of Action (hr)	Peak Effect (hr)	Duration of Activity (hr)
Rapid-acting			
Lispro	0.25 or less	0.50–1.0	3–4
Short-acting			
Regular	0.25–1.0	2–6	4–12
Intermediate-acting			
Lente	1–4	6–16	14–28
NPH	1.5–4.0	6–16	14–28
NPH 70% with regular 30%	0.5	4–8	24
Long-acting			
Ultralente (human)	3–8	4–10	9–36
Ultralente (bovine)	3–8	8–28	24–40

* Human insulins may produce a faster peak effect and a shorter duration of activity than bovine or beef insulins. Activity may be prolonged in renal failure.

of action of the most commonly used preparations are listed in Table 8–3. Lispro is a rapid-acting insulin analog. Regular is a short-acting insulin. Intermediate-acting insulins include lente and NPH. Insulin preparations with a predetermined proportion of NPH mixed with regular, such as 70% NPH to 30% regular, are considered intermediate acting. The only long-acting insulin is ultralente. Lispro, the new rapid-acting insulin, is injected 15 minutes before a meal and reaches a peak in 30 minutes to 1 hour; the duration of action is only 3–4 hours. It may be more convenient and safer than regular insulin for patients who cannot control or predict the timing of their meals. Because Lispro wears off rapidly, longer-acting insulins must also be used to provide adequate control between meals.

D. Conventional insulin treatment refers to the practice of treating with one or two injections a day of intermediate-acting insulin, with or without smaller added doses of rapid-acting insulin.

E. Initiation of insulin therapy: generally 20–40 U/day are appropriate in initial treatment. The estimated daily requirement can be divided into thirds, with two thirds given before breakfast and one third given before the evening meal. The morning dose is split into two-thirds intermediate-acting insulin and one-third rapid-acting insulin, and the evening dose is split evenly between the intermediate-acting and rapid-acting insulins.

F. When adjusting insulin doses, adjust only one insulin at a time. Insulin can be adjusted on a daily to weekly basis by 10–20% increments until daily blood sugars approach the 120-mg/dL range or slightly higher in the elderly patient.

G. Soon after initiation of treatment, many patients with type 1 diabetes experience a "honeymoon period" with a marked decrease in insulin requirements that lasts several months.

H. When using two different types of insulin, care should be taken when they are drawn from the same syringe to avoid cross-contamination of the bottles.

I. Regular insulin should be drawn up first if mixing regular and NPH in the same syringe.

J. Phosphate-buffered insulins (e.g., NPH insulin) should not be mixed with lente insulins.

K. Almost all insulins used in adults are prepared as 100 U/mL, or U-100.
L. Disposable syringes with fine 27- to 29-gauge hypodermic needles are the preferred tools for insulin administration.
M. Bottles of NPH and ultralente insulins should be agitated gently before administration.
N. Subcutaneous tissue of the abdominal wall, anterior thighs, and arms may be used for injection. Sites should be clean, and areas of infection, inflammation, lipodystrophy, or scarring should be avoided.

7. Bedside blood glucose monitoring in hospitals
   A. Useful in managing hospitalized patients with diabetes because results can be obtained quickly and therapeutic decisions can be made, improving management
   B. Enhances patient comfort

8. Intensive insulin therapy
   A. Refers to treatment regimens in which the specific aim is to continuously maintain normal to near-normal diurnal plasma glucose fluctuations in hopes of preventing late complications.
   B. Multiple daily injection (MDI) regimens are generally required to maintain normalization of blood glucose.
   C. MDI regimens can improve blood glucose control, reduce wide and erratic changes in blood glucose levels, provide additional flexibility in a patient's daily routine, and enable the patient to exercise more control over diabetes management.
   D. Requires close self–blood glucose monitoring.
   E. Goal-oriented, comprehensive approach to therapy that consists of frequent blood glucose self-monitoring and a systematic approach to quantifying food and matching insulin to food intake.

9. Continuous subcutaneous insulin infusion (CSII)
   A. CSII can be an alternative to multiple daily insulin injections for achieving near-normal levels of blood glucose and permits the greatest degree of lifestyle flexability, and can therefore facilitate achieving glycemic goals. The reasons for this are that (1) the insulin pump uses only regular insulin, making insulin absorption from subcutaneous tissues more predictable; and (2) insulin delivery is similar to that found in nondiabetic individuals in that there is a continuous basal insulin delivery supplemented by preprandial increases in plasma insulin levels.
   B. Patients must be willing to assume substantial responsibility for their day-to-day care and understand and demonstrate use of the insulin pump and self-monitoring of blood glucose.
   C. Interruption of insulin delivery can result in rapid deterioration of diabetic control.
   D. Pump malfunction, loss of battery charge, or leakage from the catheter can result in cessation of insulin delivery.
   E. Infection can develop at the infusion site where the needle is inserted.
   F. The insulin pump delivers insulin at a continous basal rate via a bolus, which is a larger amount of insulin taken 20–30 minutes before a meal. The 24-hour basal rate is usually 40–50% of the patient's total daily dose. The meal boluses can be calculated as a percentage of the total daily dose as follows: breakfast, 20%; lunch, 10%; dinner, 15%; and bedtime, 5%.

10. Combined therapy
    A. Sulfonylurea, metformin, acarbose, and rezulin: Combination therapy of a sulfonylurea with either metformin, acarbose, or rezulin is very

effective in type 2 patients who have or develop an inadequate glycemic response to either oral antidiabetic agent alone.

  B. Oral hypoglycemic/antidiabetic drugs and insulin therapy: Many patients with type 2 DM have insulin resistance and a progressive decrease in beta cell function. They may respond initially to oral hypoglycemic agents but later develop secondary failure.

    1) A trial of combination sulfonylurea and insulin therapy may be used in some patients with type 2 DM who are no longer responsive to oral hypoglycemic agents.

    2) A possible combination would be oral hypoglycemic sulfonylureas during the day to control postprandial glycemic rises and intermediate-acting insulin at night to control overnight hepatic glucose production.

    3) Rezulin can be very effective in combination with insulin.

11. IV insulin

  A. Can be given as a bolus or a continuous infusion.

  B. IV insulin bolus produces its maximum effect at 10–30 minutes and may last to 1–2 hours.

  C. An insulin infusion may be prepared by adding 100 U of regular insulin to 500 mL of 0.45% saline.

12. Therapeutic intervention for proteinuria/microalbuminuria

  A. Includes optimizing glycemic control

  B. Low-protein diet (especially for gross proteinuria)

  C. Angiotensin converting enzyme (ACE) inhibitors (use cautiously in renal insufficiency)

  D. Control of hypertension if present

13. Antiplatelet therapy in DM

  A. Treat high-risk patients. Use enteric-coated aspirin (81-325 mg a day) to prevent vascular incidents

14. Surgical management of the diabetic patient

  A. Surgical procedures, including emotional stress, the effects of general anesthesia, and the trauma of the procedure, can markedly increase plasma glucose in diabetics and induce DKA in type 1 patients.

  B. The two most important aspects of preoperative evaluation are to establish adequate metabolic control and to optimize cardiovascular status. If there is any evidence of silent ischemia or silent infarction seen on electrocardiogram, surgery should be postponed until after complete cardiovascular evaluation. (See Table 8–4 for preoperative surgical evaluation.)

  C. For elective surgery, the evaluation should be completed a few days before the scheduled operation so that changes in management can be made.

  D. Surgery should be done early in the day.

  E. A general schema for management is given in Table 8–5.

  F. The optimal glycemic range is 125–200 mg/dL because this range minimizes risk of hypoglycemia.

  G. Postoperatively, in all patients who have received insulin infusion, blood glucose should be checked every 2 hours until stable glycemia is achieved and then every 4 hours.

  H. In type 1 patients, the usual preoperative insulin dose is started as soon as the patient begins to eat again.

  I. In type 2 patients, oral agents are resumed when the patient is able

---

TABLE 8–4.   Preoperative Assessment of the Diabetic Patient

History
Angina, infarction, claudation, hypertension
Control of diabetes

Physical Examination
Blood pressure
Cardiovascular examination, including heart sounds, peripheral pulses, bruits
Neurologic examination, including peripheral and autonomic

Laboratory
ECG
Fasting blood sugar
Glycosylated hemoglobin
Electrolytes, creatinine
Urine to check for ketones/protein

---

to tolerate diet. Monitor blood glucose every 4 hours until stable glycemia is achieved.

15. Diabetic ketoacidosis: An acute metabolic disorder involving severe insulin insufficiency and resulting in a significant elevation of blood glucose and metabolic changes as the body attempts to find alternate sources of energy. There are approximately 45,000 cases annually, with an overall mortality rate of 5–10% (see Table 8–6). The mortality rate increases in elderly patients, reaching between 15% and 28%.
    A. DKA occurs as a complication of DM; see Table 8–6 for the differential diagnosis of DKA versus hyperosmolar hyperglycemic nonketotic coma (HHNK).
    B. More likely to occur in type 1 patients.
    C. DKA occurs most often in patients with DM who were previously undiagnosed or in any patient with diabetes who is sufficiently stressed.
    D. Precipitating factors leading to DKA include insufficient to interrupted insulin therapy, infection, and other stress, such as trauma, surgery, CVA, MI, and pregnancy.
    E. DKA often presents with weight loss, polyuria, and polydipsia. Common symptoms include vomiting and abdominal pain (see Table 8–7).

TABLE 8–5.   Surgical Management of the Diabetic Patient*

Minor Surgery
Type 2: Hold oral agents until after procedure and resume with the resumption of oral intake.
Type 1: One half of usual morning dose (NPH or lente), remainder with resumption of oral regular as needed. (If blood sugar is >200 mg/dL on insulin, infusion may be considered.)

Major Surgery
Type 2: If well controlled by diet or oral medication, manage as above with measured blood sugars every 4 hr and insulin/glucose infusion for blood sugar >200 mg/dL.
Type 2 on insulin and type 1: Insulin/glucose infusion.
    Insulin infusion 1–3 units/hr
    10% dextrose in 0.45% normal saline at 100 mg/hr (20 mEq/KCl)
    Check glucose and adjust insulin drip every 1–2 hr

---

* From Reusch, J., & Sussman, K. (1996). Management of hyperglycemia emergencies and other hyperglycemic states. In RC Bone (ed.). *Current Practice of Medicine* (Vol. 4). New York: Churchill Livingstone, section 4, p. 15.5, with permission.

TABLE 8–6.   Differential Diagnosis of DKA versus HHNK*

	DKA	HHNK
Population at risk	Type 1 DM <40 years	Type 2 DM >40 years
Symptoms	12–20% new onset <2 days polyuria, polydipsia, nausea, vomiting	50% no prior diagnosis >5 days polyuria, polydipsia, decreased mental status
Laboratory studies		
Glucose	<800 mg/dL	>800 mg/dL
Sodium	Normal or ▼	Normal or ▲
Potassium	▲, normal, ▼	▲, normal, ▼
Bicarbonate	<15	Normal
Ketones	Positive	Negative/trace
pH	<7.3	Normal
Osmolarity	<350 mOsm/L	>350 mOsm/L
Prognosis (in most cases HH)	5–10% mortality	30–50% mortality

* Adapted from Reusch, J., & Sussman, K. (1996). Management of hyperglycemia emergencies and other hyperglycemic states. In RC Bone (ed.). *Current Practice of Medicine* (Vol. 4.). New York: Churchill Livingstone, section 4, p. 15, with permission.

HH, hyperosmolar hyperglycemic.

TABLE 8–7.   Symptoms and Signs of Diabetic Ketoacidosis*

Symptoms	Signs
Polyuria, polydipsia	Tachycardia
Nausea and vomiting	Hypothermia
Anorexia	Dehydration
Fatigue	Kussmaul respirations
Weakness	Acetone breath
Abdominal pain	"Acute abdomen"
Dyspnea	Hypotonia/hyporeflexia
	Altered mental status
	Focal neurologic signs

* From Reusch, J., & Sussman, K. (1996). Management of hyperglycemia emergencies and other hyperglycemic states. In RC Bone (ed.). *Current Practice of Medicine* (Vol. 4). New York: Churchill Livingstone, section 4, p. 15.3, with permission.

TABLE 8–8.   Diagnostic Criteria for Diabetic Ketoacidosis*

Hyperglycemia (300–800 mg/dL)
Acidemia (pH 6.8–7.3)
Bicarbonate deletion <15
Positive ketones
Incidental increased liver function tests, elevated leukocyte count (with or without infection), increased amylase
Hypertriglyceridemia
Electrolyte abnormalities
Free water deficit

* From Reusch, J., & Sussman, K. (1996). Management of hyperglycemia emergencies and other hyperglycemic states. In RC Bone (ed.). *Current Practice of Medicine* (Vol. 4). New York: Churchill Livingstone, section 4, p. 15.3, with permission.

F. Later symptoms include lethargy or somnolence and, if untreated, progression to coma.

G. Diagnosis (see Table 8–8) requires:
1) Demonstration of hyperglycemia (usually >300 mg/dL)
2) Serum positive for ketones
3) Metabolic acidosis, blood pH <7.3, and serum bicarbonate <15 mEq/L
4) Electrolyte abnormalities
5) Free water deficit

H. Lab findings
1) Glycosuria
2) Ketonemia
3) Low arterial blood pH
4) Low plasma bicarbonate
5) Hyperkalemia

I. Treatment: Patients usually will be managed by the endocrinologist and/or internist; however, the ACNP may be involved collaboratively with the physician. The ACNP can educate patients to recognize early symptoms of DKA. Urine ketones should be measured in patients with signs of infection or when blood glucose is unexpectedly persistently high.
1) Fluid management: Restoration of intravascular volume should be prompt and guided by considerations of cardiac and renal function. Initial fluids should include 0.9% saline, and the first liter of fluid should be given within 1 hour. Patients in shock may warrant more rapid infusion. Usually fluid deficits are 3–5 L.
2) Frequent assessment of the heart rate, blood pressure (BP), and urine output.
3) Foley catheter insertion to monitor output.
4) Bicarbonate therapy: Use of bicarbonate is not recommended unless the plasma pH is <7.1 or severe hyperkalemia is present. A solution of sodium bicarbonate 1–2 ampules (44 mEq/50-mL ampule) in a liter of 0.45% saline can be infused until the blood pH reaches 7.2.
5) Potassium replacement is needed because there is a total body potassium loss from polyuria as well as from vomiting.
6) Hyperkalemia may be seen initially because of metabolic acidosis; however, once acidosis improves, serum potassium returns to the cells and hypokalemia can be observed.
7) Potassium in doses of 20–30 mEq/hr should be infused within 2–3 hours after beginning therapy or sooner if initial serum potassium is inappropriately low.
8) Insulin treatment reverses ketogenesis and restores normal nutrient utilization.
9) Initial dose should be initiated with regular insulin 10–15 U (or 0.15 U/kg) IV as a bolus, followed by a continuous IV insulin infusion of 10 U/hr (or 0.1 U/kg/hr). Insulin drip should not be stopped abruptly; because of the risk of recurrent DKA, SQ insulin should be started while the patient is on insulin drip and then doses of insulin drip tapered.

16. Hyperosmolar hyperglycemic nonketotic coma: A syndrome characterized by impaired consciousness, sometimes accompanied by seizures, extreme dehydration, and extreme hyperglycemia that is not accompanied by ketoacidosis.

A. HHNK is a complication of type 2 DM and has a mortality rate of 30–50%.
B. HHNK is most commonly a complication of previously undiagnosed or medically neglected type 2 DM.
C. May occur as a result of severe stress and may follow stroke or excessive carbohydrate intake.
D. Patients often present with obtundation or coma and severe dehydration.
E. Laboratory evaluation will show:
   1) Hyperglycemia, often >600 mg/dL.
   2) Absence of significant ketonemia.
   3) Plasma osmolarity >320 mOsm/L.
   4) Associated findings may include severe azotemia and lactic acidosis.
F. Therapy of HHNK should include:
   1) Restoration of volume and osmolarity.
   2) Management of hyperglycemia.
   3) Methods of treatment resemble those for DKA.

17. Hypoglycemia
A. May be complication from therapy using sulfonylureas or insulin. Absolute hypoglycemia is defined as a plasma glucose level <45 mg/dL but, in diabetic patients, hypoglycemia symptoms can occur at higher plasma glucose levels and often correlate with the rapidity of the fall in glucose levels.
B. Is diagnosed by a classic triad of symptoms known as the "Whipple" triad.
   1) Symptoms consistent with hypoglycemia
   2) Confirmation of a low plasma glucose concentration
   3) Relief of symptoms when plasma glucose concentrations are raised to normal levels
C. Usually results from:
   1) A change in the content or timing of meals
   2) An increase in physical activity
   3) A medication overdosage
D. Characterized by:
   1) Mild
      a. Irritability
      b. Tremors
      c. Diaphoresis
      d. Tachycardia
      e. Confusion
   2) Severe
      a. Seizure
      b. Stupor
      c. Coma
E. Elderly diabetic patients who become hypoglycemic may be at greater risk for myocardial infarction or cerebrovascular accident.
F. Treatment: Manifestations of hypoglycemia are rapidly relieved by glucose administration. If more severe hypoglycemia has produced unconsciousness or stupor:
   1) Administer 50 mL of 50% glucose solution by rapid intravenous infusion.
   2) If intravenous therapy is not available, inject 1 mg of glucagon intramuscularly.

18. Other considerations
    A. Somogyi effect: Patients with type 1 diabetes may develop nocturnal hypoglycemia, which may stimulate a surge of counterregulatory hormones to produce high blood glucose levels in the A.M.
    B. Dawn phenomenon: Occurs in both type 1 and type 2 diabetic patients. Characterized by reduced tissue sensitivity to insulin developing between 5:00 A.M. and 8:00 A.M. When the dawn phenomenon occurs alone, it may produce only mild hyperglycemia in the early morning; when it is associated with the Somogyi effect, the hyperglycemia may be more severe.
    C. Insulin allergy: Immediate-type hypersensitivity is a rare condition in which local or systemic urticaria is due to histamine release from tissue mast cells sensitized by adherence of anti-insulin IgE antibodies.
    D. Immune insulin resistance: All insulin-treated patients develop a low titer of circulating IgG anti-insulin antibodies that neutralize to a small extent the action of insulin. This results in extremely high insulin requirements.
    E. Lipodystrophy at injection sites: Atrophy of subcutaneous fatty tissue leading to disfiguring and depressed areas resulting from an immune reaction is becoming rarer with the development of pure insulin preparations.

PATIENT EDUCATION

1. For all newly diagnosed diabetic patients, explain nature of diabetes and its potential acute and chronic complications.
2. Importance of regular testing, self-monitoring of glucose levels.
3. Advise patients on personal hygiene, including care of the feet, teeth, and skin.
4. Individual instruction on diet and drug therapy—referral to dietician.
5. Advise diabetics who smoke to quit the habit.
6. Explain importance of follow-up appointment in clinic after discharge from the hospital.
7. Instruct patients to carry packets of table sugar or candy at all times for use at the onset of hypoglycemic symptoms.
8. Instruct patient to wear Medic Alert identification.
9. Educate patient on early signs of DKA and to seek medical evaluation promptly.
10. Explain importance of annual eye examinations.
11. Refer patients to the American Diabetes Association, which can serve as a continuing source of instruction (1-800-342-2383).

Review Questions

8.1 In asymptomatic patients, diabetes is established when:
    A. There is a postprandial blood glucose level >250 mg/dL
    B. There is a plasma glucose level >140 mg/dL after an overnight fast on two occasions
    C. There is a plasma glucose level >160 mg/dL after an overnight fast on two occasions
    D. There is a fasting plasma glucose level >126 mg/dL

8.2 Hemoglobin A_{1c} measures:
   A. Plasma glucose control during the preceding 3 months
   B. Plasma glucose control during the preceding 30 days
   C. Plasma glucose control during the preceding 3 days
   D. Postprandial blood glucose levels

8.3 A patient has been started on metformin for type 2 diabetes. You would tell your patient that the most common side effects of this drug are:
   A. Hypoglycemia
   B. Headaches
   C. Nausea and abdominal discomfort
   D. Constipation

8.4 A 57-year-old man has a history of diabetes mellitus and coronary artery disease (CAD) that was diagnosed 10 years ago. His past medical history is significant for hypertension, CAD, and gouty arthritis. He takes human insulin: 22 U NPH and 10 U regular before breakfast; 12 U NPH and 6 U regular before dinner. Other medications include allopurinol, aspirin, isosorbide dinitrate, and captopril. His blood glucose pattern (in milligrams per deciliter) as determined by self-monitoring is:

7:00 A.M.	11:00 A.M.	4:00 P.M.	9:00 P.M.
216	110	140	122
242	116	129	105

Which of the following insulin dose adjustments would be the most appropriate?
   A. Increase A.M. NPH insulin
   B. Increase P.M. NPH insulin
   C. Increase P.M. regular insulin
   D. Increase P.M. regular and NPH insulin

8.5 A 40-year-old woman with a history of type 1 diabetes mellitus develops confusion, slurred speech, and headache. Her medications include nifedipine, propranolol, and NPH insulin 20 U and regular insulin 5 U every A.M. Physical exam reveals a blood pressure of 110/70 mm Hg and a pulse of 110 beats per minute. The patient is lethargic but arousable and diaphoretic. Her skin is pale. Plasma glucose level is 40 mg/dL. Which of the following would be the most appropriate initial treatment?
   A. 50 mL of 50% dextrose intravenously
   B. 50 mL of 10% dextrose intravenously
   C. Orange juice
   D. Hard sugar candy

Answers and Rationales

8.1   **D** In asymptomatic patients, a diagnosis of diabetes is established when there is a plasma glucose level >126 mg/dL after no caloric intake for 8 hours on two occasions.

8.2   **A**   Glycohemoglobin has several constituents, the major one being hemoglobin A^{1c}. Because the life span of the red blood cell is about
15–17 weeks, glycohemoglobin concentration provides an index of
glycemic control over a 6- to 12-week period.

8.3   **C**   Frequent side effects of metformin include nausea and abdominal
discomfort. A rare but serious adverse effect of metformin is lactic
acidosis. Liver and kidney function tests are recommended before
starting the patient on the drug and every 6–12 months thereafter.

8.4   **B**   The patient's blood glucose pattern shows morning hyperglycemia.
Because the peak effect of regular insulin occurs after 2–4 hours and
that of NPH insulin occurs after 6–14 hours, a larger evening dose
of NPH insulin is needed to lower the patient's morning hyperglycemia.

8.5   **A**   The patient described has manifestations of hypoglycemia, and the
initial treatment should be to administer 50 mL of 50% dextrose
intravenously. The diagnosis of hypoglycemia is made if Whipple's
triad is present. The components of this triad include (1) symptoms
consistent with hypoglycemia, (2) documentation of a low plasma
glucose level, and (3) a satisfactory response of symptoms to glucose
administration.

References

Abrahamson, M., & Flier, J. (1996). Diabetes mellitus and hypoglycemia. In S. Korenman (ed.). *Current Practice of Medicine* (Vol. 1). New York: Churchill Livingstone,
Section IV, pp. 14.1–14.8.

American Diabetes Association (1994). Revised recommendation. *Diabetes Care 17,*
490–518.

American Diabetes Association. (1996). Standards of medical care for patients with
diabetes mellitus. *Diabetes Care 19*(Suppl. 1), S8–S15.

American Diabetes Association. (1997). Hospital admission guidelines for diabetes mellitus. *Diabetes Care 20*(Suppl. 1), S52.

Atkinson, M.A., & Maclaren, N.K. (1994). Mechanisma of disease: The pathogenesis of
insulin-dependent diabetes mellitus. *N Engl J Med 314,* 278–285.

Baily, C.J. (1992). Biguanides and NIDDM. *Diabetes Care 15,* 755–784.

Cefalu, W.T. (1991). Diabetic ketoacidosis. *Crit Care Clin 7,* 89–108.

Jack, D. (1997). Type II diabetes: How to use the new oral medications. *Geriatrics 51*(4),
33–37.

Karam, J. (1997). Diabetes mellitus and hypoglycemia. In L. Tierney, S. McPhee, & M.
Papadakis (eds.). *Current Medical Diagnosis and Treatment* (36th ed.). Stamford,
CT: Appleton & Lange, pp. 1069–1097.

Miller, M. (1996). Type II diabetes: A treatment approach for the older patient. *Geriatrics
51*(8), 43–49.

Orland, M. (1995). Diabetes mellitus. In *The Washington Manual* (28th ed. [20]). Boston:
Little, Brown & Co., pp. 437–463.

Porte, D., & Sherwin, R. (1997). Classification and diagnosis of diabetes. In L. Braverman & R. Utiger (eds.). *Ellenberg and Rifkin's Diabetes Mellitus* (7th ed.). Stamford, CT: Appleton & Lange, pp. 346–356.

Service, F.J. (1993). Hypoglycemias. *Clin Endocrinol Metab 76,* 269–272.

Diabetes Insipidus

DEFINITION

Diabetes insipidus is an uncommon disease characterized by an increase in thirst and the passage of large quantities of urine of low specific gravity. It is caused by a deficiency of or resistance to vasopressin.

ETIOLOGY

1. Deficiency of vasopressin
   A. Primary diabetes insipidus: May be familial, occuring as a dominant trait, or sporadic ("idiopathic").
   B. Secondary diabetes insipidus: Caused by damage to the hypothalamus or pituitary stalk by anoxic encephalopathy, surgical or accidental trauma, or infection, such as tuberculosis, syphilis, or sarcoidosis. Metastases to the pituitary are more likely to cause diabetes than are pituitary adenomas.
   C. Vasopressinase-induced diabetes insipidus: May be seen in the last trimester of pregnancy and in the puerperium. It is often associated with pre-eclampsia or hepatic dysfunction.
2. Nephrogenic diabetes insipidus: May be congenital or acquired. The congenital form is rare, usually inherited, most commonly affects males, and has been linked to a defect in the renal vasopressin receptor resulting from an abnormal gene for the vasopressin receptor located on the X chromosome. Acquired forms are seen in some patients with pyelonephritis, renal amyloidosis, myeloma, potassium depletion, or chronic hypercalcemia.

SIGNS AND SYMPTOMS

1. Onset may be insidious or abrupt and may occur at any age.
2. Intense thirst.
3. Enormous quantities of fluid may be ingested, varying from 4 to 20 L/day.
4. Very dilute urine; specific gravity usually <1.005 with large urine volumes.
5. Nocturia almost always present.
6. Dehydration and hypovolemia may develop rapidly if fluids are not replaced.
7. Muscular pains.

PHYSICAL FINDINGS

1. Tachycardia
2. Orthostatic hypotension
3. Lethargy
4. Dry mucous membranes

DIFFERENTIAL DIAGNOSIS

1. Compulsive psychogenic water drinking
2. Intravenous fluid administration
3. Central nervous system sarcoidosis
4. Diabetes mellitus
5. Polyuria caused by Cushing's syndrome

DIAGNOSTIC TESTS AND FINDINGS

1. A 24-hour urine collection for volume, glucose, and creatinine.
2. Serum glucose, BUN, creatinine, potassium sodium. Because the patient may be dehydrated, there may be hypernatremia, increased plasma osmolality, and elevation of BUN and creatinine.
3. Vasopressin challenge test: Desmopressin acetate is given in an initial dose of 0.05–0.1 mL intranasally with measurement of prior and subsequent urine volumes. Serum sodium must be obtained immediately in the event of symptoms of hyponatremia. The dosage of desmopressin is doubled if the response is marginal. Patients with true central diabetes insipidus will notice a distinct reduction in their thirst and polyuria.
4. Serum vasopressin, when measured during fluid restriction, usually will be elevated in nephrogenic diabetes insipidus and low in central diabetes insipidus.
5. In nonfamilial central diabetes insipidus, magnetic resonance imaging (MRI) of the pituitary and hypothalamus to look for mass lesions.

MANAGEMENT AND TREATMENT

Patients with diabetes insipidus should initially be evaluated by either the endocrinologist or internist; however, the ACNP may be involved in the patient's care in collaboration with the physician.

1. Correct hypernatremia or volume depletion.
   A. Treatment depends on degree of volume depletion.
   B. If evidence of marked orthostatic hypotension is present, treatment should initially be with isotonic saline.
2. Hormonal
   A. Desmopressin acetate (DDAVP) is the treatment for central diabetes insipidus.
   B. Usually given intranasally but can be given subcutaneously or intravenously.
   C. It is a synthetic analog of arginine vasopressin and has prolonged antidiuretic activity, lasting for 12–24 hours.
   D. Usual adult dosage is 0.05–0.1 mL intranasally every 12–24 hours.
   E. Also available as a parenteral preparation containing 4 μg/mL. It is given intravenously, intramuscularly, or subcutaneously in doses of 1–4 μg every 12–24 hours as needed to treat thirst or hypernatremia.
   F. Can be given as an oral preparation, starting at a dose of 0.1 mg daily and increasing to a maximum of 0.2 mg every 8 hours.
   G. Caution must be taken to avoid volume overload and/or hyponatremia when desmopressin acetate is used. Serum sodium or osmolality measurement serves as a useful guide to assessment of volume status (Fig. 8–1).
3. Other measures
   A. Mild cases require no treatment other than adequate fluid intake.
   B. Reduction of aggravating factors such as glucocorticoids will improve polyuria.
   C. Both central and nephrogenic diabetes insipidus respond partially to hydrochlorothiazide 50–100 mg daily.
   D. Chlorpropamide is sometimes effective for central diabetes insipidus and can improve thirst; however, use with caution secondary to hypoglycemia.

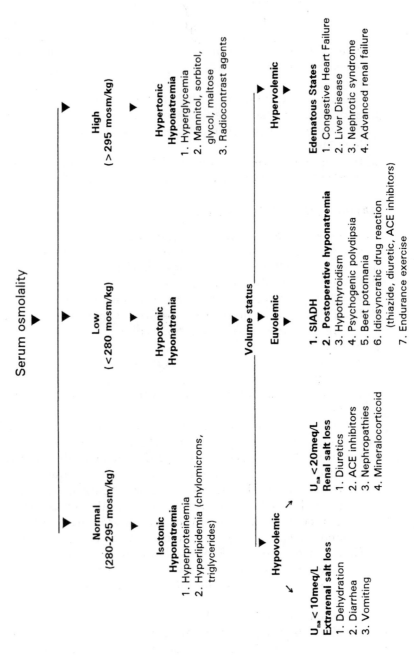

FIGURE 8–1. Evaluation of hyponatremia using the serum osmolality. (From Papadakis, M. [1997]. Fluid and electrolyte disorders. In L. Tierney, S. McPhee, & M. Papadakis [eds.]. *Current Medical Diagnosis and Treatment* [36th ed.]. Stamford, CT: Appleton & Lange, pp. 800–806, with permission.)

E. Nephrogenic diabetes insipidus may respond to combined treatments of indomethacin-hydrochlorothiazide, indomethacin-desmopressin, or indomethacin-amiloride.
F. Psychotherapy is required for most patients with complusive water drinking.
G. Avoid thioridazine and lithium because they cause polyuria.
H. Daily monitoring of body weight and periodic measurement of serum sodium are helpful in assuring that fluid intake is appropriate.

PATIENT EDUCATION

1. Explain to patient that chronic diabetes insipidus itself does not reduce life expectancy.
2. Explain importance of drug therapy and potential side effects.
3. Instruct patient on daily weights if indicated.
4. Explain need for psychotherapy if indicated.
5. Explain importance of follow-up in clinic.

Review Questions

8.6 Mr. Jones is a 30-year-old man who complains of intense thirst and nocturia. He reports consuming up to 10 L of fluids a day. Urinalysis reveals very dilute urine with a specific gravity of 1.000. Differential diagnosis would include all but which of the following?
A. Diabetes insipidus
B. Complusive psychogenic water drinking
C. Diabetes mellitus
D. Adrenal insufficiency

8.7 Which of the following tests would be most helpful to you in determining whether a patient has diabetes insipidus?
A. Vasopression challenge test
B. Rapid cosyntropin stimulation test
C. Fluid challenge
D. Glucose tolerance test

8.8 A 35-year-old female patient has a history of tuberculosis with damage to the hypothalamus. She would most likely have which type of diabetes insipidus?
A. Secondary or acquired diabetes insipidus
B. Primary or idiopathic diabetes insipidus
C. Acute diabetes insipidus
D. Chronic diabetes insipidus

8.9 Initial management of a patient with diabetes insipidus includes which of the following?
A. Correct volume depletion with IV fluids
B. Start an insulin drip
C. Correct hyponatremia with fluid restriction
D. Treat and control hypertension

8.10 Which of the following is FALSE regarding the drug desmopressin acetate?

A. Is the treatment for central diabetes insipidus
B. Is usually given intranasally
C. Has short antidiuretic activity lasting 6 hours
D. Usual adult dosage is 0.05–0.1 mL

Answers and Rationales

8.6   **D**   All of the conditions are included in the differential diagnosis of poly-uria and nocturia with the exception of adrenal insufficiency.

8.7   **A**   The vasopressin challenge test. Desmopressin acetate is given in-tranasally with measurement of prior and subsequent urine vol-umes. Patients with true central diabetes insipidus will notice a dis-tinct reduction in their thirst and polyuria.

8.8   **A**   Secondary or acquired diabetes insipidus is due to damage to the hypothalamus or pituitary stalk by a variety of pathologic lesions, including tuberculosis.

8.9   **A**   Initial management would include correcting volume depletion with IV fluids because dehydration and hypotension are present.

8.10   **C**   Desmopressin acetate has prolonged antidiuretic activity lasting for 12–24 hours.

References

Fitzgerald, P. (1997). Endocrinology. In L. Tierney, S. McPhee, & M. Papadakis (eds.). *Current Medical Diagnosis and Treatment* (36th ed.) Stamford, CT: Appleton & Lange, pp. 1013–1015.

Lippmann, B. (1995). Fluid and electrolyte management. In *The Washington Manual* (28th ed.). Boston: Little, Brown & Co., pp. 50–51.

Miller, M. (1996). Neuroendocrinology. In S. Korenman (ed.). *Current Practice of Medicine* (Vol. 1). New York: Churchill Livingstone, section IV, pp. 1.1–1.8.

Adrenal Insufficiency

DEFINITION

Adrenal insufficiency (AI) is characterized by impaired adrenal function, which leads to inadequate cortisol and aldosterone production.

ETIOLOGY

1. Primary adrenal insufficiency (Addison's disease) usually results from pro-gressive destruction of the adrenal glands.
   A. Most common cause is autoimmune adrenalitis, accounting for approxi-mately 70% of cases.
   B. Tuberculosis is responsible for approximately 20% of all cases.
   C. Other causes include fungal or cytomegalovirus infection, metastasis of malignant neoplasms to the adrenals.
   D. Certain medications associated with AI include ketoconazole, aminoglu-tethamide, metyrapone, trilostane, suramin, etomidate, rifampin, and phenytoin.

2. Secondary adrenal insufficiency is associated with deficient adrenocorticotropic hormone (ACTH) secretion from the pituitary gland because of dysfunction of the hypothalamus and/or the anterior pituitary gland.
   A. May be attributed to prolonged exposure to high doses of exogenous corticosteroids.
   B. Iatrogenic causes account for the majority of cases of AI.
   C. Can also occur if there is destruction or dysfunction of the hypothalamus and/or anterior pituitary gland.
3. Acute adrenal crisis
   A. Any of the various forms of chronic AI can evolve into acute adrenal crisis.
   B. Most often precipitated by stressful events such as trauma, severe infection, or surgery.
   C. The reduced adrenal reserve results in acute deficiency of glucocorticoids and in primary adrenal disease, as well as deficiency of mineralocorticoids.
   D. May follow a sudden withdrawal of adrenocortical hormone in a patient with chronic insufficiency.
   E. May follow bilateral adrenalectomy or removal of a functioning adrenal tumor that suppressed the other adrenal.
   F. If untreated, may result in death.

SIGNS AND SYMPTOMS

The severity in the presentation of AI depends on the rate of onset and the degree of the insufficiency as well as the precipitating cause. The majority of patients have a slowly increasing degree of insufficiency with a progressive worsening of signs and symptoms.
1. Primary adrenal insufficiency
   A. Weakness
   B. Fatigability
   C. Anorexia
   D. Nausea and vomiting
   E. Malaise
   F. Salt craving
   G. Abdominal pain or discomfort
   H. Diarrhea
   I. Myalgias
   J. Weight loss
   K. Hyperpigmentation
   L. Vitiligo
   M. Mental status changes, including depression, apathy, and confusion
2. Secondary adrenal insufficiency
   A. Similar to that of primary AI
   B. Hyperpigmentation is absent
3. Adrenal crisis
   A. Nausea and vomiting
   B. Fever
   C. Dehydration
   D. Severe abdominal pain
   E. Pain in lower back and/or legs
   F. Headache

   G. Diarrhea
   H. Circulatory shock

PHYSICAL FINDINGS

1. Primary
   A. Hypotension
   B. Hyperpigmentation
   C. Vitiligo
   D. Tachycardia
2. Secondary
   A. Hypotension
   B. Cushingoid features may suggest exogenous glucocorticoid therapy
3. Adrenal crisis
   A. Hypotension
   B. Confusion or coma
   C. Cyanosis
   D. Dehydration
   E. Fever
   F. Tachycardia

DIFFERENTIAL DIAGNOSIS

1. Occult malignancy
2. Gastrointestinal disease
3. Diabetes mellitus
4. Hypoparathyroidism

DIAGNOSTIC TESTS AND FINDINGS

1. Primary
   A. Low serum sodium (<130 mEq/L).
   B. High serum potassium (>5 mEq/L).
   C. Elevated BUN.
   D. Elevated plasma ACTH level in association with a low plasma cortisol level is diagnostic (see Table 8–9).
   E. The rapid cosyntropin stimulation test: Cosyntropin 0.25 mg is injected IV before 9:00 A.M. Normal preinjection plasma cortisol ranges from 5–25 μg/dL and doubles at 60–90 minutes. Patients with Addison's disease have low or normal values that do not rise.
2. Secondary: To distinguish between secondary and primary—plasma ACTH concentration is high in primary AI.
3. Acute crisis
   A. Low serum sodium.
   B. Elevated serum potassium.
   C. Elevated BUN.
   D. Eosinophil count may be high.
   E. Elevated hemoglobin and hematocrit (in volume depletion).
   F. Arterial blood gases: Low bicarbonate (metabolic acidosis).
   G. Low plasma cortisol.
   H. ACTH: Markedly increased in primary adrenal insufficiency (generally >200 pg/mL) and decreased in secondary adrenal insufficiency.

TABLE 8–9. Diagnostic Tests for Adrenal Insufficiency*

Rapid ACTH stimulation test: 250 μg IV cosynthopin (synthetic ACTH) (1–24)	Usually used at least 12 hr after any prior steroid use
Baseline, 30-min, 60-min blood samples for cortisol (or 45-min only)	If post-ACTH cortisol is <6–20 μg/dL from baseline level, adrenal insufficiency is confirmed
8 A.M. cortisol level	If 8 A.M. cortisol is low (<5 μg/dL), adrenal insufficiency is suspected
ACTH level (with abnormal ACTH stimulation of cortisol)	If ACTH is elevated (>52 pg/mL), primary adrenal insufficiency is confirmed If ACTH is low (<9 pg/mL), either normal or secondary adrenal insufficiency

* Adapted from Kohlmeier, L., & Feldman, D. (1996). Adrenal cortex glucocorticoids. In RC Bone (ed.). *Current Practice of Medicine* (Vol. 1). New York: Churchill Livingstone, section 4, p. 5.13, with permission.

    I. Short ACTH test: Decreased baseline plasma cortisol, decreased plasma cortisol at 30 minutes and 60 minutes after receiving IV ACTH. Normally, serum cortisol rises to at least 20 μg/dL; however, patients with acute adrenal insufficiency are unable to stimulate a normal increase in serum cortisol.

4. Other diagnostic tests
    A. Computed tomography (CT) scan of the abdomen: May show enlargement of adrenals as a result of metastatic disease or granulomatous disease. May show small, noncalcified adrenals in autoimmune Addison's disease.
    B. CT scan of the head to rule out tumor or mass and assess shape and size of pituitary gland.
    C. Chest x-ray to look for tuberculosis, fungal infection, or malignancy.
    D. Tuberculin skin test.
    E. Serum free thyroxine index (FTI), serum thyroid-stimulating hormone (TSH) level, thyroid anti-microsomal antibody test

MANAGEMENT AND TREATMENT

The ACNP should refer any patient suspected of having adrenal insufficiency to an endocrinologist for initial evaluation and management.
1. Primary adrenal insufficiency
    A. Replacement therapy should include a combination of glucocorticoids and mineralocorticoids.
    B. Hydrocortisone 15–25 mg in two divided doses daily.
    C. Fludrocortisone 0.1–0.2 mg orally once a day.
    D. Doses need to be increased during times of stress, including infections, surgery, and illness.
    E. If symptoms are unresponsive to hydrocortisone, prednisone may be used. Starting dose is 7.5 mg daily in two divided doses. Adjust dose based on symptoms.
    F. Monitor complete blood count (CBC) and SMA-7 every 6 months on outpatient basis.
    G. ACTH and thyroid function tests should be checked annually on outpatient basis.

2. Secondary adrenal insufficiency: Similar to primary AI; however, does not require replacement of mineralocorticoids because aldosterone is produced.
3. Acute adrenal crisis
    A. Intravenous fluids: D_5 0.9 normal saline rapidly infused until hypotension is corrected.
    B. Hydrocortisone 100 mg IV every 6–8 hours.
    C. Decrease the dose of hydrocortisone gradually over several days as symptoms and any precipitating illness resolve, then change to oral maintenance therapy.
    D. Mineralocorticoid replacement is not needed until the dose of hydrocortisone is less than 100 mg/day (replace only in primary AI).
4. Refer patients to the National Adrenal Foundation for information (1-516-487-4992).

PATIENT EDUCATION

1. Educate on lifetime hormone replacement therapy as well as providing information about stress doses of replacement therapy.
2. Educate patient on signs and symptoms of adrenal insufficiency and self-injection technique for administration of hydrocortisone.
3. Instruct patients that they need to keep an emergency kit of hydrocortisone with a syringe and needle with them at all times.
4. Stress importance of wearing a Medic Alert bracelet.
5. Explain to patients with primary AI that they may need to increase dietary sodium.
6. Explain the prognosis for survival is good and patients with appropriate management will live a normal life.
7. Explain to patient that it often takes up to 3 months to adjust medications and that some symptoms may persist until that time.

Review Questions

8.11 Primary adrenal insufficiency most often results from:
    A. Fungal infections
    B. Cytomegalovirus
    C. Tuberculosis
    D. Autoimmune adrenalitis

8.12 Acute adrenal crisis can result from all of the following except:
    A. Trauma, severe infection
    B. Increase of glucocorticoids
    C. Withdrawal of adrenocortical hormone
    D. Bilateral adrenalectomy

8.13 A 40-year-old female patient presents to the emergency room with complaints of severe weakness, nausea and vomiting, and weight loss for the past month. Serum sodium is 127 mEq/L, serum potassium 5.2 meq/L, and BUN 35. Blood pressure is 86/60. Differential diagnosis for this patient includes adrenal insufficiency. Which of the following would you expect to find on physical exam in a patient with adrenal insufficiency?
    A. Skin rash, jugular neck vein distention
    B. Gait disturbances, increased reflexes

    C. Hyperpigmentation, tachycardia

    D. Bradycardia, coarse hair

8.14 Which of the following laboratory findings would you expect to find in a patient with adrenal insufficiency?

    A. High serum sodium, low serum potassium, elevated plasma ACTH, and low plasma cortisol level

    B. Low serum sodium, high serum potassium, elevated plasma ACTH, and low plasma cortisol level

    C. Elevated BUN, low serum sodium, and high serum potassium

    D. Low BUN, low serum sodium, and high serum potassium

8.15 Replacement therapy for primary adrenal insufficiency includes:

    A. Combination of glucocorticoids and mineralocorticoids

    B. Mineralocorticoids

    C. Glucocorticoids

    D. Thyroxine

Answers and Rationales

8.11 **D** The most common cause of primary adrenal insufficiency is autoimmune adrenalitis, which accounts for 70% of cases.

8.12 **B** Adrenal crisis can result from trauma, severe infection, withdrawal of adrenocortical hormone, bilateral adrenalectomy, or a decrease in glucocorticoids.

8.13 **C** Classic findings of a patient with adrenal insufficiency are hypotension, hyperpigmentation, and tachycardia.

8.14 **B** Low serum sodium, high serum potassium, elevated plasma ACTH, and low plasma cortisol level can be seen in adrenal insufficiency.

8.15 **A** Replacement therapy includes a combination of glucocorticoids and mineralocorticoids because they are both deficient in primary adrenal insufficiency.

References

Fitzgerald, P. (1997). Endocrinology. In L. Tierney, S. McPhee, & M. Papadakis (eds.). *Current Medical Diagnosis and Treatment* (36th ed.). Stamford, CT: Appleton & Lange, pp. 1047–1049.

Grossman, P. (1992). Adrenocortical insufficiency. *Topics Emerg Med 14*, 1–6.

Leshin, M. (1982). Acute adrenal insufficiency: Recognition, management and prevention. *Urol Clin North Am 9*, 299.

Miller, M. (1996). Neuroendocrinology. In S. Korenman (ed.). *Current Practice of Medicine* (Vol. 1). New York: Churchill Livingstone, section IV, pp. 1.1–1.8.

Werbel, S., & Ober, P. (1993). Acute adrenal insufficiency. *Endocrinol Metab Clin North Am 22*, 303–323.

Pheochromocytoma

DEFINITION

Pheochromocytoma is a rare disease characterized by paroxysmal or sustained hypertension resulting from a tumor located in either or both adrenals or anywhere along the sympathetic nervous chain, and rarely in such aberrant locations as the thorax, bladder, or brain.

ETIOLOGY

1. A tumor of chromaffin cells that secrete catecholamines, which causes hypertension.
2. Occurs equally in both sexes.
3. In about 10% of cases the tumor involves both adrenals.
4. Are usually benign; about 10% are malignant.
5. Maximum incidence is between the third and fifth decades of life.
6. Presence of pheochromocytoma may be unrecognized for many years, and in many cases not diagnosed in life.
7. Untreated pheochromocytoma leads to morbidity and mortality through the chronic presence of hypertension or through sudden death associated with pheochromocytoma crisis. Pheochromocytoma crisis may occur spontaneously or with pregnancy, delivery, anesthesia, surgery, or trauma.

SIGNS AND SYMPTOMS

1. Attacks of severe headache, perspiration, palpations
2. Tachycardia
3. Abdominal pain
4. Nervousness and irritability
5. Flushing
6. Chest pain
7. Vomiting
8. Sense of impending doom
9. Some patients may be asymptomatic

PHYSICAL FINDINGS

1. Hypertension, which is the most prominent feature
2. Hypertension may be paroxysmal or persistent
3. Cardiac enlargement on chest x-ray
4. Postural tachycardia
5. Postural hypotension
6. Occasionally retinal hemorrhage or papilledema
7. Psychosis or confusion
8. Pulmonary edema
9. Heart failure

DIFFERENTIAL DIAGNOSIS

1. Thyrotoxicosis
2. Essential hypertension
3. Myocarditis
4. Anxiety disorder
5. Glomerulonephritis
6. Acute abdomen
7. Cocaine or amphetamine use
8. Unstable angina

9. Hypertension crisis caused by foods containing tyramine in patients taking MAO inhibitors

DIAGNOSTIC TESTS AND FINDINGS

1. A 24-hour urine sample for vanillylmandelic acid (VMA) catecholamines, metanephrines, and creatinine detects most pheochromocytomas, especially when samples are obtained during an attack (see Table 8–10). Patients with pheochromocytomas generally will have more than 2.2 μg of metanephrine per milligram of creatinine and more than 5.5 μg of VMA per milligram of creatinine. Many drugs and chemicals and some foods can affect the tests for pheochromocytoma.
2. Direct assay of epinephrine and norepinephrine in blood and urine during or following an attack is the most sensitive test for pheochromocytoma.
3. Clonidine suppression test: A positive test result that shows suppression of norepinephrine is strongly predictive of absence of pheochromocytoma, but a negative result in the presence of marginally increased catecholamines cannot be considered presumptive evidence for the presence of a chromaffin tumor. This diagnostic test may be dangerous and should be carried out only by an experienced endocrinologist.
4. CT and MRI can be helpful in the confirmation and localization of the tumor.
5. Normal thyroxine (T_4) and TSH.

MANAGEMENT AND TREATMENT (Table 8–11)

Management team should consist of the endocrinologist, surgeon, and internist. The ACNP may be involved in the care in collaboration with the physician.
1. Definitive treatment is surgical removal of the tumor.
2. Control blood pressure before surgery with α-blockade. The drug of choice is phenoxybenzamine, with a starting dose of 10 mg bid. It is reasonable to aim for a diastolic blood pressure between 90 and 100 mm Hg.
3. The need for β-blockade is indicated by tachycardia.
4. Monitor ECG until it becomes stable preoperatively.
5. Intraoperative severe hypertension is managed with phentolamine 1–5 mg IV or nitroprusside 0.5–10 μg/kg/min.

TABLE **8–10. Excretion Rates of Catecholamines and Catecholamine Metabolites in Normal Subjects and in Patients with Pheochromocytoma***

	Normal† (gm/hr)	Pheochromocytoma‡ (gm/hr)
Catecholamines (free epinephrine plus norepinephrine)	2.5 ± 0.8	10–120
Metanephrine plus normetanephrine (free plus conjugated)	16 ± 5	30–420
Normetanephrine (free and conjugated)	10 ± 5	30–720
Vanillylmandelic acid	240 ± 120	500–3500

* From De Quattro, V., & Lee, D. (1996). Pheochromocytoma. In RC Bone (ed.). *Current Practice of Medicine* (Vol. 1). New York: Churchill Livingstone, section 4, p. 7.3, with permission.
† Mean ± standard deviation.
‡ Presumptive until proved otherwise.

TABLE 8-11.   Therapy for Patients with Pheochromocytoma*

α-Blockade

Phentolamine 1–5 mg IV: drug of choice for surgery for rapid control of hypertension (many choose nitroprusside)

Phenoxybenzamide 20–80 mg/day: preoperative and long-term treatment

Specific α_1-blockade: prazosin, doxazosin, terzosin (less complete control than with phenoxybenzamine)

β-Blockade

Propranolol: 10–40 mg PO qid after α-blockade

α- and β-receptor blockade

Labetalol: 300 mg/day or more

Vasodilator

Nonspecific nitroprusside, magnesium sulfate

Calcium channel blockade: nifedipine, diltiazem

Converting enzyme inhibitor: captopril, enalapril

Malignant or Inoperable

Methylparatyrosine (1–2 gm/day)

Vincristine, cyclophosphamide, dacarbazine (as a regimen)

Tumoricidal [^{131}I]MIBG

---

* Adapted from De Quattro, V., & Lee, D. (1996). Pheochromocytoma. In RC Bone (ed.). *Current Practice of Medicine* (Vol. 1). New York: Churchill Livingstone, section 4, p. 7.7, with permission.
MIBG, metaiodobenzyguanidine.

6. Metastatic pheochromocytomas may be treated with combination chemotherapy. Median survival is about 4.5 years.

PATIENT EDUCATION

1. Explain disease process in detail.
2. Explain symptoms to patients and what to do during an "attack."
3. Explain importance of medication to control symptoms.
4. If surgery is planned, provide preoperative teaching and explain expected postoperative course.

Review Questions

8.16 Signs and symptoms of pheochromocytoma include which of the following?
   A. Bradycardia, weakness, confusion
   B. Severe headache, palpations, hypertension
   C. Lethargy, disorientation, stupor
   D. Salt craving, diarrhea, fever

8.17 Which of the following laboratory tests would be most helpful in making a diagnosis in a patient suspected of having a pheochromocytoma?
   A. CT of the abdomen
   B. Vanillylmandelic acid, electrolytes
   C. Electrolytes, fasting blood glucose
   D. Urinary catecholamines, metanephrines, and vanillylmandelic acid

8.18 Before surgery for a pheochromocytoma, patients should be treated with which of the following to control hypertension?

    A. Calcium channel blockers
    B. ACE inhibitors
    C. α-adrenergic blockers
    D. Nitrites

8.19 Which of the following is NOT true of pheochromocytoma?
    A. It is usually benign
    B. Occurs equally in both sexes
    C. Hypertension is the most prominent feature
    D. It is a common disease

8.20 Intraoperative severe hypertension can be managed with which of the following medications?
    A. Nitroprusside 0.5–10 μg/kg/min
    B. Clonidine 0.2 mg PO
    C. Verapamil 80 mg PO
    D. Minipress 2 mg PO

Answers and Rationales

8.16   **B**   Severe headache, palpations, and hypertension are frequently seen in pheochromocytoma.

8.17   **D**   Urinary catecholamines, metanephrines, and vanillylmandelic acid would be most helpful for diagnosis.

8.18   **C**   Before surgery, hypertension should be controlled with α-adrenergic blockers.

8.19   **D**   Pheochromocytoma is a rare disease usually seen between the third and fifth decade of life.

8.20   **A**   Intraoperative severe hypertension can be managed with nitroprusside 0.5–10 μg/kg/min or phentolamine 1–5 mg intravenously.

References

Bravo, E., Tarazi, R., Fouad, F., et al. (1981). Clonidine suppression test: A useful aid in the diagnosis of pheochromocytoma. *N Engl J Med 305*, 623–626.

DeQuattro, V., & Lee, D. (1996). Pheochromocytoma. In S. Korenman (ed.). *Current Practice of Medicine* (Vol. 1). New York: Churchill Livingstone, section IV, pp. 7.1–7.9.

Engleman, K., & Sjoerdsma, A. (1964). Chronic medical therapy for pheochromocytoma. *Ann Intern Med 61*, 229–241.

Gifford, R. (1994). Pheochromocytoma. *Endocrinol Metab Clin North Am 23*, 387–404.

Shapiro, B., & Fig, L. (1989). Management of pheochromocytoma. *Endocrinol Metab Clin North Am 18*, 443–470.

Syndrome of Inappropriate Secretion of Antidiuretic Hormone

DEFINITION

Syndrome of inappropriate secretion of antidiuretic hormone (SIADH) is characterized by an increased or continued release of antidiuretic hormone (ADH).

Normally, ADH is released in response to hypoxia and reduced blood pressure sensed by pressure receptors in the atria and pulmonary artery. In SIADH, the negative feedback system that normally controls the release of ADH fails. It is one of the most common causes of hyponatremia.

ETIOLOGY/INCIDENCE

1. Release of ADH occurs without osmolality-dependent or volume-dependent physiologic stimulation.
2. Occurs in oat cell carcinoma of the lung because of ectopic production of ADH.
3. Other causes or risks
   A. Hypoxia or other events that decrease left atrial filling pressures, such as pneumonia, tuberculosis, chronic pulmonary disease, cardiac failure, or positive-pressure breathing with mechanical ventilation
   B. Central nervous system disease or injury, such as Guillain-Barré syndrome, head trauma, meningitis, or tumors
   C. Various drugs such as chlorpropamide, carbamazepine, vasopressin, oxytocin, vincristine, cyclophosphamide, morphine, nicotine, barbiturates, and anesthetic agents (see Table 8–12)
   D. Hypopituitarism and ectopic ADH tumors
   E. Postoperative experiences such as stress, nausea, and hypoxia
   F. Administration of excess amounts of hypotonic fluids
   G. Acquired immunodeficiency syndrome (AIDS) patients with pulmonary or central nervous system (CNS) infections

T A B L E 8–12.   **Causes of Drug-Induced SIADH**

Increased ADH Production
Antidepressants
  Amitriptyline
  Clomipramine
  Desipramine
  Imipramine
  Monamine oxidase inhibitors
  Fluoxetime
Antineoplastics
  Cyclophosphamide
  Vincristine
  Vinblastine
Carbamazepine
Clofibrate
Neuroleptics
  Thiothixene
  Thioridazine
  Fluphenazine
  Haloperidol
  Trifluoperazine

Potentiated ADH Action
Carbamazepine
Chlorpropamide, tolbutamide
Cyclophosphamide
NSAIDs
Somatostatin and analogues

NSAIDs, nonsteroidal anti-inflammatory drugs.

SIGNS AND SYMPTOMS

1. Early
    A. Confusion
    B. Disorientation
    C. Lethargy
2. Late (serum sodium <115 mEq/L)
    A. Stupor
    B. Convulsions
    C. Neuromuscular hyperexcitability
    D. Prolonged coma and death

PHYSICAL FINDINGS

1. Mental status changes as described above
2. No peripheral edema
3. Gait disturbances

DIFFERENTIAL DIAGNOSIS

1. Hypothyroidism
2. Adrenal insufficiency
3. Thiazide diuretic therapy
4. Psychogenic polydipsia
5. Excessive chronic intake of beer
6. Idiosyncratic ACE inhibitor reactions

DIAGNOSTIC TESTS/FINDINGS

1. Hyponatremia (serum sodium concentration <130 mEq/L).
2. Decreased serum osmolality (<280 mOsm/kg) with inappropriately increased urine osmolality (>150 mOsm/kg). (See Figure 8–1 for evaluating hyponatremia using the serum osmolality.)
3. Normal thyroid function tests.
4. Urine sodium usually over 20 mEq/L.
5. Other changes frequently seen are low BUN (<10 mg/dL) and low plasma uric acid level (<4 mg/dL).

MANAGEMENT/TREATMENT

1. See Table 8–13 for management of hyponatremia resulting from SIADH.
2. Acute treatment of SIADH should be in those patients who are symptomatic or when the hyponatremia is severe (generally serum sodium <115 mEq/L).
    A. Brain damage may occur from overly rapid correction of serum sodium. Generally increase the serum sodium by 0.5–1 mEq/L/hr, aiming not to exceed 130 mEq/L in the first 48 hours.
    B. Hypertonic (3%) saline with furosemide for patients who are symptomatic. Replace potassium as needed.
3. Asymptomatic patients with SIADH
    A. Water restriction of 0.5–1 L/day. Gradual increase of serum sodium will occur over days.

TABLE 8–13.   Management of Hyponatremia Resulting from SIADH*

Treatment Modality	Mechanism of Action	Potential Adverse Complications
Acute		
IV 3% saline solution 300–500 mL over 4–6 hr, followed by 100 mL/hr	Elevation of serum sodium Reduction of cerebral edema	Cerebral pontine myelinolysis Congestive heart failure
IV furosemide, 1 mg/kg body weight	Increased free water excretion in excess	Hypokalemia, hypomagnesemia
Chronic		
Correction of underlying cause	Removal of stimulus for water retention	
Water restriction: 800–1000 mL/24 hr	Reduction of extracellular body water	Thirst stimulation
Butorphanol 4 mg 2 times per day	Inhibition of ADH secretion	CNS effects: confusion, hallucination
Lithium carbonate 600–1200 mg/day	Inhibition of ADH action via adenylate cyclase–cyclic AMP	CNS effects: confusion, dysarthria
Demeclocycline 600–1200 mg/day	Inhibition of ADH action via adenylate cyclase–cyclic AMP	Azotemia, photosensitivity Nephrotoxicity in patients with hepatic disease or congestive heart failure
ADH inhibitors (not yet clinically available)	Competitive antagonism at renal V2 receptor	None known

* From Miller, M. (1996). Neuroendocrinology. In RC Bone (ed.). *Current Practice of Medicine* (Vol. 1). New York: Churchill Livingstone, section 4, p. 1.6, with permission.

    B. Saline (0.9%) with furosemide can be used in those with a serum sodium <120 mEq/L.

    C. Demeclocycline 300–600 mg twice daily antagonizes the effect of ADH and may be helpful for patients who cannot adhere to water restriction or need additional therapy.

PATIENT EDUCATION

1. Emphasize the importance of fluid restriction.
2. Explain the nature and course of the disease.
3. Explain the importance of follow-up after discharge.
4. Explain the importance of medication compliance.

Review Questions

8.21 SIADH is characterized by which of the following?
    A. Increased or continued release of ADH
    B. Decreased release of ADH
    C. Hypernatremia
    D. Hyperkalemia

8.22 Individuals at risk for SIADH include all but which of the following?
   A. Patients with oat cell carcinoma of the lung
   B. Patients with head trauma, meningitis, or tumors
   C. Patients with diabetes
   D. Patients with AIDS with pulmonary infections

8.23 A 40-year-old female patient has a serum sodium of 122 mEq/L. Thyroid function tests are normal and her BUN is 4. Other tests that would best help you in determining the etiology of the hyponatremia include:
   A. Fasting blood glucose, serum potassium
   B. Plasma osmolality, urine osmolality
   C. CBC, uric acid
   D. ACTH, cortisol level

8.24 Mr. Smith is a 70-year-old man who is status postcrainotomy for clipping of an aneurysm. You are involved in managing his postoperative care. His serum sodium is 115 mEq/L, and he complains of nausea and vomiting. His urine sodium is 30 mEq/L and there is a decreased osmolality with inappropriately increased urine osmolality of 190 mOsm/kg consistent with SIADH. Initial treatment for this patient would include:
   A. Starting intravenous fluids of hypertonic 3% saline
   B. Increasing water intake to 2 L/day
   C. Demeclocycline 300 mg bid
   D. Restricting fluid intake to 1200 mL/day

8.25 Which of the following is TRUE about the treatment of SIADH?
   A. Patients usually respond to fluids being increased
   B. Brain damage may occur from overly rapid correction of serum sodium
   C. Sodium level should be corrected rapidly
   D. Diuretics can be used for chronic treatment

Answers and Rationales

8.21   **A**   SIADH is characterized by increased or continued release of ADH.
8.22   **C**   Individuals at risk for SIADH include patients with oat cell carcinoma of the lung, head trauma, meningitis, or tumors and AIDS patients with pulmonary infections.
8.23   **B**   Checking plasma osmolality and urine osmolality would be most helpful. Expect to find a decrease in plasma osmolality (<285 mOsm/kg) with inappropriately increased urine osmolality (>300 mOsm/kg) in SIADH.
8.24   **A**   Initial treatment of SIADH in symptomatic patients is hypertonic 3% saline.
8.25   **B**   Brain damage may occur from overly rapid correction of serum sodium.

References

Bartter, F., & Schwartz, W. (1967). The syndrome of inappropriate secretion of antidiuretic hormone. *Am J Med 42*, 790–806.
Miller, M. (1988). Disorders of water metabolism. In J. Hershman (ed.). *Endocrine Pathophysiology* (3rd ed.). Philadelphia: Lippincott-Raven, pp. 299–323.

Papadakis, M. (1997). Fluid and electrolyte disorders. In L. Tierney, S. McPhee, & M. Papadakis (eds.). *Current Medical Diagnosis and Treatment* (36th ed.). Stamford, CT: Appleton & Lange, pp. 800–806.

Thyroid Function Tests

Suspicion of thyroid dysfunction based on the history and physical findings should be followed by ordering specific thyroid tests.

The *serum thyroxine* (T_4) test measures the total amount of thyroxine in serum. The normal range is about 4.5–11 μg/dL serum. Serum T_4 is elevated in hyperthyroidism and low in hypothyroidism.

The *serum triiodothyronine* (T_3) level is a measurement of the total amount of T_3 in serum by radioimmunoassay. The normal range is about 80–180 ng/dL. It is a useful test for mild hyperthyroidism, because T_3 rises earlier and more markedly than does T_4 in all common forms of hyperthyroidism. In hypothyroidism, serum T_3 is within the normal range in at least one third of patients, so it is not a sensitive test for this diagnosis.

Free T_4 is measured by equilibrium dialysis, a tedious method, or newer direct immunoassay methods. It is reduced in hypothyroidism and increased in hyperthyroidism. The T_3 uptake (T_3U) indicates the degree of saturation of the thyroid hormone-binding proteins and is used for calculation of a free T_4 index (FT_4I) ($FT_4I = T_4 \times T_3U$).

Serum thyroid-stimulating hormone is measured by sensitive methods using monoclonal antibodies. The normal range is about 0.4–4 mU/L. Serum thyroid-stimulating hormone is particularly useful in the diagnosis of primary hypothyroidism because elevated thyroid-stimulating hormone occurs early with minimal thyroid dysfunction. In pituitary-hypothalamic hypothyroidism, the serum thyroid-stimulating hormone is low or sometimes normal. The normal level of thyroid-stimulating hormone in this circumstance is attributed to secretion of thyroid-stimulating hormone with reduced biologic activity. In hyperthyroidism, serum thyroid-stimulating hormone is low.

Thyrotropin-releasing hormone may be administered to test the adequacy of pituitary thyroid-stimulating hormone secretion. The peak thyroid-stimulating hormone response to thyrotropin-releasing hormone is usually proportional to the baseline thyroid-stimulating hormone level. In hyperthyroidism, the low serum thyroid-stimulating hormone does not rise after thyrotropin-releasing hormone, because the pituitary cannot overcome the negative feedback inhibition of the high circulating levels of T_4 and T_3. With the improved sensitivity of serum thyroid-stimulating hormone measurements, there is no need to measure the thyroid-stimulating hormone response to thyrotropin-releasing hormone for the evaluation of thyroid disease (Hershman, 1996).

Thyroxine-binding globulin (TBG) is a glycoprotein involved in both storage and synthesis of thyroid hormones. The amount of thyroid hormone attached to binding proteins will determine the amount of hormone that is free to be used by tissue and cells. Normal levels are 16–24 μg/dL. Causes of reduced TGB levels include nephrotic syndrome, hepatic disease, severe acidosis, steroid therapy, and congenital TBG deficiency. Causes of increased TBG levels include pregnancy, oral contraceptives, liver disease, hypothyroidism, and congenital TBG increase.

In addition, there are many drugs that can alter thyroid hormone levels (see Table 8–14).

**TABLE 8–14. Drug Effects on Thyroid Hormone Levels
and Laboratory Results**

Drug Effects on	Possible Laboratory Changes
TSH secretion	$\downarrow$ TSH
Dopamine	$\downarrow$ TSH
Glucocorticoids	$\downarrow$ TSH
Octreotide	
T_4 secretion	
Iodine	$\downarrow T_4$ or $\uparrow T_4$
Amiodarone	$\downarrow T_4$ or $\uparrow T_4$
Lithium	$\downarrow T_4$ or $\uparrow T_4$
TBG levels of binding capacities	
Estrogens	$\uparrow$ TBG ($\downarrow T_3$UR and $\uparrow T_4$)
Tamoxifen	$\uparrow$ TBG ($\downarrow T_3$UR and $\uparrow T_4$)
Androgens	$\uparrow$ TBG ($\uparrow T_3$UR and $\downarrow T_4$)
Glucocorticoids	$\uparrow$ TBG ($\uparrow T_3$UR and $\downarrow T_4$)
T_4 metabolism, increases	
Phenytoin	$\downarrow T_4$
Phenobarbital	$\downarrow T_4$
Carbamazepine	$\downarrow T_4$
Rifampin	$\downarrow T_4$
GI absorption of oral T_4 in hypothyroid patient	
Cholestyramine	$\downarrow T_4$ and $\uparrow$ TSH
Colestipol	$\downarrow T_4$ and $\uparrow$ TSH
Ferrous sulfate	$\downarrow T_4$ and $\uparrow$ TSH
Aluminum hydroxide	$\downarrow T_4$ and $\uparrow$ TSH
Sucralfate (carafate)	$\downarrow T_4$ and $\uparrow$ TSH

GI, gastrointestinal; T_3UR, triiodothyronine uptake ratio.

Reference

Hershman, J. (1996). Thyroid dysfunction. In RC Bone (ed.). *Current Practice of Medicine* (Vol. 1). New York: Churchill Livingstone, section IV, pp. 3.1–3.7.

Hyperthyroidism

DEFINITION

Hyperthyroidism, or "thyrotoxicosis," denotes a series of clinical disorders associated with increased circulating levels of free thyroxine or triiodothyronine. Thyrotoxicosis can present at any age and can often mimic other diseases or escape recognition for months or even years.

ETIOLOGY

The various causes of thyrotoxicosis include the following (see Table 8–15).
1. Graves' disease (toxic diffuse goiter)
    A. The most common form of thyrotoxicosis.
    B. Is an autoimmune disease.
    C. Patients with Graves' disease have thyroid-stimulating immunoglobulins that activate the TSH receptor and specifically stimulate the activity of the thyroid, causing an increase in hormone production.
    D. More common in women; onset usually between the ages of 20 and 40.

TABLE 8–15. **Thyroidal Radioiodine Uptake and Imaging in the Differential Diagnosis of Causes of Thyrotoxicosis**

Causes of Thyrotoxicosis	Fractional Uptake in 24 hours (%)	Pattern of Distribution of Radionuclide in Thyroid
Graves' disease	35–95	Homogeneous
Toxic nodular goiter (uni- or multinodular)	20–60	Restricted to regions of autonomy
Subacute thyroiditis	0–2	Little or no uptake
Silent thyroiditis	0–2	Little or no uptake
Iodine-induced thyrotoxicosis	0–50	Heterogeneous or no uptake
Factitious or iatrogenic thyrotoxicosis	0–2	Little or no uptake
Struma ovarii	0–2	Uptake in ovary
Follicular carcinoma	0–5	Uptake in tumor metastases
TSH-induced thyrotoxicosis	30–80	Homogeneous

  E. Characterized by a diffuse goiter and hyperthyroidism, often infiltrative ophthalmopathy, and rarely infiltrative dermopathy.
  2. Toxic nodular goiter
   A. The most common cause of thyrotoxicosis in the elderly.
   B. Goiter follicles are no longer fairly uniform and evenly overactive, but differ widely in size, structure, and function. Because some areas of the thyroid proliferate more than others, this type of goiter becomes nodular with time. The goiters contain follicles with widely varying individual hormone production ranging from virtually none to excessive.
   C. Thyrotoxicosis in nodular goiter is a very slowly progressing, insidiously evolving complication.
  3. Subacute thyroiditis: May be caused by viral infection causing a large, tender thyroid gland in which leakage of thyroid hormone causes transient hyperthyroidism, which is then followed by a hypothyroid phase that is also transient. During thyrotoxicosis, thyroid radioactive iodine uptake (RAIU) is low.
  4. Thyrotoxicosis factitia
   A. Results from administration of excessive thyroid hormone.
   B. Lab results will vary depending on which preparations were ingested.
  5. Jodbasedow disease: Occurs in patients with multinodular goiters after intake of large amounts of iodine in the form of radiographic contrast materials or drugs, especially amiodarone.
  6. Hashimoto's thyroiditis/chronic lymphocytic thyroiditis: Most common cause of goitrous hypothyroidism in western countries. The goiter is usually moderate in size (two to three times normal size) and is caused by lymphocytic infiltration and cell damage. Hypothyroidism may be caused by thyroid cell damage or thyroid-stimulating hormone–blocking antibodies. Like Graves' disease, it is an autoimmune disease.
  7. Struma ovarii: Thyroid tissue is contained in about 3% of ovarian dermoid tumors and teratomas. This thyroid tissue may autonomously secrete thyroid hormones as a result of a toxic nodule or in Graves' disease or toxic multinodular goiter.
  8. TSH hypersecretion by the pituitary: Overproduction of thyroid hormone can result from excess TSH secreted by a pituitary tumor.
  9. Painless thyroiditis/silent thyroiditis: Common in the postpartum period

and causes transient hyperthyroidism followed by transient hypothyroidism before recovery to euthyroidism.

10. Thyroid storm: A rare disorder where an extreme form of thyrotoxicosis develops. Usually there is a precipitating factor such as infection, gastroenteritis, severe trauma, or surgery.

SIGNS AND SYMPTOMS

1. General
   A. Nervousness
   B. Increased activity
   C. Increased sweating
   D. Heat intolerance
   E. Palpitations
   F. Fatigue
   G. Increased appetite
   H. Weight loss
   I. Insomia
   J. Weakness
   K. Frequent bowel movements (occasionally diarrhea)
   L. Menstrual irregularities
2. In the elderly
   A. May have atypical presentation or minimal symptoms.
   B. Rarely complain of loose stools. Instead may note a correction of a pre-existing constipation problem.
   C. Often there is a reduction in appetite.
   D. Reduction in muscle mass may be prominent.
   E. Decline in functional ability and activities of daily living.
   F. If history of congestive heart failure, may present with worsening of symptoms.
   G. Atrial fibrillation may be seen.
   H. Complaints of either a new or worsening angina.
   I. Myopathy—usually more proximal.
3. Thyroid storm
   A. Nausea/vomiting
   B. Marked weakness
   C. Diarrhea

PHYSICAL FINDINGS

1. General
   A. Moist, warm skin
   B. Tachycardia
   C. Atrial fibrillation
   D. Fine resting tremors
   E. Hyperreflexia
   F. Clubbing and swelling of the fingers
   G. Goiter firm and symmetric (seen in Hashimoto's)
   H. Goiter often with a bruit (seen only in Graves')
   I. Exophthalmos (seen only in Graves')
   J. Pretibial myxedema (seen in Graves')
   K. Stare, lid lag, lid retraction

2. Thyroid storm
   A. Tachycardia
   B. Fever
   C. Agitation or psychosis
   D. May present with cardiovascular collapse and shock

DIFFERENTIAL DIAGNOSIS

1. Anxiety
2. Neurosis or mania
3. Severe anemia
4. Pheochromocytoma
5. Myasthenia gravis
6. Diabetes mellitus
7. Addison's disease

DIAGNOSTIC TESTS/FINDINGS

1. Serum T_3, T_4, thyroid resin uptake, and free thyroxine are usually all increased. Sometimes the T_4 level may be normal. In the elderly, T_3 is elevated in only 50% of cases.
2. A sensitive TSH assay is the best test for thyrotoxicosis and will be suppressed except in the rare cases of pituitary inappropriate secretion of thyrotropin. A TSH level greater than 0.1 μU/mL excludes clinical hyperthyroidism. If plasma TSH is less than 0.1 μU/mL, the plasma T_4 index should be measured to determine the severity of hyperthyroidism and a baseline for therapy. If the plasma T_4 or T_4 index is elevated, the diagnosis of clinical hyperthyroidism is established.
3. Other lab abnormalities may include hypercalcemia, increased alkaline phosphatase, anemia, and decreased granulocytes.
4. TSH receptor antibody (TSH-R Ab) levels are usually high, but TSH-R Ab measurement is not ordinarily required for diagnosis.
5. Antithyroglobulin or antimicrosomal antibodies are usually elevated in Graves' disease and Hashimoto's thyroiditis.
6. Serum anti-nuclear antibodies are elevated without any evidence of lupus erythematosus or other collagen-vascular disease.
7. Increased erythrocyte sedimentation rate is seen in patients with subacute thyroiditis.
8. A high RAIU is seen in patients with Graves' disease and toxic nodular goiter (see Table 8–15).
9. A low radioactive iodine uptake is seen in patients with subacute thyroiditis (see Table 8–15).
10. MRI of the orbits is the imaging method of choice to visualize Graves' ophthalmopathy affecting the extraocular muscles; however, CT scanning and ultrasound can also be used.

TREATMENT/MANAGEMENT

The methods used to treat thyrotoxicosis will vary according to the cause and severity of the hyperthyroidism, the patient's age, the clinical situation, and the desires of the patient. Some forms of hyperthyroidism, such as silent thyroiditis or subacute thyroiditis, are transient and require only symptomatic therapy. There are three methods for definitive therapy: radioactive iodine, antithyroid drugs, and subtotal thyroidectomy. Measurement of plasma TSH is useless in assessing the initial response to therapy, because it remains suppressed until after the patient becomes euthyroid. Regardless of which therapy is used, all patients with Graves' disease require lifelong follow-up for recurrent hyperthyroidism or development of hypothyroidism.

1. Radioactive iodine (^{131}I)
   A. The administration of radioiodine is a simple, highly effective treatment. It is concentrated in the thyroid, impairing hormone synthesis and cell replication. A pregnancy test should be performed before therapy in women of child-bearing age because treatment is contraindicated. The ideal goal is to achieve a euthyroid patient. Methods for calculating the dose vary from a fixed dose to a calculated dose determined from the size of the thyroid in grams and the percentage uptake of the iodine. Most patients with Graves' disease are treated with about 8–10 mCi, while the dose for a toxic multinodular goiter usually is two to three times larger.
   B. Referral is made to a nuclear medicine physician, who administers the dose.
   C. Hypothyroidism is the main complication and occurs in the majority of patients, often years later.
   D. Follow-up is needed with free T_4 and sensitive TSH measurements.
2. Antithyroid drugs
   A. The thionamide antithyroid drugs, propylthiouracil (PTU) and methimazole (Tapazole), are given to block new hormone synthesis.
   B. No parenteral preparations are available; therefore, drugs must be given by mouth or by nasogastric tube.
   C. PTU should be started in a dose of 1200–1500 mg/day given as 200–250 mg q4h.
   D. Methimazole should be started in a dose of 120 mg/day given as 20 mg q4h.
   E. Side effects of antithyroid drugs are varied but most fall into a category that would be considered to be allergic (see Table 8–16). Agranulocytosis is the most frequent major side effect and is defined as a granulocyte count <250 × 10^9 cells/L. Agranulocytosis typically presents with fever and evidence of infection, usually in the oropharynx. Patients should be warned that if they develop a sore throat or febrile illness, they should stop the drug until a white blood cell count (WBC) is checked. Routine monitoring of WBC is not useful for detecting agranulocytosis, which usually develops suddenly.
   F. Follow-up should be conducted at 4-week intervals with assessment of clinical findings and plasma T_4. If there is no decrease in plasma T_4 following 4–8 weeks of therapy, the dose should be increased.
   G. Maintenance doses can be continued for 1 year or many years. There is no general agreement on the optimal duration of therapy. Some patients are treated until euthyroidism is restored. Studies have shown drug therapy for 1.5–2.0 years improves the chance of achieving a long-term remission, in contrast with treatment for only 6 months.
3. Propranolol
   A. Propranolol (Inderal) or other β-adrenergic antagonists relieve symptoms of hyperthyroidism such as palpitations, tremor, and anxiety. Propranolol can be used to improve well-being while definitive therapy of

TABLE 8–16.	Side Effects of Antithyroid Drugs*

Minor
Common (1–5%)
Rash
Urticaria
Arthralgia
Fever
Transient leukopenia

Rare
Gastrointestinal
Abnormalities of taste and smell
Arthritis

Major
Rare (0.2–0.5%)
Agranulocytosis

Very Rare
Aplastic anemia
Thrombocytopenia
Hepatitis (PTU)
Cholestatic hepatitis (methimazole)
Vasculitis, systemic lupus-like syndrome
Hypoprothrombinemia
Hypoglycemia (due to anti-insulin antibodies)

* From Cooper, D. (1996). Treatment of thyrotoxicosis. In L. Braverman & R. Utiger (eds.). *Werner and Ingbar's the Thyroid: A Fundamental and Clinical Text* (7th ed.). Philadelphia: Lippincott-Raven, p. 718, permission.

hyperthyroidism is being administered, or until transient forms of hyperthyroidism subside. The initial dose is 20–40 mg PO daily, and is adjusted to alleviate symptoms and tachycardia.
  B. Verapamil at an initial dose of 40–80 mg PO tid may be used to control tachycardia in patients with contraindications to β-adrenergic antagonists.
4. Surgery: Subtotal thyroidectomy provides long-term control of hyperthyroidism in most patients. Because of the risk of surgical morbidity and mortality, it is reserved for those patients who should not receive radioiodine, cannot tolerate antithyroid drugs, or have very large goiters (100–400 gm).
  A. Those undergoing surgery should be prepared by being treated with a thionamide until euthyroid and with a saturated solution of potassium iodide (SSKI) 40–80 mg orally twice daily. Both drugs are discontinued after surgery.
  B. Propranolol 20–40 mg orally four times a day is started 1–2 weeks before surgery to control tachycardia.
  C. Follow-up: Patients are evaluated at 4- to 6-week intervals with assessment of clinical findings and plasma T_4 until thyroid function stabilizes within normal range or symptomatic hypothyroidism develops. If symptomatic hypotension develops, thyroxine therapy should be initiated (see "Hypothyroidism").
5. Thyroid storm: Thyroid storm is a medical emergency that requires prompt treatment. Supportive measures and treatment of the underlying causative factor are essential (see Table 8–17).
  A. A thiourea drug is given: propylthiouracil 600 mg or methimazole 60 mg stat and half this dose 6h.

TABLE 8–17.   Management of Thyroid Crisis*

Therapy Directed against the Thyroid Gland
Inhibition of new hormone synthesis
   Antithyroid drugs of thionamide type (PTU, methimazole)
   Lithium carbonate (?)
Inhibition of hormone secretion
   Oral iodine: potassium iodide (SSKI), Lugol's solution, ipodate
   Lithium carbonate

Therapy to Avoid Decompensation of Normal Homeostatic Mechanisms
Treatment of hyperthermia
   Acetaminophen
   Cooling
Correction of dehydration and poor nutrition
   Fluids and electrolytes
   Glucose (calories)
   Vitamins
Supportive therapy
   Oxygen
   Vasopressors
   Treatment of congestive heart failure, if present (digoxin, diuretics)
   Corticosteroids

Therapy Directed against Thyroid Hormone Action in the Periphery
Inhibition of T_4-to-T_3 conversion
   Ipodate, iopanoate, amiodarone (?)
   Corticosteroids
   Propranolol
   PTU
β-Adrenergic blockade
   Propranolol
   Selective β_1-blocking agents
Removal of excess circulating hormone
   Plasmapheresis
   Dialysis
   Hemoperfusion adsorption (?)
   Cholestyramine (?)

Treatment Directed against a Precipitation or Coexistent Illness

* From Wartofsky, L. (1996). Management of thyroid crisis. In L. Braverman and R. Utiger (eds.) *Werner and Ingbar's the Thyroid: A Fundamental and Clinical Text* (7th ed.). Philadelphia: Lippincott-Raven.

B. Sodium iodide 1 gm stat and 1 gm daily for 14 days or SSKI 0.5 mL bid or sodium iodide 1 gm intravenously over 8 hours.

C. Propranolol 40–80 mg every 4–6 hours PO or 0.5–2 mg IV q4h.

D. Hydrocortisone 50 mg intravenously q6h and decreased as the clinical situation improves.

E. Avoid aspirin because it causes a rise in free T_4 levels.

F. Definitive treatment with radioactive iodine or surgery is delayed until the patient is euthyroid.

PATIENT EDUCATION

1. Educate patient on disease process and importance of taking medications as directed.

2. Instruct patients to immediately stop taking antithyroid medication if they develop fever or sore throat and to see their physician.

3. If patient is scheduled for surgery, provide preoperative teaching and explain expected postoperative course.

Review Questions

8.26 Hyperthyroidism results from which of the following?
  A. Elevated T_4 and/or elevated T_3
  B. Low T_4 and or low T_3
  C. Elevated TSH
  D. Low TSH

8.27 Mrs. Anderson is a 40-year-old woman who reports menstrual irregularities and believes she is experiencing an early menopause. She reports feeling fatigued and restless at times. Physical findings reveal a thin woman with fine hair, moist warm skin, and a goiter with a bruit present. Heart rate is 110; BP is 140/80 mm Hg. These findings are consistent with:
  A. Hypothyroidism
  B. Graves' disease
  C. Myxedema
  D. Thyroid cancer

8.28 The initial treatment of choice for symptoms of palpitations, tachycardia, and tremor seen in thyroid storm is:
  A. Ativan 0.5 mg PO bid
  B. Levothyroxine 50 μg/day
  C. Radioactive iodine
  D. Inderal (propanolol) 20 mg PO qid

8.29 Symptoms of agranulocytosis in patients taking PTU or methimazole include:
  A. Nausea and vomiting, diarrhea
  B. Abdominal discomfort, chest pain, palpitations
  C. Fever, chills, bleeding gums
  D. Tremor, palpitations, anxiety

8.30 Radioactive iodine (^{131}I) uptake and scan will show increase uptake in all but which of the following?
  A. Graves' disease
  B. Subacute thyroiditis
  C. Toxic nodular goiter
  D. Iodine-deficient state

Answers and Rationales

8.26 **A** Elevated T_4 and/or elevated T_3 results in hyperthyroidism.

8.27 **B** The findings are consistent with Graves' disease.

8.28 **D** Initial treatment of symptoms of palpitations, tachycardia, and tremor is Inderal 20 mg PO qid.

8.29 **C** Agranulocytosis is a serious side effect of the drugs PTU and methimazole. Symptoms include fever, chills, and bleeding gums.

8.30 **B** In subacute thyroiditis there will be a decreased uptake of radioactive iodine (^{131}I) on scan.

Hypothyroidism

DEFINITION

Primary hypothyroidism, a deficiency of thyroid hormone production and secretion, is invariably accompanied by increased thyrotropin (TSH) secretion. Much less often, decreased thyroidal stimulation by TSH, which is referred to as central or secondary hypothyroidism, causes deficiency of thyrotropin-releasing hormone. Hypothyroidism is the second most common endocrine disorder, following diabetes mellitus.

ETIOLOGY

1. Primary
   A. Accounts for 90% of cases.
   B. May result from diseases or treatments that destroy thyroid tissue or interfere with thyroid hormone biosynthesis (see Table 8–18).
   C. In areas where iodine intake is adequate, the most common causes are chronic autoimmune thyroiditis (Hashimoto's disease) and radiation-induced hypothyroidism. The latter may be caused either by radioactive iodine treatment of thyrotoxicosis or external radiation therapy directed to the neck in patients with lymphoma or head and neck cancer. Goiter caused by iodine deficiency is still a major health problem in many areas of the world; however, is no longer a problem in the United States. Iodine in salt, bread, and other foodstuffs is an effective prophylactic measure.
2. Central or secondary
   A. Can be the consequence of an anatomic or functional disorder of the pituitary gland, the hypothalamus, or both (see Table 8–19).
   B. Pituitary adenoma is the most frequent cause of central hypothyroidism, accounting for more than half the cases.

T A B L E 8–18.　**Causes of Hypothyroidism***

Primary Hypothyroidism
Destruction of thyroid tissue
　Chronic autoimmune thyroiditis: atrophic and goitrous forms
　Radiation: ^{131}I therapy for thyrotoxicosis, external radiotherapy to the neck for lymphoma or head and neck cancer
　Subtotal and total thyroidectomy
　Infiltrative diseases of the thyroid (amyloidosis, scleroderma)
　Defective thyroid hormone biosynthesis
　Iodine deficiency
　Drugs with antithyroid actions: lithium, iodine, iodine-containing drugs, and iodine-containing radiographic contrast agents

Central Hypothyroidism
　Pituitary disease
　Hypothalamic disease

Transient Hypothyroidism
　Silent thyroiditis†
　Subacute thyroiditis
　After withdrawal of thyroid hormone therapy in euthyroid patients

---

* From Braverman, L., & Utiger, R. (1996). Introduction to hypothyroidism. In L. Braverman & R. Utiger (eds.). *Werner and Ingbar's the Thyroid: A Fundamental and Clinical Text* (7th ed.). Philadelphia: Lippincott-Raven, p. 737, with permission.
† Including postpartum thyroiditis.

T A B L E 8–19.   Causes of Central Hypothyroidism*

Pituitary Disorders	Hypothalamic Disorders
Tumors	Tumors
Pituitary adenomas (functioning and nonfunctioning)	Suprasellar extension of pituitary adenomas
Craniopharyngiomas	Craniopharyngiomas
Meningiomas	Meningiomas
Dysgerminomas	Gliomas and other brain tumors
Metastatic tumors	Metastatic tumors
Ischemic necrosis	Traumas
Postpartum (Sheehan's syndrome)	Ischemic necrosis
Severe shock	Iatrogenic
Diabetes mellitus	Radiation therapy
Aneurysm of internal carotid artery	Surgery
Iatrogenic	Infections
Radiation therapy	Abscesses
Surgery	Tuberculosis
Infectious diseases	Syphilis
Abscesses	Toxoplasmosis
Tuberculosis	Sarcoidosis
Syphilis	Histiocytosis
Toxoplasmosis	Congenital malformations
Sarcoidosis	Basal encephalocele
Histiocytosis (Hand-Schüller-Christian)	Septo-optic dysplasia
Hemosiderosis	Idiopathic
Chronic lymphocytic hypophysitis	
Pituitary aplasia or hypoplasia	
Genetic abnormality in TSH synthesis	
Idiopathic	

* From Martino, E., et al. (1996). Central hypothyroidism. In L. Braverman & R. Utiger (eds.). *Werner and Ingbar's the Thyroid: A Fundamental and Clinical Text* (7th ed.). Philadelphia: Lippincott-Raven, p. 780, with permission.

3. Individuals who should be screened for hypothyroidism include those with a history of autoimmune disease or Graves' or Hashimoto's thyroiditis and a family history of thyroid disease. In addition, patients with the presence of a goiter or dementia, those taking medications known to affect thyroid function, or those with general disability and failure to thrive also mandate thyroid function screening. A relatively high yield may be expected from the screening of elderly with hypercholesterolemia, those with open-angle glaucoma, and women in general.

SIGNS AND SYMPTOMS (Table 8–20)

The clinical manifestations of hypothyroidism are influenced by the age of the patient, the presence of other disease, and the rate at which hypothyroidism develops. Older patients tend to have fewer symptoms and signs of hypothyroidism that tend to be less specific.
1. Physical findings
   A. Thin and brittle nails
   B. Coarse hair
   C. Delayed return phase of deep tendon reflexes
   D. Nonpitting peripheral edema and periorbital edema
   E. Bradycardia
   F. Adynamic ileus may be seen

TABLE **8–20.   Clinical Manifestations of Hypothyroidism***

Symptoms
Fatigue
Lethargy
Sleepiness
Mental impairment
Depression
Cold intolerance
Hoarseness
Dry skin
Decreased perspiration
Weight gain
Decreased appetite
Constipation
Menstrual disturbances
Arthralgia
Paresthesia

Signs
Slow movements
Slow speech
Hoarseness
Bradycardia
Dry skin
Nonpitting edema (myxedema)
Hyporeflexia
Delayed relaxation of reflexes

Symptoms and Signs Associated with Specific Causes of Hypothyroidism
Diffuse or nodular goiter
Symptoms and signs of pituitary or hypothalamic tumor
  Headache
  Visual impairment
  Deficiency or excess of pituitary hormones other than TSH

---

* From Braverman, L. & Utiger, R. (1996). Introduction to hypothyroidism. In L. Braverman & R. Utiger (eds.). *Werner and Ingbar's the Thyroid: A Fundamental and Clinical Text* (7th ed.). Philadelphia: Lippincott-Raven, p. 737, with permission.

G. Hypoventilation

H. Unexplained weight gain

2. Myxedema coma: Coma may rarely develop in patients with untreated or inadequately treated hypothyroidism. This entity is known as myxedema coma; however, this term in clinical practice is used more broadly and includes patients who, although not in coma yet, demonstrate a clear deterioration of their mental status, exhibiting lethargy, psychotic symptomatology, confusion, and disorientation. The majority of patients with myxedema coma are over 60 years of age. Myxedema coma is rare and has a high mortality rate.

A. Onset of coma is usually gradual.

B. Somnolence may be present.

C. Increasing fatiguability.

D. Use of narcotic or sedative drugs is a known precipitating factor.

E. Recent use of antipsychotic agents may precipitate coma.

F. Dilantin may precipitate coma.

G. Impending coma can present with seizures and, if inappropriately diagnosed, phenytoin may be used. Phenytoin leads to increased T_4 and T_3

catabolism, thus precipitating coma. Another agent associated with increased T_4 and T_3 catabolism is rifampin.

H. Other precipitating factors to be considered include infections such as pneumonia, urosepsis, and exposure to cold temperatures.

I. Hypoventilation, hypotension, and hypothermia are frequently encountered.

DIFFERENTIAL DIAGNOSIS

1. Hypothyroidism
   A. Nephrotic syndrome
   B. Depression and other psychiatric disorders, such as psychosis or structural CNS disease
   C. Menstrual disorders
   D. Amyloidosis
   E. Pernicious anemia
2. Myxedema coma: Euthyroid sick syndrome—encountered in elderly patients with severe infections and hypotension, and occasionally in patients with chronic illnesses.

DIAGNOSTIC TESTS/FINDINGS

1. Primary hypothyroidism
   A. TSH is the best initial diagnostic test. A normal value excludes primary hypothyroidism, and a markedly elevated value (>20 μU/mL) confirms the diagnosis. If plasma TSH is moderately elevated (<20 μU/mL), plasma T_4 index should be measured. A low T_4 index confirms clinical hypothyroidism, while a normal T_4 index with an elevated plasma TSH indicates subclinical hypothyroidism, which may account for symptoms such as fatigue and weight gain.
   B. Older patients may have hypercholesterolemia.
2. Central or secondary hypothyroidism
   A. Low TSH and T_4 levels
   B. Evaluate for other pituitary hormone deficits and for a mass lesion of the pituitary or hypothalamus
3. Myxedema coma
   A. Hyponatremia.
   B. Hypoglycemia.
   C. Elevated creatinine phosphokinase.
   D. QRS complex and/or T-wave abnormalities.
   E. Arterial blood gases usually show decreased P_{O_2} and increased P_{CO_2} indicative of respiratory failure.
   F. Chest x-ray may show the heart to be enlarged, which usually indicates pericardial effusion.
   G. Low T_4, free T_4, and FTI.
   H. High TSH.

MANAGEMENT/TREATMENT

1. Hypothyroidism: The treatment of hypothyroidism is with thyroid hormone replacement. Levothyroxine is the preferred agent because it is the predomi-

nant hormone secreted by the thyroid, and is converted to T_3 in the periphery by a regulated enzymatic mechanism.

A. Elderly patients with hypothyroidism may have underlying coronary heart disease; therefore, therapy should be started at a lower dose of 25 μg/day and gradually increased every 4–6 weeks, keeping TSH normal.

B. Younger patients may start with 50–100 μg/day with doses titrated based on TSH results.

C. Maintenance: Once the patient is feeling completely well, the dose is kept fairly constant. Frequent serum TSH levels are not necessary and may be obtained every 1–2 years on an outpatient basis.

2. Myxedema coma

A. Patients are managed by an endocrinologist and/or internist in the intensive care unit; however, the ACNP may be working collaboratively with the physician.

B. Infection is often present and must be treated.

C. Assisted mechanical ventilation may be necessary to correct hypercapnia.

D. Thyroxine (levothyroxine) replacement must be administered promptly.

E. Levothyroxine sodium 400 μg IV and repeated daily in a dose of 100 μg IV.

F. Hydrocortisone 100 mg as an initial bolus, followed by 25–50 mg 98 h, should be given if adrenal insufficiency is suspected.

G. Patients should be warmed by blanket, but not rapidly because of risk of cardiac arrhythmias.

PATIENT EDUCATION

1. Explain nature of disease to patients.
2. Instruct patients not to stop taking thyroid medication once symptoms improve and that it is a lifelong replacement.
3. Explain importance of follow-up appointment in clinic after discharge.

Review Questions

8.31 The most common cause of primary idiopathic hypothyroidism is:
   A. Graves' disease
   B. Hashimoto's disease
   C. Pheochromocytoma
   D. Diabetes

8.32 Physical findings commonly seen in hypothyroidism include:
   A. Coarse hair, thin brittle nails
   B. Malnourished appearance, alopecia
   C. Tachycardia, hyperreflexia
   D. Confusion, stupor

8.33 The most sensitive test to confirm a diagnosis of hypothyroidism is:
   A. RAIU
   B. T_4
   C. TSH
   D. T_3

8.34 On review of systems in a 60-year-old obese woman, she reports fatigue, cold intolerance, and dry skin. Thyroid function tests are as follows: TSH, 15 μU/mL T$_4$, 3 μg/dL; T$_3$, 90 ng/dL. Past medical history is positive for CAD. Based on the above data, your initial management would be to start:
   A. Levothyroxine 25 μg daily
   B. Levothyroxine 100 μg daily
   C. Hydrocortisone 100 mg
   D. Hydrocortisone 100 mg and levothyroxine 50 μg daily

8.35 Patient education for hypothyroidism would include instructing patients that:
   A. After 2 months they may discontinue their thyroid medication.
   B. Weekly blood tests will need to be done while on thyroid medication.
   C. Do not stop taking thyroid medication once symptoms improve; it is a lifelong replacement.
   D. They may adjust their thyroid medication according to their symptoms.

Answers and Rationales

8.31 **B** The most common cause of primary idopathic hypothyroidism is Hashimoto's disease.

8.32 **A** Physical findings commonly seen in hypothyroidism include coarse hair and thin, brittle nails.

8.33 **C** The most sensitive test to confirm a diagnosis of hypothyroidism is TSH.

8.34 **A** In elderly patients or those with heart disease, start with a lower dose of thyroid replacement—generally 0.025 μg.

8.35 **C** Instruct patients not to stop taking thyroid medication once symptoms improve and that it is a lifelong replacement.

References

Braverman, L., & Utiger, R. (1996). Introduction to hyperthyroidism. In L. Braverman & R. Utiger (eds.). *Werner and Ingbar's the Thyroid: A Fundamental and Clinical Text* (7th ed.). Philadelphia: Lippincott-Raven, p. 737.

Fitzgerald, P. (1997). Endocrinology. In L. Tierney, S. McPhee, & M. Papadakis (eds.). *Current Medical Diagnosis and Treatment* (36th ed.). Stamford, CT: Appleton & Lange, pp. 1007–1033.

Hershman, J. (1996). Thyroid dysfunction. In RC Bone (ed.). *Current Practice of Medicine* (Vol. 1). New York: Churchill Livingstone, section IV, pp. 3.1–3.7.

Mandel, S., Brent, G., & Larsen, P. (1993). Levothyroxine therapy in patients with thyroid disease. *Ann Intern Med 119*, 492–502.

Utiger, R. (1989). Hypothyroidism. In L. J. DeGroot et al. (eds.). *Endocrinology.* (Vol. 1, 2nd ed.). Philadelphia: W.B. Saunders Co., pp. 702–721.

CHAPTER 9

Hematologic and Oncologic Disorders

Mary Pat Lynch, RN, MSN, CRNP, AOCN

Breast Cancer

DEFINITION

Adenocarcinoma comprises the majority of primary breast cancers, located most commonly in the upper outer quadrant of the breast. Common types of breast tumors include infiltrating ductal carcinoma (most common) and invasive lobular carcinoma (5–10% of all breast cancers). Uncommon types include tubular, medullary, and mucinous adenocarcinomas.

ETIOLOGY/INCIDENCE

1. The most common form of cancer in women in the United States, occurs in approximately one in nine women.
2. The incidence increases with age: Over 70% of breast cancers occur in women over age 50.
3. Estimated new cases of breast cancer in U.S. women for 1997 is 180,200.
4. Also occurs rarely in men; estimated 1400 new cases in U.S. men in 1997.
5. Cause is unknown, but risk factors include:
   A. Family history (however, only 10% of breast cancer cases are familial)
   B. Age over 50
   C. Early menarche, late menopause
   D. Benign breast disease with atypical hyperplasia on breast biopsy
   E. First full-term pregnancy after age 30
   F. Alteration in *BRCA* 1 or *BRCA* 2 gene (responsible for 5–10% of familial breast cancers)

SIGNS AND SYMPTOMS

1. Lump or thickening in the breast: Usually hard, painless, may be fixed
2. Spontaneous, unilateral, persistent nipple discharge, especially bloody discharge
3. Change in skin texture (skin dimpling) or color in the breast
4. Axillary mass

5. Asymmetry of the breasts
6. Nipple retraction or inversion

PHYSICAL FINDINGS

1. Hard, painless mass in breast
2. Dimpling or thickening of the breast skin
3. Expression of bloody discharge from the nipple
4. Redness, ulceration, edema, or dilated veins in the breast (seen in inflammatory breast cancer)
5. Enlargement of lymph nodes in axilla or supraclavicular area

DIFFERENTIAL DIAGNOSIS

1. Benign breast disease: Eight of ten lumps biopsied are benign
2. Paget's disease
3. Primary lymphoma of the breast
4. Mastitis

DIAGNOSTIC TESTS/FINDINGS

1. Mammography detects a cancer 85% of the time.
2. Ultrasound is useful to distinguish between cyst and solid tumor.
3. Definitive diagnosis is made by histological examination of tissue.
   A. Needle aspiration biopsy: To determine if lump in question is a cyst.
   B. Stereotactic needle core biopsy: Immobilizes breast from fixed horizontal and vertical coordinates to calculate the exact position of the lesion.
   C. Needle localization under mammography for nonpalpable masses: Followed by excisional biopsy.
   D. Excisional biopsy: Removal of lump and small amount of surrounding tissue.
4. If the tumor is malignant, an axillary lymph node dissection should be done.
5. Tumor characteristics associated with high risk for recurrence and poor prognosis:
   A. Presence of axillary lymph node metastases: Found in 40–50% of patients.
   B. Hormone receptor status (estrogen and progesterone): Receptor-positive tumors have better prognosis.
   C. Tumor size >3 cm.
6. Staging studies, based on common sites of metastasis, may include:
   A. Chest x-ray
   B. Liver function tests (LFTs)
   C. Computed tomography (CT) scan of abdomen if LFTs are abnormal
   D. Bone scan
   E. Magnetic resonance imaging (MRI) of brain if symptomatic
   F. Additional studies based on symptoms and physical findings
   G. Tumor markers (e.g., carcinoembryonic antigen [CEA], CA 15-3)

MANAGEMENT/TREATMENT

Refer to oncologist for diagnostic work-up and treatment plan. The ACNP will work in close collaboration with the physician in managing the patient and may work more independently in symptom management.

1. Early-stage breast cancer
   A. Breast conservation surgery (lumpectomy) plus radiation therapy is as effective as modified radical mastectomy.
   B. Axillary node dissection is usually done at time of surgery.
2. Systemic treatment of breast cancer with hormonal therapy or chemotherapy is used to treat patients with:
   A. Axillary node involvement
   B. Poor-prognosis, node-negative disease
   C. Advanced local-regional disease
   D. Distant metastases
3. Adjuvant therapy is given to prevent or delay the development of metastatic disease: Given to patients with no demonstrable residual tumor after initial treatment with surgery or radiation.
   A. Hormone therapy with tamoxifen for 5 years for postmenopausal, hormone receptor–positive, node-positive patients.
   B. Chemotherapy is usually given to premenopausal, hormone receptor–negative, node-positive patients.
   C. Most commonly used chemotherapy agents include doxorubicin (Adriamycin), cyclophosphamide (Cytoxan), methotrexate, and 5-fluorouracil (5-FU), paclitaxel (Taxol), docetaxel (Taxotere) in various combinations: AC (Adriamycin, Cytoxan); CMF (Cytoxan, methotrexate, 5-FU); CAF (Cytoxan, Adriamycin, 5-FU).
   D. Doses are based on body surface area (weight and height) and calculated individually for each patient.
   E. IV antiemetics and IV hydration are given with emetogenic regimens.
   F. In myelosuppressive regimens, nadir occurs 7–10 days after chemotherapy when white blood cell count (WBC) reaches the lowest point, with highest risk for sepsis (see "Febrile Neutropenia").
4. Treatment of metastatic disease
   A. Incurable with either chemotherapy or hormone therapy.
   B. Treatment is palliative and to prolong survival.
   C. Patients with hormone receptor–positive disease and non-life-threatening metastatic disease are treated with hormone therapy initially: Tamoxifen 20 mg PO qd, megasterol acetate (Megace) 40 mg PO qid, or anastrozole (Arimidex) 1 mg PO qd.
   D. More aggressive disease is treated with chemotherapy.
   E. Common sites of metastases include bone, liver, lungs, brain, and skin.
   F. High-dose chemotherapy with bone marrow and peripheral blood stem cell rescues is being investigated as a treatment option for patients with high-risk, advanced disease.
   G. Bone and brain metastases may be treated with irradiation.

PATIENT EDUCATION

1. Provide information about diagnostic procedures and tests.
2. Maintain a positive and supportive environment for patient and family.
3. Provide information about disease process, postoperative care, rehabilitation issues, signs of recurrence.
4. Explain rationale for treatment, specific treatment regimen schedule, anticipated side effects.
5. Allow patient and family to verbalize fears and concerns.
6. Instruct chemotherapy patients to call with temperature greater than 101°F, because of risk of sepsis during neutropenia.

7. Inform patients of high probability of ovarian failure and early menopause in premenopausal women who are treated for breast cancer.

Review Questions

9.1 A patient is recovering from a lumpectomy with axillary node dissection for breast cancer. In discussing the need for future treatment, the ACNP explains that all of the following characteristics are associated with a high risk for recurrence EXCEPT:
A. Presence of axillary lymph node metastases
B. Estrogen receptor positivity
C. Tumor size >3 cm
D. Premenopausal status

9.2 The ACNP is ordering diagnostic studies in a woman with metastatic breast cancer whom the oncologist believes is relapsing 6 months after chemotherapy. The ACNP knows that the three most common sites of metastasis from breast cancer are:
A. Liver, bone, lungs
B. Adrenal glands, liver, bone
C. Brain, bone, diaphragm
D. Lungs, brain, bone marrow

9.3 All of the following are characteristic of malignant breast tumors EXCEPT:
A. Immobile
B. Painful
C. Irregular
D. Unilateral

9.4 The ACNP, in collaboration with the oncologist, sees a 42-year-old woman who is S/P lumpectomy with axillary node dissection. In discussing further treatment with the patient, they review the following information. The tumor was 2 cm, with one of ten axillary lymph nodes positive. The tumor was also estrogen receptor negative. The most appropriate treatment is:
A. Do nothing
B. High-dose chemotherapy with bone marrow transplant
C. Tamoxifen
D. Adjuvent chemotherapy

9.5 The single most important prognostic indicator of survival and recurrence of breast cancer is:
A. The woman's age at diagnosis
B. How quickly the treatment is initiated once diagnosis is made
C. The number of axillary nodes involved
D. How sensitive the tumor is to conventional chemotherapy

Answers and Rationales

9.1   **B** Estrogen receptor–negative tumors are associated with a higher risk for recurrence than estrogen receptor–positive tumors.

9.2   **A** These are the three most common sites. Other sites include the pleura, pituitary, adrenal and thyroid glands, kidneys, ovaries, and brain.

9.3   **B**   Benign breast tumors are often painful but malignant tumors are usually painless.

9.4   **D**   Because the patient had one positive lymph node, adjuvant treatment is indicated. Tamoxifen would not benefit an estrogen receptor–negative patient. She would probably benefit from chemotherapy. If her tumor is chemosensitive and she develops advanced disease, bone marrow transplant may be an option in the future.

9.5   **C**   The most important prognostic indicators for the woman with breast cancer are axillary node status, tumor size and the tumor's degree of invasiveness. The presence of cancer in any of the axillary lymph nodes reduces the overall survival rate, and the actual number of nodes involved is the single most important prognostic indicator of disease recurrence.

References

DeVita, V.T., Hellman, S., & Rosenberg, S.A. (1993). *Cancer: Principles and Practice of Oncology* (4th ed.). Philadelphia: J.B. Lippincott Co.

Fisher, D.S., Knobf, M.T., & Durivage, H.T. (1993). *Cancer Chemotherapy Handbook* (4th ed.). St. Louis: C.V. Mosby Co.

Gross, J., & Johnson, B.L. (1994). *Handbook of Oncology Nursing* (2nd ed.). St. Louis: C.V. Mosby Co.

Groenwald, S.L., Frogge, M.H., Goodman, M., et al. (1995). *Comprehensive Cancer Nursing Review* (2nd ed.). Boston: Jones and Bartlett Publishers.

McCorkle, R., Grant, M., Frank-Stromborg, M., et al. (1996). *Cancer Nursing: A Comprehensive Textbook* (2nd ed.). Philadelphia: W.B. Saunders Co.

Murphy, G.P., Lawrence, W., & Lenhard, R.E. (1995). *American Cancer Society Textbook of Clinical Oncology* (2nd ed.). Atlanta: American Cancer Society.

Varricchio, C. (1997). A Cancer Sourcebook for Nurses (7th ed.). Atlanta: American Cancer Society.

Gynecologic Malignancies

ENDOMETRIAL CANCER

DEFINITION

Endometrial or uterine cancer is the predominant cancer of the female genital tract, occurring primarily in postmenopausal women.

ETIOLOGY/INCIDENCE

1. Estimated 34,900 new cases in the United States in 1997.
2. Affects mostly postmenopausal women.
3. Risk factors include obesity, diabetes, hypertension, nulliparity, chronic anovulation, irregular menses, prolonged exogenous estrogen consumption, late menopause, pelvic irradiation, infertility, history of breast or ovarian cancer.

4. Approximately 80% are diagnosed with localized disease, leading to low mortality rates: Survival rates are 76% for stage I, 50% for stage II, 30% for stage III, and 9% for stage IV.

SIGNS AND SYMPTOMS

1. Postmenopausal or irregular vaginal bleeding is the hallmark sign.
2. Pelvic pain, lumbosacral or hypogastric pain in advanced disease.
3. Foul, purulent vaginal discharge.
4. In advanced cases, ascites, pelvic/abdominal mass, bowel symptoms.

PHYSICAL FINDINGS

1. Enlarged and softened uterus
2. Nodularity/induration of the adnexa and parametria
3. Possible tumor extension into the cervix, os, vagina
4. Rarely, supraclavicular/inguinal lymphadenopathy

DIFFERENTIAL DIAGNOSIS

1. Endometrial hyperplasia
2. Endometriosis
3. Uterine sarcoma
4. Gestational trophoblastic tumor
5. Uterine myoma
6. Uterine polyps

DIAGNOSTIC TESTS/FINDINGS

1. Thorough pelvic exam and pap smear
2. Endometrial biopsy, the most reliable diagnostic test
3. Dilatation and curettage if biopsy negative and symptoms persist
4. Complete blood count (CBC) and chemistries
5. Chest x-ray
6. Intravenous pyelography (IVP), cystoscopy, proctosigmoidoscopy to rule out local spread if bladder/rectal involvement suspected
7. Ultrasound, CT, MRI of pelvis
8. Serum CA 125: Elevated levels in 80% of patients with advanced disease

MANAGEMENT/TREATMENT

1. Refer to gynecologic oncologist for diagnostic work-up and treatment plan. The ACNP will work in close collaboration with the physician in managing the patient and may work more independently in symptom management.
2. Standard treatment is total abdominal hysterectomy and bilateral salpingo-oophorectomy (TAH-BSO) with selective pelvic and para-aortic lymphadenopathy, possible omentectomy, and resection of tumor implants: Surgery alone is sufficient for patients with little risk of recurrence.
3. Adjuvant radiation therapy is used for patients with risk factors, including:
   A. Cell types associated with poor outcome, including papillary serous, squamous undifferentiated, and clear cell
   B. Adnexal involvement

C. Abdominal spread

D. Pelvic and aortic node metastases

4. Advanced uterine cancer is treated with combination of surgery, radiation, chemotherapy, and progestin therapy.

A. One of the most difficult cancers to treat if metastasis or recurrence has occurred.

B. Synthetic progestational agents are most common systemic treatment for advanced disease.

C. Side effects include fluid retention, phlebitis, thrombosis.

D. Megasterol acetate (Megace) or IM medroxyprogesterone acetate are also used.

E. Chemotherapy has a limited role: few types have demonstrated activity greater than progestin therapy; drugs commonly used include doxorubicin (Adriamycin), cisplatin, cyclophosphamide (Cytoxan).

PATIENT EDUCATION

1. Explain the disease, treatment, and rationale and importance of follow-up.
2. Emotional support for patient and family.
3. Assessment and evaluation of sexual concerns, including fertility, childbearing, intimacy, body image.

OVARIAN CANCER

DEFINITION

Malignancy of the ovaries is the fifth leading cause of cancer death and the most common cause of death from gynecologic cancers in women in the United States.

ETIOLOGY/INCIDENCE

1. Estimated 26,800 new cases in the United States in 1997.
2. Risk factors include family or personal history of ovarian, breast, or colon cancer; nulliparity; first full-term pregnancy after age 35; early menarche; late menopause.
3. Seventy-five percent of patients have metastatic disease at presentation.

SIGNS AND SYMPTOMS

1. Often asymptomatic, typically no early manifestations
2. Abdominal pain
3. Abdominal swelling and fullness
4. Bloating/dyspepsia
5. Pelvic pressure
6. In advanced disease, anorexia, severe pain, weight loss, nausea/vomiting, symptoms of obstruction

PHYSICAL FINDINGS

1. Abdominal distention
2. Ascites

3. Enlargement of supraclavicular, inguinal, or axillary lymph nodes
4. Dilated cervix as a result of extrinsic compression

DIFFERENTIAL DIAGNOSIS

1. Ovarian cyst
2. Endometriosis
3. Cancer of the fallopian tube

DIAGNOSTIC TESTS/FINDINGS

1. Transvaginal ultrasound with color-flow Doppler
2. CT or MRI of the abdomen and pelvis
3. Laparoscopy
4. Serum CA 125: Elevated levels found in 80–85% of ovarian cancer patients
5. Chest x-ray
6. IVP to rule out urinary tract/ureteral obstruction
7. Barium enema, upper gastrointestinal (GI) series if patient has GI symptoms
8. Routine blood chemistries
9. Lactate dehydrogenase (LDH), β-human chorionic gonadotropin (HCG), α-fetoprotein (AFP) when germ cell tumors are suspected
10. CA 19-9 in combination with CA 125: Use remains controversial

MANAGEMENT/TREATMENT

1. Refer to gynecologic oncologist for diagnostic work-up and treatment plan. The ACNP will work in close collaboration with the physician in managing the patient and may work more independently in symptom management.
2. Stage I: Few diagnosed at this stage
   A. TAH-BSO, omentectomy, pelvic and para-aortic lymph node sampling
   B. Adjuvant radiation therapy
   C. Surgery alone offers 90% survival
3. Stage II: Locally advanced disease, few diagnosed at this stage, several options
   A. Surgical resection and cytoreduction
   B. Intraperitoneal ^{32}P radium implant
   C. Whole abdominal radiation
   D. Chemotherapy with single agents (cisplatin or carboplatin) or in combination (e.g., platinum-based drug with paclitaxel [Taxol])
4. Stage III, IV: Regional lymph node involvement, peritoneal metastases outside pelvis, distant metastases
   A. Cytoreductive surgery to reduce tumor burden and residual disease
   B. Chemotherapy with platinum-based drugs and Taxol
   C. Radiation therapy
   D. High-dose chemotherapy with bone marrow or peripheral blood stem cell rescue
5. Recurrent or persistent disease
   A. Second-look surgery
      1) Performed on patients with complete clinical response to initial therapy

2) Determines whether patient has a complete remission and therapy can be stopped
3) Assesses response, whether change in therapy is needed

B. Secondary cytoreductive surgery to attempt to prolong survival
C. Benefits of salvage chemotherapy are limited

PATIENT EDUCATION

1. Explain the disease, treatment, and rationale and importance of follow-up.
2. Stress importance of annual Pap smear and pelvic exam for screening.
3. Genetic counseling for hereditary cancers.
4. Emotional support for patient and family.
5. Assessment and evaluation of sexual concerns, including fertility, childbearing, intimacy, body image.

Review Questions

9.6 A 65-year-old Caucasian woman presents to the emergency room (ER) with heavy vaginal bleeding and passage of several large clots earlier in the day. The ACNP performs a physical exam, which reveals an enlarged, softened uterus and nodularity of the adnexa. The ACNP suspects:
   A. Endometrial cancer
   B. Ovarian cancer
   C. Cervical cancer
   D. Vaginal cancer

9.7 Which of the following women would be at highest risk for endometrial cancer?
   A. A woman with multiple sexual partners
   B. A woman who is infertile as a result of anovulation
   C. A woman on birth control pills for 20 years
   D. A woman who has had six children

9.8 A 32-year-old woman with ovarian cancer is admitted with abdominal distention, ascites, and shortness of breath. She had undergone a TAH-BSO 1 year ago for stage II disease, followed by radiation therapy. She now appears to have recurrent disease. The most appropriate first step for the ACNP is:
   A. Paracentesis
   B. Chest x-ray
   C. Refer to gynecologic oncologist for restaging and treatment options
   D. Consult surgery for secondary cytoreduction

9.9 When managing this patient in collaboration with the oncologist, the ACNP would order which of the following tumor markers as part of the restaging work-up?
   A. CA 125
   B. CEA
   C. CA 15-3
   D. AFP

Answers and Rationales

9.6   **A**   Postmenopausal bleeding and a softened, enlarged uterus are consistent with endometrial cancer.

9.7   **B**   Women who are nulliparous as a result of anovulation have an increased risk of endometrial cancer. Multiple sexual partners increases the risk of cervical cancer. Birth control pills have not been shown to increase the risk of endometrial cancer.

9.8   **C**   Management of this patient should be under the direction of a specialist in the field of gynecologic oncology. The ACNP may work collaboratively with the physician in developing a plan of treatment but should not work independently to do so. After referral, a paracentesis may be indicated for palliation, and a chest x-ray may be appropriate to evaluate for lung metastases. After restaging the patient, the gynecologic oncologist may consider cytoreductive surgery for this patient.

9.9   **A**   The CA 125 marker is elevated in 80–85% of ovarian cancer patients, making it a useful marker to evaluate regression and progression of disease. The CEA marker is elevated in a number of cancers, making it less specific. The CA 15-3 marker is commonly associated with breast cancer. AFP is associated with embryonal tumors.

References

DeVita, V.T., Hellman, S., & Rosenberg, S.A. (1993). *Cancer: Principles and Practice of Oncology* (4th ed.). Philadelphia: J.B. Lippincott Co.

Fisher, D.S., Knobf, M.T., & Durivage, H.T. (1993). *Cancer Chemotherapy Handbook* (4th ed.). St. Louis: C.V. Mosby Co.

Gross, J., & Johnson, B.L. (1994). *Handbook of Oncology Nursing* (2nd ed.). St. Louis: C.V. Mosby Co.

Groenwald, S.L., Frogge, M.H., Goodman, M., et al. (1995). *Comprehensive Cancer Nursing Review* (2nd ed.). Boston: Jones and Bartlett Publishers.

McCorkle, R., Grant, M., Frank-Stromborg, M., et al. (1996). *Cancer Nursing: A Comprehensive Textbook* (2nd ed.). Philadelphia: W.B. Saunders Co.

Murphy, G.P., Lawrence, W., & Lenhard, R.E. (1995). *American Cancer Society Textbook of Clinical Oncology* (2nd ed.). Atlanta: American Cancer Society.

Varricchio, C. (1997). *A Cancer Sourcebook for Nurses* (7th ed.). Atlanta: American Cancer Society.

Multiple Myeloma

DEFINITION

Multiple myeloma is the most common plasma cell disorder. These are a group of diseases characterized by the overproduction of immunoglobulins.

ETIOLOGY/INCIDENCE

1. Represents 1% of all hematologic malignancies.
2. Peak occurrence is between 50 and 70 years.

3. In the United States, more common in blacks than whites by 14:1.
4. Exact etiology is unknown; associated factors include:
   A. Frequent chromosomal abnormalities have been observed.
   B. Chronic low-level exposure to radiation has been associated with increased incidence.
   C. Chronic antigenic stimulation (e.g., recurrent infections and drug allergies) may be associated.
5. The lymphoid stem cell differentiates into either T lymphocytes or B lymphocytes.
   A. T lymphocytes regulate the immune response and participate in cell-mediated immunity.
   B. B lymphocytes are responsible for humoral immunity and mature into plasma cells that manufacture large numbers of immunoglobulins.
6. In multiple myeloma, there is overproduction of the M protein, one of the immunoglobulins.
7. The M protein, despite large quantities being produced, is unable to produce antibody necessary for maintaining humoral immunity.
8. Untreated, symptomatic patients have a median survival of 7 months; treatment extends survival to 2–3 years.

SIGNS AND SYMPTOMS

1. May have long asymptomatic period
2. Bone pain
3. Decreased mobility
4. Signs and symptoms of infections
5. Fatigue
6. Bleeding
7. Blurred vision (with hyperviscosity syndrome)
8. Irritability
9. Headache
10. Confusion

PHYSICAL FINDINGS

1. May have no abnormal findings in early stage
2. Fever
3. Fatigue
4. Weakness
5. Hypotension
6. Oliguria
7. Change in mental status

DIFFERENTIAL DIAGNOSIS

1. Bone metastases from solid tumor
2. Other myelodysplastic syndrome
3. Leukemia

DIAGNOSTIC TESTS/FINDINGS

1. Diagnosis confirmed by bone marrow biopsy: Increase in plasma cells (>10%).

2. Presence of M protein either in urine or serum.
3. Osteolytic lesions on bone survey.
4. Elevated serum B_2 microglobulin has prognostic value.
5. Anemia.
6. Thrombocytopenia.
7. Elevated blood urea nitrogen (BUN) and creatinine.
8. Hypercalcemia.
9. Positive Bence-Jones protein (light chain immunoglobulins) in urine.
10. Increased serum viscosity.

MANAGEMENT/TREATMENT

1. Refer to oncologist for diagnostic work-up and treatment plan. The ACNP will work in close collaboration with the oncologist and may work independently in symptom management.
2. Asymptomatic, indolent patients are followed without treatment.
3. When clinical symptoms arise, systemic chemotherapy is started: Melphalan and prednisone PO is first-line treatment, with a 30–60% response rate, median survival 24–36 months.
4. About 30–40% will not respond to first-line treatment; those who do will eventually relapse.
5. Second-line treatment is VAD chemotherapy (vincristine, doxorubicin [Adriamycin], dexamethasone IV).
   A. An 84% response rate, improved survival.
   B. Side effects include steroid toxicity, neurologic and hepatic toxicity.
6. Interferon for maintenance therapy for patients who have responded to two courses of induction: Side effects include anorexia, fatigue, hepatic toxicity, neurologic changes.
7. Radiation therapy for palliation of bone lesions, pain control: Myeloma is highly radioresponsive.
8. Hemibody radiation therapy for refractory myeloma palliation: Side effects include nausea, bone marrow suppression, pneumonitis.
9. Bone marrow transplant is under investigation as a treatment option.

PATIENT EDUCATION

1. Inform patient and family about the nature of the disease and treatment regimens.
2. Instruct patient and family in signs and symptoms of infection and when to call physician.
3. Review side effects and dosing schedules of chemotherapy regimens.
4. Consistently review pain control methods and evaluate effectiveness.
5. Educational materials are available from the National Cancer Institute, the American Cancer Society, and the Leukemia Foundation.

Review Questions

9.10 A 70-year-old African American man with indolent, previously untreated multiple myeloma is admitted with intractable pain of the legs and back.

The ACNP suspects destructive osteolytic lesions. The most appropriate diagnostic test would be:
A. Bone scan
B. Lumbar-sacral spine films
C. Bone survey
D. CT scan

9.11 The patient is found to have multiple discrete "punched out" lesions. The ACNP consults the oncologist for a treatment plan. The most appropriate first-line treatment would be:
A. Vincristine, doxorubicin, decadron IV chemotherapy
B. Melphalan and prednisone oral chemotherapy
C. Bone marrow transplant
D. Hemibody irradiation

9.12 Multiple myeloma is a hematologic malignancy characterized by:
A. An abnormal overproduction of plasma cells and M protein
B. Overproduction of lymphocytes and monocytes
C. Anemia unresponsive to transfusions
D. Malignant transformation of T lymphocytes

Answers and Rationales

9.10 **C** Lytic lesions will not appear on bone scan. Lumbar-sacral spine films might miss lesions in other areas of the body. A bone survey is more appropriate in order to find all lesions, including those that may be asymptomatic.

9.11 **B** In a previously untreated patient, the first-line and least toxic treatment would be melphalan and prednisone. VAD chemotherapy is usually given as a second line of treatment. Bone marrow transplant is still experimental in multiple myeloma, and a 70-year-old gentleman would not be eligible because of high toxicity levels. Hemibody irradiation is palliative for intractable pain.

9.12 **A** Multiple myeloma is characterized by abnormal overproduction of plasma cells and M protein.

References

DeVita, V.T., Hellman, S., & Rosenberg, S.A. (1993). *Cancer: Principles and Practice of Oncology* (4th ed.). Philadelphia: J.B. Lippincott Co.

Fisher, D.S., Knobf, M.T., & Durivage, H.T. (1993). *Cancer Chemotherapy Handbook* (4th ed.). St. Louis: C.V. Mosby Co.

Gross, J., & Johnson, B.L. (1994). *Handbook of Oncology Nursing* (2nd ed.). St. Louis: C.V. Mosby Co.

Groenwald, S.L., Frogge, M.H., Goodman, M., et al. (1995). *Comprehensive Cancer Nursing Review* (2nd ed.). Boston: Jones and Bartlett Publishers.

McCorkle, R., Grant, M., Frank-Stromborg, M., et al. (1996). *Cancer Nursing: A Comprehensive Textbook* (2nd ed.). Philadelphia: W.B. Saunders Co.

Murphy, G.P., Lawrence, W., & Lenhard, R.E. (1995). *American Cancer Society Textbook of Clinical Oncology* (2nd ed.). Atlanta: American Cancer Society.

Varricchio, C. (1997). *A Cancer Sourcebook for Nurses* (7th ed.). Atlanta: American Cancer Society.

Adult Leukemias

DEFINITION

Adult leukemias are hematologic malignancies that affect the bone marrow and lymph tissues.

ETIOLOGY/INCIDENCE

1. Estimated 28,300 new cases in the United States in 1997.
2. Symptoms are caused by excessive proliferation of leukocytes in blood-forming organs (bone marrow, spleen, lymph nodes) and crowding of the bone marrow, resulting in a decrease in the number of normal leukocytes, erythrocytes, and thrombocytes.
3. Acute leukemias are characterized by a block in differentiation, resulting in a massive accumulation of immature cells or blasts.
4. Chronic leukemias have unregulated proliferation and overexpansion of mature cells.

ACUTE MYELOGENOUS LEUKEMIA

DEFINITION

Acute myelogenous leukemia (AML), also known as acute nonlymphoblastic leukemia (ANLL), is the result of an abnormality in the pluripotent myeloid stem cell. The rapid accumulation of leukemic cells in the marrow causes crowding that both inhibits the growth of normal blood cells and forces immature blood cells into the peripheral circulation.

ETIOLOGY/INCIDENCE

1. Incidence increases with age.
2. Classified into seven groups (M1–M7) based on morphologic, histochemical, and immunologic findings.
3. Etiology is unknown; linked to radiation and toxin exposure.
4. Fatal in months if untreated.
5. About 70–80% remission with aggressive therapy.
6. About 25–30% long-term survival.

SIGNS AND SYMPTOMS

1. Fatigue
2. Shortness of breath
3. Bleeding and easy bruising
4. Oropharyngeal complaints
5. Rarely, headache, nausea/vomiting

PHYSICAL FINDINGS

1. Infiltration of skin, gingiva, other soft tissue
2. Petechiae
3. Cranial neuropathy
4. Change in mental status

DIFFERENTIAL DIAGNOSIS

1. Infection
2. Myelodysplastic syndrome
3. Primary thrombocytosis
4. Polycythemia vera
5. Lymphoma
6. Leukemoid reaction

DIAGNOSTIC TESTS/FINDINGS

1. Leukocytosis with circulating blasts on peripheral smear
2. Anemia
3. Thrombocytopenia
4. Neutropenia
5. Hyperuricemia (because of rapid turnover of cells)
6. Elevated LDH level
7. Positive disseminated intravascular coagulation (DIC) profile

MANAGEMENT/TREATMENT

1. Refer to oncologist for diagnostic work-up and treatment plan. The ACNP will work in close collaboration with the physician in managing the patient and may work more independently in symptom management.
2. Therapy is aimed at eradication of leukemic clone and re-establishment of normal hematopoiesis: Complete remission (CR) is defined as restoration of normal peripheral counts and <5% blasts in the bone marrow.
3. Induction chemotherapy (cytosine arabinoside [Ara C] for 7 days and an anthracycline such as daunorubicin, doxorubicin, or mitoxantrone for 3 days).
   A. Therapy assessed with bone marrow biopsy and aspirate on day 14.
   B. Induction treatment repeated if there are residual leukemic cells in marrow.
   C. About 20–30% are cured with chemotherapy alone.
4. Postremission therapy is given to prevent recurrence; can include:
   A. Consolidation: Very high doses of same drugs used in induction.
      1) Toxic side effects are substantial, including extended myelosuppression, cerebellar dysfunction, hepatic dysfunction.
      2) Two or more courses given.
   B. Intensification: Uses different drugs than those used in induction.
   C. Maintenance: Uses lower doses of same or other drugs at monthly intervals for prolonged time (not currently recommended for AML).
5. Allogeneic bone marrow transplant in first remission gives 60% long-term survival.
6. Oral differentiating agents (*trans*-retinoic acid) look promising.

7. Cranial irradiation and intrathecal chemotherapy for leukemic meningitis.
8. Altered mental status, dyspnea, retinal hemorrhage, priapism resulting from leukostasis are emergent situations treated by cranial irradiation, hydroxyurea, and/or leukopheresis.
9. Tumor lysis syndrome treated with vigorous hydration and allopurinol (see "Oncologic emergencies").

PATIENT EDUCATION

1. Teach patient and family about the nature of the disease, treatment course, and side effects of treatment.
2. Maintain supportive environment for patient and family.
3. Instruct patient and family about signs and symptoms of infection, bleeding, when to contact health care provider.
4. Identify past and present coping strategies, patient and family perceptions of the illness.
5. Teaching for bone marrow transplant if indicated.
6. Educational materials can be obtained from the Leukemia Society, American Cancer Society, National Cancer Institute.

ACUTE LYMPHOCYTIC LEUKEMIA

DEFINITION

Acute lymphocytic leukemia (ALL) is a malignant disease of the lymphoid progenitor cells. Although the defect does not involve the myeloid cell lines, the secondary effect of the high leukemic cell burden on the bone marrow interferes with normal hematopoietic activity.

ETIOLOGY/INCIDENCE

1. Uncommon in adults; accounts for 80% of childhood leukemias.
2. About 60–80% remission rates with aggressive therapy.
3. Forty percent long-term survival.
4. Etiology is unknown; increased risk with radiation exposure, Down's syndrome, ataxia telangiectasia, Fanconi's anemia.
5. Classified into three groups (L1, L2, L3).

SIGNS AND SYMPTOMS

1. Abrupt onset of malaise
2. Bony pain
3. Fatigue
4. Bruising
5. Rarely, headache

PHYSICAL FINDINGS

1. Petechiae
2. Ecchymosis
3. Cranial nerve palsies (imply central nervous system [CNS] involvement)

4. Hepatosplenomegaly
5. Lymphadenopathy
6. Mediastinal mass
7. Bulky abdominal lymphadenopathy

DIFFERENTIAL DIAGNOSIS

1. Infection
2. Myelodysplastic syndrome
3. Primary thrombocytosis
4. Polycythemia vera
5. Lymphoma
6. Leukemoid reaction

DIAGNOSTIC TESTS/FINDINGS

1. Neutropenia with circulating lymphoblasts
2. Anemia
3. Thrombocytopenia
4. Elevated uric acid and LDH
5. Tumor lysis syndrome and DIC are rare

MANAGEMENT/TREATMENT

1. Refer to oncologist for diagnostic work-up and treatment plan. The ACNP
   will work in close collaboration with the physician in managing the patient
   and may work more independently in symptom management.
2. Treatment divided into three phases: induction, CNS prophylaxis, and postremission treatment.
   A. Induction in adults usually consists of vincristine, prednisone, and L-
      asparaginase, plus an anthracycline (daunorubicin, doxorubicin, or mi-
      toxantrone).
   B. CR is achieved in 70–75%.
   C. Treatment initiated in hospital; once in remission, can be treated as
      outpatient.
3. Meningeal leukemia occurs in 50% of ALL patients who do not receive CNS
   prophylaxis.
   A. Signs and symptoms include headache, blurred vision, nausea and vom-
      iting, cranial nerve palsies.
   B. CNS prophylaxis involving cranial radiation therapy and intrathecal
      methotrexate should start within a few weeks of the start of treatment.
   C. Side effects of treatment include somnolence, chemical meningitis, para-
      paresis, leukoencephalopathy.
4. Postremission therapy.
   A. Maintenance treatment uses same drugs as induction with or without
      the addition of methotrexate ± 6-mercaptopurine.
   B. With prolonged maintenance therapy (2–3 years), cure rates of 40% have
      been reported.
   C. Without maintenance therapy, relapse occurs in 2–3 months.
   D. If relapse occurs after completion of maintenance therapy, second remis-
      sion can be achieved in up to 50% with high-dose chemotherapy: Idaru-
      bicin and high-dose cytosine arabinoside have induced second remission
      in 65% of patients.

    E. Patients with unfavorable prognosis should be referred for bone marrow transplant.

    F. Allogeneic bone marrow transplant in first remission remains controversial.

PATIENT EDUCATION

1. Teach patient and family about the nature of the disease, treatment course, and side effects of treatment.
2. Maintain supportive environment for patient and family.
3. Instruct patient and family about signs and symptoms of infection, bleeding, when to contact health care provider.
4. Identify past and present coping strategies, patient and family perceptions of the illness.
5. Teaching for bone marrow transplant if indicated.
6. Educational materials can be obtained from the Leukemia Society, American Cancer Society, National Cancer Institute.

CHRONIC MYELOGENOUS LEUKEMIA

DEFINITION

Chronic myelogenous leukemia (CML) is a disorder of the myeloid stem cell. It is characterized by an increased production of granulocytes and marked splenomegaly. It is also known as chronic granulocytic leukemia (CGL).

ETIOLOGY/INCIDENCE

1. Incidence increases with age; males have a rate 1.7 times as high as females.
2. Exposure to radiation promotes evolution of CML.
3. Philadelphia chromosome is diagnostic marker found in 90% of cases.
4. Three clinical periods (with median survivals):
   A. Stable or chronic phase (3–4 years)
   B. Accelerated phase (6–24 months)
   C. Blast crisis (8–16 weeks)

SIGNS AND SYMPTOMS

1. Fatigue
2. Fever
3. Malaise
4. Decreased exercise tolerance
5. Weight loss
6. Night sweats
7. Early satiety
8. Left upper quadrant fullness or pain

PHYSICAL FINDINGS

1. Fever
2. Splenomegaly

3. Chloroma (isolated foci of tumor cells, in any soft tissue)
4. Hepatomegaly

DIFFERENTIAL DIAGNOSIS

1. Infection
2. Myelodysplastic syndrome
3. Primary thrombocytosis
4. Polycythemia vera
5. Lymphoma
6. Leukemoid reaction

DIAGNOSTIC TESTS/FINDINGS

1. Leukocytosis with eosinophils, hypogranulated basophils, large platelets.
2. Moderate anemia and thrombocytopenia.
3. Increased number of blasts and basophils in peripheral blood suggest progression.
4. Elevated uric acid and LDH.
5. Pseudohyperkalemia.
6. Low leukocyte alkaline phosphatase in stable-phase CML.

MANAGEMENT/TREATMENT

1. Refer to oncologist for diagnostic work-up and treatment plan. The ACNP will work in close collaboration with the physician in managing the patient and may work more independently in symptom management.
2. Treatment in chronic phase is palliative, with oral chemotherapy agents (hydroxyurea, busulfan) and α-interferon.
3. Blast crisis: Re-establishment of chronic phase is unlikely; aggressive chemotherapy generally ineffective; life expectancy less than 1 year.
   A. Blast crisis is treated like AML, with cytosine arabinoside and an anthracycline.
   B. If lymphoblastic transformation has occurred, vincristine and predisone are added.
4. Allogeneic bone marrow transplant offers only potential cure when performed in the chronic phase.
   A. About 50–60% long-term survival but 20% mortality in first 100 days after transplant.
   B. Not all patients are eligible.

PATIENT EDUCATION

1. Teach patient and family about the nature of the disease, treatment course, and side effects of treatment.
2. Maintain supportive environment for patient and family.
3. Instruct patient and family about signs and symptoms of infection, bleeding, when to contact health care provider.
4. Identify past and present coping strategies, patient and family perceptions of the illness.
5. Teaching for bone marrow transplant if indicated.

6. Educational materials can be obtained from the Leukemia Society, American Cancer Society, National Cancer Institute.

CHRONIC LYMPHOCYTIC LEUKEMIA

DEFINITION

Chronic lymphocytic leukemia (CLL) is a disorder affecting the lymphoid cell line, characterized by an accumulation of normal but functionally ineffective lymphocytes. As the disease progresses, the lymphocytes accumulate in the marrow, spleen, liver, and lymph nodes.

ETIOLOGY/INCIDENCE

1. Most common form of adult leukemia.
2. Ninety percent of cases affect persons over age 50.
3. Twice as common in males as in females.
4. Etiology remains unknown; only leukemia not associated with radiation or toxin exposure.
5. Classified as stage 0 to stage IV based on physical findings and laboratory abnormalities.
6. Prognosis is determined by clinical stage; varies from 1 to over 10 years.

SIGNS AND SYMPTOMS

1. Asymptomatic, with incidental finding of lymphocytosis
2. Fatigue
3. Shortness of breath
4. Night sweats
5. Bleeding
6. Malaise
7. Anorexia
8. Early satiety
9. Abdominal discomfort

PHYSICAL FINDINGS

1. Lymphadenopathy (mobile, discrete, nontender)
2. Splenomegaly
3. Hepatomegaly

DIFFERENTIAL DIAGNOSIS

1. Infection
2. Myelodysplastic syndrome
3. Primary thrombocytosis
4. Polycythemia vera
5. Lymphoma
6. Leukemoid reaction

DIAGNOSTIC TESTS/FINDINGS

1. Lymphocytosis with small, mature-appearing lymphocytes
2. "Smudge cells" on smear
3. Positive CD5 (aberrant expression of a normal T-cell antigen)
4. Anemia
5. Thrombocytopenia
6. Hypogammaglobulinemia in approximately 50% on serum protein electrophoresis
7. Elevated uric acid, LDH

MANAGEMENT/TREATMENT

1. Refer to oncologist for diagnostic work-up and treatment plan. The ACNP will work in close collaboration with the physician in managing the patient and may work more independently in symptom management.
2. Early stage (lymphocytosis only): Observation.
3. Symptomatic patients: Chemotherapy with oral alkylating agents (chlorambucil or cyclophosphamide) or fludarabine, cladribine.
4. Radiation therapy to sites of bulky, painful disease.
5. Splenectomy in selective patients to decrease pain, thrombocytopenia.
6. Allogeneic bone marrow transplant under investigation.
7. Gamma globulin replacement to decrease number of bacterial infections.
8. Corticosteroids to control leukocytosis and cytopenias mediated by the immune system.
9. Treatment of advanced CLL with anemia and thrombocytopenia involves combination chemotherapy with cyclophosphamide, vincristine, doxorubicin, and prednisone (CHOP).

PATIENT EDUCATION

1. Teach patient and family about the nature of the disease, treatment course, and side effects of treatment.
2. Maintain supportive environment for patient and family.
3. Instruct patient and family about signs and symptoms of infection, bleeding, when to contact health care provider.
4. Identify past and present coping strategies, patient and family perceptions of the illness.
5. Teaching for bone marrow transplant if indicated.
6. Educational materials can be obtained from the Leukemia Society, American Cancer Society, National Cancer Institute.

Review Questions

9.13 The ACNP examines a 32-year-old man who presents to the ER with a 1-month history of fatigue, fever, and night sweats and a 10-lb weight loss. Physical exam is significant for splenomegaly. Laboratory data reveal leukocytosis, normal hemoglobin and platelets, and elevated LDH and uric acid. The ACNP suspects leukemia. The most likely diagnosis is:
   A. AML
   B. CML

C. ALL

D. CLL

9.14 The presence of the Philadelphia chromosome is indicative of which type of leukemia?

A. AML

B. CML

C. ALL

D. CLL

9.15 The ACNP is examining a patient with chronic myelogenous leukemia who presented to the ER with left upper quadrant pain. The patient also reports early satiety and vague abdominal fullness. She is currently being treated with hydroxyurea. These symptoms are most likely to be related to:

A. Drug toxicity

B. Bowel obstruction

C. Splenomegaly

D. Hypercalcemia

9.16 The most appropriate next step that the ACNP should take is:

A. Consult surgery for splenectomy

B. Refer to oncologist for diagnostic work-up and treatment plan

C. Order an obstruction series

D. Discuss further chemotherapy options

9.17 What differentiates an acute leukemia from a chronic leukemia?

A. Number of white blood cells

B. Frequency of infections

C. Degree of differentiation of white blood cells

D. Lymphadenopathy

Answers and Rationales

9.13 **B** CML has a higher incidence in males and usually has a normal hemoglobin and platelet count, unlike AML and ALL. CML occurs in a younger population, unlike CLL.

9.14 **B** Philadelphia chromosome is indicative of CML.

9.15 **C** Splenomegaly is a classic sign of CML, and is characterized by fullness and pain in the upper quadrant as well as early satiety as the enlarged spleen compresses the stomach.

9.16 **B** The most appropriate action for the ACNP to take is to refer the leukemic patient to a specialist for appropriate diagnostic work-up and treatment plan.

9.17 **C** The white blood cells in acute leukemia are primarily immature cells, whereas those in chronic leukemia tend to be more mature or differentiated cells. Patients with both types of leukemia are likely to have lymphadenopathy and are at risk of infections.

References

DeVita, V.T., Hellman, S., & Rosenberg, S.A. (1993). *Cancer: Principles and Practice of Oncology* (4th ed.). Philadelphia: J.B. Lippincott Co.

Fisher, D.S., Knobf, M.T., & Durivage, H.T. (1993). *Cancer Chemotherapy Handbook* (4th ed.). St. Louis: C.V. Mosby Co.

Gross, J., & Johnson, B.L. (1994). *Handbook of Oncology Nursing* (2nd ed.). St. Louis: C.V. Mosby Co.

Groenwald, S.L., Frogge, M.H., Goodman, M., et al. (1995). *Comprehensive Cancer Nursing Review* (2nd ed.). Boston: Jones and Bartlett Publishers.

McCorkle, R., Grant, M., Frank-Stromborg, M., et al. (1996). *Cancer Nursing: A Comprehensive Textbook* (2nd ed.). Philadelphia: W.B. Saunders Co.

Murphy, G.P., Lawrence, W., & Lenhard, R.E. (1995). *American Cancer Society Textbook of Clinical Oncology* (2nd ed.). Atlanta: American Cancer Society.

Varricchio, C. (1997). *A Cancer Sourcebook for Nurses* (7th ed.). Atlanta: American Cancer Society.

Lymphomas

DEFINITION

Lymphomas are malignancies involving the cells of the lymphatic system, also termed lymphoproliferative disorders. They are divided into Hodgkin's disease (HD), which is curable, and the non-Hodgkin's lymphomas (NHL), which constitute a very large, heterogeneous group of tumors that vary in responsiveness and curability. The distinctions between HD and NHL are important because their clinical courses, prognoses, and treatment modalities are substantially different.

HODGKIN'S DISEASE

DEFINITION

Neoplasm that arises from the uncontrolled proliferation of the cellular components of the lymphoreticular system.

ETIOLOGY/INCIDENCE

1. Estimated 7500 new cases in the United States in 1997.
2. Accounts for approximately 14% of all malignant lymphomas.
3. Incidence rates rise sharply after age 10, peak in late 20s, then decline until age 45. After age 45, incidence steadily rises with age.
4. Epstein-Barr virus has been suggested as a possible etiologic agent.
5. Usually spreads contiguously from one lymph node region to another.
6. Four major histologic classifications:
   A. Lymphocyte predominant (5–10%)
   B. Nodular sclerosis (30–60%)
   C. Mixed cellularity (20–40%)
   D. Lymphocyte depleted (<5%)

SIGNS AND SYMPTOMS

1. "B" symptoms—fever, malaise, night sweats, weight loss, pruritis: Occur in about 40% of patients.
2. Cough

3. Dyspnea
4. Dysphagia
5. Left upper quadrant pain
6. Jaundice
7. Genitourinary dysfunction

PHYSICAL FINDINGS

1. Lymphadenopathy: Usually supradiaphragmatic, frequently in cervical area; firm, rubbery, freely moveable
2. Wheezing
3. Superior vena cava syndrome (see "Oncologic Emergencies"): Facial, trunk, upper extremity edema; neck and chest vein distention
4. Hepatosplenomegaly
5. Jaundice
6. Ascites

DIFFERENTIAL DIAGNOSIS

1. Acquired immunodeficiency syndrome (AIDS)
2. Infection (acute or chronic)
3. Systemic lupus erythematosus
4. Serum sickness
5. Leukemia
6. Rheumatoid arthritis
7. Hyperthyroidism
8. Hypoadrenocorticism
9. Hypopituitarism
10. Metastatic cancer

DIAGNOSTIC TESTS/FINDINGS

1. Lymph node biopsy: Removed with capsule intact
   A. Presence of Reed-Sternberg cell on biopsy
   B. Needle biopsies yield limited tissue, not helpful
2. CT scans of chest, abdomen, pelvis to evaluate lymph nodes and liver
3. Staging laparotomy with splenectomy, removal of suspicious nodes, liver and bone marrow biopsies: Usually done if CT scans are negative
4. Gallium scan
5. Bipedal lymphangiogram: No longer commonly used
6. CBC: Leukocytosis with lymphocytopenia, eosinophilia
7. Elevated erythrocyte sedimentation rate (ESR)
8. Elevated serum alkaline phosphatase levels: Suggests liver or bone involvement
9. Hypergammaglobulinemia in early disease: Immunoglobulin levels may decrease in advanced disease

MANAGEMENT/TREATMENT

1. Refer to oncologist for diagnostic work-up and treatment plan. The ACNP will work in close collaboration with the physician in managing the patient and may work more independently in symptom management.

2. More than 75% are curable.
3. Treat regions of known disease and the presumed next site of involvement.
4. Early stages are treated with limited radiation therapy: Complications of radiation therapy include hypothyroidism, pericarditis, pneumonitis, sterility, myelosuppression.
5. Advanced stages are treated with aggressive chemotherapy ± radiation therapy.
    A. Common chemotherapy regimens include alternating MOPP (nitrogen mustard, vincristine, procarbazine, and prednisone) with ABVD (doxorubicin, bleomycin, vinblastine, and dacarbazine) in three alternating cycles of each.
    B. Complications of chemotherapy include myelosuppression, nausea and vomiting, alopecia, paresthesias, pulmonary fibrosis, and rarely cardiomyopathy and sterility.
6. Surgery to remove large nodes is not indicated.

PATIENT EDUCATION

1. Provide support by educating the patient about potential physical and psychological side effects of the treatment.
2. Acknowledge fear and provide supportive environment.
3. Teach patient about signs and symptoms of infection.
4. Teach patient good oral hygiene to prevent mucositis.
5. Evaluate patient for alterations in body image with decreased libido, sterility.
6. Long-term survivorship may be complicated by fatigue, depression, infertility, and anxiety.
7. Patient education materials are available from the National Cancer Institute and the American Cancer Society.

NON-HODGKIN'S LYMPHOMA

DEFINITION

The non-Hodgkin's lymphomas are a diverse group of malignancies derived from different developmental and functional subdivisions of the lymphoreticular system. They exhibit a wide range of immunologic and biologic characteristics.

ETIOLOGY/INCIDENCE

1. Estimated 53,600 new cases in the United States in 1997.
2. The incidence of NHL is escalating in the United States because of the increasing numbers of AIDS patients who have developed NHL. It is the fifth most common cancer in the United States.
3. Multicentric in origin with tendency to spread widely.
4. Progressive increase in incidence with age.
5. Etiology of most types unknown; possible causal relationships have been suggested with immunosuppression, viruses, cytogenetic abnormalities.
6. Pattern of dissemination less orderly than in HD.

7. Working histologic classification divided into three groups with subgroups:
   A. Low grade
      1) Small lymphocytic
      2) Follicular small cleaved lymphocytic
      3) Mixed follicular small cleaved cell and large cell
   B. Intermediate grade
      1) Follicular, predominantly large cell
      2) Diffuse cleaved small cell
      3) Diffuse large cell
   C. High grade
      1) Diffuse large cell immunoblast
      2) Lymphoblastic
      3) Small noncleaved (Burkitt's/non-Burkitt's)

SIGNS AND SYMPTOMS

1. Asymptomatic
2. Painless swelling of lymph nodes
3. "B" symptoms: Initial complaint in 20%
   A. Night sweats
   B. Fever
   C. Weight loss
4. Cough
5. Dyspnea
6. Chest pain
7. Abdominal pain

PHYSICAL FINDINGS

1. No physical findings
2. Painless lymphadenopathy
3. Abdominal mass
4. Hepatomegaly

DIFFERENTIAL DIAGNOSIS

1. AIDS
2. Infection (acute or chronic)
3. Systemic lupus erythematosus
4. Serum sickness
5. Leukemia
6. Rheumatoid arthritis
7. Hyperthyroidism
8. Hypoadrenocorticism
9. Hypopituitarism
10. Metastatic cancer

DIAGNOSTIC TESTS/FINDINGS

1. Lymph node biopsy
2. Bone marrow biopsy
3. CT scans of chest, abdomen, and pelvis to evaluate for lymphadenopathy

4. Gallium scan
5. No benefit from staging laparotomy; most patients have advanced disease at presentation
6. Coomb's-positive autoimmune hemolytic anemia: More common in NHL than HD
7. Elevated ESR
8. Elevated liver function tests
9. Serum protein electrophoresis and serum immunoelectrophoresis: Detection of paraprotein

MANAGEMENT/TREATMENT

1. Refer to oncologist for diagnostic work-up and treatment plan. The ACNP will work in close collaboration with the physician in managing the patient and may work more independently in symptom management.
2. Chemotherapy is the primary treatment modality because NHL disseminates early and widely by hematogenous routes rather than, by orderly, continuous node extension: Treatment is based on cell type.
3. Radiation therapy is used for localized disease and as adjunct to chemotherapy.
4. Primary role of surgery is to establish the diagnosis.
5. Low-grade NHL
   A. Ninety percent of patients have stage III or IV disease.
   B. Indolent but progressive; not curable.
   C. Median survival is 7.5–9 years with minimal therapy.
   D. Combination chemotherapy regimens are used when patient is symptomatic: CHOP.
   E. Generally highly responsive to radiation therapy, used to control disease.
   F. Autologous bone marrow transplant is being investigated.
6. Intermediate- and high-grade NHL
   A. More aggressive disease, rapid course.
   B. Median survival is 1–2 years with minimal treatment.
   C. Aggressive combination chemotherapy results in high percentage of long-term survival with some cures: Common regimens include CHOP, MACOP-B (methotrexate with leukovorin rescue, doxorubicin, cyclophosphamide, vincristine, prednisone, bleomycin).
   D. Bone marrow transplant is most effective salvage treatment for relapsing patients who achieved remission with initial treatment.
   E. Factors associated with poor prognosis include:
      1) B symptoms (fever, weight loss, night sweats)
      2) More than 2 extranodal sites
      3) Spleen involvement
      4) Elevated LDH
      5) Stage III or IV

PATIENT EDUCATION

1. Provide support by educating the patient about potential physical and psychological side effects of the treatment.
2. Acknowledge fear and provide supportive environment.
3. Teach patient about signs and symptoms of infection.
4. Teach patient good oral hygiene to prevent mucositis.

5. Evaluate patient for alterations in body image with decreased libido, sterility.
6. Long-term survivorship may be complicated by fatigue, depression, infertility, and anxiety.
7. Patient education materials are available from the American Cancer Society and the National Cancer Institute.

Review Questions

9.18 All of the following statements are TRUE in reference to Hodgkin's disease EXCEPT:
   A. Incidence peaks in the late 20s
   B. Confirmed by the presence of Reed-Sternberg cells
   C. Highly curable
   D. Multicentric in origin with tendency to spread widely

9.19 Chemotherapy-induced granulocytopenia usually reaches its nadir:
   A. 3–5 days after chemotherapy
   B. 5–6 days after chemotherapy
   C. 7–10 days after chemotherapy
   D. 14–21 days after chemotherapy

9.20 Which of the following is true about low-grade non-Hodgkin's lymphoma?
   A. Is likely to be a localized disease at diagnosis
   B. The recommended treatment may be to do nothing
   C. Should be treated aggressively to achieve a cure
   D. Is usually treated with high-dose chemotherapy

9.21 The ACNP is reviewing the staging of a newly diagnosed patient with high-grade non-Hodgkin's lymphoma in collaboration with the oncologist. In order to determine if the patient has "B" symptoms, the review of systems should include questions about:
   A. Fevers, enlarged lymph nodes, weight loss
   B. Night sweats, enlarged lymph nodes, weight loss
   C. Fevers, night sweats, weight loss
   D. Fever, weight loss, itching

9.22 Which of the following cancers has shown a significant increase in association with the increase in AIDS cases in the United States?
   A. Hodgkin's disease
   B. Non-Hodgkin's lymphoma
   C. Breast cancer
   D. Acute lymphocytic leukemia

Answers and Rationales

9.18   **D** Hodgkin's disease usually spreads contiguously from one lymph node group to another. Non-Hodgkin's lymphomas are multicentric and spread widely.

9.19   **C** Chemotherapy-induced granulocytopenia reaches its nadir about 7–10 days after chemotherapy.

9.20 **B** Patients with low-grade lymphomas usually have widespread disease at diagnosis that is considered incurable. The initial treatment may be to do nothing if the patient is asymptomatic and has indolent disease. Aggressive, high-dose chemotherapy is used for intermediate- to high-grade lymphomas because they are fast-growing tumors that are more likely to respond to chemotherapy.

9.21 **C** "B" symptoms consist of fever, night sweats, and weight loss. Lymphoma patients are likely to have lymphadenopathy; however, it is not a "B" symptom. Pruritis is a common symptom with Hodgkin's disease.

9.22 **B** Non-Hodgkin's lymphoma is an AIDS-defining illness and its incidence has increased significantly over the past decade in the United States. Hodgkin's disease and breast cancer are seen in AIDS patients, but not in large numbers.

References

DeVita, V.T., Hellman, S., & Rosenberg, S.A. (1993). *Cancer: Principles and Practice of Oncology* (4th ed.). Philadelphia: J.B. Lippincott Co.

Fisher, D.S., Knobf, M.T., & Durivage, H.T. (1993). *Cancer Chemotherapy Handbook* (4th ed.). St. Louis: C.V. Mosby Co.

Gross, J., & Johnson, B.L. (1994). *Handbook of Oncology Nursing* (2nd ed.). St. Louis: C.V. Mosby Co.

Groenwald, S.L., Frogge, M.H., Goodman, M., et al. (1995). *Comprehensive Cancer Nursing Review* (2nd ed.). Boston: Jones and Bartlett Publishers.

McCorkle, R., Grant, M., Frank-Stromborg, M., et al. (1996). *Cancer Nursing: A Comprehensive Textbook* (2nd ed.). Philadelphia: W.B. Saunders Co.

Murphy, G.P., Lawrence, W., & Lenhard, R.E. (1995). *American Cancer Society Textbook of Clinical Oncology* (2nd ed.). Atlanta: American Cancer Society.

Varricchio, C. (1997). *A Cancer Sourcebook for Nurses* (7th ed.). Atlanta: American Cancer Society.

Anemia

DEFINITION

Anemia is a reduction in either the red blood cell (RBC) volume or the concentration of hemoglobin in the blood. Anemia is not a diagnosis itself, but rather an objective sign of the presence of disease.

ETIOLOGY/INCIDENCE

1. RBCs originate in the bone marrow of the sternum, ribs, vertebrae, pelvis, and proximal ends of the femur and humerus.
2. A feedback mechanism initiated by decreased oxygen tension at the level of the kidney causes an increased release of erythropoietin from the kidney, which stimulates the production of RBCs.
3. Anemias can be divided into three categories according to the size of the RBC as determined by the mean corpuscular volume (MCV):
   A. Microcytic (small size)

B. Normocytic (normal size)

C. Macrocytic (large size)

4. Anemias can also be classified by the reticulocyte count:

A. Low reticulocyte count (state of decreased production)

B. High reticulocyte count (state of increased destruction)

DIAGNOSTIC TESTS/FINDINGS

The following diagnostic tests are used in all types of anemia. (See Table 9–1 for normal values.)

1. Hemoglobin and hematocrit

2. Reticulocyte count

A. Indicates bone marrow response to anemia

B. Normal values 0.5–2.5%

C. Reticulocyte index (RI) corrects for the degree of anemia: RI = 1/2 (reticulocyte count × patient hematocrit/normal hematocrit)

D. Low reticulocyte count suggests decreased RBC production

E. High reticulocyte count suggests increased RBC destruction

3. MCV

A. Indicates size of RBC

B. May have small and large cells present simultaneously

4. Red cell distribution width (RDW)

A. Measures similarity of sizes

B. Anisocytosis = variation in RBC size

5. RBC morphology (shape abnormalities)

A. Spherocytes (hereditary spherocytosis, immunohemolytic anemias)

B. Teardrop cells (myeloproliferative disorders, pernicious anemia, thalassemia)

C. Schistocytes (traumatic and microangiopathic hemolysis)

D. Sickle cells (sickle cell disease)

E. Target cells (liver disease, sickle cell disease, thalassemia, hemoglobin C)

F. Burr cells (uremia)

G. Spur cells (acanthocytosis, spur cell anemia)

TABLE 9–1.   Laboratory Assessment of Anemia: Normal Values* (Adults)

Laboratory Test	Normal Value
Red blood cell count	M: 4.7–6.0 million/mm^3; F: 4.2–5.4 million/mm^3
Hemoglobin	M: 13.5–18.0 gm/dL; F: 12–16 gm/dL
Hematocrit	M: 42–52%; F: 37–47%
Mean corpuscular volume	78–100 fL
Mean corpuscular hemoglobin	27–31 pg
Red cell distribution width	11.5–14%
Reticulocyte count	0.5–1.85% of erythrocytes
Ferritin	M: 20–300 ng/mL; F: 15–120 ng/mL
Serum iron	M: 75–175 μg/dL; F: 65–165 μg/dL
Total iron-binding capacity	250–450 μg/dL
Serum erythropoietin level	M: 17.2 mU/mL; F: 18.8 mU/mL
Coombs' test (direct & indirect)	Negative
Serum B$_{12}$	190–900 ng/mL
Serum folate	≥3.5 μg/L

* Adapted from Wallach, J. (1996). *Interpretation of Diagnostic Tests* (6th ed.). Boston: Little, Brown & Co., with permission.

6. Mean corpuscular hemoglobin concentration (MCHC): RBC color
   A. Hypochromia (iron deficiency, sideroblastic anemia)
   B. Hyperchromia (megaloblastic anemia, spherocytosis)
7. Ferritin: Measures the body's storage of iron
8. Hemoglobin electrophoresis: If hemoglobinopathies are suspected
9. Serum B_{12} and folate levels
   A. Check in patients with macrocytic anemias
   B. Schilling test if B_{12} deficiency is found
10. Renal, liver, thyroid function tests: If anemia of chronic disease if found
11. Coombs' test (a.k.a. Direct antiglobulin test [DAT]) in all patients with suspected hemolysis
    A. Direct
    B. Indirect
12. Bone marrow aspiration and biopsy if cause of anemia cannot be determined
13. GI work-up to rule out malignancy in any adult male or postmenopausal female with iron deficiency

IRON-DEFICIENCY ANEMIA

DEFINITION

Iron-deficiency anemia is a microcytic, hypochromic anemia with a low reticulocyte count, caused by insufficient iron for hemoglobin synthesis.

ETIOLOGY/INCIDENCE

1. Most frequent cause of anemia in the world.
2. The result of inadequate intake (<1–2 mg/day), inadequate absorption (after partial gastrectomy), or excessive loss of iron (menorrhagia, gastritis, polyps, GI polyps or neoplasm, esophageal varices, hemorrhoids).
3. Most frequently occurs in young children, women during reproductive years, and the elderly.

SIGNS AND SYMPTOMS

Depend on etiology, degree and rapidity of onset of anemia.
1. Pallor
2. Fatigue
3. Shortness of breath, dyspnea on exertion
4. Pica (desire to eat nonfood substances such as ice, clay, starch)
5. Burning of tongue
6. Paresthesias
7. Brittle nails

PHYSICAL FINDINGS

1. Pallor
2. Koilonychia (spoon nails)
3. Glossitis

4. Papillary atrophy of the tongue
5. Angular cheilitis

DIFFERENTIAL DIAGNOSIS

1. Thalassemia
2. Anemia of chronic disease
3. Sideroblastic anemia
4. Lead toxicity

DIAGNOSTIC TESTS/FINDINGS

See Tables 9–1 and 9–2 for common diagnostic tests for anemia.
1. Decreased hemoglobin, hematocrit and reticulocyte count
2. Low MCV and MCHC
3. Increased RDW
4. Decreased ferritin
5. Low or normal serum iron concentration
6. Increased total iron-binding capacity (TIBC)
7. GI work-up in any male or postmenopausal female to rule out GI malignancy

MANAGEMENT/TREATMENT

1. Replete iron with $FeSO_4$ 325 mg tid for 6 months.
2. Transfusions usually not needed.
3. Response indicated by increase in reticulocyte count in 1–2 weeks, correction of anemia in 2–4 months, reaccumulation of iron stores in 4–6 months.
4. Refer to hematologist if patient fails to respond to iron supplementation.
5. Consult physician if positive fecal occult blood, unexplained bleeding.

PATIENT EDUCATION

1. Take iron between meals for better absorption.
2. Side effects include nausea, constipation, diarrhea, and black stools.

T A B L E 9–2. **Laboratory Assessment of Anemia: Result of Tests**

| | Laboratory Test | | | | | | | |
Type of Anemia	MCV	Retic	Ferritin	Iron	TIBC	Bili	B_{12}	Folate
Iron deficiency	D	D	D	D/N	I	N	N	N
Thalassemia	D	I/N	I/N	I/N	N	I	N	N/D
Sideroblastic	D	D	I	I	NA	NA	NA	NA
Aplastic anemia	N	D	NA	NA	NA	NA	NA	NA
Chronic disease	D/N	D/N	I/N	D	D	N	N	N/D
B_{12} deficiency	I	D/N	I	I	N	N	D	N
Folate deficiency	I	D/N	I	I	N	N	N	D
Acute blood loss	N	I	NA	NA	NA	NA	NA	NA
Sickle cell	N	I	NA	NA	NA	NA	NA	NA
G6PD deficiency	N	I	NA	NA	NA	I	NA	NA
Hemolytic—warm	N	I	NA	NA	NA	I	NA	NA
Hemolytic—cold	N	I	NA	NA	NA	NA	NA	NA

MCV, mean corpuscular volume; Retic, reticulocyte count; TIBC, total iron-binding capacity; Bili, bilirubin; I, increased; D, decreased; N, normal; NA, not applicable.

3. Foods high in iron include organ and lean meats, egg yolk, shellfish, apricots, peaches, prunes, grapes, raisins, green leafy vegetables, iron-fortified breads and cereals.

THALASSEMIAS

DEFINITION

The thalassemias are a group of genetic disorders characterized by abnormal hemoglobin synthesis, most commonly occurring as a result of reduced or absent production of α or β chains.

ETIOLOGY/INCIDENCE

1. Inherited, autosomal recessive disorders.
2. Second most common cause of microcytic anemia.
3. α-thalassemia is more common in blacks and Asians.
4. β-thalassemia is more common in Mediterranean populations (Italians, Greeks, Arabs, Sephardic Jews).

SIGNS AND SYMPTOMS

Severity of the anemia and symptoms can range from mild to severe.
1. Pallor
2. Fatigue
3. Shortness of breath, dyspnea on exertion
4. Headache
5. Angina

PHYSICAL FINDINGS

1. Pallor or bronze appearance
2. Splenomegaly
3. Hepatomegaly
4. Tachycardia
5. Systolic murmur if anemia is moderate or severe

DIFFERENTIAL DIAGNOSIS

1. Iron-deficiency anemia
2. Anemia of chronic disease
3. Lead toxicity

DIAGNOSTIC TESTS/FINDINGS

1. Decreased hemoglobin and hematocrit
2. Decreased MCV
3. Normal or increased serum iron
4. Normal or increased ferritin
5. Normal TIBC

6. Normal or increased reticulocyte count
7. Hemoglobin electrophoresis: Decreased α or β hemoglobin chains

MANAGEMENT/TREATMENT

1. No treatment for mild or moderate forms.
2. Refer patients with severe forms to hematologist.
3. Iron supplementation contraindicated; overload may occur in all types.
4. Refer for genetic counseling.

PATIENT EDUCATION

1. Encourage good nutrition without additional iron supplementation.
2. Explain genetic risks.
3. Teach signs and symptoms of iron overload, including weakness, loss of body hair, palmar erythema, weight loss, thinning and darkening of skin.

APLASTIC ANEMIA

DEFINITION

Aplastic anemia is a life-threatening condition in which the production of all blood cells have stopped and pancytopenia results.

ETIOLOGY/INCIDENCE

1. Possible causes include intrinsic stem cell defect, growth factor defect, immune suppression of marrow.
2. Classified as acquired, hereditary, or idiopathic.
   A. Causes of acquired aplastic anemia include chemicals (benzene and related compounds), drugs (see Table 9–3), radiation, viruses.
   B. Hereditary types include Faconi's anemia.
   C. Sixty-five percent of cases are idiopathic.
3. Median survival with untreated severe aplastic anemia is 3–6 months.

SIGNS AND SYMPTOMS

1. Fatigue
2. Bleeding
3. Infections

TABLE 9–3. Drugs Associated with Moderate Risk of Aplastic Anemia

Gold salts
Penicillamine
Phenylbutazone
Oxyphenbutazone
Carbamazepine
Hydantoins
Chloramphenicol
Quinacrine
Acetazolamide

PHYSICAL FINDINGS

1. Pallor
2. Petechiae
3. Fever

DIFFERENTIAL DIAGNOSIS

1. Pure red cell aplasia
2. Hypoplastic myelodysplastic syndrome
3. Paroxysmal nocturnal hemoglobinuria
4. Hypoplastic acute lymphocytic anemia

DIAGNOSTIC TESTS/FINDINGS

1. Pancytopenia
2. Decreased reticulocyte count
3. Markedly hypocellular marrow

MANAGEMENT/TREATMENT

1. Refer to hematologist/oncologist for treatment.
2. Bone marrow transplant is curative.
3. Minimal or no transfusions in potential transplant recipients.
4. Patients ineligible for transplant get supportive care with blood transfusions and platelet transfusions if bleeding.
5. Neutropenic precautions, broad spectrum antibiotics for fever.
6. Immunosuppressive therapy with antithymocyte globulin and/or cyclosporin is not curative; 50% response rate.

PATIENT EDUCATION

1. Explain need for bone marrow transplantation as treatment for disease.
2. Immediate human leukocyte antigen (HLA) typing of patient and siblings as possible marrow donors.
3. Instruct on neutropenic and bleeding precautions.

ANEMIA OF CHRONIC DISEASE

DEFINITION

Anemia of chronic disease (ACD) is a normocytic, normochromic anemia with low reticulocyte count, associated with chronic infection, inflammatory disease, or neoplastic disease.

ETIOLOGY/INCIDENCE

1. Etiology and mechanisms of ACD are not clearly understood. Proposals include:
   A. Iron is not released from its storage form.

B. Inadequate release of erythropoietin from the kidney in response to anemia.

C. Ability of erythroid precursors to respond to erythropoietin is impaired. Most common type of anemia found in hospitalized patients.

SIGNS AND SYMPTOMS

1. Fatigue
2. Weakness
3. Dyspnea on exertion
4. Fewer and milder symptoms than most other anemias
5. Other signs and symptoms related to underlying disease

PHYSICAL FINDINGS

1. Pallor

DIFFERENTIAL DIAGNOSIS

1. Aplastic anemia
2. Pure red cell aplasia
3. Malignant invasion of the bone marrow
4. Drug-induced marrow suppression or hemolysis
5. Anemia of chronic renal failure

DIAGNOSTIC TESTS/FINDINGS

1. Decreased hemoglobin but, if <9 gm/dL, consider other causes
2. Normochromic and normocytic, but hypochromic, microcytic features develop as ACD progresses
3. Decreased reticulocyte count
4. Decreased serum iron
5. Decreased or normal TIBC
6. Normal or increased serum ferritin

MANAGEMENT/TREATMENT

1. No treatment may be necessary.
2. Iron is contraindicated.
3. Refer to appropriate specialist when work-up reveals underlying inflammatory, infectious, or neoplastic disease for treatment.
4. Blood transfusions if symptomatic; not usually necessary in this mild anemia.
5. Erythropoietin 100–150 U/kg SQ three times per week.
   A. Start $FeSO_4$ 325 mg TID PO with erythropoietin, as ferritin will drop quickly with treatment.

PATIENT EDUCATION

1. Importance of adequate nutritional intake and adequate rest
2. Education on etiology and treatment of the underlying chronic disease
3. Instruction for self-injection with erythropoeitin

VITAMIN B$_{12}$ DEFICIENCY ANEMIA

DEFINITION

Vitamin B$_{12}$ deficiency causes a megaloblastic, macrocytic, normochromic anemia.

ETIOLOGY/INCIDENCE

1. Deficiency usually results from impaired absorption of B$_{12}$. There are several types:
   A. Pernicious anemia: Caused by a failure of secretion of intrinsic factor by the gastric mucosa as a result of atrophy.
   B. Gastrectomy syndrome: Develops within 5–6 years after a partial or total gastrectomy, as a result of cessation of secretion of intrinsic factor.
   C. Dietary: Insufficient intake; occurs rarely, usually in vegetarians who also avoid dairy products and eggs.
2. Common in Caucasians of Northern European descent.
3. Most present around age 60; can occur in younger patients.

SIGNS AND SYMPTOMS

1. Weakness
2. Sore throat
3. Paresthesias of extremities, including numbness, tingling, burning
4. Swelling of legs
5. Dizziness
6. Dementia in advanced stages of B$_{12}$ deficiency

PHYSICAL FINDINGS

1. Decreased position sense
2. Poor or absent vibratory sense in lower extremities
3. Ataxia
4. Increased or decreased deep tendon reflexes
5. Mental status changes
6. Smooth, beefy, red tongue
7. Sclera and skin may be slightly icteric
8. Systolic murmur

DIFFERENTIAL DIAGNOSIS

1. Folate deficiency
2. Anemia of chronic disease
3. Myelodysplastic syndrome

DIAGNOSTIC TESTS/FINDINGS

1. Increased MCV ($>$100)
2. Decreased or normal reticulocyte count
3. Decreased B$_{12}$ level ($<$0.1 μg/mL)
4. Normal or increased serum folate

ʰhilling test: Measures urinary radioactivity after ingestion of oral dose of
ᵈioactive cobalamin

ᴳEMENT/TREATMENT

1. Vitamin B_{12} 100 μg IM daily over 2 weeks, then weekly till hemoglobin
   normalized. Should receive a total of 2000 μg during the first 6 weeks.
2. When repleted, B_{12} 100 μg monthly for rest of life.
3. Reticulocyte count should increase in 3–5 days, hemoglobin should normalize in 1–2 months.
4. Transfusion may be required if prompt alleviation of anemia is necessary.
5. Refer patients with other immunologic problems.
6. Consult physician if pernicious anemia is suspected and further testing is
   indicated (e.g., gastric analysis, bone marrow biopsy, GI radiographic
   studies).
7. Monitor serum potassium levels; severe hypokalemia may develop after B_{12}
   deficiency.

PATIENT EDUCATION

1. Teach patient about the nature of the disease.
2. Explain and reinforce need for lifelong B_{12} replacement.
3. Teach patient/family to administer injections.
4. Warm patient of increased risk for gastric cancer in patients with pernicious
   anemia.

FOLATE DEFICIENCY ANEMIA

DEFINITION

Folic acid deficiency causes a macrocytic, normochromic, megaloblastic anemia.

ETIOLOGY/INCIDENCE

1. Folic acid is needed for DNA synthesis, RBC maturation, and maintenance
   of gastric mucosa.
2. Inadequate diet is principle cause of folic acid deficiency. Other causes in-
   clude:
   A. Impaired absorption (e.g., sprue)
   B. Increased requirements (e.g., pregnancy, infancy, chronic hemolytic
      anemia)
3. Folic acid reserves are small, deficiency can develop rapidly.
4. Alcohol can depress serum folate levels.
5. Drugs that may cause decreased folic acid levels include:
   A. Phenytoin (Dilantin)
   B. Antimalarials
   C. Estrogen
   D. Chloramphenicol
   E. Phenobarbitol

SIGNS AND SYMPTOMS

1. Fatigue
2. Dyspnea on exertion
3. Dizziness
4. Pallor
5. Weakness
6. Headache
7. Angina

PHYSICAL FINDINGS

1. No overt signs if anemia is mild
2. Pallor
3. Brittle nails
4. Fine hair
5. Angular cheilitis
6. Tachycardia
7. Systolic murmur

DIFFERENTIAL DIAGNOSIS

1. Pernicious anemia
2. Myelodysplastic syndrome
3. Acute megaloblastic anemia
4. Megaloblastic anemia caused by drugs; for example:
   A. Methotrexate
   B. Pyrimethamine
   C. Trimethoprim
   D. Sulfasalazine
   E. Triamterene
   F. Acyclovir
   G. 5-Fluorouracil
   H. Zidovudine
   I. Hydroxyurea
   J. Cytarabine
   K. Phenytoin
   L. Phenobarbitol

DIAGNOSTIC TESTS/FINDINGS

1. Normal or decreased reticulocyte count
2. Increased MCV
3. Decreased serum folate level
4. Normal serum B_{12}
5. Leukopenia and thrombocytopenia are frequently present
6. Presence of megaloblastic cells and oval macrocytes on peripheral smear

MANAGEMENT/TREATMENT

1. Folate 1 mg PO daily; duration depends on etiology of deficiency.
2. Up to 5 mg PO daily may be used if deficiency is related to sprue.

Check hemoglobin and reticulocyte count for response in 1–2 weeks, then every 6–12 months while on treatment.
When possible, elimination of underlying cause.
Evaluate for B_{12} deficiency as well.
.. Consult physician if coexisting iron deficiency, thalassemia trait, or inflammation suspected.

PATIENT EDUCATION

1. Teach dietary sources of folic acid, including asparagus, bananas, fish, green leafy vegetables, peanut butter, oatmeal, red beans, beef liver, wheat bran: Encourage daily intake from these foods.
2. Instruct in preparation because overcooking can destroy folic acid.

SICKLE CELL ANEMIA

DEFINITION

Sickle cell anemia is a chronic, hereditary, hemolytic anemia characterized by sickle-shaped RBCs.

ETIOLOGY/INCIDENCE

1. Marked by periods of well-being interspersed with episodes of deterioration; severity of symptoms varies widely among patients.
2. Autosomal recessive genetic disorder, homozygous for hemoglobin (Hb) SS.
3. Abnormal hemoglobin (Hb S) develops in place of normal hemoglobin (Hb A).
4. Patients with sickle cell trait are heterozygous, with about one fourth of their hemoglobin in abnormal Hb S form; the rest is normal Hb A.
5. Prevalent in Africans and African-Americans; also found at lower frequency in persons of Mediterranean ancestry.

SIGNS AND SYMPTOMS

1. Sickle cell trait patients are essentially asymptomatic except in cases of severe hypoxia.
2. Vaso-occlusive crises are seen in sickle cell patients.
   A. Precipitated by hypoxia, infection, high altitudes, stress, surgery, blood loss, dehydration; occasionally occur spontaneously.
   B. Sudden onset of excruciating pain in back, chest, extremities, lasting from a few hours to a few days

PHYSICAL FINDINGS

1. Acute: May be no physical findings
   A. Tachycardia
   B. Flow murmurs
2. Chronic
   A. Skin ulcers
   B. Splenomegaly

C. Hematuria
D. Hepatomegaly
E. Priaprism
F. Visual loss

DIFFERENTIAL DIAGNOSIS

1. Acute pulmonary infarction
2. Acute hepatitis
3. Cholycystitis

DIAGNOSTIC TESTS/FINDINGS

1. Normocytic, normochromic anemia
2. Variation in red cell size and shape
3. Elevated reticulocyte count
4. Sickled cells and target cells on smear
5. Leukocytosis
6. Thrombocytosis
7. Hemoglobin electrophoresis: Presence of hemoglobin S in sickle cell anemia, Hb S and Hb A in sickle cell trait

MANAGEMENT/TREATMENT

1. Refer to specialist for management of sickle cell anemia.
2. Therapy includes supportive care with:
   A. IV fluids
   B. Analgesics
   C. Antibiotics
   D. Oxygen
   E. Hydroxyurea
3. Experimental treatment includes bone marrow transplant.

PATIENT EDUCATION

1. Review the basis of disease and reasons for supportive care.
2. Education on pain control.
3. Genetic counseling for sickle cell trait.

GLUCOSE-6-PHOSPHATE DEHYDROGENASE DEFICIENCY ANEMIA

DEFINITION

Glucose-6-phosphate dehydrogenase deficiency is an inherited red cell enzyme deficiency that causes episodic hemolysis after exposure to oxidants or infection.

ETIOLOGY/INCIDENCE

1. Oxidant challenge leads to formation of denatured hemoglobin, making red cells less deformable and liable to splenic destruction.

TABLE 9-4. Drugs to Be Avoided in G6PD Deficiency

Sulfa drugs
Primaquine phosphate
Quinacrine
Nitrofurantoin (Furadantin)
Nalidixic acid (NegGram caplets)
Phenazopyridine hydrochloride (Pyridium)

2. Sex-linked disorder; found in 11% of African-American males.
3. See Table 9–4 for list of inciting drugs.
4. Drug-induced hemolysis occurs 1–3 days after drug exposure.

SIGNS AND SYMPTOMS

1. Abdominal or back pain
2. Dark urine

PHYSICAL FINDINGS

1. Signs of infection
2. Jaundice
3. Hematuria
4. Splenomegaly
5. Ankle ulcers

DIFFERENTIAL DIAGNOSIS

1. Pyruvate kinase deficiency
2. Hereditary spherocytosis
3. Acquired hemolytic anemia

DIAGNOSTIC TESTS/FINDINGS

1. Anemia ranges from severe to normal hemoglobin.
2. RBCs have normal morphology in absence of hemolysis.
3. Increased bilirubin during hemolysis.
4. Increased lactate dehydrogenase during hemolysis.
5. Positive G6PD screen.

MANAGEMENT/TREATMENT

1. Avoidance of oxidant drugs.
2. Transfusions only given in severe cases of G6PD deficiency.
3. Iron therapy avoided unless iron deficient.
4. Refer to hematologist for management of hemolytic episode.

PATIENT EDUCATION

1. Teach patient which drugs to avoid.
2. Instruct patient that febrile illnesses may precipitate hemolysis.

3. Severe hemolysis may occur after ingestion of fava beans.
4. Genetic counseling.

MICROANGIOPATHIC HEMOLYTIC ANEMIA

DEFINITION

Microangiopathic hemolytic anemia (MHA) is caused by intravascular hemolysis resulting from fragmentation of normal red cells passing through abnormal arterioles.

ETIOLOGY/INCIDENCE

1. Usually starts with intravascular coagulation with deposition of platelets and fibrin in small arterioles.
2. Red cells stick to fibrin and are fragmented by force of blood flow.
3. Results in both intravascular and extravascular hemolysis.
4. Underlying disorders include:
   A. Invasive carcinomas
   B. Complications of pregnancy
   C. Malignant hypertension
   D. Thrombotic thrombocytopenic purpura
   E. Hemolytic uremic syndrome
   F. Antineoplastic drugs, including mitomycin, bleomycin, daunorubicin with cytosine arabinoside, cisplatin
   G. Post-transplantation of kidney or liver, post–allogeneic or autologous bone marrow transplant
   H. Generalized vasculitis
   I. Localized vascular abnormalities
   J. Disseminated intravascular coagulation

SIGNS AND SYMPTOMS

1. Related to the underlying process
2. Dyspnea on exertion
3. Chest pain
4. Fatigue and weakness
5. Oliguria
6. Anuria

PHYSICAL FINDINGS

1. Related to the underlying process
2. Petechiae
3. Edema
4. Pallor

DIFFERENTIAL DIAGNOSIS

1. Paroxysmal nocturnal hemoglobinuria
2. Paroxysmal cold hemoglobinuria
3. Autoimmune hemolytic anemia

DIAGNOSTIC TESTS/FINDINGS

1. Increased reticulocyte count
2. Increased serum LDH
3. Decreased serum haptoglobin level
4. Schistocytes, helmet cell, burr cells on peripheral smear
5. Iron deficiency due to urinary loss of iron
6. Direct Coomb's test is usually negative
7. Lab findings due to causative disease

MANAGEMENT/TREATMENT

1. Directed toward management of underlying process: Refer to appropriate specialist.
2. RBC transfusions.
3. Platelet transfusions if bleeding due to thrombocytopenia.
4. Heparin use is controversial.

PATIENT EDUCATION

1. Related to underlying disease process
2. Explanation of need for diagnostic work-up to find underlying process

AUTOIMMUNE HEMOLYTIC ANEMIA—WARM ANTIBODIES

DEFINITION

This anemia is an acquired hemolytic anemia with shortened RBC survival as the result of warm-reacting host antibodies that react with autologous RBCs.

ETIOLOGY/INCIDENCE

1. May be classified as primary (idiopathic) or secondary to an underlying disease.
    A. Fifty-five percent of cases are idiopathic.
    B. In primary acquired hemolytic anemia (AHA), the autoantibody is often specific for a single RBC membrane protein, suggesting an aberrant immune response has occurred to an autoantigen.
    C. In secondary AHA, the autoantibody most likely develops from an immunoregulatory defect.
    D. Secondary causes include chronic lymphocytic leukemia, Hodgkin's disease, lymphoma, systemic lupus erythematosus, infection, nonlymphoid neoplasms, chronic inflammatory diseases, drugs (e.g., methyldopa).
2. May also be classified by the nature of the antibody, either warm, cold, or mixed.
3. Warm-antibody AHA is the most common type.
4. Occurs at all ages; incidence rises with age.

SIGNS AND SYMPTOMS

Symptoms are usually slow in onset, but rapidly developing anemia can occur.
1. Jaundice
2. Fatigue

3. Weakness
4. Dyspnea on exertion
5. Signs and symptoms of underlying disease

PHYSICAL FINDINGS

1. Pallor
2. Jaundice
3. Splenomegaly
4. Tachycardia

DIFFERENTIAL DIAGNOSIS

1. Hereditary spherocytosis
2. Microangiopathic hemolytic anemia
3. Paroxysmal nocturnal hemoglobinuria
4. Transfusion reaction
5. Cold-reactive autoimmune hemolytic anemia

DIAGNOSTIC TESTS/FINDINGS

1. Normocytic, normochromic anemia, ranges from mild to severe.
2. Positive direct antiglobulin test (a.k.a. Coombs' test): Diagnosis of AHA requires demonstration of immunoglobulin or complement bound to RBC.
3. Increased reticulocyte count.
4. Indirect Coombs' test is positive in 60% of cases.
5. Spherocytes on peripheral smear.
6. Elevated LDH.
7. Decreased haptoglobin levels.
8. Increased bilirubin.

MANAGEMENT/TREATMENT

1. Patients with minimal hemolysis and stable hemoglobin require no treatment: Observe for progression.
2. Consult hematologist for recommendations.
3. RBC transfusion not usually required for slowly developing anemia but may be lifesaving for rapid hemolysis: Transfused RBCs are destroyed as fast as or faster than host RBCs.
4. Glucocorticoids quickly slow or stop hemolysis in two thirds of patients:
   A. Oral prednisone 60–100 mg/day
   B. IV methylprednisolone 300 mg/day for critically ill
   C. When hemoglobin stabilizes, taper steroids over 2–3 months
5. Relapses are common; monitor patient closely: Refer to hematologist for long-term follow-up.
6. Splenectomy is used for patients who cannot be tapered off prednisone (approximately one third of patients).
7. Patients who fail to respond to steroids and splenectomy may benefit from immunosuppressive drugs: Cyclophosphamide 60 mg/m^2 or azathioprine 80 mg/m^2 daily up to 6 months, then tapered.

PATIENT EDUCATION

1. Explain that AHA tends to have an unpredictable course with remissions and relapses.
2. Teaching related to dosing, schedule, and side effects of steroids and immunosuppressive drugs.
3. Pneumococcal vaccine should be given prior to splenectomy.
4. In secondary AHA, the prognosis is related to the underlying disease.

AUTOIMMUNE HEMOLYTIC ANEMIA—COLD ANTIBODIES

DEFINITION

This anemia is an autoimmune hemolytic anemia caused by autoantibodies that bind red cells best at temperatures below 37°C.

ETIOLOGY/INCIDENCE

1. Cold agglutinins are IgM autoantibodies that agglutinate red cells.
2. Classified as either primary (chronic cold agglutinin disease) or secondary: Secondary is usually due to *Mycoplasma* or infectious mononucleosis.
3. Peak incidence for chronic syndrome is over age 50.
4. Some patients develop Waldenström's macroglobulinemia, a B-cell lymphoproliferative disorder.
5. Cold agglutinin-mediated hemolysis accounts for 10–20% of all cases of AHA.
6. Hemolysis is generally chronic, but acute episodes can occur upon chilling.

SIGNS AND SYMPTOMS

1. Pallor
2. Weakness
3. Fatigue
4. Dyspnea on exertion
5. Peripheral vaso-occlusive symptoms
6. Symptoms of infection, including cough, fever

PHYSICAL FINDINGS

1. Acrocyanosis
2. Splenomegaly occasionally seen
3. Signs of mycoplasma infection, including fever
4. Pallor

DIFFERENTIAL DIAGNOSIS

1. Raynaud's phenomenon
2. Drug-induced hemolytic anemia
3. Mixed-type autoimmune hemolysis
4. Paroxysmal cold hemoglobinuria
5. Paroxysmal nocturnal hemoglobinuria

DIAGNOSTIC TESTS/FINDINGS

1. Mild to moderate normocytic anemia.
2. Increased reticulocyte count.
3. Direct antiglobulin test (a.k.a. Coombs' test) is positive with anticomplement reagents.
4. Peripheral smear shows rare spherocytes, autoagglutination, polychromasia.
5. Diagnosed by demonstrating cold antibody in serum; serum titers can be >1:100,000.
6. Increased LDH.
7. Increased bilirubin.

MANAGEMENT/TREATMENT

1. Refer to hematologist for management and long-term follow-up.
2. Keeping the patient warm is important and may be the only treatment needed for mild conditions.
3. Chlorambucil and cyclophosphamide are useful for more severe chronic cases.
4. Very high-dose glucocorticoids may be useful in the severely ill.
5. Plasmapheresis may provide temporary relief.

PATIENT EDUCATION

1. Reassure patient that postinfectious syndromes are self-limited, resolving in few weeks.
2. Teach patient with chronic syndrome that it is usually a stable condition with long-term survival.
3. Instruct patient to keep warm.

Review Questions

9.23 A 17-year-old African American girl with sickle cell anemia is admitted in sickle cell crisis, for hydration and pain control. Sickle cell anemia is caused by:
   A. Replacement of hemoglobin A with hemoglobin CS
   B. Transposition of glutamic acid on hemoglobin A molecule
   C. Abnormal hemoglobin S in place of hemoglobin A
   D. Sickle cell trait

9.24 A 45-year-old Caucasian man has been hospitalized for 2 months following a hemicolectomy for Crohn's disease. The postoperative course has been complicated by a wound infection with methcillin-resistant *Staphylococcus aureus*. The ACNP notes that the patient has developed normocytic anemia when checking his CBC. In normocytic anemia of chronic disease:
   A. Treatment is symptomatic only.
   B. Long-term B_{12} and folate supplementation is needed.
   C. Treatment is focused on the associated disease.
   D. Serum iron and TIBC are the most specific and sensitive diagnostic tests.

9.25 In managing this patient with ACD, the ACNP knows that which of the following are true?
A. A hemoglobin of less than 9 gm/dL confirms the diagnosis.
B. Symptoms associated with the anemia may be masked by symptoms of the underlying disease.
C. ACD is manifested by more severe signs than most other common anemias.
D. ACD is never associated with reversible causes.

9.26 An ACNP is teaching a woman with iron deficiency about her disease. The ACNP instructs the woman that:
A. Return of normal blood values will occur within 1 week of iron supplementation.
B. Iron supplements will need to be taken for the rest of her life.
C. Taking iron preparations with milk will enhance absorption.
D. Iron supplementation should be taken between meals.

9.27 In alcoholics with anemia:
A. Pernicious anemia is more common than folate deficiency.
B. Iron deficiency and folate deficiency may coexist
C. Alcohol interferes with iron absorption.
D. All of the above.

9.28 A 24-year-old Asian woman who is S/P autologous bone marrow transplant 2 months ago is admitted with a decreased hemoglobin, elevated reticulocyte count, and elevated LDH. The ACNP suspects the most likely cause to be:
A. Autoimmune hemolytic anemia
B. Microangiopathic hemolytic anemia
C. Aplastic anemia
D. Cold agglutinin hemolytic anemia

9.29 The ACNP confirms her diagnosis by which of the following test results?
A. Positive direct Coombs' test
B. Presence of schistocytes on peripheral smear
C. Increased serum haptoglobin level
D. Presence of cold antibody in serum

9.30 A 40-year-old African American woman presents to the ER with complaints of chest pain and shortness of breath. The work-up reveals a microcytic anemia and a low reticulocyte count. The ACNP considers the most likely diagnosis to be:
A. Thalassemia
B. Lead toxicity
C. Iron deficiency
D. Vitamin B_{12} deficiency

9.31 When examining a new patient in the hospital, the ACNP finds impaired vibratory and position sense as well as spastic weakness. Upon questioning, the patient also reports paresthesias in his fingers and toes. When reviewing the laboratory data, the ACNP finds a hemoglobin of 10. What is the most likely cause of this patient's anemia?
A. Vitamin B_{12} deficiency
B. Folate deficiency

C. Iron deficiency

D. Sickle cell disease

9.32 A 50-year-old white man is admitted to the hospital with a hemoglobin of 6 gm/dL and a high reticulocyte count, as well as complaints of fatigue and dyspnea on exertion. All of the following are possible causes of the anemia EXCEPT:

A. Acute blood loss

B. Hereditary hemolytic anemia

C. Acquired hemolytic anemia

D. Aplastic anemia

Answers and Rationales

9.23 **C** Sickle cell patients carry the abnormal hemoglobin S, which causes sickling of the cells, increase in blood viscosity, vascular stasis, and tissue damage. Patients with hemoglobin SC have the sickle cell trait, with less than half the hemoglobin in each RBC from hemoglobin S. This protects against the sickling except in the most severe circumstances.

9.24 **C** Anemia of chronic disease occurs in patients with an inflammatory, infectious, or neoplastic disease of >6 months' duration. The treatment is aimed at eradicating the underlying process, thereby resolving the anemia. Serum iron and TIBC will be decreased in most patients with a chronic illness, making them less specific tests. B_{12} and folate deficiencies cause a macrocytic anemia, not a normocytic anemia.

9.25 **B** ACD is a diagnosis of exclusion; there is no one confirmatory test. It is a mild anemia and therefore the symptoms may be mild, masked by the symptoms of the underlying disorder, or the patient may be asymptomatic. ACD may be associated with infection, inflammation, or malignancy, all of which may be reversible in some cases.

9.26 **D** Iron absorption is optimal when the supplement is taken on an empty stomach.

9.27 **B** Folate deficiency is more common than pernicious anemia in alcoholics. Poor nutrition can lead to a simultaneous iron and folate deficiency.

9.28 **B** Post-transplant patients are at risk for microangiopathic hemolytic anemia. Aplastic anemia is a hypoproliferative anemia and therefore would not have an elevated reticulocyte count.

9.29 **B** Coombs' test is usually negative in MHA but positive in AHA and cold agglutinin hemolytic anemia (CAHA). Schistocytes are seen in MHA; spherocytes are seen in AHA and rarely seen in CAHA. Haptoglobin level is decreased in all three.

9.30 **C** Iron deficiency is the most common cause of anemia in the world. A microcytic anemia with decreased RBC production is most likely due to iron deficiency.

9.31 **A** Vitamin B_{12} deficiency is the only anemia to cause neurologic toxicities such as paresthesias and weakness.

9.32 **D** Aplastic anemia is characterized by a low reticulocyte count.

References

Erickson, J.M. (1996). Anemia. *Semin Oncol Nurs 12*, 2–14.

Lee, G.R., Bithell, T.C., Foerster, J., et al. (1993). *Wintrobe's Clinical Hematology* (6th ed.). Philadelphia: Lea & Febiger.

Wallach, J. (1996). *Interpretation of Diagnostic Tests* (6th ed.). Boston: Little, Brown & Co.

Williams, W.J., Beutler, E., Erslev, A.J., et al. (1996). *William's Hematology* (5th ed.). New York: McGraw-Hill.

Common Hematologic Problems

DISSEMINATED INTRAVASCULAR COAGULATION

DEFINITION

Disseminated intravascular coagulation is an alteration in the normal clotting mechanism that manifests itself as diffuse clotting occurring simultaneously with hemorrhage—an oncologic emergency.

ETIOLOGY/INCIDENCE

1. The normal clotting cascade is a tightly controlled homeostatic mechanism that protects the body when injury has occurred.
2. DIC is a secondary complication that requires some type of triggering event.
3. Occurs as acute or chronic forms: Acute DIC is often accompanied by multi–organ system dysfunction, such as shock, respiratory failure, and renal failure, caused directly by the inciting illness.
4. Occurs in approximately 15% of cancer patients; associated with intravascular hemolysis from transfusion reactions, overwhelming viral or bacterial sepsis and shock (especially gram-negative sepsis), and release of thrombin from malignant cells.
5. Results from a generalized activation of the coagulation system causing consumption of clotting factors, including fibrinogen and platelets, and initiation of fibrinolytic pathway.
   A. Fibrinogen and fibrin are broken down by fibrinolysis, resulting in appearance of fibrin split products (a.k.a. fibrin degradation products).
   B. As fragments circulate, they interfere with formation of fibrin and also coat the platelets, decreasing their adhesive ability.
   C. Results in continued anticoagulation along with fibrinolysis.
   D. Can cause generalized, often catastrophic bleeding as well as gross and microscopic thrombosis.

SIGNS AND SYMPTOMS

1. Easy bruising
2. Petechiae
3. Prolonged bleeding from injection sites
4. Epistaxis
5. Hematuria

6. Change in mental status
7. Markedly decreased urine output

PHYSICAL FINDINGS

1. Petechiae
2. Ecchymosis
3. Bleeding from injection sites, incisions
4. Hypotension
5. Tachycardia
6. Hematuria
7. Acrocyanosis (generalized sweating with cold, mottled fingers and toes)
8. Retinal hemorrhages

DIFFERENTIAL DIAGNOSIS

1. Coagulopathy of liver disease
2. Primary fibrinolysis
3. Myelodysplasia
4. Drug-induced thrombocytopenia
5. Idiopathic thrombocytopenic purpura (ITP)
6. Thrombotic thrombocytopenic purpura (TTP)

DIAGNOSTIC TESTS/FINDINGS

1. Presence of thrombocytopenia with three of the following abnormalities confirms the diagnosis:
   A. Increased fibrinogen, fibrin split products (fibrin degradation products)
   B. Prolonged prothrombin time (PT)
   C. Prolonged partial thromboplastin time (PTT)
   D. Prolonged thrombin time (TT)
   E. Decreased fibrinogen level
   F. Elevated D-dimers
2. Decreased hemoglobin/hematocrit (with active bleeding).
3. Inspection of peripheral smear for fragmentation of RBCs.
4. Lab values are variable for chronic DIC.
   A. Increased production may compensate for consumption and platelet count; clotting times and fibrinogen level may be normal.
   B. Usually increased concentrations of fibrin degradation products and D-dimer.

MANAGEMENT/TREATMENT

1. Consult physician for appropriate diagnostic work-up and treatment plan. The ACNP may manage the patient collaboratively with the active consultation of the physician.
2. Remove the precipitating factor or underlying cause: Rapid and appropriate treatment of underlying disorder is of utmost importance.
3. Supportive measures include:
   A. Control active bleeding.
   B. Platelet transfusions for thrombocytopenia.
   C. Cryoprecipitate for hypofibrinogenemia.

    D. Prevent organ failure with pressors, dialysis, respiratory and ventilator management.

    E. Adequate hydration for renal perfusion.

    F. Thrombocytopenic precautions.

       1) Avoid IM injections, rectal medications/exams/temperatures.

       2) Minimize invasive procedures.

       3) Avoid drugs that interfere with platelet function (e.g., aspirin).

4. Administration of heparin in some cases.

    A. Inactivates thrombin, which will inhibit the clotting process and thereby inhibit fibrinolysis.

    B. In most forms of acute DIC, has not been shown to decrease mortality rates.

    C. May improve lab parameters but may aggravate bleeding.

    D. DIC caused by malignancy often responds to IV heparin followed by long-term SQ heparin.

    E. Antifibrinolytic therapy is generally contraindicated.

    F. For chronic DIC, heparin dose of 500–750 U/hr via continuous infusion without loading bolus may be sufficient.

    G. For acute DIC, heparin bolus 10,000 U IV followed by 1000 U/hr continuous infusion.

    H. Check PTT 4 hours after starting and 4 hours after each change in dosage, then at least qd.

PATIENT EDUCATION

1. Inform patient and family about the disorder and need for intensive monitoring, supportive measures.

2. Teach patient and family about thrombocytopenic precautions.

    A. Soft toothbrush, no flossing, nonastringent mouthwash

    B. Fluids and high-fiber diet to prevent constipation

    C. No straining at stool, no rectal medications or temperatures

    D. Electric razor only

    E. Hold pressure at cuts for at least 5 minutes

    F. Provide safe physical environment

IDIOPATHIC THROMBOCYTOPENIC PURPURA (ITP)

DEFINITION

Idiopathic thrombocytopenic purpura is an acquired disease of children and adults characterized by a low platelet count, a normal marrow, and absence of evidence for other disease.

ETIOLOGY/INCIDENCE

1. In children, ITP is acute in onset and resolves spontaneously within 6 months, but in adults, ITP is insidious in nature and rarely resolves spontaneously.

2. Thrombocytopenia appears to be due to splenic sequestration and destruction of platelets.

    A. Most patients have either normal or diminished platelet production.

    B. Anti-platelet antibodies bind to megakaryocytes and may cause ineffective thrombocytopoiesis.

3. In 15–20% of patients, thrombocytopenia is associated with an underlying disease and may be considered secondary ITP: Paraproteins in patients with lymphoma, multiple myeloma, and Waldenström's macroglobulinemia can cause thrombocytopenia.

SIGNS AND SYMPTOMS

1. Greater than 2-month history of purpura
2. Petechiae, often in dependent regions
3. Menorrhagia
4. Epistaxis
5. Gingival bleeding
6. Hematuria
7. Occult GI bleeding
8. Overt bleeding is rare

PHYSICAL FINDINGS

1. Petechiae, often in dependent regions.
2. Purpura.
3. Gingival bleeding.
4. Ecchymosis.
5. A palpable spleen strongly suggests ITP is *not* the cause of thrombocytopenia.

DIFFERENTIAL DIAGNOSIS

1. Acute infection
2. Myelodysplasia
3. Chronic DIC
4. Drug-induced thrombocytopenia
5. Congenital thrombocytopenia

DIAGNOSTIC TESTS/FINDINGS

1. Decreased platelet count (<20,000).
2. Review blood smear to rule out pseudothrombocytopenia.
3. WBC and hemoglobin usually normal.
4. Coagulation studies normal.
5. Bleeding time normal.
6. Increased megakaryocytes in the bone marrow.

MANAGEMENT/TREATMENT

1. Spontaneous remissions are rare in adults but occur frequently in children.
2. Consult physician for appropriate diagnostic work-up and treatment plan. The ACNP may manage the patient collaboratively with the active consultation of the physician.
3. Refer to hematologist for long-term management.
4. Asymptomatic mild or moderate thrombocytopenia.
   A. Follow without treatment.
   B. Evaluate for underlying cause (e.g., hypersplenism).

5. Severe thrombocytopenia with acute bleeding.
   A. Platelet transfusions for platelet counts <20,000 and bleeding.
      1) Recheck count 6 hours after transfusion.
      2) Single-donor platelets are preferable.
   B. Intravenous IgG, single infusion 0.4–0.1 gm/kg, followed immediately by platelet transfusion.
   C. High-dose glucocorticoids (e.g., methylprednisolone 1 gm IV daily for 3 days).
   D. Aminocaproic acid to help control acute bleeding.
6. Splenectomy offers complete, permanent responses in two thirds of patients: Short course of radiation therapy to spleen for those who cannot tolerate surgery.
7. Chronic, refractory ITP.
   A. Intravenous IgG may be helpful, especially when a situation requires a transient increase in the platelet count.
   B. Given 2 gm/kg over 2–5 days; platelet count will usually increase after several days and return to pretreatment level in several weeks.
   C. Maintenance therapy with single infusion of 60 gm when count falls below 20,000.

PATIENT EDUCATION

1. Teach patient and family about thrombocytopenic precautions.
   A. Soft toothbrush, no flossing, nonastringent mouthwash
   B. Fluids and high-fiber diet to prevent constipation
   C. No straining at stool, no rectal medications or temperatures
   D. Electric razor only
   E. Hold pressure on cuts for at least 5 minutes
   F. Provide a safe physical environment
2. Preoperative teaching for splenectomy.
3. Postoperative instruction about increased risk of infection, especially pneumococcal infections for patients undergoing splenectomy.

Review Questions

9.33 A 66-year-old Caucasian man with lung cancer is admitted for sepsis. During his work-up, the ACNP notes petechiae and easy bruising and suspects DIC. All of the following statements about DIC are true EXCEPT:
   A. Results from activation of the clotting system, causing consumption of clotting factors.
   B. Diffuse clotting occurs simultaneously with hemorrhage.
   C. Associated lab results include increased platelet count, increased fibrinogen, and prolonged PT and PTT.
   D. Heparin may improve lab parameters but aggravate bleeding.

9.34 The ACNP is following a postoperative patient in collaboration with the surgeon. Upon review of a routine CBC, the patient is found to have a platelet count of 15,000. Review of systems is noncontributory, all other lab studies (including coagulopathy studies) are within normal limits, and the physical exam is normal. The most likely diagnosis is:

A. DIC
B. ITP
C. TTP
D. Cancer

9.35 The ACNP is caring for a patient with DIC in the intensive care unit. Possible therapeutic options include all of the following except:
A. Heparin
B. ε-Aminocaproic acid (EACA or Amicar)
C. Vitamin K
D. Platelet transfusion

9.36 The symptoms of DIC seem paradoxical because:
A. Both platelet function and platelet number are implicated in DIC
B. Patients may have fever along with hypothermia
C. DIC may be both the cause and effect of malignancy
D. Thrombosis and hemorrhage may occur simultaneously

Answers and Rationales

9.33 **C** A patient with DIC has a decreased platelet count.

9.34 **B** ITP is characterized by thromboctyopenia, a normal bone marrow, and absence of evidence of other disease.

9.35 **C** Vitamin K might be administered to a patient experiencing hypocoagulability but not the hypercoagulability caused by DIC. All of the other therapies may provide short-term relief of DIC while the underlying causative condition is determined and corrected.

9.36 **D** DIC results from an underlying disease process that triggers abnormal thrombin formation. Thrombin is both a powerful coagulant and an agent of fibrinolysis; thus small clots and clotting factors are being consumed. The result is hemorrhage because the body is unable to respond to vascular or tissue injury.

References

Lee, G.R., Bithell, T.C., Foerster, J., et al. (1993). *Wintrobe's Clinical Hematology* (6th ed.). Philadelphia: Lea & Febiger.

Wallach, J. (1996). *Interpretation of Diagnostic Tests* (6th ed.). Boston: Little, Brown & Co.

Williams, W.J., Beutler, E., Erslev, A.J., et al. (1996). *William's Hematology* (5th ed.). New York: McGraw-Hill.

Oncologic Emergencies

FEBRILE NEUTROPENIA

DEFINITION

Neutropenia is commonly defined as an absolute neutrophil count (ANC) of <1000 cells/mm^3. The frequency of infection increases as the ANC falls below 500 and the longer the patient remains neutropenic.

ETIOLOGY/INCIDENCE

1. Considered a potentially life-threatening emergency; fatality rates during the first 48 hours range from 18–40%.
2. One of the most common causes of morbidity and mortality in patients with cancer.
3. Many cancer patients are immunocompromised as a result of the disease or its treatment.
4. Multimodality treatment of cancer may render patients vulnerable to opportunistic infections.
5. Infection may be difficult to assess because the normal response does not occur.
6. Gram-negative bacteria are the most common and most significant cause of infection in cancer patients: Other causes include gram-positive bacteria, viruses, fungus, protozoa.
7. Mortality has been reported as high as 20–40%, higher with multimicrobial sepsis.
8. Half of neutropenic patients have unexplained fever.
9. More than 80% of infections are from the patient's endogenous flora, usually acquired during hospitalization.
10. Most common sites of infection include:
    A. Respiratory tract
    B. Alimentary tract
    C. Genitourinary tract
    D. Skin and mucous membranes
    E. Central nervous system
    F. Systemic
11. Risk of infection is increased by:
    A. Comorbid conditions
    B. Poor performance status
    C. Poor nutritional status
    D. Implanted medical devices
    E. High-dose, combination, and dose-intensive chemotherapy
12. Prolonged neutropenia (>7 days) increases risk of fungal infections.

SIGNS AND SYMPTOMS

May include any of the following:
1. Fever; temperature of ≥100.5°F is considered fever in neutropenic cancer patient.
2. Confusion or somnolence.
3. Productive cough.
4. Headache.
5. Dysuria.
6. Vaginal discharge.
7. Skin lesions with swelling and tenderness.
8. Diarrhea.

PHYSICAL FINDINGS

Include, but are not limited to, any of the following:
1. Fever
2. Change in mental status.

3. Open lesions (e.g., stomatitis).
4. Edema, erythema, and/or tenderness of skin, especially pressure areas and biopsy sites.
5. Sinus tenderness.
6. Decreased breath sounds, crackles, egophony, bronchial breath sounds.
7. Hypotension and tachycardia (suggestive of sepsis).
8. Abdominal tenderness.
9. Costovertebral angle tenderness.
10. Many patients may exhibit no abnormal physical findings.

DIFFERENTIAL DIAGNOSIS

1. Nonneutropenic fever and infection
2. Tumor fever
3. Neutropenia without infection

DIAGNOSTIC TESTS/FINDINGS

1. Decreased WBC
   A. ANC <1000 cells/mm^3
   B. ANC = total WBC × % segmented neutrophils and bands
2. Blood chemistries to evaluate electrolytes, renal and hepatic function
3. Arterial blood gas if sepsis is suspected: Acid-base state, metabolic or respiratory causes
4. Chest x-ray to rule out pneumonia
   A. Neutropenic patients may not develop pulmonary infiltrates commonly seen in pneumonia; bone marrow cannot mobilize the white blood cells to mount a response.
   B. Pulmonary infiltrates will often appear on follow-up x-rays when WBC has risen.
5. Blood cultures
   A. One set of aerobic and one set of anaerobic cultures.
   B. Taken from at least two different sites.
   C. Patients with vascular access devices should have one set taken from each lumen.
6. Urinalysis and urine culture, even if asymptomatic
7. Stool for WBC, ova and parasites, culture, *Clostridium difficile* antigen if patient has diarrhea
8. Lumbar puncture if CNS source is suspected
9. Culture of skin lesions
10. Patient with persistent febrile neutropenia without a source identified
    A. Fungal and viral cultures
    B. Grams stains of lesions or body fluids
    C. Culture for acid-fast bacilli

MANAGEMENT/TREATMENT

1. Initial treatment focuses on hemodynamic stabilization and eradication of organism.
2. Once fever work-up is complete, a course of empiric antibiotics is started without waiting for culture results. When results are available, therapy can be modified to treat the identified organism.

    A. Usually consists of broad-spectrum antibiotics directed at both gram-positive and gram-negative organisms.

    B. Current recommendations include either:

        1) Two β-lactam antibiotics (e.g., azetreonam + ceftazidime)

        2) A β-lactam and an aminoglycoside antibiotic (piperacillin + tobramycin)

        3) Monotherapy with an extended-spectrum cephalosporin (e.g., ceftazidime) or carbapenum (e.g., imipenum)

            a. Commonly used β-lactams include extended-spectrum penicillins, extended-spectrum cephalosporins, monobactams.

            b. Antibiotic regimens vary widely with institution and geographic location.

            c. Use of a third drug has not been shown to increase efficacy.

    C. Empiric therapy is commonly continued until resolution of the neutropenia.

3. Neutropenic patients with persistent fever that fails to respond to antibacterials usually require empiric treatment with antifungal agents (e.g., amphotericin B, at least 1 mg/kg/day; total dose determined upon clinical status, infection resolution, marrow recovery).

PATIENT EDUCATION

1. Educate patient and family about risk of infection while undergoing myelosuppressive treatment, including time of greatest risk.
2. Instruct patient to call for fever >100.5°F or any symptoms of infection: Consistently reinforce importance with each visit.
3. Institute self-care measures to prevent infection, including stringent handwashing, avoiding persons with acute illnesses, eating only fresh fruits and vegetables that can be peeled, skin and mouth care.

SUPERIOR VENA CAVA SYNDROME

DEFINITION

The compression of the superior vena cava (SVC) by tumor leads to a characteristic pattern of upper extremity manifestations. If untreated, superior vena cava syndrome (SVCS) can lead to airway obstruction. SVCS is an oncologic emergency.

ETIOLOGY/INCIDENCE

1. Occurs in 3–4% of the oncology population.
2. May be the presenting sign of a malignancy.
3. The SVC is the main vessel for venous return from the upper thorax: A thin-walled vessel with low intravascular pressure.
4. SVC compression can occur by:
    A. External compression by tumor or lymph node
    B. Direct invasion of vessel wall by tumor
    C. Thrombosis of vessel
5. Lung cancer and lymphoma are the two most frequent causes.
6. SVC obstruction causes increased venous pressure and congestion.

7. Severity of symptoms related to rapidity of onset and adequacy of collateral circulation.
8. Rapidly developing SVCS may be fatal.

SIGNS AND SYMPTOMS

1. Shortness of breath.
2. Swelling of the face, chest, upper extremities.
3. Cough.
4. Hoarseness.
5. Stridor.
6. Increased intracranial pressure may cause headache, dizziness, visual disturbances, occasional change in mental status.

PHYSICAL FINDINGS

1. Facial edema
2. Edema of the chest and upper extremities
3. Neck and chest vein distention
4. Tachypnea
5. Cyanosis of the upper extremities

DIFFERENTIAL DIAGNOSIS

1. Thrombus formation around a central venous catheter
2. Anaphylaxis

DIAGNOSTIC TESTS/FINDINGS

1. Chest x-ray shows a mediastinal mass, mediastinal widening or adenopathy.
2. CT scan if chest x-ray is negative.
3. Biopsy to discover histology of lesion.
   A. Lymph node
   B. Via bronchoscopy, thoracotomy, mediastinoscopy

MANAGEMENT/TREATMENT

1. Refer to radiation oncology for treatment. ACNP may co-manage symptoms with oncologist and radiation oncologist.
2. In quickly progressing acute SVCS, radiation to the mediastinum may begin without tissue diagnosis, but this is a rare exception.
3. With more slowly progressing SVCS, a tissue diagnosis is obtained and the underlying disease is treated initially: Type of chemotherapy depends on the underlying malignancy.
4. Patients with good prognosis and chronic or recurrent SVCS may require surgical approach with SVC bypass graft and stent placement.
5. Maintenance of adequate airway by positioning patient with head elevated and avoidance of invasive or constrictive procedures involving upper extremities.
6. Resolution of symptoms should occur within 1–3 days of start of syndrome when radiation or chemotherapy has begun.
7. More than 50% have either partial or complete response to treatment.

PATIENT EDUCATION

1. Instruct patient to position with head of bed elevated to allay anxiety and maximize breathing.
2. Reassure that alterations in appearance will resolve with successful treatment.

ACUTE TUMOR LYSIS SYNDROME

DEFINITION

Acute tumor lysis syndrome (ATLS) occurs when a large number of rapidly proliferating cells are lysed, releasing their intracellular minerals and uric acid into the blood, causing acute hyperuricemia, hyperkalemia, hyperphosphatemia, and hypocalcemia with or without acute renal failure. ATLS is an oncologic emergency.

ETIOLOGY/INCIDENCE

1. Most commonly seen in patients with high-grade lymphomas or ALL.
    A. Rapidly growing tumors are treated with chemotherapy or radiation therapy.
    B. As cells die and lyse, large amounts of intracellular electrolytes and chemicals enter the bloodstream.
2. ATLS may also occur without treatment, when massive, rapidly growing and dividing tumors themselves break down and undergo profound cell destruction.
3. When the cell membrane is ruptured, released nucleic acids are converted by the liver into uric acid, while potassium and phosphorus are released into the bloodstream, causing high levels of these and a decrease in calcium.
4. The degree of metabolic abnormality depends on the adequacy of renal function.
5. Precipitation of uric acid and/or crystallization of calcium phosphorus in the renal tubules can cause acute renal failure.

SIGNS AND SYMPTOMS

1. Hyperkalemia
    A. Weakness
    B. Paresthesias
    C. Muscle cramps
    D. Diarrhea
    E. Nausea
2. Hyperphosphatemia
    A. Oliguria
    B. Anuria
3. Hypocalcemia
    A. Muscle twitching
    B. Tetany
    C. Paresthesias
    D. Convulsions

4. Hyperuricemia
   A. Nausea, vomiting, diarrhea
   B. Lethargy
   C. Flank pain
   D. Hematuria
   E. Oliguria
   F. Anuria

PHYSICAL FINDINGS

1. Hyperkalemia
   A. Bradycardia
   B. Muscle weakness
   C. Flaccid paralysis
2. Hyperphosphatemia
   A. Oliguria
   B. Anuria
3. Hypocalcemia
   A. Twitching
   B. Tetany
   C. Arrhythmias
4. Hyperuricemia
   A. Oliguria
   B. Anuria
   C. Lethargy

DIFFERENTIAL DIAGNOSIS

1. Hyperkalemia alone
2. Hyperphosphatemia alone
3. Hypocalcemia alone
4. Hyperuricemia alone
5. Acute renal failure due to other causes
6. Brain metastases
7. Syndrome of inappropriate secretion of antidiuretic hormone (SIADH)

DIAGNOSTIC TESTS/FINDINGS

1. Increased potassium (>5 mEq/L)
2. Increased phosphorus (>2.6 mEq/L)
3. Increased uric acid (>8 mg/dL)
4. Decreased calcium (<9 mg/dL)
5. Possibly increased BUN and creatinine
6. Electrocardiogram: Possible bradycardia, ventricular arrhythmias, heart block

MANAGEMENT/TREATMENT

Oncologic emergencies should be referred to the physician for diagnostic work-up and treatment plan. The ACNP may be part of the management in close collaboration with the oncologist.

1. Prophylaxis
   A. For patients at risk, prevention with vigorous hydration for 1–2 days prior to chemotherapy; continue for several days after chemotherapy to decrease uric acid concentration in the urine and enhance renal excretion.
      1) Maintain urine output of at least 100 mL/hr.
      2) Monitor fluid balance by assessing intake and output, weight, observing for edema.
   B. Diuretics such as furosemide (Lasix), along with IV hydration, induce diuresis and cause excretion of potassium and phosphorus: Monitor electrolytes carefully; may need to replace magnesium or potassium if deficits appear.
   C. Allopurinol 300 mg PO qd used to decrease uric acid concentration and prevent acute renal failure.
2. Treatment
   A. Renal failure may still occur despite these measures, especially in patients with pre-existing renal compromise.
   B. Add an alkaline diuresis with 5% dextrose IV + 50–100 mEq of sodium bicarbonate per liter; maintain urine pH at 7 or greater.
      1) As urine becomes more alkaline, uric acid becomes more soluble, decreasing precipitation and stone formation.
      2) Complications include increased calcium phosphate deposits in renal tubules and exacerbation of hypocalcemia.
   C. If all measures fail to increase urine output, hemodialysis may be used.
   D. Hyperkalemia is managed by restricting potassium and avoiding pharmacologic agents that cause potassium retention. Kayexelate may be used to decrease potassium as well.
   E. Hyperphosphatemia is managed by limiting dietary phosphate and administering oral phosphate-binding antacids (aluminum hydroxide 30–60 ml PO q4–6h).
   F. Hypocalcemia is best managed by lowering the serum phosphate level.
   G. The occurrence and resolution of ATLS is dependent on the tumor's responsiveness to cytotoxic therapy.
   H. ATLS usually resolves within 7 days following treatment, but may recur.

PATIENT EDUCATION

1. Inform high-risk patients of the syndrome, including signs and symptoms as well as treatment.
2. Reassure patient that ATLS is treatable and usually resolves as the tumor responds to therapy.
3. Explain the need for close monitoring, careful intake and output, and reporting of symptoms.

Review Questions

9.37 A patient who is being treated for breast cancer with chemotherapy is admitted with a fever of 101°F. She reports that her last chemotherapy treatment was given 1 week ago. She complains of increased fatigue, decreased appetite, mouth sores, and mild nausea. Further review of systems is negative. The ACNP finds that her physical exam is significant for fever and erythematous ulcers on the oropharynx. She is considered neutropenic if her absolute neutrophil count is:

A. <3000
B. <2000
C. <1500
D. <1000

9.38 This patient is found to have an ANC of 800. The ACNP would order all of the following diagnostic studies for this patient EXCEPT:

A. Chest x-ray
B. Urinalysis and urine culture
C. Two sets of blood cultures
D. Lumbar puncture

9.39 When the diagnostic work-up has been completed on this patient, the ACNP should:

A. Wait for culture results, then treat as indicated
B. Begin empiric antibiotic coverage with a β-lactam and an aminoglycoside antibiotic
C. Begin empiric antibiotic coverage with two β-lactam antibiotics and an antifungal agent
D. Begin empiric antibiotic coverage with an aminoglycoside antibiotic

9.40 The ACNP could order any of the following antibiotics for this febrile neutropenic woman EXCEPT:

A. Azetreonam + ceftazidime
B. Gentamycin + piperacillin
C. Imipenum
D. Tobramycin

9.41 The most common sites of infection in a patient with febrile neutropenia include all of the following EXCEPT:

A. Respiratory tract
B. Gastrointestinal tract
C. Heart
D. Genitourinary system

9.42 A 22-year-old man is admitted with newly diagnosed ALL. The ACNP knows that this patient is at risk for which of the following oncologic emergencies?

A. SVCS
B. SIADH
C. ATLS
D. Cardiac tamponade

9.43 All of the following are true in reference to ATLS except:

A. Patients with rapidly multiplying tumors are at highest risk for this syndrome.
B. The major threat is a rapid increase in serum potassium.
C. Patients at risk should be well hydrated and be receiving allopurinol before starting chemotherapy.
D. All cancer patients are at risk for ATLS.

9.44 A 66-year-old man with lung cancer presents to the ER with shortness of breath, facial edema, trunk and upper extremity edema, neck and chest vein distention, cough, hoarseness, and stridor. The ACNP suspects which oncologic emergency?

A. Cardiac tamponade
B. SVCS
C. DIC
D. Spinal cord compression

9.45 The ACNP consults with the patient's oncologist for a treatment plan for this patient. The initial plan might include all of the following except:
A. Treatment of underlying disease with chemotherapy
B. Radiation therapy to the mediastinum
C. Close monitoring of cardiopulmonary status
D. Surgical SVC bypass graft

Answers and Rationales

9.37　**D**　Neutropenia is commonly defined as an absolute neutrophil count of <1000 cells/mm^3.

9.38　**D**　Lumbar puncture is usually done only if CNS source is suspected, and this patient had no signs or symptoms of CNS involvement. The other studies are done routinely, even if no urinary tract or respiratory tract symptoms are noted.

9.39　**B**　Empiric coverage must begin immediately following a fever work-up in a neutropenic patient. Current recommendations for antibiotic coverage include either two β-lactams or a β-lactum and an aminoglycoside. Addition of a third drug has not been shown to increase efficacy.

9.40　**D**　Tobramycin does not provide broad enough coverage by itself; febrile neutropenia requires the addition of a broad-spectrum β-lactam to an aminoglycoside. However, imipenum does provide broad coverage and can be used as a single agent.

9.41　**C**　The heart is not a common site of infection in the neutropenic patient. Other common sites include the skin and mucous membranes and the central nervous system.

9.42　**C**　ALL is a rapidly growing and dividing tumor that is extremely chemosensitive. When this patient is treated with aggressive induction chemotherapy, the destruction and lysis of large numbers of tumor cells put him at risk for ATLS.

9.43　**D**　Patients who are receiving cytotoxic therapy for tumors with rapid growth, not all cancer patients, are at risk for ATLS.

9.44　**B**　The symptoms are caused by elevated venous pressure and congestion. Although some of these signs may be seen with cardiac tamponade, they are the classic signs seen with SVCS.

9.45　**D**　Surgical approaches are reserved for patients with good prognosis who have chronic or recurrent superior vena cava syndrome and have exhausted other treatment options. Surgery is not a first line of therapy.

References

DeVita, V.T., Hellman, S., & Rosenberg, S.A. (1993). *Cancer: Principles and Practice of Oncology* (4th ed.). Philadelphia: J.B. Lippincott Co.

Fisher, D.S., Knobf, M.T., & Durivage, H.T. (1993). *Cancer Chemotherapy Handbook* (4th ed.). St. Louis: C.V. Mosby Co.

Gross, J., & Johnson, B.L. (1994). *Handbook of Oncology Nursing* (2nd ed.). St. Louis: C.V. Mosby Co.

Groenwald, S.L., Frogge, M.H., Goodman, M., et al. (1995) *Comprehensive Cancer Nursing Review* (2nd ed.). Boston: Jones and Bartlett Publishers.

McCorkle, R., Grant, M., Frank-Stromborg, M., et al. (1996). *Cancer Nursing: A Comprehensive Textbook* (2nd ed.). Philadelphia: W.B. Saunders Co.

Murphy, G.P., Lawrence, W., & Lenhard, R.E. (1995). *American Cancer Society Textbook of Clinical Oncology* (2nd ed.). Atlanta: American Cancer Society.

Varricchio, C. (1997). *A Cancer Sourcebook for Nurses* (7th ed.). Atlanta: American Cancer Society.

CHAPTER 10

Gastrointestinal Disorders

Cydney G. Hirsch, RN, MN, CS-ANP, CCRN
Deborah Caswell, RN, MN, ANP-C, CCRN

Bowel Ischemia

DEFINITION

Bowel ischemia is defined as focal or widespread necrosis of the small or large intestine as a result of a critical decrease in blood and oxygen supply to the mesentery. This can be due to an acute or chronic process.

ETIOLOGY/INCIDENCE

1. Bowel ischemia accounts for approximately 0.1% of all hospital admissions.
2. Decrease in incidence of nonocclusive ischemia may be due to increased use of systemic vasodilators, such as nitrates and calcium channel blockers.
3. Mortality of bowel ischemia is 70–90% despite advances in medical diagnosis and treatment.
4. Occurs most often in patients more than 50 years of age with systemic and/or cardiovascular disease.
5. Patients at increased risk are those with history of cardiac arrythmias, especially atrial fibrillation, recent transmural myocardial infarction, or previous peripheral arterial embolization. The elderly population are at increased risk from any disease process that leads to third spacing with hypovolemia and hypoperfusion.
5. Arterial thrombosis has the poorest survival rate (5%).
6. Approximately 40% of acute ischemic events are caused by emboli; 50% are associated with low flow states and arterial thrombosis; and 10% or fewer are due to venous occlusion.

PATHOPHYSIOLOGY

1. Arterial blood is supplied to the bowel by the celiac, superior mesenteric, and inferior mesenteric arteries. The superior mesenteric artery (SMA) is the main blood supply to the bowel. Occlusion of the celiac and/or inferior mesenteric is well tolerated if supply to the superior mesenteric artery is not

compromised. Occlusion of the superior mesenteric artery results is bowel ischemia and death. A gradual decrease in the flow of blood through the SMA allows adequate collateral formation.

2. Acute mesenteric ischemia is caused by sudden termination or marked reduction of flow in the SMA, which produces extensive bowel necrosis. Mortality increases rapidly if therapy is delayed longer than 12 hours after onset of symptoms and approaches 100% by 48 hours.
   A. Occlusive ischemia results in sudden termination of flow to the SMA that is due to embolization from a remote source or by spontaneous primary thrombosis of atherosclerotic vessel. Most common contributing factors are atrial fibrillation, prosthetic cardiac valves, atherosclerosis, and hypercoagulable states.
   B. Nonocclusive ischemia is also known as low-flow ischemia. This commonly occurs in critically ill patients with compromised cardiac output or who are receiving vasoconstrictive medications, and is characterized by progressive ischemia of the intestine that leads to infarction, sepsis, and septic shock. Reflects mesenteric vasospasm in response to systemic hypoperfusion in an attempt to shunt blood to maintain cerebral and cardiac circulation.
   C. Mechanism of injury from acute mesenteric ischemia is poorly understood. It is thought that a portion of injury occurs during the period of ischemia, with further damage occurring during the period of restored blood flow. Re-perfusion results in vascular damage as well as distant tissue injury, encouraging multisystem organ failure.
3. Chronic mesenteric ischemia is almost always caused by an atherosclerotic process involving three proximal visceral arteries, all of which must be involved to produce symptoms. There is usually no threat to viability of bowel, but inadequate flow is unable to sufficiently perfuse bowel. This is also known as intestinal angina.
4. Colonic ischemia results from a sudden fall in the blood supply from either iatrogenic causes or spontaneous occlusion.
   A. Iatrogenic causes are usually the result of ligation of the inferior mesenteric artery during aortic aneurysmectomy or aortic replacement for occlusive atherosclerotic disease. When this occurs, ischemia usually progresses to frank gangrene.
   B. Spontaneous occlusion has uncertain etiology, although it is thought to involve low colonic flow. Changes produced are transient and reversible.

SIGNS AND SYMPTOMS

1. Acute abdominal pain is the only consistent finding. Pain varies in severity, nature, and location.
2. Acute ischemia
   A. Patients appear seriously ill.
   B. Condition is characterized by sudden onset of severe, unrelenting abdominal pain that is often out of proportion to the physical signs and is unrelieved by narcotics. Pain is usually severe periumbilical that begins poorly localized and visceral, progresses to severe, unrelenting pain.
   C. Vomiting is present in 50–75% of patients, diarrhea in 25–40%. Reflects forceful gut emptying in response to continuing ischemia.
3. Chronic mesenteric ischemia
   A. Predominant symptom is postprandial pain that is crampy in nature

and occurs 15–30 minutes after meals and may last hours. May cause "food fear" to avoid pain.
  B. Weight loss is common and often significant. May be presenting symptom.
  C. Food fear may be present.
  D. Other signs of atherosclerotic disease may be evident.
  4. Colonic ischemia
  A. Clinical presentation may vary greatly, especially in the early stages of disease. Patients do not appear ill.
  B. Presentation is characterized by mild, crampy pain in the left lower quadrant with tenderness and some guarding.
  C. May present with rectal bleeding or diarrhea.

PHYSICAL FINDINGS

1. Bowel sounds vary depending on extent of bowel affected. Hyperactive bowel sounds may be heard early in acute ischemia.
2. Tenderness to palpation over abdomen may be only mild or diffuse. Guarding and other signs of peritoneal irritation may be present if peritonitis or necrosis is present.
3. Abdominal bruit is heard in 60–85% of patients with chronic mesenteric ischemia.
4. Occult blood detected in stool in 75% of patients.
5. In acute ischemia the vital signs may be normal initially. Tachycardia may be present but is not helpful in making diagnosis.
6. Progression of disease process results in systemic manifestations of sepsis and septic shock. Presence of localized tenderness and rigidity usually indicates infarction has occurred.

DIFFERENTIAL DIAGNOSIS

1. Gastroenteritis
2. Pneumonia
3. Appendicitis
4. Inflammatory bowel disease
5. Pancreatitis
6. Systemic lupus erythematosus
7. Cholecystitis
8. Diverticulitis
9. Abdominal aortic aneurysm
10. Myocardial infarction
11. Black widow spider bite
12. Ectopic pregnancy
13. Peptic ulcer disease
14. Intestinal obstruction
15. Blunt abdominal trauma

DIAGNOSTIC TESTS/FINDINGS

1. Leukocytosis is present in more than 90% of patients, often exceeding 20,000/mm^3. A predominance of immature cells is characteristic. Elderly patients may not present with elevation.

2. Metabolic acidosis is common. Approximately 50% of patients will have significant uncompensated metabolic acidosis.
3. Electrolytes may reflect acidosis, hypovolemia, malnutrition.
4. Mild hyperamylasemia is noted in 25–50% of patients, as well as elevated transaminases as a result of intestinal infarction.
5. Radiology plain films are indicated to exclude other causes of abdominal pain. Radiographic findings may be interpreted as abnormal in up to 75% of patients but are rarely diagnostic of acute visceral ischemia. Nearly 50% of patients with acute visceral ischemia present with a pattern interpreted as consistent with mechanical small bowel obstruction. Other findings may range from "thumb printing" from extramural edema or hemorrhage to pneumatosis or portal vein gas.
6. Mesenteric arteriography is procedure of choice and should be obtained as soon as bowel ischemia is suspected. Arteriography will define site and type of occlusion.
   A. "Meniscus" sign located 4–6 cm from origin of superior mesenteric artery is the classic angiographic finding in mesenteric arterial occlusion resulting from embolus.
   B. Acute mesenteric ischemia resulting from venous occlusion is diagnosis frequently made by inference. Findings are reflux of contrast into aorta, opacification of few peripheral arteries, intense opacification of the thickened bowel wall, and no evidence of mesenteric portal-venous system.
   C. Nonocclusive mesenteric ischemia findings include arterial narrowing with slow filling of distal branches, regular abrupt tapering of arterial branches, and diffuse arterial spasm.
   D. Chronic mesenteric ischemia angiographic findings include obstructive lesions of both the celiac and axis and superior mesenteric artery.
7. Computed tomography (CT) scan will demonstrate portal and main superior mesenteric venous thrombosis.

MANAGEMENT/TREATMENT

1. Surgical consult is mandatory for all patients suspected of having mesenteric ischemia or infarction.
2. Hospital admission is necessary. Goal of therapy for acute occlusion is rapid resuscitation and prompt operation. Specific attention should be placed on increasing cardiac output and oxygen delivery.
3. Eliminate all agents that cause mesenteric vasoconstriction.
4. Patients must receive nothing by mouth (be NPO) in preparation for surgical procedure.
5. Prompt intravenous fluid hydration is indicated to replace fluid losses resulting from vomiting, diarrhea, or third spacing.
6. Nasogastric tube is indicated if patient is vomiting or has signs of peritonitis, and/or in preparation for surgery.
7. Oxygen indicated to increase oxygen delivery to tissues.
8. Antibiotics are indicated if peritonitis or sepsis is present. Preoperative antibiotic is necessary if patient is going to emergency surgery. Antibiotic should be broad-spectrum antibiotic that covers gram-negative rods and anaerobic bacteria (i.e., piperacillin sodium/tazobactam sodium [Zosyn] 3.375 gm IV q6h).
9. Vasodilator therapy has been shown to improve survival in patients with nonocclusive disease. Intra-arterial therapy: injection into the superior mesenteric artery of vasodilators (60 mg papaverine or 25 mg tolazoline bolus followed by 0.75–1.0 mg/min continuous infusion of papaverine).

10. Anticoagulation recommended following surgical intervention for ischemic bowel. Heparin infusion titrated to keep partial thromboplastin time (PTT) two times normal in the immediate postoperative period, followed by warfarin titrated to keep International Normalized Ratio (INR) of 2.0–3.0 for up to 6 months.

PATIENT EDUCATION

1. Teach patient/family disease course and expected outcome.
2. As patient may be critically ill, family must be included in any and all teaching/discussions and decisions.
3. Preoperative teaching should include procedure, time factors, postoperative expectations regarding pain, level of consciousness, activity.
4. Medication teaching should include purpose, dosage, side effects, toxic effects, and length of time drug will be required.
5. Dietary precautions should be taught for patients on long-term anticoagulation.

Review Questions

10.1 A 72-year-old male patient is admitted to the emergency department with complaints of sudden onset, severe abdominal pain. He denies smoking history, peptic ulcer disease, diabetes mellitus, and renal failure. Past medical history includes atrial fibrillation, for which he takes digitalis; congestive heart failure; and colon cancer, for which he had colectomy 2 years prior. His vital signs are stable except for tachycardia of 132 bpm. Moderate abdominal tenderness to palpation with no rigidity or guarding. No abdominal distention present; hyperactive bowel sounds present. The next diagnostic/treatment intervention to take would be:
A. Draw blood for complete blood count (CBC) with differential, arterial blood gas, electrolytes, phosphorus, aspartate aminotransferase (AST), alanine transaminase (ALT), amylase, lactate dehydrogenase (LDH) and alkaline phosphatase
B. CT scan with contrast, CBC, electrolytes
C. Increase IV pain medications and obtain patient-controlled analgesia with morphine sulfate; surgical consult
D. Obtain CBC with differential, start dopamine 5 μg/kg/min, start cefoxitin 2 gm IVPB q6h, type and cross six units packed red blood cells

10.2 Laboratory results show leukocytosis of 16,000 with 92 lymphocytes. Transaminases are slightly elevated. Abdominal pain is becoming more severe, is unrelieved by narcotics. Arterial blood gas shows a moderate, uncompensated metabolic alkalosis. Given the patient's history and presenting symptoms, the diagnostic test of choice would be:
A. X-ray of kidney, ureter, bladder (KUB)
B. Spiral CT scan to differentiate soft tissue versus intraperitoneal fluid collection, abscess
C. Angiography
D. Endoscopy

10.3 The most likely diagnosis for this patient, given the history and symptoms thus far, is:
   A. Severe diverticulitis
   B. Acute mesenteric ischemia
   C. Perforated peptic ulcer
   D. Ruptured abdominal aortic aneurysm

10.4 The decision is made to take the patient to emergency surgery. The preoperative antibiotic of choice would be:
   A. Zosyn 3.375 mg IV
   B. Ancef 1 gm
   C. Ciprofloxacin 400 mg IV
   D. Neomycin 12 gm PO for bowel sterilization

10.5 A patient presents to a clinic with a history of 30-lb weight loss over the last year. Past medical history is significant for 30-pack-year smoking history, type II diabetes, myocardial infarction 5 years ago. Medications include glipizide, Cardizem, Lasix, amitriptyline, diazepam, and Pravachol. She states she does not eat "because after I eat I have really bad pain in my stomach." During the physical examination, special attention should be placed on:
   A. Oral examination because of smoking history and increased incidence of carries associated with diabetes
   B. Assessment of pulmonary status with forced expiratory volume because of known correlation between weight loss and pulmonary carcinoma.
   C. Funduscopic examination checking for arteriovenous nicking and cotton wool spots
   D. Assessment of evidence of atherosclerotic disease

Answers and Rationales

10.1 **A** The CBC will indicate whether an infectious process is present and if significant blood loss has occurred, and may give some clue to the volume status. Arterial blood gas will assist in the diagnosis of mesenteric ischemia and will reveal the elevation of transaminases. CT scan with contrast is not indicated at this point. Pain may be controlled but should be delayed until after the physical examination. There is no need to start vasopressor medication because there is not yet hypotension. Dopamine may not be the vasopressor of choice because of history of heart disease. Type and cross would be indicated if the patient was bleeding or if surgery was anticipated; however, it is too early in the diagnostic process to make that decision.

10.2 **C** The history of atrial fibrillation, sudden-onset abdominal pain that is severe, essentially negative abdominal exam, leukocytosis, and metabolic acidosis make acute mesenteric ischemia the probable diagnosis. The definitive diagnostic tool for this pathology is angiographic examination. KUB is likely to provide information that there is a pathologic process going on in the gut; however, most often mesenteric ischemia may be seen as bowel obstruction. If the working diagnosis is mesenteric ischemia, the diagnostic process should not be held up by nondiagnostic tests. Spiral CT may assist in showing venous thrombosis of the mesentery but is not considered first line for acute mesenteric ischemia. There is no indication for endoscopy in mesenteric ischemia.

10.3 **B** Given the patient's history and symptoms, acute mesenteric ischemia is the most likely diagnosis (see rationale for question 2).

10.4 **A** Zosyn is a broad-spectrum antibiotic that is effective on enteric pathogens, specifically gram-negative rods and anaerobes. Ancef, a first-generation cephalosporin, is not effective for anaerobe coverage. The quinolone antibiotics such as Cipro also have poor anaerobic coverage. There is no place in the management of acute mesenteric ischemia for neomycin.

10.5 **D** The triad of symptoms associated with chronic mesenteric ischemia is weight loss, intestinal angina, and presence of atherosclerotic occlusive disease elsewhere (e.g., peripheral vascular, cerebrovascular, cardiovascular).

References

Briones, T. (1991). The gastrointestinal system. In G. Alspach, (ed.). *American Association of Critical Care Nurses Core Curriculum for Critical Care Nursing*. Philadelphia: W.B. Saunders Co., pp. 748–828.

Bugliosi, T., Meloy, T., & Vukov, L. (1990). Acute abdominal pain in the elderly. *Ann Emerg Med 19*, 1383.

Ekers, M. (1988). Mesenteric ischemia. In V. Fahey, (ed.). *Vascular Nursing*. Philadelphia: W.B. Saunders Co., pp. 331–341.

Hansen, K. (1996). Mesenteric ischemia syndromes. In R. Dean, J. Yao, & D. Brewster (eds.). *Current Diagnosis and Treatment in Vascular Surgery*. Norwalk, CT: Appleton & Lange., pp. 263–275.

McQuaid, K. (1996). Alimentary tract. In L. Tierney, S. McPhee, & M. Papadakis (eds.). *Current Medical Diagnosis and Treatment*. Stamford, CT: Appleton & Lange.

Intestinal Obstruction

DEFINITION

Intestinal obstruction can be partial or complete and exist when there is a failure, reversal, or impairment of the normal passage of intestinal contents.

ETIOLOGY/INCIDENCE

1. Most common cause of intestinal obstruction is adhesions, almost exclusively in postoperative patients.
2. Hernias, whether internal (inguinal, femoral, umbilical, ventral, incisional) or external (abdominal wall), can cause obstruction. Strangulation of hernia is surgical emergency.
3. Neoplasms can cause obstruction but usually have primary origin from intra-abdominal site, such as colon, pancreas, stomach, or gynecologic site.
4. Other causes include intussusception, volvulus, gallstones, foreign body, bezoar, inflammatory bowel disease, intestinal worms, traumatic injury, radiation injury.

5. Large bowel obstruction is most commonly due to cancer of the colon or volvulus. Partial obstruction can be caused by diverticulitis.
6. Intestinal obstruction accounts for approximately 20% of all admissions for acute abdominal conditions.
7. Risk factors for intestinal obstruction include previous abdominal surgery, hernia, chronic constipation, diverticular disease.

SIGNS AND SYMPTOMS

1. Cramping periumbilical pain occurs initially at intervals lasting a few seconds to a few minutes. This progresses to constant, diffuse pain as distention develops.
2. Vomiting follows onset of pain. Timing dependent on location of obstruction. Proximal obstruction will result in vomiting within minutes of onset of pain; vomiting will follow onset of pain by hours in distal obstruction.
3. Obstipation soon develops, although initially may pass contents distal to obstruction.
4. Abdominal distention is minimal in proximal obstruction but may be pronounced in distal obstruction.

PHYSICAL FINDINGS

1. Mild tenderness is present. Mass may be palpable. Rigidity, severe tenderness is suggestive of strangulation or perforation. Mass may be seen in femoral or inguinal area, suggesting incarcerated or strangulated hernia.
2. Abdominal distention may be present as above.
3. Bowel sounds may be high pitched, tinkling with peristaltic rushes.
4. Visible peristalsis may be noted.
5. Occult or gross fecal blood may be present.
6. Dehydration may be evident with continued vomiting and intraluminal loss of fluids.
7. Fever is suggestive of strangulation or perforation.

DIFFERENTIAL DIAGNOSIS

1. Adynamic ileus
2. Chronic intestinal pseudo-obstruction
3. Pancreatitis
4. Acute gastroenteritis
5. Appendicitis
6. Acute mesenteric ischemia

DIAGNOSTIC TESTS/FINDINGS

1. Leukocytosis may be present. Significant increase indicates perforation or strangulation. Hematocrit may be elevated as a result of dehydration.
2. Electrolytes may reflect dehydration.
3. Laboratory tests are of no diagnostic value generally.
4. Supine and upright plain films of abdomen demonstrate dilated loops of bowel and air-fluid levels in a ladder-like pattern. Free air beneath the diaphragm is an ominous sign indicating bowel perforation.
5. Barium enema may be used in cases in which there is uncertainty about

the diagnosis; barium will confirm the presence and location of small bowel obstruction.

MANAGEMENT/TREATMENT

1. Surgical consult is indicated because nearly all complete obstructions require surgical intervention.
2. Nasogastric tube is indicated for decompression and to relieve vomiting.
3. Isotonic fluids should be given intravenously for rehydration and to correct electrolyte disorders (i.e., normal saline with 10–20 mEq of potassium to run at 75–100 mL/hr).
4. Consider use of antibiotics that cover gram-positive, gram-negative, and anaerobic organisms in the perioperative period (e.g., cefoxitin 1 gm IV q6h).
5. Patient should be maintained NPO.
6. Use of cathartics or gastrointestinal stimulants are contraindicated because they may result in perforation.

PATIENT EDUCATION

1. Inform patient of interventions, purpose, and duration.
2. Teach patient cause of disease, onset, course, and prognosis: Perforation leads to life-threatening infection and surgery may be necessary to repair.
3. If partial bowel resection is necessary, ostomy may have to be performed with reanastomosis at a later date.
4. If ostomy is necessary, teach patient care, purpose, duration, and danger signs to watch for.
5. Teach drug, dosage, purpose, frequency, side effects, signs of toxicity if patient is to be discharged on medication.

Review Questions

10.6   The most common risk factor for occurrence of bowel obstruction is:
   A. Acute gastroenteritis with severe vomiting
   B. History of abdominal surgical intervention
   C. Chronic constipation
   D. Barium enema

10.7   A 59-year-old male patient presents complaining of severe, crampy abdominal pain that is intermittent but becoming more frequent and seems to be occurring in waves. Denies nausea, vomiting, diarrhea. He was discharged from the hospital 20 days ago after surgical treatment for diverticulitis. Physical examination reveals tender abdomen that is very distended. Your preliminary diagnosis is:
   A. Proximal bowel obstruction
   B. Recurrent diverticulitis
   C. Mesenteric ischemia
   D. Distal bowel obstruction

10.8   The test that will be most useful in confirming your diagnosis is:
   A. Arterial blood gas, which will reflect metabolic acidosis

B. Hematocrit, which will reflect chronic gastrointestinal (GI) blood loss
C. Supine and upright films of abdomen, which will reflect dilated loops of bowel and air-fluid levels in a ladder-like pattern
D. CT scan, which will show edematous changes in the bowel wall with mucosal thickening

10.9 The patient suddenly develops nausea with vomiting; rigid, exquisitely tender abdomen, and fever. You suspect which of the following has happened?
A. Your preliminary diagnosis was wrong and the patient actually had acute gastroenteritis
B. The patient is developing signs of peritonitis; you suspect bowel perforation has occurred and you call a surgical consult stat
C. The patient's diverticulitis has flared up again; give him some morphine for pain
D. The patient had irritable bowel syndrome and needs psychological support

10.10 A 36-year-old male construction worker was admitted from the emergency room (ER) with abdominal pain and distention that began about 12 hours ago. He began vomiting about 6 hours prior to presentation. He denies nausea, diarrhea, fever. He has severe tenderness to palpation. Physical examination reveals no surgical scars on abdomen, mass noted in scrotum that is painful to palpation. Most likely diagnosis and treatment for this patient is:
A. Diverticulitis; treat with bowel rest, cefoxitin 1 gm IV q6h
B. Mesenteric infarction, which is a surgical emergency: surgical consult stat
C. Fulminant ulcerative colitis; treat with IV hydration, methylprednisolone 20 mg IV tid, imipenem 500 mg IV q6h
D. Incarcerated inguinal hernia; surgical consult is needed if hernia is not reducible

---

Answers and Rationales

10.6 **B** History of recent abdominal surgical intervention is indicative of obstruction resulting from adhesions from postoperative scarring, most common cause of bowel obstruction.
10.7 **D** Distal bowel obstruction will cause early distention and late vomiting. Proximal obstruction will cause minimal or late distention with early vomiting.
10.8 **C** Metabolic acidosis would be a sign of bowel infarction. Hematocrit drop would reflect chronic GI blood loss, but there is no history of this mentioned. CT scan may be useful but is more expensive test when supine and upright films will usually confirm diagnosis.
10.9 **B** Abdominal rigidity, severe pain, and fever are signs of peritonitis, a surgical emergency.
10.10 **D** The patient has an inguinal hernia that has become incarcerated. If the hernia cannot be reduced, it will become strangulated, at which point it becomes a surgical emergency.

References

Dambro, M. (1996). *Griffith's 5 Minute Clinical Consultant.* Baltimore: Williams & Wilkins.

Gerbo, R. (1996). Small and large bowel obstruction. In R.E. Rakel (ed.). *Saunders Manual of Medical Practice.* Philadelphia: W.B. Saunders Co., pp. 337–338.

McQuaid, K. (1996). Alimentary tract. In L. Tierney, S. McPhee, & M. Papadakis (eds.). *Current Medical Diagnosis and Treatment.* Stamford, CT: Appleton & Lange, pp. 489–575.

Inflammatory Bowel Disease

Inflammatory bowel disease includes ulcerative colitis, Crohn's disease, and granulomatous colitis (Crohn's disease of the colon). Only ulcerative colitis and Crohn's disease are addressed in this portion of the chapter (Table 10–1).

ULCERATIVE COLITIS

DEFINITION

Ulcerative colitis is defined as idiopathic, diffuse inflammatory disease of the bowel mucosa characterized by inflammation and destruction; usually involves left colon.

ETIOLOGY/INCIDENCE

1. Can affect any age but typically begins in adolescence or young adulthood. Peak incidence is between 15 and 37.
2. Whites are affected most often, with highest prevalence in Jews.
3. Risk of disease is increased 10-fold by having first-degree relative with disease.
4. Exact etiology is unknown; thought to be idiopathic.
5. Rectum is involved most often, with inflammation extending proximally, and uninterrupted, for a variable distance.
6. Significant relationship between ulcerative colitis and cancer of the colon.

TABLE 10–1. **Major Differences Between Ulcerative Colitis and Crohn's Disease***

Extent of disease	Ulcerative Colitis	Crohn's Disease
	Mucosa	Entire wall
Ulceration	Extensive, superficial	Patchy, deep
Mesentery	Normal	Thickened
Granulomata	Absent	Present (25–75%)
Distribution	Symmetric	Eccentric
"Skip" areas	Never	Common
Diseased rectum	Always	10–20%
Small intestine disease	Never	Usual
Results of surgery	Cure	Frequent recurrence

* From Bullock, B., & Rosendahl, P. (1986). *Pathophysiology: Adaptations and Alterations in Function.* Boston: Little, Brown & Co., with permission.

PATHOPHYSIOLOGY

Ulcerative colitis begins as an inflammatory intestinal disorder affecting the mucosal lining of the colon and rectum. The chronic inflammatory process can cause diffuse bleeding throughout mucosa. As a result of chronic inflammation, the colon wall becomes thickened. The bowel fills with bloody mucoid stool that produces crampy pain, rectal urgency, and diarrhea. Approximately 50% of patients have disease confined to the rectosigmoid region (proctosigmoiditis); in 30% disease extend to the splenic flexure (left-sided colitis); and in fewer than 20% it extend more proximally (extensive colitis).

SIGNS AND SYMPTOMS

1. Cardinal symptoms are bloody diarrhea, lower abdominal cramps, and urgency.
2. Mild disease presents with:
   A. History of gradual onset of infrequent diarrhea (less than five stools/day) with intermittent rectal bleeding and mucus.
   B. Rectal inflammation leads to feeling of fecal urgency and tenesmus.
   C. Left lower quadrant cramps relieved by defecation are common.
3. Moderate disease presents with:
   A. Four to six loose stools per day with more frequent bleeding
   B. More severe diarrhea
4. Severe cases present with:
   A. Six to 10 bloody stools per day
   B. Fatigue, orthostatic dizziness
   C. Weight loss of greater than 10 lb
5. Extracolonic manifestations include:
   A. Arthritis or arthralgia
   B. Eye symptoms, including pain, blurred vision, photophobia
   C. Mouth sores
   D. Skin problems, redness, sores

PHYSICAL FINDINGS

1. Mild disease may include:
   A. Vital signs within normal range
   B. Laboratory values within normal range
   C. Mild tenderness to abdominal palpation
2. Moderate disease may include:
   A. Low-grade fever of 99–100°F; slight tachycardia
   B. Anemia with hematocrit between 30 and 40 mg/dL
   C. Sedimentation rate 20–30 mm/hr
   D. Albumin level 3–3.5 gm/dL
   E. Weight loss of <10 lb
   F. Mild to moderate tenderness to abdominal palpation
3. Severe disease may include:
   A. Severe anemia
   B. Hypovolemia
   C. Impaired nutrition with hypoalbuminemia (<3.0 gm/dL)
   D. Fever >100°F; tachycardia >100 bpm
   E. Weight loss of >10 lb
   F. Abdominal pain and tenderness

   4. Stools contain blood, pus, or mucus
   5. Extracolonic manifestations:
     A. Scleral injection, uveitis
     B. Erythema nodosum or pyoderma gangrenosum
     C. Apthous ulcers of mouth
     D. Arthritis
     E. Jaundice, hepatomegaly, splenomegaly
     F. Hepatobiliary problems, such as sclerosing cholangitis
     G. Hematologic manifestations, such as iron-deficiency anemia, thrombosis

DIFFERENTIAL DIAGNOSIS

1. Irritable bowel syndrome
2. Crohn's disease
3. Ischemic colitis
4. Radiation colitis
5. Diverticulitis
6. Colon cancer
7. Infectious diarrhea
8. Infectious colitis; human immunodeficiency virus (HIV)-associated diarrhea
9. Gonorrhea, herpes, chlamydia, syphilis should be considered in the sexually active patient

DIAGNOSTIC TESTS/FINDINGS

1. CBC may show anemia of chronic blood loss; leukocytosis during exacerbation, elevated sedimentation rate are reflective of disease severity.
2. Electrolyte abnormalities may reflect hypokalemia, prerenal azotemia.
3. Stool studies show leukocytes, occult blood.
4. Proctosigmoidoscopy is most important diagnostic modality. Best performed without cleansing preparations so as not to distort the appearance of the bowel mucosa.
   A. Acute phase: The mucosa appears friable and inflamed with loss of normal vascular pattern, progression of disease leads to mucopus and erosions.
   B. Chronic phase of disease is characterized by granular mucosa and inflammatory pseudopolyps.
5. Colonoscopy should not be performed in patients with severe disease because of risk of perforation.
6. Plain abdominal radiographs in patient with severe colitis to look for significant colonic dilatation (sign of toxic megacolon).
7. Barium enema is useful in determining extent of involvement but may exacerbate the disease and should never be performed during acute or relapsing phase of the illness.
8. In chronic, longstanding disease, typical radiographic changes include shortening of the bowel, loss of haustra, narrowing of the lumen, and rigidity.

MANAGEMENT/TREATMENT

1. No specific therapy available for ulcerative colitis. Goal of management is symptom relief and suppression of inflammation. Without therapy, 75% of patients will have a disease relapse.

2. Mild to moderate attacks
   A. Eat a regular diet with restrictions on caffeine and gas-producing vegetables.
   B. Fiber supplements decrease diarrhea and rectal symptoms (psyllium 3.4 gm bid or methylcellulose 2 gm tid).
   C. Antidiarrheal agents such as loperamide 2 mg or diphenoxylate with atropine 1 tablet may be given up to four times daily. These are particularly useful at night or when taken prophylactically for occasions when patients may not have reliable access to toilet facilities.
   D. Disease extending above the sigmoid colon is best treated with oral agents. Sulfasalazine 500 mg bid, increase gradually over 1–2 weeks to 1.5–2 gm bid. Mesalamine 800 mg tid can be used for patients who are unable to tolerate sulfasalazine.
   E. Patients who fail to improve on this therapy should be started on topical therapy with hydrocortisone foam or enemas (80–100 mg bid) as first therapy. Prednisone 20–30 mg qd is utilized if topical therapy fails to improve after 2 weeks.
   F. Steroids may be tapered after 2 weeks, tapering no more than 5 mg/wk.
3. Severe attacks
   A. Admit to hospital for stabilization and treatment.
   B. No oral intake. Nutritionally depleted patients should be started on parenteral nutrition.
   C. Fluid volume resuscitation with crystalloid or blood products as appropriate. Electrolyte imbalances should be corrected as well. Isotonic saline with added electrolytes can be used for initial replacement.
   D. Methylprednisolone IV, 20–30 mg tid or as continuous infusion over 24 hours.
   E. Hydrocortisone enema, 100 mg over 30 minutes bid administered as a drip.
   F. Intravenous antibiotics with suitable coverage for gram-negative rods and anaerobes should be instituted. Zosyn 3.375 gm IV q6h or ceftizoxime 2 gm IV q6h may be used.
   G. Frequent abdominal examinations are necessary to look for evidence of worsening distention or pain.
   H. Plain abdominal radiograph on admission to look for evidence of colonic dilation.
   I. Stool specimens should be sent for bacterial culture and ova and parasite exam.
   J. Observe for signs of toxic megacolon or fulminate colitis. These include:
      1) History of fulminant course with rapid progression of symptoms over 1–2 weeks.
      2) Appear very ill with hypovolemia, hemorrhage requiring transfusion.
      3) Abdominal distention with tenderness.
      4) Toxic megacolon is characterized by colonic dilation of more than 6 cm on plain films with signs of toxicity.
   K. Nasogastric tube for decompression may be needed, especially in the case of fulminant colitis or toxic megacolon.
   L. Obtain gastroenterology and surgical consult on all patients with severe disease or evidence of fulminant colitis or toxic megacolon.
4. Surgery is performed on 25% of patients. Indications for surgery include hemorrhage, perforation, documented carcinoma, fulminant colitis, or toxic megacolon that does not improve within 48–72 hours; high-grade dysplasia;

and in refractory disease requiring steroids to manage symptoms. Surgical options include:

A. Total colectomy offers complete cure of bowel disease and remission of most peripheral symptoms.

B. Proctocolectomy with ileostomy is traditional procedure, being the safest and fastest. Disadvantages include presence of ileostomy with incontinence, stoma drainage management, skin excoriations, potential need for stoma revisions.

C. Total proctocolectomy with continent ileostomy (Koch pouch). Requires permanent ileostomy that does not require wearing appliance.

D. Total colectomy, rectal mucosectomy, ileal reservoir, and ileoanal anastomosis is attractive to younger patients with fecal incontinence because it provides an opportunity to retain continence and avoid a stoma.

5. Maintenance therapy

A. Do not use steroids as maintenance therapy.

B. Sulfasalazine 1–2 gm bid with folic acid 1 mg qd.

C. Olsalazine 500 mg bid is effective in patients who cannot tolerate sulfasalazine.

PATIENT EDUCATION

1. Pathophysiology and chronicity of disease: Ulcerative colitis is chronic disease with variable course. Aggravating and alleviating factors should be taught, with patient told to be aware of other factors in own disease course.

2. Excoriation of skin around perianal area may be a problem, especially if leakage is present. Protective barriers can be used in this case.

3. Diet teaching to avoid or limit intake of caffeine (including chocolate), gas-producing vegetables, carbonated beverages, high-fat foods, and lactose-containing foods. Patient should be alert to which food items increase symptoms.

4. Risk of colorectal cancer greatly increased. Follow-up testing should be part of yearly physical examination.

5. Pregnancy should be planned.

6. Medication purpose, dosage, side effects, signs of toxicity.

7. Frequent follow-up is needed in the early phases of illness both for close monitoring of disease progression and for psychological support.

8. Educational materials are available through Crohn's and Colitis Foundation of America, 386 Park Avenue South, 17th Floor, New York, NY 10016 (1-800-343-3637).

CROHN'S DISEASE

DEFINITION

Crohn's disease is chronic, relapsing disease of the alimentary tract (mouth to anus) manifested by discontinuous mucosal fissure ulcers, transmural inflammation, and often granulomas in the segment. Crohn's disease primarily involves the small intestine (usually terminal ileum) or large intestine, or both. Typically, the inflammation extends through all layers of gut wall and often involves mesentery and regional lymph nodes.

ETIOLOGY/INCIDENCE

1. Cause of disease is unknown but thought to be multifactorial.
2. Familial tendency, with 15% of patients having first-degree relative with disease. All monozygotic twins develop disease in similar sequence, severity.
3. Affinity for Caucasians, especially Jews.
4. Has environmental predisposition, with industrial areas having higher incidence and rapid increase.
5. Predominant age 15–25 years.
6. More common in females.
7. Most often the distal ileum and proximal colon are involved.
8. Colon disease present in 30% of patients; skip areas allow for differentiating from ulcerative colitis.
9. Regional enteritis present in 30% of patients that is associated with formation of strictures.
10. Smoking may be a risk factor. Prevalence of smokers is higher among patients with Crohn's disease than among those with ulcerative colitis.

PATHOPHYSIOLOGY

Crohn's disease is characterized by recurrent, nonspecific inflammation of the entire intestine. Process involves the mucosa and surrounding musculature. Terminal ileum is the most common site. Deep fissures form in the intestinal wall; bowel becomes congested, thickened, and rigid, with adhesions involving the peri-intestinal fat. Lymphoid dilations and deposits occur in all levels of bowel involvement. Functional disruption of the mucosa ensues. Large segment involvement can cause fluid imbalances. Crohn's disease has tendency to cause strictures, fistulas, and abscesses because the granulomatous inflammatory process may extend through all layers of the bowel wall.

SIGNS AND SYMPTOMS

1. Patients may present with a variety of symptoms as a result of variable location of involvement and severity of inflammation.
2. Clinician should take note of symptoms such as history of fever, presence of abdominal pain, general sense of well-being, number of liquid stools per day, and previous surgical history.
3. Characterized by intermittent bouts of diarrhea, low-grade fever, and colicky or steady abdominal pain located primarily in right lower quadrant; occur in approximately 80% of patients.
4. Will usually have periods of normal bowel function interspersed with periods of diarrhea.
5. Fatigue, weight loss, vomiting, perianal discomfort, and bleeding are also common complaints.
6. Constipation may be an early manifestation of obstruction.
7. Extracolonic manifestations include:
   A. Arthritis or arthralgia
   B. Eye symptoms, including pain, blurred vision, photophobia
   C. Mouth sores
   D. Skin problems, redness, sores

PHYSICAL FINDINGS

1. Some patients have no physical findings while others have highly variable findings.
2. Abdominal tenderness, particularly in right lower quadrant, along with diarrhea are cardinal symptoms, occurring in 80% of patients.
3. Chronic inflammatory disease presents with:
   A. Abdominal tenderness, especially in right lower quadrant
   B. May have mass, especially in right lower quadrant, that represents thickened or matted loops of inflamed intestine.
4. Disease may progress to include:
   A. Intestinal obstruction caused by narrowing of the small bowel as a result of inflammation, spasm, or fibrotic stenosis.
   B. Abdominal or perianal fistulas with purulent discharge are noted in about 10% of patients.
5. Fever not uncommon.
6. Extracolonic manifestations
   A. Scleral injection, uveitis
   B. Erythema nodosum or pyoderma gangrenosum (idiopathic, chronic, debilitating skin diseases associated with systemic disease; characterized by presence of irregular, boggy, blue-red ulcers with undermined borders surrounding purulent necrotic bases)
   C. Apthous ulcers of mouth; not as common as in ulcerative colitis
   D. Arthritis
   E. Jaundice, hepatomegaly, splenomegaly
   F. Hepatobiliary problems, such as sclerosing cholangitis
   G. Hematologic manifestations, such as iron-deficiency anemia, thrombosis

DIFFERENTIAL DIAGNOSIS

1. Ulcerative colitis
2. Ischemic colitis
3. Pseudomembranous colitis
4. Radiation colitis
5. Infectious colitis
6. Irritable bowel syndrome
7. Colorectal cancer
8. Hemorrhoids
9. Diverticulitis
10. Gastroenteritis
11. Appendicitis
12. Celiac disease

DIAGNOSTIC TESTS/FINDINGS

1. Poor correlation between laboratory studies and patient's clinical picture.
2. Complete blood count may show anemia of chronic illness, mucosal blood loss, iron-deficiency anemia, pernicious anemia, leukocytosis.
3. Sedimentation rate and C-reactive protein level are elevated in many patients during acute inflammatory stages.
4. Electrolytes, blood urea nitrogen (BUN), and creatinine may reflect metabolic acidosis, prerenal azotemia.

5. Albumin level may reflect intestinal protein loss, malabsorption, or chronic inflammation.
6. Liver function studies: Abnormal values would suggest sclerosing cholangitis.
7. Stool for leukocytes, routine pathogens, ova and parasites, *clostridium difficile*.
8. Colonoscopy to diagnose extent and severity of disease, to obtain biopsies, screen for colon cancer. Typical findings include ulcers, strictures, and segmental involvement with areas of normal-appearing mucosa interspersed with areas of inflammation.
9. Upper GI and small bowel series shows segmental narrowing (classic finding in Crohn's disease), areas with loss of normal mucosal pattern interspersed with areas of normal mucosa, fistula formation, and narrow band of barium flowing through inflamed or scarred terminal ileum (string sign).

MANAGEMENT/TREATMENT

1. Treatment must be tailored to individual because disease onset and course are highly variable. Goal is to improve symptoms and control disease process.
2. Low-residue diet is helpful when obstructive symptoms or cramping and diarrhea are present; otherwise diet restriction not necessary unless symptomatic from specific element such as lactose intolerance.
3. Supplement diet with a multivitamin preparation that contains five times the normal daily vitamin requirements plus iron, calcium, magnesium, and zinc.
4. Enteral therapy with elemental diet such as Vivonex with partial bowel rest is effective to induce remission. Relapse rate after return to normal diet is high without steroid therapy, however.
5. Total parenteral nutrition (TPN) is used to provide bowel rest during acute phases for patients with compromised nutrition.
6. For patients with colonic involvement
   A. Sulfasalazine 1.5–2.0 gm bid is effective but has little benefit for small intestine disease.
   B. Olsalazine 500 mg bid can be used for the sulfa-allergic patient.
   C. If a response is noted, continue therapy for 4–6 months, then stop if symptoms have ceased.
   D. Metronidazole 250–500 mg tid should be used if there is unsatisfactory response to sulfasalazine/olsalazine. Continue for 4-week trial; if improvement is noted, medication should be continued to 4–6 months and then discontinued if symptoms have ceased.
7. Perianal disease: Metronidazole 500 mg tid; may need prolonged course of treatment.
8. Ileal disease
   A. Olsalazine 500 mg bid may be tried for 4- to 6-week therapy, although the effectiveness of 5-aminosalicylic acid (5-ASA) drugs is not yet proven in ileal disease.
   B. Prednisone 40–60 mg/day for severe cases and for those that are nonresponsive to 5-ASA therapy.
   C. Azathioprine 50 mg/day is used for patients with fistulas, refractory symptoms, or persistent requirement for high-dose steroid therapy. Treatment is continued for 12 months and then cessation is attempted. Long-term therapy is sometimes necessary.

9. Prednisone 40–60 mg qd for acute exacerbations, tapered over 2 months. Prednisone in low dose may be needed for suppression therapy.
10. Antidiarrheals, such as diphenoxylate-atropine 1 to 2 tablets or loperamide 2–4 mg two to four times a day, may be used for chronic diarrhea.
11. Admission and consult is indicated for intractable symptoms resulting from fixed stricture, fistulas, severe unresponsive disease, massive bleeding, intra-abdominal abscess. Surgical referral may be necessary. Majority of patients require surgery at some point during disease course. Surgery is not curative as it is with ulcerative colitis; disease usually reoccurs, often at site of anastomosis.
12. Maintenance therapy with steroids and sulfasalazine has not been shown to be effective in decreasing disease recurrence.

PATIENT EDUCATION

1. Teach onset and course of disease, including special problems, chronicity, aggravating and alleviating factors. Include need to notify health care provider if symptoms of exacerbation are experienced.
2. Medications teaching, including purpose, dosage, frequency, side effects, toxicity.
3. Diet teaching for disease management should include:
   A. Bowel rest during acute, fulminating disease.
   B. Elimination of high-residue foods during exacerbations and in patients with low-grade obstruction.
   C. Elimination of lactose, milk protein, and gluten have been helpful in some patients. Trial of dietary elimination of each can be encouraged to determine if these elements cause discomfort.
   D. Dietary fat should be limited to 70 gm/day during periods of active disease or when there is steatorrhea.
   E. Be aware of other foods or beverages that cause discomfort and eliminate those from diet.
4. Emphasize importance of adequate rest in preventing disease recurrences and speeding resolution of exacerbations.
5. Stress may aggravate disease. If patient finds this to be true, stress management techniques should be taught, or refer for stress management counseling.
6. Encourage smoking cessation. Referral to smoking cessation counselor or group may be indicated.
7. Pregnancy should be planned.
8. Increased risk of colon cancer with need for surveillance with annual physical examination.
9. Educational materials are available through Crohn's and Colitis Foundation of America, 386 Park Avenue South, 17th Floor, New York, NY 10016; (1-800-343-3637).

Review Questions

10.11 The difference between Crohn's disease and ulcerative colitis is that ulcerative colitis:

A. Is a functional disorder of visceral perception
B. Involves the entire alimentary tract
C. Is an inflammatory disorder affecting the mucosal lining of the colon and rectum
D. All of the above

10.12 A 23-year-old Caucasian female presents complaining of bloody diarrhea, severe abdominal pain, and fatigue. States she has had urgency for approximately 2 weeks prior. Your preliminary diagnosis for this patient is ulcerative colitis or Crohn's disease. How will you validate a final diagnosis?
A. Refer for proctosigmoidoscopy, which will show friable bleeding mucosa characteristic of ulcerative colitis with no intermittent areas of normal mucosa that would be typical of Crohn's disease
B. CBC with differential will show leukocytosis in Crohn's disease with decreased hematocrit reflecting chronic GI blood loss
C. Barium enema will differentiate the mucosal lesions during the acute exacerbation but is of no use during remission
D. The only way to differentiate is by stool leukocytes, which will show change in morphology of white cells on fecal smear

10.13 A 33-year-old female is admitted with acute, severe exacerbation of ulcerative colitis. Symptoms include 10-lb weight loss in the last 3 weeks, bloody diarrhea for 2 weeks, right lower quadrant pain and abdominal cramping, and severe tenesmus that awakens her frequently during the night. She also states that she has been afraid to eat due to fear of increasing the pain and diarrhea. She is allergic to penicillin and sulfa. Your treatment plan should include:
A. CBC, platelet count, coagulation profile, serum albumin, routine urinalysis, barium enema, high-fiber diet to control diarrhea, and Demerol 25–50 mg IV for pain.
B. Type and cross for four units of red cells, upper gastrointestinal tract series (UGI) with small bowel follow-through, nasogastric tube to low intermittent suction, Tylenol # 3 for pain, sulfasalazine 750 mg qid with folic acid supplementation
C. Surgical consult because tenesmus is a sign of abscess formation following microperforation of the colon, usually in the area of the splenic flexure
D. CBC with differential, serum albumin, electrolytes, plain abdominal films, methylprednisolone 20 mg tid, Zosyn 3.375 mg IV q6h, referral for gastroenterology and surgical consult

10.14 A 33-year-old male is admitted to the hospital from the emergency department, where he was seen for a 3-week history of diarrhea, and intermittent fever, with colicky abdominal pain that seems to be primarily in the right lower quadrant. Has begun to have bloody diarrhea in the last week. He states he is having five to eight liquid stools a day, mostly bloody. He denies recent travel, cannot recall what he ate prior to the onset of the diarrhea, and is not aware that anyone else in his family has the same symptoms, although he says his sister was diagnosed recently with some kind of bowel disorder but he cannot recall the name of the disorder. The most appropriate series of test that should be ordered include:
A. CBC; stool for culture, ova and parasites, *C. difficile*; plain films of abdomen, UGI, and small bowel follow-through

B. CBC; stool for culture, ova and parasites, *C. difficile*; angiogram with embolization of bleeders
C. CBC, routine urinalysis, serum albumin, barium enema
D. CBC, UGI and barium enema, proctosigmoidoscopy

10.15 The diagnosis of Crohn's disease affecting the distal ileum is made. The medication most appropriate for this young man would be:
A. Sulfasalazine 2 gm bid
B. Olsalazine 500 mg tid
C. Metronidazole 500 mg tid
D. Ampicillin 500 mg IV qid

Answer and Rationales

10.11 **C** Ulcerative colitis is an inflammatory disorder affecting the mucosal lining of the colon and rectum. Crohn's disease can affect the entire alimentary tract, can skip areas, and most frequently occurs in the terminal ileum.

10.12 **A** Ulcerative colitis affects the mucosal lining of the colon and rectum, which can cause diffuse bleeding throughout the mucosa. Crohn's disease affects the mucosa as well as the surrounding musculature, forming deep fissures. Bowel becomes congested, thickened, and rigid, with adhesions involving the peri-intestinal fat. Barium enema may be helpful in establishing extent of disease but should never be used in acute disease.

10.13 **D** CBC will provide assessment of anemia resulting from acute and chronic blood loss; and leukocytosis may be evident in acute exacerbations. Serum albumin will assist in assessing nutritional state. Electrolyte abnormalities such as hypokalemia or prerenal azotemia may be evident; dehydration may also be reflected in electrolyte values. Plain films of the abdomen are required in acute states to rule out toxic megacolon. Medication treatment for acute ulcerative colitis includes treatment with IV steroids such as methylprednisolone, as well as a broad-spectrum antibiotic with coverage for bowel flora (gram-negative rods and anaerobes), such as Zosyn. All patients with severe ulcerative colitis should have gastroenterology and surgical consult.

10.14 **A** Initial work-up should include stool evaluation to rule out other causes of diarrhea, such as bacterial or viral gastroenteritis. Complete blood count is indicated to determine anemia, leukocytosis. Other diagnostic tests, such as plain film of abdomen, are helpful in ruling out other pathology as well. UGI and small bowel follow-through in Crohn's disease will often show segmental involvement of large and small bowel, often with strictures, fistulas, and ulcers.

10.15 **B** Olsalazine 500 mg is the first-line drug for treatment of uncomplicated Crohn's disease of the small bowel. If the inflammation is not responsive to the olsalazine, prednisone may be added. Sulfasalazine has not been shown effective in treatment of Crohn's disease of the ileum.

References

Briones, T. (1991). The gastrointestinal system. In G. Alspach (ed.). *American Association of Critical Care Nurses Core Curriculum for Critical Care Nursing*. Philadelphia: W.B. Saunders Co., pp. 748–835.

Bullock, B., & Rosendahl, P. (1986). *Pathophysiology: Adaptations and Alterations in Function*. Boston: Little, Brown & Co.

Greenwald, B. (1996). Ulcerative colitis. In R.E. Rakel (ed.). *Saunders Manual of Medical Practice*. Philadelphia: W.B. Saunders Co.

James, S. (1996). Crohn's disease. In R.E. Rakel (ed.). *Saunders Manual of Medical Practice*. Philadelphia: W.B. Saunders Co., pp. 341–343.

McQuaid, K. (1996). Alimentary tract. In L. Tierney, S. McPhee, & M. Papadakis (eds.). *Current Medical Diagnosis and Treatment*. Stamford, CT: Appleton & Lange, pp. 489–575.

Ruyman, F., & Richter, J. (1995). Management of inflammatory bowel disease. In A. Goroll, L. May, & A. Mulley (eds.). *Primary Care Medicine: Office Evaluation and Management of the Adult Patient* (3rd ed.). Philadelphia: J.B. Lippincott Co., pp. 416–424.

Tooson, J., & Varilek, G. (1995). Inflammatory diseases of the colon. *Postgrad Med 98*, 46.

Irritable Bowel Syndrome

DEFINITION

Irritable bowel syndrome (IBS) is a functional disturbance of intestinal motility and visceral perception that is triggered or exacerbated by psychological stress and luminal irritants.

ETIOLOGY/INCIDENCE

1. Patients have a reduced sensory threshold for stimuli such as rectal or ileal distention. This has been proven by balloon dilation at certain points in small and large intestine, reproducing pain.
2. IBS very common; up to 20% of population have IBS but most never seek medical attention.
3. Age at presentation/onset of disease ranges from 20 to 50 years.
4. Patients with IBS commonly have past history that is significant for allergies, headache, kidney disease, joint pain.

PATHOPHYSIOLOGY

Psychopathologic view is one of visceral perception and motor activity disturbance usually related to psychological disturbance. Nonpropulsive colonic contractions and slow-wave myoelectric patterns at 2–3 cycles/min make up approximately 40% of electrical and contractile activity at rest in patients with IBS compared to 10% in patients with normal bowel functioning. Constipation occurs when these contractions become excessive, prolonging transit time and impeding propulsion of stool. Diarrhea occurs when the increase in contractility localized to the small bowel and proximal colon develops a pressure gradient, causing accelerated movement of intestinal contents.

SIGNS AND SYMPTOMS

1. Criteria for IBS include continuous or recurrent symptoms for at least 3 months of:
   A. Abdominal pain or discomfort relieved by defecation or associated with a change in the frequency of consistency of stool and/or
   B. Irregular pattern of defecation at least 25% of the time (three or more of the following):
      1) Altered passage of stool
      2) Altered stool form
      3) Altered stool passage (straining, urgency, feeling of incomplete evacuation)
      4) Passage of mucus
      5) Bloating or feeling of abdominal distention
2. Patients who present with pain generally are not bothered by pain at night.
3. Symptoms begin soon after eating breakfast.
4. Patients who seek medical attention for IBS tend to have higher incidence of psychopathology, including anxiety, depression, hypochondriasis.

PHYSICAL FINDINGS

1. Physical examination in most patients is normal.
2. Abdominal tenderness, especially in the lower abdomen, is common but is typically not pronounced.

DIFFERENTIAL DIAGNOSIS

Irritable bowel syndrome is diagnosis of exclusion. Important to rule out other etiologies.
1. Colonic neoplasia
2. Inflammatory bowel disease
3. Pelvic inflammatory disease
4. Cholecystitis/biliary colic
5. Infectious gastroenteritis
6. Malabsorption, enzyme deficiencies
7. Hypothyroidism, hypercalcemia may be cause of constipation

DIAGNOSTIC TESTS/FINDINGS

1. Complete blood count, electrolytes, sedimentation rate, serum albumin, and stool occult blood test should all be normal. Minimal examination should consist of complete blood count, erythrocyte sedimentation rate.
2. Patients with diarrhea should have stool for ova and parasites, leukocytes, enteric pathogens; and 24-hour stool collection (weight >300 gm/dL is atypical for IBS).
3. Urinalysis should be obtained to rule out renal/urinary tract disease.
4. Patients under age 40 should have flexible sigmoidoscopy to rule out inflammatory bowel disease. Air insufflation will often reproduce the symptoms.
5. Patients over age 40 should consider barium enema or colonoscopy.

MANAGEMENT/TREATMENT

Management depends on predominate symptom exhibited.
1. Diagnosis is typically one of exclusion. Physician consult may be necessary to assist in obtaining appropriate diagnostic evaluation.
2. Diet modification may include limiting or eliminating lactose, fructose, sorbitol. Malabsorption of these will cause distention, bloating, flatulence, and diarrhea.
3. Trial of high-fiber diet is recommended for most patients. Some patients do not tolerate this, and fiber supplements such as psyllium may be better tolerated.
4. Anticholinergic agents such as Bentyl 10–20 mg PO 30–40 minutes prior to meals and at bedtime may help patients with gas, bloating. Treatment aimed at eliminating postprandial pain.
5. Opioid and other antidiarrheal agents may be useful in patients with frequent loose stool; usually best when used prophylactically when stressful situation is anticipated or when diarrhea would be inconvenient.
6. Prokinetic agents such as cisapride 10–20 mg PO qid may be useful for patients with refractory diarrhea.
7. Simethicone 2–4 tablets with meals helps to control gas.
8. Amitriptyline 25–75 mg PO tid or once a day at bedtime may be useful for patients with chronic continuous abdominal pain. This group of patients have a high incidence of psychiatric disturbances.
9. Anxiolytics and narcotics are contraindicated in this population.

PATIENT EDUCATION

1. Development of trusting, ongoing provider-patient relationship is most important factor in successful management of IBS, and is related to reduced number of return visits.
2. Explanation of the functional nature of this problem, that symptoms are indeed a real functional disturbance related to psychological stressors, will reassure patient that disease is not "all in his head."
3. Explanation of disease pattern, exacerbating factors will assist patient in coping with symptoms.
4. Assure patients that chronic nature of symptoms does not mean progression to more serious illness.
5. Encourage patient to concentrate on maintaining normal functioning rather than on elimination of symptoms.
6. Teach purpose, dosage, frequency, side effects, and signs of toxicity of all medications.
7. Teach diet measures that may assist in eliminating or alleviating symptoms.

Review Questions

10.16 Irritable bowel syndrome is defined as:
    A. A functional disturbance of intestinal motility and visceral perception triggered by psychological stress
    B. Diffuse inflammation of the bowel mucosa

    C. Chronic inflammatory disease of the alimentary tract

    D. An acute, self-limited disease with symptoms that include diarrhea, nausea, and vomiting

10.17 The diagnosis of IBS is best made by:

    A. Eliciting the assistance of psychologist for personality assessment of patient

    B. Finding loss of haustral markings on barium study

    C. A careful history and exclusion of other possible pathology

    D. Abdominal CT scan finding of fluid in peritoneal space

10.18 A 27-year-old female presents in the emergency room with complaints of chronic abdominal pain, bloating, and occasional diarrhea. She states that she is currently working full time and attending graduate school. She has been under a great deal of stress because of finals and a big deadline at work happening concurrently. Family history includes sister with irritable bowel syndrome. Her only other health problem is severe allergies. She denies nocturnal diarrhea, bloody stools, weight loss, or fever. Initial diagnostic tests that should be done include:

    A. Chest x-ray, CBC with differential, chemistry panel, swallowing study to assess motility, CT scan of abdomen

    B. CBC with differential, chemistry panel, barium enema, upper endoscopy, and upright film of abdomen

    C. Upper GI series, prealbumin, serum iron, transferrin, and thyroid function tests

    D. CBC, sedimentation rate; albumin; stool for occult blood

10.19 The treatment plan for this patient should include:

    A. Anticholinergics, Imodium, low-protein diet

    B. Diet modification, teaching regarding management of symptoms, Bentyl

    C. Imodium 2–4 mg every 4–6 hours until symptoms begin to disappear and then 2 mg q6h for 24 hours followed by 2 mg qd for 2 weeks

    D. Surgical consult for evaluation of need for proctocolectomy or ileal anal pull-through

10.20 This patient was referred to GI clinic for follow-up. Symptoms continue with some relief reported. However, patient states that the pain is continuing to be chronic and is disrupting her life. She is quite distressed and tearful. She states she feels nothing will ever help her. One option that has had some success in this population is:

    A. Psychotherapy

    B. Amitriptyline 25 mg tid

    C. Drinking a glass of milk prior to meals

    D. Colace 100 mg bid

Answers and Rationales

10.16 **A** Irritable bowel syndrome is a true malfunction of the visceral sensitivity to pressure, which results in increase or decrease in colonic transit.

10.17 **C** Irritable bowel syndrome is a diagnosis of exclusion. Careful history to elicit timing and character of symptoms and a thorough physical examination to rule out other pathology are essential for the accurate diagnosis of this syndrome.

10.18 **D** In a patient 20–50 years of age with a presumed diagnosis of irritable bowel syndrome, a limited series of examinations is needed to rule out other pathology. Patients less than 40 years of age should have flexible sigmoidoscopy, patients over age 40 should have barium enema or colonoscopy if they have not previously.

10.19 **B** Anticholinergics may be useful in this patient with abdominal pain and bloating as her predominate symptoms by ameliorating post-prandial pain. Diet modifications may include elimination of those foods containing agents that can cause bloating, flatulence, and diarrhea, such as sorbitol, lactose, fructose, caffeine. Teaching patient to anticipate and control symptoms will help to alleviate symptoms and aid in maintaining normal lifestyle in face of chronic illness.

10.20 **B** Amitriptyline has been shown useful in patients with chronic continuous abdominal pain because of high incidence of psychological disturbances in this group.

References

Connor, S., D'Andrea, K., Piper, J., et al. (1989). *Comprehensive Review Manual for the Adult Nurse Practitioner.* Glenview: Scott, Foresman, and Company

McQuaid, K. (1996). Alimentary tract. In L. Tierney, S. McPhee, & M. Papadakis (eds.). *Current Medical Diagnosis and Treatment.* Stamford, CT: Appleton & Lange, pp. 489–575.

Ruyman, F., & Richter, J. (1995). Approach to the patient with functional gastrointestinal disease. In A. Goroll, L. May, & A. Mulley, (eds.). *Primary Care Medicine: Office Evaluation and Management of the Adult Patient* (3rd ed.). Philadelphia: J.B. Lippincott Co., pp. 425–433.

Steinhart, M. (1992). Irritable bowel syndrome: How to relieve symptoms enough to improve daily function. *Postgrad Med 91*, 315.

Sutton, F. (1996). Irritable bowel syndrome. In R.E. Rakel (ed.). *Saunders Manual of Medical Practice.* Philadelphia: W.B. Saunders Co., pp. 347–349.

Uphold, V., & Graham, M. (1994). *Clinical Guidelines in Adult Health.* Gainesville, FL: Barmarrae Books.

Appendicitis

DEFINITION

Inflammation of the vermiform appendix caused by fecaliths, calculi, hyperplasia or submucosal lymphoid follicles, tumors, strictures, or foreign bodies.

ETIOLOGY/INCIDENCE

1. Most common abdominal surgical emergency: 250,000 cases annually in United States.
2. Most common in young adults, with 70–80% of cases in patients 10–30 years of age (male > female, 3:2).
3. Children account for 10% of cases, with most cases occurring between ages of 6 and 14.

4. Highest incidence in spring and summer.
5. Risk factors
    A. Adolescence in males
    B. Familial tendency
    C. Intra-abdominal tumors
    D. Low-fiber diet

PATHOPHYSIOLOGY

1. Primary event is obstruction of the lumen of the appendix. Appendiceal mucosa secretion continues despite obstruction. This along with rapid proliferation of intestinal bacteria results in distention of appendix, which in turn stimulates visceral pain fibers.
2. Gangrenous appendix and perforation is result of progressive distention with rising intraluminal pressure that compromises vascular supply. Usually results if left untreated for 36 hours.

SIGNS AND SYMPTOMS

1. Classic presentation is characterized by nausea, anorexia, obstipation, fever (usually no more than 1°C increase), and periumbilical epigastric pain that progresses to localization of pain to right lower quadrant.
2. Pain begins as dull, diffuse periumbilical pain; may be associated with cramping. Progression of inflammation over next 4–12 hours causes involvement of adjacent peritoneum with shift of pain to right lower quadrant. Abdominal pain is most important symptom, occurring in >90% of patients.
3. Constipation, obstipation more common than diarrhea, but diarrhea occurs in one sixth of patients.
4. Vomiting occurs in one half to two thirds of patients, especially children.
5. Elderly patients may have atypical presentation, however—rapid progression toward perforation and abscess formation.
6. Rupture may present with sudden decrease in severity of pain. Pain will return as diffuse peritonitis sets in.
7. Atypical presentation not uncommon owing to variable location of appendix.

PHYSICAL FINDINGS

1. Right lower quadrant (RLQ) tenderness is most significant early sign, occurring in approximately 95% of patients.
2. Rebound tenderness at McBurney's point (1.5–2 inches from the iliac crest, along line drawn from crest to umbilicus). Point of maximal tenderness may be other than RLQ depending on location of appendix.
3. Diagnostic physical signs
    A. Rosvig's sign: RLQ pain on palpation of left lower quadrant
    B. Obturator sign: Right lower quadrant pain elicited by flexing right leg and internally rotating right hip while patient is lying supine
    C. Psoas sign: Right lower quadrant pain elicited by hyperextension of right hip while patient lying on left side.
4. Voluntary guarding noted early in course, usually localized. Involuntary guarding becomes present as peritoneal inflammation becomes widespread.
5. Tenderness may be found on pelvic or vaginal exam. All women with lower abdominal pain should undergo pelvic and rectal examination as part of their diagnostic examination.

6. Low-grade fever. If fever greater than 100.5°F, should consider perforation or other diagnosis.

DIFFERENTIAL DIAGNOSIS

1. Ectopic pregnancy
2. Diverticulitis
3. Cholecystitis
4. Gastroenteritis
5. Pelvic inflammatory disease
6. Crohn's disease
7. Rupture of ovarian follicle (mittelschmerz)
8. Mesenteric adenitis
9. Pyelonephritis
10. Renal calculi
11. Acute salpingitis

DIAGNOSTIC TESTS/FINDINGS

1. Complete blood count: Leukocytosis between 10,000 and 18,000/μL. Polymorphonuclear predominance is present with shift to left on differential. Increase greater than 20,000/μL should raise suspicion of perforation. Elevated white blood cell count (WBC) most valuable laboratory test in patient >60 years of age.
2. Urinalysis: Microscopic hematuria and pyuria are present in one fourth of patients, especially those with retrocecal or retroileal appendicitis.
3. Pregnancy test should be done on all females of child-bearing age.
4. Gonorrhea and chlamydia screen should be performed on female patients in whom pelvic inflammatory disease may be suspected.
5. Radiographic or pelvic ultrasound studies may be beneficial in some patients but are not advocated in patients suspected of having appendicitis.
6. Diagnostic tests should be reserved for patients in whom the diagnosis is unclear. Unnecessary diagnostic tests can delay surgery, which is definitive treatment.

MANAGEMENT/TREATMENT

1. The ACNP should obtain surgical consult as soon as possible. Definitive therapy is appendectomy, which should not be delayed in unequivocal cases.
2. IV fluids if dehydrated. Fluid resuscitation is directed at restoring both fluid volume that has been depleted and deficits in electrolytes.
3. Antibiotics should be given to all patients after cultures have been obtained and decision is made by surgeon to operate. Cefoxitin 1 gm IVPB or other single broad-spectrum cephalosporin is drug of choice for prophylaxis prior to appendectomy.
4. Pain medication after diagnosis is made and decision to operate has been made by surgical consult. Patient who is to be observed should not be given analgesia. Meperidine 25–50 mg IM, or morphine 1–2 mg IVP or 8–12 mg IM, or equivalent analgesic should be given intramuscularly or intravascularly in divided doses.
5. All patients considered to have acute appendicitis must be admitted for surgery as soon as possible.

PATIENT EDUCATION

1. Disease course and expected outcome: Explain nature of illness, expected course, and that surgery will be necessary as soon as is possible.
2. Preoperative teaching should include expected recovery, pain management, deep breathing exercises, and expected discharge.
3. Discharge teaching should include wound care instructions, allowed activity, return to usual activity, and when to return to clinic for postoperative follow-up.
4. Medication teaching should include purpose, dosages, side effects, precautions, toxicity.

Review Questions

10.21 The most common presenting symptoms for appendicitis include:
   A. Epigastric pain, leukocytosis, hematemesis
   B. Right lower quadrant pain, anorexia, nausea
   C. Diarrhea, nausea, vomiting, left lower quadrant pain
   D. Diffuse abdominal pain, constipation, high fever

10.22 A 21-year-old patient comes into the emergency department complaining of acute abdominal pain that started in her epigastric area earlier in the afternoon but over the course of the last 4–5 hours has localized in the right lower quadrant. Has had anorexia and nausea but no vomiting for the last 12 hours. She denies diarrhea, constipation. She is sexually active but denies history of sexually transmitted disease. Last menstrual period was approximately 3 weeks ago. Denies hematuria, fever. Work-up for this patient must include:
   A. Abdominal ultrasound, electrolytes, CBC, chest x-ray
   B. KUB and, if negative, CT scan of abdomen; CBC, chemistry panel
   C. CBC with differential, pelvic examination with rectal exam, pregnancy test
   D. Urinalysis, CT scan, C-reactive protein, CBC with differential

10.23 The physical examination findings that you would expect to support your preliminary diagnosis of acute appendicitis include:
   A. Positive obturator sign, positive psoas sign, tenderness over McBurney's point, and low-grade fever
   B. Rectal tenderness, cervical motion tenderness, positive Murphy's sign
   C. Positive fluid wave test, truncal telangiectasias, jaundice
   D. Hematuria, tenderness at costovertebral angle, high fever

10.24 Laboratory tests were ordered on this young woman. You would expect to find which of the following to support the diagnosis of appendicitis?
   A. Elevated LDH, AST, and ALT
   B. Leukocytosis, increase in polymorphonuclear predominance, and shift to left
   C. Leukopenia, thrombocytopenia, mononuclear cells
   D. Polycythemia, leukocytosis, shift to right of differential

10.25 The young woman now reports that "she doesn't hurt as bad any more" and wants to have something to drink. You realize that this decrease in the severity of pain may indicate:

A. Passing of fecalith and resolution of appendicitis
B. Return of peristalsis
C. Mittelschmerz
D. Rupture of appendix

Answers and Rationales

10.21 **B** Right lower quadrant pain, anorexia, and nausea are the most common presenting symptoms for appendicitis. The pain typically begins as epigastric but soon localizes to the right lower quadrant. Other presentations are not uncommon, especially in the elderly.

10.22 **C** Pelvic examination with rectal exam should always be performed in women of child-bearing age. Clinician must rule out pelvic inflammatory disease, ectopic pregnancy.

10.23 **A** Positive obturator sign, positive psoas sign, tenderness over McBurney's point, and low-grade fever are most common findings on physical examination. Appendix lies under McBurney's point in abdomen in most patients. Positive psoas and obturator signs indicate inflammation or irritation of intrapelvic area.

10.24 **B** Leukocytosis, increase in polymorphonuclear predominance, and shift to left are most common findings in appendicitis. Leukocytosis greater than 18,000/μh should raise suspicion of rupture. Leukocyte count may be normal. Leukocytosis or abnormal differential is most valuable laboratory test in elderly.

10.25 **D** Rupture of appendix will result in sudden decrease in abdominal pain, with return of pain as peritonitis begins to spread through abdomen. This is a surgical emergency.

References

Addis, D., Shaffer, N., Fowler, B.S., et al. (1990). The epidemiology of appendicitis and appendectomy in the United States. *Am J Epidemiol 132*, 910.

Bohnen, J., Solomkin, J., Dellinger, E., et al. (1992). Guidelines for clinical care: Anti-infective agents for intra-abdominal infection. A Surgical Infection Society policy statement. *Arch Surg 127*, 83.

Bongard F., Landers, D., & Lewis, F. (1985). Differential diagnosis of appendicitis and pelvic inflammatory disease: A prospective analysis. *Am J Surg 150*, 90.

Cook, M. (1996). Appendicitis. In R.E. Rakel (ed.). *Saunders Manual of Medical Practice*. Philadelphia: W.B. Saunders Co., pp. 330–331.

Davies, M., Cunningham, S., Cooke, D., et al. (1993). Is the hot appendix really hot? *Postgrad Med J 69*, 862.

Franz, M., Norman, J., & Fabri, P. (1995). Increased morbidity of appendicitis with advancing age. *Am Surg 61*, 40.

Maxwell, J., & Ragland, J. (1991). Appendicitis: Improvements in diagnosis and treatment. *Am Surg 57*, 282.

McQuaid, K. (1996). Alimentary tract. In L. Tierney, s. McPhee, & M. Papadakis (eds.). *Current Medical Diagnosis and Treatment*. Stamford, CT: Appleton & Lange.

Rothrock, S., Green, S., Dobson, M., et al. (1995). Misdiagnosis of appendicitis in nonpregnant women of childbearing age. *J Emerg Med 13*, 1.

Diverticulitis

DEFINITION

Diverticulitis is necrotizing inflammation in one or more colonic diverticula with perforation, allowing free passage of fecal matter into the peritoneal cavity.

ETIOLOGY/INCIDENCE

1. Affects adults older than age 50. Colonic diverticulosis is prevalent in over one third of patients over 60 years of age. Most are asymptomatic.
2. Most common in patients with widespread diverticulosis, which is associated with highly refined diet deficient in fiber. Very common in western cultures, uncommon in Third World countries.
3. Diverticulitis accounts for greater than 200,000 hospitalizations and greater than 50,000 surgical procedures in the United States.
4. Sigmoid and descending colon primary site in whites; ascending colon primary site in blacks and Orientals.

PATHOPHYSIOLOGY

1. Diverticulosis is believed to arise following a prolonged diet deficient in fiber. The undistended, contracted segments of colon have higher intraluminal pressures. Eventually, the colonic musculature develops hypertrophy, thickening, rigidity, and fibrosis from working against higher pressures to move small, hard stools. Colonic diverticula are characterized by herniation of the mucosa and submucosa through the colonic muscle wall.
2. Diverticulitis is thought to be due to increased pressure in diverticula that may force a fecal mass to become hardened, causing obstruction, inflammation, and perforation. Retention of undigested food residues and bacteria may cause a fecalith to form in a diverticulum, which compromises the blood supply. This results in perforation, which may range from microperforation (most common) with localized paracolic inflammation to macroperforation with either abscess or generalized peritonitis.

SIGNS AND SYMPTOMS

Clinical presentation may range from mild, with patients not seeking medical attention until several days after onset, to severe, with dramatic signs of peritonitis.

1. Abdominal pain, constant in nature, typically left lower quadrant but may be diffuse.
2. May report history of fever; however, high fever may be associated with perforation.
3. Alteration in bowel habits—most commonly constipation, although diarrhea is reported by approximately 25% of patients.
4. Nausea and vomiting are frequent and may be associated with obstruction or abscess.
5. Dysuria and frequency are common because of colonic inflammatory process causing irritation to bladder.
6. History of emotional stress common; thought to increase colonic spasm.

PHYSICAL FINDINGS

1. Moderate to marked tenderness in left lower quadrant; mass may be palpable.
2. Guarding, rebound tenderness, muscle spasm may be present with complicated diverticulitis.
3. Bowel sounds usually hypoactive; may be high pitched with early obstruction or absent with complete obstruction.
4. Temperature usually >100°F.

DIFFERENTIAL DIAGNOSIS

1. Intestinal ischemia
2. Infectious diarrhea
3. Appendicitis
4. Cancer of colon
5. Perforated duodenal ulcer
6. Inflammatory bowel disease
7. Pancreatitis
8. Sigmoid volvulus

DIAGNOSTIC TESTS/FINDINGS

1. CBC with differential: Leukocytosis may be evident; shift to left is typically seen; may see decreased hematocrit as a result of chronic GI blood loss.
2. Guaiac test may reveal occult bleeding from colonic diverticula.
3. Urinalysis may show white cells because of contiguous involvement of bladder.
4. Upright, supine, and left lateral decubitus films are among most important films to obtain initially to look for free air. May also see ileus, obstruction, distended colon, pneumoperitoneum.
5. CT scan is initial diagnostic test of choice to evaluate acute diverticulitis in severe cases and in patients with mild symptoms with presumptive diagnosis of diverticulitis who do not respond to acute medical management. Should always be considered if mass is palpable.
6. Barium enema is useful in unequivocal cases. Most reliable diagnostic finding is appearance of sinus tract or streak of barium outside the contour of colon in lumen.
7. Flexible sigmoidoscopy and barium enema are contraindicated during the initial stages of an acute attack because of risk of creating free perforation.

MANAGEMENT/TREATMENT

1. Mild diverticulitis may be treated without hospital admission in most cases by:
   A. Bed rest
   B. Clear liquid diet
   C. Antibiotics: metronidazole (Flagyl) 500 mg PO tid *plus* trimethoprim-sulfamethoxazole (Bactrim) 1 double-strength tablet PO bid for 10 days or ciprofloxacin 500 mg PO bid
2. Moderate to severe diverticulitis requires admission to hospital and referral for surgical consult for management/surgery. Approximately 20–30% of patients will require surgical management.

3. Intravenous fluids necessary to correct signs of dehydration, electrolyte imbalance.
4. Antibiotics to cover anaerobic and gram-negative bacteria (second or third-generation cephalosporin, such as cefoxitin 1–2 gm IV q6–8h, plus metronidazole 500 mg q6h. Continue antibiotics for 7–10 days.
5. Narcotic analgesics such as morphine sulfate 1–4 mg IVP q1–2h as needed for pain management.
6. Nasogastric tube is indicated for patients with acute abdomen, persistent vomiting, or ileus.
7. Diet may be increased slowly to low-residue diet with stool softener such as Colace 100 mg bid after resolution of acute inflammation.
8. Gradual increase of dietary fiber to goal of 25–35 gm/day.

PATIENT EDUCATION

1. Patient and family should be taught need to maintain adequate dietary intake of:
   A. At least 25–35 gm/day of fiber. Fiber should be obtained from fresh fruits and vegetables, high-fiber cereals, whole grain cereals, legumes.
   B. Adequate fluid intake is essential to prevent bloating from high-fiber diet and prevent constipation.
   C. Dietary fat intake should not exceed 30% of total calories.
2. Follow-up with health care provider 1 month postrecovery for evaluation of extent of disease with either flexible sigmoidoscopy or barium enema.
3. Nature, course, and onset of disease, including exacerbating factors. Diverticulitis recurs in one third of patients treated with medical management. Recurrent attacks warrant elective surgical resection, which carries a lower morbidity and mortality risk than emergency surgery.
4. Medications: Purpose, dosage side effects, toxic effects, and importance of compliance with regimen.
5. Prevention of exacerbation, such as stress reduction, relaxation techniques.

Review Questions

10.26 The most consistent presenting symptom for diverticulitis is:
   A. Sudden onset nausea, vomiting, and diarrhea
   B. Lower GI bleeding with history of emotional upset
   C. High fever, tachycardia, hypotension, severe mid-epigastric pain
   D. Pain in left lower quadrant

10.27 The cause of diverticulitis is thought to be:
   A. A weakness in the lining of duodenum that allows an outpouching to develop with strong peristalsis.
   B. A break in the intimal lining of small intestine
   C. Increased pressure in the diverticula that can cause hardening of the fecal mass leading to obstruction, inflammation.
   D. Hypertrophy of the colonic musculature with herniation of the mucosa and submucosa through the colonic muscle wall

10.28 A 63-year-old male presents to the emergency department with complaints of 2-day history of left lower quadrant pain, fever, constipation.

Denies vomiting but has had some nausea. States he also has had to "get up to go the bathroom more often than usual" but denies hesitancy or burning with urination. Physical examination reveals abdominal tenderness in the left lower quadrant with a palpable mass, hypoactive bowel sounds, and a fever of 39°C. You suspect diverticulitis. The first diagnostic tests that should be done include:

A. CBC with differential; upright, supine, and left lateral decubitus films of the abdomen; urinalysis
B. CBC with differential, CT scan, barium enema
C. CBC with differential, flexible sigmoidoscopy, barium enema
D. Serum electrolytes, arterial blood gas, barium enema

10.29 A diagnosis of diverticulitis is validated on this patient. The initial management plan includes admission to the hospital, intravenous fluid replacement. What other interventions/actions should follow?

A. Surgical consult, intravenous antibiotics
B. Narcotic analgesics, nasogastric tube
C. Metronidazole 500 mg IV q6h
D. All of the above

10.30 The most important teaching focus for prevention of further attacks would be:

A. The necessity of taking stool softener at set times each day, in the morning and before bedtime, to decrease the chance of constipation and obstructive fecalith.
B. Stress management and relaxation techniques will significantly decrease the incidence of recurrent attacks because of the resultant decrease in bowel motility and acid secretion.
C. Adequate fiber and fluid intake from dietary sources.
D. Addition of calcium channel blockers to the medication regimen for the smooth relaxation effects on the intestine.

Answers and Rationales

10.26 **D** Symptoms of diverticulitis can range from mild constant pain to high fevers, severe abdominal pain, nausea, and vomiting. The location of pain is reflective of location of infected diverticula.

10.27 **C** The fecalith formed in the diverticula compromises blood supply, which results in perforation with localized paracolic inflammation to macroperforation with either abscesses or generalized peritonitis.

10.28 **A** Barium enema and sigmoidoscopy are contraindicated during acute stage of diverticulitis.

10.29 **D** Surgical consult is needed in case of perforation, which requires surgical intervention and for assistance in management of patient. IV antibiotics and metronidazole are necessary and should cover anaerobic and gram-negative bowel flora. Narcotic analgesics are necessary to alleviate abdominal pain. Nasogastric tube is indicated if patient has vomiting, ileus.

10.30 **C** High fiber—at least 25–30 gm/day from fresh fruits and vegetable, high-fiber cereals, whole grain cereals, and legumes—increases the bulk of the stool and has been shown to decrease incidence and recurrence of diverticulitis. Adequate fluid intake is necessary to prevent bloating and constipation.

References

Brooks, M. (1996). Diverticulitis. In R.E. Rakel (ed.). *Saunders Manual of Medical Practice*. Philadelphia: W.B. Saunders Co., pp. 350–352.

Bugliosi, T., Meloy, T., & Vukov, L. (1990). Acute abdominal pain in the elderly. *Ann Emerg Med 19*, 1383.

Elfrink, R., & Miedema, B. (1992). Colonic diverticula: when complications require surgery and when they don't. *Postgrad Med 92*, 97.

McQuaid, K. (1996). Alimentary tract. In L. Tierney, S. McPhee, & M. Papadakis (eds.). *Current Medical Diagnosis and Treatment*. Stamford, CT: Appleton & Lange, pp. 489–575.

Norman, D., & Yoshikawa, T. (1983). Intra-abdominal infections in the elderly. *J Am Geriatr Soc 31*, 677.

Viral Hepatitis

DEFINITIONS

Viral hepatitis—inflammation of the hepatocytes resulting in necrosis and bile stasis. Causative viral agents are classified as enteral (hepatitis A and E) and parenteral (hepatitis B, C, D).

Cirrhosis (scarring)—widespread replacement of hepatic architecture with fibrous tissue. Associated with chronic active hepatitis B, hepatitis C infection.

HEPATITIS A

Viral Characteristics

1. Hepatitis A virus (HAV) is small RNA virus causing acute hepatitis only.
2. Serum markers: anti-HAV, anti-HAV immunoglobulin M (IgM) (persists in blood 3–12 months following infection, then disappears) (see Table 10–2).

ETIOLOGY/INCIDENCE

1. Common worldwide; 80% of population >60 yr is anti-HAV positive.
2. Children, adolescents most susceptible population.
3. Frequent cause of both sporadic and endemic disease in industrialized nations.
4. Reservoir: humans.
5. Transmission: fecal-oral route; contaminated food (shellfish), water.
6. Incubation period: 25 days (range 15–60).
7. Viral shedding occurs during prodromal asymptomatic stage.
8. No carrier state.
9. Exposure/infection confers lifelong immunity.
10. Risk factors include crowded living conditions; poor sanitation.
11. High-risk population: travelers to endemic areas in developing countries, male homosexuals, child care workers.

TABLE 10–2. **Serology and Diagnosis of Hepatitis Virus Infection***

Hepatitis Virus	Serologic Test Patterns	Diagnostic Interpretation
Hepatitis A	Anti-HAV IgM	Acute infection
	Anti-HAV IgG	Past infection
Hepatitis B	HBsAg$^+$, anti-HBc IgM	Acute infection
	HBsAg$^+$, anti-HBc IgG	Acute infection
	HBsAg$^+$, anti-HBc IgG	Chronic infection
	HBsAg$^+$, anti-HBc IgG, HBV DNA$^+$, HBeAg$^-$	Chronic *e-minus* infection
	HBsAg$^+$, anti-HBc IgG, HBV DNA$^+$, HBeAg$^+$	Chronic *replicative* infection
	HBsAg$^+$, anti-HBc IgG, HBV DNA$^+$, HBeAg$^-$	Chronic *nonreplicative* infection
	HBsAg$^-$, anti-HBc IgG, anti-HBs	Resolved infection
Hepatitis D	anti-HDV IgM, HBsAg$^+$	HDV infection
	anti-HDV IgM, HbsAg$^+$, anti-HBc$^+$	HDV co-infection
	anti-HDV IgM, HbsAg$^+$, anti-HBc$^-$	HDV superinfection
Hepatitis C	Anti-HCV IgM	HCV infection

* Adapted from Martin, P., Friedman, L.S., & Dienstag, J.J. (1991). Diagnostic approach. In A.J. Zuckerman & H.C. Thomas (eds.). *Viral Hepatitis: Scientific Basis and Clinical Management.* London: Churchill Livingstone, pp. 393–409, with permission.

12. Immunoprophylaxis available.
    A. Immune globulin: given pre-exposure to travelers to endemic areas; postexposure to contacts within 2 weeks of exposure.
    B. Hepatitis A vaccine (Harvix) recommended for high-risk populations (e.g., health care, child care workers).

DIAGNOSTIC TESTS/FINDINGS

1. Anti-HAV IgM (early in acute episode)
2. Anti-HAV IgM (later in acute episode and persists for life)
3. Liver function tests: ALT, AST, LDH, bilirubin total-to-conjugated (T/C) ratio elevated

HEPATITIS B

Viral Characteristics

1. Hepatitis B virus (HBV) is a medium-sized DNA virus causing acute and chronic disease detectable by conventional testing.
2. *HBsAg:* Surface antigen detected at onset of symptoms; clears at 4–5 months in acute episodes and persists in chronic disease.
3. *HBeAg:* Envelop antigen, secreted product of *HBV* gene detected in serum at onset of symptoms to 2–3 months in acute disease, and to 4 years in chronic disease
4. Qualitative indicator of viral replication.
5. *Anti-HBe:* Envelop antigen antibody, detectable when HBeAg is lost and implies resolution of HBV infection
6. *HBV DNA:* Quantitative indicator of replication of HBV in hepatocytes; is detectable at onset of symptoms and persists in chronic infection; used to identify patients with active disease likely to respond to interferon therapy and to monitor HBV replication during antiviral therapy.

7. *HBcAg:* Core antigen; not detectable in serum by convention methods
8. Detectable in liver by biopsy; most sensitive method of identifying viral replication in chronic active hepatitis B (CAHB).
9. *Anti-HBc IgM:* detectable 1–2 months following symptoms with peak at 3–4 months; disappears at 12 months in acute disease.
10. *Anti-HBc:* detectable at 1–2 months; peaks 5–6 months; levels out at 24 months.

ETIOLOGY/INCIDENCE

1. Major worldwide cause of cirrhosis, liver failure, and hepatocellular carcinoma (300 million people).
   A. Worldwide, maternal-fetal transmission predominates
   B. Western countries, sexual transmissions predominates
2. Causes both acute and chronic disease.
3. Reservoir: humans.
4. Transmission modes.
   A. Percutaneous routes: placenta, blood transfusion, use of common needles (e.g., intravenous drug abuse [IVDA])
   B. Nonpercutaneous routes: saliva, tears, vaginal and seminal fluids, breast milk, urine, pleural fluid, synovial fluids
5. Carrier: Individual who is HBsAg positive for 6 months or more.
6. High-risk groups: drug addicts, hemophiliacs, health care workers, dialysis patients, homosexual population.
7. Immunoprophylaxis: Hepatitis B Vaccine, a recombinant DNA preparation (Energix-B, Recombivax HB), is available in three preparations for different age groups.
   A. It is recommended for health care workers and others at occupational risk; hemophiliacs and other recipients of selected blood products; household contacts and sex partners of HBsAg-positive persons; injection drug users, sexually active homosexual or bisexual males; heterosexual individuals with more than one sex partner in previous 6 months and/or those with a recent episode of sexually transmitted disease; inmates of long-term correctional institutions.
   B. CDC recommends all newborns be vaccinated.
8. Hepatitis B immune globulin postexposure.

DIAGNOSTIC TESTS/FINDINGS

1. Acute hepatitis B
   A. HBsAg: positive
   B. Liver function tests: ALT, AST, LDH, bilirubin T/C elevated
   C. Anti-HBsAg IgM
2. CAHB
   A. Liver function tests: ALT, AST, LDH, bilirubin T/C elevated
   B. HBsAg: positive
   C. HBV DNA
   D. Anti-HBc

HEPATITIS C

Viral Characteristics

1. Hepatitis C virus (HCV) is a single-stranded RNA virus responsible for most cases of parenterally transmitted non-A, non-B hepatitis.

2. Fifty percent of individuals with active infection progress to chronic disease.
3. Twenty-five percent of those develop cirrhosis.
4. No way to differentiate acute and chronic disease.
5. Diagnosis by immunoassay for anti-HCV, which appears late (4–24 weeks, mean 15 weeks) after onset of clinical symptoms and/or elevated liver function tests (LFTs).
6. No test for HCV antigen; however, there is a HCV RNA (polymerase chain reaction [PCR]) assay that can detect hepatitis C virus RNA in the serum.
7. Hepatitis C–specific immunoprophylaxis not available.

ETIOLOGY/INCIDENCE

1. United States: Most common cause of chronic hepatitis.
2. Transmission: 15% parenteral via blood transfusion; maternal-fetal and sexual transmission infrequent.
3. High-risk groups: HIV patients, IVDA, history of blood transfusions, hemodialysis, health care workers

DIAGNOSTIC TESTS/FINDINGS

1. Liver function tests: AST, ALT, LDH, Bilirubin T/C elevated for ≥6 months
2. Anti-HCV (enzyme immunoassay 2 [EIA-2]) positive or HCV RNA (PCR) positive
3. Positive for clinical signs and symptoms

HEPATITIS D (Delta Hepatitis)

Viral Characteristics

1. Hepatitis D virus (HDV) is a small RNA virus that requires the helper function of hepatitis B virus to complete its replicative cycle; therefore, HDV infection is not encountered in the absence of HBV infection.
2. Co-infection: Simultaneous infection with acute HBV.
3. Superinfection: Superimposed on chronic HBV; can cause more severe liver disease than HBV alone.
4. Diagnosis made by detection of anti-HDV by EIA or radioimmunoassay.
   A. Chronic HDV superinfection: IgM anti-HDV detectable onset to 6 months; anti-HDV detectable throughout course of disease
   B. Acute HDV co-infection: IgM anti-HDV detectable onset to 6 months; anti-HDV detectable at onset to 12 months, then disappears from serum

ETIOLOGY/INCIDENCE

1. Prevalence in United States highest among hemophiliacs and intravenous drug abusers
2. Transmission (see "Hepatitis B")
3. Immunoprophylaxis (see "Hepatitis B")

DIAGNOSTIC TESTS/FINDINGS

1. Anti-HDV positive
2. HBV serum markers (see "Hepatitis B")

HEPATITIS E

Viral Characteristics

1. Hepatitis E virus (HEV) is an RNA virus causing acute hepatitis only.
2. Serologic testing by research methods only.
   A. HEV antigen can be identified by electron microscopy in feces, bile, liver during incubation and symptomatic phases.
   B. Anti-HEV detectable in serum using research methods.

ETIOLOGY/INCIDENCE

1. Endemic in Southeast Asia; outbreaks reported in Mexico.
2. Incidence in the United States related to visitors from endemic areas and travelers returning to the United States.
3. Transmission: Fecal-oral route due to contaminated food and water; associated with GI symptoms of diarrhea.
4. High-risk population: Pregnant women in third trimester; causes fulminant hepatitis in this group, with a 20% mortality rate.
5. Incubation/disease course resembles hepatitis A.
6. No specific treatment; or immunoprophylaxis.

DIAGNOSTIC TESTS/FINDINGS

1. Serologic testing available only by research methods.
2. Diagnosis made by history of travel to or exposure to infected individuals from endemic areas.
3. Clinical findings same as hepatitis A.

GENERAL CONSIDERATIONS

SIGNS AND SYMPTOMS

1. Prodromal (preicteric): Asymptomatic to mild nonspecific presentation
   A. Fatigue
   B. Anorexia
   C. Smell/taste changes—characteristic of hepatitis
   D. Headache
   E. Coryza
   F. Pruritis
   G. Arthralgia
   H. Fever, low grade (100–102°F)
2. Icteric phase: Duration variable
   A. Dark urine: Occurs 1–2 days prior to icteric sclera, skin
   B. Jaundice
   C. Clay-colored stools: Occurs in 20–40% of patients the first week of jaundice
   D. Pruritis: Occurs in 50% of patients; transient mild
   E. Complaint of fullness in abdomen
   F. Right upper quadrant (RUQ) tenderness; enlarged liver

DIFFERENTIAL DIAGNOSIS

1. Upper respiratory infection
2. GI infection
3. Influenza
4. Cholestatic disease
5. Hepatic/hepatobiliary carcinoma
6. Cirrhosis

MANAGEMENT/TREATMENT

1. General principles
   A. Managed in ambulatory care setting.
   B. Hospitalization for high-risk population.
      1) Elderly
      2) Chronically ill; debilitated/immunocompromised
      3) Infants, toddlers
   C. Support nutrition.
      1) No dietary restrictions
      2) Small frequent feedings to improve tolerance/intake
   D. No activity restrictions.
      1) Bed rest not required.
      2) Avoid heavy lifting/sit-ups or other activities that may aggravate or damage a tender/enlarged liver.
   E. No alcohol.
   F. Monitor administration of hepatotoxic drugs: isoniazid, erythromycin, phenytoin, phenothiazines.
   G. Manage nausea and vomiting with nonphenothiazine antiemetics.
   H. Monitor progress of disease with follow-up exam and diagnostics.
2. CAHB: Patients who are HBeAg$^+$ and HBV DNA$^+$
   A. Refer to hepatologist for evaluation and recommendation for treatment with interferon-α_{2b}.
   B. Interferon-α_{2b} is administered as follows: 5 million units subcutaneously daily or 10 million units subcutaneously three times/week for 4 months.
3. HCV infection
   A. Refer to hepatologist for evaluation and treatment.
   B. Interferon-α_{2b} has been approved for treatment of chronic hepatitis C.
   C. Antiviral use is being researched.
4. HDV infection (see "Hepatitis B")
5. Hepatitis E infection (see "Hepatitis A")

PATIENT EDUCATION

1. Hepatitis A and E
   A. Avoid intimate contact.
   B. Do not handle food or serve others.
   C. Instruct regarding handling patient's fecal material (careful handwashing and disposal).
   D. Proper water treatment/sewage disposal.
   E. Proper treatment of foods that may be contaminated (heat to 185–194°F or steam 90 seconds).

2. Hepatitis B: Precautions listed to be continued until HBsAg clears from serum
    A. Sexually transmitted diseases: Use barrier technique.
    B. ANCP advises patient to inform partners of his/her infectious status.
    C. Avoid sharing needles/syringes.
    D. Use disposable needles/syringes.
    E. Do not share personal items (razor, toothbrush).
    F. Avoid sexual behavior that co-mingles body fluids.
    G. Instruct on thorough handwashing after direct contact with body fluids.
3. Hepatitis C and D
    A. Use disposable needles/syringes.
    B. Do not share personal items (razor, toothbrush).
    C. Instruct on thorough handwashing after direct contact with body fluids.
    D. Inform health care practitioners/blood donor facilities of history of hepatitis.

Review Questions

Ms. P is a 45-year-old corporate executive who was admitted from same-day surgery for removal of a plate from tibia/fibula for a sports injury sustained 1 year prior to admission. Past medical history reflects that, while traveling in Asia, the patient was in an auto accident 12 years earlier that required two blood transfusions. She recalls no permanent sequelae from the injuries, and has no current medical problems. Physical exam is negative. On review of her preoperative laboratory tests, CBC, platelets, prothrombin time (PT), PTT, Chem 20 were normal with the exception of the following: AST, 215; ALT, 343; LDH, 235; bilirubin total, 1.6 mg/dL.

10.31 What do these values indicate?
    A. Abnormal endocrine function
    B. Clotting disorder
    C. Abnormal liver function
    D. Underlying neurohumoral dysfunction

10.32 Given the patient's past medical history and laboratory values, which of the following tests should be ordered next?
    A. Cholangiogram
    B. Hepatic artery ultrasound
    C. Serum amylase, alkaline phosphatase
    D. HBsAg, anti-HCV, anti-HAV

10.33 Which factors put this patient at risk for hepatitis?
    A. Blood transfusion outside of United States
    B. Elevated LFTs
    C. Blood transfusion prior to anti-HCV screening
    D. All of the above

10.34 Which mode/modes of transmission are common to both HBV and HCV?
    A. Fecal-oral
    B. Sexual

      C. Parenteral

      D. Fecal-oral and sexual

10.35 How would the ACNP best handle this problem if the serologies show anti-HCV?

      A. Order further testing to include liver biopsy and abdominal ultrasound

      B. Recommend that the patient begin a low-protein, low-sodium diet

      C. Refer to a hepatologist

      D. Introduce the option of liver transplantation

Answers and Rationales

10.31 **C** AST, ALT, LDH, and bilirubin are indicators of liver function.

10.32 **D** Given the elevated liver function studies, the next set of tests to order are serologies that will screen for hepatitis. HBsAg will indicate the presence of surface antigen for HBV; anti-HCV will indicate past infection with HCV; anti-HAV will indicate past infection with HAV. The results of these tests will dictate which additional serologic testing is necessary.

10.33 **D** Blood transfusion outside the United States carries a risk when donor screening is not performed. Elevated LFTs indicate abnormal liver function. Hepatitis B and C donor screening was not available worldwide 12 years ago.

10.34 **C** Both HBV and HCV are transmitted parenterally.

10.35 **C** This patient needs referral to a hepatologist, given the elevated LFTs and presence of anti-HCV. The physician will decide on differential serologies and indication for liver biopsy. It is too early to initiate dietary changes; the patient is asymptomatic. It is not appropriate to discuss liver transplantation at this time. Further work-up and information are required.

References

Advisory Committee on Immunization Practice. (1991). Hepatitis B virus: A comprehensive strategy for eliminating transmission in the United States through universal childhood vaccination. *MMWR Morb Mortal Wkly Rep 40*(RR-12), 1–25.

Dienstag, J.L. (1995). Management of hepatitis. In A.H. Goroll, L.A. May, & A.G. Mulley Jr. (eds.). *Primary Care Medicine: Office Evaluation and Management of the Adult Patient* (3rd ed.). Philadelphia: J.B. Lippincott Co., pp. 399–407.

Dienstag, J.L. (1995). Prevention of viral hepatitis. In A.H. Goroll, L.A. May, & A.G. Mulley Jr. (eds.). *Primary Care Medicine: Office Evaluation and Management of the Adult Patient* (3rd ed.). Philadelphia: J.B. Lippincott Co., pp. 319–325.

Kowdley, K.V. (1996). Update on therapy for hepatobiliary diseases. *Nurse Pract 21*(7), 73–83.

Martin, P., Friedman, L.S., & Dienstag, J.J. (1991). Diagnostic approach. In A.J. Zuckerman & H.C. Thomas (eds.). *Viral Hepatitis: Scientific Basis and Clinical Management* London: Churchill Livingstone, pp. 393–409.

Uphold, C.R., & Graham, M.V. (1994). *Clinical Guidelines in Adult Health*. Gainesville, FL: Barmarrae Books.

Acute Gastroenteritis

DEFINITION

Acute gastroenteritis is defined as an increase in stool frequency or water content and/or vomiting that involves inflammation of the mucous membrane of both the stomach and intestine.

ETIOLOGY/INCIDENCE

1. Numerous viral and bacterial agents and parasites invade intestinal tract; each is associated with unique epidemiologic and clinical characteristics.
2. May be caused by emotional stress, infections, food intolerance, inorganic or organic poisons, or drugs.
3. Travel to another country, especially if the change involves a marked difference in climate, social conditions, or sanitation standards.
4. Most episodes of acute endemic diarrhea occurring in the United States are self-limiting, lasting 7–10 days.
5. Fifty to 60% are viral in origin.
6. Less than 30% are bacterial in origin.
7. Nonbacterial gastroenteritis more common in winter months.
8. May be epidemic in family, school, community.

PATHOPHYSIOLOGY

Pathogenesis involves a wide variety of infectious and chemical agents. Enterotoxin is formed that reacts with receptors in gut or is absorbed in bloodstream. Bacterial toxin–mediated illnesses (such as those caused by *Staphylococcus aureus, Clostridium perfringens*) are not truly infections. The secretory activity of the small bowel overcomes the absorptive capacity of the distal small bowel and proximal colon, resulting in diarrhea.

SIGNS AND SYMPTOMS

1. Presentation varies with etiology. Historical clues are essential to establish diagnosis. History should include onset, character, frequency of stools, presence of blood or mucous, drug usage, diet, recent travel, and sexual preference.
2. Presenting symptoms vary with the specific diarrheal diseases.
   A. Viral: Abrupt onset, vomiting and respiratory symptoms are common, fever >101.3°F (38.5°C). Stools are loose, brown with unpleasant odor. History of chills and fever, myalgia usually present.
   B. Bacterial gastroenteritis presents with colicky or crampy abdominal pain, nausea, vomiting, diarrhea, chills.
      1) Diarrhea that begins 1–6 hours after ingesting contaminated food or beverage is suggestive of staphylococcal infection.
      2) Diarrhea that begins 8–48 hours after ingesting contaminated food or beverage is likely to be caused by *Shigella* or *Salmonella* (see Table 10–3).
   C. Symptoms of nausea and vomiting that do not clear but progress to diplopia, dysphagia, dizziness may be indications of botulism and require emergency medical consult.

TABLE 10–3. Characteristics of Acute Gastroenteritis by Etiology

Etiology	Nature of Diarrhea			Associated Symptoms and Signs	Epidemiologic Data	Laboratory Results
	W/S	OB	GB			
Viral	+/+	−	−	n, v, fever, myalgias, abdominal cramps, headache	Occurs in short-lived epidemics	WBC: nl or elevated; Stool: usually no WBC
Staphylococcus aureus	−/+	−	−	n, v, no fever	Custards; incubation: 2–8 hr	WBC: nl; Stool: no WBC
Clostridium perfringens	+/+	−	−	n, v, no fever	Steam table incubation: 8–24 hr	WBC: nl; Stool: no WBC
Bacillus cereus	+/+	−	−	n, v, no fever	Rice, sprouts	WBC: nl; Stool: no WBC
Salmonella	+/−	+	+	n, v, fever, in some cases dysentery	Eggs, turtles, poultry	Stool: WBC+, culture+
Salmonella typhi	+/+ "Pea soup"	+	−	Rose spots, HA, splenomegaly, bradycardia, fever, toxic	Water, food	Stool: monos, culture +
Shigella	+/− Dysentery	+	−	n, v, fever, toxic in severe cases	Ghettos; day care centers; Indian reservations	Stool: WBC+, culture+
Campylobacter	+/− Dysentery	+	+	n, v, fever	Poultry, pets	Stool: WBC+, culture+
Yersinia	+/+	+	−	Simulates Crohn's disease and appendicitis; joint complaints	Dairy products, meat	Stool: WBC+, culture+
Vibrio sp.	+/+	−	−	n, v, cramps, occasionally fever	Raw seafood; 2-day course	Stool culture+
Cryptosporidia	+/−	−	−	occasionally n, v, cramps, dehydration	AIDS patients, immunosuppressed	Stool for o & p +

* Adapted from Rickter, J. (1995). Evaluation and management of diarrhea. In A.H. Goroll, L.A. May, & A.G. Mulley (eds.). *Primary Care Medicine: Office Evaluation and Management of the Adult Patient, (3rd ed.).* Philadelphia: J.B. Lippincott Co., with permission.

W/S, watery/soft; OB, occult blood; GB, gross blood; +, present; −, absent; n, nausea; v, vomiting; HA, headache; AIDS, acquired immunodeficiency syndrome; o & p, ova and parasites; nl, normal; WBC, white blood cells.

D. Abdominal pain is typically diffuse or periumbilical, reflecting involvement of the small bowel. Abdominal discomfort is usually relieved by bowel movement.

E. Grossly bloody, mucoid stools are indicative of dysentery.

PHYSICAL FINDINGS

1. Generally ill appearance
2. High fever
3. Mild tenderness with palpation of the abdomen, no rigidity, guarding
4. Hyperactive bowel sounds
5. No signs of peritoneal inflammation

DIFFERENTIAL DIAGNOSIS

1. Appendicitis
2. Ulcerative colitis
3. Cystic fibrosis
4. Peptic ulcer disease
5. Pancreatitis

DIAGNOSTIC TESTS/FINDINGS

1. Stool for occult blood and fecal white cell smear. Finding of 25 or more white blood cells correlates with bacterial pathogen as etiologic agent.
2. For symptoms that last for more than 1 week, stool for ova and parasites, *Giardia* should be sent.
3. Time and amount of last void will assist in establishing volume status.
4. Immunosuppressed populations with symptoms lasting longer than 5–7 days should be referred for comprehensive work-up.

MANAGEMENT/TREATMENT

1. Treatment is aimed at symptoms because majority of cases of gastroenteritis will not respond to antibiotic therapy.
2. Bed rest for first few days of illness.
3. Diet should be initially aimed at replenishing lost fluids and resting the bowel.
   A. Clear fluids should be administered for first 24 hours or until symptoms improve.
   B. Caffeine should be avoided because it stimulates intestinal motility.
   C. Lactose-containing foods may cause bloating, flatulence.
   D. Foods that are high in carbohydrates and low in residue indicated after vomiting ceases (noodles, baked potatoes, saltine crackers).
   E. Vegetables, broiled poultry, fish can be introduced after diarrhea is improved.
4. Bismuth subsalicylate reduces volume of watery stools by 50%. Do not administer salicylates concurrently. Dosage is 30 mL or 2 tablets q30min up to maximum of eight doses.
5. Antiperistaltic agents can be useful for treating abdominal cramps and reducing frequency of stools. Loperamide 4 mg initially followed by 2 mg after each loose stool, not to exceed 16 mg/day. Diphenoxylate hydrochloride 1–2 tablets or tsp tid or qid initially; decrease dose to 1 tablet or tsp bid or tid.
6. Antibiotics are indicated if patient has fever and dysentery. Ciprofloxacin 500 mg PO bid or norfloxacin 400 mg PO bid for 3 days.
7. Patients with signs of hypovolemia may require intravenous replacement, such as normal saline with 20 mEq of potassium to run at 100 mL/hr until urine output >30 mL/hr.
8. The ACNP should refer any patient with persistent symptoms that do not clear after 2 weeks, those with bloody diarrhea, and immunosuppressed patients with symptoms lasting longer than 5 days.

PATIENT EDUCATION

1. Nutrition teaching as indicated above.
2. Need for bed rest with progression to regular activity as tolerated.

3. Disease course and expected outcome; symptoms should resolve within 24–48 hours.
4. Inform patient to return to clinic if symptoms persist beyond 3 days.
5. Medication teaching regarding dosage, frequency, side effects, signs of toxicity.

Review Questions

10.36 Pathophysiology of acute gastroenteritis is:
   A. Bacterial invasion of large intestine, which causes mucosal ulcerations and in severe cases can lead to perforation and peritonitis
   B. Related to an inability of the body to defend against invading organisms, with resultant overgrowth of endogenous flora
   C. Due to a wide variety of infectious and chemical agents in which the secretory activity of the bowel overcomes the absorptive capacity
   D. All of the above

10.37 The etiologic agent for gastroenteritis is:
   A. Bacterial
   B. Viral
   C. Chemical
   D. All of the above

10.38 A 21-year-old college student presents with complaints of severe diarrhea with 10–12 loose brown stools in the last 24 hours. Has abdominal cramping that is temporarily relieved by passing stool. Has had low-grade fever and nausea. Denies vomiting, dizziness, diplopia. She lives alone and does not know if anyone else has similar symptoms. She has not traveled to a foreign country, denies use of any recreational drugs or alcohol. Her last meal was about 36 hours ago when she had eggs Benedict for brunch at her favorite restaurant. Based on this history you suspect the etiology of her illness to be:
   A. Viral gastroenteritis
   B. *Salmonella*
   C. *Staphylococcus*
   D. Crohn's disease

10.39 A stool specimen is sent for occult blood and fecal white smear. A white blood cell count of 36 is returned. This finding is highly correlated with:
   A. Bacterial pathogen
   B. Viral pathogen
   C. *Giardia*
   D. Infectious diarrhea in an immunocompromised host; HIV test should be sent after consent is obtained

10.40 A 29-year-old male presents complaining of high fever, diarrhea, nausea, and vomiting for 24 hours. Your presumptive diagnosis is acute gastroenteritis. To assist in validating this diagnosis, your history should include:
   A. History of onset, frequency of stools, medications, diet history, recent travel, and sexual preference
   B. Recent history of upper respiratory infections
   C. Family members, friends with similar symptoms
   D. All of the above

Answers and Rationales

10.36 **C** Acute gastroenteritis is due to a wide variety of infectious and chemical agents in which the secretory activity of the bowel overcomes the absorptive capacity.

10.37 **D** Viral, bacterial, and chemical agents can cause acute gastroenteritis by interfering with the resorptive or secretory functions of the intestine.

10.38 **B** The diarrhea began about 12 hours after eating eggs Benedict. The time frame for *Salmonella* and *Shigella* is 8–48 hours after eating. The most common form of *Salmonella* is found in eggs and poultry.

10.39 **A** The finding of WBC >25 on fecal smear is indicative of bacterial pathogen.

10.40 **D** The etiology will dictate the presenting symptoms. Viral etiology will have sudden onset with fever, chills. Bacterial cause will present with abdominal pain, diarrhea that begins after ingesting contaminated food; may or may not have fever. Chemical cause will vary but does not include fever as presenting symptoms. Bloody mucoid stools are a sign of dysentery and require emergency medical consult.

References

Connor, S., D'Andrea, K., Piper, J., et al. (1989). *Comprehensive Review Manual for the Adult Nurse Practitioner.* Glenview, IL: Scott, Foresman, and Company

Fenton, B. (1996). Infectious diarrhea. In R.E. Rakel (ed.). *Saunders Manual of Medical Practice.* Philadelphia: W.B. Saunders Co., pp. 302–306.

Jacobs, R. (1996). General problems in infectious diseases. In L. Tierney, S. McPhee, & M. Papadakis (eds.). *Current Medical Diagnosis and Treatment.* Stamford, CT: Appleton & Lange, pp. 1111–1134.

Rickter, J. (1995). Evaluation and management of diarrhea. In A. Goroll, L. May, & A. Muley (eds.). *Primary Care Medicine: Office Evaluation and Management of the Adult Patient* (3rd ed.). Philadelphia: J.B. Lippincott Co, pp. 357–368.

Talal, A. (1994). Acute and chronic diarrhea: how to keep laboratory testing to a minimum. *Postgrad Med 96*, 30.

Hepatic Failure

DEFINITIONS

Cirrhosis (scarring): Irreversible widespread replacement of hepatic architecture with fibrous tissue as a result of chronic liver disease, ultimately progressing to hepatic failure.

Hepatic failure (end-stage liver disease [ESLD]): Loss of liver function resulting in a clinical syndrome characterized by hyperbilirubinemia, decreased synthetic function, portal hypertension, encephalopathy, hepatorenal syndrome. Caused by viral hepatitis (fulminant and chronic), autoimmune hepatitis, alcoholic cirrhosis, Wilson's disease (genetic defect causing excessive copper accumulation), Budd-Chiari syndrome (hypercoagulable state causing progressive clotting of the hepatic veins leading to ESLD), primary biliary cirrhosis, sclerosing cholangitis.

PATHOPHYSIOLOGY

1. Portal hypertension: Portal vein pressure >10 mm Hg caused by obstruction of and/or impedance to blood flow in the portal circulation.
   A. Causes
      1) Obstruction to blood flow inside liver as a result of thrombosis, inflammation, fibrosis of sinusoids (cirrhosis)
      2) Impedance to portal outflow (hepatic vein thrombosis)
   B. Clinical indicators
      1) Varices in esophagus, anterior abdominal wall, rectum
      2) Splenomegaly: Enlargement of spleen caused by increased pressure in splenic vein; contributes to clotting disorders due to thrombocytopenia
2. Altered synthetic function
   A. Decreased protein synthesis of key clotting factors II, VII, IX, X and plasma proteins (70% albumin) causing coagulopathy and fluid retention.
   B. Clinical indicators: elevated prothrombin time; ascites, peripheral edema. In the setting of fulminant liver failure, loss of protein synthesis results in cerebral edema, leading to death.
3. Hyperbilirubinemia (>1.2 mg/dL)
   A. Resulting from hepatocellular damage and obstruction of bile canaliculi.
   B. Clinical indicators: jaundice, pruritis
4. Encephalopathy: Caused by portal systemic shunting allowing toxins (ammonia) absorbed from the GI tract to circulate freely to the brain, resulting in a complex neurologic syndrome characterized by altered cerebral function, flapping tremor (asterixis), and electroencephalographic changes.
5. Hepatorenal syndrome: Characterized by advanced liver disease, functional renal failure manifested by elevated creatinine, oliguria, sodium and water retention, (with or without ascites and peripheral edema), hypotension, and peripheral vasodilation. Most commonly associated with portal hypertension and cirrhosis.

SIGNS AND SYMPTOMS

1. Variceal bleeds
   A. Incidence: 20–30% of patients with cirrhosis
   B. UGI: Bleeding episodes—esophageal varices
      1) Hematemesis (vomiting fresh or changed blood)
      2) Melena
      3) Associated with weakness/dizziness
   C. Rectal varices
      1) Hematochezia, bright red or maroon blood per rectum
      2) Associated with weakness/dizziness
2. Fluid retention
   A. Enlarged abdomen: Ascites
   B. Bilateral lower extremity edema
3. Encephalopathy: Symptom progression
   A. Subtle changes in personality
   B. Irritability
   C. Memory loss
   D. Sleep disturbance (nightmares, insomnia)

    E. Hyperreflexia (liver flap)

    F. Stupor

    G. Coma

4. Jaundice

    A. Dark urine

    B. Icteric sclera

    C. Yellow-green skin color

    D. Pruritis

5. Significant history

    A. Excessive alcohol intake

    B. Chronic active hepatitis B

    C. Hepatitis C

    D. Hemachromatosis

    E. Primary biliary cirrhosis

    F. Sclerosing cholangitis

PHYSICAL FINDINGS

Vary significantly.

1. Ascites—enlarged abdomen, shifting dullness, fluid wave, bulging flanks
2. Bilateral pitting lower extremity edema; sacral/flank edema; scrotal edema
3. Jaundice—dark urine, icteric sclera
4. Splenomegaly—palpable spleen
5. Liver: 70% may be firm to palpation; firm, nodular and suggesting hepatoma; or not palpable because of cirrhosis and ascites
6. Spider angiomata: Upper half of body
7. Telangiectases of exposed areas
8. Palmar erythema
9. Cheilosis, glossitis: Evidence of vitamin deficiency; associated with alcoholic cirrhosis
10. Hypogonadism and feminization prominent in men with alcoholic cirrhosis or hemochromatosis

    A. Gynecomastia (men)

    B. Testicular atrophy

    C. Amenorrhea

    D. Loss of axillary and public hair

11. Weight loss, wasting, appearance of chronic illness

DIFFERENTIAL DIAGNOSIS

1. Fulminant acute disease (toxic, drug induced, viral)
2. Chronic active hepatitis B; hepatitis C
3. Hemachromatosis: Associated with "bronzing" of the skin, arthritis, heart disease, diabetes mellitus; >50% saturation of serum transferrin or elevated serum ferritin level
4. Cholestatic disease
5. Primary biliary cirrhosis: Chronic disease manifested by cholestasis in women 40–60; associated with elevated alkaline phosphatase; complicated by portal hypertension
6. Alcoholic cirrhosis
7. Toxic and drug-induced hepatitis
8. Primary/metastatic malignant disease

DIAGNOSTIC TESTS/FINDINGS

1. LFTs
   A. AST elevated in hepatocellular disease, viral hepatitis
   B. ALT more than doubled in alcoholic cirrhosis
   C. ALT elevated in hepatocellular disease, viral hepatitis
   D. Alkaline phosphatase mildly elevated in hepatocellular disease, markedly elevated in cholestatic disease
   E. Bilirubin direct/total ratio elevated in hepatocellular jaundice
2. Urine bilirubin elevated in hepatocellular/obstructive jaundice
3. Serum albumin decreased
4. Prothrombin time (INR) elevated
5. Platelet count decreased with associated splenomegaly
6. Creatinine elevated with associated hepatorenal syndrome
7. Serum ammonia elevated with associated variceal bleeding/ encephalopathy serum albumin
8. Serum sodium decreased; associated with ascites/marked edema/low
9. Serum potassium elevated with hepatorenal syndrome, decreased with loop diuretic use
10. Hemoglobin (HgB)/hematocrit (Hct) decreased with variceal bleeds
11. Macrocytic anemia associated with alcoholic cirrhosis
12. Microcytic anemia (iron deficiency, chronic disease) associated with alcoholic cirrhosis

MANAGEMENT/TREATMENT

Most patients with ESLD are managed in the ambulatory care setting. The indications for admission include:

1. Active GI bleeding
2. Worsening encephalopathy
3. Increasing azotemia
4. Signs of infection/peritoneal irritation
5. Intractable ascites

The patients admitted are managed by the physician with the ACNP working in collaboration per practice protocols. Some of these patients may be candidates for liver transplantation (Table 10–4) or have been evaluated and are listed for liver transplantation. Admission for the above criteria will affect their status and must be communicated to the transplant center.

Diagnostics

1. Laboratory tests: Bilirubin T/C, ALT, AST, alkaline phosphatase, BUN, creatinine, electrolytes, CBC with differential, platelet count, prothrombin time, serum albumin, ammonia level. Stool for occult blood. Hepatitis serologies as needed.
2. Imaging: Plain films of abdomen for liver, spleen enlargement. Ultrasound to determine presence of occult ascites, liver size, hepatic nodules, tumor. Doppler ultrasound to evaluate patency of splenic, portal, hepatic veins. CT scan with contrast to determine lesions in liver. Cholangiogram to determine patency of biliary tree. Esophagogastroscopy to demonstrate/confirm varices or bleeding in stomach/proximal duodenum.

TABLE 10–4.   Referral Criteria: Liver Transplantation Evaluation—Adults*

Indications	Absolute Contraindications
Post necrotic cirrhosis—fulminant liver failure	Active drug/alcohol use
Primary biliary cirrhosis	
Primary sclerosing cholangitis	Extrahepatic sepsis
Alcohol-induced liver disease—demonstrated 6 months of sobriety	Metastic cancer
Hepatitis C—chronic active (CAHC)	Severe cardiopulmonary disease
Hepatitis B—HBeAg negative	
Primary hepatocellular carcinoma—no metastasis	

* Data from Weisner, R.H., (1996). Current indications, contraindications and timing for liver transplantation. In R.W. Busuttil & G.B. Klintmalm, (eds.). *Transplantation of the Liver*. Philadelphia: W.B. Saunders Co., pp. 71–84, with permission.

Management

1. General Considerations
   A. Caloric intake 2000–3000 Kcal/day
   B. Prohibit use of alcohol/hepatotoxic agents (isoniazid, Valproate, phenytoin, methyldopa, acetaminophen)
   C. Avoid use of sedative and tranquilizing agents
   D. Monitor stools for occult blood
   E. Assess for signs of encephalopathy
   F. Assess abdomen for signs of ascites
2. Ascites
   A. A 2 to 4-gm sodium diet for mild fluid retention.
   B. A 2-gm sodium diet for moderate fluid retention/ascites.
   C. Fluid restriction to 1500 mL/day if hyponatremic (Na <125 mEq/L).
   D. Diuretic therapy: Spironolactone 100 mg/day in divided doses to 400 mg maximum; furosemide 20–40 mg/day, increasing dose to reduce weight by 1 lb/day with ascites and 2 lb/day in patients with both ascites and peripheral edema. Monitor BUN/creatinine.
   E. Potassium replacement 20–40 mEq/day; use with caution in patients with elevated creatinine or on potassium-sparing diuretics.
   F. Paracentesis (treatment for tense ascites) to drain 3–6 L for comfort and to limit risk of respiratory compromise; replace with 6–8 gm albumin/L removed to protect intravascular volume. Other colloids may be used, such as dextran. (*Note:* These patients will reaccumulate peritoneal fluid in 2–3 days as a result of low serum albumin and portal hypertension.)
3. UGI: Variceal bleeding (refer to section on "Gastrointestinal Bleeds")
   A. Assess for risk
   B. B-Blockers: Propranolol 80 mg (primary prevention)
   C. Acute bleeds with hypotension: Fluid resuscitation, Sengstaken-Blakemore tube; refer to gastroenterologist/interventional radiologist for interventions listed below:
      1) Injection sclerotherapy
      2) Transjugular intrahepatic portosystemic shunt (TIPS)
      3) Splenorenal/portacaval shunt
4. Encephalopathy
   A. Dietary management: First-line intervention

1) Protein restriction: 20–30 gm/day
2) Lactulose 15–30 mL q 3–4h until patients have three or four loose stools/day
3) Metronidazole (Flagyl) 250 mg tid to inhibit nitrogen-producing gram-negative organisms
4) Neomycin 1 gm bid: Nephrotoxic—use with caution in patients at risk for hepatorenal syndrome
5) Bromocriptine (Parlodel) 2.5 mg tid: Started when serum ammonia is low, patient is receiving lactulose, but still exhibits encephalopathic behavior interfering with activities of daily living

B. Bleeding: Clotting factor deficiency
1) Monitor prothrombin time/platelet count
2) Vitamin K 10 mg SQ qd for 3 days if prothrombin time >14 seconds

C. Pruritis
1) Cholestyramine 4 gm or colestipol 5 gm in water or juice tid
2) Rifampin 300 mg orally bid

PATIENT EDUCATION

1. Stress importance of no longer using alcohol or hepatotoxic drugs.
2. Stress importance of strict dietary compliance.
3. Referral for group support for patient/family when untreated alcoholism is underlying cause of hepatic failure.
4. Inform patient/family of potential for depression to complicate late stages of liver failure.
   A. Teach family signs of depression and when to report them.
   B. Emphasize need to limit use of sedative/tranquilizing agents.
   C. Refer for mental health support/treatment.
5. Teach patient/family action and side effects of all drugs in treatment regimen.
6. Inform patient/family what signs/symptoms need to be reported immediately to health care providers.
   A. Marked increase in fluid retention (weight gain >1 lb/day); increase in dependent edema; increase in ascites/shortness of breath
   B. Brisk bleeding
   C. Signs of infection: Fever/abdominal tenderness
   D. Intractable pruritis
   E. Increase in weakness/dizziness/orthostasis
   F. Increased confusion/stupor/coma

Review Questions

Mr. K is a 62-year-old admitted in ESLD secondary to alcohol and chronic active hepatitis. This is hospitalization day 2, and you note the patient is tachypneic; has a markedly enlarged, tense, nontender abdomen; 3+ pitting at the ankle, and pretibial edema. Blood pressure (BP) is 98/60 pulse is 84 bpm, respirations are 38/min. He complains of memory loss, and irritability, is obtunded and slow to respond to questions.

10.41 These clinical findings indicate:
   A. CHF/pulmonary edema
   B. Ascites/encephalopathy
   C. Tenesmus/peritonitis
   D. Azotemia/coagulopathy

10.42 The treatment for this patient will include:
   A. Diuretic therapy
   B. Protein-restricted diet
   C. Paracentesis
   D. All of the above

Mr. K received a paracentesis. Three liters of clear amber fluid were removed. His respirations are 18/min at rest; oxygen saturation 96% on 3 L per nasal canula. It is noted that his BP is now 78/48, pulse 100 bpm.

10.43 What is the most likely cause of these symptoms?
   A. Intravascular volume depletion
   B. Acute variceal bleed
   C. Bacteremia/sepsis
   D. Cerebral edema

10.44 What is the treatment of choice?
   A. Colloid replacement
   B. Crystalloid replacement
   C. Vasopressors
   D. Blood products

10.45 Symptom progression of encephalopathy, in the setting of hepatic failure, may be seen when:
   A. The diagnosis of hepatitis is made
   B. The serum creatinine begins to climb
   C. In the setting of concomitant UGI variceal bleeds
   D. None of the above

Answers and Rationales

10.41 **B** In the setting of ESLD, the clinical indicators of ascites include enlarged abdomen that elevates diaphragm, leading to tachypnea. The symptoms of memory loss, irritability, and slow response indicate the presence of encephalopathy.

10.42 **D** This patient will benefit from diuretic therapy as indicated by the marked peripheral edema and ascites; from paracentesis because of the presence of tachypnea; and from a protein-restricted diet to decrease serum amonia levels, thereby helping to control encephalopathy.

10.43 **A** This patient has lost 3 L of fluid and most probably has a low serum albumin as a result of the ESLD, thereby contributing to intravascular volume depletion.

10.44 **A** In the setting of ESLD, characterized by tense ascites, patients run a low serum albumin and require colloid replacement following paracentesis to prevent intravascular volume depletion.

10.45 **C** Symptom progression of encephalopathy in the setting of ESLD occurs with UGI variceal bleeds. Blood in the GI tract is broken down into ammonia, elevating serum ammonia levels.

References

Friedman, L.S. (1995). Liver, biliary tract, and pancreas. In L. Tierney, S. McPhee, & M. Papadakis (eds.). *Current Medical Diagnosis and Treatment.* Stamford: CT: Appleton & Lange, pp. 555–578.

Goroll, A.H. (1995). Management of cirrhosis and chronic liver failure. In A.H. Goroll, L.A. May, & A.G. Mulley (eds.). *Primary Care Medicine: Office Evaluation and Management of the Adult Patient* (3rd ed.). Philadelphia: J.B. Lippincott Co., pp. 319–325.

Kowdley, K.V. (1996). Update on therapy for hepatobiliary diseases. *Nurse Pract 21*(7), 73–83.

Podolsky, D.K., & Isselbacher, K.J. (1994). Alcohol-related liver disease and cirrhosis. In L.I. Isselbacher, E.H. Braunwald, J.D. Wilson, J.B. Martin, A.S. Fauci, & D.L. Kasper (eds.). *Harrison's Principles of Internal Medicine* New York: McGraw-Hill, pp. 1483–1495.

Reishstein, J. (1993). Liver failure: Case study of a complex problem. *Crit Care Nurse* October, 36–47.

Weisner, R.H. (1996). Current indications, contraindications and timing for liver transplantation. In R.W. Busuttil & G.B. Klintmalm (eds.). *Transplantation of the Liver.* Philadelphia, W.B. Saunders Co., pp. 69–72.

Colorectal Cancer

DEFINITION

Colorectal cancer (CRC) is an adenocarcinoma type of neoplasm occurring in the colorectal area arising from glandular epithelium and extending into adjacent organs or spreading via lymphatics to regional lymph nodes, and then via the bloodstream.

ETIOLOGY/INCIDENCE

1. Colorectal cancer is the second most common form of cancer in the United States and has the second highest mortality rate, accounting for approximately 140,000 new cases and 55,000 deaths each year.
2. In the United States, a higher incidence is seen in the northeastern states than in the western and southern areas.
3. Survival rates for whites and blacks are estimated at 58% and 47%, respectively.
4. Sixty percent of patients with CRC have both regional and distant metastases at time of diagnosis.
5. Estimated 5-year survival is 91% in persons with localized disease, 60% in persons with regional spread, and only 6% in those with distant metastases.
6. Eleven percent of total cancer deaths are due to cancer associated with colorectal malignancies.

RISK FACTORS

1. Age
   A. Individuals over 60 years: 75 cases of CRC diagnosed per 100,000 population
   B. Individuals over 80 years: 300 cases of CRC diagnosed per 100,000 population
2. Family History
   A. First-degree relative raises personal risk two- to three-fold, with greatest risk if CRC was diagnosed at an early age (<45 years)
   B. Hereditary adenocarcinomatosis syndrome
   C. Familial colorectal cancer syndrome
3. Pre-existing disease
   A. Inflammatory bowel disease
   B. Previously resected CRC
   C. Pelvic cancer postirradiation
   D. Neoplastic colorectal polyps
   E. Crohn's colitis: May cause dysplasia, then CRC
4. Genetic
   A. Polyposis syndromes (numerous polyps in an organ)
   B. Variants include:
      1) Familial adenomatous polyposis syndrome
      2) Gardner syndrome
      3) Turcot syndrome
      4) Peutz-Jeghers syndrome
5. Diet: Subject of extensive research over past 20 years; thought to have an influence on the development of CRC
   A. Factors associated with increased risk
      1) High fat intake
      2) High protein intake
   B. Factors associated with decreased risk
      1) Selenium
      2) Calcium
      3) Increased fiber intake
6. Chemoprotective Agents: Being investigated as inhibitors of carcinogenesis
   A. Ascorbic acid
   B. Flavones, indoles found in cruciferous vegetables (brussels sprouts, cauliflower, broccoli, cabbage)

PATHOPHYSIOLOGY

Adenocarcinomas are characterized microscopically into polypoid or annular constricting lesions. Both may appear throughout the colon. However, polypoid tumors appear more frequently on the right side of the colon and present as a large mass that infrequently constricts the bowel lumen; annular constricting lesions are associated with the left colon and present as nodular infiltrating lesions that may ulcerate and present on left side, sigmoid, or rectum and appear on barium enema as an "apple core" configuration.

   The degree of progression depends on histologic classification, differentiation, and local and distant metastases. Primary cancers of the large bowel grow slowly, with doubling times >600 days (1.6 years). Once metastases occurs, the doubling rate increases.

The duration of symptoms does not correlate to degree of tumor advancement, with symptoms occurring late in the course of CRC growth. Approximately 60% of patients who present with clinical symptoms demonstrate tumor dissemination to regional nodes or distant organs.

SIGNS AND SYMPTOMS

1. Asymptomatic
   A. Positive fecal occult blood testing (FOBT) or six-test guaiac stool test.
   B. Fatigue/malaise may be presenting symptoms secondary to slow GI bleed causing anemia.
2. Right-sided colon carcinomas: Bulky mass-like lesions; present late in course of tumor growth because of the distensibility of the right colon
   A. Reported minor changes in bowel habits; frequently corrected with diet changes.
   B. Intermittent rectal bleeding frequently relieved through symptomatic treatment of hemorrhoids.
   C. Vague cramping pain or aching-pressure sensation.
   D. Acute pain may be indistinguishable from acute appendicitis or cholecystitis; may be accompanied by physical findings of bowel perforation.
3. Left-sided colon carcinomas: Constricting lesions; symptomatic earlier
   A. Initially reported sensations of fullness or cramping
   B. Progression to changes in bowel habits; obstipation and constipation
   C. Acute abdominal pain caused by intestinal obstruction or perforation
   D. Bright-red blood, hematochezia are more common with carcinoma of left colon
4. Rectal cancer
   A. Bowel habit changes are classic symptoms.
   B. Increased frequency of evacuation in morning.
   C. Incomplete evacuation/tenesmus develop.
   D. Complaints of rectal pressure and/or fullness.
   E. Decrease in stool caliber ("pencil-like").
   F. Bleeding that is bright red, either mixed with or nonsurface of stool.
   G. Pain is *not* a prominent feature of early rectal cancer.

PHYSICAL FINDINGS

1. Asymptomatic stage, physical findings are negative.
2. Palpable abdominal mass RLQ: Right-sided colon cancer.
3. Alteration in bowel sounds (hyperactive vs. hypoactive) may be indicative of obstruction or perforation.
4. Rebound tenderness may indicate bowel perforation/peritonitis.
5. Enlarged liver/spleen may indicate metastases.
6. Digital rectal exam (DRE): To detect presence of fecal occult blood and to palpate tumor (only 15–20% of colorectal carcinomas are within a 7-cm area from the anal verge).
7. Vaginal examination required to detect fistula or rectal cancer extending to the abdominal side walls, which may be detected on exam in females.

DIFFERENTIAL DIAGNOSIS

1. Constipation
2. Diverticulitis

3. Appendicitis
4. Peritonitis
5. Bowel obstruction/perforation
6. Cholecystitis

DIAGNOSTIC TESTS/FINDINGS

It is essential to evaluate each patient individually, taking into account age and risk factors when ordering initial diagnostic tests. The ACNP will collaborate with the physician when presented with a patient who requires work-up for potential CRC. Initial tests ordered may include:

1. Fecal occult blood testing to validate findings
2. CBC with differential to detect inflammation/infection, anemia
3. Liver function tests: ALT, AST, LDH, alkaline phosphatase to evaluate for cholecystitis/liver metastases

Referral to a collaborating physician is required for further diagnostic testing.
1. Colonoscopy is procedure of choice to most accurately visualize and evaluate entire large bowel from rectum to cecum and to enable biopsy of polyps and lesions.
2. Barium enema may be used to evaluate large bowel masses; diagnostic in only 70% of cases when used alone; optimally should be combined with sigmoidoscopy.
3. Routine abdominal films, flat and upright, to evaluate bowel obstruction.
4. Carcinoembryonic antigen (CEA) tested as a prognostic tool in the pretreatment phase of evaluation following diagnosis.
5. CT scan to determine spread of tumor and assess lymph node involvement.
6. Magnetic resonance imaging used to stage rectal cancer.

REFERRAL CRITERIA

1. Patients with positive physical findings
2. High-risk patients (see Table 10–5)
   A. History of colorectal cancer or adenomas in first-degree relative
   B. Personal history of large adenomatous polyps or colorectal cancer
   C. Prior diagnosis of endometrial, ovarian, or breast cancer

MANAGEMENT/TREATMENT

1. Fecal occult blood testing/DRE: Important screening procedures/examination for those at risk and individuals over age of 40
2. Flexible sigmoidoscopy or colonoscopy indicated for following:
   A. Rectal pain
   B. Bright red bleeding per rectum
   C. Hematochezia
   D. Change in bowel habits
   E. Chronic constipation
   F. Unexplained weight loss
   G. Abdominal or rectal mass
   H. Guaiac-positive stool
   I. Patients at high risk for colorectal malignancy (ulcerative colitis, familial polyposis)

TABLE 10-5. High Risk Factors for Colorectal Cancer
History positive for colorectal carcinoma
History positive for colorectal adenoma
Colorectal carcinoma in first-degree relative
Hereditary gastrointestinal polyposis syndrome
Hereditary nonpolyposis colorectal cancer syndrome
Crohn's disease
Ulcerative colitis

    J. Unexplained iron-deficiency anemia

    K. Men and women over the age of 55 years

3. Colorectal carcinoma: Referral to a general surgeon—surgery is treatment of choice

    A. Extent and type of resection is determined by tumor location, vascular supply, and distribution of lymph nodes in the region.

    B. Resections include a margin of 2–5 cm on either side of the tumor.

    C. Types of procedures include:

        1) Right hemicolectomy: Indicated for tumors of appendix, cecum, ascending colon, and hepatic flexure

        2) Transverse colectomy

        3) Left hemicolectomy, left partial colectomy: Indicated when splenic flexure and descending colon are involved

        4) Sigmoid colectomy: For neoplasms of sigmoid colon

        5) Subtotal or total colectomy: Indicated for large tumors found in either the left or right colon; can cause nutritional problems and skin breakdown around stoma

4. Rectal cancer: Referral to a surgeon

    A. Surgery selected based on tumor location and preservation of bowel continuity.

    B. Low anterior resection: Indicated for tumor in distal sigmoid upper rectum, with temporary or permanent colostomy.

    C. Abdominal perineal resection: Indicated when tumor is adjacent to sphincter, 8 cm from the anal verge; physically altering, requiring permanent colostomy; can result in impaired erectile function

PATIENT EDUCATION

1. Information regarding the disease, risk factors

2. Information regarding screening for prevention/early identification: American Cancer Society recommendations are shown in Table 10–6

3. Recognition and reporting of signs and symptoms

4. Information regarding influential dietary factors—fiber, fat, etc.

TABLE 10-6. American Cancer Society CRC Screening Recommendations		
Age	**Test**	**Frequency**
≥40	Digital rectal examination	Annually
≥50	Fecal occult blood testing	Annually
≥50	Flexible sigmoidoscopy	3–5 years

Review Questions

Ms. P is a 55-year-old woman admitted for a chief complaint of abdominal pain to rule out bowel obstruction. She denies nausea and vomiting; reports change in bowel habits over the past year characterized by sensation of fullness, cramping, and constipation. She has noted bright-red blood, at times, in her stools. She reports a 6-lb weight loss over the past 3 months and complains of fatigue and weakness. Past medical history reveals that her mother died at 68 from colon cancer. Temperature is 36.8°C, BP is 112/89, pulse is 88 bpm, respirations are 18/min. Physical exam reveals a soft, mildly distended abdomen with tenderness and a 4-cm palpable mass in the left lower quadrant. No guarding or rebound tenderness.

10.46 Initial laboratory tests will include:
   A. CBC, electrolytes, LFTs
   B. Amylase, lipase
   C. CEA
   D. Triglycerides, cholesterol, high- and low-density lipoproteins

10.47 What factor/factors most influence this patient's risk for CRC?
   A. Age >50 years
   B. History of weight loss, weakness
   C. CRC in first-degree relative
   D. Change in bowel habits

10.48 Left-sided colon carcinomas are characterized by which of the following?
   A. Sensations of fullness, cramping
   B. Constipation, hematochezia
   C. Intestinal obstruction/perforation
   D. All of the above

10.49 The screening procedure of choice for patients at high risk for colorectal cancer is:
   A. FOBT
   B. CEA
   C. Colonoscopy
   D. Barium enema
   E. Sigmoidoscopy

10.50 The ACNP who did the admission history and physician examination on Mrs. P is most likely to proceed in what manner?
   A. Order a colonoscopy and CT scan
   B. Order a CEA level
   C. Refer to a gastroenterologist regarding therapeutic management
   D. Consult with a general surgeon regarding surgical procedure of choice

Answers and Rationales

10.46 **A** Initial lab tests will include CBC to ascertain Hct, Hgb with history of bloody stools, weakness, fatigue, red blood cell count, WBC to rule out infection, anemias. LFTs to rule out liver disease, electrolytes to ascertain baseline data.

10.47 **C** This patient has a first-degree relative who died from colon cancer, making her a patient at high risk.

10.48 **D** Left-sided colon cancer is characterized by sensations of fullness, cramping progressing to constipation, hematochezia, and intestinal obstruction.

10.49 **C** Colonscopy is the procedure of choice to screen/diagnose high-risk patients.

10.50 **C** This a symptomatic high-risk patient who requires physician referral, preferably to a gastroenterologist. In collaboration with the physician, the ACNP may assist with management of this patient.

References

Alabaster, O. (1992). Colorectal cancer: epidemiological risks and prevention. In J.D. Algren, J.S. Macdonald (eds.). *Gastrointestinal Oncology*. Philadelphia: J.B. Lippincott Co., pp. 243–259.

Barry, M.J. (1995). Screening for colorectal cancer. In A.H. Goroll, L.A. May, & G.G. Mulley (eds.). *Primary Care Medicine: Office Evaluation and Management of the Adult Patient*, (3rd ed.). Philadelphia, J.B. Lippincott Co., pp. 311–313.

Beart, R.W. (1991). Colorectal cancer. In A.I. Holleb, D.J., Fink, & G.P. Murphy (eds.). *Clinical Oncology*. Atlanta: American Cancer Society, pp. 213–219.

Hampton, B. (1993). Gastrointestinal cancer: Colon, rectum, and anus. In S.L. Groenwald, M. Goodman, M.H. Frogge, & C.H. Yarbro (eds.). *Cancer Nursing Principles and Practice*. Boston: Jones and Bartlett Publishers, pp. 1045–1062.

U.S. Preventive Services Task Force. (1996). *Guide to Clinical Preventive Services* (2nd ed.). Baltimore: Williams & Wilkins, pp. 89–99.

Simon, J.B. (1993). Colonic polyps, cancer, and fecal occult blood. *Ann Intern Med 118*, 71.

Acute Cholecystitis

DEFINITIONS

Cholecystitis: Inflammation of the gallbladder; 85–90% of cases are associated with gallstone disease, and occur when a calculus becomes impacted in the cystic duct and inflammation develops behind the obstruction.

Acalculous Cholecystitis: In approximately 15% of cases gallbladder calculi are absent. Etiology appears to include multiple trauma, major burn injury, sepsis, infection, surgery, prolonged fasting, total parenteral nutrition, drugs, vasculitis, congestive heart failure, renal failure, conditions predisposing to bile stasis, increased bile viscosity, and mechanical cystic duct obstruction to outflow of the bile, including adhesion, neoplasms, and periductal adhesions. It is more common in men over 50.

Cholelithias is (gallstones): More common in women over the age of 40 who are obese. May be asymptomatic or symptomatic; higher incidence in individuals with inflammatory involvement of the terminal ileum resulting from interruption of bile salt resorption.

Choledocholithiasis: Bile duct obstruction associated with a history of biliary colic or prior jaundice; Charcot's triad of pain, fever (and chills), and jaundice is the classic picture. Mirizzi's syndrome is a clinical syndrome of cholecystitis and jaundice related to a stone from the cystic duct obstructing the common bile duct. Bile duct obstruction lasting longer than 30 days may result in liver damage, leading to cirrhosis.

ETIOLOGY/INCIDENCE

1. Gallstone disease is common and increases in frequency with aging. By age 75, about 35% of women and 20% of men develop gallstones. Most are asymptomatic.
2. Calculous cholecystitis occurs two to three times more frequently in women than men. Prevalence increases with age, peaking between ages 50 and 65 years. Acalculous cholecystitis occurs more frequently in men.
3. In the United States, the incidence of gallbladder disease is highest among American Indians of the southwest and lowest among whites and blacks. Mexican Americans are at higher risk of gallstone disease than other Hispanic populations.
4. Symptomatic disease generally occurs as uncomplicated, infrequent biliary pain.
5. Death caused by gallstones is infrequent and accounts for approximately 5000 in 2.2 million deaths/year in the United States; caused by biliary complications, including the surgery to treat complications.
6. High-risk populations include the elderly, diabetic, those with recurrent symptomatic gallstones.

SIGNS AND SYMPTOMS

Generally do not differ in calculous and acalculous disease.

1. Biliary pain develops rapidly and is often precipitated by a large or fatty meal.
2. Pain is severe, steady, and unrelieved by usual household remedies, position change, and gas passage. Radiation often occurs to the right scapula or interscapular area and is exacerbated by sudden movement, coughing, or deep inspiration. Onset is 60–90 minutes after a meal, increases over a period of a few hours, remains at a plateau, decreases over the next few hours, and may subside in 12–18 hours.
3. Vomiting occurs in 75% of cases and results in variable relief. Generally it is not as severe as that associated with acute pancreatitis or intestinal obstruction
4. Fever is usually present.

PHYSICAL FINDINGS

Generally do not differ in calculous and acalculous disease.

1. Pain localized to epigastrium or right hypochondrium.
2. Right upper quadrant abdominal tenderness is present and is associated with muscle guarding and rebound pain. A positive Murphy's sign may be elicited (i.e., pain and inspiratory arrest occurring during a deep breath while the examiner palpates the right subcostal region).

3. Palpable gallbladder is present in about 15% of cases.
4. If gallbladder is palpable, distended, and nontender, this is Courvoiser's sign.
5. Jaundice is present in about 25% of cases.
6. Cholangitis classically present with Charcot's triad: fever/chills, right upper quadrant pain, and jaundice. Ninety-five percent of these patients have common bile duct stones; however, only a minority of patients with acute cholecystitis present with common bile duct obstruction and triad symptoms.

DIFFERENTIAL DIAGNOSIS

1. Perforated peptic ulcer
2. Acute pancreatitis
3. Appendicitis
4. Angina
5. Abdominal trauma by history or physical exam
6. Perforated colon
7. Hepatitis
8. Pyelonephritis
9. Liver abscess
10. Pneumonia with pleurisy

DIAGNOSTIC TESTS/FINDINGS

1. Laboratory work-up should include complete blood count, liver function tests, amylase. These will usually be normal but should be done to rule out other diseases producing similar symptoms.
   A. WBC elevated (12,000–15,000/μL) in acute cholecystitis.
   B. Total bilirubin elevated in 8–37% of cases, usually to >5 mg/dL. The higher the bilirubin, the more likely that cystic duct obstruction is present.
   C. AST/ALT elevated in 40–75% of cases, usually to greater than five times normal.
   D. Alkaline phosphatase may be elevated, usually to less than two times normal, and may be associated with ascending cholangitis.
   E. Serum amylase may be moderately elevated.
2. Right upper quadrant abdominal ultrasound is test of choice in patients with biliary colic and suspected cholecystitis. It may show presence of gallstones but is not specific for acute cholecystitis.
3. Plain films of abdomen may show radiopaque gallstones but are not particularly useful.
4. HIDA scan of liver (hepatobiliary imaging using iminodiacetic acid compounds) may demonstrated an obstructed cystic duct, which may be cause of acute cholecystitis.

MANAGEMENT/TREATMENT

Acute care setting: Moderate to severe pain, vomiting.

1. Acute cholecystitis will generally resolve with conservative treatment in 3–6 days.
2. Withhold oral food and fluids.

3. Nasogastric tube for those with vomiting.
4. IV fluid and electrolyte replacement to maintain intravascular volume and serum electrolytes. $D_{5/0.5}$ NS at 125–250 mL/hr (moderate for geriatric population).
5. Broad-spectrum antibiotic therapy for those patients with evidence of prolonged symptoms, who are high risk (diabetic, elderly, altered resistance), and with suspected septic complications (abscess, perforation).
6. Analgesics for pain control, favoring use of meperidine (75–100 mg IM or IV q4h prn) over morphine for its antispasmodic effect on the sphincter of Oddi. (*Note:* Obtain surgical consultation prior to initiating analgesics.)

REFERRAL CRITERIA FOR SURGICAL INTERVENTION

Early cholecystectomy is the treatment of choice in the majority of stable patients with acute cholecystitis who are not critically ill and are able to tolerate the procedure.

PATIENT EDUCATION

1. Educate patients in differentiating symptoms of biliary colic from dyspepsia.
2. Educate patients regarding therapeutic alternatives.
   A. Surgical intervention: Open cholecystectomy, laparoscopic cholecystectomy
   B. Expectant management: Prophylactic cholecystectomy to decrease risk of recurrent biliary pain, biliary complication, gallbladder cancer, or death. Advise that 30% of patients with a first episode may not incur more episodes even after prolonged follow-up.
   C. Nonsurgical management—removal of gallstones but not gallbladder.
      1) Extracorpeal shock wave lithotripsy (ESWL): Advise that best candidates have a solitary radiolucent stone <2 cm.
      2) Pharmacologic dissolution: Dissolves gallstones <2 cm that are primarily comprised of cholesterol.
         a. Urosodiol (10–15 mg/kg/day): Therapy is continued for 12–24 months and requires monitoring every 6 months with a gallbladder ultrasound. Recurrence rate following cessation of medication is high. May be useful and cost-effective in older and high-risk patients.
         b. Chenodeoxycholic acid (CDCA) and ursodeoxycholic acid (UDCA) reduce the amount of cholesterol present in the bile and hence allow for dissolution of the cholesterol in formed stones. CDCA blocks hepatic synthesis of cholesterol and UDCA blocks intestinal uptake. Criteria that would favor this form of therapy include radiolucency, lack of calcification, small stones, small number of stones, floating stones, and nonoverweight patient.
      3) Contact dissolution: Requires percutaneous entry into the gallbladder and installation of methylterbutylethene (MTBE). This is still investigational but early results are promising.
3. Educate patients on health maintenance strategies:
   A. Weight reduction to ideal weight
   B. Exercise
   C. Stop smoking
4. Health-conscious eating patterns.

Review Questions

Ms. F is a 52-year-old obese woman who presents with complaints of severe steady epigastric pain that radiates to the right shoulder. It began 12 hours earlier following a late dinner. She has vomited three times with little relief. Denies hematemesis, melena. Temperature 101°F. Physical exam reveals right upper quadrant tenderness, a positive Murphy's sign, and icteric sclera.

10.51 Which of the following laboratory tests are required?
    A. Hemoglobin, Hct, platelets, prothrombin time, fibrinogen
    B. WBC, AST, ALT, bilirubin, alkaline phosphatase
    C. BUN, creatinine, ammonia, serum magnesium and phosphorus
    D. Serum glucose, sodium, potassium, chloride, CO_2
    E. All of the above

10.52 The diagnostic test of choice for this patient is:
    A. Plain films of the abdomen.
    B. Right upper quadrant abdominal ultrasound
    C. Upper GI barium swallow
    D. Oral cholecystogram
    E. None of the above

10.53 Impaction of a biliary stone in the cystic duct is the most common cause of:
    A. Autoimmune hepatitis
    B. Acute pancreatitis
    C. Cholecystitis
    D. Cystic fibrosis

10.54 A 63-year-old female patient is seen in the ER with complaints of severe RUQ pain, vomiting of about 4 hours' duration. She states that she had a similar attack a few weeks ago and was seen in the ER but the pain resolved quickly and she was sent back home. Physical exam is notable for RUQ tenderness and severe pain to palpation on inspiration. You would expect the ultrasound to show:
    A. Presence of gallstones
    B. Dilated loops of bowel with no free air under the diaphragm
    C. Fluid pockets in the retroperitoneal space as a result of pancreatic ascites
    D. Nothing significant because ultrasound is not the test of choice in a patient with these symptoms

10.55 The choice of pain control for the patient with cholecystitis is:
    A. Morphine sulfate
    B. Tylenol or a nonsteroidal anti-inflammatory drug (NSAID)
    C. Demerol
    D. Non-narcotic analgesic such as Nubain or Stadol

Answers and Rationales

10.51 **B** WBC, liver function tests, and amylase should be done to rule out other causes. WBC will be elevated in acute cholecystitis. LFTs and amylase may be elevated, especially if there is obstruction of the cystic duct.

10.52 **B** Right upper quadrant ultrasound, especially in patients with biliary colic and suspected cholecystitis, will show presence of gallstones in the dependent portion of the gallbladder. In acute cholecystitis it may show a dilated gallbladder with a thickened wall and surrounding edema.

10.53 **C** The most common cause of cholecystitis is impaction of a biliary stone in the cystic duct, thereby blocking flow, causing inflammation behind the blockage. Other causes include vascular abnormalities and pancreatitis.

10.54 **A** Gallstones will most likely be seen on an ultrasound of the abdomen. Other findings that may show up on ultrasound include dilated gallbladder with a thickened wall and surrounding edema.

10.55 **C** Demerol is the pain medication of choice for patients with acute cholecystitis. Morphine may cause spasm of the sphincter of Oddi, thus increasing pain for the patient.

References

American College of Physicians. (1993). Guidelines for the treatment of gallstones. *Ann Intern Med 119*, 620–622.

Friedman, L.S. (1995). Liver, biliary tract, and pancreas. In L. Tierney, S. McPhee, M. Papadakis (eds.), *Current Medical Diagnosis and Treatment*. Stamford, Ct: Appleton & Lange, pp. 580–582.

Goroll, A.H. (1995). Management of asymptomatic and symptomatic gallstones. In A.H. Goroll, L.A. May, A.G. Mulley (eds.), *Primary Care Medicine: Office Evaluation and Management of the Adult Patient* (3rd ed.). Philadelphia: J.B. Lippincott Co., pp. 394–399.

Opila, D. (1996). Gallstones and cholecystitis. In R.E. Rakel (ed.). *Saunders Manual of Medical Practice*. Philadelphia: W.B. Saunders Co., pp. 376–378.

Ransohoff, D.F., & Gracie, W.A. (1993). Treatment of gallstones. *Ann Intern Med 119*, 606–619.

Way, L.A. (1994). Biliary tract. In L. Tierney, S. McPhee, & M. Papadakis (eds.). *Current Surgical Diagnosis and Treatment*. Stamford, CT: Appleton & Lange, pp. 546–557.

Gastroesophageal Reflux Disease

DEFINITIONS

Gastroesophageal reflux disease (GERD) is characterized by heartburn and may be associated with regurgitation.

Heartburn: Described as retrosternal discomfort, "burning" that may move up and down the chest like a wave. When severe it may radiate to the sides of the chest, neck, and angles of the jaw. It is aggravated by bending forward, straining, lying recumbent and worse following meals. It is relieved by upright posture, swallowing, antacids. It reoccurs following meals and in response to aggravating factors.

Regurgitation: Effortless appearance of gastric or eosphageal contents in the mouth. It may cause laryngeal aspiration, described by patients as spells of coughing or choking that awaken them from sleep.

Esophagitis: Inflammation of the squamous mucosa in the distal esophagus as a result of exposure to regurgitated acid and pepsin from the stomach in association with chronic esophageal reflux disease.

Water brash: Reflex salivary hypersecretion, which may also be present as a response to peptic esophagitis; it should not be confused with regurgitation.

INCIDENCE

1. About 10% of adults suffer from daily heartburn.
2. About 30% of adults have symptoms monthly.
3. Incidence is higher in adults who are 30% over ideal body weight.

PATHOPHYSIOLOGY

Esophageal reflux results from transient relaxation of the lower esophageal sphincter. These episodes are more common after meals than at other times and are stimulated by fat in the duodenum. In the presence of slow gastric emptying, this may account for increased reflux following high-fat meals. Reflux is also stimulated by obesity, pregnancy, ascites, tight binders or girdles.

Esophagitis is a complication of reflux caused by repeated exposure to acid and pepsin from the stomach, and can result in peptic stricture.

SIGNS AND SYMPTOMS

1. History is the mainstay of diagnosis.
2. Complaints of heartburn described as retrosternal burning radiating upward occurring 30–60 minutes following meals and/or upon reclining; relieved by antacids or baking soda.
3. "Burping up bitter-tasting liquid"; may occur at night and awaken patient.
4. Patient may report staining of sheets with stomach contents.
5. Cough, "choking sensation" awakening patient from sleep.
6. Acid laryngitis, often described as "lump in throat"; atypical symptom.
7. Acid-induced asthma associated with complaints of wheezing associated with reflux; difficult to diagnose.
8. Complaints of dysphagia (difficulty with speech), odynophagia (painful swallowing), and aerophagia (excessive air swallowing) are not characteristic of GERD and require follow-up for esophageal obstruction, mass, neoplasm.

PHYSICAL FINDINGS

1. Abdomen: Generally not revealing; may have some epigastric tenderness; examine to rule out mass, hernia.
2. Assess for tight-fitting clothing associated with increased intra-abdominal pressure, which may contribute to symptoms of GERD.
3. Kyphosis associated with GERD.
4. Loss of lingual surface tooth enamel associated with severe GERD.
5. Chest: Lung auscultation to detect crackles, an indication of associated aspiration pneumonia.

DIFFERENTIAL DIAGNOSIS

1. Peptic ulcer disease
2. Esophagitis/motility disorder/stricture/biliary tract disease
3. Diaphragmatic hiatal hernia
4. Esophageal tumor
5. Cardiac chest pain/coronary artery disease

DIAGNOSTIC TESTS/FINDINGS

1. No single test is accepted as standard for clinical diagnosis of GERD.
2. Screen stool for occult blood.
3. Electrocardiogram (ECG) to rule out cardiac ischemia in patients at risk.
4. Barium swallow with UGI or endoscopy is indicated if patient has painful swallowing, dysphagia, significant weight loss, or stool positive for occult blood.
5. Endoscopy will reveal visible mucosal abnormalities such as erythemia, and friability of the squamocolumnar junction and erosions, which are graded I (mild) to IV. Grade IV lesions include severe erosions, stricture, or Barrett's esophagus, a term used when the squamous epithelium of the esophagus has been replaced by columnar epithelium, which is subject to peptic ulceration and dysplasia. Diagnosis is made by endoscopy.

MANAGEMENT/TREATMENT

1. Goals
   A. Reduce volume of refluxate
   B. Neutralize refluxate acid concentration
   C. Promote esophageal clearance
   D. Protect esophageal mucosa
2. Interventions
   A. Diet (see Table 10–7)
   B. Lifestyle modifications (see Table 10–8)
   C. Pharmacologic therapy
      1) Pharmacologic therapy for mild symptoms is initiated with antacids or a daily dose of oral histamine antagonists, and procedes to an increased dose and frequency of the H_2 antagonists, use of proton pump inhibitors, and addition of prokinetic agents depending on the clinical response.
      2) The choice of agents depends on the severity of clinical symptoms, patient's age, potential drug interactions. It is advisable that the

---

TABLE 10–7. **Diet Modification: Foods to Avoid/Reduce in GERD Patients**

Foods high in fat
Foods containing caffeine, which stimulates acid secretion
   coffee, tea, chocolate, cocoa, cola beverages
Tomato products and citrus juices
Milk products—potent stimulator of acid secretion
Spearmint/peppermint-containing products
Alcohol

TABLE **10–8.** **Lifestyle Modifications for GERD Patients**

Weight reduction if over ideal weight; as little as a 10-lb weight loss can improve symptoms.

Eat four to six small meals per day.

Avoid large evening meals; eat small evening meal at least 3 hours before bedtime.

Avoid ingestion of large quantities of liquids with meals.

Elevate head of bed with 6-inch blocks under bedposts (no pillows).

Avoid medications that irritate esophageal mucosa (NSAIDs, potassium, tetracycline).

Wear loose-fitting clothing.

ACNP become familiar with the many potential agents that may be used and their pharmacologic action. Tables 10–9, 10–10, and 10–11 list the agents used most commonly in the acute care setting.

3) Initiation of therapy with H_2 antagonists is indicated for hospitalized symptomatic patients and for patients with erosive eosphagitis diagnosed by endoscopy.

4) Use of proton pump inhibitor is initiated in patients with erosive esophagitis and those resistant to therapy with H_2 antagonists.

5) Prokinetic agents are added to the treatment regimen if the patient does not respond fully to the H_2 antagonists.

6) Limit use of medications that may decrease sphincter tone—anticholinergics, calcium channel blockers, and other smooth muscle relaxants.

3. Duration of therapy/referral: The ACNP works collaboratively with the physician managing these patients in the acute care setting. Generally these patients are hospitalized for indications other than GERD, or for complications secondary to erosive esophagitis. When treatment is initiated in the acute care setting, it is included in comprehensive discharge summary detailing therapy/response and suggested follow-up as delineated below.

A. If treatment produces a good clinical response, the patient should receive maintenance therapy with the smallest dose of histamine-receptor blocker that will control symptoms.

B. If H_2 blocker therapy fails, then institute omeprazole 20 mg qd for 1 month, increasing to 40 mg if symptoms persist. Omeprazole is also effective in treating acid laryngitis and asthma; however, it may not be given indefinitely.

TABLE **10–9.** **Histamine H_2 Receptor Antagonists***

Drug	Dosage	
Famotidine (Pepcid)	40 mg PO	daily hs *or* 20 mg PO bid A.M./hs
	20 mg IV	daily hs *or* 20 mg IV q12h
Cimetidine (Tagamet)	800 mg PO	daily hs *or* 400 mg PO bid, A.M./hs
	400 mg IV	daily hs *or* 400 mg IV bid, A.M./hs
	37.5 mg/hr	continuous infusion up to 900 mg/day
Ranitidine (Zantac)	300 mg PO	daily hs *or* 150 mg PO bid, A.M./hs
	50 mg IV	q6–8h up to 150 mg/day
	6.25 mg/hr	continuous infusion up to 150 mg/day

* Reduce output of hydrogen ions by the parietal cells.

TABLE **10–10.   Proton Pump Inhibitor***

Drug	Dosage
Omeprazole (Prilosec)	20–40 mg PO daily

* Higher rate of positive clinical response in patients who failed therapy with H_2 antagonists, antacids. Demonstrated efficacy in healing erosive esophagitis. Reduces output of hydrogen ions by parietal cells.

Note: There is a question regarding safety with long-term use of this agent.

C. Referral for antireflux surgery is suggested for patients who do not respond to medical therapy, those with debilitating symptoms, or those who are unwilling or unable to continue medication.

PATIENT EDUCATION

1. Educate regarding disease process, course, complications, reoccurrence, outcome.
2. Educate regarding symptoms to report to health care practitioners:
   A. Persistent pain after making suggested changes
   B. Increasing pain following exercise
   C. Crushing/heavy chest/upper abdomen pain
   D. Recent weight loss
   E. Pain or difficulty swallowing, coughing or vomiting of blood
   F. Pain not relieved by medications
   G. Bowel movements containing red blood or tarry/black in color
3. Educate regarding medications: effects, side effects, interactions.
4. Educate regarding diet, lifestyle modifications as delineated below. Avoid coffee, tea, cocoa, chocolate, mint, citrus, tomato products, and caffeine-containing beverages.
   A. Eat four to six small meals per day in place of three large ones.
   B. Eat evening meal 3 hours prior to retiring.
   C. Limit intake of alcohol.
   D. Maintain weight at ideal level for age/height.
   E. Avoid constricting clothing.
   F. Elevate head of bed at least 6 inches on blocks.
   G. Eat in a seated position and maintain upright position 30–60 minutes following meal.

TABLE **10–11.   Prokinetic Agents***

Drug	Dosage
Cisapride (Propulsid)†	20 mg PO bid
Metoclopramide (Reglan)‡	10 mg PO qid ac/hs

* Use to promote healing by strengthening the contraction of the lower esophageal sphincter and esophageal body, and to increase gastric emptying.

† Agent of choice; works synergistically with H_2 antagonists.

‡ Agent causes additive sedative effects with central nervous system depressants and should be used with caution, especially in the elderly.

Review Questions

Ms. D is a 74-year-old obese woman postoperative day 4 from a hip replacement. She has complained repeatedly of "burning retrosternal discomfort" that occurs at night, a problem she has had for many years. She has had an ECG and cardiac enzymes, which are negative. She is taking a soft diet. Denies nausea/ vomiting. Has passed flatus/stool. Abdomen is soft, nontender. Medications include: hydrocodone/acetaminophen (Vicodin) 5 mg/500 mg, 1–2 tablets q6h PRN for pain; enoxaparin sodium (Lovenox) 30 mg SQ bid; and alprazolam (Xanax) 0.5 mg for sleep.

10.56 What additional history is required?
　　A. What associated symptoms may accompany it?
　　B. What medications has the patient taken for these symptoms?
　　C. Does the patient ever experience difficulty or pain on swallowing?
　　D. All of the above

10.57 What factors in the scenario are likely contributors to the symptoms?
　　A. Surgical procedure, postoperative course
　　B. Age, diet
　　C. Weight, recumbency
　　D. Fluid imbalance

10.58 Given the information provided in the scenario, what is the most likely diagnosis?
　　A. GERD
　　B. IBS
　　C. Acute cholecystitis
　　D. Bowel obstruction

10.59 Pharmacologic therapy will be initiated for this patient with:
　　A. Famotidine 20 mg PO q A.M. & bedtime
　　B. Cimetidine 400 mg PO q A.M.
　　C. Sucrafate 1 gm PO qid
　　D. Metoclopramide 10 mg PO qid

10.60 Ms. D will be transferred to a rehabilitation facility on postoperative day 6. In preparation for transfer what information regarding management of GERD should be included in the discharge plan as well as in the education material reviewed with the patient?
　　A. Elevate head of bed on 6-inch blocks
　　B. Avoid fatty foods, citrus, caffine-containing products
　　C. Continue on medication regimen
　　D. Recommend four to five small meals, weight reduction
　　E. All of the above

Answers and Rationales

10.56 **D** History is the mainstay of diagnosis in GERD. This patient has had these symptoms; therefore, history of prior pharmacologic treatment is essential in order to reinstitute on hospitalization. It is essential to rule out dysphagia, odynophagia, which may indicate esophageal mass, stricture.

10.57 **C** This is an obese patient who is recumbant and immobile secondary to surgery. Both are factors most likely to contribute to GERD.

10.58 **A** This patient does not demonstrate symptoms of IBS. Symptoms and physical exam not characteristic of cholecystitis. She is passing stool/flatus and tolerant of her diet, which is inconsistent with bowel obstruction.

10.59 **A** Famotidine 20 mg PO q A.M. and at bedtime is indicated for this patient. Initiation with an H_2 antagonist is indicated given the weight, mobility, and surgical stress factors. Cimetidine 400 mg qd is not adequate dosing; the recommended daily dose for GERD is 800 mg qd or 400 mg bid. Sucralfate is not first-line intervention for a patient with past history in the acute care setting. Metoclopramide would be contraindicated for this patient given her age and the fact that she is currently on CNS depressants.

10.60 **E** It is essential that discharge orders/plan that accompany this patient to a rehabilitation facility include diet, weight reduction, medication, position in the delineated regimen to manage GERD.

References

Ellis, H.E., Jr. (1990). Diaphragmatic hiatal hernias. *Postgrad Med 88*, 112–124.

Goyal, R.K. (1994). Diseases of the esophagus. In K.J. Isselbacher, E. Braunwald, J.D. Wilson, J.B. Martin, A.S. Fauci, & D.L. Kasper (eds.). *Harrison's Principles of Internal Medicine*. New York: McGraw-Hill, pp. 1355–1363.

Pope, C.E. (1994). Acid-reflux disorders. *N Engl J Med 331*, 656–660.

Richter, J.M. (1995). Approach to the patient with heartburn and reflux. In A.H. Goroll, L.A. May, & A.G. Mulley (eds.). *Primary Care Medicine: Office Evaluation and Management of the Adult Patient* (3rd ed.). Philadelphia: J.B. Lippincott Co., pp. 344–348.

Tagg, P.I. (1996). Patient education heartburn. *Nurse Pract 21*(9), 145.

Uphold, C.R., & Graham, M.V. (1994). *Clinical Guidelines in Adult Health* Gainesville, FL. Barammae Books, pp. 380–383.

Gastrointestinal Bleeds

DEFINITIONS

Hematemesis: Vomiting of blood, either bright red or dark color, generally indicating a bleeding source proximal to the ligament of Treitz. Stomach and esophagus are the most common sites contributing to this finding. *Coffee grounds* appearance of vomitus resulting from precipitated blood clots occurs with slower, lower volume bleeds in which the blood remains longer in the stomach.

Melena: Passage of black or tarry stools. Generally results from upper GI tract bleeding but can be produced by blood entering the bowel at any point from mouth to cecum. Can be produced by as little as 50–100 mL of blood in the stomach

Hematochezia: Passage of bright-red blood from the rectum; signifies bleeding distal to the ligament of Treitz from the colon, rectum, or anus. May also occur if intestinal tract transit is rapid in the presence of rapid hemorrhage into the esophagus, stomach, or duodenum.

Occult GI bleeding: Bleeding detected by a card test for fecal hemoglobin peroxidase; may also be suggested by the presence of iron-deficiency anemia without apparent cause. The source may be anywhere in the GI tract. May be an early indicator in colorectal cancer.

Upper GI bleeding: Bleeding originating in the GI tract proximal to the ligament of Treitz, characterized by hematemesis or a positive nasogastric aspirate.

Lower GI bleeding: Intraluminal bleeding originating distal to the ligament of Treitz, characterized by hematochezia and/or melena.

ETIOLOGY/INCIDENCE

1. Upper GI Bleeding
   A. Frequency of underlying causes: 15–30% attributable to duodenal ulcer, 20–25% to gastric erosions, 20–25% to gastric ulcers, 20–25% to esophageal varices, 5–15% to Mallory-Weiss syndrome, 3–15% to esophagitis, 6% to duodenitis, >5% to gastritis, <3% to neoplasm
   B. Incidence: Results in hospitalization of >300,000 patients annually in United States or approximately 10% of admissions to a general hospital
   C. Mortality: 10–20%, with highest rates associated with esophageal varices
   D. Risk factors: Chronic NSAID/ASA use; age >75; history of excessive and/ or long-term ethanol ingestion; anticoagulation therapy; past medical history of peptic ulcer disease (PUD)
2. Lower GI bleeding
   A. Primarily occurs in elderly: causes by age as follows:
      1) Elderly: Diverticulosis, angiodysplasia, malignancy, polyps, hemorrhoids, aortoenteric fistula, rectal hemorrhoids
      2) Adults <60 years: Diverticulosis, inflammatory bowel disease, polyps, malignancy, congenital vascular malformations, hemorrhoids, rectal varicies
      3) Young adults/adolescents: Inflammatory bowel disease, polyps, Meckel's diverticulum
   B. Mortality: 10–20% with acute massive bleeding. Risk of death is increased with preoperative shock state, steroid therapy, malignancy, or rebleeding. Measures of overall disease severity (APACHE III and Organ System Failure Index) are more important predictors than severity of GI hemorrhage.

PATHOPHYSIOLOGY

Physiologic response to obvious or occult bleeding is directly related to the rapidity and amount of hemorrhage. Underlying disease and associated illness may alter the compensatory response to blood loss. Factors that may further complicate physiologic compensatory response include the patient's age, state of hydration, anemia, cardiovascular disease, and medications.

Classification of acute hemorrhage:

Class I: <15% of total blood volume—minimal clinical symptoms, mild increase in heart rate

Class II: 15–30% loss in blood volume—tachycardia, tachypnea, anxiety, decreased pulse pressure, orthostasis

Class III: 30–40% loss in blood volume—marked tachycardia, tachypnea, orthostasis progressing to measurable decrease in blood pressure, syncope, altered mental status, inadequate systemic perfusion

Class IV: >40% loss in blood volume—shock state (tachycardia, hypotension, cool pale skin); imminent danger of death

SIGNS AND SYMPTOMS

1. Fatigue and exertional dyspnea are classic presenting symptoms in individuals with chronic slow blood loss.
2. Estimates of blood loss as reported by patients are difficult to ascertain; focus on description of blood lost, color, consistency, and associated symptoms, such as lightheadedness, dizziness, weakness.
3. Report of large-volume blood loss accompanied by weakness/syncope requires assessment for orthostasis and a complete work-up.
4. Admission is indicated if BP drops 10–15 mm Hg or pulse increases >10–15 bpm.
5. Patient screening:
   A. Alcoholism, chronic liver disease, to rule out esophageal varices
   B. ASA, NSAID use, post medical history of PUD, to rule out gastric or duodenal ulcer
   C. Complaints of change in bowel habits, weight loss, dull nagging persistent RLQ pain, diarrhea/bloody diarrhea, urgency, tenesmus, to rule out diverticulosis, rectosigmoid disease, ulcerative colitis
   D. Anticoagulation use; underlying hematologic disorders that may account for GI bleeding
   E. History of malignancy
   F. Recent trauma
6. Anorexia may occur because of blood in stomach, secondary to anemia, or as a result of underlying primary disease process (e.g., gastritis).
7. Nausea/vomiting prior to bleed may indicate gastric ulcer/gastric carcinoma.
8. Abdominal pain: General guidelines
   A. Burning epigastric pain present prior to bleed may suggest PUD/gastritis/esophagitis.
   B. Diffuse abdominal pain associated with bleeding may suggest trauma/mesenteric insufficiency, ischemia/necrosis/bowel perforation.
   C. Painless large-volume bleeding suggests variceal bleeding.

PHYSICAL FINDINGS

1. Vital signs: Assess hemodynamic stability, orthostasis, trends indicating rising heart rate, decreasing blood pressure. Febrile episodes associated with GI bleeding are rare.
2. Skin: Pallor, diaphoresis reflecting hemodynamic compromise; ecchymosis, petechiae, telangiectasias, or evidence of chronic liver disease (jaundice, spider angiomata).
3. Nasopharynx: Rule out as source of bleeding.
4. Lymph nodes: Enlargement (left supraclavicular adenopathy) may indicate intraabdominal malignancy as a underlying cause of bleeding.
5. Abdomen: Palpation may reveal organomegaly, ascites, masses; abdominal pulsations accompanied by mass may indicate aortic aneurysm; in the presence of old abdominal scar, the possibility of aortic-enteric fistula exists. Gut motility is increased by intraluminal bleeds.

6. Rectal exam: Inspect for anorectal lesions; digital exam to examine stool for blood.
7. Stomach: Nasogastric tube (NGT) may be inserted to ascertain gastric contents.
8. Cardiovascular system: increased chest pain and silent myocardial infarction may be the initial presentation in the elderly following GI hemorrhage.
9. Nervous system: Volume loss and hypotension may result in confusion.

DIFFERENTIAL DIAGNOSIS

1. Hematemesis
   A. Esophageal varices
   B. Eosphagitis/ulceration
   C. Gastric or duodenal ulcer
   D. Mallory-Weiss tear
   E. Gastritis/duodenitis
   F. Gastric neoplasm
2. Melena—All causes listed above in addition to:
   A. Meckel's diverticulum
   B. Crohn's disease
   C. Small bowel neoplasms
3. Hematochezia (include upper GI lesions if significant bleeding is present)
   A. Hemorrhoid
   B. Anal fissure
   C. Colonic polyp
   D. Colorectal neoplasm
   E. Diverticular disease
   F. Inflammatory disease
   G. Angiodysplasia

DIAGNOSTIC TESTS/FINDINGS

Trends are more important than isolated values. The following tests are listed in order of priority.

1. Hematologic studies (*Note:* Hematocrit is a poor indicator of the severity of acute bleeding because it takes 24–72 hours to equilibrate with the extravascular fluid.
   A. Hemoglobin/hematocrit: Initial Hct of <28% and Hgb <11gm/dL indicate significant hemorrhage or an acute bleeding episode superimposed on chronic bleeding.
   B. Mean corpuscular volume: Low volume suggests possibility of iron-deficiency anemia caused by chronic blood loss.
   C. Platelets: May be increased or decreased; coagulopathy may develop secondary to hemorrhage, characterized by consumption of clotting factors; thrombocytosis may occur also as a result of shock.
   D. Coagulation tests: PT, PTT; important to ascertain requirement for clotting factor replacement.
2. Chemistry studies
   A. BUN/creatinine: BUN elevated (>40–85 mg/dL) in the absence of underlying renal disease (normal creatinine) may indicate significant blood loss (two or more units of blood in the GI tract).

    B. Liver function tests: AST, ALT, LDH, bilirubin, alkaline phosphatase to rule out underlying liver disease, which may be contributing to bleeding episode.

    C. Guaiac: Stool and nasogastric contents.

3. Endoscopy: Diagnostic procedure of choice for patients with moderate to severe hemorrhage; indicated in the following circumstances:

    A. Rule out esophageal varices/neoplasm

    B. Previous aortic graft

    C. Anticoagulation/thrombolytic therapy

    D. Patients who require this procedure should be referred by the ACNP to the collaborating physician. Shock on presentation

4. Colonoscopy: Procedure of choice to identify slow-bleeding lesions, polyps, diverticula, angiodysplasia, carcinoma, inflammatory bowel disease; allows biopsy and polypectomy. If bleeding is active, colon must be lavaged prior to procedure, which may be done with oral nonabsorbable lavage solutions given 1–2 hours prior to procedure. Patients who require this diagnostic procedure should be referred by the ACNP to the collaborating physician.

MANAGEMENT/TREATMENT

1. Active UGI bleeding episode: *These patients require immediate consultation and are referred to the physician.* When stabilized, they may be managed collaboratively per protocol/guidelines with the ACNP.

    A. Vital sign monitoring/pulse oximetry.

    B. Placement of two large-bore intravenous lines.

    C. Blood sent for type/screen for four units blood, CBC, coagulation studies.

    D. Oxygen administration: 3–5 L.

    E. Nasogastric tube placement with gentle lavage of room temperature saline or water.

    F. Foley catheter placement to monitor urine output; maintain at 40–60 mL/hr.

    G. Fluid resuscitation per American College of Surgeons classification (Ringer's lactate or normal saline may be used):

Class	Blood Loss (%)	Fluid Replacement
I	<15	Crystalloid
II	15–30	Crystalloid
III	30–40	Crystalloid + blood
IV	>40	Crystalloid + blood

    H. Blood transfusion: Objective is to correct shock and restore blood volume. Packed red blood cells (PRBCs) are given to maintain a hematocrit of 25–30%. In the absence of continued bleeding, the Hct should rise 3% for each unit of transfused PRBCs.

    I. Clotting factor replacement: One unit of fresh frozen plasma (FFP) should be given for each five units of PRBCs when sustained massive bleeding occurs or for patients with marked coagulopathies, platelet counts <60,000/μL.

    J. Vasopressors: Should only be used as a last resort in hypovolemic shock and only in the presence of adequate volume and blood replacement.

    K. Histamine antagonists/proton pump inhibitors are effective in reducing gastric acidity associated with gastritis and peptic ulcer disease; however, suppression of gastric acid secretion does not influence immediate outcome of acute UGI hemorrhage.

   L. Warfarin complication: FFP is given to replace coagulation factors; vitamin K 20–40 mg IV may be given, but has a delayed effect.
   M. Endoscopy/sclerotherapy: Performed by gastroenterologist
      1) Procedure of choice for rapid variceal bleeds
      2) An effective and safe emergency therapy for achieving initial hemostasis in nonvariceal GI bleeding, including peptic ulcers
   N. Arteriography/embolization: Performed by interventional radiologist. Considered as an alternative to surgery in patients with large severe UGI bleeding, who have comorbid factors (cardiopulmonary disease, severe liver disease, renal failure, or sepsis).
2. UGI variceal bleed (see "Active UGI Bleeding Episode")
   A. Fluid resuscitation per American College of Surgeons classification (see above).
   B. NGT/lavage (see above).
   C. Sengstaken-Blakemore tube.
   D. Endoscopy: To be done emergently or within 12 hr of presentation if bleeding is brisk. Done for diagnosis as well as institution of sclerotherapy.
3. Hematochezia—acute rapid lower GI bleeding: *These patients require immediate consultation and are referred to the physician.* When stabilized, they may be managed collaboratively per protocol/guidelines with the ACNP. Resuscitation protocol same as above, followed by therapeutic endoscopic procedure, which includes diagnostic colonoscopy with embolization, arteriography, and electrocoagulation as appropriate.
4. Melena: May occur from upper and lower GI source; patient's history and physical exam will determine diagnostic/therapeutic interventions; UGI sources are generally more likely.
5. Occult bleeding
   A. Goal of intervention is to rule out asymptomatic neoplasms at the curable stage.
   B. Colonoscopy is the diagnostic procedure of choice.
   C. If colonoscopy is negative and the symptoms persist, then UGI/small bowel evaluation is required.

ADMISSION/REFERRAL CRITERIA

1. Recent or ongoing brisk bleeding accompanied by orthostatic symptoms, marked fatigue, syncope.
2. Patients with pre-existing conditions (ischemic heart disease) that may be aggravated by anemia, blood loss.
3. Patients who are candidates for endoscopic evaluation will benefit from referral to a gastroenterologist.

PATIENT EDUCATION

1. Recognize/report symptoms of melena, hematochezia, hematemesis
2. Importance of routine screening for fecal occult blood if over 50 yr
3. Importance of baseline colonoscopy or sigmoidoscopy if over 55 yr
4. Importance of reporting fatigue, weakness, malaise that interferes with activities of daily living
5. Importance of adhering to prescribed therapeutic regimen

Review Questions

Mr. G is a 78-year-old widower admitted for progressive weakness, fatigue, and a Hgb of 8.5 gm/dL. The patient reports dark black stools over the past month. Denies nausea/vomiting, melena, or hematemesis. He complains of epigastric burning discomfort prior to meals and has been treated for peptic ulcer in the past. He does not drink alcohol. He takes Motrin for "aches and pains" and is on no other medication. BP 134/84, pulse 102 bpm, respirations 181 min, temperature 37.2°C.

10.61 In the setting of suspected GI bleeding, it is essential to *initially* screen for which of the following?
A. ASA/NSAID use
B. Alcohol consumption
C. Anticoagulant use
D. Fatigue/malaise/dizziness
E. All of the above

10.62 The initial laboratory tests ordered for this patient will include:
A. CBC/type and screen for blood
B. LFTs
C. Chest x-ray, abdominal series
D. UGI

10.63 When ordering IV fluids for this patient, key factors that will influence the volume/rate ordered by the ACNP will include:
A. Cost of colloid versus crystalloid replacement
B. Age, cardiovascular/renal function
C. Neurologic/endocrine function
D. Prior history of peptic ulcer disease

10.64 The highest rate of mortality resulting from upper gastrointestinal bleeds is associated with:
A. Aortoenteric fistula
B. Gastric ulcers
C. Acute mestenteric artery infarction
D. Esophageal varices
E. Fulminant hepatic failure

10.65 The most significant laboratory test findings in hospitalized patients with suspected GI bleeding will reveal:
A. Sharp elevation in the liver function studies
B. Progressive normalization of serum amylase
C. Decreasing trend in the hemoglobin and hematocrit
D. Sharp increase in urine specific gravity
E. Sharp decrease in fibrinogen levels

Answers and Rationales

10.61 **E** Major risk factors for patients presenting with UGI bleeds include ASA/NSAID use, alcohol consumption, anticoagulant use, and complaints of fatigue/malaise/dizziness.

10.62 **A** The initial laboratory test will include CBC to determine the Hgb and Hct as well as evidence of chronic anemia. This patient will also require a type and screen of blood because of the presenting symptoms of weakness/fatigue, tachycardia, and low hemoglobin.

10.63 **B** The key factors that must be considered when ordering the volume and rate of fluid replacement for geriatric population are cardiovascular and renal status. These patients often need a slower rate of replacement or concominant use of diuretics to prevent intravascular volume overload leading to pulmonary congestion. Renal function must also be considered to account for the patient's ability to mobilize and excrete fluid.

10.64 **D** Overall mortality of UGI hemorrhage is 10–20%, with the highest rates associated with esophageal varicies.

10.65 **C** The most significant laboratory test finding in hospitalized patients with GI bleeding is the decreasing trend of hemoglobin and hematocrit. These values are monitored q4–6h during a bleed and following therapeutic intervention.

References

Giesecke, A.H., Grande, C.M., & Whitten, C.W. (1990). Fluid therapy and the resuscitation of traumatic shock. *Crit Care Clin 6*, 66–72.

Kollef, M.H., Canfield, D.A., & Zuckerman, G.R. (1995). Triage consideration for patients with acute gastrointestinal hemorrhage admitted to a medical intensive care unit. *Crit Care Med 23*, 1048–1054.

Podolsky, D.K., & Isselbacher, K.J. (1994). Alcohol-related liver disease and cirrhosis. In I.J. Isselbacher, E.L. Braunwald, J.D. Wilson, et al. (eds.). *Harrison's Principles of Internal Medicine*. New York: McGraw-Hill, pp. 1489–1491.

Reinus, J.F., & Brandt, L.J. (1990). Upper and lower gastrointestinal bleeding in the elderly. *Gastroenterol Clin North Am. 19*, 293–318.

Richter, J.M., & Isselbacher, K.J. (1994). Gastrointestinal bleeding. In L.J. Isselbacher, E. Braunwald, J.D. Wilson, (eds.). *Harrison's Principles of Internal Medicine*. New York: McGraw-Hill, pp. 223–226.

Weinstein, D.F., & Richter, J.M. (1995). Evaluation of gastrointestinal bleeding. In A.H. Goroll, L.A. May, A.G. Mulley (eds.). *Primary Care Medicine: Office Evaluation and Management of the Adult Patient* (3rd ed.). Philadelphia: J.B. Lippincott Co., pp. 352–356.

Clostridium difficile–Associated Diarrhea

DEFINITION

Clostridium difficile–associated diarrhea (CDAD) is an antibiotic-induced diarrhea caused by an overgrowth of *C. difficile* resulting in release of toxins that cause mucosal damage and inflammation. CDAD may also be induced by antineoplastic agents, especially methotrexate and fluorouracil, because of their ability to disrupt the intestinal mucosal lining with alterations in bowel flora.

ETIOLOGY/INCIDENCE

1. Five percent of healthy adults carry toxigenic *C. difficile* in their feces, usually in low numbers.

2. *Clostridium difficile* infection is responsible for virtually all cases of pseudo-membranous colitis and for up to 20% of cases of antibiotic-associated diarrhea without colitis.
3. Hospitalized patients are the most susceptible. The bowel is made susceptible to infection by the use of clindamycin, broad-spectrum penicillins, and cephalosporins. *Clostridium difficile* forms heat-resistant spores that persist in the environment for months or years and are transmitted to susceptible hosts via fecal-oral routes.
4. Infection results from oral ingestion of the spores, which survive the acid environment of the stomach and convert to vegetative forms in the colon.
5. It is transmitted via hospital workers and exposure to contaminated environmental surfaces (toilets, counters, bedpans, bedding), with higher rates of infection being reported among acute care patients in double rooms as compared with those in single rooms.
6. Incubation period is 4–10 days; infection may develop up to 3 weeks after cessation of antibiotic therapy.
7. Relapse is common, particularly in the elderly and immunocompromised patients.

PATHOPHYSIOLOGY

It is thought that the growth of *C. difficile* can be inhibited in vitro by gut organisms that include lactobacilli, *Bacteroides* organisms, group D entero-cocci, *Escherichia coli*, and *Peptostreptococcus* products. When these organisms are eradicated from the gut as a result of broad-spectrum antibiotic therapy, the host becomes susceptible to overgrowth and infection by *C. difficile*. *Clostridium difficile* produces toxin A and toxin B. Their mechanisms of action are not completely understood, but they disrupt cell membranes, microfilaments, and protein synthesis, resulting in pseudomembranous colitis (PMC). The disease may be induced by a short course of antibiotic therapy, including procedure or operative prophylaxis as well as extended treatment.

Clinical presentations include the following, in increasing order of severity:

1. Asymptomatic carrier
2. Antibiotic-associated colitis without pseudomembrane formation
3. Pseudomembranous colitis
4. Fulminant colitis

The most severe forms of the disease are the least common.

SIGNS AND SYMPTOMS

1. History reveals treatment with broad-spectrum antibiotics within 2 days to 6 weeks prior to symptoms.
2. History reveals recent treatment with antineoplastic agents referred to above.
3. Most patients report mild to moderate watery diarrhea, three to four times per day with lower abdominal cramps.
4. Sense of fecal urgency.
5. Abdominal pain.
6. Watery, green, foul-smelling or bloody diarrhea may occur, with the latter being characteristic of the more severe colitis.

PHYSICAL AND LABORATORY FINDINGS

1. Mild cases
   A. Physical examination may be normal or reveal mild left lower quadrant tenderness.
   B. Temperature >38°C (100.4°F) with or without leukocytosis.
   C. Test for fecal leukocytes may or may not be positive.
   D. Positive fecal culture for *C. difficile*.
   E. Cytotoxin B stool assay positive.
2. Severe to fulminant cases of PMC (rare occurrence)
   A. Temperature ≥39.5°C (103.1°F)
   B. Marked abdominal tenderness, with or without signs of perforation
   C. Abdominal distention with evidence of paralytic ileus; nausea, vomiting
   D. Leukocytosis ($\geq 35 \times 10^9$/L)
   E. Dehydration, hypovolemia, hypoalbuminemia
   F. Cytotoxin B stool assay positive
   G. Positive test for fecal leukocytes
   H. Positive fecal culture for *C. difficile*

DIFFERENTIAL DIAGNOSIS

CDAD in hospitalized patients is diagnosed by a history of recent broad-spectrum antibiotic use and the presence of *C. difficile* toxins in the stool.

1. Inflammatory bowel disease
2. Ischemic colitis
3. Antineoplastic agent side effects or induced colitis
4. Traveler's diarrhea

DIAGNOSTIC TESTS/FINDINGS

1. Cytotoxin B stool assay positive—gold standard for diagnosis.
2. Stool toxin assays (enzyme-linked immunosorbent assay [ELISA]) positive for toxin A and toxin B; less expensive, sensitivity 80–90%; however, do not detect all cases of PMC.
3. CBC: Leukocytosis ($\geq 35 \times 10^9$/L) may be present in the more severe cases.
4. Stool culture for *C. difficile* positive.
5. The ACNP will consult with the collaborating gastroenterologist if suspicion of PMC is high. Further diagnostic testing may be ordered as follows:
   A. Colonoscopy is ordered by the gastroenterologist when PMC is suspected. It provides the most rapid diagnosis in severe cases; biopsy may be required if pseudomembranes are not present.
   B. Abdominal CT: May reveal, in PMC, marked thickening of the colonic wall in the sigmoid and descending colon, megacolon, pericolonic inflammation.
   C. Plain abdominal radiographs, in PMC, may reveal mucosal "thumbprinting" indicating evidence of edema; severe PMC may reveal loops of dilated small intestine indicating paralytic ileus.

MANAGEMENT/TREATMENT

Initial Treatment

1. Discontinue antibiotic therapy if possible or rearrange the regimen to alternative compounds.

2. Up to 25% of mild cases improve in 2–4 days following cessation of antibiotic therapy.
3. Metronidazole (Flagyl) 250–500 mg PO q8h for 10 days for patients who are mildly or moderately ill.
4. Patients who are seriously ill and unable to tolerate oral medication may be given metronidazole via NGT with intermittent clamping.
5. Metronidazole (Flagyl) HCl 500 mg IV q8h for 10 days may be used for those patients who do not tolerate oral/NGT medication; however, its reliability has not been proven.
6. Vancomycin (Vancocin) 125 mg PO q6h for 10 days is equally effective; expensive, and preferred for oral treatment of the seriously ill or immunocompromised patient; however, it carries a risk of having the patient develop vancomycin-resistant enterococcus in the gut.
7. Fluid/electrolyte replacement as needed.
8. Patients with positive ELISA for *C. difficile* toxin may benefit from the one of the following agents to bind the toxins:
   A. Cholestyramine (Questran) 4 gm three to four times a day for 3–10 days
   B. Kaolin-pectin (Kaopectate) 30 mL PO four times a day, 3–10 days
   C. Sucralfate (Carafate) 1 gm PO four times a day, 3–10 days
   Note: When one of these agents is added to the treatment regimen, it must be given at least 2 hours before or after all oral medications, including antibiotics because it will also bind to or absorb the medications, thereby inhibiting pharmacologic action.
9. Use of antiperistaltic agents is contraindicated in PMC because they may lead to intestinal stasis, retention of toxins, and complications, especially in the older population.

Relapse Treatment

1. Up to 20% of patients relapse within 1–2 weeks of termination of initial therapy.
2. Reinstitute metronidazole therapy promptly.
3. Recurrent relapses will respond to a 4- to 6-week course of vancomycin accompanied by a slow taper over 1–2 months to ensure success.
4. Use of oral anion exchange resins, as noted above, to bind the toxins while administering lactobacillus preparations to assist with colonic flora reconstitution may also benefit these patients.

PATIENT EDUCATION

1. Educate regarding disease process, course, complications, reoccurrence and outcome; when to report the above to health care practitioner.
2. Educate regarding medications, side effects.
3. Education regarding recognition of symptoms of dehydration.
4. Encourage intake of sufficient fluids.
5. Educate regarding fecal-oral transmission; hand-washing technique, toileting hygiene.
6. Educate regarding prophylactic use of agents to preserve colonic flora—lactobacilli, *S. boulardii*—if future antibiotic use is required.

Review Questions

Mr. W is a well-developed 35-year-old male, with a negative medical history who was admitted to the hospital with cellulitis of the left arm secondary to a cat bite. He has received treatment with IV broad-spectrum antibiotics for 72 hours. Over the past 24 hours he reports four to five watery, yellow-brown stools accompanied by mild, cramping lower abdominal pain. He denies nausea, vomiting; temperature is 38°C. Physical examination reveals mild left lower quadrant tenderness. Stool is negative for occult blood.

10.66 The most likely cause of this patient's symptoms would be:
   A. Cellulitis-induced sepsis
   B. Allergic reaction to the animal bite
   C. Irritable bowel syndrome precipitated by anxiety
   D. Antibiotic-induced diarrhea

10.67 The diagnostic test of choice for this patient is:
   A. Stool culture for ova/parasites
   B. Stool culture for bacteria/fungus
   C. Blood cultures for bacteria, fungus, virus
   D. Cytotoxin B stool assay

10.68 In collaboration with the infectious disease physician, it is decided to begin treatment empirically. The first-line management is:
   A. Discontinue IV antibiotics
   B. Institute fluid and electrolyte replacement
   C. Metronidazole (Flagyl) 500 mg PO q8h
   D. Diphenoxylate HCl 2.5 mg/2.5 mg atropine sulfate (Lomotil), 2 tablets after each loose stool

10.69 The ACNP, in preparation, for discharge of Mr. W, has arranged for home IV antibiotic therapy for 2 weeks. Given the prescribed home IV antibiotic treatment regimen, it is recommended that the patient also be discharged on which of the following medications/dietary regimens?
   A. Metronidazole (Flagyl) 500 mg PO tid for 14 days
   B. Kaolin-pectin 30 ml PO qid as needed
   C. Lactobacillus dietary supplements
   D. All of the above

10.70 This patient will be directed to call the ANCP if which of the following symptoms persist.
   A. Diarrhea, fever
   B. Back pain
   C. Headache, blurred vision
   D. Lower extremity swelling

Answers and Rationales

10.66 **D** Antibiotic-induced diarrhea in hospitalized patients occurs as a result of an overgrowth of *C. difficile*, resulting in release of toxins that cause mucosal damage and inflammation. Patients who present with cellulitis-induced sepsis spike fevers >38°C accompanied by chills and rigors. The patient has no prior history of irritable bowel syndrome; stool is negative for blood. Allergic reaction to the animal bite would not include diarrhea.

10.67 **D** The gold standard for diagnosis of *C. difficile* is a positive cytotoxin B tool assay. Stool culture for ova/parasites is indicated in patients who are at risk for traveler's diarrhea. Stool culture for bacteria/fungus may be ordered if the cytotoxin B stool assay is negative. Blood cultures are not indicated given the clinical presentation.

10.68 **C** Metronidazole 500 mg PO q8h may be instituted empirically once a stool specimen has been obtained for assay. Discontinuing the antibiotics for this patient is not an option. Fluid and electrolyte replacement may be needed if the diarrhea persists but is not the priority intervention. Diphenoxylate HCL/atropine sulfate (Lomotil) is contraindicated in patients with CDAD. Decreasing gut motility increases the risk of toxin retention, intestinal stasis.

10.69 **D** Metrondidazole 500 mg PO q8h should be continued for the duration of IV antibiotic therapy. Use of kaolin-pectin to absorb toxins may be helpful in preventing relapse. Use of lactobacillus dietary supplements to recolonize and preserve intestinal flora is indicated to prevent relapse.

10.70 **A** The reoccurrence or persistence of diarrhea, fever may indicate progression of CDAD. Fever accompanied by rigors, chills may also indicate systemic infection from cellulitis. Back pain, headache, blurred vision, lower extremity swelling are not symptoms expected in this clinical scenario.

References

Czachor, J.S. & Herchline, T.E. (1996). Infectious diarrhea in immunocompetent hosts: Part II. CDAD and traveler's diarrhea. *Hosp Physician 60*, 26–33.

Fekety, R., & Shah, A.B. (1993). Diagnosis and treatment of *Clostridium difficile* colitis. *JAMA 269*, 71–75.

Gerding, D.N., Johnson, S., & Peterson, L.R. (1995). *Clostridium difficile*–associated diarrhea and colitis. *Infect Control Hosp Epidemiol 16*, 459–477.

Hunter, W.J., Venters, J., & Hunter, D.A. (1994). Management of *Clostridium difficile*: A troublesome cause of GI complications. *Hosp Formul 29*, 454–461.

Kelly, C.P., Pothoulakis, C., & LaMont, J.T. (1994). *Clostridium difficile* colitis. *N Engl J Med 330*, 257–262.

Pancreatitis

DEFINITION

Pancreatitis is a pancreatic inflammatory disease associated primarily with dysfunction of the exocrine function of the gland. It is classified as acute and chronic by clinical criteria that distinguish between restoration of normal function in acute disease and permanent residual damage in chronic disease. In most patients, acute pancreatitis is a mild disease that subsides spontaneously within several days (3–7) upon institution of treatment.

ETIOLOGY/INCIDENCE

Acute pancreatitis affects 1 in 10,000 people annually. In the alcoholic population the incidence rises to 1 in 100. Biliary tract disease (gallstones) and alcohol are associated with 65–90% of all cases of acute pancreatitis. Other causes include surgery (abdominal, nonabdominal), endoscopic retrograde cholangiopancreatography (ERCP), trauma (blunt abdominal type), hypertriglyceridemia, drugs (azathioprine, sulfonamides, thiazide diuretics, furosemide, oral contraceptives [estrogen]), viral infections (e.g., mumps, cytomegalovirus, hepatitis), and bacterial infections (e.g., *Mycoplasma*, tuberculosis).

In the United States acute pancreatitis is more commonly related to alcoholism, whereas in England it is most commonly related to biliary tract disease. The overall prevalence of acute pancreatitis in the United States is 0.5%.

Chronic pancreatitis develops in about 10% of patients.

PATHOPHYSIOLOGY

Acute inflammation triggers activation of exocrine pancreatic enzymes, leading to autodigestion and extravasation to surrounding tissues. The pathologic presentation includes edematous pancreatitis, which is generally a mild and self-limited disorder, and necrotizing pancreatitis, in which the degree of necrosis correlates with the severity of the attack. Hemorrhagic pancreatitis is related to interstitial hemorrhage found in pancreatitis as well as pancreatic trauma and pancreatic carcinoma.

Chronic pancreatitis develops in a subset of patients, especially those with a history of high alcohol ingestion. The constant inflammation and irritation results in progressive fibrosis and destruction of functioning glandular tissue. Differentiation of chronic from recurrent pancreatitis is important in that recurrent pancreatitis is initiated by a specific event. Chronic pancreatitis, characterized by pain and ultimately by pancreatic insufficiency, is a self-perpetuating disease.

SIGNS AND SYMPTOMS

1. Abdominal pain: *Hallmark symptom*, varying from mild, tolerable discomfort to severe, constant, and incapacitating distress.
   A. Steady, boring character
   B. Epigastric and/or periumbilical area, often radiating to back, chest, flanks, and lower abdomen
   C. Pain more intense in supine position
   D. Relief obtained by sitting with trunk flexed and legs drawn up
2. Nausea, vomiting, anorexia.
3. Abdominal distention.
4. Sweating, weakness.
5. Fever.
6. History of heavy alcohol intake with recent precipitating episode.
7. Recent history of biliary tract disease; cholelithiasis, ERCP.
8. May have history of heavy meal immediately preceding the attack, or history of milder similar episodes or biliary colic in the past.
9. Steatorrhea occurs when 90% of pancreas is destroyed.
10. Diabetes mellitus is a late manifestation indicating endocrine function failure; hyperglycemic episodes may be fatal.

PHYSICAL FINDINGS

1. Distressed, anxious patient especially in severe attacks.
2. Tender upper abdomen, often without guarding, rigidity, or rebound.
3. Fever of 38.4–39°C (101.1–102.2°F).
4. Tachycardia, pallor, cool clammy skin, hypotension, tachypnea may be present and symptomatic of shock.
5. Mild jaundice may be present.
6. Palpable upper abdominal mass (phlegmon, pseudocyst, pancreatic mass) occasionally present.
7. Bowel sounds may be diminished or absent when associated with ileus.
8. Nausea and vomiting usually present.
9. Basal consolidation of the lung with minimal pleural effusion on left side. Crackles may be present.
10. Rare findings include bluish discoloration of flanks at the costovertebral angle caused by extravasation of blood in acute hemorrhagic pancreatitis (Grey Turner sign).
11. Blush discoloration of the periumbilical region (Cullen's sign) is due to intraperitoneal hemorrhage and indicates acute hemorrhagic pancreatitis.
12. Xanthomas may present and are indicative of hyperlipidemia.
13. Signs of hypocalcemia may be present, including Chvostek's sign, which is spasms of facial muscle elicited by tapping facial nerve in region of parotid gland; Trousseau's sign, which is spasmodic contractions of muscles provoked by pressure upon the nerves that supply them.

DIFFERENTIAL DIAGNOSIS

1. Peptic ulcer
2. Perforated viscus
3. Acute cholecystitis and biliary colic
4. Acute intestinal obstruction
5. Acute mesenteric ischemia; vascular occlusion
6. Renal colic
7. Myocardial infarction
8. Dissecting aortic aneurysm
9. Pneumonia

DIAGNOSTIC TESTS/FINDINGS

Laboratory Tests

Serum amylase and lipase are the only laboratory tests that are diagnostic of pancreatitis. Other tests that should be drawn for prognostic evaluation and intervention include CBC, electrolytes, glucose, BUN, creatinine, liver function tests, and blood gas studies.

1. Serum amylase elevated greater than four times normal is suggestive of acute pancreatitis. Serum amylase elevation occurs early in course; usually elevated within 24 hours of symptom onset in 90% of cases. Return to normal is variable depending on severity of case. Elevation of amylase may be due to other causes.

2. Serum lipase elevation is more specific indicator of pancreatitis but elevation is delayed.
3. CBC may reflect leukocytosis; 10,000–30,000/L indicative of inflammatory process. Hematocrit elevated, indicating hemoconcentration in severe cases as a result of loss of fluid into retroperitoneal space and peritoneal cavity.
4. Serum bilirubin (>4.0 mg/dL), AST, alkaline phosphatase may be elevated in 10% of cases but return to normal in 7–10 days.
5. Hyperglycemia/glycosuria: 10–20% of cases as a result of decreased insulin release, increased glucagon release, and increased output of adrenal glucocorticoids and catecholamines.
6. Proteinuria, casts (present in 25% of cases).
7. Hypocalcemia occurs in 25% of cases; pathogenesis unknown but may indicate saponification (conversion into soapy substance) and correlates with severity of disease.
8. Serum protein and albumin levels may be decreased.
9. Hypokalemia may be present.
10. Coagulation studies may reflect coagulapathy, specifically elevated PT.
11. Hypertriglyceridemia: Rare finding; however, when present, indicates a probable history of alcoholism with a recent bout of drinking or pre-existing hypertriglyceridemia.

Radiologic/Imaging Studies

1. CT scan: Contrast enhanced is the imaging study most useful in demonstrating an enlarged pancreas, in detecting pseudocysts and phlegmon, as well as differentiating from other intra-abdominal catastrophes such as carcinoma, obstruction.
2. Plain films of the abdomen: May indicate gallstones, a "sentinel loop" (a segment of air-filled intestine in the left upper quadrant), the "colon cutoff sign" (a gas-filled segment of the transverse colon abruptly ending at the area of pancreatic inflammation), or linear focal atelectasis of the left lower lobe of the lung with or without pleural effusion. Calcified pancreas is indicative of chronic pancreatitis.
3. Biliary tract ultrasound: To rule out gallstone disease, a treatable cause of pancreatitis. Will show pseudocyst, enlargement, abscess.
4. Radionuclide biliary excretion scan can help to differentiate between alcoholic pancreatitis and biliary pancreatitis if bilirubin <10 mg/dL.
5. ERCP will demonstrate dilated main pancreatic duct with strictures, intraductal stones, or pseudocyst.

Electrocardiogram

ST-T wave changes may occur but usually differ from those of myocardial infarction. Abnormal Q waves do not occur a result of pancreatitis.

MANAGEMENT/TREATMENT

Severe pancreatitis should be referred to general surgeon for management as soon as possible.

Pancreatic Rest Program (Mild to Moderate Acute Pancreatitis)

1. No food or fluids by mouth 2–4 days; clear liquids 3–6 days; full diet as tolerated 5–7 days. No food or fluids by mouth until the patient is largely free from pain and has bowel sounds.
2. Bed rest.
3. Nasogastric suction for those with moderately severe pain or ileus.
4. Pain control using meperidine 75–150 mg IM q3–4h or on patient-controlled analgesia machine. Meperidine should be used over morphine because it decreases spasm in the sphincter of Oddi. Patients with impaired hepatic or renal function may need decreased doses.
5. Intravenous fluids and colloids to maintain normal intravascular volume. Volume replacement may be accomplished with normal saline or normal saline and dextrose with 20 mEq of potassium/L, to run at 75–100 mL/hr.
6. Antibiotic use when infection or risk for infection (demonstrated areas of necrosis) has been identified. A broad-spectrum intravenous antibiotic such as piperacillin tazobactam (Zosyn) 3.375 gm IV q6h should be used.
7. TPN may be instituted for patients with severe protracted disease who are unable to eat.
8. Monitor laboratory values—liver function tests, serum amylase, electrolytes (hypocalcemia, hypomagnesemia), hemoglobin, hematocrit, glucose, BUN, creatinine.
9. Calcium gluconate given intravenously for evidence of hypocalcemia with tetany.
10. Insulin supplementation may be required for hyperglycemia.

Chronic Pancreatitis

1. Treatment is symptomatic for pain, steatorrhea, and diabetes.
2. Pain is treated with abstinence from alcohol, non-narcotic analgesics, narcotic analgesics for severe intractable pain, low-fat diet.
3. Steatorrhea is treated with oral enzyme supplements with meals, low-fat diet, and medium-chain triglyceride supplementation.
4. Diabetes is treated with insulin injection as indicated by blood sugar measurement.
5. Referral is necessary for pseudocyst and pancreatic ascites.

REFERRAL CRITERIA

The ACNP should refer any patient with:
1. Three or more of Ranson's criteria on admission (see Table 10–12)
2. Evidence of worsening clinical state following the first 48 hours of treatment

COMPLICATIONS

1. Prerenal azotemia or acute tubular necrosis may result from severe fluid shifts that occur with moderate to severe pancreatitis. Renal symptoms usually become evident within 24 hours of onset of acute pancreatitis, lasting 10 days to 2 weeks. Treatment for renal symptoms is supportive; some patients may require short-term dialysis.

TABLE 10–12.   Acute Pancreatitis: Assessment of Severity Ranson's Criteria*

Age over 55
WBC >16,000/μL
Blood glucose >200 mg/dL
Base deficit >4 mEq/L
Serum LDH >350 IU/L
AST >250 IU/L

Development of the following findings in the first 48 hours
   indicates worsening prognosis
   Hct ↓ >10%
   BUN ↑ 5 mg/dL
   P_aO_2 <60 mm Hg
   Serum calcium <8 mg/dL
   Estimated fluid sequestration >6 L

---
* Adapted from Greenberger, N.J., Toskes, P.P., & Isselbacher, K.J. (1994). Acute and chronic pancreatitis. In L.J. Isselbacher, E. Braunwald, J.D. Wilson, et al. (eds.). *Harrison's Principles of Internal Medicine.* New York: McGraw-Hill, pp. 1520–1527, with permission.

---

2. Sterile or infected pancreatic necrosis may occur in 10% of cases. Necrosis is the primary cause of mortality in pancreatitis. Necrosis is associated with high fevers, leukocytosis, and progression to shock. Pancreatic necrosis is absolute indication for operative intervention.
3. Adult respiratory distress syndrome may occur 3–7 days after onset of pancreatitis in patients who required large volumes of fluid for hemodynamic support. Treatment for this is outlined in other sections.
4. Pancreatic pseudocyst (encapsulated fluid collection with high enzyme content) occur commonly with pancreatitis. Some patients may have multiple cysts. Those <6 cm in diameter resolve spontaneously. Pseudocysts require no intervention unless infection develops.

PATIENT EDUCATION

1. Educate regarding the function of the pancreas and its role in digestion.
2. Educate patient regarding the connection between alcohol abuse and pancreatitis.
3. Inform of the necessity of alcohol abstinence during the course and recovery from episode. Referral may be necessary in those who demonstrate untreated alcoholism.
4. Inform the patient who is recovering from mild/moderate inflammation that reoccurrence is uncommon when the underlying cause is treated.
5. Patients with hypertriglyceridemia as the underlying cause will need to comply with the following suggestions to prevent reoccurrence:
   A. Weight loss to ideal weight
   B. Lipid-restricted diet
   C. Exercise
   D. Avoidance of alcohol and drugs that elevate serum triglycerides (vitamin A, thiazides, β-blockers, estrogens)
   E. Control of diabetes if present
6. Patient with chronic pancreatitis should be taught:
   A. Prevention measures, such as low-fat diet, avoidance of alcohol
   B. Signs of exocrine insufficiency, such as digestive problems, weight loss

    C. Signs of endocrine insufficiency (abnormal glucose)

    D. Need for pancreatic enzyme supplements

Review Questions

Mr. S is a 39-year-old male who is anxious and in acute distress. He presents to the clinic with a recent history of heavy alcohol intake and a chief complaint of epigastric pain described as severe, constant, and boring in character, with radiation to the back. The pain is alleviated somewhat by sitting up and leaning forward. He has had intractable nausea and vomiting over the past 36 hours.

10.71 The most likely diagnosis for this patient is:
    A. Acute pancreatitis
    B. Acute cholecystitis
    C. Gastroesophageal reflux disease
    D. Colon cancer

10.72 The management of mild to moderate acute pancreatis includes:
    A. NPO 2–4 days
    B. Bed rest
    C. Pain management
    D. IV fluids/TPN support as needed
    E. All the above

10.73 Acute pancreatitis is most frequently associated with:
    A. Alcohol-related liver and biliary tract disease
    B. Alcohol-related liver and peptic ulcer disease
    C. Peptic ulcer disease and hepatitis
    D. Gastric ulcer disease and diverticulitis

10.74 The management of acute pancreatitis may include:
    A. High-fat diet
    B. Demerol 100–150 mg IM
    C. Cholinergic drugs
    D. Low-calcium diet

10.75 The most helpful laboratory finding for diagnosis of acute pancreatitis is:
    A. Bilirubin, total and direct
    B. Amylase
    C. Acid phosphate
    D. AST

Answers and Rationales

10.71 **A** The history of recent heavy alcohol intake along with the history of relief when sitting up and leaning forward, as well as the location and quality of the pain, would suggest pancreatitis, cholesystitis, carcinoma with obstruction. The addition of the other history and physical findings allows pancreatitis to be the suspected diagnosis.

10.72 **E** Treatment for mild to moderate pancreatitis includes bowel rest, which translates to nothing by mouth with parenteral nutrition support if needed, pain management preferably with demerol, and bed rest.

10.73 **A** Acute pancreatitis is most frequently associated with alcohol-related liver and biliary tract disease.

10.74 **C** Demerol has less effect on the sphincter of Oddi than the other narcotic analgesics.

10.75 **B** The serum amylase will rise within 24 hours of onset of acute pancreatitis. The rate of return to normal values varies depending on the severity of the disease. The level of serum amylase does not correlate with prognosis.

References

Brown, A. (1991). Acute pancreatitis: Pathophysiology, nursing diagnoses and collaborative problems. *Focus Crit Care AACN 18*(2), 121–130.

Friedman, L.S. (1995). Liver, biliary tract, and pancreas. In L. Tierney, S. McPhee, & M. Papadakis (eds.). *Current Medical Diagnosis and Treatment*. Stamford, CT: Appleton & Lange, pp. 587–590.

Greenberger, N.J., Toskes, P.P., & Isselbacher, K.J. (1994). Acute and chronic pancreatitis. In L.J. Isselbacher, E. Braunwald, J.D. Wilson, et al. (eds.). *Harrison's Principles of Internal Medicine*. New York: McGraw-Hill, pp. 1520–1527.

Richter, J.M. (1995). Management of pancreatitis. In A.H. Goroll, L.A. May, & A.G. Mulley (eds.). *Primary Care Medicine: Office Evaluation and Management of the Adult Patient* (3rd ed.). Philadelphia, J.B. Lippincott Co., pp. 412–415.

Peptic Ulcer Disease

DEFINITION

Peptic ulcer is a break in the gastric or duodenal mucosa that extends through the muscularis mucosae and is usually over 5 mm in diameter. Peptic ulcers are five times more common in the duodenum, with over 95% located in the bulb or pyloric channel (Table 10–13). In the stomach, approximately 60% of benign ulcers are located in the antrum. Twenty-five percent are located at the junction of the antrum and body on the lesser curvature.

Stress-induced gastritis is caused from damage from gastric secretions as a result of increased mucosal susceptibility from conditions of extreme physical stress. The true incidence may be 80–100% of critically ill patients. Stress gastritis is characterized by multiple erosions of proximal stomach.

ETIOLOGY/INCIDENCE

1. Over 4 million people affected annually.
2. In the past men were three to four times more likely to develop disease; however, recent studies indicate women develop gastric ulcers as frequently as men.
3. Most common in middle-aged to elderly adults but occurs in all ages, including infants.
4. Approximately 3000 deaths/year result from duodenal ulcer (6% mortality with perforation).

TABLE 10-13.   Characteristics of Duodenal, Gastric, and Stress Ulcers

	Duodenal Ulcer	Gastric Ulcer	Stress Ulcer
Incidence	Duodenal/gastric ulcer ratio approximately 4:1. Most common age group 25–50, with men being affected 4 times more than women.		Related to severe physiologic stress such as trauma, sepsis, burns, head injuries. No age or sex differences. Found in 100% of critically ill patients who undergo endoscopic exam.
Pathogenesis	Hyperacidity is most important factor. Diseases associated include hyperparathyroidism, chronic pulmonary disease, chronic pancreatitis, alcoholic cirrhosis. Also associated with alcohol, tobacco. Blood group O has higher frequency. Associated with high stress levels.	Disruption of mucosal barrier is most important factor. HCl production is normal to low in most patients. Ulcerogenic drugs also associated include alcohol, tobacco, chronic bile reflux.	Head injuries: Hypersecretion of HCl. All others: Most likely associated with gastric ischemia.
Location	Duodenal bulb: 90%	Antrum and lesser curvature: 90%	Multiple, diffuse erosions more commonly located in stomach.
Clinical features	Pain-food relief pattern of pain. Weight loss seldom affects occurrence. Seasonal exacerbations have been seen. Night pain common.	Food may relieve or exacerbate the pain. Anorexia, weight loss are common. Night pain less common.	Are asymptomatic until serious complication such as hemorrhage or perforation. Usually not associated with pain.

5. Elderly women are high risk for NSAID-associated gastric ulcers with perforation and hemorrhage.

PATHOPHYSIOLOGY

1. The integrity of the gastric mucosa is maintained by a balance between aggressive factors—acid, pepsin—and normal defense mechanisms of gastric and duodenal mucosa—mucosal and bicarbonate secretion, mucosal blood flow, cell restitution, prostaglandins.
2. PUD occurs from an imbalance between aggressive and defensive factors as a result of external factors.
   A. NSAIDs disrupt defense by inhibiting gastric mucosal prostaglandin synthesis.
   B. *Helicobacter pylori* infection disturbs defense factors, making the mucosa more susceptible to the effects of acid and pepsin.
   C. Zollinger-Ellison syndrome is caused by gastrin-secreting tumors (gastrinomas) that cause hypergastrinemia and acid hypersecretion. Less than 1% of PUD is caused by this syndrome.
3. NSAID-induced disease

A. Is not generally associated with new duodenal ulcer disease, but rather with pre-existing disease.
B. Chronic NSAID users increase risk of gastric ulcers 40-fold and are three times more likely to suffer serious GI complications (hemorrhage, perforation) from the ulcers.
C. Smoking, alcohol use, alcohol-related disease, and pre-existing PUD greatly increase risk of ulcer and ulcer complications in NSAID-treated patients.
4. Helicobacter pylori infection
A. Gram-negative bacterium that infects gastric mucus layer of all patients with duodenal ulcer and most patients with gastric ulcer disease.
B. Lives on gastric mucosa. Organism has been found in over 95% of cases of duodenal ulcer and ulcer recurrence and causes type B gastritis.
C. Majority of individuals infected with *H. pylori* do not develop ulcer disease, but pre-existing infection increases the risk of developing gastric ulcer threefold and duodenal ulcer fourfold.
D. Eradication speeds ulcer healing and greatly reduces rates of recurrence.
E. Cures of PUD have been associated with eradication of *H. pylori* infection.
F. Studies have indicated NSAID use does not predispose to *H. pylori* infection.

SIGNS AND SYMPTOMS (see Table 10–13)
Clinical presentation of duodenal and gastric ulcer are similar and nonspecific.
1. Dyspepsia
A. Characterized by vague group of symptoms including heartburn, nausea, bloating; exacerbated by food and change in position.
B. PUD is the most common single cause of this symptom and must be ruled out when present.
2. Pain: Classic symptom
A. Epigastric pain well localized to epigastrium and not severe; described as gnawing, dull, aching, "hunger-like"; may radiate to back.
B. Characterized by rhythmicity, fluctuates in intensity throughout day and night, and periodicity with symptomatic episodes lasting several weeks with pain-free intervals of months to years.
C. Approximately 50% of patients report relief of pain with food or antacids, especially duodenal ulcers, and a recurrence of pain 2–4 hours later.
D. Nocturnal pain occurs with a higher frequency in duodenal ulcers but is not a specific or consistent symptom.
E. Sudden acute onset of pain, or pain that was once relieved by food or antacids and no longer is, may indicate perforation.
3. Nausea: May occur and is more highly associated with gastric ulcers
4. Anorexia
A. May occur secondary to anemia, blood in stomach, or underlying primary disease process (e.g., gastric carcinoma)
B. May also occur in elderly secondary to vomiting and exacerbation of discomfort with meals
5. Vomiting and weight loss
A. Significant vomiting does not present with uncomplicated disease.
B. When present, it may indicate gastric outlet obstruction or gastric malignancy.
6. Weakness and malaise: Associated with slow bleeding and anemia

PHYSICAL FINDINGS

PUD

1. Abdominal exam
   A. Unremarkable in uncomplicated disease.
   B. May reveal mild, localized epigastric tenderness to deep palpation.
   C. More severe tenderness suggests possibility of complicated disease such as pancreatitis or gastric or duodenal perforation.
   D. Rebound tenderness suggests peritonitis secondary to perforation and/ or penetration.
2. Musculoskeletal exam
   A. Back pain may be a manifestation of referred pain secondary to gastric ulcer or posterior penetrating ulcer or perforation.
   B. Shoulder pain may be present with gastric ulcers as a result of irritation of left diaphragm by penetration of an ulcer high on greater curvature near cardia.
3. Melena
   A. Most likely to be present with PUD
   B. Duodenal ulcer twice as likely as gastric ulcer to present with melena
4. Hematemesis: Presents with melena when gastric ulcers are present
5. Hematochezia
   A. Occurs if bleeding is excessive and especially if continuous bright red blood per rectum appears.
   B. Bright red blood per rectum with an upper GI source indicates a blood loss of 1000 mL with orthostatic BP changes or hypotension.

Stress Gastritis

Physical findings significant for stress gastritis include hematemesis, bloody nasogastric aspirate, or other evidence of gastrointestinal bleeding. Intravascular volume depletion and shock may be seen.

DIFFERENTIAL DIAGNOSIS

1. Gastroesophageal reflux disease
2. Chronic cholecystitis
3. Biliary tract/liver disease
4. Chronic pancreatitis
5. Nonulcer dyspepsia
6. Gastritis
7. Neoplasms

DIAGNOSTIC TESTS/FINDINGS

Laboratory Tests

Extensive tests are unnecessary for stable symptomatic patients.

1. Detection of *H. pylori* (essential in all patients with peptic ulcer disease): Urease test is the best endoscopic diagnostic test; also histopathology, culture, urea breath, serum *H. pylori* antibodies. Campylobacter-like organism test useful in confirming presence of *H. pylori*.

2. CBC with differential and platelet count: Minimum initial test
    A. WBC count may be normal or elevated in cases of perforation or penetration.
    B. Hct may be decreased; however, anemia is inconsistent with PUD alone. Hct <28% represents significant hemorrhage or an acute bleeding episode superimposed on chronic bleeding; however, even with significant bleeding the Hb and Hct may remain normal for several hours.
    C. Hypochromic microcytic anemia secondary to blood loss may be present.
3. Electrolytes
    A. Sodium increase may be due to extracellular fluid depletion secondary to vomiting.
    B. Potassium decrease may be seen secondary to protracted vomiting.
    C. Chloride decrease from protracted vomiting.
    D. Calcium may be elevated in the presence of Zollinger-Ellison syndrome, or excessive ingestion of calcium-containing antacids, or ulcer disease complicating hyperparathyroidism.
4. BUN/creatinine
    A. In the absence of renal disease, a BUN level >40 mg/dL with a normal creatinine level may be indicative of significant blood loss.
    B. BUN level >85 mg/dL with a normal creatinine level may indicate a loss of two or more units of blood into the GI tract.
5. Amylase: May be increased in perforation and in posterior penetrating duodenal ulcers.
6. Gastrin: Serum gastrin useful in recurrent, refractory, or complicated PUD and in patients with a family history of PUD to screen for Zollinger-Ellison syndrome. Gastrin level will be increased with gastric ulcer but not duodenal.

Radiologic Tests

1. Upper GI series with contrast
    A. Procedure of choice to establish the etiology of abdominal pain or confirm diagnosis of ulcer disease in suspicious cases unless bleeding is present.
    B. Unable to always identify lesions <5 mm, and may miss gastric ulcers that are shallow, as may occur in NSAID-induced ulceration.
2. Endoscopy
    A. Considered superior to barium study for detection of gastric ulcer, malignancy, and *H. pylori*, because brushings, biopsy, and cultures can be performed.
    B. Recommendations are to individualize test selection, with use of endoscopy for those with recurrent disease to rule out *H. pylori* infection and for elderly persons who may present with a gastric ulcer requiring biopsy to rule out carcinoma.

MANAGEMENT/TREATMENT

1. Goals: Speed healing, reduce pain, prevent complications and recurrences; minimize costs and side effects of interventions
2. Duration of therapy
    A. Medical therapy is required for a minimum of 4 weeks, the time required to heal duodenal ulcers in 90% of patients.
    B. Resolution of pain is therapeutic end point but correlates poorly with complete healing.

    C. Patients may require an additional 2–4 weeks of therapy if there is any question regarding complete healing or past medical history of PUD reoccurrence.

    D. Large gastric ulcers require up to 12 weeks of treatment.

3. Nonpharmacologic interventions

    A. Diet: No dietary restrictions necessary; recommend limiting intake of coffee and caffeine-containing beverages

    B. Smoking

        1) Impedes healing of peptic ulcers and response to H_2 receptor antagonists.

        2) Compliance with cessation is required.

    C. Avoidance of mucosa-irritating agents

        1) Avoid use of NSAIDs; aspirin is the most irritating of this classification.

        2) Limit or cease alcohol intake because it may impair healing or cause complications.

        3) Use of prophylactic regimens if prednisone >30 mg/day is required for prolonged periods.

    D. Alleviating stress-producing situations: Consider referral for counseling for those with difficult home or work environments

4. Pharmacologic interventions

    A. Active *H. pylori* infection–associated ulcer

        1) First line: Ranitidine (Zantac) 150 mg bid for 6–8 weeks, plus triple therapy with:

            a. Metronidazole (Flagyl) 250 mg qid for 2 weeks or clarithromycin 500 mg tid

            b. Tetracycline 500 mg q6h for 2 weeks

            c. Bismuth subsalicylate 2 tablets qid

            (May substitute amoxicillin if the combination is not tolerated.)

        2) Alternative

            a. Omeprazole (Prilosec) 40 mg daily for first 2 weeks, then 20 mg daily for 2–4 weeks, *plus*

            b. Clarithromycin (Biaxin) 500 mg tid for the first 2 weeks

            c. Consider adding a second antibiotic: amoxicillin 500 mg qid or metronidazole 250 mg qid for first 2 weeks.

    B. Antacids (see Table 10–14)

        1) Antacid therapy is given for its buffering capacity and is indicated if patient is reliable, wants to minimize cost, systemic effects, and drug-drug interactions.

        2) Use magnesium-aluminum hydroxide liquid with high acid-neutralizing capacity and low sodium content (Maalox TC or Mylanta Double Strength) 140 mEq/dose for duodenal ulcers; 50 mEq/dose for gastric ulcers 2 hours pc and hs. Monitor side effects.

        3) May substitute aluminum hydroxide or decrease dose of magnesium-aluminum hydroxide if diarrhea develops.

    C. Histamine H_2 receptor antagonists

        1) Cimetidine (Tagamet) 400 mg PO bid; watch for drug potentiation if patient is on propranolol, warfarin, benzodiazepines, phenytoin, theophylline. May cause confusion and should be used with caution in the elderly.

        2) Famotidine (Pepcid) 20 mg bid. Causes less drug interaction and central nervous system side effects.

TABLE **10–14.**   **Medications Commonly Used in Gastrointestinal Disorders***

Generic (Trade) Name	Action	Indications	Contraindications	Adult Dose	Common Side Effects
Dihydroxyaluminum sodium carbonate (Rolaids antacid tablets)	Neutralizes gastric acid accompanied by the release of carbon dioxide	Heartburn: Gastric acidity	Sodium-restricted diet; concurrent use of tetracycline	Chew 1–2 tablets; repeat hourly; do not exceed 24 tablets in 24 hours or exceed 2 weeks' use at maximum dose	None listed
Calcium carbonate, precipitated, USP (500 mg)	Antacid	Peptic ulcer; gastritis, gastric hyperacidity; hiatal hernia; peptic esophagitis	Renal disease; hypercalcemia; concurrent use with large amounts of milk; severe debilitation	Chew tablets as symptoms occur; repeat hourly as needed; do not exceed 16 tablets in 24 hours or exceed 2 weeks' use at maximum dose	None listed
Aluminum and magnesium hydroxide (Maalox, Mylanta, Riopan, Gelusil H)	Antacid; acid binding	Peptic ulcer; occasional heartburn	Concurrent use of tetracycline, kidney disease; sodium content necessitates use with caution in cardiac patients (Riopan low in sodium)	2–4 tsp qid; not to exceed 16 tsp/day	Diarrhea, constipation
Aluminum hydroxide (Amphojel, Gelusil)	Antacids	Peptic ulcer; gastritis; esophagitis; hiatal hernia; gastric hyperacidity	Concurrent tetracycline use	2 tsp. 5–6 times a day between meals	Constipation

* Adapted from Connor, S., D'Andrea, K., Piper, J., et al. (1989). *Comprehensive Review Manual for the Adult Nurse Practitioner.* Glenview, IL: Scott, Foresman and Company, with permission.

3) Nizatidine (Axid) 300 mg PO once daily; alternatively may give 150 mg PO bid.
4) Ranitidine (Zantac) 150 mg PO hs.

D. Sucralfate
   1) Aluminum hydroxide and sulfated sucrose complex that acts as a mucosal barrier, inhibiting pepsin activity and binding bile salts.
   2) A 1-gm dose administered bid.
   3) Indicated for those not tolerating antacids or H_2 blockers and not bothered with problems of constipation.
   4) *Caution:* Will inhibit absorption of drugs given at the same time.

E. Prostaglandin analog (misoprostol)
   1) Proved less effective that H_2 blockers for treatment of peptic ulcers.
   2) Only agent that is approved by the Food and Drug Administration for prevention of gastric ulcers in patients requiring chronic NSAID therapy.
   3) Because of high cost and GI side effects (diarrhea) at efficacy dosing (100–200 μg qid), its use is recommended for only those patients described above.

    F. Omeprazole
1) "Proton pump" inhibitor that reduces 24-hour acid production by more than 90%; 60-minute half-life, duration 24 hours.
2) A 20- to 30-mg dose administered once daily before breakfast.
3) Effective agent used to heal duodenal ulcers in 4 weeks as opposed to 8-week conventional therapy.
4) Increases serum drug levels of warfarin, benzodiazepines, phenytoin.
5) Efficacy for long-term use has not yet been established.
    G. Anticholinergics
1) Decreases gastric motility.
2) Because of frequency of dosing plus side effects, these agents have generally fallen out of favor as a first-line drug for treatment of PUD.
3) Combination tablets containing phenobarbital + hyoscyamine sulfate + atropine sulfate + hyoscine hydrobromide are dosed 1–2 tablets tid–qid
4) Side effects include blurred vision, dry mouth, urinary hesitancy, flushing

5. Treatment of stress gastritis that results in severe hemorrhage: Managed with a variety of surgical and nonsurgical therapies; surgical consultation is required. Prevention is most important.

FOLLOW-UP AND REFERRAL

1. Eradication of *H. pylori* decreases the 1-year recurrence rate to <10% on no therapy.
2. Maintenance therapy is not required in patients who have uncomplicated ulcers and who have had *H. pylori* infection eradicated. It should be considered in patients older than 60, smokers, and patients with recurrent, refractory, or complicated ulcers, particularly those in whom *H. pylori* has not been eradicated.
3. Duodenal ulcer: Cancer risk small.
4. The ACNP refers for the following:
    A. Follow-up radiologic or endoscopic evaluation recommended when persistence or recurrence of pain, symptoms of gastric outlet obstruction, and/or evidence of bleeding occur.
    B. Gastric ulcer: Endoscopic examination and biopsy are required if there is suspicion of refractory gastric ulcer (persistent pain after 8 weeks despite full treatment regimen) and in patients over 40.
    C. Patient with symptoms of complications, such as perforation/bleeding.

PATIENT EDUCATION

1. Instruct on medications; action, side effects, and most effective dosing.
2. Instruct on course of disease/symptoms of complications.
    A. Majority of ulcers heal in 4 weeks; can take up to 8–12 weeks.
    B. Follow-up is required.
    C. Recurrence rate is high (30–90% in 5 years).
    D. Symptoms for recognition of perforation/bleeding.
3. Diet management.
    A. Avoid eating before bedtime.
    B. Avoid eating foods that are not tolerated.
    C. Bland, frequent feedings are not necessary.

    D. Avoidance of spices and acidic foods is not necessary; however, recommend limiting intake of caffeine-containing beverages.
4. Stress management.
5. Smoking cessation.
6. Cease or limit alcohol intake.
7. Restrict use of NSAIDs.
8. Educate on need to consult with health care provider regarding ulcer prophylaxis if patient requires future steroid or NSAID therapy.

Review Questions

Mr. M is a 52-year-old patient you are evaluating for discharge following a successful first rib resection for thoracic outlet syndrome. He reports complaints of pain in his stomach for the past 3 weeks. He describes the pain as dull, gnawing, "hunger-like." He has been taking Rolaids, which afford him temporary relief. He has had three previous episodes of stomach pain lasting 3–4 weeks each time over the past 14 months. He denies chest pain, nausea, vomiting, melena, weight loss, fatigue, malaise, fever. This episode is similar to the others, and he wants information regarding a better treatment because of the reoccurrence.

10.76 The abdominal examination will most likely reveal:
    A. Marked tenderness in RLQ with tenesmus
    B. Enlarged, tender spleen and liver
    C. Severe rebound tenderness
    D. Unremarkable findings

10.77 Minimum baseline laboratory tests for the abdominal complaints will include:
    A. CBC; SMA 20
    B. Amylase, ALT, AST, LDH, alkaline phosphatase
    C. PT, PTT, platelet count
    D. CBC with differential

10.78 Pharmacologic therapy for this patient following detection of *H. pylori* will include:
    A. Rantidine 150 mg P/O bid for 4–6 weeks
    B. Metronidazole 250 mg qid for 2 weeks
    C. Tetracycline 500 mg qid for 2 weeks
    D. Bismuth subsalicylate 2 tablets qid for 4 weeks
    E. All of the above

10.79 Nonpharmacologic interventions for uncomplicated duodenal ulcer disease include:
    A. Restrict intake of alcohol, NSAIDs, ASA, caffeine
    B. Endoscopic examination with brushings and biopsy
    C. UGI with barium swallow
    D. Triple therapy for 6–8 weeks

10.80 The length of therapy for this patient will be:
    A. When the patient reports resolution of pain
    B. A minimum of 8 weeks because of the vascular disease

    C. Two weeks of antibiotics; 4–6 weeks of H$_2$ antagonists.

    D. Determined by endoscopic brushings and biopsy

Answers and Rationales

10.76 **D** Abdominal examination is generally unremarkable in patients with uncomplicated peptic ulcer disease.

10.77 **D** The minimum baseline laboratory test in patients presenting with uncomplicated peptic ulcer disease is a CBC with differential. Extensive testing is not required in otherwise stable patients with initial presenting symptoms.

10.78 **E** Triple therapy for *H. pylori* includes, in addition to rantidine, metronidazole, tetracycline, and bismuth subsalicylate.

10.79 **A** Nonpharmacologic interventions for uncomplicated duodenal ulcer disease include restriction of alcohol intake, NSAIDs, ASA, caffeine.

10.80 **C** Initial triple therapy includes 2 weeks of antibiotics and 4–6 weeks of histamine antagonists.

References

Anderson, M.L. (1994). Helicobacter pylori infection: When and in whom is treatment important? *Postgrad Med 96*, 40–49.

Connor, S., D'Andrea, K., Piper, J., et al. (1989). *Comprehensive Review Manual for the Adult Nurse Practitioner.* Glenview, IL: Scott, Foresman, and Company

Fantry, G. (1996). Peptic ulcer disease. In R.E. Rakel (ed.). *Saunders Manual of Medical Practice.* Philadelphia: W.B. Saunders Co., pp. 319–321.

Freston, M.S., & Freston, J.W. (1990). Peptic ulcers in the elderly: Unique features and management. *Geriatrics 45*, 39–45.

Goroll, A.H. (1995). Management of peptic ulcer disease. In A.H. Goroll, L.A. May, A.G. Mulley (eds.). *Primary Care Medicine: Office Evaluation and Management of the Adult Patient* (3rd ed.). Philadelphia: J.B. Lippincott Co., pp. 382–391.

McQuaid, K.R. (1995). Alimentary tract. In L. Tierney, S. McPhee, & M. Papadakis (eds.), *Current Medical Diagnosis and Treatment.* Stamford, CT: Appleton & Lange, pp. 512–519.

NIH Consensus Conference: *Helicobacter pylori* in peptic ulcer disease. (1994). *JAMA 272*, 65–69.

Pope, J. (1996). Gastritis. In R.E. Rakel (ed.). *Saunders Manual of Medical Practice.* Philadelphia: W.B. Saunders Co., pp. 327–329.

Rosen, S.D., & Rogers, A.I. (1990). Clinical recognition and evaluation of peptic ulcer disease. *Postgrad Med 88*, 42–55.

Peritonitis

DEFINITION

Peritonitis is the inflammation of the endothelial lining of the abdominal cavity and abdominal viscera. Inflammation may be either acute or chronic.

TABLE 10-15. Causes of Secondary Peritonitis	
Acute pancreatitis	Hepatic abscesses
Acute salpingitis	Mesenteric ischemia
Appendicitis	Multiple trauma, blunt or penetrating
Bowel obstruction	Perinephric abscess
Cholecystitis	Postsurgical complications
Diverticulitis, perforated	Ruptured tubal pregnancy
Gastroduodenal ulcer	Tubo-ovarian abscess

ETIOLOGY/INCIDENCE

1. Primary peritonitis: Bacterial agent gains contact with peritoneum through either the vascular system or the fallopian tubes. Usually yields a single microbe.
2. Secondary peritonitis is most important complication of wide variety of acute abdominal disorders (see Table 10-15).
3. Gangrene of bowel, rapid absorption of toxins increases the severity of the process.
4. Trauma, blunt or penetrating: Peritonitis may occur days after initial injury, and without visceral perforation.
5. Peritonitis from surgery may occur if bile leakage develops, a localized infection spreads, or an anastomosis breaks down.

PATHOPHYSIOLOGY

The peritoneal cavity contains <50 mL of sterile transudate to prevent friction between the viscera during peristalsis. Additionally, bidirectional fluid and electrolyte exchange occurs through the semipermeable mesothelial layers of the visceral and parietal peritoneum. The surface area of the peritoneum is comparable to that of the skin, providing a large amount of absorption area. A variety of inflammatory cells (macrophages, mast cells, eosinophils, and basophils) are present in the mesentery, providing peritoneal defense. The initiation of an inflammatory stimulus, such as bacteria, mast cells, and macrophages, releases histamine and prostaglandins, which lead to vasodilation with increased vascular permeability. A large amount of exudative fluid high in fibrin, complement, clotting factors, and immunoglobulins is released into the peritoneal cavity. Generation of chemotaxins such as leukotriene B_4, and C_{5a} leads to influx of neutrophils and bacterial destruction. Fibroblastic exudate is deposited on the peritoneum and plasters the adjacent bowel, mesentery, and omentum to the inflamed area, forming a watertight seal. Failure of this *localization* or *walling-off* occurs when there is continuous contamination or the original contamination is massive, resulting in diffuse peritonitis.

Chemical reaction from spillage of digestive enzymes occurs when stomach, pancreas, or upper small bowel are origin of leak. Lower small bowel and colonic spillage result in peritoneal inflammation from the entry of bacterial content into the peritoneal cavity.

SIGNS AND SYMPTOMS

1. Abdominal pain, tenderness: Location of pain and tenderness depends on the underlying cause and whether the inflammation is localized or generalized. In localized peritonitis, such as seen in uncomplicated appendicitis or

diverticulitis, the physical findings are limited to the area of inflammation. Widespread peritoneal inflammation results in generalized peritonitis with diffuse abdominal tenderness.

2. History of low-grade fever, may have intermittent spikes.
3. Chills, nausea, vomiting.
4. Diarrhea, urinary urgency may be present with pelvic abscess.
5. Subphrenic abscess may present with dyspnea, referred shoulder pain.
6. History of possible cause of contamination and/or cause of infection of the peritoneum should be assessed.
7. Patients who are immunosuppressed, chronically ill, older age, or immediately postoperative may present with mild to moderate symptoms.

PHYSICAL FINDINGS

1. Abdominal pain, rigidity and fever initially, followed by abdominal distention and paralytic ileus, are essentials of diagnosis. Abdominal pain associated with movement, including respirations.
2. Malaise, prostration, vomiting are seen in proportion to disease severity.
3. Abdominal palpation reveals diffuse or localized tenderness with peritoneal signs (guarding, rigidity, rebound tenderness). Tenderness to light percussion over inflamed peritoneum is characteristic.
4. Muscles overlying inflamed areas usually become spastic; marked rigidity may be present with generalized peritonitis.
5. Diminished to absent peristalsis and progressive abdominal distention are cardinal signs (occur when inflammation markedly inhibits intestinal motility).
6. Mass indicative of abscess, phlegmon, or ileus may be present.
7. Signs of recent operative event may be present.
8. Bibasilar atelectasis may be heard with auscultation, especially with subphrenic abscess.
9. Patient may be found lying with knees flexed.
10. Hypotension, tachycardia, tachypnea; may progress to septic shock without rapid intervention.

DIFFERENTIAL DIAGNOSIS

Differential diagnosis is extensive and includes all causes of acute abdomen, peritonitis, and systemic sepsis.

DIAGNOSTIC TESTS/FINDINGS

1. CBC with differential will demonstrate leukocytosis, especially polymorphonuclear cells. Presence of leukopenia is ominous predictor.
2. Serum electrolytes may reflect large fluid shifts.
3. Liver and kidney function tests are indicated to determine baseline and/or degree of organ involvement.
4. Arterial blood gases should be drawn to provide baseline data and to determine oxygen utilization.
5. Culture of urine, blood, and sputum should be done prior to starting any empiric antibiotics. If peritoneal fluid is available, cultures should be done on this as well.

6. Chest x-ray will show presence of pneumonia, free air, pleural effusion, bibasilar atelectasis (which may be indicative of inflammatory process).
7. Abdominal series may show obstruction or ileus, organ displacement, air within the bowel wall, or free air under the diaphragm.
8. Ultrasound is useful to diagnose acute cholecystitis, pancreatitis, fluid collections, abscesses. This study may be limited by overlying bowel, skin incisions, etc.; however, it is inexpensive and does not expose the patient to radiation.
9. CT scan is more specific (95–100% sensitivity); however, is expensive and does expose patient to ionizing radiation. May be used for guidance for percutaneous drainage of abscess.
10. Radionuclide scan may be used as adjunct to CT scan for isolating occult intra-abdominal abscess.

MANAGEMENT/TREATMENT

1. Fluid resuscitation is necessary because of massive sequestering of fluid in the peritoneal or retroperitoneal spaces and in the bowel. Intravenous fluid should be replaced with solution appropriate to patient situation and amount of replacement required. Normal saline, lactated Ringer's, or normal saline with 5% dextrose may be utilized. Colloids may be utilized if clinically indicated.
2. Fluid status must be monitored with daily weights, Foley catheter, hemodynamic measurements. Central venous pressure or Swan-Ganz catheter may be utilized if clinically indicated.
3. Antibiotic intervention should be initiated as soon as appropriate cultures are obtained. Standard treatment for intra-abdominal pathogens varies with severity, etiology, and provider preference. Accepted therapies are listed below.
   A. For mild to moderate peritonitis:
      1) Second-generation cephalosporin such as cefuroxime (Ceftin) 750–1500 mg IV q8h
         or
      2) Third-generation penicillin such as ampicillin/sulbactam (Unasyn) 1–2 gm IV q6h
   B. For severe or tertiary peritonitis:
      1) Extended-spectrum penicillin such as piperacillin tazobactam (Zosyn) 3.375 gm IV q6h
         or
      2) Aminoglycoside such as gentamicin (Garamycin) 1 mg/kg q8h with additional coverage for anaerobic bacteria, such as metronidazole (Flagyl) 500 mg q6h PO or IV
      3) A third-generation cephalosporin such as ceftazidime (Fortaz) 1–2 gm IV q8h may be combined with antiaerobic coverage for patients with impaired renal function.
4. Surgical consult is *mandatory* for any patient with peritonitis because definitive treatment relies on operative removal of the primary septic focus with débridement of any necrotic tissue that may be involved. Percutaneous drainage may be possible for well-localized or retroperitoneal abscesses.
5. Pain management should be accomplished by intravenous analgesia. Morphine sulfate 1–10 mg qh IV via patient-controlled analgesia (PCA) pump is most commonly utilized.

6. Ventilatory support should be based on clinical status of patient and may be via supplemental oxygen. Intubation tray should be readily available for use should the situation demand mechanical ventilatory support.

7. Postoperative care should be based on clinical situation, with attention being paid to nutrition, fluid balance, and cardiorespiratory function.

PATIENT EDUCATION

1. Teach patient/family disease course and expected outcome.

2. Because patient may be critically ill, family must be included in any and all teaching/discussions and decisions.

3. Preoperative teaching should include procedure, time factors, postoperative expectations regarding pain, level of consciousness, activity.

4. Medication teaching should include purpose, dosage, side effects, toxic effects, and length of time drug will be required.

Review Questions

10.81. Peritonitis is defined as the inflammation of the endothelial lining of the abdominal cavity. The most significant and most common physiologic response is:

A. Fluid sequestration in the bowel walls, retroperitoneal and peritoneal spaces resulting in intravascular fluid depletion

B. Decrease in the glomerular filtration rate resulting in hyperproteinemia and acute tubular necrosis

C. Pulmonary insufficiency caused by increase in vascular permeability followed by hemoglobin leakage into the peritoneal space; this results in an increase in physiologic oxygen demand created by the septic event, which overwhelms the oxygen supply available, leading to tissue hypoxia.

D. All of the above

10.82. A 35-year-old male was admitted to the surgical intensive care unit from the emergency department, S/P gunshot wound to the abdomen. CT scan showed no perforation of the abdominal viscera. Vital signs were stable. The patient was awake, alert, and oriented. Decision was made that no surgical intervention was needed at this time. Fluid management was initiated in the ER and patient appeared euvolemic. Pain management was successfully accomplished with morphine PCA. Additional interventions for this patient should include:

A. Nasogastric tube for gastric decompression and to prevent aspiration

B. Glucocorticoids to decrease the peritoneal inflammatory response, thereby decreasing the likelihood of peritonitis

C. Unasyn 2 gm q6h for 24 hours

D. Serial hemoglobins to prospectively follow any occult bleeding that may be occurring as a result of unknown injuries from bullet trajectory

10.83. Blood work drawn on hospital day 3 reveals leukocytosis with a WBC of 17.7. Patient's temperature is 38.5°C (101°F). Physical exam reveals decreased breath sounds at bases bilaterally, abdominal tenderness with some guarding, especially at wound site. Bowel sounds are present. Chest x-ray shows bibasilar atelectasis. The most likely reason for the leukocytosis and fever is:

A. Dehydration with hemoconcentration resulting from the massive fluid shifts involved in peritoneal injury
B. Pneumonia
C. Peritonitis
D. B and C

10.84. A 24-year-old female with a 3-day history of abdominal pain was admitted for observation. The patient states that she was seen in an ER of another facility 2 days ago with abdominal pain, nausea, diarrhea; she was diagnosed with gastroenteritis and sent home with a prescription for Compazine. She states the pain continued for about 12 hours, then she felt much better. At this time she ate a cheeseburger with fries and a milkshake. About 5 hours ago she began to have chills and fever with abdominal pain that increased in intensity. She now presents with a very tender abdomen, temperature of 39°C, nausea, vomiting. Physical examination reveals rigid abdomen, positive rebound, positive psoas. CBC shows WBC of 23.5. The most likely diagnosis is:

A. Peritonitis from ruptured appendix
B. Acute cholecystitis that relapsed as a result of ingestion of meal that was very high in fat
C. Pelvic inflammatory disease
D. Relapse of gastroenteritis, which should be supported with fluid resuscitation

---

Answers and Rationales

10.81 **A** The inflammatory response that occurs in the peritoneum as a result of peritonitis is similar to a burn in the degree of fluid shifts that occur.

10.82 **C** Coverage for this patient should include antibiotic appropriate for intra-abdominal pathogens as well as pathogen introduced from bullet entry.

10.83 **D** Peritonitis in trauma patients without visceral penetration may be due to externally introduced pathogen and is most likely to occur on hospital day 3. Bibasilar atelectasis may be from hypoventilation resulting from pain or immobility, or from exudate from intra-abdominal process. More definitive study is called for.

10.84 **A** The most likely diagnosis is peritonitis from ruptured appendix.

References

Bleiweis, M., & Klein, S. (1996). Surgical infections. In F. Bongard & D. Sue (eds.). *Current Medical Diagnosis and Treatment*. Stamford, CT: Appleton & Lange, pp. 156–169.

Bohnen, J.M. (1996). Duration of antibiotic treatment in surgical infections of the abdomen: Postoperative peritonitis. *Eur J Surg Suppl 576*, 50–52.

Christou, N.V., Turgeon, P., Wassef, R., et al. (1996). Management of intra-abdominal infections: The case for intraoperative cultures and comprehensive broad-spectrum antibiotic coverage. The Canadian Intra-abdominal Infection Study Group. *Arch Surg 131*, 1193–1201.

Graninger, W., Zedtwitz-Liebenstein, K., Laferl H., et al. (1996). Quinolones in gastrointestinal infections. *Chemotherapy 42* (Suppl. 1), 43–53.

Ohmann, C., & Hau, T. (1997). Prognostic indices in peritonitis. *Hepatogastroenterology 44*, 937–946.

Quinn, J.P. (1997). Rational antibiotic therapy for intra-abdominal infections. *Lancet 349*, 517–518.

CHAPTER 11

Infections and Common Problems in Acute Care

Debra L. Tribett, RN, MS, CS, LNP
Kim Wilkins, MS, RD, CNSD
Maryann T. Hardesty, RN, MSN, ANP
Joan E. Davies, RN, MSN, NP
Barbara M. Bates-Jensen, RN, MN, CETN
Kathy Stull Rodgers, RN, MSN, CCRN, CEN

Fever

DEFINITION

Fever is an elevation in core body temperature resulting from an elevation in the set point of hypothalamic thermal regulators. Normal circadian temperature rhythm causes daily variations with a morning low point and a high point in the late afternoon to early evening. Normal temperature variance is about 0.6°C (1.0°F). This pattern still can be observed during fever.

A temperature of >38.3°C (101.0°F) on several occasions and lack of a specific diagnosis after 3 days of hospital investigation or three outpatient visits is the updated definition of the classic diagnosis of fever of unknown origin (FUO). Fever that is not present upon admission but develops after 48 hours in the hospital is a considered a nosocomial fever.

In the acute or critically ill patient, a new-onset core temperature of ≥38.3°C (101.0°F) should prompt a thoughtful investigation of its etiology. Temperatures of >38.9°C (102°F) in the intensive care unit (ICU) patient are more likely infectious in origin, whereas temperature less than this value more likely is attributable to noninfectious causes.

Hyperthermia is an elevated core body temperature when the hypothalamic set point is at normothermic levels. It is a result of inhibited or inadequate heat loss mechanisms, as in heat stroke. In susceptible individuals, malignant hyperthermia can also be caused by anesthetic agents that produce a rapid uncoupling of oxidative phosphorylation. Body temperature >41°C (>105.8°F) is rarely physiologically mediated and suggests hyperthermia.

There is no way to rapidly differentiate fever from hyperthermia. Patient history, clinical situation, and physical exam must be considered when making the diagnosis.

ETIOLOGY/INCIDENCE

1. Fevers are induced by endogenous or exogenous pyrogens.
2. Endogenous pyrogens or pyrogenic cytokines are produced by the host in response to injury, inflammation, infection, or antigenic challenge. Examples include:
   A. Interleukin-1
   B. Interferons (α, β, γ)
   C. Tumor necrosis factor
   D. Interleukin-6
   E. Interleukin-11
   F. Ciliary neurotropic factor
   G. Leukemia inhibitory factor
3. Exogenous pyrogens are microbial products, toxins, and the microbes themselves. Examples include:
   A. Endotoxin from the walls of gram-negative bacteria
   B. Enterotoxins from gram-positive bacteria (*Staphylococcus aureus*, groups A and B streptococcus)
4. In adults, 70% of patients have fever as a result of:
   A. Infections (localized or systemic); the most common cause of fever
   B. Malignancy
      1) Hodgkin's disease
      2) Non-Hodgkin's lymphoma
      3) Leukemia
      4) Renal cell carcinoma
      5) Hepatoma
      6) Atrial myxomas
   C. Autoimmune disorders
5. Other noninfectious causes of fever in adults:
   A. Central nervous system (CNS)
      1) Bleeding
      2) Seizure
   B. Cardiovascular/pulmonary
      1) Myocardial infarction
      2) Dressler's syndrome
      3) Pulmonary infarction/embolism
      4) Pericarditis
      5) Myocarditis
      6) Atelectasis
   C. Metabolic
      1) Substance withdrawal
      2) Fabry's disease
      3) Hyperthyroidism
      4) Adrenal insufficiency
      5) Heat stroke
   D. Hematologic
      1) Deep vein thrombosis
      2) Bleeding
      3) Sickle cell disease
   E. Gastrointestinal
      1) Pancreatitis
      2) Cholecystitis

      3) Hepatitis (infectious, noninfectious)

      4) Inflammatory bowel disease

      5) Ischemic colitis

  F. Miscellaneous

      1) Drug fever

      2) Sarcoidosis

      3) Familial Mediterranean fever

      4) Burns

      5) Invasive procedures (e.g., bronchoscopy)

      6) Factitious fever

6. It is important to remember the following in evaluation of fever.

  A. Fever does not always indicate an infection is present.

  B. Infection does not always present with a fever, particularly in the elderly patient.

  C. The degree of elevation of the fever does not necessarily correlate with the severity of an infectious process.

  D. The longer the fever lasts, the less likely it is due to infection.

7. Specific patient populations have different etiologies for cause of fever:

  A. Postoperative fever can be characterized by the four Ws:

      1) Wind: Pulmonary origin, likely atelectasis within 3 postoperative days

      2) Water: Urinary tract, likely resulting from urinary catheterization

      3) Wound: Infection of the surgical field if within the first 4 postoperative days, incisional or deeper tissues after 4 days

      4) Walk: Deep vein thrombosis, suppurative phlebitis, or pulmonary emboli

  B. Patients in the ICU may have one or more simultaneous causes of fever. Infections are the most common cause of fever in this patient population; however, many other noninfectious etiologies must be considered when evaluating a new febrile episode (see Table 11–1).

8. The most common cause of fever in the ICU patient is infection. Infection is often nosocomial in origin. The most common types and sites of nosocomial infection in the ICU patient are:

  A. Catheter-related urinary tract infections.

  B. Pneumonia associated with intubation and mechanical ventilation.

  C. Postoperative surgical wound and intra-abdominal infections.

  D. Bacteremia from intravascular devices. Percutaneously placed non-cuffed central venous catheters are most often associated with bacteremia. Infection rates are highest when these catheters are used for hemodialysis or are multilumen all-purpose central lines. Centrally placed pulmonary artery catheters are associated with lower rates of infection.

  E. Antibiotic-associated diarrhea caused by *Clostridium difficile*.

  F. Sinusitis in nasally intubated patients.

SIGNS AND SYMPTOMS

1. Patients may present with fever and localizing symptoms such as:

  A. Head, ears, eyes, nose, and throat (HEENT)

      1) Discharge from eyes, ears, nose

      2) Pain—temporal, ear, periorbital, maxillary, swallowing, pharynx

      3) Lesions of face, mouth, mucosa

      4) Loss of hearing

TABLE 11–1.   Causes of Fever in the ICU Patient

System	Infectious	Noninfectious
Central nervous	Meningitis Encephalitis	Infarction Hemorrhage Seizures
Cardiovascular	Endocarditis Catheter-associated bacteremia Local catheter thrombophlebitis Pacemaker infection	Myocardial infarction Dressler's syndrome Postpericardiotomy syndrome Postperfusion syndrome Deep vein thrombosis

Upper/lower
  respiratory
	Pneumonia
	Empyema
	Tracheobronchitis
	Sinusitis
	Otitis media
	Parotitis
	Pharyngitis
		Atelectasis
		Chemical pneumonitis
		Pulmonary infarction/emboli
		ARDS (fibroproliferative
		  stage)

Gastrointestinal	Intra-abdominal abscess Cholecystitis/choleangitis Peritonitis Diverticulitis Antibiotic-associated colitis	Gastrointestinal hemorrhage Acalculus cholecystitis Nonviral hepatitis Pancreatitis Inflammatory bowel disease Ischemic colitis
Renal	Urinary tract infection Pyelonephritis	
Musculoskeletal	Osteomyelitis Septic arthritis	Gout/pseudogout
Skin/soft tissue	Cellulitis Wound infection Decubitus ulcer	Hematoma Intramuscular injections Burns
Endocrine/ metabolic		Adrenal insufficiency Hyperthyroidism/thyroiditis Substance withdrawal
Hematologic/ immunologic	Bacteremia	Neoplasm/metastasis Transfusion reaction Collagen vascular disease Vasculitis Graft-versus-host reaction
Miscellaneous		Drug fever Postprocedure IV contrast reaction

ARDS, acute respiratory distress syndrome.

    B. CNS
        1) Headache
        2) Photophobia
        3) Stiff neck
        4) Confusion
        5) Lethargy
    C. Respiratory
        1) Cough—productive or nonproductive
        2) Dyspnea
        3) Pleuritic chest pain

      4) Sputum production
      5) Hemoptysis
  D. Cardiovascular: Chest pain characteristic of pericarditis
  E. Gastrointestinal
      1) Nausea
      2) Vomiting
      3) Diarrhea
      4) Abdominal pain
  F. Genitourinary
      1) Frequency
      2) Urgency
      3) Hesitancy
      4) Dysuria
      5) Flank pain
      6) Hematuria
      7) Discharge from penis/vagina
      8) Lesions on genitalia
  G. Skin/hair/nails
      1) Rash
         a. Macular/papular
         b. Vesicular/bullous
         c. Petechial/purpuric
      2) Jaundice
      3) Hair loss
      4) Redness, swelling, pain in soft tissues
      5) Open lesions or wounds
  H. Musculoskeletal
      1) Low back pain referred to lower extremities
      2) Joint pain, swelling, redness
2. Patients may present with fever and secondary symptoms:
  A. Chills
  B. Sweats
  C. Malaise
  D. Myalgias
  E. Weight loss
  F. Swollen, painful glands

HISTORY

1. Documentation of actual temperature elevation is important to rule out factitious fever.
2. A single temperature spike that returns to normal without treatment is usually not a clinically significant event. Transient bacteremia from a procedure can cause an isolated spike in temperature.
3. The pattern of fever has little significance in the diagnosis of prolonged fever. There are two diseases in which the pattern of fever helps make the diagnosis. These exceptions are:
  A. Malaria has a synchronized paroxysmal pattern.
      1) Tertian: Fever every other day
      2) Quartan: Fever on day 1, day 4, etc.
  B. Cyclic neutropenia has a 21-day cyclic pattern of fever that corresponds with neutropenia.

4. Patients with acute-onset fever and localizing symptoms are generally easier to diagnose that those with chronic febrile illness. A complete history with review of systems is an essential part of making the diagnosis for the etiology of fever.

5. Patients or their family members should be questioned to determine the following information:
   A. Recent travel, especially outside the United States, to determine exposure to infections endemic to specific geographic areas (e.g., malaria, hemorrhagic fevers)
   B. Exposure to domestic or wild animals
   C. Bites from humans, animals, mosquitoes, or ticks
   D. Intravenous drug use with possible exposure to bacterial infections, human immunodeficiency virus (HIV), hepatitis B and/or C
   E. Alcoholism (potential risk for withdrawal, tuberculosis [TB], aspiration pneumonia)
   F. Sexual history, to determine exposure to sexually transmitted infections
   G. Ethnic group, to determine risk factors for certain malignancies or autoimmune disorders
   H. Occupation, to assess biohazard exposure or blood/body fluid exposure
   I. Current medications, examples of medications commonly associated with fever:
      1) Cardiovascular—α-methyldopa, quinidine, procainamide, hydralazine
      2) Antimicrobials—β-lactam agents, trimethoprim-sulfamethoxazole, vancomycin, isoniazid, amphotericin B
      3) CNS—carbamazapine, diphenylhydantoin
      4) Immune-modulating agents/colony-stimulating factors
   J. Dietary habits, to identify ingestion of unpasteurized dairy products, raw meats or seafood, or well water
   K. Previous transfusion of blood or blood products
   L. Recent surgery or invasive procedure, such as bronchoscopy
   M. Presence of prosthetic device (joint, graft, valve, shunt, pacemaker, defibrillator)
   N. Recent trauma
   O. Risk for immunocompromise, which increases risk for opportunistic infections or malignancies:
      1) Transplant recipient
      2) Recent chemotherapy/radiation therapy
      3) Chronic steroid usage
      4) HIV disease
      5) Inherited immunodeficiency
      6) Chronic illness, such as diabetes, renal failure, liver disease
      7) Splenectomy
   P. History of immunizations

PHYSICAL FINDINGS

A thorough physical exam may identify subtle findings. All physical findings are important to determine the etiology of fever. Physical exam may need to be repeated frequently during the evaluation of fever.
   1. Vital signs
      A. Tachycardia

       1) Appropriate heart rate for febrile response is 10 bpm for every degree over 101°F added to 100.

       2) Relative bradycardia (<100) in the absence of β-blockers or intrinsic conduction defects, is associated with drug hypersensitivity reactions and certain infections (typhoid, rickettsial infections)

  B. Hypotension

  C. Pulsus paradoxus

  D. Tachypnea

2. HEENT

  A. Erythema, external ear canal

  B. Bulging tympanic membrane/exudate/erythema

  C. Red, swollen, nasal mucosa

  D. Sinuses tender to palpation

  E. Oral/labial ulcers/lesions

  F. Koplik's spots: Cluster of tiny bluish white papules with an erythematous areola on buccal mucosa opposite premolar teeth seen in patients with measles

  G. Tonsils swollen, erythematous, with exudate present

  H. Displaced uvula with redness, swelling, bulging of tonsil/pillar

  I. Goiter

  J. Thyroid tender to palpation

  K. Temporal tenderness

  L. Alopecia

  M. Corneal ulceration

  N. Conjunctival lesions

  O. Funduscopic lesions

3. CNS

  A. Nuchal rigidity

  B. Mental status changes

  C. Focal neurologic abnormality

4. Respiratory

  A. Adventitious breath sounds (crackles, rhonchi, wheezes)

  B. Dullness to percussion

  C. Increased tactile fremitus

  D. Egophony

  E. Whispered pectoriloquy

  F. Pleural friction rub

5. Cardiovascular

  A. Friction rub

  B. Murmur

  C. Muffled heart sounds

6. Gastrointestinal

  A. Organomegaly

  B. Ascites

  C. Tenderness

  D. Rebound

  E. Guarding

7. Genitourinary

  A. Enlarged kidney

  B. Suprapubic tenderness

  C. Genital ulcers

  D. Cervical discharge

    E. Cervical motion tenderness

    F. Prostate tender, enlarged, or nodular

    G. Adnexa tender, painful to palpation

    H. Perirectal tenderness, fluctuance

8. Skin/hair/nails

    A. Rash—macular, papular, vesicular, or bullous

    B. Petechiae/purpura

    C. Jaundice

    D. Redness, induration, tenderness of soft tissue

    E. Janeway lesions: Small erythematous or hemorrhagic, nonpainful macules or nodules of palms or soles associated with bacterial endocarditis

    F. Osler's nodes

    G. Subungual splinter hemorrhages linear in middle of nail bed

    H. Ulcers

9. Lymph: Localized or generalized lymphadenopathy

10. Musculoskeletal

    A. Costovertebral angle tenderness

    B. Spinal tenderness

    C. Joints red, warm, tender, or deformed

DIFFERENTIAL DIAGNOSIS

1. Seventy percent of fever in adults can be attributed to:

    A. Infection

    B. Neoplasm

        1) Hodgkin's disease

        2) Non-Hodgkin's lymphoma

        3) Leukemia

        4) Renal cell carcinoma

        5) Hepatoma

        6) Atrial myxoma

    C. Autoimmune diseases

        1) Systemic lupus erythematus (SLE)

        2) Rheumatoid arthritis

        3) Vasculitis

        4) Graft-versus-host reaction

        5) Gout

        6) Polymyalgia rheumatica

        7) Polyarteritis rheumatica

        8) Erythema multiforme

2. Other causes, particularly in the ICU patient population, include:

    A. Infection of the following types:

        1) Catheter-related urinary tract

        2) Pneumonia associated with intubation and mechanical ventilation

        3) Postoperative surgical wound and intra-abdominal abscess

        4) Bacteremia from intravascular devices

        5) Antibiotic-associated diarrhea

        6) Sinusitis in nasally intubated patients

    B. Noninfectious

        1) Myocardial infarction

        2) Dressler's syndrome

        3) Deep vein thrombosis

      4) Posterior fossa syndrome
      5) CNS hemorrhage
      6) Seizures
      7) Pulmonary emboli/infarction
      8) Gastrointestinal (GI) hemorrhage
      9) Acalculous cholecystitis
    10) Pancreatitis
    11) Inflammatory bowel disease
    12) Ischemic colitis
    13) Gout
    14) Burns
    15) Alcohol/drug withdrawal
    16) Drug reaction
    17) Transfusion reaction
    18) Adrenal insufficiency
    19) Hyperthyroidism/thyroiditis
3. Hyperthermia
  A. Vigorous exercise
  B. Heat stroke
  C. Malignant hyperthermia
  D. Neuroleptic malignant syndrome
4. Drug reaction
5. Factitious or self-induced fever

DIAGNOSTIC TESTS/FINDINGS

The patient's history, signs, and symptoms lead to a clinical impression that guides the use of diagnostic tests. Patients without focal signs and symptoms provide a challenge. Those in the ICU require additional evaluation based on their high risk for the development of infection and the nature of the therapies utilized in their care.

Laboratory Testing

1. Complete blood count with differential
  A. Elevated white blood cell count (WBC): >15,000 cells/mm^3 often seen with bacterial infection: ≥25,000–30,000 cells/mm^3 seen with TB, empyema, abscess, leukemia, other malignancy.
  B. Elevated WBC with eosinophilia may be present in drug reaction.
  C. Leukopenia in viral disease.
  D. Atypical lymphocytes in Epstein-Barr virus or cytomegalovirus (CMV) mononucleosis or other viral infection.
  E. WBC <2,500 cells/mm^3 in acutely ill patient is an ominous sign and may indicate severe bacterial sepsis.
  F. Absolute granulocyte count ≤500 cells/mm^3 in immunocompromised patient is associated with bacteremias or fungal infection.
  G. Low hemoglobin and hematocrit are seen in chronic illness.
  H. Low platelet counts in sepsis-associated disseminated intravascular coagulation, alcoholism, drug reaction.
  I. Thrombocytosis in empyemas, abscesses, malignancies.
2. Urinalysis
  A. Urinalysis dipstick positive for leukocyte esterase or nitrite should prompt a microscopic analysis for pyuria (WBC >5/hpf).

B. Dipstick will give a positive result for >5 red blood cells (RBC)/hpf detected on microscopic analysis but will also be positive for free hemoglobin or myoglobin. Hematuria with WBC and bacteria suggests a urinary tract infection. Hematuria may be indicative of malignancy (prostate, bladder, kidney). Other systemic diseases causing glomerulonephritis, such as SLE or subacute bacterial endocarditis (SBE), are associated with hematuria. Positive dipstick should be confirmed by microscopic analysis.

C. Proteinuria by dipstick is seen with protein levels of approximately 100 μg/mL at trace levels. Normal urinary excretion is <150 mg/day. Systemic diseases causing proteinuria can include SLE, SBE, HIV disease, and malignancy such as adenocarcinoma or lymphoma.

3. Cultures: Growth of organisms from a presumably sterile site is almost always significant.

A. Urinalysis microscopic analysis for pyuria (WBC >5/hpf) should prompt urine culture. Results of $\geq 10^5$ cfu/mL are associated with urinary tract infection in a symptomatic female, $\geq 10^3$ cfu/mL in a symptomatic male, or $\geq 10^2$ cfu/mL in a catheterized patient are diagnostic for bacteriuria.

B. Blood cultures obtained at the onset of fever:

1) Obtain at least 10 to 15 mL of blood from one peripheral site and divide into aerobic and anaerobic media. This is defined as one blood culture. A second sample of 10 to 15 mL should be obtained 10 minutes after the first from a second venipuncture site and be divided into aerobic and anaerobic media.

2) If the patient has poor peripheral vasculature, draw one set of cultures peripherally and one set simultaneously from the most recently inserted catheter.

3) More than two sets of cultures in a 24-hour period are unnecessary.

C. For suspected catheter-related cause of fever:

1) Gram's stain and culture expressed purulent drainage from catheter site.

2) Obtain paired quantitative blood cultures form a peripheral site and from the suspected catheter (as described above).

3) Removal of suspected catheter and culture of tip. For pulmonary artery (PA) catheters, both the introducer and PA tip should be cultured.

D. Sputum

1) Gram's stain

2) Culture and sensitivity

3) Acid-fast bacilli smear and culture

4) Tests for *Legionella* (culture, direct fluorescent antibody test)

E. Stool cultures should be obtained in specific patient populations.

1) Diarrhea upon admission from the community should prompt evaluation for enteric pathogens, ova and parasites, fecal leukocytes, occult blood.

2) Patients with diarrhea and a recent travel history to developing countries need extensive evaluation directed toward the likely pathogens that occur in their area of travel.

3) HIV-positive patients need stool analysis directed toward identification of cryptosporidium, CMV, *Mycobacterium avium-intracellulare* complex (MAC), fecal leukocytes, enteric pathogens, and *C. difficile*.

4) Hospitalized ICU patient with fever and (more than two diarrhea

stools/day needs evaluation for *C. difficile* toxin by enzyme immuno-assay.) Send one sample per day and, if the first specimen is negative, up to two additional specimens.

    5) Patients with a recent history of antibiotic therapy with persisting diarrhea should be evaluated for *C. difficile*.

  F. Oral/lesion/throat cultures

    1) Rapid strep antigen

    2) Bacterial

    3) Viral culture for suspected herpes lesions

  G. Pelvic examination with endocervical cultures for *Chlamydia* and gonor-rhea. Vaginal secretions for Gram's stain, KOH, and wet mount. Culture of external lesions for herpes.

4. Acute-phase reactants may be elevated.

  A. Fibrinogen

  B. Haptoglobin

  C. C-reactive protein

5. Erythrocyte sedimentation rate is usually elevated beyond normal range with infections, inflammatory disease, or malignancy. The trend of results can be followed to detect improvement (return toward normal) or worsening (continued elevation) in patient's condition, but it is not a disease-specific test. The normal/abnormal value ranges are dependent on the laboratory method of test used.

6. Antibody titers to specific organisms can be diagnostic in many infectious diseases. The presence of immunoglobulin M (IgM) is indicative of a current/recent infection. IgG levels will rise later in the infectious process and persist to show past exposure to an organism.

7. Based on history, risk factors, and presenting signs and symptoms, HIV testing with enzyme-linked immunosorbant assay (ELISA) and confirmed positive reaction with Western blot.

8. Immunologic testing for autoantibodies to detect autoimmune diseases:

  A. Rheumatoid factor

  B. Antinuclear antibodies (ANA)

  C. Anti-Smith (Anti-Sm)-Highly diagnostic for SLE

  D. Antineutrophil cytoplasmic antibody: associated with Wegener's granu-lomatosis

  E. Anti-SS-A and Anti-SS-B: May be produced in Sjögren's syndrome

9. Arterial blood gases in suspected pneumonia patient.

Diagnostic Testing

1. Chest x-ray to detect infiltrates, consolidation, pleural effusion, atelectasis, tumor, cavitary lesions.

2. Upper GI series with small bowel follow-through and barium enema in patient with FUO.

3. Radionuclide scanning can detect:

  A. Abscesses

  B. Many neoplastic diseases, such as bone tumors, lymphoma

  C. Osteomyelitis

4. Computed tomography (CT) scan can detect:

  A. Intra-abdominal abscess

  B. Lymph nodes in retroperitoneal, retrosternal, and mesentary

   C. Defects in spleen, liver, kidney, adrenals, pancreas, heart, pelvis
   D. Preferred to detect sinusitis in ICU patients
5. Magnetic resonance imaging (MRI) is usually superior to CT in identifying causes of FUO in nervous system.
6. Ultrasound is the initial choice for evaluation of the pelvis, kidneys, biliary tree, and pancreas.
7. Echocardiogram is useful to detect vegetation of heart valves.

Invasive Procedures

The ACNP may refer the patient for invasive procedures. Some of these procedures may be performed by the ACNP with appropriate training and in accordance with state nurse practice acts.

1. Biopsy of tissue to obtain culture and histologic specimens of a variety of tissues may be necessary based on results of other tests. This may include liver, bone marrow, skin, lymph node, kidney, muscle, nerve, or intestine.
2. Bronchoscopy, laparoscopy, mediastinoscopy, endoscopy, or colonoscopy for direct inspection and tissue sampling.
3. Lumbar puncture for patients with fever, headache, CNS symptoms with analysis of cerebrospinal fluid (CSF) for:
   A. Opening pressure (normal is 50–180 mm H_2O in the lateral decubitus position)
   B. Cell count with differential:
      1) Normal WBC 0–5/μL. An elevated number is termed pleocytosis and results from inflammatory process, hemorrhage, neoplasm, or trauma. A predominance of neutrophils or mononuclear cells in association with pleocytosis helps to identify types of infection, malignancy, or hemorrhage.
      2) Normal RBC count is 0. The presence of red cells can be indicative of a traumatic tap or hemorrhage.
   C. Chloride
   D. Glucose
   E. Total protein
   F. Culture and sensitivity
   G. India ink or cryptococcal antigen
   H. Venereal Disease Research Laboratory (VDRL) test
4. Thoracentesis if pleural effusion is present sent for:
   A. WBC with differential
   B. Lactate dehydrogenase (LDH)
   C. pH
   D. Protein
   E. Glucose
   F. Gram stain
   G. Acid fast bacili stain
   H. Culture
5. Skin testing Purified protein derivative (PPD) skin test controls (e.g., mumps, *Candida*) to determine:
   A. Exposure to TB
   B. Anergy associated with malignancy, HIV disease, or depressed immunologic response secondary to poor nutritional status

MANAGEMENT/TREATMENT

1. Symptomatic
   A. Fever increases the demand for oxygen and can aggravate pre-existing cardiac or pulmonary insufficiency. Oxygen consumption is increased by 13% for every 1°C C temperature rises above 37°C.
   B. Use of antipyretics should be considered in patients who have history of cardiac or pulmonary disease and for those who have limited metabolic reserves.
   C. Choices of antipyretics include:
      1) Acetaminophen 650 mg oral or rectal suppository every 4 hours
      2) Nonsteroidal anti-inflammatory agents (e.g., naproxen 275, 375, or 500 mg orally every 12 hours)
      3) Aspirin 650 mg orally every 4 hours
      4) Corticosteroids (e.g., prednisone 10 mg orally every 6 hours)
   D. Oxygen therapy
2. Supportive
   A. IV hydration to compensate for insensible losses if patient cannot take oral fluids.
   B. Nutritional support to prevent catabolism (see "Nutritional Management in Acute Care," below).
3. Definitive
   A. Antibiotic treatment of bacterial infections (see guidelines in next section of this chapter).
   B. For noninfectious etiologies of fever, treatment would be guided by the underlying disease and the patient condition. For example, chemotherapy, radiation, surgery, or a combination of therapies may be planned for a patient determined to have a malignancy.

PATIENT EDUCATION

1. Patients are often very apprehensive regarding their symptoms of recurring fevers. It is important to explain to them the possible cyclic nature of fever, the etiology of rigors, and concept of defervesence.
2. In preparation for discharge and home care, the correct method for taking temperature and reading a thermometer may need to be taught to the patient/significant other charged with monitoring temperature on an outpatient basis.
3. Discuss with the patient the level of temperature at which the patient/significant other should contact the health care provider.
4. Discuss the proper use of antipyretics, particularly if patient is on a suppressive rather than episodic regimen for temperature control.
5. Explain the purpose, procedure, and risks of any diagnostic tests required during the work-up of fever.
6. Once empiric or definitive therapy is instituted, explain the name, purpose, dose, side effects, method for administration, and length of therapy for drugs utilized. This may be inappropriate in the critically ill patient but useful to the significant other/family. When outpatient therapy is utilized, specific instructions of when and how to contact health care provider are necessary.
7. Discuss the signs and symptoms of improvement or worsening of condition to report to health team members.

8. Discuss results of diagnostic tests and their implications for confirming an etiology for fever.
9. Discuss with the patient and significant others options for treatment when a diagnosis for the etiology of fever is determined.
10. For patients who are at high risk for infection, provide recommendations for vaccines and prophylaxis against infection (see Chapter 13).

Review Questions

11.1 Which of the following is characteristic of fever of unknown origin?
   A. Fever with negative cultures
   B. Temperature of >101°F with a lack of diagnosis
   C. Temperature that develops 48 hours after admission
   D. Hyperthermia in the morning and afternoon, normothermia during the day

11.2 The proper technique for blood cultures is:
   A. One culture at the time of onset of fever
   B. One culture at the onset of fever and 12 hours later
   C. Two cultures—one at the onset of fever and one 10 minutes after the first
   D. Two cultures—one at the onset of fever and one 12 hours later

11.3 Which of the following statements related to fever is correct?
   A. Fever always accompanies an infection.
   B. Circadian effects will cause highest temperatures in the morning.
   C. The amount of temperature elevation correlates with the severity of infection.
   D. Fever does not always indicate an infection.

11.4 Which of the following patients should have a stool culture ordered?
   A. Patient with a new onset of diarrhea with a 2-day history of antibiotics
   B. A hospitalized ICU patient with fever and more than 2 diarrhea stools/day
   C. Patient with diarrhea and known colitis
   D. Patient with diarrhea recently returned from Europe

11.5 A patient presents with fever and has small, erythematous, nonpainful macules on the palms of the hands. Based on this presentation, which test would be most useful for a diagnosis?
   A. Sedimentation rate
   B. CBC
   C. Echocardiogram
   D. Antibody titers

Answers and Rationales

11.1   **B**   A temperature of >38.3°C (101°F) on several occasions and lack of a specific diagnosis after 3 days of hospital investigation or three outpatient visits is the updated definition of the classic diagnosis of fever of unknown origin.

11.2   **C**   The proper technique for drawing blood cultures is (1) obtain 10 to 15 mL of blood from one peripheral site, and (2) obtain a second sample of 10 to 15 mL 10 minutes after the first from a second venipuncture site.

11.3   **D**   Many situations of inflammation or malignancy can cause fever as a symptom without infection. Patients may have hypothermia as a presentation of severe infection. Usual circadian rhythm causes highest temperatures in the evening.

11.4   **B**   Stool cultures should be obtained from people who present with diarrhea and recent travel to developing countries, a patient with a recent history of antibiotic therapy with persisting diarrhea, and any hospitalized ICU patient with fever and more than two diarrheal stools/day.

11.5   **C**   Janeway lesions—small, erythematous, nonpainful macules on the palms or soles—and fever are associated with bacterial endocarditis. An echocardiogram is the best test to determine vegetations on the heart valves.

References

Bartlett, J.G., & Mundy, L.M. (1995). Community acquired pneumonia. *N Engl J Med 333*, 1618–1624.

Cunha, B.A., & Shea, K.W. (1996). Fever in the intensive care unit. *Infect Dis Clin North Am 10*, 185–209.

Dinarello, C.A., & Wolf, S.M. (1995). Pathogenesis of fever and the acute phase response. In G.L. Mandell, J.E. Bennett, & R. Dolin (eds.). *Principles and Practice of Infectious Disease* (4th ed.). New York: Churchill Livingstone, pp. 530–536.

Gelfand, J.A., & Wolf, S.M. (1995). Fever of unknown origin. In G.L. Mandell, J.E. Bennett, & R. Dolin (eds.). *Principles and Practice of Infectious Diseases* (4th ed.). New York: Churchill Livingstone, pp. 536–547.

Irizarry, L. (1996). Fever. In R.H., Rubin, C., Voss, D.J., Derkin, et al. (eds.). *Medicine: A Primary Care Approach.* Philadelphia: W.B. Saunders Co., pp. 69–75.

Maki, D.G. (1995). Nosocomial infection in the intensive care unit. In J.E. Parillo & R.C. Bone (eds.). *Critical Care Medicine: Principles of Diagnosis and Management.* St. Louis: C.V. Mosby Co., pp. 893–954.

O'Grady, N.P., Barie, P.S., Bartlett, J., et al. (1998). Practice parameters for evaluating new fever in critically ill adult patients. *Crit Care Med 26*, 392–408.

Stapczynski, J.S. (1996). The febrile adult. In A.B. Wolfson & P.M. Paris (eds.). *Diagnostic Testing in Emergency Medicine.* Philadelphia: W.B. Saunders Co., pp. 112–128.

Use of Antibiotics for Hospital and Community Acquired Infections

DEFINITION

Traditionally, the environment to which the patient is exposed influences the type of microorganisms suspected in causing an infection. The source of an infection is generally defined as community acquired or hospital (nosocomial) acquired. However, in today's health care environment, the distinction between community and hospital acquired is less distinct. As the population changes, more elderly patients, patients with chronic illness, and immunocompromised patients are in the community. This broadens the spectrum of organisms that may be seen in community-acquired infections. With more outpatient surgery and shortened hospital stays, nosocomial etiologies for infection may not manifest themselves until the patient is back in the community. Home intravenous therapy is a common situation, adding intravenous device infections to the list of possible community-acquired infection. Nosocomial etiologies for infection vary from hospital to hospital or even between units in the same facility.

The term *antibiotic* has traditionally referred to a substance produced by a microorganism to suppress the growth of other microorganisms. The term *antimicrobial agent* is a broader term including both natural antibiotics and synthetic agents. Most agents used today are either synthetic or semisynthetic in origin.

1. Antimicrobial agents rely on host defenses to help in the elimination of pathogens and can be categorized as:
    A. Bactericidal: Have the ability to kill organisms
        1) Better choice of drug for patients with impaired host defense.
        2) Examples of types of infections requiring this type of drug include endocarditis, meningitis.
    B. Bacteriostatic: Have the ability to prevent organisms from growing
        1) Adequate for uncomplicated infection
        2) Examples—tetracycline, erythromycin
2. Antimicrobial agents may be used in three general modes.
    A. Therapeutic/definitive: A drug is prescribed to treat an established clinical infection where the identity of the infecting organism is known (i.e., an organism is identified by a culture).
    B. Prophylactic: A drug is prescribed to all members of a given population prior to an event to prevent the occurrence of clinical infection.
        1) Medical situations examples:
            a. Close contacts of patients with bacterial meningitis are given antibiotics.
            b. Prior to dental procedures, patients with abnormal or prosthetic valves are given antibiotics to prevent bacterial endocarditis.
            c. Patients with HIV are given antibiotics to prevent some opportunistic infections from occurring.
        2) Preoperatively or intraoperatively antibiotics are given:
            a. To prevent wound infections
            b. When contamination of the surgical site is probable
    C. Preemptive/empiric: Drug is administered to a group at highest risk of serious infection on the basis of either a laboratory marker or clinical epidemiologic characteristics that define a significant risk of serious clinical infection.
        1) Initial coverage with broad-spectrum agent that treats all the likely pathogens prior to defining the infecting organism(s).
            a. Single broad-spectrum agent
            b. Combination therapy
            c. Estimated 75% of bacterial infections receiving antibiotic therapy get initial empiric coverage
        2) Switch to definitive therapy as soon as microorganism is identified; however, it is estimated that pathologic organism may not be clearly identified in 50% of situations.

CONSIDERATIONS FOR CHOICE OF ANTIBIOTIC

1. Identity of the infecting organism
   A. Gram's stain of specimens (exudates, body fluids or tissues): A fast, simple, inexpensive method to identify bacteria and fungi.
      1) Gram-positive organisms stain dark blue.
      2) Gram-negative organisms stain red.
      3) The appearance of the organism (cocci, rod, bacilli) coupled with the results of staining can help to identify the type of organism prior to its growth in a culture.
      4) The presence of polymorphonuclear leukocytes may be detected in some specimens and aid in the diagnosis of infection (e.g., presence in a stool Gram's stain in a patient with diarrhea indicates possible bacterial infection).
   B. Culture of a specific microorganism.
      1) Obtain all specimens for cultures prior to antibiotic administration.
      2) Culture all likely sources of infection based on individual patient signs and symptoms.
   C. Use bacteriologic statistics by applying knowledge of the organism most likely to cause infection in a given clinical setting. The "best guess" of causative organism is based on the site of suspected infection. (See "Etiology/Incidence" in this section for site-specific information on common infecting organisms.)
2. Antimicrobial susceptibility of the infecting organism isolated from a culture
   A. Minimum inhibitory concentration (MIC): The lowest concentration of antimicrobial agent that prevents visible growth after an 18 to 24-hour incubation period.
   B. Minimum bacterial concentration (MBC): The lowest concentration of antimicrobial agent that totally suppresses growth after overnight incubation.
   C. Consider geographic differences in patterns of susceptibility.
      1) Community versus hospital.
      2) Emergence of resistant organisms.
      3) Refer to the institution antibiogram for patterns of occurrence and resistance.
   D. The laboratory report of sensitivities includes a listing of the antibiotics to which a cultured organism is susceptible and resistant. This report may also include daily antibiotic cost to assist the clinician in making both appropriate and cost-effective choices.
3. Host factors
   A. Allergy or a previous severe adverse reaction to an agent generally precludes its use. However, it is important to determine the nature of the reaction. Patients often use the term *allergy* to refer to a side effect of a medication that occurred during its use.
      1) Nausea, vomiting, or diarrhea after oral administration of a drug does not prevent its use.
      2) Anaphylaxis, Stevens-Johnson syndrome, or interstitial nephritis would preclude use of a drug.
      3) Desensitization to a drug (penicillin) may be accomplished under controlled circumstances when use of a specific agent is necessary to treat a specific infection.

B. Age
   1) Higher gastric pH in children <3 years and patients >60 years.
   2) Impaired renal excretion in neonates and elderly patients may require a dose reduction in some antibiotics.
   3) Sulfonamides may produce increased levels of unbound bilirubin by displacing it from albumin, predisposing neonates to kernicterus.
   4) Hypersensitivity is more common in elderly than in young patients because of likelihood of previous exposure and sensitization.
   5) Specific drug toxicities to developing tissues in children (tetracycline, quinolones) or to a fetus.
C. Genetic or metabolic abnormalities
   1) Glucose-6-phosphate dehydrogenase deficiency: Antimicrobial-induced hemolysis induced by drugs such as sulfonamides, pyrimethamine; more common in black males
   2) Diabetes
      a. Drug interactions with oral sulfonamides (especially the long-acting types)
      b. Impaired absorption of antibiotics administered by intramuscular route
D. Renal and hepatic function
   1) Renal excretion is the most important route of elimination for most antimicrobial drugs; therefore, dose adjustments must be made if renal function is impaired, particularly for aminoglycosides and vancomycin.
   2) Antimicrobial drugs primarily excreted or detoxified by the liver (erythromycin, clindamycin, chloramphenicol) should be used with caution in patients with impaired hepatic function.
E. Pregnancy
   1) All antimicrobials cross the placenta to some degree, thereby exposing the fetus to the adverse effects of drugs.
   2) Cephalosporins, ampicillin, erythromycin are unlikely to be teratogenic and are safe in pregnancy.
   3) Tetracycline negatively affects fetal dentition and can be toxic to the mother.
   4) Metronidazole, ticarcillin, rifampin, fluoroquinolones should be avoided in pregnancy to protect the developing fetus.
F. Nursing mother
   1) Under usual circumstances the concentration of antibiotics in breast milk is low but still may be high enough to cause significant adverse reactions in the nursing infant.
G. Site of infection
   1) Determines choice of agent and route by which drug is administered.
   2) Adequate dose of agent (ideally a concentration equal to or greater than the MIC of the infecting organism) must be delivered to the site.
   3) Penetration of drug into certain tissues of the body is difficult.
      a. Crossing blood-brain barrier
      b. Bone
      c. Cardiac valves
      d. Devitalized tissue
      e. Gallbladder
      f. Prostate

     4) Local factors influence activity of drug (even at therapeutic concentrations).
- a. Inactivation by purulent material (aminoglycosides, vancomycin)
- b. Hemoglobin binding of drug in hematoma formation (penicillins, tetracycline)
- c. Low oxygen tension (aminoglycosides)
- d. Low pH (aminogycosides, erythromycin, clindamycin)
- e. Presence of a foreign body (artificial joint, prosthetic heart valve, shunts)

     5) Route of administration.
- a. Oral preferred (peak serum level 1–2 hours postadministration)
- b. Parenteral recommended in seriously ill
  - i. Intramuscular (peak serum level 0.5–1 hour postinjection)
  - ii. Intravenous (peak serum level after a 20 to 30 min infusion occurs at the end of infusion)

H. Host defenses
1) Absence of white blood cells predisposes patient to bacterial infection.
2) Absolute neutrophil count of <500–1000 cells/mm^3 is a critical value.
3) Splenectomized patients are at high risk for infections with encapsulated bacteria (pneumococcal, meningococcal, or *Haemophilus* infections).
4) Bactericidal agents are necessary in patients with impaired host defenses.
5) Acquired immunodeficiency syndrome (AIDS) patient: Therapy is rarely curative, only suppressive because of impaired cellular immunity.

I. Disorders of the nervous system
1) Patient with seizure disorders maybe at increased risk for seizure with high-dose penicillin G.
2) Patient with renal insufficiency may develop neurotoxicity from penicillin and other β-lactam antibiotics.
3) Patients with myasthenia gravis or other neuromuscular problems may be at more risk for neuromuscular blocking effects of aminoglycosides.
4) Patients receiving neuromuscular blocking agents are susceptible to neuromuscular toxicity of aminoglycosides.

ETIOLOGY/INCIDENCE

A thorough history from the patient is essential when attempting to apply bacteriologic statistics to determine possible etiologies for infections. The suspected site of an infection and the usual microorganisms causing infection at that site are primary considerations when initiating antibiotic therapy.

    It is beyond the scope of this text to review all possible infections. Common organisms are listed for selected sites of infection that the ACNP may encounter when patients present to the hospital with an infection. In the intensive care unit, it is estimated that 75% of patients receive antimicrobial therapy for treatment of either a primary illness or a nosocomial infection.

1. Community-acquired infection
  A. Skin/skin structures
    1) *Staphylococcus aureus*
    2) Group A streptococcus

B. Vascular devices
1) *Staphylococcus aureus*
2) *Staphylococcus epidermidis*
C. Urinary tract: 85% caused by *Escherichia coli*
D. Meningitis
1) *Streptococcus pneumoniae* (pneumococcus)
2) *Neisseria meningitidis* (meningococcus)
3) *Listeria monocytogenes* (in older patients)
E. Pneumonia
1) Typical
   a. *Streptococcus pneumoniae*
   b. *Haemophilus influenzae*
   c. *Staphylococcus aureus*
   d. *Moraxella catarrhalis*
   e. Aerobic gram-negative bacilli
2) Atypical
   a. Viral
   b. *Mycoplasma pneumoniae*
   c. *Chlamydia pneumoniae*
   d. *Legionella*
F. Gastrointestinal
1) Gastroenteritis
   a. *Salmonella*
   b. *Shigella*
   c. *Campylobacter jejuni*
   d. *Vibrio cholerae*
   e. *E. coli* 0157-H7
   f. *Cyclospora*
   g. *Yersinia enterocolitica*
2) Gastric/duodenal ulcer: *Helicobacter pylori*
3) Gallbladder
   a. Enterobacteriaceae (*Klebsiella, Proteus, Enterobacter, Serratia*)
   b. Enterococci
   c. *Bacteroides* species
   d. *Clostridium*
G. Bone
1) *Staphylococcus aureus*
2) *Pseudomonas* species (following a tennis shoe punctured by nail)
H. Joint
1) *Staphylococcus aureus*
2) Group A streptococcus
3) Enterobacteriaceae (*Klebsiella, Proteus, Enterobacter, Serratia*)
4) *Pseudomonas* species
5) *Neisseria gonorrhoeae*
I. Genitourinary: Pelvic inflammatory disease
1) *Neisseria gonorrhoeae*
2) *Chlamydia trachomatis*
3) *Bacteroides* species
4) Enterobacteriaceae (*Klebsiella, Proteus, Enterobacter, Serratia*)
5) Streptococci
J. Infective endocarditis: Native valve
1) *Streptococcus viridans*

      2) Other streptococci, nutritionally variant (deficient)

      3) Enterococci

      4) Staphylococci

2. Nosocomial infection

  A. Skin/skin structures

      1) Pressure ulcers: Usually polymicrobial

         a. *Streptococcus pyogenes* (groups A, C, G)

         b. Enterococci

         c. Anerobic streptococci

         d. Enterobacteriaceae (*Klebsiella, Proteus, Enterobacter, Serratia*)

         e. *Pseudomonas* species

         f. *Bacteroides* species

         g. *Staphylococcus aureus* (methicillin resistant [MRSA])

      2) Whirlpool folliculitis: *Pseudomonas aerugenosa*

  B. Vascular device: Immunocompromised patients will have additional risks for:

      1) *Candida* species

      2) *Pseudomonas* species

  C. Urinary tract: Related to use of urinary catheters

      1) Thirty percent caused by *E. coli*

      2) Enterococci

      3) *Pseudomonas aerugenosa*

      4) Enterobacteriaceae (*Klebsiella, Proteus, Enterobacter, Serratia*)

      5) *Candida*

  D. Meningitis: Postneurosurgical or posttraumatic

      1) *Staphylococcus aureus*

      2) Enterobacteriaceae (*Klebsiella, Proteus, Enterobacter, Serratia*)

      3) *Pseudomonas* species

      4) *Streptococcus pneumoniae*

  E. Pneumonia: The microorganisms responsible for pneumonia are vastly different in nosocomial pneumonia, especially in the ICU patient. The microorganisms are predominately aerobic gram-negative bacilli and are relatively antibiotic resistant.

      1) *Pseudomonas aeruginosa*

      2) *Klebsiella* species

      3) *Enterobacter* species

      4) *Acinetobacter* species

      5) *Staphylococcus aureus*

      6) Enterococci

  F. Gastrointestinal infection secondary to the use of antibiotic therapy: *Clostridium difficile*

  G. Surgical wound infection: Usually related to the flora at the site of the surgery and if the surgery is clean or contaminated.

      1) Clean surgery with or without a prosthesis:

         a. Staphylococci

         b. Streptococci

      2) Clean surgery involving the gut can also include:

         a. *E. coli*

         b. *Bacteroides fragilis*

      3) Contaminated wounds (stabs, gunshot) are potentially polymicrobic.

  H. Bone: Post open fracture or postoperative

      1) *Staphylococcus aureus*

       2) *Pseudomonas* species
       3) Enterobacteriaceae (*Klebsiella, Proteus, Enterobacter, Serratia*)
  I. Joint: Postoperative, prosthetic replacement
       1) *Staphylococcus epidermidis*
       2) *Staphylococcus aureus*
       3) Enterobacteriaceae (*Klebsiella, Proteus, Enterobacter, Serratia*)
       4) *Pseudomonas* species
  J. Infective endocarditis: Prosthetic valve
       1) Early (<2 months postoperative)
          a. *Staphylococcus epidermidis*
          b. *Staphylococcus aureus*
          c. Rare Enterobacteriaceae, diptheroids, fungi
       2) Late (>2 months postoperative)
          a. *Staphylococcus epidermidis*
          b. *Streptococcus viridans*
          c. Enterococci
          d. *Staphylococcus aureus*
3. Bacteremia: Defined as presence of viable bacteria in the blood (ACCP/SCCM, 1992) and determined by organism growth from a blood culture
  A. May be a consequence of a definable site of infection, for example:
       1) Biliary
       2) Urinary tract
       3) Peritonitis
       4) Pneumonia
  B. Intravascular catheter infection
       1) *Staphylococcus epidermidis*
       2) *Staphylococcus aureus*
  C. May be a result of translocation of intestinal flora into the bloodstream.
4. Sepsis: Systemic inflammatory response to infection (Members, 1992). Patients may present clinically with signs and symptoms of sepsis but blood cultures are negative. In the situation of a septic patient with no site of infection identified, empiric therapy may be started based on the age and immune system status of the patient (See "Septic Shock," later in this chapter).

DIAGNOSTIC TESTS/FINDINGS

General points related to the initiation and monitoring use of antimicrobial therapy.

1. Obtain creatinine and blood urea nitrogen (BUN) to determine baseline renal function.
2. Calculate creatinine clearance to determine need for antibiotic dose reduction.
  A. Males: Ideal body weight = 50 kg + 2.3 kg/inch over 5 ft.

$$\frac{(140\text{-age})(\text{ideal body weight in kg})}{(72)\ (\text{serum creatinine in mg/dL})}$$

  B. Females: Ideal body weight = 45.5 kg + 2.3 kg/inch over 5 ft; calculate as per males, then multiple by 0.85.
  C. Decreased creatinine clearance may necessitate a change in maintenance doses of antibiotic.

     1) Reduce dose and give at same interval
     2) Keep dose same and give at less frequent interval
3. Follow complete blood count (CBC) for return to normal patient baseline.
4. Follow sedimentation rate for return to normal or patient baseline.
5. Monitor serum chemistry for fluid, electrolyte, glucose abnormalities.
6. Monitoring of selected drug level for peak/trough values. This is very important when renal function is changing, as in a hemodynamically unstable patient. Only trough levels are needed in patients with stable renal function, in whom high trough levels are responsible for drug toxiciy. Peak levels are important to determine adequacy of dosage. After an initial loading dose of antibiotic, peak and trough levels are usually obtained on the first or second maintenance dose of antibiotics. If the patient's renal function is rapidly deteriorating, as evidenced by a rising creatinine, levels must be monitored to adjust dosage to avoid toxicities.
   A. Aminoglycosides
     1) Elevated trough levels result in oto- or nephrotoxicity.
     2) Peak levels to achieve effective treatment:
       a. Gentamicin or tobramycin 4–10 μg/mL
       b. Amikacin >20 μ/mL
   B. Vancomycin
     1) Therapeutic peak level 20–40 μ/mL.
     2) Peak levels should not exceed 40 μ/mL to avoid ototoxicity.

MANAGEMENT/TREATMENT

1. The ACNP would consult with the physician when developing an antibiotic treatment plan for treating infection.
2. The ACNP must follow the local prescriptive authority regulations when ordering antimicrobial therapy.
3. The "best guess" for empiric antibiotic coverage until a specific organism can be identified is the starting point for prescription of antibiotics in many clinical settings. Multiple acceptable regimens often exist for a suspected organism at a specific location. For the ACNP, a pocket reference guide to antimicrobial therapies is suggested as a resource for selection of empiric antibiotic therapies. This type of reference usually lists primary suggested regimens and alternative selections to choose from in situations of allergy or when other host-related factors preclude use of the primary regimen.
4. Hospitals and physician practice groups often have clinical pathways prescribing preferred antibiotic therapies to be used in specific patient populations. The ACNP must be familiar with standard protocols for antibiotics in the setting where he or she practices.
5. For disease-specific therapy, refer to the appropriate chapter in this text.
6. Combination antibiotic therapy is utilized to:
   A. Treat life-threatening infections
   B. Treat polymicrobial infections
   C. Obtain synergistic effect of drugs (enhanced antimicrobial acitivity)
   D. Prevent emergence of resistant strains
   E. Permit lower dose of one of the antimicrobials used
7. Disadvantages of combination antibiotic therapy:
   A. Potential toxicities from multiple agents
   B. Increased cost
   C. Possible antagonism of agents

8. Duration of antibiotic therapy is based on clinical response of the patient. In general, initial recommendations are based on site of infection and type of organism being treated. Some general examples include:
   A. Urinary tract
      1) Uncomplicated female cystitis: 3 days
      2) Complicated: 10–14 days
      3) Uncomplicated male gonococcal urethritis: 24 hours
   B. Pneumonia: 10–14 days (up to 21 days)
   C. Skin/skin structure: 10–14 days
   D. Endocarditis
      1) *Streptococcus viridens*: 2–4 weeks
      2) Staphylococcal: 4–6 weeks
   E. Meningitis until patient afebrile for 5 days (7–10 days)
   F. Osteomyelitis: 6 weeks
   G. Septic arthritis: 3 weeks
   H. Pharyngitis—streptococcal: 10 days
9. Resistant organisms are an ominous trend that results in few therapeutic options for patients with infection caused by these organisms. Preventing the nosocomial spread of these organisms is a patient management challenge in hospitals today. Hospital policy must be followed, but strict isolation for patients determined to have infections with resistant organisms, such as methicillin-resistant staphylococci and vancomycin-resistant enterococci, is necessary to prevent spread to other patients.
   Alternative therapies are based on the site/type of infection and sensitivities of the organism isolated from culture.
   A. Penicillin-resistant pneumococci
      1) Meningitis
         a. Third-generation cephalosporin (cefotaxime or ceftriaxone)
         b. Imipenem
         c. Vancomycin
         d. Chloramphenicol
      2) Pneumonia/bacteremia
         a. Second- or third-generation cephalosporin
         b. Vancomycin
         c. Imipenem
      3) Otitis media
         a. Oral
            i.   Clindamycin
            ii. Macrolide
            iii. Trimethoprim/sulfamethoxazole (TMP-SMX)
         b. Parenteral
            i.   Third-generation cephalosporin
            ii. Imipenem
            iii. Vancomycin
   B. MRSA
      1) Colonization of nares:
         a. Topically applied mupirocin
         b. Oral agents if susceptibility testing done prior to therapy
            i.   Minocycline
            ii. TMP-SMX
            iii. Rifampin
      2) Intravenous vancomycin drug of choice for infections.

3) Other drugs may be used in combination with vancomycin, alone, or in combination with one another if patient is intolerant of vancomycin.
   a. Gentamicin
   b. Rifampin
   c. TMP-SMX
   d. Minocycline
   e. Ciprofloxacin
C. Vancomycin-resistant enterococci
   1) β-lactamase-producing enterococcal strains
      a. Imipenem
      b. Amoxicillin-clavulanic acid
      c. Ampicillin-sulbactam
      d. Piperacillin-tazobactam
   2) Amoxicillin resistant *E. faecium*: vancomycin
   3) Potentially useful agents that are bacteriostatic drugs
      a. Tetracycline
      b. Chloramphenicol
      c. Ciprofloxacin
      d. Rifampin

PATIENT EDUCATION

Appropriate patient education will be determined by the condition of the patient and the circumstances (outpatient versus inpatient). Information may be relayed to family members or significant others involved in patient care.

1. Explain the purpose of all tests performed to determine underlying cause of infection, their results, and implications for therapy.
2. Instruct the patient on antimicrobial agents (this information is increasingly important if patient is to continue on outpatient IV therapy or continue on oral medications).
   A. Name
   B. Dose
   C. Dosing interval
   D. Anticipated side effects
   E. Drug/food/alcohol interactions
   F. Duration of therapy
   G. Monitoring of drug levels if required
3. Explain signs and symptoms indicating improvement or deterioration in condition.
4. If intravenous therapy is indicated at home, complete patient/family education regarding care, use, and safety related to IV access.
5. Identify the designated intervals for follow-up visits.
6. Explain important symptoms to report and when and how to notify health care providers.
7. Discuss future needs for antibiotic prophylaxis and under which circumstances it is needed.
8. In cases of contagious or resistant organisms, explain the rationale for isolation precautions to the patient, family, or any visitors. They must be taught appropriate measures and monitored for compliance.

Review Questions

11.6   In which group of patients should the dosage of some antimicrobials be decreased?
A. Trauma, elderly, pediatric
B. Elderly, neonates, impaired renal function
C. Impaired hepatic function, cardiac, neonates
D. Pregnant, sepsis, pediatric

11.7   Which lab values are imperative prior to starting an antibiotic regimen?
A. Potassium, CBC, platelets
B. Creatinine, BUN, CBC
C. Creatinine clearance, CBC, cultures
D. Sedimentation rate, electrolytes, blood cultures

11.8   Which drug level is needed for patients with stable renal function?
A. Trough
B. Peak
C. Loading
D. Maintenance

11.9   The systemic agent of choice for a MRSA infection is:
A. Mupirocin
B. Penicillin G
C. Azithromycin
D. Vancomycin

11.10   Antibiotic coverage for what organism is considered in a trauma patient with open fractures of the femur and tibia?
A. Enterobacteriaceae
B. Staphylococcus aureus
C. Staphylococcus epidermidis
D. Streptococci

Answers and Rationale

11.6   **B**   Impaired renal excretion in neonates and the elderly may require a reduction in dosage of some antibiotics. Renal excretion is important in some antimicrobials; therefore, dose adjustments must be made if renal function is impaired.

11.7   **B**   General points related to the initiation and monitoring of antibiotics are to obtain a creatinine and BUN to determine baseline renal function. Follow CBC for return to normal or baseline.

11.8   **A**   Trough drug levels are needed for patients with stable renal function.

11.9   **D**   Vancomycin is the systemic agent of choice for MRSA; mupirocin can be used topically for this resistant organism.

11.10   **B**   The most common organism creating infections in open bone fractures is *Staphylococcus aureus*.

References

American College of Chest Physicians/Society of Critical Care Medicine Consensus Conference Committee. (1992). American College of Chest Physicians/Society of Critical Care Medicine Consensus Conference: Definitions for sepsis and organ failure and guidelines for the use of innovative therapies in sepsis. *Crit Care Med 20*, 864–874.

Chamber, H.F., & Sande, M.A. (1996). Antimicrobial agents: general considerations. In J.G. Hardman, L.E. Limbird, P.B. Molinoff, et al. (eds.). *Goodman & Gilman's The Pharmacological Basis of Therapeutics* (9th ed.). New York: McGraw-Hill, pp. 1029–1056.

Fraimow, H.S., & Abrutyn, E. (1995). Pathogens resistant to antimicrobial agents. *Infect Dis Clin North Am 9*, 497–525.

Maki, D.G. (1995). Nosocomial infection in the intensive care unit. In J.E. Parrillo & R.C. Bone (eds.). *Critical Care Medicine: Principles of Diagnosis and Management*. St. Louis: C.V. Mosby Co., pp. 893–954.

Mollering, Jr., R.C. (1995). Principles of anti-infective therapy. In G.L. Mandell, J.E., Bennett, & R. Dolin (eds.). *Principles and Practice of Infectious Diseases* (4th ed.). New York: Churchill Livingstone, pp. 199–210.

Neu, H.C. (1994). Principles of antimicrobial use. In T.M. Brody, J. Larner, K.P. Minneman, et al. (eds.). *Human Pharmacology: Molecular to Clinical* (2nd ed.). St. Louis: C.V. Mosby Co., pp. 617–630.

Rubin, R.H., & Teplick, R.S. (1995). Antimicrobial therapy. In J.E. Parrillo & R.C. Bone (eds.). *Critical Care Medicine: Principles of Diagnosis and Management*. St. Louis: C.V. Mosby Co., pp. 955–967.

Sanford, J.P., Gilbert, D.N., & Sande, M.A. (1996). *Guide to Antimicrobial Therapy* (26th ed.). Dallas, TX: Antimicrobial Therapy, Inc.

Septic Shock

DEFINITION

Septic shock is a form of distributive shock. The pathogenesis of septic shock is currently thought to be the result of the release of inflammatory mediators in response to infection. The host's immune system generates a systemic inflammatory response resulting in hemodynamic instability, causing maldistribution of blood flow to body tissues.

In 1992 the American College of Chest Physicians and Society of Critical Care Medicine held a consensus conference that generated definitions of the following terms:

Systemic inflammatory response syndrome (SIRS): The systemic inflammatory response to a variety of clinical insults that is manifested by two or more of the following conditions:
1. Temperature >38°C or <36°C
2. Heart rate of >90 bpm
3. Respiratory rate of >20 breaths/min or $Paco_2$ <32 mm Hg
4. White blood cell count >12,000 cells/mm^3, <4000 cells/mm^3, or >10% bands

Sepsis: The systemic inflammatory response to infection manifested by two or more of the following conditions as a result of infection:
1. Temperature >38°C or <36°C
2. Heart rate of >90 bpm

3. Respiratory rate of >20 breaths/minute or $Paco_2$ <32 mm Hg
4. White blood cell count >12,000 cells/mm^3, <4000 cells/mm^3, or >10% bands

Severe sepsis: Sepsis associated with organ dysfunction, hypoperfusion, or hypotension. Hypoperfusion and perfusion abnormalities may be evidenced by but are not limited to lactic acidosis, oliguria, or an acute alteration in mental status.

Septic shock: Sepsis with hypotension (systolic blood pressure [BP] <90 mm Hg or a reduction of >40 mm Hg from baseline), despite adequate fluid resuscitation, along with perfusion abnormalities that may include but are not limited to lactic acidosis, oliguria, or an acute alteration in mental status. Patients who are on inotropic or vasopressor agents may not be hypotensive at the time that perfusion abnormalities are measured.

Multiple organ dysfunction syndrome: Presence of altered organ function in an acutely ill patient such that homeostasis cannot be maintained without intervention.

ETIOLOGY/INCIDENCE

1. The exact incidence of septic shock is not known because it is not a reportable disease to the Centers for Disease Control and Prevention (CDC) and because of variability in definition of the syndrome. However, over the past decade the National Hospital Discharge Survey had reported steady increases in the number of patients with the discharge diagnosis of septicemia (ICDM-9 code 038). This increase is attributed to a variety of factors associated with recent innovation in medical practice:
   A. More frequent use of invasive medical procedures
   B. Increased use of prosthetic devices
   C. Growing numbers of patients with impaired immune system function, patients with organ transplants, AIDS, and cancer treatment with chemotherapy
   D. Increased survival of patients prone to sepsis (the elderly, patients with cancer)
   E. Increased use of antibiotics with disruption of normal flora and predisposition to colonization by more resistant organisms
2. It is estimated that septic shock develops in 40% of cases of sepsis.
3. Septic shock is the most common cause of death in medical and surgical intensive care units. Mortality of septic shock has remained high over the last 10 years (25–60%).
4. Septic shock is primarily a nosocomial illness. It occurs as a complication of other medical problems and contributes to the morbidity and mortality of a variety of diseases.
5. Gram-negative and gram-positive bacteria are commonly cultured from the blood; however, fungi, protozoa, and viruses are implicated in sepsis.

SIGNS AND SYMPTOMS

The presentation of sepsis varies depending on the underlying condition of the patient.

1. Immune-competent patients may present with a variety of *symptoms* based on the primary site of infection:

A. Fever or hypothermia

B. Chills/rigors

C. Weakness/malaise

D. Nausea/vomiting/diarrhea

E. Headache/nuchal rigidity/photophobia

F. Localized area of redness, pain, swelling of the skin

G. Abdominal pain/guarding

H. Dysuria/flank pain

I. Dyspnea/cough/sputum production/chest pain

2. Elderly or immunocompromised patients may fail to exhibit some of these symptoms, thereby confounding the diagnosis. Patients may exhibit subtle changes in sensorium or hyperventilation, or report nonspecific symptoms, including pain.

PHYSICAL FINDINGS

1. Physical findings may vary depending on the following:
   A. Underlying state of the immune system
   B. Location of infection
   C. Initiation of therapy, such as IV fluids prior to physical examination

2. Physical findings in *sepsis*:
   A. Core body temperature >38°C or <36°C
   B. Tachycardia >90 bpm
   C. Tachypnea >20 breaths/min
   D. Skin may be cold, clammy, and cyanotic or hot and dry
   E. Peripheral pulses may be diminished or bounding
   F. Mental confusion/lethargy
   G. Oliguria of <0.5 mL/kg

3. When sepsis progresses to *severe sepsis*, the patient demonstrates hypotension.
   A. Systolic BP <90 mm Hg *or*
   B. Unexplained systolic BP decrease of >40 mm Hg from baseline

DIFFERENTIAL DIAGNOSIS

1. Shock of other etiologies
   A. Hypovolemic
   B. Cardiogenic
   C. Obstructive (pericardial tamponade, massive pulmonary emboli)

2. Distributive shock of other etiologies
   A. Toxic shock syndrome
   B. Anaphylactic
   C. Neurogenic
   D. Adrenal crisis
   E. Thyroid storm

DIAGNOSTIC TESTS/FINDINGS

1. Complete blood count with differential:
   A. WBC >12,000 cells/mm^3
   B. WBC <4000 cells/mm^3
   C. >10% bands

2. Chemistry panel:
   A. BUN, creatinine will elevate with decreased renal perfusion.
   B. Transaminases (alanine transaminase aspartate transaminase, γ-glutamyl transpeptidase) alkaline phosphatase, and bilirubin will elevate with decreased liver perfusion.
   C. Other electrolyte disorders may be result of underlying condition or compensatory mechanisms for a shock state.
3. Arterial blood gases:
   A. Early: Respiratory alkalosis ($Paco_2$ <32 mm Hg)
   B. Late: Metabolic acidosis with or without hypoxemia
4. Serum lactic acid: Elevated
5. Hematologic parameters:
   A. Decreased platelets
   B. Prolonged prothrombin time and partial thromboplastin time
   C. Decreasing fibrinogen
   D. Presence of fibrin degradation products
   E. Presence of d-dimer
   F. Morphologic abnormalities on peripheral blood smear, such as schistocytes, platelet destruction
6. Electrocardiogram (ECG):
   A. Sinus tachycardia >90 bpm
   B. Premature ventricular beats
   C. Dysrhythmias
7. Chest radiograph:
   A. Pulmonary infiltrates as one etiology of septic shock
   B. Noncardiogenic pulmonary edema (capillary leak) as a result of septic shock
8. Hemodynamic monitoring:
   A. Systolic BP <90 mm Hg or a reduction of >40 mm Hg from baseline
   B. Decreased mean arterial pressure (MAP)
   C. Decreased systemic vascular resistance
   D. Decreased left and right ventricular ejection fraction
   E. Cardiac output/cardiac index is normal or elevated
   F. Right atrial pressure low or normal
   G. Pulmonary artery occlusion pressure (PAOP) low or normal
   H. High mixed venous oxygen saturation
9. Blood cultures should be obtained to identify an etiologic microbial agent; however, 50% of clinically septic patients may have negative cultures.
   A. Draw at least two 10 to 15-mL samples, preferably from separate peripheral venipuncture sites.
   B. If two venipunctures from peripheral sites cannot be obtained, draw one specimen from a peripheral site and draw one sample from the most recently inserted catheter.
10. Cultures should be obtained of urine, sputum, wounds, joint fluid, or CSF dependent on the underlying condition of the patient. Gram's stains (especially of CSF, sputum, and joint fluid) may be utilized as a rapid assessment for identification of microorganisms.
11. Additional radiologic studies such as ultrasounds (abdomen, hepatobiliary, genitourinary) or CT scans of abdomen, chest, or head may be needed to identify nidus of infection.
12. Pulse oximetry data may not be reliably obtained because of peripheral vasoconstriction. Arterial blood gas measurement are the most reliable indicators of arterial oxygen content and acid-base status.

MANAGEMENT/TREATMENT

The priorities in shock management must be implemented simultaneously and, ideally in the critical care environment, with continuous ECG monitoring.

1. Support airway and breathing.
   A. Supplemental oxygen to provide an arterial oxygen saturation of >90%.
   B. Maintain adequate oxygen delivery by maintaining adequate hemoglobin and hematocrit and cardiac output.
   C. May require intubation, mechanical ventilation, and positive end-expiratory pressure.
2. Volume resuscitation:
   A. Establish reliable large-bore IV access.
   B. Colloid, crystalloid, or blood and blood products can be utilized based on the underlying condition of the patient. The underlying principle of rapid administration is probably more important than the type of solution.
   C. Administration of 500–1000 mL of fluid over 15–60 minutes may be necessary.
   D. Goals of fluid administration are MAP of >60 mm Hg and PAOP of >15 mm Hg.
   E. It is common for patients with severe sepsis to require in excess of 10 L of fluid; subsequent resuscitation complications include weight gain ("third spacing"), pulmonary and peripheral edema.
3. Hemodynamic monitoring is recommended when rapid restoration of BP is not achieved with fluid administration in order to confirm diagnosis and for guiding additional therapy.
   A. Arterial catheter
   B. Pulmonary artery catheter
   C. Calculation of hemodynamic profiles
4. Vasoactive agents are essential when fluid resuscitation alone has not stabilized the hemodynamic status of the patient.
   A. Dopamine starting at low dose (1–5 μg/kg/min) and titrated to maintain MAP >60 mm Hg.
   B. If dopamine dose at 10–20 μg/kg/min fails to achieve effective hemodynamic support or results in dysrhythmias, norepinephrine is suggested.
   C. In conjunction with norepinephrine, dopamine should be reduced to a low renal perfusion dose of 2–4 μg/kg/min.
   D. If cardiac dysrhythmias persist, phenylephrine may be utilized, although cardiac irritability can still occur, especially with concurrent metabolic abnormalities of sepsis.
   E. Less than 10% of patients with septic shock have uncompensated myocardial depression with low cardiac output. In this subgroup of patients, dobutamine may be used in combination with norepinephrine, dopamine, or epinephrine.
5. Obtain all appropriate cultures and initiate empiric broad-spectrum antibiotic coverage.
   A. Immune-competent patient: Utilize IV antibiotic coverage with
      1) One drug with coverage of gram-positive bacteria + one drug with coverage of gram-negative bacteria *or*
      2) One broad-spectrum agent with coverage against both gram-positive and gram-negative bacteria.

B. Immunocompromised patient with neutropenia:
1) Third-generation cephalosporin + aminoglycoside *or*
2) Antipseudomonal penicillin + aminoglycoside
3) Vancomycin is indicated if possibility of a catheter-associated infection
C. Apply principles of antibiotic selection outlined in this section. When the offending organism is determined, selective antibiotic therapy should be started to prevent resistance or suprainfection.
6. Continue to search for and eliminate the source of infection.
A. Surgical removal of abscess or necrotic tissue
B. Removal of infected foreign body
C. Drainage of infected fluids (i.e., septic joint, abdominal fluid collections)
7. Monitor for organ system dysfunction and institute supportive therapy.
A. Monitor urinary output and use fluids, diuretics, or low-dose dopamine to preserve renal function and urinary output.
B. Institute nutritional support (enteral preferable if tolerated).
C. Stress ulcer prophylaxis. (*Caution:* Increased gastric pH may increase the risk of gastrointestinal aspiration.)
D. Prevention of deep vein thrombosis.
E. Minimize risk for nosocomial infection and monitor closely for signs of new or recurrent infection.
F. Pulmonary toilet to mobilize secretions.
8. Utilize pain medication and sedation as appropriate for painful procedures and to manage anxiety and allow for sleep.
9. New therapies are being developed to neutralize microbiologic toxins and modulate the host mediator response. These therapies are still considered experimental and none is an acceptable alternative to the measures indicated in this section.

PATIENT EDUCATION

Based on the underlying condition of the patient, opportunities for patient education may be limited.

1. Explain procedures and monitoring used in the critical care management of the patient.
2. Give explanations of current condition to the patient (when possible) and to designated family members/significant others.
3. Allow patient and family contact as much as possible.
4. Because of the high mortality of septic shock, the patient's family should be made aware of the possibility of a fatal outcome.
5. Assisting the patient's family with the grieving process may be necessary.

Review Questions

11.11 A patient develops a temperature of 38°C, with a heart rate of 106 bpm and WBC of 15,000 cells/mm^3. The patient has developed:
A. SIRS
B. Sepsis

    C. Severe sepsis

    D. Septic shock

11.12 A patient's BP remains 80/40, mm Hg, heart rate 130 bpm, despite aggressive fluid resuscitation; pH = 7.10 and urinary output 10 mL/2 hours. The patient has developed:

    A. SIRS

    B. Sepsis

    C. Severe sepsis

    D. Septic shock

11.13 An 80-year-old female is admitted from an extended care facility with mental status changes, BP 90/palpated, and temperature 34°C. She has an indwelling catheter following recent surgery. Which of the following is the best choice of intervention?

    A. Obtain a urine culture and wait for results to select antibiotic therapy.

    B. Request a urology consultation.

    C. Obtain two blood cultures and a urine culture, and start broad-spectrum antibiotics.

    D. Remove and culture the catheter and obtain a neurology consult.

11.14 The hemodynamic goal of fluid resuscitation for a patient in septic shock is:

    A. MAP 70, PAOP 12

    B. MAP 60, PAOP 10

    C. MAP 80, PAOP 20

    D. MAP 75, PAOP 12

11.15 Which of the following pharmacologic regimens would be recommended for a patient in septic shock with hypotension, recurrent ventricular dysrhythmias, and a cardiac index of 2.5?

    A. Fluids, phenylephrine, amrinone

    B. Dopamine, norepinephrine, dobutamine

    C. Dopamine, norepinephrine, milrinone

    D. Norepinephrine, phenylephrine, dobutamine

Answers and Rationales

11.11 **A** A temperature of >38°C, heart rate >90 bpm, and WBC >12,000 cells/mm^3 are diagnostic of SIRS.

11.12 **D** Hypotension despite aggressive fluid resuscitation, lactic acidosis, and oliguria are diagnostic of septic shock.

11.13 **C** It is best to obtain multiple blood cultures and other appropriate cultures prior to starting broad-spectrum antibiotic coverage in a case of suspected sepsis/septic shock.

11.14 **C** The goal of fluid resuscitation is MAP >60 and PAOP >15.

11.15 **B** Dopamine is the first drug of choice as a vasoactive substance. If dopamine fails to achieve a hemodynamic effect, norepinephrine should be added. In patients with septic shock and decreased cardiac output, dobutamine should be added.

References

Bone, R.C. (1996). Sir Isaac Newton, sepsis, SIRS, and CARS. *Crit Care Med 24*, 1125–1128.

Beal, A.L., & Cerra, F.B. (1994). Multiple organ failure syndrome in the 1990's: systemic inflammatory response and organ dysfunction. *JAMA 271*, 226–233.

Clochesy, J.M. (1996). Patients with systemic inflammatory response syndrome. In J.M. Clochesy, C. Breu, S. Cardin, et al. (eds.). *Critical Care Nursing* (2nd ed.). Philadelphia: W.B. Saunders Co., pp. 1359–1370.

Kellum, J.A., & Decker, J.M. (1996). The immune system: Relation to sepsis and multiple organ failure. *AACN Clin Issues 7*, 339–350.

Members of the American College of Chest Physicians/Society of Critical Care Medicine Consensus Conference Committee. (1992). American College of Chest Physicians/Society of Critical Care Medicine Consensus Conference: Definitions for sepsis and organ failure and guidelines for the use of innovative therapies in sepsis. *Crit Care Med 20*, 864–874.

Natanson, C., Hoffman, W.D., & Parrillo, J.E. (1995). Septic shock and multiple organ failure. In J.E. Parrillo & R.C. Bone (eds.). *Critical Care Medicine: Principles of Diagnosis and Management.* St. Louis: C.V. Mosby Co., pp. 355–374.

Sanford, J.P., Gilbert, D.N., & Sande, M.A. (1996). *Guide to Antimicrobial Therapy.* Dallas, TX: Antimicrobial Therapy, Inc.

Immunologic Disorders: Acquired Immunodeficiency Syndrome

DEFINITION

Human immunodeficiency virus (HIV) leads to a chronic, progressive disease of the immune system. The spectrum of HIV infection ranges from asymptomatic infection to the acquired immunodeficiency syndrome. The 1993 CDC definition of AIDS incorporates presumptive and definitive diagnoses (constitutional symptoms, opportunistic infection, malignancy) with or without positive HIV serology and CD4 counts, into a matrix of nine mutually exclusive categories (see Table 11–2).

ETIOLOGY/INCIDENCE

1. HIV is one of a group of RNA retroviruses causing a syndrome characterized by a gradual, progressive deterioration of the immune system. The T-lymphocyte helper/inducer cells, known as T4 or CD4 cells, are predominately affected, although effects on the function of others cells, such as B lymphocytes, monocytes/macrophages, and microglial cells and oligodendrocytes, have been documented.
2. Modes of transmission of HIV include sexual, parenteral, and vertical transmission. Risk groups for HIV infection include:
   A. Male homosexuals or bisexuals
   B. Intravenous drug users
   C. Infants of an infected mother
   D. Recipient of contaminated blood or blood products (predominately prior to 1985)
   E. Sexual partner of a member of a high-risk group
   F. Occupational exposure

TABLE 11–2.   1993 Revised CDC AIDS Surveillance Case Definitions for Adolescents and Adults

CD4 Cell Categories	Clinical Category A: Asymptomatic, PGL, or Acute HIV Infection	Clinical Category B (Not A or C)	Clinical Category C: AIDS Indicator Conditions
1: ≥500/mm^3 (≥29%)	A1	B1	C1
2: 200–499/mm^3 (14–28%)	A2	B2	C2
3: <200/mm^3 (<14%)	A3	B3	C3

Clinical Category A Conditions
Asymptomatic HIV infection
Persistent generalized lymphadenopathy (PGL)
Acute primary HIV infection with accompanying illness or history of acute infection

Clinical Category B Conditions
Bacillary angiomatosis
Candidiasis, oropharyngeal (thrush)
Candidiasis, vulvovaginal persistent, frequent, or poorly responsive to therapy
Cervical dysplasia (moderate or severe)/cervical cancer in situ
Constitutional symptoms, such as fever (38.5°C) or diarrhea lasting >1 month
Oral hairy leukoplakia
Herpes zoster (shingles) involving at least two distinct episodes or more than one dermatome
Idiopathic thrombocytopenic purpura
Listeriosis
Pelvic inflammatory disease, particularly if complicated by tubo-ovarian abscess
Peripheral neuropathy

Clinical Category C Conditions
Candidiasis of esophagus, bronchi, trachea, or lungs
Invasive cervical cancer
Coccidioidomycosis, disseminated or extrapulmonary
Cryptococcosis, extrapulmonary
Cryptosporidiosis, chronic intestinal (>1 month duration)
Cytomegalovirus disease (other than liver, spleen, or nodes)
Cytomegalovirus retinitis with loss of vision
HIV-related encephalopathy
Herpes simplex: chronic ulcers >1 month duration, bronchitis, pneumonitis, or esophagitis
Histoplasmosis, disseminated or extrapulmonary
Isosporiasis, chronic intestinal >1 month duration
Kaposi's sarcoma
Lymphoma: Burkitt's, immunoblastic, or primary of the brain
Mycobacterium avium complex or *M. kansasii* disseminated or extrapulmonary
M. tuberculosis, any site pulmonary or extrapulmonary
Mycobacterium, other species or unidentified species disseminated or extrapulmonary
Pneumocystis carinii pneumonia
Recurrent pneumonia
Progressive multifocal leukoencephalopathy
Recurrent salmonellosis sepsis
Toxoplasmosis of the brain
HIV wasting syndrome

3. A total of 573,800 persons ≥13 years old have been documented to have AIDS in the United States between 1981 and 1996.
4. In 1996, for the first time deaths from AIDS have decreased substantially. This is attributed to improved survival of AIDS patients receiving combination therapy with antiretroviral therapy and increased use of prophylactic drugs to prevent opportunistic infections.
5. Recent trends (1992 through 1996) reveal that non-Hispanic blacks, Hispanics, and women account for increasing proportions of persons reported with AIDS.

SIGNS AND SYMPTOMS

Signs and symptoms may be absent for a mean of 10 years after initial HIV infection. When symptoms occur, they may be nonspecific or, in the situation of advanced immunosuppression, related to development of an opportunistic infection or malignancy. Virtually every symptom can be attributable to other diseases. The combination of complaints in a high-risk patient is more suggestive and may include:

1. Fever of ≥4 weeks
2. Night sweats
3. Unexplained weight loss
4. Malaise/fatigue
5. Chronic diarrhea
6. Anorexia/nausea/vomiting
7. Rash/skin lesions
8. Persistent swollen glands
9. Mouth ulcers/lesions
10. Odynophagia
11. Visual disturbances
12. Joint pain
13. Cough
14. Shortness of breath/dyspnea at rest or exertional
15. Vaginal discharge, burning, itching
16. Myalgias
17. Difficulty concentrating/memory loss
18. Pain/paresthesias in lower extremities

PHYSICAL FINDINGS

The physical exam may be totally normal in the HIV-positive patient. As the disease progresses, signs of wasting, opportunistic infections, and/or malignancy may appear. The HIV patient may develop any finding that could be seen in an adult patient population. The following list includes *common* findings in HIV patients, particularly seen with progression of the disease.

1. Weight loss
   A. Loss of body fat
   B. Decrease in muscle mass
   C. Temporal wasting
   D. Cachexia

2. Oral infections/lesions
   A. Candidiasis
      1) Pseudomembranous (thrush)
      2) Erythematous
      3) Hyperplastic
      4) Angular cheilitis
   B. Recurrent aphthous ulcers
   C. Oral hairy leukoplakia
   D. Herpetic lesions
      1) Primary infection of mucous membranes
      2) Herpes labialis
      3) Cytomegalovirus lesions of mucous membranes
      4) Herpes zoster involving trigeminal nerve
   E. Oral warts associated with human papillomavirus (HPV)
   F. Periodontal disease
      1) Linear gingival erythema
      2) Necrotizing ulcerative periodontitis
   G. Salivary gland disease
   H. Kaposi's sarcoma lesions
   I. Non-Hodgkin's lymphoma presenting as a swelling or ulcer
3. Generalized lymphadenopathy
4. Skin lesions characteristic of:
   A. Herpes zoster ("shingles")
   B. Kaposi's sarcoma
   C. Seborrheic dermatitis
   D. Eosinophilic folliculitis
   E. Molluscum contagiosum
   F. *Staphylococcus aureus* skin infection, such as folliculitis
   G. Bacillary angiomatosis
   H. Petechiae
5. Genital lesions associated with sexually transmitted diseases
   A. Condyloma acuminatum
   B. Herpes simplex
   C. Primary syphilis chancre
   D. Urethral discharge
   E. Molluscum contagiosum
6. Female patients
   A. Recurrent vaginal yeast infection
   B. Pap smear indicative of invasive carcinoma
7. Vision/retinal abnormalities
   A. Visual field loss
   B. Cotton wool spots
   C. Exudate and hemorrhage
8. Respiratory
   A. Findings consistent with interstitial pneumonia
      1) Tachypnea
      2) Nonproductive cough
      3) Normal adventitious breath sounds
   B. Findings consistent with lobar pneumonia
      1) Tachypnea
      2) Productive cough
      3) Abnormal breath sounds—crackles, rhonchi, wheezes

9. Abdominal
   A. Hepatomegaly
   B. Splenomegaly
10. Neurologic
    A. Neuropsychological testing abnormalities: Slowed verbal response, difficulties with complex sequencing, problem solving, performance with time pressure and visual-motor integration
    B. Cognitive deterioration: Problems with concentration and memory
    C. Abnormal peripheral sensations, particularly in lower extremities
    D. Motor dysfunction: Imbalance, incoordination, difficulty with complex motor tasks
    E. Neurologic testing abnormalities: Problems with rapid alternating movements, ataxia, hyperreflexia
11. Cardiovascular
    A. Tachycardia, usually associated with other signs and symptoms of underlying illness (fever, infection such as pneumonia, hypovolemia)
    B. Hypotension/postural changes

DIFFERENTIAL DIAGNOSIS

1. A high index of suspicion based on history of risk behaviors
2. Depending on the presenting signs and symptoms
   A. Infection (tuberculosis, mononucleosis, cytomegalovirus, secondary syphilis, occult abscess, hepatitis, endocarditis, pneumonia)
   B. Connective tissue disease
   C. Drug reaction
   D. Malignancy
   E. Endocrine disorder (hyperthyroidism, adrenal insufficiency)
   F. Neurologic disease (any condition causing mental status change or neuropathy: alcoholism, liver disease, renal dysfunction, vitamin deficiency, CNS malignancies, multiple sclerosis, demylinating disorders)
   G. GI disease (malabsorptive syndromes, inflammatory bowel disease)

DIAGNOSTIC TESTS/FINDINGS

1. Laboratory findings with HIV infection (see Table 11–3)
   A. HIV serologic testing for presence of anti-HIV antibody. An initial positive screening test using ELISA is confirmed using the Western blot. The sensitivity and specificity of this combination approaches 99%, and it is the most commonly used for diagnosis. This method can be falsely negative if the exposure is too recent for antibody production (within 6–12 weeks).
   B. The HIV polymerase chain reaction (PCR) can detect presence of virus when the HIV ELISA in the immediate postexposure period is still negative. This test is usually reserved for clarification of indeterminate results of ELISA and Western blot testing. Identification of HIV indicates infection.
   C. The measurement of absolute and percentage of CD4 subset of total lymphocyte count has traditionally been used to determine the level of HIV damage to the immune system and as a guide for the initiation of antiretroviral therapy and prophylaxis against opportunistic infection. Values may be normal (>500 cells/mm^3) early after infection with HIV

TABLE 11–3.   Laboratory Findings with HIV Infection

Test	Significance
HIV ELISA	Screening test for HIV infection. Sensitivity >99.9%. Repeatedly reactive test must be confirmed with Western blot.
Western blot	Confirmatory test for HIV infection. Combined with ELISA, has specificity of >99.9%. Indeterminate results may be seen early in HIV infection, HIV-2 infection, autoimmune disease, pregnancy, or recent tetanus toxoid immunization.
Absolute CD4 lymphocyte count	Predictor of HIV progression. AIDS defined when <200 cells/μL.
CD4 lymphocyte percentage	May be more reliable than absolute count. AIDS defined with percentage <14%.
HIV plasma viral load by RTA PCR, NASBA or bDNA	High viral load leads to poor clinical outcome. Lowering viral load results in clinical improvement. Therapy recommended for patients with >5,000–10,000 copies/mL and considered for any detectable levels.

or severely depleted (0–50 cells/mm^3) in advanced AIDS. A CD4 cell count of <200 cells/mm^3 regardless of clinical presentation meets the CDC definition of AIDS.

   D. Measurement of quantitative HIV-1 plasma viral load using the RTA PCR, NASBA or bDNA method provides evidence of HIV disease progression. It is now the marker for initiation of or changes in antiretroviral therapy and, in conjunction with the CD4 count, for the institution of prophylaxis against opportunistic infection. Values may be <400 copies/mL if the patient is receiving effective multidrug therapy or in the millions of virions in advanced disease.

   E. The CBC is obtained in the initial evaluation of HIV-positive patients and periodically for monitoring side effects of medications and disease manifestations. Anemia, leukopenia, and thrombocytopenia are common abnormalities. A macrocytic anemia (elevated mean corpuscular hemoglobin) is seen secondary to antiretroviral therapy.

2. Baseline diagnostic testing obtained in initial evaluation of HIV patient

   A. A serum chemistry panel is advocated in the initial evaluation of patients with HIV infection because of the high incidence of concurrent illness. It also serves as a baseline for monitoring effects of medication regimens.

   B. Screening VDRL or rapid plasma reagin with a confirmatory fluorescent treponemal antibody test on positive results.

   C. Hepatitis serology:
      1) Hepatitis B surface antigen (HBsAg)
      2) Hepatitis B core antibody (anti-HBc)
      3) Hepatitis C antibody (anti-HCV)

   D. *Toxoplasma gondii* IgG to determine past exposure.

   E. PPD skin test with standard Mantoux test. A response of ≥5 mm is positive in HIV-positive patient.

   F. Chest x-ray for detection of asymptomatic lung infections and as a baseline for future comparison.

   G. Pap smear: A high rate of cervical dysplasia with rapid progression to carcinoma is seen in HIV-positive women. Patients with cellular abnor-

malities should be referred to a gynecologist for colposcopy and possible biopsy.
H. Antibody testing for CMV if the patient is at low risk for CMV. Over 90% of IV drug users, homosexual men, and hemophiliacs are seropositive.

MANAGEMENT/TREATMENT

Pharmacologic therapy in HIV disease involves use of antiretroviral drugs to combat HIV, prophylaxis against and treatment of opportunistic infections.

1. Antiretroviral therapy recommendations are rapidly changing based on new evidence of HIV pathogenesis and viral replication and as new agents receive Food and Drug Administration (FDA) approval. Ideally antiretroviral therapy should be initiated prior to irreversible immunologic damage.
   A. Initiation of antiretroviral therapy:
      1) Symptomatic HIV disease
      2) Asymptomatic with CD4 cell count 350–500 cells/mm^3 when HIV RNA assays are not available.
      3) Viral load of >5000–10,000 HIV RNA copies/mL regardless of CD4 counts
      4) Consider therapy for any patient with detectable plasma HIV RNA who requests therapy and is willing to comply with therapy.
   B. Choice of drugs for initial antiretroviral therapy involves use of three drugs. Two drugs in the nucleoside reverse transcriptase inhibitors (NRTI) category and one protease inhibitor (PI). (See Table 11–4 for FDA-approved antiretroviral drugs and their dosages.)
   C. The primary alternative regimen in patients in whom PI drugs are not possible to use, includes two NRTI drugs and one non-nucleoside reverse transcriptase inhibitor (NNRTI).
2. The HIV virus mutates and develops resistance to antiretroviral drug therapy over time. It is essential to monitor the patient for signs of drug resistance evidenced by a decline in clinical condition, increase in viral load, or decrease in CD4 cell count.
   A. Reasons for changing antiretroviral therapy:
      1) Treatment failure indicated by increase in viral load, decrease in CD4 cell count, or clinical disease progression
      2) Drug-induced toxicity, intolerance or nonadherence to regimen
      3) Current use of a suboptimal drug regimen, such as monotherapy or dual therapy.
   B. Factors to consider when changing drug therapy:
      1) Reason for change
         a. For toxicity or intolerance, choose a drug that the patient will be able to tolerate and be willing to take.
         b. For treatment failure, a more potent regimen is needed, with a different mechanism of action and no cross-resistance.
      2) Prior treatment history with antiretroviral agents
      3) Currently available drug options
      4) Stage of HIV disease
      5) Underlying conditions, such as peripheral neuropathy
      6) Concomitant medications and potential interactions
      7) Cost of medications and resources available to patient for costly therapy

TABLE 11–4. **Antiretroviral Therapy**

Class/Drug	Usual Daily Dose	Common Side Effects	Monitoring*
Nucleoside Analogues			
Zidovudine (AZT) (Retrovir)	300 mg bid or 200 mg tid	Anemia, neutropenia, nausea, malaise, headache, insomnia	CBC with differential
Didanosine (ddI) (Videx)	>60 kg: 200 mg bid <60 kg: 125 mg bid	Peripheral neuropathy, pancreatitis, dry mouth, hepatitis	CBC with differential, aminotransferases, amylase, triglycerides, neurologic exam monthly
Zalcitabine (ddC) (Hivid)	0.75 mg tid	Peripheral neuropathy, apthous ulcers, hepatitis, pancreatitis	Aminotransferases, amylase, monthly neurologic exam
Stavudine (d4T) (Zerit)	>60 kg: 40 mg bid <60 kg: 30 mg bid	Peripheral neuropathy, pancreatitis, hepatitis	Aminotransferases, amylase, monthly neurologic exam
Lamivudine (3TC) (Epivir)	150 mg bid	Rash, peripheral neuropathy	Monthly neurologic exam
Non-nucleoside reverse transcriptase inhibitors			
Nevirapine (Viramune)	200 mg qd for 2 weeks, then 200 mg bid	Rash, hepatitis	Aminotransferase
Delavirdine (Rescriptor)	400 mg tid	Rash	
Protease Inhibitors			
Saquinavir (Invirase) (Fortovase)	600 mg tid with food 1200 mg tid with food	Nausea, abdominal pain, diarrhea, headache	Aminotransferases, triglycerides, glucose
Ritonavir (Norvir)	Day 1: 300 mg bid Day 2–3: 400 mg bid Day 4: 500 mg bid Then 600 mg bid	Nausea, vomiting, diarrhea, circumoral & peripheral paresthesias, asthenia, ↑ cholesterol, ↑ triglycerides	Aminotransferases, triglycerides, cholesterol, glucose
Indinavir (Crixivan)	800 mg tid on an empty stomach. Drink 48 oz fluids qd	Kidney stones; asymptomatic ↑ indirect bilirubin	Aminotransferases, bilirubin, glucose
Nelfinavir (Viracept)	750 mg tid with food	Nausea, diarrhea, asthenia, rash	Aminotransferases, glucose

* The HIV virus mutates and develops resistance to antiretroviral drug therapy over time. It is essential to monitor the patient for signs of drug resistance evidenced by a decline in clinical condition, increase in viral load, or decrease in CD4 cell count.

C. Stopping antiretroviral therapy may be appropriate in patients with very advanced AIDS. The difficulty in taking drugs, the quality of the patient's life, and toxicities must be weighed against the benefit that drug therapy offers in each individual patient situation.

D. Recommendations for primary HIV infection (the first 4–7 weeks after HIV infection has occurred, when rapid viral replication occurs) are based on limited research but suggest treatment with at least two nucleoside analogs and a protease inhibitor for a minimum of two years.

E. Recommendations from the CDC for occupational exposures are based on the route of exposure (percutaneous, mucous membrane, skin) and the type of source material (blood, fluid containing or likely to contain blood, fluid unlikely to contain blood).

1) Percutaneous exposures to gross blood are further categorized as:

a. *High* risk (deep injury with hollow-bore needle used in vascular site of patient with terminal HIV disease); zidovudine (AZT) and lamivudine (3TC) + indinavir at the same dose used in treating HIV disease is recommended

b. *Increased* risk (large-volume exposure or terminal HIV disease): AZT and 3TC is recommended

c. No increased risk: Offer AZT and 3TC

2) Exposure to blood via mucous membranes or skin: offer AZT and 3TC ± indinavir

3) Exposure to other fluids contaminated with blood via mucous membranes or skin: offer AZT and 3TC

F. Vertical transmission prophylaxis includes perinatal treatment of all HIV-infected mothers with AZT 300 mg bid starting at 14 weeks' gestation and continuing until onset of labor. During labor, give AZT by IV infusion with 2 mg/kg for 1 hour followed by 1 mg/kg/hr until delivery.

1) Treat the newborn, regardless of treatment of the mother, with AZT 2 mg/kg q6h for 6 weeks; start 8–12 hours after birth.

2) Bottle feeding of the newborn should be encouraged if at all possible.

3. Opportunistic infection (OI) is an infection whose incidence and severity are increased among HIV-infected persons because of their immunosuppressed state. The OI emerges with decline in CD4 cell counts, usually occurring at levels below 200 cells/mm^3. (See Table 11–5.) Infection may occur secondary to an initial contact with an organism but is often the result of reactivation of latent infection.

A. Primary prophylaxis against OI is initiated to prevent a first episode of infection and, once initiated, must be continued for the life of the patient. Recent potent drug therapy regimens using protease inhibitors have shown dramatic improvement in immune system function and CD4 counts. Recommendations are to continue prophylaxis based on the lowest-documented CD4 count.

B. Secondary prophylaxis is initiated to prevent recurrence of an OI. Following active disease from OI, patients generally stay on secondary prophylaxis regardless of improvement in their CD4 counts.

C. *Pneumocystis carinii* pneumonia (PCP)

1) Risk

a. Major AIDS design diagnosis and cause of death

b. CD4 count <200/mm^3

2) Presentation

a. Cough

b. Lack of sputum production

c. Progressive dyspnea

d. Fever

3) Diagnosis

a. Chest x-ray: Bilateral interstitial infiltrates

b. Pao$_2$ <80 mm Hg

TABLE 11–5. Relationship Between CD4 Cell Counts and Opportunistic Infections

CD4 Cell Count	Opportunistic Infection
>500/μL	*Mycobacterium tuberculosis*
<200/μL	*Pneumocystis carinii* pneumonia
<100/μL	Toxoplasmosis, deep fungal infection
<50/μL	Disseminated MAC
	Cytomegalovirus

    c. Pulse oximetry shows activity-induced oxygen desaturation
    d. Elevated LDH
    e. Induced sputum or bronchoscopy secretions demonstrate oocytes
  4) Prophylaxis recommended for
    a. Patient with history of PCP
    b. CD4 count <200/mm^3
    c. Oral candidiasis, unexplained fever ≥2 weeks' duration
  5) Preferred prophylactic regimen: TMP-SMZ one double-strength (DS) tablet PO qd
  6) Alternative therapies include:
    a. TMP-SMZ one DS tablet PO three times a week
    b. Dapsone 100 mg PO qd or 50 mg PO bid
    c. Dapsone 200 mg + pyrimethamine 75 mg + leucovorin 25 mg PO q wk
    d. Aerosolized pentamidine 300 mg q mo via Respirgard II nebulizer
  7) Treatment of active disease
    a. TMP 15 mg/kg/day + SMZ 75 mg/kg/day PO or IV in three or four divided daily doses for 21 days
    b. Moderate to severe disease (Pao$_2$ <70 mm Hg) should receive prednisone 40 mg PO bid for 5 days, 40 mg PO qd for 5 days then 20 mg PO qd for the rest of their TMP-SMZ therapy
D. Toxoplasmosis
  1) Risk
    a. Relapse of latent infection in patients with positive serology
    b. CD4 count <100/mm^3
  2) Presentation
    a. Headache
    b. Confusion
    c. Fever
  3) Diagnosis
    a. Positive serology
    b. CT or MRI with one or more space-occupying lesions of the brain
    c. Institute empiric treatment, follow scans and clinical presentation rather than performing brain biopsy
  4) Prophylaxis
    a. Serology-negative patients should prevent infection by avoiding eating rare or improperly cooked red meat, avoiding oral contact with soil, and using protective measures if changing cat litter.
    b. Serology-positive patients should institute medication when CD4 count reaches 100/mm^3.
  5) Preferred agent: TMP-SMZ one DS tablet PO qd

      6) Alternative therapy

        a. TMP-SMZ one DS tablet PO three times a week

        b. Dapsone 50 mg PO qd + (pyrimethamine 50 mg + leucovorin 25 mg) PO q wk

        c. Dapsone 200 mg PO q wk + (pyrimethamine 75 mg + leucovorin 25 mg) PO q wk

      7) Treatment of active disease for at least 6 weeks followed by lifelong suppressive therapy. Initial treatment may use:

        a. Pyrimethamine + folinic acid + sulfadiazine

        b. Pyrimethamine + folinic acid + clindamycin

E. MAC

    1) Risk

      a. MAC is widely dispersed in the environment; no person-to-person transmission implicated

      b. CD4 count <50/mm^3

    2) Presentation

      a. Fever

      b. Fatigue

      c. Malaise

      d. Night sweats

      e. Abdominal pain

      f. Diarrhea

      g. Neutropenia

      h. Anemia

      i. Elevated alkaline phosphatase

    3) Diagnosis

      a. Isolation of MAC from blood culture

      b. Isolation from biopsy of liver, bone marrow, lymph node, or GI tract

    4) Prophylaxis considered for CD4 count <50/mm^3

    5) Preferred regimens:

      a. Clarithromycin 500 mg PO bid

      b. Azithromycin 1200 mg PO q wk

    6) Alternative therapy: Rifabutin 300 mg PO qd

    7) Treatment of active disease involves multidrug therapy using clarithromycin or azithromycin + ethambutol + rifabutin

F. *Mycobacterium tuberculosis* (TB)

    1) Risk

      a. Latent reactivation

      b. Thirty to 50% of cases are primary TB

      c. CD4 count <500/mm^3

    2) Presentation

      a. Asymptomatic with positive PPD ≥5 mm on screening

      b. Atypical clinical findings in advanced HIV disease

        i. Lower lobe infiltrates

        ii. Infrequent cavitary lesions

        iii. Mediastinal lymphadenopathy

        iv. Extrapulmonary infection (lymph node, meningeal)

    3) Diagnosis

      a. Screening PPD annually

      b. Chest x-ray

      c. Sputum culture for acid-fast bacilli

      d. Biopsy of extrapulmonary site

4) Prophylaxis for patients with no active disease and:
   a. Positive PPD of ≥5 mm induration
   b. History of positive PPD with inadequate chemoprophylaxis
   c. High-risk contacts of person with active TB
5) Preferred regimen for 12 months
   a. Isoniazid (INH) 300 mg PO qd *and*
   b. Pyridoxine 50 mg PO qd
6) Alternative therapy regimens
   a. INH 900 mg twice weekly by direct observation therapy
   b. Rifampin 600 mg PO qd
7) Treatment of active disease requires multidrug therapy combining at least four drugs and directly observed treatment. Multidrug-resistant strains of TB are prevalent and therapy should be adjusted according to sensitivity of the organism. First-line TB therapy drugs include:
   a. INH
   b. Rifampin
   c. Pyrazinamide
   d. Ethambutol
   e. Streptomycin
G. CMV
   1) Risk
      a. Major cause of severe complications in multiple organ systems in late-stage HIV infection
      b. CD4 count $<50/mm^3$
   2) Presentation
      a. Retinitis may be asymptomatic and detected during routine retinal exam, or symptomatic with complaints of visual disturbances
      b. GI—esophagitis, gastritis, colitis
      c. CNS—encephalitis
      d. Peripheral nervous system—radiculitis
   3) Diagnosis
      a. Positive serology
      b. Culture of urine, buffy coat, tissue obtained by biopsy
   4) Prophylaxis is not generally recommended for most patients.
      a. For seronegative patients requiring transfusion, the use of CMV-negative blood.
      b. Oral ganciclovir is FDA approved for prophylaxis but conflicting data about its efficacy and disadvantages to its use (poor bioavailability, expense) make its use an option but not a standard of care at this time.
   5) Preferred regimen for active disease uses IV drug therapy for the life of the patient using one of the following agents, which have potential serious toxicities:
      a. Ganciclovir (for retinitis an intraocular form is available)
      b. Foscarnet
      c. Cidofovir
H. *Candida*
   1) Risk
      a. Superficial *Candida* infection is extremely high. Oropharyngeal candidiasis is often the first manifestation of HIV disease and is a marker for disease progression.

b. More serious fungal infections occur with CD4 count <50–100/mm³.

2) Presentation
   a. Oropharyngeal candidiasis
   b. Vulvovaginal candidiasis
   c. Esophagitis

3) Diagnosis
   a. Oral candidiasis is usually diagnosed by characteristic white plaques on mucosal surface.
   b. Scraping of suspected area shows *Candida* pseudohypae as well as budding yeast.
   c. Endoscopy documents esophagitis.

4) Primary prophylaxis is not currently recommended for fungal infections for most patients based on multiple factors:
   a. No evidence of increased survival benefit
   b. Development of *Candida* resistance to azole drugs
   c. Problematic drug interactions with other HIV medications

5) Preferred regimen for active disease administered by route appropriate for site of infection:
   a. Nystatin
   b. Clotrimazole troche
   c. Fluconazole

6) Alternative therapy
   a. Amphotericin B
   b. Itraconazole

I. Herpes simplex

1) Risk
   a. Primary infection, oral or genital
   b. Recurrance of prior infection

2) Presentation
   a. Genital ulcers
   b. Oral lesions
   c. Esophagitis
   d. Disseminated

3) Diagnosis by direct observation and culture

4) Prophylaxis to suppress reactivation with acyclovir 400 mg PO bid

5) Preferred treatment for active disease with acyclovir oral or IV for more severe infection

6) Alternative therapy
   a. Famciclovir for genital herpes
   b. Foscarnet IV for acyclovir-resistant strains
   c. Valacyclovir not recommended for primary treatment or suppressive therapy in the HIV patient

4. Malignancy in HIV infection is probably linked to the immunosuppressive state and the loss of immune-mediated tumor surveillance. There is no prophylaxis available to prevent malignancy. Today, patients with AIDS who have had primary prophylaxis against OI may develop cancer as their first opportunistic event.

A. Kaposi's sarcoma (KS)
   1) Most common in homosexual men.
   2) Association with human herpesvirus 8.

3) Nodular lesions contain characteristic spindle cells, lymphocytes, plasma cells, and atypical endothelial cells.

4) Lesions are purple in light-skinned persons and dark brown or black in dark-skinned persons.

5) Multiple lesions may occur on skin, mucous membranes (particularly common on the palate), visceral organs. Lesions may be few in number in a scattered distribution or can involved large surface areas of extremities or torso.

6) Suspect KS in inguinal nodes if HIV patient presents with unilateral lower extremity edema.

7) Diagnosis from punch biopsy of lesion.

8) Treatment:
   a. Local therapy
      i. Topical liquid nitrogen
      ii. Intralesional vinblastine
      iii. Radiation
      iv. Laser surgery
   b. Systemic therapy regimens
      i. Adriamycin, bleomycin, and either vinblastine or vincristine
      ii. Etoposide (VP-16)
      iii. Liposomal daunorubicin
      iv. α-Interferon

B. Non-Hodgkin's lymphoma occurs later in HIV disease when CD4 cell counts are low.

1) Types of lymphoma
   a. Large-cell lymphoma
   b. Burkitt-like lymphomas
   c. Primary CNS lymphoma

2) Patients usually present with disseminated disease. Patients require cytotoxic therapy. Although a 50% complete remission rate occurs, most patients soon relapse. A median survival of 5–8 months with chemotherapy is seen. Chemotherapy regimen with cyclophosphamide, Adriamycin, vincristine, and corticosteroids ± radiation may be used.

3) Patients with an already compromised immune system from HIV disease who are treated with cytotoxic agents suffer from severe bone marrow suppression.
   a. Neutropenia may be treated with colony-stimulating factors.
   b. Anemia may be treated with erythropoietin or transfusion of packed red blood cells.
   c. Thrombocytopenia may be treated with platelet transfusion.

4) Development of OI is likely and requires the appropriate drug regimen based on the type of OI.

5) Side effects from the chemotherapy (nausea, vomiting, hair loss) are managed with supportive therapies.

C. Cervical cancer is an AIDS-defining illness in HIV-infected women.

1) Higher risk of cervical intraepithelial neoplasia (CIN) in women with HIV.

2) There is also a higher incidence of human papillomavirus in this group.

3) High rate of cervical dysplasia and reports of rapidly progressive cervical cancer in HIV-positive women.

4) Routine monitoring of Pap smears in HIV-positive women are performed to detect abnormalities. Referral to a gynecologist for colposcopy and biopsy for results showing atypia or CIN I–III.

5) High-grade lesions require treatments such as cryotherapy, loop excision, laser, or conization.

6) Recurrence rate after standard therapy is increased in HIV-positive women.

PATIENT EDUCATION

Multiple areas of focus for patient education exist and depend upon the patient's location on the HIV disease spectrum and current lifestyle.

1. Counseling on prevention of spread of HIV disease to others.
   A. Safer sex practices (limit number of partners, always use condoms, no exchange of body secretions)
   B. Household contact and management of situations involving blood or body secretions
   C. Risk behavior reduction for IV drug users
   D. Prevention of pregnancy
2. Explanation of anticipated course of illness/prognosis.
   A. Monitoring of condition
   B. Laboratory testing (CD4 cell counts and viral load)
3. Avoidance of exposure to opportunistic infection.
   A. Sexual
   B. Environmental and occupational
   C. Pet related
   D. Food and water related
   E. Travel related
4. Opportunistic infections.
   A. Signs, symptoms, and seeking health care
   B. Prophylaxis
5. Antiretroviral therapy.
   A. Options for therapy
   B. Side effects and their management
   C. Monitoring therapy
6. Confidentiality versus notification of HIV status.
   A. Notify sexual partners and/or needle-sharing partners.
   B. Notify health care providers.
   C. Health care workers may need to notify their employers based on institutional guidelines.
   D. Repercussions of notification.
7. Counseling on general wellness and health maintenance.
   A. Diet (may need nutritional assessment and counseling to avoid eating raw meat or eggs to prevent disease exposure)
   B. Exercise (based on status, exercise is encouraged in moderation)
   C. Smoking cessation
   D. Alcohol use (no more than one drink per day)
   E. Avoid any use of recreational drug
   F. Routine eye exam and retinal exam every 6 months with CD4 count $<100/mm^3$.
   G. Gynecologic exam and Pap smear every 6 months

8. Referral to resources.
   A. Financial assistance/special entitlement programs
   B. Clinical trials
   C. Support groups (HIV, drug, alcohol)
   D. Substance abuse programs for addicted patients
9. Patients with advanced AIDS may need referrals to:
   A. Home care agencies
   B. Hospice
   C. Pain service or clinic for management of chronic neuropathy or other pain
   D. Legal services for advance directives, wills, disability claims
10. Supportive counseling of patient, partners, families in regard to the psychological impact of disease and dying.

Review Questions

11.16 Which of the following tests is most definitive for the diagnosis of AIDS?
   A. CD4 count
   B. HIV plasma load by RTA PCR
   C. HIV ELISA
   D. Western blot

11.17 Which pharmacologic regimen is recommended to a health care worker exposed to HIV-infected blood through a mucous membrane route?
   A. AZT and 3TC
   B. AZT, 3TC, and indinavir
   C. AZT only
   D. 3TC only

11.18 A newly diagnosed HIV patient is in your care. The patient has a positive PPD result of 5 mm induration and a normal chest x-ray. Which of the following represents preferred treatment of this patient?
   A. INH 300 mg PO qid + pyridoxine 50 mg PO qd for 12 months
   B. INH 900 mg three times a week + rifampin 600 mg PO qd
   C. Rifabutin 300 mg PO bid + streptomycin 500 mg once a week
   D. Directly observed therapy with a five-drug regimen

Answers and Rationales

11.16 **D** The Western blot is the confirmatory test for HIV infection. The ELISA is a screening test that has to be confirmed with a Western blot. The CD4 and the RTA PCR counts are predictors of HIV progression.

11.17 **A** A health care worker exposed to blood via mucous membranes or skin should be offered AZT and 3TC ±indinavir.

11.18 **A** One year of prophylaxis is recommended for the HIV-positive patient with a positive PPD of ≥5 mm and no evidence of active tuberculosis.

References

Bartlett, J.G. (1996). *The Johns Hopkins Hospital 1996 Guide to Medical Care of Patients with HIV Infection.* Baltimore: Williams & Wilkins.

Bartlett, J.G., & Feinberg, J. (1996). Management of opportunistic infections in patients with HIV infection: Update. *Infect Dis Clin Pract 4,* 267–276.

Carpenter, C.J., Fischl, M.A., Hammer, S.M., et al. (1997). Antiretroviral therapy for HIV infection in 1997 updated recommendations of the International AIDS Society–USA panel. *J Amer Med Assoc 277,* 1962–1969.

Centers for Disease Control. (1992). 1993 Revised classification system for HIV infection and expanded surveillance case definition for AIDS among adolescents and adults. *MMWR Morbid Mortal Wkly Rep 41,* 1–19.

Centers for Disease Control and Prevention. (1996). Update: Provisional public health service recommendations for chemoprophylaxis after occupational exposure to HIV. *MMWR Morbid Mortal Wkly Rep 45,* 468–472.

Centers for Disease Control and Prevention. (1996). Ten leading nationally notifiable infectious diseases—United States, 1995. *MMWR Morbid Mortal Wkly Rep 45,* 883–884.

Centers for Disease Control and Prevention. (1996). *HIV/AIDS Surveillance Report, 8.*

Centers for Disease Control and Prevention. (1997). USPHA/ISDA guidelines for the prevention of opportunistic infections in persons infected with human immunodeficiency virus. *MMWR Morbid Mortal Wkly Rep 46,* 1–46.

Centers for Disease Control and Prevention. (1997). Update: Trends in AIDS incidence, deaths, and prevalence—United States, 1996. *MMWR Morbid Mortal Wkly Rep 46,* 165–173.

Greenspan, D., & Greenspan, J.S. (1996). HIV-related oral disease. *Lancet 348,* 729–733.

Masur, H., Whitcup, S.M., Carwright, C., et al. (1996). Advances in the management of AIDS-related cytomegalovirus retinitis. *Ann Intern Med 125,* 126–145.

Tribett, D. (1995). Human immunodeficiency virus (HIV) and acquired immunodeficiency syndrome (AIDS). In N.A. Urban, K.K. Greenlee, J.M. Krumberger, et al. (eds.). *Guideline for Critical Care Nursing.* St. Louis: C.V. Mosby Co., pp. 574–586.

Tschachler, E., Bergstresser, P.R., & Stingl, G. (1996). HIV-related skin disease. *Lancet 348,* 659–663.

Pain Management

Pain management should be an important aspect of a health professional's commitment to total patient care. The goal is to relieve pain with a minimum of side effects.

DEFINITION

According to the International Association for the Study of Pain, pain is "an unpleasant sensory and emotional experience associated with actual or potential tissue damage, or described in terms of such damage" (Storey, 1996).

BASIC CONCEPTS OF PAIN MANAGEMENT

1. Principles of effective management
   A. Prevention is better than treatment. Established pain is difficult to control.

B. Regularly reassess efficiency of pain management and side effects.

C. Consider patient preferences regarding methods and routes of administration.

D. Address psychological factors and functional deficits.

E. Consider a multidisciplinary approach.

2. Patients who may require additional consideration:
   A. Those who are cognitively impaired
   B. Those who are psychotic
   C. The pediatric and the elderly
   D. Those who do not speak English
   E. Those with cultural differences regarding pain and its meaning

3. Somatic pain versus visceral pain

	Somatic Pain	Visceral Pain
Site	Well localized	Poorly localized
Radiation	Follows distribution of somatic nerve	Diffuse radiation
Character	Sharp, definite	Dull, vague
Relation to stimulus	Hurts where stimulus is	May be referred
Time	Often constant	Often periodic

4. General principles for pharmacologic management
   A. Choose an appropriate drug.
   B. Choose a short-acting drug.
   C. Utilize one drug at a time and start with low doses (particularly in the young and old).
   D. Increase the dose until relief is obtained or side effects occur, or until maximum dose is reached.

5. Medications and recommended dosages
   A. Nonsteroidal anti-inflammatory drugs (NSAIDs)
      1) Acetaminophen 325–650 mg PO q4–6h
      2) Ibuprofen 200–600 mg PO q6h
      3) Naproxen 250–375 mg bid
   B. Anticonvulsants
      1) Carbamazepine 50–100 mg PO qhs/bid starting dose
      2) Gabapentin 150–300 mg qd
      3) Phenytoin 100 mg PO qhs/bid starting dose
   C. Tricyclic antidepressants
      1) Amitriptyline 10–25 mg PO qhs
      2) Nortriptyline 10–25 mg PO qhs
      3) Desipramine 10–25 mg PO q A.M.
   D. Selective serotonin reuptake inhibitor
      1) Fluoxetine 20 mg; may increase to 20 mg bid
      2) Paroxetine 20 mg; may increase if needed by 20 mg up to 50 mg
   E. Antiarrhythmic: Mexiletine 150 mg PO tid, with range from 450 to 900 mg qd
   F. Psychostimulants: Methylphenidate 2.5 mg PO qd, then qd and q noon, titrating to desired dose with range of doses from 10 to 40 mg qd
   G. Opioids: See Table 11–6
   H. Patient-controlled analgesia (PCA) either intravenously or epidurally. ACNP should consult with anesthesiologist for starting dose and titration. This includes continuous infusion rate, bolus rate, and lockout intervals. This may vary according to different institutional protocols.

TABLE 11–6. Equal Analgesic Dose of Opioids for Pain Management

	Oral	Rectal	IM/SC
Morphine	30	30b	10
Codeine	200	NA	60
Oxycodone (hydrocodone)	15	NA	NA
Dilaudid (hydromorphone)	4	3	1.5
Methadone	10	NA	5
Fentanyl patch (75 mg/hr patch = 30 mg oral morphine q4h)			

Patient Status	Suggested Analgesic
No pain orders; patient expresses need for a pain medication	Acetaminophen 325 mg 1–2 tab q4–6h *or* ibuprofen 400 or 600 mg q6h
Patient taking maximum dose of acetaminophen (4 gm/day) or NSAIDs (equivalent to 2400 mg ibuprofen/day) and additional pain relief is needed	Hydrocodone bitartrate with APAP 5/500 mg (Vicodin) 1–2 tab q4–6h *or* oxycodone 5 mg 1–3 tab q4–6h
Patient taking maximum dose of Vicodin (4 gm acetaminophen) or oxycodone and additional pain relief is needed	Morphine sulfate 15–30 mg 1–2 tab q4–6h *or* dilaudid (1.3 mg/10 mg of morphine)
Patient can no longer take medications PO	Morphine solution (20 mg/mL) may be given sublingually as an equivalent morphine PO dose; second choice is PR or IM
Patient allergic to all opioids	Methadone 5–20 mg q6–8h

ACUTE PAIN/POSTOPERATIVE PAIN

DEFINITION

Acute pain is usually easily identified with a cause and signals tissue damage, causing immobility essential for tissue healing. Anxiety is frequently associated with acute pain. Examples of causes of acute pain include:

1. Acute disease—surgery, posttraumatic pain, burns, myocardial infarction, acute pancreatitis, renal colic, biliary colic
2. Chronic disease: Can have acute exacerbations such as cancer with compression fractures from bone metastasis, AIDS, vascular disease with seasonal exacerbations
3. May be cutaneous, somatic, or visceral

Occurrence of Incidents That May Involve Acute Pain

1. Estimated 64,000,000 patients with injuries/year
2. Estimated 49,000,000 patients with acute disease/year
3. Estimated 23,000,000 patients undergo surgery/year

Significance of Proper Management of Acute/Postoperative Pain

1. Postoperatively, patients are at increased risk for deep venous thrombi, pulmonary emboli, myocardial infarction, and vascular occlusion resulting from hypercoaguability.

2. Mainstay of postoperative pain management was intramuscular injections of Demerol and morphine, which was ineffective because of route and method of administration.
3. Today, PCA pumps and epidural infusions not only control pain more effectively, they also decrease hypercoaguability as a result of pain. Additionally, this sense of control increases patient satisfaction and perception of adequate pain management.

Effects of Postoperative Pain

1. Respiratory system
   A. Respiratory dysfunction after surgery or trauma to chest leads to muscle splinting.
   B. Causes decreased tidal volume, vital capacity, and alveolar ventilation.
   C. Can lead to atelectasis, hypercarbia, hypoxia.
   D. Elderly, smokers, and those with respiratory disease at higher risk for postoperative respiratory complications.
   E. Manifested by splinting of abdominal and thoracic muscles, grunting on expiration, rapid respiratory rate, and decreased tidal volume.
2. Cardiovascular system
   A. Acute pain increases sympathetic activity, which leads to increase in heart rate, peripheral resistance, blood pressure, and cardiac output.
   B. Increase in myocardial oxygen consumption and risk of hypoxemia.
   C. Alpha receptors in the coronary vasculature may respond with vasoconstriction, raising the risk of myocardial ischemia, angina, and myocardial infarction.
   D. Peripherally, decreased limb blood flow, which is serious in patients undergoing vascular grafting operations.
3. Musculoskeletal system
   A. Pain may precipitate muscle spasms that increase pain, developing a vicious cycle.
   B. Persistent postoperative pain limits mobility, which impairs muscle metabolism, which may lead to muscle atrophy and delayed return of function.
4. Gastrointestinal and urinary systems
   A. Increased sympathetic activity increases intestinal secretions and smooth muscle tone, which decreases intestinal motility.
   B. Gastric stasis and paralytic ileus may occur as side effect from opioids.
   C. Increased urinary sphincter activity leads to urinary retention.

MANAGEMENT/TREATMENT

1. Treatment of acute pain is aimed at interrupting the nociceptive signals.
2. Successful management of postoperative/acute pain begins with preoperative assessment of pain levels and patient education regarding expected outcomes of pain management.
3. Nonpharmacologic management involves cognitive/behavior options such as relaxation exercises, imagery, and music therapy by referral to psychology services and/or recreational therapy.
4. Pharmacologic management involving nonsteroidal anti-inflammatory agents, opioids, PCA infusions, spinal analgesia (epidural opioid and/or local anesthetic infusion), and/or local nerve blockade.

5. Physical therapy options such as massage, heat, and cold therapy.
6. Physical therapy may use transcutaneous electrical nerve stimulation (TENS), which consists of selective stimulation of cutaneous receptors with low-intensity electrical current applied via skin electrodes. This appears to decrease pain perception by the individual by disrupting the transmission of the pain impulse.
7. Special considerations should be given to the geriatric patient.

CHRONIC PAIN

DEFINITION

Chronic pain persists for over 1 month beyond the usual course of an acute illness or injury. It may include pain that recurs at intervals over a long period of time, or pain that is a result of a chronic pathologic process. Chronic pain is to be distinguished from chronic pain syndrome, which involves complaints of pain, chronic anxiety and depression, and probable permanent lifestyle changes.

UNIQUE FEATURES OF CHRONIC PAIN

1. Cause of chronic pain tends to be multifactorial.
2. Cumulative effect of chronic pain is often maladaptive behavior.
3. Often accompanied by depression.
4. Functional decline is usually present.

SIGNS AND SYMPTOMS

1. Presents with complex collection of symptoms and signs that may not have a direct connection to the injury or tissue damage that initiated the pain.
2. Psychological findings—depression, anxiety, frustration, anger, decreased self-worth, decreased self-esteem.
3. Impact on activities of daily living—sleep disturbances, change in appetite, inactivity, bowel/bladder dysfunction.
4. Changes in personal relationships—altered family dynamics, decreased libido, decreased involvement in social activities.
5. Impact on health maintenance—increased number of health care visits, frequent use of medications.
6. Social concerns—financial stresses, inability to work, legal issues.

Goals for Management of Chronic Pain

1. Increased tolerance for physical activity
2. Decreased suffering and pain
3. Decreased use of the health care system
4. Decreased use of medications
5. Return to work or other role in society

MANAGEMENT/TREATMENT

1. Treatment of choice is prevention, which requires early and adequate acute pain treatment.

2. Pharmacologic (see below)
3. Physical therapy, such as exercise, range of motion, and TENS unit.
4. Referral to pain clinic, anesthesiologist, or neurosurgeon for blockade procedures such as trigger point injections, epidural steroid injection (i.e., low back pain), efferent sympathetic interruption (i.e., reflex sympathetic dystrophy).
5. Mental health referral for possible individual or marital counseling, training in biofeedback/relaxation techniques, or treatment of psychiatric co-morbidities as indicated.

Pharmacological Treatment

1. NSAID: Suggested for rheumatoid arthritis, fibromyalgia
2. Tricyclic antidepressants such as amitriptyline, desipramine HCl, and nortriptyline HCl: Suggested for burning, neuropathic pain (e.g., diabetic peripheral neuropathy)
3. Anticonvulsants such as carbamazepine, phenytoin, and gabapentin: Suggested for lancinating neuropathic pain (such as trigeminal neuralgia)
4. Antiarrhythmic agents such as mexiletine: Suggested for pain that is not relieved by other classifications of medications
5. Topical agents such as capsaicin cream: Suggested for postherpetic neuralgia
6. Selective serotonin reuptake inhibitors such as fluoxetine HCl and paroxetine HCl: May help with neuropathic pain, especially if associated with depression
7. Opioids: Generally avoided but may be used in selected patients if monitored carefully

Side Effects/Patient Education Issues

1. NSAIDs: Increase risk of ulcer disease, bleeding, and renal dysfunction. Need to monitor renal function (especially in the elderly), avoid acetyl salicylic acid (aspirin) and warfarin.
2. Opioids—sedation, cognitive impairment, constipation, nausea, vomiting, pruritus, ileus, respiratory depression.
3. Tricyclic antidepressants—anticholinergic side effects (dryness of mouth, urinary retention, constipation, delirium), postural hypotension, and cardiac arrhythmias.

NEUROPATHIC PAIN

DEFINITION

Neuropathic pain is a type of chronic pain that results from trauma or disease that causes damage by transection, avulsion, or demylination to the peripheral nerves, posterior roots, spinal, cord or certain areas of the brain. Common examples of neuropathic pain include:

1. Postherpetic neuralgia
2. Phantom limb
3. Trigeminal neuralgia

4. Multiple sclerosis
5. Neuroma

Characteristics of Neuropathic Pain

1. Continuous, spontaneous: In the skin (burning, cutting, pricking sensation), in the muscles or bone (throbbing, crushing sensation)
2. Paroxysmal: Short duration, shooting, electric-like sensation
3. Allodynia: Produces a pain inconsistent with the stimulus
4. Hyperalgesia: Painful sensation of abnormal severity following noxious stimulation

Neuropathic Pain and Normal Pain Can Coexist

1. Failed lumbar disc can cause neuropathic pain secondary to compression injury to spinal nerve or root, and normal pain is due to activation of periosteal nociceptors in the facet joint and activation of nociceptors innervating pain sheath.
2. Cancer tumors can produce normal pain by activating nociceptors in muscle, viscera, and bone secondary to mechanical compression and distention. When nerve, plexus, root, or spinal cord is involved, neuropathic pain may result.

Postherpetic Neuralgia

DEFINITION

Presence of pain more than 1 month after the onset of the eruption of zoster or pain existing after crusting of skin lesions.

ETIOLOGY/INCIDENCE

1. Ten to 70% of patients develop postherpetic neuralgia.
2. Increased incidence in females, the elderly, and those patients with ophthalmic zoster.
3. Pain results from injury to the peripheral nerves and central nervous system signal processing.
4. Peripheral neurons discharge spontaneously, have decreased activation threshold and exaggerated responses to stimuli.
5. Hyperexcitability of the dorsal horn results in exaggerated central nervous system response to input.

SIGN AND SYMPTOMS

1. Pain may be described as similar to pain preceding outbreak of zoster.
2. Described as deep, aching, or burning.
3. Altered sensitivity to touch (paresthesia).
4. Exaggerated response to stimuli (hyperesthesia).
5. May be provoked by trivial stimuli (allodynia).
6. Escalated pain by repeated stimulation (windup).
7. Area of pain surrounds the area of zoster scarring and may be quite wide.
8. Pain interrupts sleep, mood, and work, affecting quality of life.

MANAGEMENT/TREATMENT

1. Nonpharmacologic treatment
   A. Physical therapy consult for possible TENS unit trial.
   B. Psychology consult for possible hypnosis, biofeedback, or behavioral counseling if appropriate. It is thought that these techniques can help decrease anxiety, improve the ability to relax, and offer alternative coping mechanisms for the individual living with pain.
2. Pharmacologic treatment
   A. Topical medications such as lidocaine 5% gel have been mentioned in the research literature, while the use of capsaicin has been controversial.
   B. Mild analgesics such as aspirin and ibuprofen afford limited relief.
   C. Narcotics usually not effective and should be used cautiously.
   D. Tricyclic antidepressants work by blocking the reuptake of norepinephrine and serotonin and relieve pain by increasing the inhibition of spinal neurons involved in pain perceptions.
   E. Anticonvulsant drugs decrease the lancinating component of neuropathic pain.
3. Persistent pain
   A. Referral to pain management specialty clinic/anesthesiologist for possible nerve block, implantable medication pump
   B. Referral to neurosurgery clinic for possible procedures such as electrical stimulus of the thalamus, counterirritation

PATIENT EDUCATION

1. Inform patient that pain control may take several weeks to reach maximum benefits.
2. Teach about side effects of medication and drug interactions.
3. Contact American Pain Society (708-966-5595) for list of pain clinics/specialists.
4. Contact Varicella-Zoster Virus Research Foundation (212-472-3181) for newsletter and support group information.

Phantom Pain

DEFINITIONS

Phantom pain: Painful sensations referred to the missing limb
Stump pain: Pain at the site of the extremity amputation
Phantom limb: Any sensation of the missing limb except pain

ETIOLOGY/INCIDENCE

1. Variable reports from 0.02% to 100% in the research literature.
2. Usually in the first postoperative week 50–75% will report phantom pain.
3. May be delayed in onset.

SIGNS AND SYMPTOMS

1. Characteristics of phantom pain
   A. Usually distal in phantom limb
   B. Varied reports of quality of pain
   C. Varied reports regarding length of time pain exists
2. Characteristics of stump pain
   A. Localized to the stump, usually posterior aspect of the scar.
   B. Can occur despite healing of the incision.

   C. Chorea of the stump can occur, ranging from painful, hardly visible myo-
       clonic jerks to severe clonic contractions of the stump.
   D. Long-term stump pain predisposes to phantom pain.
3. Aggravating factors
   A. Emotional distress
   B. Pressure or touch applied to the stump
   C. Stimulation of other body parts
   D. Wearing a prosthesis
   E. Weather changes
4. Relieving factors
   A. Rest
   B. Distraction
   C. Cold or heat
   D. Using a prosthesis
   E. Elevation and/or massage of stump

MANAGEMENT/TREATMENT

1. Nonpharmacologic treatment
   A. Physical therapy consult for possible TENS unit trial, ultrasound, mas-
       sage, and instruction to the patient and the family regarding the value
       of passive movement to prevent trophic changes and vascular congestion.
   B. Psychology consult for possible instruction in relaxation techniques, hyp-
       nosis, or biofeedback techniques.
   C. May consider referral to clinic that performs acupuncture (thought to
       assist with balancing an individual's energy pathway). For additional
       information, contact the American Association of Acupuncture and Ori-
       ental Medicine (610-433-2448).
2. Pharmacologic treatment
   A. No specific classification of medication is solely indicated.
   B. Anticonvulsants such as carbamazepine strongly suggested as being
       most effective for unknown reason.
   C. Antidepressants such as fluoxetine in low doses.
   D. Opioids may be tried; however, usually not as effective for neuropathic
       pain.
3. Invasive treatment: Surgical consult for stump revision for neuromas may
    be considered; however, neuromas may reoccur.

CANCER PAIN

Pain associated with cancer is frequently undertreated. Flexibility is the key
to treatment because changes in diagnosis, stage of disease, response to pain
interventions, and personal preferences must be considered. Because cancer
pain exhibits features of both acute and chronic pain, treatment should employ
multiple modalities.

Barriers to Cancer Pain Management

1. Clinician's inadequate knowledge
   A. Pain management options
   B. Poor assessment and reassessment
   C. Fear of addiction
   D. Fear of side effects

2. Patient's belief system
   A. Reluctance to report pain
   B. Fear that pain means disease is worse
   C. Fear of addiction
   D. Fear of side effects

Assessment is Crucial!

1. Initial assessment
   A. History, including functional abilities
   B. Physical exam
   C. Psychosocial
   D. Diagnostic findings
2. Pain assessment
   A. Quality of pain: Use of descriptive phrases such as "burning, sharp, agonizing" to describe the sensory perception of the individual's pain.
   B. Intensity: Also known as the severity rating, usually on a scale of 0–10.
   C. Location: The area where the pain is felt (may need body map), and radiates.
   D. Duration: The length of time per episode of pain; may help if patient is able to keep a journal.
   E. Precipitating and palliating features.
   F. Associated symptoms (e.g., anxiety, depression, nausea, dyspnea).
   G. Determine goals for pain control with patient/family (e.g., complete pain relief vs. maintain mentally alert or functional status).
   H. Reassess often, particularly after drug/dose/route change is initiated for efficiency and side effects.
   I. Check for behavior changes suggesting pain in patients who are cognitively impaired.

Common Cancer Pain

1. Bone pain
   A. Most common causes are multiple myeloma or metastatic carcinoma of the lung, breast, and prostate.
   B. Must rule out nonneoplastic causes such as osteoporotic fractures and focal osteonecrosis.
   C. Most common areas of bony metastases are the spine, pelvis, ribs, and proximal long bones.
   D. Back pain may be indicator of epidural compression.
2. Spinal cord compression
   A. May be caused by posterior extension of vertebral body metastasis to the epidural space or by tumor extension.
   B. Untreated leads to neurologic compromise, including paraplegia or quadriplegia.
   C. Back pain, especially if rapidly progressing in a crescendo pattern, is particularly ominous for epidural compression.
   D. Back or radicular pain that is exacerbated by recumbency, cough, sneeze, or strain is suggestive of epidural compression.
   E. Weakness, sensory loss, autonomic dysfunction (e.g., urinary retention), and reflex abnormalities.

F. Effective treatment, involving corticosteroids, radiation therapy, or neurosurgical decompression, may decrease the amount of neurologic involvement depending on the amount of impairment noted at onset of the treatment.

3. Peripheral nerve injury: May be the result of chemotherapy, radiation, or surgical interventions for treatment of cancer

4. Postchemotherapy pain syndromes
   A. Chronic painful peripheral neuropathy (e.g., vincristine)
   B. Avascular (aseptic) necrosis of femoral or humeral head
      1) May occur spontaneously or as a complication of corticosteroid therapy.
      2) May be unilateral or bilateral.
      3) Femoral head involvement is more common with pain in hip, thigh, or knee.
      4) Humeral head involvement presents with pain in shoulder, upper arm, or elbow.
      5) Pain is exacerbated by movement and relieved with rest.
      6) Pain precedes radiologic changes by weeks to months.
      7) Treatment may include analgesics, decrease or discontinuation of steroids, and possible joint replacement.
   C. Plexopathy: caused by infusion of chemotherapy

5. Hormonal therapy
   A. Chronic gynecomastia and breast tenderness as result of antiandrogen therapies for prostate cancer.
   B. Increased association with diethylstilbestrol, less common with flutamide and cyproterone.
   C. Primary or secondary breast cancer must be ruled out, particularly in the geriatric population.

6. Chronic postradiation pain syndromes
   A. Brachial and lumbosacral plexopathies
      1) Weakness and sensory changes in the C5, C6 plexuses.
      2) Radiation changes and lymphedema are usually seen.
      3) Usually progressive, although patients may plateau.
   B. Chronic radiation myelopathy
      1) Late complication of spinal cord irradiation (latency period of 12–14 months).
      2) Most common presentation is partial transverse myeolopathy at the cervicothoracic level.
      3) Pain typically precedes the development of progressive motor dysfunction.
      4) Pain is usually localized at area of spinal cord damage or below, described as burning.
   C. Chronic radiation enteritis/proctitis
      1) Occur as a delayed complication in 2–10% of those patients who have abdominal or pelvic radiation therapy.
      2) Rectum and rectosigmoid more commonly involved than the small bowel.
      3) Signs and symptoms include bloody diarrhea, tenesmus, or cramping pain caused by proctitis or obstruction from stricture formation.
      4) Colicky abdominal pain associated with nausea and/or malabsorption may indicate small-bowel radiation damage.

MANAGEMENT/TREATMENT

1. Nonpharmacologic treatment
   A. Physical therapy consult for cutaneous stimulation such as heat pad, coldpack, massage, and exercise to strengthen weak muscles and improve joint function
   B. Nursing orders or family instruction regarding frequent repositioning
   C. Immobilization to manage acute pain or to stabilize fractures
   D. Appropriate referrals for TENS acupuncture
   E. Psychology referral for behavioral techniques such as relaxation, imagery, biofeedback
   F. Patient education and psychotherapy support regarding disease process and pain management options available
   G. Referral to social worker for support groups for patient and caregivers; referral to chaplain for spiritual counseling if desired
2. Pharmacologic treatment
   A. Essential to individualize the regimen to the patient.
   B. Stepwise approach recommended by the World Health Organization (WHO) (see Fig. 11–1).
   C. Use simplest dosage schedules with least invasive route first.
   D. If mild to moderate pain, use step 1 of the WHO analgesic ladder.
   E. If pain continues or becomes moderate to severe, use step 2 of the WHO analgesic ladder.
   F. If pain is moderate to severe, use step 3 of the WHO analgesic ladder.
   G. Use different drug in same category before changing category of medications.
   H. Use routine (not prn) dosing schedules, with breakthrough pain medication available as needed.

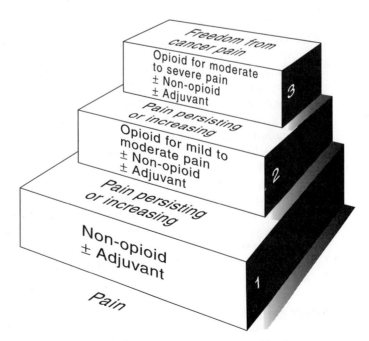

FIGURE 11–1. WHO three-step analgesic ladder. (Adapted from World Health Organization. [1997] with permission.)

3. Categories of medications
   A. Acetaminophen/NSAID
      1) Available in oral tablets, caplets, liquids, or suppository form with exception of ketorolac, which is approved for parenteral use.
      2) Not for use for those patients with thrombocytopenia or at risk for platelet dysfunction.
      3) May cause renal failure, hepatic dysfunction, bleeding, or gastric ulceration.
      4) Use cautiously in those patients taking Coumadin, methotrexate, digoxin, oral antidiabetic agents, and sulfa drugs because of potential for altered efficacy or toxicity.
      5) Use cautiously in the geriatric patient.
   B. Opioids
      1) Opioid tolerance and physical dependence does not indicate addiction.
      2) Potential to become opioid tolerant during long-term therapy may require increasing dose of opioids during pain management.
      3) Full agonists such as morphine will not reach a dose "ceiling"; therefore, doses may be progressively increased until pain is relieved or side effects occur.
      4) Morphine is available in sustained-release, immediate-release, oral solution, and rectal suppositories.
      5) Meperidine is considered useful only for brief period because of its short duration of action and its toxic metabolite.
      6) Mixed agonist-antagonists have dose-related ceiling effect and are limited in their use for cancer pain.
      7) Methadone useful for patients allergic to opioids but long half-life may cause prolonged duration of side effects.
   C. Adjuvant drugs
      1) Corticosteroids for reduction of cerebral or spinal cord edema; antiemetic, anti-inflammatory action; appetite stimulation; and treatment of epidural compression.
      2) Anticonvulsants (e.g., carbamazepine) or antidepressants (e.g., amitriptyline) for neuropathic pain.
      3) Neuroleptics for sedation and antiemetic effect.
      4) Psychostimulants to reduce opioid-induced sedation and increase appetite (e.g., methylphenidate).
      5) Placebos should not be used in pain management.
4. Management of side effects (see "Hospice Care")
5. Invasive techniques for pain management
   The ACNP should consider:
   A. Oncology consult for possible radiation therapy: local, whole body, or single injection such as strontium-89
   B. Surgical consult for curative excision or palliative debulking of tumor
   C. Anesthesia consult for nerve block, epidural injection, PCA, or implantation of pumps to deliver medications continuously
   D. Neurosurgical consult for ablation of nerve pathways, or electrical stimulation therapy

PATIENT EDUCATION

1. Instruct patient/family in pain management regimen, including side effects.
2. Encourage use of a log to determine outcome of pain management regimen.

3. Encourage reporting of side effects and functional changes related to pain management regimen.
4. Reassess often, including patient and/or family in changes in regimen.
5. Encourage individual and group support.

HOSPICE CARE

DEFINITION

Hospice care is also known as palliative care. According to the World Health Organization, palliative care "is the active total care of patients whose disease is not responsive to curative treatment. Control of pain, of other symptoms, and of psychological, social, and spiritual problems is paramount. The goal of palliative care is achievement of the best possible quality of life for patients and their families" (Storey, 1996).

Aspects of Palliative Care

1. Affirms life and regards dying as a normal process
2. Does not hasten or postpone death
3. Provides relief from pain
4. Offers psychological and spiritual support to the patient and family
5. Assists with the bereavement process
6. Is compatible with radiotherapy, chemotherapy, and palliative surgery when the symptomatic benefits outweight the disadvantages

MANAGEMENT/TREATMENT

1. See *"Cancer Pain."*
2. When conversion from one medication to another is needed, calcuate amount of routine and breakthrough pain medication taken over 24 hours for baseline information.
3. See Table 11–6 for equal analgesic doses.

Common Side Effects in Pain Management/ Palliative Care

1. Dyspnea
   A. Combination of physical, psychosocial, and spiritual origins may be present.
   B. If bronchospasm is present, consider nebulized bronchodilators or oral steroids.
   C. If rales are noted, reduce artificial feedings, stop IV fluids, consider diuretics, consider antibiotics for pneumonia if patient/family request.
   D. If effusion is present, thoracentesis may be considered palliative.
   E. If airway obstruction is present, consider risk of aspiration and change to pureed diet to prevent aspiration.
   F. If thick secretions are present, thin with nebulized saline or dry them with nebulized atropine. These drugs also help with "death rattle."
   G. If anemia is present, occasionally a blood transfusion can increase energy and reduce dyspnea.

      H. If anxiety is a problem, consider repositioning, bedside fan, calm music, relaxation techniques; use of benzodiazepines may be helpful.

      I. Consider whether interpersonal, social, or financial problems may be contributing to dyspnea.

      J. Consider if patient would like to receive chaplain services or spiritual counseling.

2. Nausea and vomiting

      A. Check medication profile for medications such as NSAIDs that may cause nausea.

      B. Consider adding H_2-blocking drug if peptic ulceration is considered.

      C. If increased intracranial pressure is suspected, consider dexamethasone.

      D. If nausea appears related to motion sickness, consider cyclizine or meclizine.

      E. Maintain effective bowel management program to avoid obstipation.

      F. More severe nausea may require occasional suppository such as prochlorperazine with routine metoclopramide given 30 minutes prior to meals and at bedtime.

      G. If nausea becomes intractable, may require a combination of antiemetics such as haloperidol and hydroxyzine, or subcutaneous dexamethasone.

      H. Nausea associated with chemotherapy may respond to ondansetron.

      I. Frequent, small meals may be tolerated better than three large meals.

3. Anorexia

      A. Loss of appetite and cachexia are distressing symptoms to the patient and the family.

      B. Causes may include unrelieved pain, nausea, oral candidiasis, depression, constipation, retention, xerostomia, gastritis, peptic ulcers.

      C. Appetite stimulants such as megestrol, medroxyprogesterone, and dexamethasone.

      D. Discuss artificial tube feedings and total parenteral nutrition with the patient and family if desired, remembering that nasogastric and gastrostomy tube feedings are associated with high risk of aspiration pneumonia and that total parenteral nutrition has not been shown to increase survival.

      E. Recognize that the family of the hospice patient may feel strongly that withholding fluids and feedings is hastening death and they may feel feeding is a comfort issue.

4. Constipation

      A. Always review patient's medication profile and oral intake to ensure that stool softeners are ordered, such as docusate sodium, docusate/cosanthrol, and sorbitol. Metamucil may not be an appropriate choice if patient is not taking adequate fluids.

      B. Prevalent in hospice patients because of low fluid and fiber intake combined with opioid analgesic and decreased mobility.

      C. If hard fecal impaction is found, softening with an oil retention enema prior to digital removal will be needed.

      D. If soft impaction is suspected, bisacodyl suppositories or enemas may be needed.

      E. Bowel management program must be initiated and followed as closely as pain management regimen, particularly when changes are made in medication regimen.

      F. Bulk-forming agents such as psyllium should be avoided when inadequate amount of fluids are being taken.

G. May begin bowel management program with docusate or docusate with casathranol.

H. Consider bisacodyl tablets or suppositories on a routine basis (q3d if no bowel movement).

I. If additional bowel care is needed, consider higher dose docusate or low-dose sorbitol.

J. If constipation is severe, sodium phosphate by mouth may be considered; soapsuds enema, enema with higher volume delivered higher up into the colon may be needed.

K. Do not forget the social and psychological aspects of constipation; occasionally use of a bedside commode may facilitate bowel management.

5. Restlessness and delirium

A. Common in final stage of life.

B. May be due to pain, anxiety, constipation, or urinary retention.

C. May be related to drug interactions.

D. May be due to electrolyte or glucose abnormality.

E. May be related to liver disease.

F. May be due to hypoxia.

G. May be indicative of brain metastases.

H. If unable to find cause, may need neuroleptic agent.

I. Haloperidol by mouth or subcutaneously may be effective.

J. In patients with AIDS dementia, oral thioridazine or chlorpromazine may be more effective.

K. In severe agitated delirium, benzodiazepines may be necessary, such as lorazepam PO or sublingually.

Burnout Prevention

1. Not only an issue for the family and caregivers of the hospice patient, but also an issue for the health care professionals who care for them both.
2. Be aware of and acknowledge its existence.
3. Begin a support group for those interested.
4. Continued reading on burnout prevention should be done.

GERIATRIC CONSIDERATIONS

Etiology/Incidence

The experience of pain in the geriatric population is considered common because of the increased frequency of illness and injury. Frequent sources of pain include osteoarthritis, headaches, vertebral compression fractures, low back pain, postherpetic neuralgia, peripheral vascular disease, and cancer. However, the elderly tend to underreport their pain.

Psychological Reasons Why Pain is Underreported

1. Geriatric patients "don't want to bother anyone."
2. Belief in ageism or that pain is a natural part of aging.
3. Fear of overmedication and addiction.
4. Pain is considered a weakness, especially for men.
5. Implications of increased pain could be frightening.
6. Complaints of exhaustion and constipation are more immediate concerns to the elderly.

Possible Manifestations of Pain

1. Facial or vocal changes
2. Aggressive behavior
3. Increase in body movement
4. Changes in ability to perform activities of daily living
5. Irritability
6. Sudden confusion

MANAGEMENT/TREATMENT

1. Initial treatment approach
   A. History should include current functional ability.
   B. Discuss psychological concerns and beliefs regarding pain and its purpose.
   C. Institute nonpharmacologic treatment.
   D. When using pharmacologic agents, use agents with greatest benefit and least toxicity.
   E. Start with low doses and titrate to response and tolerance.
   F. Assess on regular basis and make adjustments as needed.
   G. Communicate with patient and family to decrease anxiety as needed.
2. Nonpharmacologic pain management strategies
   A. Physical therapy, including stretching and strengthening exercises to reduce muscle spasms and improve joint function.
   B. Heat pad, coldpack, and physical massage may be helpful.
   C. Physical therapy consult for TENS unit.
   D. Psychology consult for biofeedback, relaxation, and hypnosis.
   E. Recreational therapy consult may decrease pain by increasing mobility and giving diversion to pain perception.
3. Pharmacologic agents and precautions
   A. NSAIDs
      1) Use shorter half-life drugs such as ibuprofen, fenoprofen.
      2) Good for bone pain secondary to tumor metastasis.
      3) For severe pain, narcotics and NSAIDs work synergistically through different mechanisms.
      4) Avoid using in patients who are being anticoagulated.
      5) Should be administered with food.
      6) Caution to avoid overusage.
      7) May increase incidence of ulcers, impaired renal function, cognitive impairment, and headaches.
   B. Narcotics
      1) Geriatric patients more sensitive to therapeutic doses than younger patients because of prolonged duration of action.
      2) Start low and be cautious with titration (start with minimum recommended dose).
      3) Monitor bowel movements and start on bowel program.
      4) May increase incidence of cognitive disturbances, respiratory depression, paradoxical excitement, and agitation.
      5) Meripidine should not be used in the geriatric patient because declining renal function causes accumulation of metabolite, which may cause delerium and seizures.

C. Tricyclic antidepressants
1) Anticholinergic side effects such as confusion, delirium, cognitive impairment, dry mouth, blurred vision, tachycardia, and urinary retention are common in geriatric population.
2) Low doses to avoid side effects; single dose at half-strength at bedtime may be sufficient.
D. Benzodiazepines
1) May be used to decrease anxiety with pain; however, beware of increase half-life in geriatric population.
2) May cause sedation, drowsiness, and decreased cognitive abilities.

Review Questions

11.19 Which one of the following statements is not a principle of effective pain management?
A. Assess and reassess efficiency of pain management regimen often and regularly.
B. Consider patient preferences regarding methods and routes of pain administration.
C. Assume that the patient who is cognitively impaired will not be able to report pain.
D. Consider a multidisciplinary approach for more effective pain management.

11.20 Mrs. Y, a 65-year-old woman who is scheduled for a cholecystectomy, and is nervous about her surgery because of previous experiences regarding poor pain management with previous surgeries. Which of the following management options should be considered first?
A. Cognitive/behavior options such as relaxation exercises, imagery, and music therapy
B. Pharmalogic management such as NSAIDs, opioids, PCA infusions, or spinal analgesia
C. Preoperative assessment and patient education regarding pain management
D. Physical therapy options such as massage, heat, cold, and TENS unit

11.21 Mr. K is a 78-year-old man who presents to your clinic with postherpetic neuralgia of over 6 months' duration. He has tried ibuprofen and Tylenol with Codiene without relief. He also cannot tolerate tricyclic antidepressants because of difficulty with urination. He complains of sleeping poorly and notes his appetite has decreased, with a weight loss of 5 lb over the last month. He comes to you wanting relief of his chronic pain. What would be your next choice for management of his pain?
A. Consider anticonvulsant drugs such as carbamazepine or gabapentin
B. Consider psychological consult to evaluate for depression
C. Consult to physical therapy for trial of TENS unit
D. Have patient contact Varicella-Zoster Virus Research Foundation for information regarding support groups
E. All of the above

11.22 Mrs. P is a 74-year-old woman on your unit with a diagnosis of breast cancer with metastases to the spine and brain. She has been doing fairly well on oxycodone 10 mg PO q6h routinely with 5 mg PO q4–6h PRN for breakthrough pain. She is also on ibuprofen 600 mg q6h. Nursing staff reports that she is experiencing increased pain and is having difficulty swallowing her medications. Based on this information, you would consider:

A. Calculating total amount of routine and breakthrough oxycodone in previous 24 hours, converting to equal analgesic doses of morphine either sublingual, subcutaneous, or rectal

B. Assess for causes of increased pain, including epidural compression, obstipation, infection, anxiety

C. Consult anesthesiology for possible epidural/PCA pump for improved pain management

D. All of the above

11.23 In the geriatric patient with pain, which of the following statements is incorrect?

A. NSAIDs may increase incidence of ulcers, impaired renal function, cognitive impairment, and headaches

B. Meperidine is a safe choice for occasional acute pain relief in the geriatric patient

C. "Start low and go slow" is a good reminder in prescribing pain medications for geriatric patients

D. Many geriatric patients believe pain is part of aging

Answers and Rationales

11.19 **C**   Cognitively impaired individuals may report pain via nonverbal cues such as changes in behaviors, facial expressions, grimaces, changes in functional ability.

11.20 **C**   Although all the options listed are appropriate if indicated, preoperative assessment and patient education regarding pain and its management has been shown to positively influence the outcome of pain management.

11.21 **E**   All of the choices would be appropriate management options for care. Mr. K's complaints of alterations in sleep and appetite may be signs of depression associated with chronic pain. TENS unit may provide relief of his pain, and support groups may provide him with reassurance and increased knowledge regarding the chronicity of his pain.

11.22 **D**   All of the options would be appropriate considerations for care. It would be important to assess for other possible causes for reports of increased pain rather than assuming that it is related to the diagnosis of cancer.

11.23 **C**   Use of meperidine should be avoided in the geriatric patient because of possibility of renal impairment, increased delirium, and increased seizure activity.

References

Acute Pain Management Guideline Panel. (1992). *Acute Pain Management in Adults: Operative Procedures. Quick Reference Guide for Clinicians* (AHCPR Publ. No. 92-0019). Rockville, MD: Agency for Health Care Policy and Research.

Bennett, G. (1994). Neuropathic pain. In P.D. Wall & R. Melzack (eds.). *Textbook of Pain.* New York: Churchill Livingstone, pp. 201–224.

Cherny, N., & Portenoy, R. (1994). Cancer pain: Principles of assessment and syndromes. In P.D. Wall & R. Melzack (eds.). *Textbook of Pain.* New York: Churchill Livingstone, pp. 787–824.

Cousins, M. (1994). Acute and postoperative pain. In P.D. Wall & R. Melzack (eds.). *Textbook of Pain.* New York: Churchill Livingstone, pp. 357–387.

Dossey, B. (1994). Imagery: Awakening the inner healer. In B.M. Dossey, L. Keegan, C.E. Guzzetta, et al. (eds.). *Holistic Nursing: A Handbook for Practice.* Gaithersburg, MD: Aspen, pp. 573–605.

Ferrell, B. (1995). Pain evaluation and management in the nursing home. *Ann Intern Med 123,* 681–687.

Gaston-Johansson, F., Johansson, F., & Johansson, C. (1996). Pain in the elderly: prevalence, attitudes, and assessment. *Nurs Home Med 4*(11), 325–331.

Grichnik, K., & Ferrante, F. M. (1991). The difference between acute and chronic pain. *Mt Sinai J Med 58,* 217–220.

Hopf, H., & Weitz, S. (1994). Postoperative pain management. *Arch Surg 129,* 128–131.

Jacox, A., Carr, D.B., Payne, R., et al. (1994). *Management of Cancer Pain: Adults Quick Reference Guide No. 9* (AHCPR Publ. No. 94-0593). Rockville, MD: Agency for Health Care Policy and Research.

Jensen, T., & Rasmussen, P. (1994). Phantom pain and other phenomena after amputation. In P.D. Wall & R. Melzack (eds.). *Textbook of Pain.* New York: Churchill Livingstone, pp. 651–667.

Kost, R., & Straus, S. (1996). Postherpetic neuralgia—pathogenesis, treatment, and prevention. *N Engl J Med 335,* 32–42.

Manning, D. (1994). Physiology and anatomy of pain and pain states. In *American Pain Society: Meeting the Chronic Pain Challenge.* Los Angeles: American Pain Society, pp. 1–12.

Tangeman, J., & Jones, W. (1996). Geriatric pain management. *Strategies Geriatr 1*(3), 1–5.

Salerno, E., & Willens, J. (1996). *Pain Management Handbook.* St. Louis, MD: C.V. Mosby, Co.

Stacey, B. (1996). Effective management of chronic pain. *Postgrad Med 100,* 281–290.

Storey, P. (1994). *Primer of Palliative Care.* Gainesville, FL: Academy of Hospice Physicians.

Wall, R. (1990). Use of analgesics in the elderly. *Clin Geriatr Med 6,* 345–364.

Nutritional Management in Acute Care

POTENTIAL NUTRITIONAL CHARACTERISTICS OF ACUTELY ILL PATIENTS

1. Malnutrition
   A. An imbalance between nutritional intake and nutritional needs
   B. May be acute or chronic
   C. May exist in lean as well as obese individuals

D. Results in impaired growth and tissue repair, depressed immune function, impaired organ function, and increased mortality
E. Risk factors
1) Twenty percent below ideal weight
2) Recent weight loss of 10% or more
3) Excess alcohol intake
4) Chronic disease
5) Nothing by mouth for >7 days
6) Increased needs
7) Protracted nutrient losses
8) Medications (steroids, immunosuppressives, antitumor agents)
9) Very young, very old
2. Hypermetabolic state
A. An increase in basal metabolic rate related to injury or illness to allow mobilization of substrates to support inflammation, immune function, and tissue repair
B. Results in increased oxygen consumption, increased CO_2 production, increased energy expenditure, hyperglycemia, inability to mobilize fat stores for energy
C. Occurs at the expense of lean body mass
D. Usually self-limiting; may progress to multiorgan system failure
E. Occurs with surgery, skeletal trauma, blunt trauma, head trauma, sepsis, and burns

NUTRITIONAL GOALS FOR THE ACUTELY ILL PATIENT

1. Use the gastrointestinal tract whenever possible.
2. Provide adequate calories and protein for energy expenditure and tissue synthesis; meet vitamin, minerals, and fluid needs.
3. Avoid overfeeding.
4. Avoid complications associated with feeding.

ASSESSMENT OF NUTRITIONAL STATUS

The ACNP must perform a nutrition assessment to identify individuals at nutritional risk (those patients with malnutrition or hypermetabolism) and determine which patients may benefit from nutrition education. The following factors are considered:

1. Medical, nutrition, social, and psychosocial histories
2. Physical and clinical data
3. Laboratory data

NUTRITIONAL NEEDS OF THE ACUTELY ILL

Nutritional needs are determined by the dietician, taking into account the patient's nutritional status, nutritional goals, and disease processes.

1. Energy needs
A. General rule for estimation of calorie needs of nonventilated, noncritically ill patients (use the lowest of ideal or actual weight):
1) Maintenance: 30 calories/kg

2) Repletion: 35 or more calories/kg
3) Weight loss: 25 calories/kg

B. General rule for estimation of calorie needs for critically ill, stressed patients: 25–30 calories/kg (use lowest of ideal or actual weight)

C. Factors that increase energy needs
1) Hyperthermia
2) Anxiety
3) Dialysis
4) Dressing changes
5) Muscle spasms
6) Chest physical therapy
7) Suctioning
8) Medications (epinephrine, dopamine)
9) Growth
10) Pregnancy/lactation

D. Factors that decrease energy needs
1) Sleep
2) Age
3) Starvation
4) Hypothermia
5) Hypothyroidism
6) Anesthesia
7) Barbiturates
8) Muscle relaxants
9) Paralytics

2. Protein needs

A. General rule for estimation of protein needs in stable patients (use lowest of ideal or actual weight):
1) Maintenance: 1.0–1.2 gm/kg
2) Repletion: 1.3–1.5 gm/kg

B. General rule for estimation of protein needs in critically ill, stressed patients: 1.5 or more gm/kg (without renal or hepatic dysfunction; use lowest of ideal or actual weight)

C. Clinical conditions that may necessitate increased protein delivery
1) Wounds
2) Steroids
3) Catabolic state

D. Clinical conditions that may necessitate decreased protein delivery
1) Renal dysfunction, not on dialysis
2) Some types of liver dysfunction

3. Vitamin and mineral needs

A. In general, 100% of U.S. Recommended Daily Allowance for vitamins and minerals should be provided to all patients.

B. Patients with specific disease states or receiving certain pharmacologic therapy may require additional supplementation.

C. Oversupplementation should be avoided.

4. Fluid needs

A. General guideline: 1 mL/calorie or 30–35 mL/kg body weight

B. Conditions which may necessitate increased fluid delivery
1) Temperature (fluid needs increase about 150 mL/day for each degree of body temperature over 37°C)
2) Excessive perspiration

      3) Increased GI output (diarrhea, fistula output)
      4) Draining wounds
      5) Burns
  C. Conditions that may necessitate decreased fluid delivery
      1) Congestive heart failure, cardiac cachexia
      2) Renal failure (anuric, may or may not receive dialysis; patients on continuous dialysis therapies and peritoneal dialysis may not require fluid restriction)
      3) Hepatic failure with evidence of fluid overload

WHEN TO START FEEDING THE ACUTELY ILL PATIENT

The length of time patients are allowed to be without nutrition varies among practitioners and institutions. The ACNP needs to be aware of the institution's guidelines. General guidelines for the ACNP include:

1. Patients with normal nutritional status upon admission, with inadequate calorie and protein intake for 5–7 days, should be evaluated for nutrition support.
2. Patients with malnutrition upon admission, with inadequate calorie and protein intake for 3–5 days, should be evaluated for nutrition support.
3. Critically ill, hypermetabolic patients should begin nutrition support as soon as the patient has passed through the "ebb" or shock phase of the metabolic response to injury.

CHOOSING THE MODE OF NUTRITION

The ACNP should always consider the preferred feeding route as oral. If intake is insufficient to meet needs, the patient should be considered for enteral feeding. Parenteral nutrition should be limited to patients without a functional gastrointestinal tract.

1. Oral diet
  A. Preferred feeding route is oral.
  B. Consult with the dietician to obtain orders for appropriate diet and to arrange for meal plan, snacks, and nutrition supplements as needed.
  C. Avoid overly restrictive diets, which may result in suboptimal oral intake; diet modifications should be limited to those medically necessary.
  D. Consult with swallowing therapist (usually occupational or speech pathologist therapist) as needed.
2. Enteral feeding
  A. Benefits of enteral feeding
      1) More effective utilization of nutrients
      2) Blunts the hypermetabolic response
      3) Promotes preservation of GI integrity and function
      4) Maintains gut barrier function
      5) Reduces gut-related sepsis and septic complications
      6) May reduce cost
  B. Contraindications for enteral feeding
      1) Intestinal ileus or hypomotility
      2) Severe diarrhea
      3) Jejunal or high-output ileal fistula (>500 mL/24 hr)

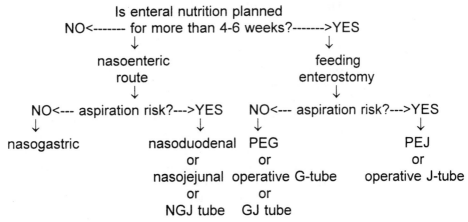

FIGURE 11–2. Route of enteral nutrition. (PEG, percutaneous endoscopic gastrostomy; PEJ, percutaneous endoscopic jejunostomy.)

    4) Acute pancreatitis
    5) Early stages of short bowel syndrome
    6) Near-total intestinal resection
    7) Intractable vomiting
  C. Feeding route (Fig. 11–2)
    1) Nasogastric
      a. Short-term intervention (<6 weeks)
      b. Requires intact gag reflex
      c. Requires normal gastric emptying
    2) Nasointestinal
      a. Short-term intervention (<6 weeks)
      b. Decreases, but does not eliminate, pulmonary aspiration risk
      c. Allows early postoperative feeding
      d. May be used concurrently with gastric suctioning to allow feeding in the presence of delayed gastric emptying (double-lumen tubes allow feeding into the small bowel while the stomach is decompressed using the gastric portion of the tube; commonly referred to as "NGJ" tubes)
    3) Gastrostomy
      a. Long-term feeding (>6 weeks)
      b. Requires normal gastric emptying
      c. Percutaneous endoscopic gastrostomy does not require surgery
      d. Operative gastrostomy can be placed at time of surgery
    4) Jejunostomy
      a. Long-term feeding (>6 weeks)
      b. Decreases, but does not eliminate, pulmonary aspiration risk
      c. Allows early postoperative feeding
      d. May be used concurrently with gastric suctioning to allow feeding in the presence of delayed gastric emptying (double-lumen tube; commonly referred to as "GJ" tube)
  D. Formula selection
    1) Selection of enteral formula is based upon the patient's nutritional and fluid needs, nutritional status, gastrointestinal function, and disease state.

2) The ACNP should consult with the dietician for formula recommendations.

E. Initiation and progression of enteral feeding

  1) The ACNP should consult with the dietician for recommendations regarding feeding initiation and progression.

  2) General guidelines:

   a. Gastric feedings may begin once gastric residuals are <300–600 mL/24 hr (normal gastric secretions are about 1500 mL/24 hr).

   b. In general, intestinal feedings can start immediately because paralytic ileus affects only the stomach and colon. Patient should be hemodynamically stable. Intestinal feeding can take place even in the presence of gastric ileus; audible bowel sounds, passage of flatus or stool are not necessary to begin intestinal feeding.

   c. Radiographic confirmation of tube placement should be obtained prior to feeding.

   d. Isotonic feedings should be initiated at full strength; a general rule for progression is 25 mL every 8 hours until goal rate is obtained.

   e. Hypertonic formulas should be initiated at isotonic strength and advanced to full strength and then to goal rate by 25 mL every 8 hours.

F. Enteral feeding administration methods the ACNP should consider include:

  1) Continuous feedings

   a. Infuse slowly over 24 hours.

   b. Most hospitalized patients receive continuous feedings.

  2) Intermittent feedings

   a. Indicated for noncritically ill patients, home patients, or rehab patients; allow greater freedom from equipment; may be associated with increased gastrointestinal intolerance

   b. Types of intermittent feedings:

    i. Intermittent feeding: Feedings are given in volume of 100–400 mL over 20–40 minutes every 2–4 hours; can usually be initiated with 120 mL isotonic formula every 4 hours and advanced 60 mL every 8 hours until goal volume is achieved.

    ii. Bolus feeding: Feedings are given in volume of 250–500 mL over several minutes every 4–6 hours; can be initiated and advanced as stated above for intermittent feeding.

  3) Cyclic feeding: Feedings are delivered at an increased rate over 8–16 hours, usually overnight, by infusion pump. Patients can transition to cyclic feedings by gradually increasing the feeding rate and decreasing the number of hours. Also called nocturnal or compressed feeding

G. Management of common complications associated with enteral feeding

  1) Metabolic complications (see Table 11–7)

  2) Gastrointestinal complications (see Table 11–8)

  3) Diarrhea (see Table 11–9)

  4) Infectious complications (see Table 11–10)

  5) Mechanical complications (see Table 11–11)

H. Sanitation precautions

  1) Change tube feeding delivery container and tubing every 24 hours.

  2) Flush feeding tube with 30 mL water every 4 hours and whenever feeding is interrupted.

TABLE 11–7. **Metabolic Complications of Enteral Feeding**

Problem	Possible Cause	Interventions
Hypercapnia	Overfeeding; excess carbohydrate	Reassess energy needs; provide formula with balanced distribution of protein, fat, & carbohydrate
Hypervolemia	Renal failure; excess intake; hepatic or cardiac insufficiency; rapid refeeding	↓ fluid intake; diuretic therapy; use formula with less free water; refeed slowly
Hypovolemia	GI fluid losses; osmotic diuresis; inadequate intake; diabetes insipidus; fever; high-protein formula	↑ fluid intake; replace losses; ↓ protein intake if excessive
Hyperglycemia	Refeeding syndrome; sepsis; metabolic stress; diabetes; steroid induced	Correct underlying disorder; oral hypoglycemic or insulin therapy; ↑ % calories as fat; fiber-containing formula (Jevity, Ultracal)
Hypoglycemia	Sudden cessation of feeding in patients receiving insulin or hypoglycemic agent	Taper feeding gradually; when feeding interrupted, replace with glucose-containing IV fluid
Hypernatremia	Fluid losses; excess intake	Replace fluid losses; ↓ intake
Hyponatremia	GI losses; fluid overload; diuretics; SIADH	↑ or ↓ Na depending on cause; ↓ fluid intake; use concentrated formula (Deliver 2.0; TwoCal HN)
Hyperkalemia	Metabolic acidosis; renal failure; excess intake	↓ K intake; medication to decrease K
Hypokalemia	GI losses; diuretics; anabolism; refeeding syndrome; amphotericin B	↑ K intake; can add KCl elixir to feeding bag
Hyperphosphatemia	↓ renal function	↓ Phos intake; Phos binders
Hypophosphatemia	Diuretics; anabolism; refeeding syndrome; increased losses; insulin administration	Minimize Phos-binding medications; ↑ Phos intake; supplement when <2 mg/dL
Hypermagnesemia	Renal insufficiency	↓ Mg intake
Hypomagnesemia	GI losses; malabsorption; drug induced (cisplatin, amphotericin, diuretics, cyclosporin); alcoholism; refeeding syndrome	↑ Mg intake
Hypocalcemia	Hypoalbuminemia; chronic renal failure	Evaluate ionized Ca; ↑ Ca intake
Hypozincemia	GI losses; wound losses; diuretics	Zinc supplementation
Essential fatty acid deficiency	Prolonged use of low-fat formula	Add modular fat source to formula (e.g., 5 mL canola oil daily); provide IV fat

SIADH, syndrome of inappropriate secretion of antidiuretic hormone.

    3) Observe sterile technique when diluting feeding and filling delivery container.

    4) Do not hang more than 8 hours of formula at a time.

I. Aspiration precautions

    1) Elevate head of bed 30 degrees minimum.

    2) Check gastric residuals every 4 hours. Good scientific literature does

TABLE 11–8.   Gastrointestinal Complications of Enteral Feeding

Problem	Possible Cause	Interventions
Gastric retention	Diabetic gastroparesis; motility disorder; drug induced	Use isotonic formula (Isocal, Nutren 1.0, Osmolite) avoid fiber; avoid high-fat formula; feed continuously; advance slowly; check tube position; elevate head of bed 30–45 degrees; monitor residuals & hold per protocol; if unable to check residuals, monitor for distention, nausea; evaluate medications; ambulate if allowed; consider prokinetic agent (metoclopramide; propulsid) consider intestinal feeding with simultaneous gastric suctioning
Abdominal cramping, gas	Gastric retention; cold formula; rapid administration	Use room-temp formula; change to continuous feeding; decrease fat; consider more elemental formula (Vital HN; Vivonex TEN)
Constipation (bowel movement >3–4 days)	Fecal impaction; inadequate fluid; inadequate fiber; inadequate activity	Disimpact; provide free water; use fiber-containing formula (Ultracal, Jevity; Nutren 1.0 with fiber); ambulate if allowed

TABLE 11–9.   Managing Diarrhea in Tube-Fed Patients*

Cause	Intervention
Concurrent drug therapy	Minimize drugs associated with diarrhea; minimize high-osmolality or sorbitol-containing elixirs
Antibiotic-induced colitis	Check for & treat *C. difficile;* consider Lactinex granules to provide *Lactobacillus*
Hypoalbuminemia	Provide isotonic formula (Isocal, Nutren 1.0); advance slowly; consider albumin replacement
Pancreatitis, short bowel	Provide low-fat, elemental formula (Vivonex TEN, Criticare HN, Alitraq); provide pancreatic enzymes
Inadequate fiber intake	Provide fiber-containing formula (Ultracal, Jevity, Nutren 1.0 with Fiber); provide psyllium hydrocolloid (Metamucil)
Hyperosmolar feeding	Provide formula at isotonic strength (~300 mOsm)
Fat malabsorption	Provide low-fat formula (Vivonex TEN, Criticare HN, Vital HN)
Fecal impaction or constipation	Disimpact; provide adequate free water; provide fiber-containing formula
Intestinal atrophy from prolonged bowel rest	Avoid with early enteral feeding; provide isotonic formula; advance slowly; avoid high-fat formula (Deliver, TwoCal HN, Nutren 2.0)
Bacterial contamination	Hang maximum 12-hour supply of formula; change bag & tubing every 24 hours; refrigerate open formula and discard after 24 hours; use clean technique in handling formula & administration set

* Diarrhea is defined as greater than three loose stools or 300 mL/24 h.

TABLE 11–10. **Infectious Complications Associated with Enteral Feeding**

Problem	Possible Cause	Prevention/Interventions
Aspiration pneumonia	Displacement of tube; delayed gastric emptying	Verify tube placement; check residuals and hold feeding for at least 4 hours; consider intestinal feeding; add food coloring to feeding; check pulmonary secretions for glucose
Vomiting & diarrhea	Formula contamination	Hang maximum 12-hour supply of formula; change bag & tubing every 24 hours; refrigerate open formula and discard after 24 hours; use clean technique in handling formula & administration set

not exist to justify a specific parameter of when to hold a feeding; standards vary by institution from twice the hourly feeding rate to 100 mL to monitor for abdominal distention.

3) Observe patients with small-diameter tubes in which residuals cannot be aspirated for signs of abdominal distention or nausea.

4) Verify feeding tube position by abdominal auscultation every 4 hours.

5) Avoid maneuvers that increase intra-abdominal pressure.

J. Medication administration

1) Flush feeding tube with 30 mL water before and after medication administration.

2) Use crushed and liquid medications when possible to minimize clogging.

3) In general, do not mix medications with formula or add medications to the feeding bag.

4) Administer each medication separately and flush the tube with at least 5 mL water between each drug.

5) Consult pharmacist regarding drug administration.

TABLE 11–11. **Mechanical Complications Associated with Enteral Feeding**

Problem	Possible Cause	Prevention/Intervention
Clogged tube	Inadequate irrigation; undissolved formula; formula-medication interaction; crushed medication; formula viscosity excessive for tube size	Flush tube every 4 hours with 20–30 mL water for continuous feedings and before & after each bolus feeding; blenderize formula thoroughly; flush tube with 20–30 mL water before & after medication administration; use elixir medication when possible; consult with pharmacist regarding medication administration; use elemental formula with needle catheter jejunostomies. To declog: try meat tenderizer, Viokase solution (consult pharmacist), cola, cranberry juice
Nasopharyngeal erosion	Large-bore tube; prolonged tube placement	Use small-bore polyurethane or silicon tube; provide proper care of nose & mouth; consider gastrostomy tube for feeding >6 weeks

6) Bulk-forming agents, such as metamucil, are likely to cause clogging if not thoroughly dissolved in water.

7) The administration of phenytoin (Dilantin) with a continuous feeding may result in subtherapeutic concentrations of the drug. The feeding should be discontinued 1–2 hours before and after phenytoin is administered. The feeding schedule should be increased to meet the patient's nutritional needs for a 24-hour period.

8) The administration of warfarin (Coumadin) with a continuous feeding may result in subtherapeutic concentrations of the drug; in such situations, holding the feeding before and after each dose may assist in achieving therapeutic drug levels.

3. The ACNP may consult with the dietician and pharmacist when ordering total parenteral nutrition (TPN).

A. Indications for TPN
1) Complete mechanical intestinal obstruction
2) Intestinal ileus or hypomotility
3) Severe unresolvable diarrhea
4) Proximal high-output fistula (>500 mL/24 hr)
5) Severe acute pancreatitis
6) Early stages of short bowel syndrome
7) Near-total bowel resection
8) Severe enterocolitis
9) Intractable vomiting

B. Contraindications for TPN
1) Treatment anticipated for <5 days in patients without severe malnutrition
2) Functioning GI tract
3) Inability to obtain venous access
4) Prognosis that does not warrant aggressive nutrition support

C. Administration of TPN is a complex medical intervention and requires an interdisciplinary approach. The ACNP should consult with the dietician and pharmacist when ordering TPN. An in-depth discussion of TPN is beyond the scope of this chapter. General guidelines for the ACNP include the following:

1) Formulas with greater than D_{10} require central access.
2) Glucose should be monitored with fingersticks every 6 hours.
3) Fat administration should be infused slowly to avoid hyperlipidemia; 10% fat emulsion administration should not exceed 100 mL/hr; 20% fat emulsion administration should not exceed 50 mL/hr.
4) Patients receiving the sedative propofol (Diprivan) may receive excess fat; the drug is administered in a lipid emulsion, and in large quantities provides large amounts of fat. Consult the dietician or pharmacist for recommendations.
5) When serum triglycerides levels are checked to monitor fat tolerance, the blood should be drawn approximately 6 hours after the fat infusion ends to allow time for adequate clearance. A general rule of thumb is to decrease or hold lipid infusion when triglycerides exceed 300–400 mg/dL.
6) Intravenous fat and propofol contain 15 mmol phosphorus/L; this may be relevant in patients with hyperphosphatemia.
7) Vitamin K and iron are not routinely included in TPN. Patients receiving long-term TPN may require supplementation of these nu-

TABLE 11–12. Metabolic Complications Associated with TPN

Problem	Possible Cause	Interventions
Hypercapnia	Overfeeding; excess carbohydrate	Reassess energy needs (avoid; overfeeding); provide solution with balanced distribution of fat & carbohydrate
Hypervolemia	Excess intake; renal failure; hepatic or cardiac insufficiency; rapid refeeding	↓ fluid intake; diuretic therapy; refeed slowly; dialysis in extreme situations
Hypovolemia	Inadequate intake; ↑ fluid losses (fever, GI or renal losses, sweating, hyperventilation); diabetes insipidus; high protein intake	↑ fluid intake; replace losses; ↓ protein intake if excessive
Hyperglycemia	Refeeding syndrome; sepsis; metabolic stress; diabetes; steroid induced; pancreatitis; hypokalemia; chromium deficiency; excess dextrose infusion; peritoneal dialysis	Correct underlying disorder; insulin therapy; ↑ % calories as fat
Hypoglycemia	Sudden cessation of feeding, especially in patients receiving insulin	Taper feeding slowly; when feeding is interrupted replace with D_{10}
Hypernatremia	↑ fluid losses (fever, GI or renal losses, sweating, hyperventilation); inadequate fluid intake; excess Na intake	↑ fluid intake; replace fluid losses; ↓ Na intake
Hyponatremia	Excess fluid intake; diuretic therapy; SIADH	↓ fluid intake; ↑ or ↓ Na intake depending on cause; use concentrated TPN solution
Hyperkalemia	Excess intake; metabolic acidosis; renal failure; hyperglycemia	↓ K intake; K binders; control glucose
Hypokalemia	Inadequate intake; ↑ losses (diuretic therapy, GI or renal losses); anabolism; refeeding syndrome; drug induced (amphotericin B)	↑ K intake
Hyperphosphatemia	Excess intake; ↓ renal function	↓ Phos intake; Phos binders
Hypophosphatemia	Inadequate intake; ↑ losses (GI or renal, diuretic therapy); anabolism; refeeding syndrome	↑ Phos intake; supplement when <2 mg/dL; minimize Phos binders
Hypermagnesemia	Excess intake; renal insufficiency	↓ Mg intake
Hypomagnesemia	↑ losses (diuretic therapy, GI or renal losses); malabsorption; drug induced (cisplatin, amphotericin, cyclosporin); alcoholism; anabolism; refeeding syndrome	↑ Mg intake
Hypercalcemia	Renal failure; tumor lysis syndrome; excess vitamin D intake; prolonged immobilization	Supplement Phos; evaluate vitamin D intake
Hypocalcemia	Hypoalbuminemia; chronic renal failure; vitamin D deficiency; blood transfusions	Evaluate ionized Ca; calculate corrected Ca; ↑ Ca intake

Table continues

TABLE 11-12. (Continued)

Problem	Possible Cause	Interventions
Azotemia	Dehydration; excess protein intake; catabolism of protein stores because of inadequate nonprotein calorie intake	↑ fluid intake; ↓ protein intake; ↑ nonprotein calories
Hypozincemia	↑ losses (GI or wound losses, diuretics)	Zinc supplementation
Hypertriglyceridemia	Excess fat infusion; familial hyperlipidemia; medication induced (i.e., cyclosporin); pancreatitis; draw time error	↓ lipid administration; lengthen time of administration; discontinue lipid if necessary; measure triglycerides 6–8 hours after lipid administration
Essential fatty acid deficiency	Prolonged use of low- or no-fat solution	Administer lipids (provide minimum 8–10% calories as fat)
Metabolic acidosis	GI losses; renal failure	↑ acetate and ↓ chloride in TPN
Metabolic alkalosis	GI losses	↓ acetate and ↑ chloride in TPN
Trace element deficiencies	GI losses (copper & zinc); liver disease (copper)	Provide standard trace element package; monitor serum levels in long-term patients

SIADH, syndrome of inappropriate secretion of antidiuretic hormone.

trients; consult with the dietician or pharmacist for recommendations.
8) H_2 blockers may be added to TPN formula.
9) TPN solutions with a dextrose concentration of >10% should not be abruptly discontinued because of the risk of hypoglycemia. TPN may be tapered 25 mL every 8 hours; to taper the solution when acutely needed, decrease the infusion rate by 50% every 15 minutes. Blood glucose by finger stick should be checked when the infusion is stopped and 30 and 90 minutes later; TPN solutions may be replaced with D_{10} to help maintain adequate glucose levels.

D. Complications of parenteral nutrition
  1) Metabolic complications (see Table 11–12)
  2) Hepatobiliary and gastrointestinal complications (see Table 11–13)

ORDERING TRANSITIONAL FEEDING

1. TPN to enteral feeding
   A. In general, titrate tube feeding up as tolerated and TPN down, keeping total volume constant.
   B. Document tolerance of enteral feeding prior to discontinuing TPN.
   C. Do not discontinue TPN too soon.
2. TPN to oral diet
   A. Assess need for swallow evaluation.
   B. Begin with 1–2 oz clear liquids every 30 minutes. Advance to soft solids as soon as tolerated.
   C. Cut TPN rate in half and maintain until patient is eating at least 50%.

TABLE 11–13. Hepatobiliary and Gastrointestinal Complications Associated with TPN Feeding

Problem	Possible Cause	Interventions
Fatty liver (↑ LFTs)	Etiology unclear; excess calories or carbohydrate; essential fatty acid deficiency; continuous TPN administration; pre-existing liver disease	↓ calorie/carbohydrate intake (avoid overfeeding); give essential fatty acid; change to cyclic TPN
Cholestasis (↑ total bilirubin, phos)	Etiology unclear; excess carbohydrate; lack of enteral stimulation of bile secretion	↓ carbohydrate intake (avoid overfeeding); provide oral or enteral & alkaline feeding when possible
Gastrointestinal atrophy	Disuse of GI tract	Use GI tract as early as possible; provide small amount of enteral or oral feeding when possible for GI tract stimulation

LFTs, liver function tests.

    D. Consider nocturnal TPN.
    E. Initiate calorie count.
3. Enteral feeding to oral diet
    A. Assess need for swallow evaluation.
    B. Begin with full liquid or soft solids.
    C. Consider nocturnal tube feeding.
    D. Consider bolus feeding after meal to replace uneaten portion of meal.
    E. Do not discontinue tube feeding too soon.
    F. Initiate calorie count.

MONITORING RESPONSES TO NUTRITION INTERVENTIONS

1. Serum proteins
    A. Albumin
        1) Carrier protein of zinc, magnesium, calcium, fatty acids; necessary for maintenance of oncotic pressure
        2) Indicator of long-term nutrition status
        3) Half-life of 20 days
        4) Minimal use in patients with short lengths of stay
        5) Affected by many nonnutrition factors
        6) Interpretation
            a. Normal: >3.5 gm/dL
            b. Mild depletion: 3.0–3.5 gm/dL
            c. Moderate depletion: 2.5–3.0 gm/dL
            d. Severe depletion: <2.0 gm/dL
    B. Prealbumin
        1) Functions as a carrier protein for retinol-binding protein and as a transport protein for thyroxine
        2) Indicator of short-term nutrition status
        3) Half-life of 2 days
        4) Less sensitive to hydration than albumin

5) Affected by nonnutrition factors
6) Interpretation
   a. Normal: >18 mg/dL
   b. Mild depletion: 10–18 mg/dL
   c. Moderate depletion: 5–10 mg/dL
   d. Severe depletion: <5 mg/dL
7) In presence of adequate nutrition should see increase of 1 mg/day or at least 4–5 mg/wk
8) Recommended weekly for all nutritionally compromised patients

C. Transferrin
1) Carrier protein for iron
2) Half-life of 8–10 days
3) Affected by many nonnutrition factors
4) More useful in liver disease than albumin
5) Interpretation
   a. Normal: >200 mg/dL
   b. Mild depletion: 150–200 mg/dL
   c. Moderate depletion: 100–150 mg/dL
   d. Severe depletion: <100 mg/dL

2. Nitrogen balance study
A. Compares nitrogen intake (obtained from 24-hour calorie count) with nitrogen loss (obtained from 24-hour urine collection for urea along with an adjustment factor for insensible losses).
   1) Healthy adult: Nitrogen balance
   2) Anabolism: Positive nitrogen balance
   3) Catabolism: Negative nitrogen balance
B. Indicated when protein status is not improving or there is a high degree of uncertainty regarding protein needs.
C. Contraindicated when there are large nonurine losses of nitrogen, as in GI losses, draining wounds, or renal or liver dysfunction. It is possible to measure the nitrogen content of nonurine fluids, as well as using urea kinetics in anuric patients, to assess nitrogen loss in these situations; however, these measurements are generally not used in the acute care setting.

3. Indirect calorimetry
A. Allows measurement of patient's oxygen consumption, carbon dioxide production, resting energy expenditure, and respiratory quotient using a metabolic cart or a bedside calorimeter that integrates with the ventilator, allowing the collection of 24-hour data.
B. Useful in patients when there is a high degree of uncertainty regarding energy needs, including failure to wean from ventilator, multiple organ failure, severe malnutrition, obesity, eating disorders.
C. Requires patient to breath room air and tolerate canopy or be ventilator dependent and lie quietly at rest for study.

COMPLICATIONS OF OVERFEEDING

1. Overfeeding patients, particularly with TPN, is not uncommon in the hospital setting.
2. A weight gain of in excess of 0.45 kg/day likely represents fluid retention.
3. Potential complications, in addition to volume overload, include:
   A. Excessive CO_2 production

B. Increased minute ventilation
C. Respiratory failure
D. CO_2 retention leading to metabolic acidosis
E. Hyperglycemia
F. Lipogenesis
G. Fat gain rather than lean body mass gain
H. Fatty liver
I. Abnormal liver enzymes
J. Uremia
K. Dehydration
L. Hypokalemia
M. Hypophosphatemia

REFEEDING SYNDROME

1. Syndrome characterized by the rapid decline of phosphorus, potassium, and magnesium upon feeding a malnourished patient.
2. Patients at risk for refeeding syndrome include acutely ill patients with poor nutritional intake for >7 days, chronic malnutrition, chronic alcoholism, and anorexia nervosa, and obese patients with unintentional weight loss.
3. Left uncorrected, hypophosphatemia (<1 mg/dL) can result in respiratory muscle weakness and ventilatory failure; refeeding syndrome may also lead to cardiac failure and neuromuscular dysfunction.
4. Prevention and management.
   A. Correct all electrolyte abnormalities before feeding.
   B. Advance feeding slowly (25 mL every 24 hours).
   C. Monitor electrolytes daily, replace as needed.
   D. Monitor blood glucose.
   E. Assess fluid status with daily weights, intake and output records.

PATIENT EDUCATION

1. Identify educational needs of the patient and/or family and provide education as needed.
2. Discuss with the patient rationale for the type of diet modifications or nutrition support provided.
3. Provide written education materials for review and reinforcement.
4. Review the plan for nutrition support during the acute illness and follow-up care.

Review Questions

11.24 The benefits associated with early enteral feeding include all but which of the following?
   A. Blunts the catabolic response of injury
   B. Eliminates the risk of pulmonary aspiration
   C. Helps to maintain gut barrier function
   D. May reduce cost

11.25 In which of the following situations is a 24-urine collection for urea for a nitrogen balance study, alone, a useful measure of protein requirements?
A. A critically ill patient undergoing daily dialysis
B. A severely injured burn patient
C. A patient with respiratory failure on mechanical ventilation
D. A patient with a large amount of drainage from an enterocutaneous fistula

A 64-year-old male is admitted to the hospital with altered mental status and severe dyspnea. The patient is diagnosed with pneumonia and requires mechanical ventilation. The patient's medical history includes chronic obstructive pulmonary disease, insulin-dependent diabetes, and gastroparesis. The patient appears thin and, according to the family, ate very little for 3 days prior to admission. The baseline prealbumin is 9.7 mg/dL. On hospital day 2 the patient is hemodynamically stable and is tolerating clamping of the nasogastric tube for 4 hours with minimal gastric residual.

11.26 What is the preferred mode of nutrition support for the above described patient?
A. Enteral feeding with a fiber-containing formula
B. Parenteral nutrition via a centrally placed catheter
C. Enteral feeding with an isotonic formula containing no fiber
D. No feeding indicated at this time; reassess for enteral feeding in 3–5 days

11.27 Enteral feeding is initiated but the patient is unable to reach his goal of 80 mL/hr because of gastric residuals >150 mL and has had two episodes of emesis. The patient did tolerate the feeding at 50 mL/hr. What is the appropriate intervention for this patient?
A. Discontinue enteral feeding and begin parenteral nutrition.
B. Temporarily reduce the feeding rate to 50 mL/hr, initiate a motility agent, and monitor for constipation.
C. Discontinue the current formula and order a high-fat concentrated formula to allow less volume to be given.
D. Discontinue feeding and retry in 48 hours.

11.28 The patient is successfully extubated. He is stable, alert, and requesting the nasogastric tube be discontinued. No swallowing difficulty is anticipated. The patient's blood sugars have been under good control. Which of the following is not indicated for this patient?
A. Order a full liquid diet with enteral feeding to be held 2 hours before each meal.
B. Consider transition to nocturnal enteral feeding and allow oral diet during the day.
C. Order a 3-day calorie count.
D. Discontinue the nasogastric tube and order a clear liquid diet.

Answers and Rationales

11.24 **B** Enterally fed patients, including intestinally fed patients, are at risk for pulmonary aspiration of enteral formula.

11.25 **C** Patients with end-stage renal failure retain nitrogen; patients with large wounds and significant gastrointestinal losses lose nitrogen. These sources of nitrogen are not captured in a 24-hour urine collection. The test, therefore, would underestimate nitrogen losses in these patients.

11.26 **C** Enteral feeding is indicated because the patient has a functional gastrointestinal tract and has been without nutrition for 5 days. Formulas containing fiber or high in fat content should be avoided because of the history of gastroparesis.

11.27 **B** The feeding rate should be decreased to the last tolerated rate. Because the patient has a history of gastroparesis, a motility agent is probably indicated. Additionally, constipation should be ruled out because this is a common cause of high gastric residuals in hospitalized patients. Formulas high in fat are likely to further delay gastric emptying. Parenteral nutrition should not be initiated until all attempts at enteral feeding have been exhausted.

11.28 **D** Nutrition support should not be discontinued until the patient has demonstrated the ability to meet 50–75% of his nutritional needs via the oral route.

References

ASPEN Board of Directors. (1986). Guidelines for the use of total parenteral nutrition in the hospitalized adult patient. *J Parenter Enteral Nutr 10*, 441–445.

ASPEN Board of Directors. (1987). Guidelines for the use of total parenteral nutrition in the hospitalized adult patient. *J Parenter Enteral Nutr 11*, 435–439.

Barton, R.G. (1994). Nutrition support in critical illness. *Nutr Clin Pract 9*, 127–140.

Bell, S.J., Pasulka, P.S., & Blackburn, G.L. (1989). Enteral formulas. In A. Skipper (ed.). *Dietitian's Handbook of Enteral and Parenteral Nutrition.* Rockville, MD: Aspen Publishers, pp. 279–291.

Grant, J.P. (1986). Nutritional assessment in clinical practice. *Nutr Clin Pract 2*, 3–11.

Hopkins, B. (1992). Assessment of nutritional status. In M.M. Gottschlich, L.E. Matarese, & E.P. Shronts (eds.). *Nutrition Support Dietetics Core Curriculum* (2nd ed.). Silver Spring, MD: American Society of Parenteral and Enteral Nutrition, pp. 15–70.

Ideno, K.T. (1992). Enteral nutrition. In M.M. Gottschlich, L.E. Matarese, & E.P. Shronts (eds.). *Nutrition Support Dietetics Core Curriculum* (2nd ed.). Silver Spring, MD: American Society of Parenteral and Enteral Nutrition, pp. 71–104.

Lenssen, P. (1989). Monitoring and complications of parenteral nutrition. In A. Skipper (ed.). *Dietitian's Handbook of Enteral and Parenteral Nutrition.* Rockville, MD: Aspen Publishers, pp. 347–373.

Skipper, A. (1989). Monitoring and complications of enteral feeding. In A. Skipper (ed.). *Dietitian's Handbook of Enteral and Parenteral Nutrition.* Rockville, MD: Aspen Publishers, pp. 293–309.

Skipper, A., & Marian, M.J. (1992). Parenteral nutrition. In M.M. Gottschlich, L.E. Matarese, & E.P. Shronts (eds.). *Nutrition Support Dietetics Core Curriculum* (2nd ed.). Silver Spring, MD: American Society of Parenteral and Enteral Nutrition, pp. 105–125.

UCLA Medical Center, Department of Nutrition. (1996). *Guidelines for Nutrition Care.* Los Angeles: UCLA Medical Center.

Winkler, M.F., & Lysen, L.K. (1993). *Suggested Guidelines for Nutrition and Metabolic Management of Adult Patients Receiving Nutrition Support* (2nd ed.). Chicago, IL: American Dietetic Association.

Pressure Ulcer Wound Care

DEFINITION

The acute care nurse practitioner is likely to provide care for several types of chronic wounds, including pressure ulcers, arterial/ischemic ulcers, venous disease ulcers and diabetic neuropathic ulcers, as well as nonhealing surgical wounds. Differential diagnosis of chronic wound etiology is essential for directing appropriate interventions. This section focuses on the pressure ulcer and may be useful as a model for addressing other types of chronic wounds.

Pressure ulcers are areas of local tissue trauma usually developing where soft tissues are compressed between bony prominences and any external surface for prolonged periods. A pressure ulcer is a sign of local tissue necrosis and death. Pressure ulcers are most commonly found over bony prominences subject to external pressure. More than 95% of all pressure ulcers develop over five classic locations: the sacral/coccygeal area, greater trochanter, ischial tuberosity, heel, and lateral malleolus. Pressure exerts the greatest force at the bone-tissue interface; therefore, there may be significant muscle and subcutaneous fat tissue destruction underneath intact skin.

ETIOLOGY/INCIDENCE

1. In acute care settings, incidence ranges from 2.7% to 29.5% and prevalence ranges from 3.5% to 29.5%. Extensive surveys of acute care hospitals in 1990 found prevalence rates of 9.2% among 148 facilities, and in 1994 a prevalence of 11.1% among 177 facilities.
2. Certain populations have higher rates of pressure sore development: elderly patients admitted for femoral fracture, critical care patients, spinal cord–injured patients, and hospitalized patients bedbound or chairbound for a week.
3. Pressure ulcers are the result of mechanical injury to the skin and underlying tissues, causing hypoxia, ischemia, and necrosis. The primary forces involved are pressure and shear.
   A. *Pressure* is the perpendicular force or load exerted on a specific area, causing ischemia and hypoxia of the tissues. High-pressure areas in the supine position are the occiput, sacrum, and heels. In the sitting position, the ischial tuberosities exert the highest pressure, and the trochanters are affected in the sidelying position. Immobility, inactivity, and decreased sensory perception all affect the duration and intensity of the pressure over the bony prominence.
   B. *Shear* is a parallel force. Shear causes ischemia by displacing blood vessels laterally and impeding blood flow to tissues. Shear acts to stretch and twist tissues and blood vessels at the bone-tissue interface, affecting the deep blood vessels and deeper tissue structures. The most common example of shear is the bed patient in semi-Fowler's position. The patient's skeleton slides down toward the foot of the bed but the sacral skin stays in place (with the help of friction against the bed linen). This produces stretching, pinching, and occlusion of the underlying vessels, producing ulcers with large areas of internal tissue damage or undermining and less damage at the skin surface.
4. Secondary forces involved in pressure ulcer formation are friction, moisture, nutrition, and age. These forces act to decrease the tolerance of tissues to pressure and external forces.

A. *Friction* occurs when two surfaces move across one another. Friction acts on the tissue tolerance to pressure by abrading and damaging the epidermal and upper dermal layers of the skin that increases the skin's susceptibility to pressure injury. Additionally, friction acts with gravity to cause shear.

B. *Moisture* contributes to pressure ulcer development by removing oils on the skin, making it more friable, as well as interacting with body support surface friction. Constant moisture on the skin leads to maceration of the tissues. Excess moisture may be due to wound drainage, diaphoresis, and fecal or urinary incontinence. Urinary and fecal incontinence are common risk factors associated with pressure ulcer development. Incontinence contributes to pressure ulcer formation by creating excess moisture on the skin and by chemical damage to the skin. Fecal incontinence has the added detrimental effect of bacteria in the stool, which can contribute to infection as well as skin breakdown.

C. *Malnutrition* is associated with pressure ulcer development. Low serum albumin levels (<2.5 mg/dL) are associated both with having a pressure ulcer and developing a pressure ulcer.

D. *Age,* itself, may be a risk factor for pressure ulcer development. The skin and support structures undergo changes in the aging process. There is a loss of muscle, a decrease in serum albumin levels, diminished inflammatory response, decreased elasticity, and reduced cohesion between the dermis and epidermis.

PATHOPHYSIOLOGY

Several cellular responses to pressure and shear occur in the development of pressure ulcers.

1. Vessel occlusion
2. Tissue hypoxia
3. Tissue ischemia
4. Anaerobic metabolism
5. Buildup of metabolic wastes
6. Increased protein accumulation in interstitial space
7. Capillaries leak because of increased permeability
8. Tissues become edematous
9. Perfusion worsens

SIGNS AND SYMPTOMS

1. The clinical presentation of a pressure ulcer is a predictable cutaneous chain of events dependent on the severity of the tissue insult.
   A. Reactive hyperemia—normal tissue response to compression
   B. Blanchable erythema in light-skinned persons
   C. Nonblanchable erythema in light-skinned persons
   D. Indicators in dark-skinned persons—induration, purple-blue hue to skin, edema, warmth, pain
   E. Early pressure sore
   F. Chronic deep ulcer
2. The first clinical sign of pressure ulcer formation—*blanchable erythema*—presents as a patch of flat, nonraised area of discoloration of the

skin larger than 1 cm. This discoloration presents as redness or erythema that varies in intensity from pink to bright red in light-skinned patients. In dark-skinned patients, the discoloration appears as a deepening of normal ethnic color or as a purple hue to the skin. Other characteristics include slight edema and increased temperature of the area. In light-skinned patients, the severity of the tissue insult can be evaluated by testing for blanchability of tissues. After finger pressure is applied to the area, complete blanching occurs following by quick return of redness once the finger is removed. In dark-skinned patients, it is difficult to discern blanching. Use of temperature is a more valuable assessment of the severity of the tissue damage in the dark-skinned patient. Initial skin trauma and discoloration will exhibit an elevated skin temperature when compared to healthy tissues. The beginning clinical indicators of pressure ulceration all relate to the signs of inflammation in the tissues.

3. *Nonblanchable erythema* involves more severe damage and is commonly the first stage of pressure ulceration. The color of the skin is more intense. It varies from dark red to purple or cyanotic in both light- and dark-skinned patients. Dark-skinned patients exhibit deepening of normal skin color, a purple or gray hue to the skin, and changes in skin texture, with induration and an "orange peel" appearance. Skin temperature is now cool compared to healthy tissues, and the area may feel indurated. In light-skinned patients, nonblanchable erythema is detected by testing for blanching of tissues. The damage to tissues is more severe and is indicated by the inability of the tissues to blanch.

4. The result of further deterioration in the tissues is evidenced as the epidermis is disrupted, with subepidermal *blisters, crusts, or scaling* present.

5. The *early pressure ulcer* reflects continued tissue insult and progressive injury. The early ulcer is superficial with indistinct margins and a red shiny base. It is usually surrounded by nonblanchable erythema. Superficial ulcers begin at the skin surface and progress to deeper layers. Deep ulcers do not originate at the skin surface; they begin at the bony prominence–soft tissue interface and spread to involve the skin structures.

6. The *chronic deep ulcer* usually has a dusky red wound base and does not bleed easily. It is surrounded by nonblanchable erythema or deepening of normal ethnic tone; there is induration and warmth, and the ulcer is possibly mottled in color. Undermining and tunneling may be present with a large necrotic cavity. The terms *slough* and *eschar* refer to different levels of necrosis and are described according to color and consistency. Slough is described as yellow (or tan) and either thin, mucinous, or stringy. Eschar is described as brown or black and soft or hard and indicates a full-thickness loss of skin. Eschar is usually surrounded by a ring of blanchable erythema.

7. History: Immobility, inactivity, decreased sensory deprivation (e.g., cerebral vascular accident, spinal cord injury, diabetes), malnutrition, incontinence, altered mental status, orthopedic procedures, prolonged bed rest, critical illness.

8. Location: Bony prominences, most commonly sacral/coccygeal area, greater trochanters, ischial tuberosities, and heels.

9. Appearance
   A. Color: Variable. If significant necrotic debris present, will have erythema surrounding ulcer. If chronic, ulcer will have hemosiderin stain-

ing at ulcer borders (appears as hyperpigmentation or purple color to wound margins).

B. Surrounding skin: Usually normal unless continuing pressure injury exists; then blanchable and nonblanchable erythema may be present.

C. Depth: Variable.

D. Wound margins: Usually regular and well defined; in early stages will be irregular and diffuse.

E. Exudate: Variable.

F. Edema: Variable; in later stages, pitting or nonpitting and induration possible.

G. Skin temperature: Normal. In early stages increased warmth to touch, in later stages cool to touch.

H. Granulation tissue: Usually present and red color in proliferative phase of healing.

I. Infection: Not usually present; signs of inflammation will be present when necrotic tissue is present.

J. Necrosis: When ulcer presents with more severe tissue insult, necrosis will be present in chronic, later stages; may be yellow slough or black eschar.

10. Perfusion

A. Pain: Unknown; may be minimal or procedural in nature

B. Peripheral pulses: Present and palpable (unless concomitant peripheral vascular disease)

PHYSICAL FINDINGS

Pressure ulcers are staged upon diagnosis of the lesion and must be evaluated with an assessment tool at regular intervals to monitor for healing.

1. Pressure ulcers are commonly classified according to grading or staging systems based on the depth of tissue destruction. The stage is determined on initial assessment by noting the deepest layer of tissue involved. The ulcer is not restaged unless deeper layers of tissue become exposed. The ulcer is not "downstaged" or "backstaged" to document healing. Table 11–14 provides the pressure ulcer staging criteria.

2. Pressure ulcer assessment includes:

A. Location

B. Size

C. Stage

D. Condition of wound edges

E. Presence of undermining or tunneling

F. Necrotic tissue characteristics

G. Exudate characteristics

H. Surrounding tissue conditions

I. Granulation tissue

J. Epithelialization characteristics

3. Pressure ulcer assessment should be performed weekly and whenever a significant change is noted in the wound. Assessment should not be confused with monitoring the wound at each dressing change.

4. Monitoring the wound can be performed by less skilled caregivers; however, assessment should be performed on a routine basis by health care professionals.

TABLE 11–14. Pressure Ulcer Staging Criteria

Pressure Ulcer Stage	Definition
Stage I*	Nonblanchable erythema of intact skin; the heralding lesion of skin ulceration. In individuals with darker skin, discoloration of the skin, warmth, edema, induration, or hardness may also be indicators.
Stage II	Partial-thickness skin loss involving epidermis or dermis, or both. The ulcer is superficial and presents clinically as an abrasion, blister, or shallow crater.
Stage III	Full-thickness skin loss involving damage to or necrosis of subcutaneous tissue, which may extend down to but not through underlying fascia. The ulcer presents clinically as a deep crater with or without undermining of adjacent tissue.
Stage IV	Full-thickness skin loss with extensive destruction, tissue necrosis, or damage to muscle, bone, or supporting structures (such as tendon, joint capsule).

* The National Pressure Ulcer Advisory Panel has recently considered an alternative definition of the Stage I pressure ulcer. The definition under review is as follows: An observable pressure-related alteration of intact skin whose indicators, as compared to an adjacent or opposite area on the body, may include changes in skin color (red, blue, purple tones), skin temperature (warmth or coolness), skin stiffness (hardness, edema), and/or sensation (pain).

5. The Pressure Sore Status Tool (PSST), a research-based instrument for assessment and documentation of pressure ulcers, incorporates the necessary indices for pressure ulcer assessment, provides for quantification of observations, and allows for tracking the condition of the ulcer over time. The PSST is recommended for use as a method of assessment and monitoring of pressure ulcers. The PSST is meant to be used once a pressure ulcer has developed; it is not a risk assessment tool. It is recommended that the pressure ulcer be scored initially for a baseline assessment and at regular intervals to evaluate therapy. Once a lesion has been assessed for each item on the PSST, the 13 item scores can be added to obtain a total score for the wound. The total score can then be monitored to see at a glance regeneration or degeneration of the wound. Total scores range from 13 (skin intact but always at risk) to 65 (profound tissue degeneration). The tool is included at the end of this chapter.

6. Assessment of Status
   A. PSST contains 15 items: 2 nonscored items, location and shape of the wound; and 13 items rated on a modified Likert scale, with 1-best for the item and 5-worst for the item. The 13 items can be summed for a total score (range 13–65), that can be used as an indicator of overall wound status.
   B. Items examined with the PSST
      1) Size
         a. Uses length × width = surface area
         b. Uses gross changes in size
      2) Depth
         a. Uses National Pressure Ulcer Advisory Panel, Agency for Health Care Policy and Research (AHCPR), and Wound, Ostomy and Continence Nurses (WOCN) terminology for staging
         b. Uses full and partial thickness definitions
      3) Edges
         a. Most important?
         b. Attached versus nonattached

       c. Flush, even with skin surface
       d. Well-defined versus diffuse
    4) Undermining
       a. Quantifies percentage of wound involved
       b. Number of centimeters around wound
       c. Undermining = cave; tunneling = subway
    5) Necrotic tissue type and amount
       a. Determine predominant color
       b. Black, hard is bad; soggy, black is less severe
       c. Yellow slough: Look at moisture content of material, stringy or mucinous appearance
       d. Adherence to wound bed and edges
       e. Quantify percentage of wound covered
    6) Exudate type and amount
       a. Difficult to assess
       b. Evaluate after cleansing with normal saline
       c. Quantify amount of dressing involved in drainage
    7) Surrounding tissue characteristics
       a. Skin color surrounding wound
       b. Peripheral tissue edema
       c. Peripheral tissue induration
       d. Palpate from healthy tissues to wound edge
       e. Look for purple, gray, black skin color changes indicating tissue hypoxia/ischemia
    8) Granulation tissue
       a. Quantify percentage of wound base covered/filled
       b. Type of granulation tissue
       c. Remember partial-thickness wounds heal only with epithelialization! No granulation tissue-necrotic wound or nonproliferating wound
    9) Epithelialization
       a. Quantify percentage
       b. Measure amount of epidermal resurfacing that has occurred in wound; remember partial-thickness wounds can epithelialize from all over wound, not just edges

DIFFERENTIAL DIAGNOSIS AND TREATMENT CONSIDERATIONS

Differential diagnosis of pressure ulcers involves determining the etiology of the wound and intervening appropriately. Pressure ulcers of the lower extremities must be differentiated from venous ulcers, arterial/ischemic ulcers, and neuropathic ulcers. Pressure ulcers on the sacral/coccygeal area must be differentiated from perineal dermatitis. Treatment varies according to type of ulcer.

1. Venous ulcers
   A. History: Previous deep vein thrombosis and varicosities, obesity, phlebitis, traumatic injury to site, congestive heart failure, orthopedic procedures, previous vascular ulcers
   B. Location: Medial aspect of lower leg and ankle, superior to medial malleolus

   C. Appearance
     1) Color: Red and ruddy
     2) Surrounding skin: Erythema, brown staining (hemosiderin deposits)
     3) Depth: Usually partial thickness and shallow
     4) Wound margins: Irregular
     5) Exudate: Moderate to heavy (dependent on amount of edema present in extremities)
     6) Edema: Pitting or nonpitting, induration, cellulitis possible
     7) Skin temperature: Normal, warm to touch
     8) Granulation tissue: Present and red color
     9) Infection: Not usually present
   D. Perfusion
     1) Pain: Minimal
     2) Peripheral pulses: Present and palpable (unless edema hinders palpation)
     3) Capillary refill: Normal, <3 seconds
   E. Treatment considerations
     1) Elevation of legs.
     2) Compression therapy to provide at least 30 mm Hg compression at the ankle (examples include short stretch bandages, therapeutic support stockings, Unna's boot, Profore three- or four-layer wraps or compression pumps).
     3) Topical therapy goals: Absorb exudate and maintain moist wound environment.
     4) See "Chronic Venous Insufficiency" in Chapter 3 for further information.
 2. Arterial/ischemic ulcers
   A. History: Diabetes, cerebral vascular accident, smoking intermittent claudication, vascular procedures, hypertension, hyperlipidemia, arteriosclerosis/atherosclerosis, traumatic injury to site
   B. Location: Toe tips and/or web spaces, phalangeal heads around lateral malleolus, areas exposed to repeated trauma or pressure
   C. Appearance
     1) Color: Pale on elevation, dependent rubor
     2) Surrounding skin: Shiny, taut, thin, evidence of tissue and skin atrophy, hair loss on lower extremities
     3) Depth: Deep
     4) Wound margins: Even and regular
     5) Exudate: Minimal
     6) Edema: Variable
     7) Skin temperature: Decreased, cool to touch
     8) Granulation tissue: Rarely present; if present, pale pink color
     9) Infection: Frequent
     10) Necrosis: Eschar, gangrene may be present
   D. Perfusion
     1) Pain: Intermittent claudication—resting, positional (relieved with dependent position), nocturnal
     2) Peripheral pulses: Absent or diminished
     3) Capillary refill: Delayed, >3 seconds
     4) Ankle/brachial index: >0.8
   E. Treatment considerations
     1) Improve tissue perfusion: Revascularization procedures, no smoking,

no caffeine, no constrictive garments or compression, avoidance of cold.

2) Medications to improve red blood cell transit through narrowed vessels, such as rheologic agents.

3) Hydration.

4) Trauma prevention: Footwear at all times.

5) Topical therapy

a. Dry uninfected ulcer—keep dry.

b. Dry infected ulcer—referral for surgical débridement with aggressive antibiotic therapy.

c. Open ulcer—moist wound healing, nonocclusive dressings *or* cautious use of occlusive dressings, aggressive treatment of any infection.

6) See "Arterial Occlusive Disease" in Chapter 3 for further information.

3. Neuropathic ulcers

A. History: Diabetes, Hansen's disease

B. Location: Plantar aspect of foot, metatarsal heads, heels

C. Appearance

1) Color: Normal skin color

2) Surrounding skin: May have callus formation; fissures and cracks in skin present

3) Depth: Variable

4) Wound margins: Well defined

5) Exudate: Variable

6) Edema: Cellulitis, erythema, induration common

7) Skin temperature: Normal, warm to touch

8) Granulation tissue: Frequently present

9) Infection: Frequent

10) Necrosis: Variable; gangrene uncommon

11) Reflexes: Diminished

12) Altered gait, orthopedic deformities common

D. Perfusion

1) Pain: Painless; diminished sensitivity to touch; insensate foot

2) Peripheral pulses: Present and palpable

3) Capillary refill: Normal, <3 seconds

E. Treatment considerations

1) Pressure relief for heel ulcers

2) Orthotic consultation for appropriate footwear

3) Off-loading for plantar ulcers

4) Tight glucose control

5) Aggressive infection control: Débride necrotic tissue, antibiotic coverage, orthopedic consult for exposed bone

6) Topical therapy: Moist wound healing, nonocclusive dressings *or* cautious use of occlusive dressings, absorb exudate

4. Perineal dermatitis

A. History: Urinary or fecal incontinence

B. Location: Buttocks, including sacral/coccygeal area and perineal area

C. Appearance

1) Color: Ulcers are multiple, appearing over the entire buttocks and sacral/coccygeal areas (not confined to the bony prominence). Buttocks will have diffuse erythema with uneven borders, extending beyond bony prominence of sacrum or coccyx.

2) Surrounding skin: Denuded and erosions evident (particularly with fecal incontinence); flaking and scaling may also be present.

3) Depth: Usually partial thickness and shallow.

4) Wound margins: Irregular.

5) Exudate: Minimal.

6) Skin temperature: Normal, warm to touch.

7) Granulation tissue: Partial-thickness ulcers, so no granulation tissue will be present.

8) Infection: Concomitant yeast infection may be present.

9) Necrosis: Not typically present.

10) Pain: Moderate to severe depending on level of denudation and erosion of the skin.

D. Treatment considerations

1) Manage the incontinence (underpads, adult briefs or pads, external catheters, indwelling catheter if severe, fecal incontinence collector for diarrhea states; avoid rectal tube).

2) Behavior management strategies for incontinence, including prompted voiding or scheduled voiding.

3) Pharmacologic intervention if appropriate, such as antidiarrheal agents for diarrhea, anticholinergics for urge urinary incontinence.

4) Aggressive treatment of yeast infection if present.

5) Topical therapy goals: Maintain moist wound environment, protect skin from incontinence.

DIAGNOSTIC TESTS/FINDINGS

The primary concern for the patient with a pressure ulcer is accurate identification of infection and management of bacterial colonization. It is critical to understand that all pressure ulcers are colonized with bacteria and most do not require culturing or antibiotic treatment. To decrease the potential of wound infection or high bacterial burdens in the wound, the following guidelines are offered.

1. A. Minimize potential with adequate débridement and cleansing.

B. Do not use swab cultures to diagnose wound infections; use needle aspiration or tissue biopsy. Stotts (1995) recommends a swab procedure using a 1-cm area of ulcer and swabbing for 5 minutes.

C. Consider initiating 2-week trial of topical antibiotics (e.g., silver sulfadiazine, triple antibiotic) for clean ulcers that are not healing after 2–4 weeks of *appropriate, optimal* management.

D. Evaluate for osteomyelitis.

E. Do not use topical antiseptics (e.g., Betadine, acetic acid, Dakin's solution, hydrogen peroxide) to reduce bacteria in wound tissue.

F. Use appropriate systemic antibiotics for those with septicemia, cellulitis, or osteomyelitis.

G. For infection control, clean technique is appropriate for pressure ulcer care (e.g., clean gloves, clean dressings).

H. Sterile technique should be used for débridement of pressure ulcers.

I. Wounds with necrotic tissue are likely to have both aerobic and anaerobic organisms present (e.g., *Bacteroides*—anaerobe).

J. Wounds without necrosis are likely to have primarily aerobic organisms present, such as *Pseudomonas aeruginosa* or *Staphylococcus aureus*.

2. When to culture (positive cultures indicated if $>10^5$ pathog
   A. Signs and symptoms of systemic infection (elevated V
      present.
   B. Wound shows signs and symptoms of inflammation (er
      induration, pain) and wound is not filled with necrotic
   C. Wound is nonhealing with appropriate treatment.
   D. There is evidence of bone or joint involvement (osteomylitis).
   E. For superficial infection (bacterial burden approaching 10^5 without signs
      and symptoms of deeper tissue invasion, a 2-week course of topical anti-
      biotics such as mupirocin (Bactroban) or metronidazole (topical Flagyl)
      may be helpful.
   F. MRSA presents special concerns for patients with wounds. *Staphylococ-
      cus aureus* is part of normal skin flora and can be found on the skin
      of approximately 20–50% of healthy adults and can persist in wounds.
      Patients at highest risk for developing MRSA colonization and infection
      are those with history of injection drug abuse, presence of chronic dis-
      ease, previous antimicrobial therapy, previous hospitalization, admis-
      sion to an intensive care unit, or prolonged stay in a health care institu-
      tion. All forms of *S. aureus*, including MRSA, can quickly invade and
      infect breaks in skin integrity, making wounds one of the most common
      sites of *S. aureus* infection and a site commonly colonized with *S. aureus*
      or MRSA.
   G. Mupirocin (Bactroban) is specific for MRSA and can be used topically
      for wounds infected with the organism. This agent must not be used
      inappropriately so that it is effective when really needed for MRSA or-
      ganisms.

MANAGEMENT/TREATMENT

1. Basic prevention interventions
   A. Repositioning—q2h
   B. Small shifts in position
   C. Thirty-degree laterally inclined position
   D. Use of pillows, chairs
   E. Skin inspection and care
   F. Inspect bony prominences
   G. Use lukewarm water and mild soap for cleansing
   H. Protect from moisture
   I. Do not massage bony prominences
   J. Lubricate to prevent dryness
   K. Avoid exposure to cold and low humidity
   L. Perform risk assessment (use Braden scale, Norton scale, or other tools)
      on admission to facility, once a week, and whenever condition changes
      (e.g., after surgery, after transfer to different units)
2. Early intervention strategies
   A. Prevention of causative/contributing factors
   B. Underlying cause influences treatment choices
   C. Friction versus shear versus pressure
   D. Measures to reduce pressure
      1) Head of bed at 30 degrees or lower to decrease shear, bottom of bed
         raised to elevate legs.
      2) Avoid 90-degree sidelying, use 30-degree laterally inclined position.

3) Keep heels off surface.
4) Do not use donuts.
5) Use turn-and-lift sheets to reduce friction.
6) Use of pillows between bony prominences.
7) Pressure relief/reduction for wheelchairs and in sitting positions.
E. Minimize friction and shearing
1) Transparent dressings
2) Turn-and-draw sheets
3) Position in bed
4) Cornstarch
F. Minimize moisture and manage incontinence
G. Maximize nutrition
1) Monitor serum albumin, total lymphocyte count, and other nutritional markers.
2) Provide supplemental vitamin C, zinc, iron to promote healing.
3) Provide for adequate calorie and protein intake.
3. Manage tissue loads—support surfaces
A. Pressure reduction devices: Lower tissue interface pressures, but do not *consistently* maintain interface pressures below capillary closing pressures, in all positions, on all locations. *Indicated for patients who are assessed to be at risk for pressure sore development, who can be turned, and who have skin breakdown involving only one surface.*
1) Static devices: Do not move; reduce pressure by spreading the load over a larger area. Examples: foam-air,- gel-, water-filled mattresses.
2) Dynamic devices: Move, use electricity to alter inflation and deflation and thus decrease pressure. Examples: Alternating air pressure pads.
3) Overlays: Devices that are applied on top of the standard mattress. *Most* are *pressure reducing* devices, and require a one-time charge, setup fee, daily rental fee, or a combination of fees. Most are single-use items and may present environmental issues for disposal. Height of bed is increased, so transfers and linen change may be complicated. Static or dynamic. Some provide air movement to reduce moisture buildup. Examples: Foam-, gel-, water-, air-filled mattress; alternating pressure pads; low air-loss overlays.
4) Replacement mattresses: Designed to reduce the interface pressures and replace the standard hospital mattress. Most are made of foam and gel combinations. Some are air-filled chambers and foam structures. All are covered with bacteriostatic cover that can be maintained with standard cleaning.
B. Pressure relief devices: *Consistently* reduce tissue interface pressures to a level below capillary closing pressure, in any position and in most locations. *Indicated for patients who are assessed to be at high risk for pressure sore development and who cannot turn independently* or *have skin breakdown involving more than one surface.*
1) Low air-loss therapy: A bed frame with a series of connected air-filled pillows. The amount of pressure in each pillow can be controlled and can be calibrated to provide maximum pressure reduction for the individual patient.
2) Air-fluidized therapy: Also called high air-loss therapy; consists of a bed frame containing silicone-coated beads and incorporating both air and fluid support. The beads become fluid when air is pumped through, making them behave like a liquid. Bactericidal properties

because of alkalinity (pH 10), temperature, and entrapment of n. organisms by the beads.

3) Kinetic therapy: Beds designed to counter the effects of immobility by continuous passive motion. Believed to improve respiratory function and oxygenation, prevent urinary stasis, and reduce venous stasis. Multiple body systems involved in the therapy.

4) Obesity accommodation: Beds designed to handle obese patients.

4. Débridement

A. Sharp, mechanical, enzymatic, autolytic with no sepsis.

B. Sharp with sepsis or advancing cellulitis.

C. Arterial/ischemic wounds: Do not débride unless certain of collateral circulation or surgery to improve circulation.

D. Black heels: Inspect daily; if signs and symptoms of pathology appear, débride.

E. Mechanical: Wet-to-dry gauze; nonselective, painful, causes greater tissue damage, usually not done correctly, labor intensive and costly, *not recommended*.

F. Enzymatic: Several ointments used; selective, should see wound predominantly clean in 14 days, should be stopped when wound bed is clean.

1) Elase and Elase-Chloromycetin (fibrinolysin and deoxyribonuclease)
   a. Action: Attacks DNA and fibrin of blood clots and fibrinous exudates
   b. Dosage: One to three times a day
   c. Duration of action: 6–8 hours
   d. Notes: Hypersensitivity for people with bovine sensitivity; superinfection with chloromycetin; more effective if applied more frequently rather than thicker; available in powder and can be used to pack wounds but very expensive

2) Santyl (collagenase)
   a. Action: Digests collagen, lysis of collagen in necrotic tissue and collagen fibers anchoring necrotic tissue to wound base
   b. Dosage: Once a day.
   c. Duration of action: 24 hours.
   d. Notes: pH range is 6–8; can be used with triple antibiotic to also treat infection; detergents, antiseptics, and heavy metals will inactivate the enzyme. Strong emphasis on its use in AHCPR guidelines.

3) Panafil and Panafil White (papain and urea; white also has chlorophyllin copper)
   a. Action: Enzyme débrider and emollient, kerotolytic
   b. Dosage: Once a day
   c. Duration of action: 24 hours
   d. Notes: pH range 3–12; can be used under pressure dressings; hydrogen peroxide, detergents, antiseptics, and heavy metals will inactivate the enzyme; may experience transient burning on application

4) Granulex Spray (trypsin 0.1 mg, balsam Peru, castor oil)
   a. Action: Proteolytic pancreatic enzyme, capillary bed stimulant, and emollient; *will not* débride moderate to large amounts of necrotic debris
   b. Dosage: Two to three times a day

      c. Notes: Do not use on fresh arterial clots; *external use only*; transient burning with initial application

  G. Sharp: Selective; gives acute wound edges if performed on one-time basis; may be one time or sequential; may be performed by advanced practice nurses such as enterostromal therapy or wound nurses, nurse practitioners, clinical nurse specialists (dependent on state board of nursing requirements by state and certification of competency) or physicians; may be performed in operating room or at bedside. Stop débriding if it causes pain, if it causes bleeding, if you don't know what you're cutting. Use sequential sharp débridement in conjunction with other methods such as autolytic or enzymatic dressings in between sharp débridement procedures.

  H. Autolytic: Selective, conservative; should see softening, lifting of eschar by 14 days; can use thin film dressing, hydrocolloid, hydrogel, or other moist wound-healing dressing.

5. Cleansing
  A. Cleanse at each dressing change.
  B. Use minimal force with gauze, cloth, or sponge cleansing.
  C. Do not use skin cleansers or antimicrobial solutions to clean ulcer (e.g., povidone-iodine, iodophor, sodium hypochlorite or Dakin's solution, hydrogen peroxide, acetic acid).
  D. Use normal saline to cleanse most wounds.
  E. Irrigation pressures during cleansing should range from 4 to 15 psi (35-ml syringe with 19-gauge angiocath needle = 8 psi).
  F. Whirlpool is only indicated for ulcers with thick exudate, slough, or necrotic tissue; discontinue when ulcer is clean.

6. Dressings
  A. Use dressings that support moist wound healing. (See Table 11–15 for basic dressing characteristics).
  B. Choose a dressing that protects skin surrounding ulcer.
  C. Manage exudate.
  D. Eliminate dead space, loosely fill all cavities.
  E. As wounds heal/degenerate, treatment options change to meet the wound's needs.
  F. Appropriate treatment for appropriate ulcers (see "Differential Diagnosis").
  G. Consistent product usage: Use for minimum of 10 days to evaluate effectiveness; use products correctly.

7. Adjunctive therapy
  A. Electrical stimulation for unresponsive stage III and IV ulcers; involve physical therapy in wound care.
  B. Not enough clinical studies to support recommendations for other adjunctive therapies (e.g., hyperbaric oxygen; ultrasound; ultraviolet light; nonantibiotic systemic medications such as rheologic agents, vasodilators or fibrolytic agents, growth factors).

PATIENT EDUCATION

1. Assist patient in identifying specific risk factors for pressure ulcer development.
2. Teach immobility, inactivity, and decreased sensory perception strategies.
  A. Passive repositioning

TABLE 11-15.   Topical Treatment for Pressure Ulcers: Wound Dressings

Product	Definition and Example	Use	Reimbursement Codes, Utilization Guidelines	Notes
Skin Sealants	Skin Prep (Smith & Nephew United, Inc.)	Prevent friction, protect from adhesives, seal in powders	HCPC Code: A6250	Not alcohol wipe, contains alcohol, should not be used under most hydrocolloids
Gauze—woven: nonimpregnated, sterile and nonsterile, with or without adhesive borders, pads, rolls	Woven natural cotton fibers	Protection, absorbency (minimal)	Pads with or without adhesive borders—HCPC Codes: A6216-21; A6402-4; Utilization Guide: with borders, 2 pads 1×/day; without borders, 2 pads 3×/day Rolls (elastic, nonelastic)—HCPC Codes: A6263-64, A6405-6	May lint, more abrasive, adheres to tissues, primary or secondary dressing, nonadhesive
Gauze—nonwoven: nonimpregnated, sterile and nonsterile, with or without adhesive borders, pads, rolls	Rayon & polyester blends used for soft bulk, polyester alone used for increased strength Nu Gauze (Kendall), Sof-Wick (J&J Medical)	Protection, absorbency (minimal to moderate)	Pads with or without adhesive borders—HCPC Codes: A6216-21; A6402-4; Utilization Guide: with borders, 2 pads 1×/day; without borders, 2 pads 3×/day Rolls (elastic, nonelastic)—HCPC Codes: A6263-64, A6405-6	Lints less, absorbs and wicks away moisture, does not stick to wounds, soft, bulky

Table continues

T A B L E   **11–15.**   *(Continued)*

Product	Definition and Example	Use	Reimbursement Codes, Utilization Guidelines	Notes
Gauze—impregnated: water or saline, or other than water or saline, with or without adhesive borders, pads, rolls	Adaptic (J&J Medical), Xeroform (Sherwood Medical)	Protection, nonadherent, moist wound contact	Pads with or without adhesive borders—HCPC Codes: A6222-30; Utilization Guide: with borders, 2 pads 1×/day; without borders, 2 pads 3×/day Rolls—HCPC Code: A6266	Be sure impregnated with substance nonharmful to healing wound, nonadherent, limited absorbent capacity
Composite dressings	Combine one dressing group with another to address wound characteristics (e.g., gauze/foam and transparent film dressing properties, hydrocolloid and alginates) Viasorb (Sherwood, Geck and Davis Medical), CombiDerm (Convatec), BAND-AID Island Dressing (Johnson & Johnson)	Absorbent, wicks away excess moisture, nonadherent to wound bed, use depends on the combination of properties	HCPC Code: KO203-05; Utilization Guide: 3×/wk	May be difficult to apply, nonadherent to wound bed, can be confusing to the caregiver as combines various properties
Transparent film dressings	Polyurethane and polyethylene membrane film coated with a layer of acrylic hypoallergenic adhesive, moisture vapor transmission rates (MVTR) vary Op-Site (Smith & Nephew United, Inc), Tegaderm (3M), Bioclusive	Partial-thickness wounds, promotes epithelialization, moist wound healing, semipermeable, bacterial barrier, autolysis, wound visible, protects against friction, adhesive	HCPC Codes: KO257-59; Utilization Guide: 3×/wk	May re-injure area on removal, nonabsorbent, can lead to wound edge maceration, tendency to remove prematurely, not indicated for moderate to heavy exudate

Hydrocolloid: regular, thin, paste, granules	Gelatin, pectin, carboxymethyl-cellulose in a polyisobutylene adhesive base with a polyurethane or film backing DuoDERM (ConvaTec), Restore (Hollister Inc.), Comfeel (Kendall Healthcare), RepliCare (Smith & Nephew United, Inc.)	Moist wound healing, absorbs low to moderate wound fluid, autolysis, thermal insulation, bacterial barrier, reduces pain, translucent to opaque, increased wear time, easy to apply, controls odor, impermeable to semipermeable	HCPC Code: KO234-41; Utilization Guide: 3×/wk	Not indicated for heavy exudate, limited absorbent abilities when used alone, use with other products increases absorbent abilities, odor on removal, opaque, melt down and stick to linens, some difficult to remove, possible sensitivity to adhesive backing, use with close supervision on immunosuppressed patients, diabetics, extensive burns, infected lesions
Hydrogels: sheets, wafers amorphous gels, impregnated gauze	May or may not be supported by a fabric net, high water content, varying amounts of gel-forming material (glycerin, co-polymer, water, propylene glycol, humectant) Elasto Gel (Southwest Technologies), Vigilon (Bard), Clear Site (New Dimensions in Medicine), Carrington Wound Gel (Carrington Labs)	Moist wound healing, absorb low to moderate drainage, autolysis, nonadhesive, may have adhesive borders, semipermeable or impermeable depending on backing, thermal insulation, reduces pain, carrier for topical medication, rehydrate wound, conformable	No borders—HCPC Code: KO242-44; Utilization Guide: 7×/wk Borders—HCPC Code: KO245-47; Utilization Guide: 3×/wk Gel filler—HCPC Code: KO248; Utilization Guide: 3 oz/mo Filler/Dry—HCPC Code: KO249; Utilization Guide: 7×/wk	Can dry out, may macerate surrounding tissues, require secondary dressing or tape, does not cause reinjury upon removal, cooling effect, Candidiasis may present from inappropriate usage.

Table continues

TABLE 11-15. (Continued)

Product	Definition and Example	Use	Reimbursement Codes, Utilization Guidelines	Notes
Exudate absorbers—wound fillers: beads, flakes pastes, powders	Consists of co-polymer starch, dextranomer beads or hydrocolloid paste that swells on contact with wound fluid to form a gel: dextranomers, polysaccharides, starch, natural polymers, and colloidal particles Allevyn Cavity Wound Dressing (Smith & Nephew United, Inc.), Debrisan (J&J), Bard Absorption Dressing (Bard Home Health Division)	Moisture retentive, absorptive, obliterate dead space, autolysis, can be used with topical medications	Gel/pastes—HCPC Code: A6261 Dry forms—HCPC Code: A6262	Non-adhesive, requires a secondary dressing, may have burning sensation on application, may have odor, may require mixing, requires wound irrigation for nontraumatic removal
Enzyme débriding agents: ointments	Chemical or enzymatic débriding agents in an ointment or cream base Elase (Fugisawa); Santyl (Knoll Pharmaceuticals); Panifil (Rystan)	Débridement of necrotic tissue, must score hard eschar before using agent, should be discontinued when granulation tissue is present in the wound bed	Prescription needed Utilization Guide: depends on agent used; can be 1×/day, bid, tid, or qid	Use with caution on patients with coagulation disorders; do not use soap, detergents, other acidic solutions, or metallic ion solutions (e.g., PhisoHex, Burrow's solution, Betadine) because they inhibit enzyme activity; most work best with damp secondary dressing; require secondary dressing
Alginates: pads, ropes	Calcium-sodium salts of alginic acid (naturally occurring polymer in seaweed) Sorbsan (Dow B. Hickam), Kaltostat	Autolysis, moisture retentive, absorptive (moderate to large), eliminate dead space, can be used with topical medications, can be used on infected wounds	HCPC Code: KO196-99; Utilization Guide: 1×/day	Nonadherent, hemostatic properties, requires irrigation, no reinjury on removal, requires secondary dressing, may dry out, should not be used on wounds with

Lubricating/ stimulating agents: sprays, ointments, creams	Hydrating creams, ointments, and sprays with various ingredients Granulex, Proderm (Dow B. Hickam), Dermagran Ointment/Spray (DermaSciences, Inc.)	Moist wound healing, autolysis (limited), reduces pain		Nonadherent, easy application, requires secondary dressing, requires 2–3 dressing changes per day, nonabsorptive, can use to impregnate gauze
Foams: wafers, pillows, with film coverings, surfactant impregnated or charcoal layer	Inert material that is hydrophilic and nonadherent, modified polyurethane foam LYOfoam (Acme United Corp.), Epi-Lock (Calgon Vestal Labs.), Allevyn (Smith & Nephew United, Inc.)	Moist wound healing, absorptive (moderate to large), autolysis, can be used with topical medications, can be used on infected wounds, thermal insulation, conformable, thick or thin	HCPC Code: KO209-14; Utilization Guide: 3×/wk Fillers—HCPC Code: KO215; Utilization Guide: 1×/day	Nonadhesive, requires taping, nontraumatic removal, opaque, waterproof, inert
Collagens: pads, powders, pastes	Bovine collagen attached to nylon mesh (a pad), powder or paste (supplied in syringe); composite collagen available as 90% collagen and 10% alginate ChroniCure (Dermasciences), Fibracol (Johnson & Johnson).	Small to moderate exudate, slight absorption, no adherence to wound bed, some left on wound 7 days, can be used with other topicals, indicated for contaminated, infected, wounds	HCPC Code: A6020	Nonadhesive, requires secondary dressing to hold in place or tape, nontraumatic removal, sensitivities to bovine materials may be experienced, dry wounds require additional saline before application

        1) Demonstrate one-person turning.
        2) Demonstrate two-person turning.
        3) Frequency of turning/repositioning.
        4) Full shifts in position versus small shifts in position.
        5) Avoidance of 90-degree sidelying position; demonstrate 30-degree laterally inclined position.
        6) Passive range of motion exercises and frequency.
    B. Pillow bridging
        1) Use of pillows to protect heels
        2) Pillows between bony prominences
    C. Pressure reducing/relieving support surface
        1) Management of support surface in use
        2) Devices for sitting
        3) Up in chair: How long, number of times per day
3. Teach nutrition strategies.
    A. Provide adequate nutrition.
        1) Small, frequent meals (6 a day) high-calorie/high-protein meals
        2) Nutritional supplements: Amount, type of supplement, number of times per day
    B. Provide adequate hydration: Eight 8-oz glasses of noncaffeine fluids/day unless contraindicated
    C. Provide vitamin, mineral supplements: vitamin C, zinc, iron as ordered
4. Teach friction and shear strategies.
    A. Use of turn-and-draw sheets
    B. Use of cornstarch, lubricants, pad protectors, thin film dressings or hydrocolloid dressings over friction risk sites
    C. General skin care
        1) Skin cleansing
        2) Skin moisturizing: Product, site(2) to apply, number of times per day
5. Teach moisture/incontinence management strategies.
    A. Use of absorbent products
        1) Pad when lying in bed
        2) Brief or panty pad when up in chair or walking
    B. Use of ointments, creams and skin barriers prophylactically in perineal and perianal areas: Product, number of times per day
    C. Use of behavioral management strategies for incontinence
        1) Scheduled toileting: Number of hours between
        2) Prompted voiding
    D. General skin care
        1) Skin cleansing: Cleanser, soap, frequency
        2) Skin moisturizing: Product(s), site(s) to apply, number of times per day
        3) Skin inspection daily
6. Reinforce importance of follow-up with health care provider.

PRESSURE SORE STATUS TOOL
Instructions for use

General Guidelines:

Fill out the attached rating sheet to assess a pressure sore's status after reading the definitions and methods of assessment described below. Evaluate once a week and whenever a change occurs in the wound. Rate according to each item by picking the response that best describes the wound and entering that score in the item score column for the appropriate date. When you have rated the pressure sore on all items, determine the total score by adding together the 13-item scores. The HIGHER the total score, the more severe the pressure sore status. Plot total score on the Pressure Sore Status Continuum to determine progress.

Specific Instructions:

1. **Size:** Use ruler to measure the longest and widest aspect of the wound surface in centimeters; multiply length × width.

2. **Depth:** Pick the depth, thickness, most appropriate to the wound using these additional descriptions:

   1 = tissues damaged but no break in skin surface.
   2 = superficial, abrasion, blister or shallow crater. Even with, &/or elevated above skin surface (e.g., hyperplasia).
   3 = deep crater with or without undermining of adjacent tissue.
   4 = visualization of tissue layers not possible due to necrosis.
   5 = supporting structures include tendon, joint capsule.

3. **Edges:** Use this guide:

Indistinct, diffuse	= unable to clearly distinguish wound outline.
Attached	= even or flush with wound base, <u>no</u> sides or walls present; flat.
Not attached	= sides or walls <u>are</u> present; floor or base of wound is deeper than edge.
Rolled under, thickened	= soft to firm and flexible to touch.
Hyperkeratosis	= callous-like tissue formation around wound & at edges.
Fibrotic, scarred	= hard, rigid to touch.

4. Undermining: Assess by inserting a cotton tipped applicator under the wound edge; advance it as far as it will go without using undue force; raise the tip of the applicator so it may be seen or felt on the surface of the skin; mark the surface with a pen; measure the distance from the mark on the skin to the edge of the wound. Continue process around the wound. Then use a transparent metric measuring guide with concentric circles divided into 4 (25%) pie-shaped quadrants to

5. Necrotic Tissue Type: Pick the type of necrotic tissue that is <u>predominant</u> in the wound according to color, consistency and adherence using this guide:

White/gray non-viable tissue	= may appear prior to wound opening; skin surface is white or gray.
Non-adherent, yellow slough	= thin, mucinous substance; scattered throughout wound bed; easily separated from wound tissue.
Loosely adherent, yellow slough	= thick, stringy, clumps of debris; attached to wound tissue.
Adherent, soft, black eschar	= soggy tissue; strongly attached to tissue in center or base of wound.
Firmly adherent, hard/black eschar	= firm, crusty tissue; strongly attached to wound base <u>and</u> edges (like a hard scab).

6. Necrotic Tissue Amount: Use a transparent metric measuring guide with concentric circles divided into 4 (25%) pie-shaped quadrants to help determine percent of wound involved.

7. Exudate Type: Some dressings interact with wound drainage to produce a gel or trap liquid. Before assessing exudate type, gently cleanse wound with normal saline or water. Pick the exudate type that is <u>predominant</u> in the wound according to color and consistency, using this guide:

Bloody	= thin, bright red
Serosanguineous	= thin, watery pale red to pink
Serous	thin, watery, clear
Purulent	= thin or thick, opaque tan to yellow
Foul purulent	= thick, opaque yellow to green with offensive odor

8. Exudate Amount: Use a transparent metric measuring guide with concentric circles divided into 4 (25%) pie-shaped quadrants to determine percent of dressing involved with exudate. Use this guide:

None	= wound tissues dry.
Scant	= wound tissues moist; no measurable exudate.
Small	= wound tissues wet; moisture evenly distributed in wound; drainage involves ≤ 25% dressing.
Moderate	= wound tissues saturated; drainage may or may not be evenly distributed in wound; drainage involves > 25% to ≤ 75% dressing.
Large	= wound tissues bathed in fluid; drainage freely expressed; may or may not be evenly distributed in wound; drainage involves > 75% of dressing.

9. Skin Color Surrounding Wound: Assess tissues within 4cm of wound edge. Dark-skinned persons show the colors "bright red" and "dark red" as a deepening of normal ethnic skin color or a purple hue. As healing occurs in dark-skinned persons, the new skin is pink and may never darken.

10. Peripheral Tissue Edema: Assess tissues within 4cm of wound edge. Non-pitting edema appears as skin that is shiny and taut. Identify pitting edema by firmly pressing a finger down into the tissues and waiting for 5 seconds, on release of pressure, tissues fail to resume previous position and an indentation appears. Crepitus is accumulation of air or gas in tissues. Use a transparent metric measuring guide to determine how far edema extends beyond wound.

11. Peripheral Tissue Induration: Assess tissues within 4cm of wound edge. Induration is abnormal firmness of tissues with margins. Assess by gently pinching the tissues. Induration results in an inability to pinch the tissues. Use a transparent metric measuring guide with concentric circles divided into 4 (25%) pie-shaped quadrants to determine percent of wound and area involved.

12. Granulation Tissue: Granulation tissue is the growth of small blood vessels and connective tissue to fill in full thickness wounds. Tissue is healthy when bright, beefy red, shiny and granular with a velvety appearance. Poor vascular supply appears as pale pink or blanched to dull, dusky red color.

13. Epithelialization: Epithelialization is the process of epidermal resurfacing and appears as pink or red skin. In partial thickness wounds it can occur throughout the wound bed as well as from the wound edges. In full thickness wounds it occurs from the edges only. Use a transparent metric measuring guide with concentric circles divided into 4 (25%) pie-shaped quadrants to help determine percent of wound involved and to measure the distance the epithelial tissue extends into the wound.

© 1990 Barbara Bates-Jensen

PRESSURE SORE STATUS TOOL   NAME _____

Complete the rating sheet to assess pressure sore status. Evaluate each item by picking the response that best describes the wound and entering the score in the item score column for the appropriate date.

Location: Anatomic site. Circle, identify right (R) or left (L) and use "X" to mark site on body diagrams:

_____	Sacrum & coccyx	_____	Lateral ankle
_____	Trochanter	_____	Medial ankle
_____	Ischial tuberosity	_____	Heel Other Site _____

Shape: Overall wound pattern; assess by observing perimeter and depth. Circle and <u>date</u> appropriate description:

_____	Irregular	_____	Linear or elongated
_____	Round/oval	_____	Bowl/boat
_____	Square/rectangle	_____	Butterfly Other Shape _____

Item	Assessment	Date	Date	Date
		Score	Score	Score
1. Size	1 = Length × width < 4 sq cm 2 = Length × width 4–16 sq cm 3 = Length × width 16.1–36 sq cm 4 = Length × width 36.1–80 sq cm 5 = Length × width > 80 sq cm			
2. Depth	1 = Non-blanchable erythema on intact skin 2 = Partial thickness skin loss involving epidermis &/or dermis 3 = Full thickness skin loss involving damage or necrosis of subcutaneous tissue; may extend down to but not through underlying fascia; &/or mixed partial & full thickness &/or tissue layers obscured by granulation tissue 4 = Obscured by necrosis 5 = Full thickness skin loss with extensive destruction, tissue necrosis or damage to muscle, bone or supporting structures			
3. Edges	1 = Indistinct, diffuse, none clearly visible 2 = Distinct, outline clearly visible, attached, even with wound base 3 = Well-defined, not attached to wound base 4 = Well-defined, not attached to base, rolled under, thickened 5 = Well-defined, fibrotic, scarred or hyperkeratotic			
4. Under-mining	1 = Undermining < 2 cm in any area 2 = Undermining 2–4 cm involving < 50% wound margins 3 = Undermining 2–4 cm involving > 50% wound margins 4 = Undermining > 4 cm in any area 5 = Tunneling &/or sinus tract formation			
5. Necrotic Tissue Type	1 = None visible 2 = White/gray non-viable tissue &/or non-adherent yellow slough 3 = Loosely adherent yellow slough 4 = Adherent, soft, black eschar 5 = Firmly adherent, hard, black eschar			
6. Necrotic Tissue Amount	1 = None visible 2 = < 25% of wound bed covered 3 = 25% to 50% of wound covered 4 = > 50% and < 75% of wound covered 5 = 75% to 100% of wound covered			

© 1990 Barbara Bates-Jensen

Item	Assessment	Date	Date	Date
		Score	Score	Score
7. Exudate Type	1 = None or bloody 2 = Serosanguineous: thin, watery, pale red/pink 3 = Serous: thin, watery, clear 4 = Purulent: thin or thick, opaque, tan/yellow 5 = Foul purulent: thick, opaque, yellow/green with odor			
8. Exudate Amount	1 = None 2 = Scant 3 = Small 4 = Moderate 5 = Large			
9. Skin color Surrounding Wound	1 = Pink or normal for ethnic group 2 = Bright red &/or blanches to touch 3 = White or gray pallor or hypopigmented 4 = Dark red or purple &/or non-blanchable 5 = Black or hyperpigmented			
10. Peripheral Tissue Edema	1 = Minimal swelling around wound 2 = Non-pitting edema extends < 4 cm around wound 3 = Non-pitting edema extends ≥ 4 cm around wound 4 = Pitting edema extends < 4 cm around wound 5 = Crepitus &/or pitting edema extends ≥ 4 cm			
11. Peripheral Tissue Induration	1 = Minimal firmness around wound 2 = Induration < 2 cm around wound 3 = Induration 2-4 cm extending < 50% around wound 4 = Induration 2-4 cm extending ≥ 50% around wound 5 = Induration > 4 cm in any area			
12. Granulation Tissue	1 = Skin intact or partial thickness wound 2 = Bright, beefy red; 75% to 100% of wound filled &/or tissue overgrowth 3 = Bright, beefy red; < 75% & > 25% of wound filled 4 = Pink, &/or dull, dusky red &/or fills ≤ 25% of wound 5 = No granulation tissue present			
13. Epithelialization	1 = 100% wound covered, surface intact 2 = 75% to < 100% wound covered &/or epithelial tissue extends > 0.5 cm into wound bed 3 = 50% to < 75% wound covered &/or epithelial tissue extends to < 0.5 cm into wound bed 4 = 25% to < 50% wound covered 5 = < 25% wound covered			
TOTAL SCORE				
SIGNATURE				

PRESSURE SORE STATUS CONTINUUM

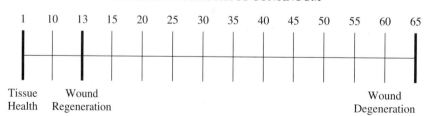

Plot the total score on the Pressure Sore Status Continuum by putting an "X" on the line and the date beneath the line. Plot multiple scores with their dates to see-at-a-glance regeneration or degeneration of the wound.
© 1990 Barbara Bates-Jensen

Review Questions

11.29 A 70-year-old male is S/P cerebral vascular accident and has a stage III pressure ulcer on his right trochanter, with 75% of the ulcer filled with yellow, stringy slough. Which initial intervention would be most appropriate in the management of this wound?
   A. Intravenous antibiotics
   B. Cleanse with normal saline and cover with dry gauze dressing
   C. Enzymatic debridement
   D. Alginate dressing

11.30 An 81-year-old female is admitted from a nursing home with pneumonia, urinary incontinence, and a stage II pressure ulcer on the sacral/coccygeal area. What laboratory tests or supplemental treatments might be helpful in treating this patient's wound?
   A. Obtain and monitor serum albumin levels; provide supplemental vitamin C, zinc, and iron.
   B. Monitor CBC and electrolytes; folic acid supplementation.
   C. Obtain thyroid function tests; administer oral antibiotics.
   D. Obtain wound culture and sensitivity and begin broad-spectrum topical antibiotic treatment.

11.31 Mrs. J is a 60-year-old female with a history of multiple sclerosis who has been bedbound for the past 5 years. She has a large, foul-smelling, stage IV pressure ulcer on the coccyx that has purulent drainage, is 75% covered with necrotic debris and surrounding erythema. There is mild peripheral tissue edema, and induration is present and extends approximately 3 cm from the wound margin. Virtually no granulation tissue or epithelialization is present. She has a temperature of 101°F. The ACNP should consider which of the following interventions to further evaluate the patient?
   A. Wound culture and sensitivity; use aerobic swab and be sure to swab the necrotic tissue; CBC, blood cultures
   B. X-ray to rule out osteomyelitis; immediate débridement of nonviable necrotic tissue; systemic antibiotics (broad-spectrum coverage); CBC; tissue biopsy or needle aspiration of wound once bulk of necrotic debris is removed
   C. Intravenous antibiotics (broad-spectrum coverage); wound cultures and sensitivity; CBC and electrolyte panel, serum albumin level
   D. X-ray to rule out osteomyelitis and CBC

11.32 The ACNP is evaluating a 70-year-old patient who has a lower leg venous ulcer. Which of the following WILL NOT optimize venous return?
   A. Four-layer wrap
   B. Unna's boot
   C. Pressure gradient support stocking
   D. Antiembolism stockings

11.33 Wound débridement is contraindicated in which of the following cases?
   A. Stage III pressure ulcer on the ankle with 50% yellow, stringy slough present; peripheral pulses palpable; ankle/brachial index >0.5
   B. Arterial/ischemic ulcer on lateral malleolus covered with 50% necrotic tissue; peripheral pulses not palpable; ankle/brachial index <0.5; significant pain in ulcer

C. Pressure ulcer on sacrum covered with soggy, black eschar; slight surrounding edema and induration
D. Venous ulcer on medial calf with 50% covered with stringy, yellow fibrinous material; peripheral pulses palpable; ankle/brachial index >0.5; no complaints of pain in ulcer

Answers and Rationales

11.29 **C** The first principle of wound care is to remove necrotic debris. The only choice given for débridement in this scenario is enzymatic débriding agents. Other choices would include autolytic débridement using moisture-retentive dressings and sequential sharp débridement in conjunction with enzymatic or autolytic dressings.

11.30 **A** Serum albumin levels help monitor nutritional status (provide an index to nutrition over the last 3 weeks). Supplemental vitamin C, zinc, and iron have been shown to improve healing when levels are below normal.

11.31 **B** Débridement of nonviable necrotic tissue will often suffice in preventing wound infection. It is useless to obtain swab cultures of a wound filled with necrosis. Tissue biopsy or needle aspiration are the recommended methods of determining wound infection. Systemic antibiotics are more effective in eliminating true infection than topical antibiotics.

11.32 **D** Antiembolism stockings do not provide the needed 30 mm Hg compression required to treat venous disease.

11.33 **B** There are several contraindications to sharp débridement in this case; the first is the nature of the ulcer. Always use caution in débridement of arterial lesions. The ankle/brachial index indicates significant ischemia and is a direct contraindication to débridement, as is the lack of pulses.

References

Allman, R.M., Laprade, C.A., Noel, L.B., et al. (1986). Pressure sores among hospitalized patients. *Ann Intern Med 105*, 337–342.

Alterescu, V. (1989). The financial costs of inpatient pressure ulcers to an acute care facility. *Decubitus 2*(3), 14–23.

Alvarez, O.M. (1988). Moist environment for healing: Matching the dressing to the wound. *Ostomy/Wound Management Winter*, 64–83.

Bates-Jensen, B. (1990). New pressure ulcer status tool. *Decubitus 3*(3), 14–15.

Bates-Jensen, B. (1994). An analytical tool to enhance wound healing. *Nurs Home Pract 2*(6), 6–12.

Bates-Jensen, B. (1994). The Pressure Sore Status Tool: an outcome measure for pressure sores. *Topics Geriatr Rehabil 9*(4), 17–34.

Bates-Jensen, B. (1995). Indices for pressure ulcer assessment: The Pressure Sore Status Tool. *Adv Wound Care 8*(3, Suppl.), 28–25.

Bates-Jensen, B. (1997). Incontinence management. In L.C. Parish, J.A. Witkowski, & J.T. Crissey, (eds.). *The Decubitus Ulcer in Clinical Practice*. Berlin: Springer, pp. 189–199.

Bates-Jensen, B.M., Vredevoe, D.L., & Brecht, M.L. (1992). Validity and reliability of the Pressure Sore Status Tool. *Decubitus* 5(6), 20–28.

Bennett, L., Kavner, D., Lee, B.Y., et al. (1969). Skin stress and blood flow in sitting paraplegic patients. *Arch Phys Med Rehabil 65*, 186.

Bennett, M.A. (1995). Report of the task force on the implications for darkly pigmented intact skin in the prediction and prevention of pressure ulcers. *Adv Wound Care* 8(6), 34–35.

Bergstrom, N., Bennett, M.A., Carlson, C.E., et al. (1994). *Pressure Ulcer Treatment Guideline: Reference Guide for Clinicians, No. 15* (AHCPR Publ. No. 95-0653). Rockville, MD: Agency for Health Care Policy and Research.

Bergstrom, N., Demuth, P.J., & Braden, B.J. (1987). A clinical trial of the Braden Scale for predicting pressure sore risk. *Nurs Clin North Am 22*(2), 417.

Braden, B.J., & Bergstrom, N. (1987). A conceptual schema for the study of the etiology of pressure sores. *Rehabil Nurs 12*(1), 8.

Brennan, S.S., Foster, M.E., & Leaper, D.J. (1986). Antiseptic toxicity in wounds healing by secondary intention. *J Hosp Infect 8*, 263–267.

Brown-Etris, M. (1995). Measuring healing in wounds. *Adv Wound Care 8*(3, Suppl.), 28–53.

Bryant, R.A., Shannon, M.L., Pieper, B., et al. (1992). Pressure ulcers. In R.A. Bryant (ed.). *Acute and Chronic Wounds: Nursing Management.* St. Louis: Mosby–Year Book, pp. 105–152.

Cooper, D.M. (1992). Wound assessment and evaluation of healing. In R.A. Bryant (ed.). *Acute and Chronic Wounds: Nursing Management.* St. Louis: Mosby–Year Book, pp. 69–90.

Doughty, D.B. (1992). Principles of wound healing and wound management. In R.A. Bryant (ed.). *Acute and Chronic Wounds: Nursing Management.* St. Louis: Mosby–Year Book, pp. 31–61.

Eaglestein, W., Mertz, P., & Alvarez, O. (1984). Effect of topically applied agents on healing wounds. *Clin Dermatol 2*, 112–115.

Gilson, G.M. (1991). *Topical Agents for Open Wounds.* Charleston, SC: Support Systems International, Inc.

Harding, K.G. (1990). Wound care: putting theory into clinical practice. *Wounds 2*(1), 21–31.

Lineaweaver, W. (1985). Cellular and bacterial toxicities of topical antimicrobials. *Plast Reconstr Surg 75*, 394–396.

Panel for the Prediction and Prevention of Pressure Ulcers in Adults. (1992). *Pressure Ulcers in Adults: Prediction and Prevention: Clinical Practice Guideline, No. 3* (AHCPR Publ. No. 92-0047). Rockville, MD: Agency for Health Care Policy and Research.

Robson, M., Phillips, L.G., Thomason, A., et al. (1992). Platelet-derived factors BB for treatment of chronic pressure ulcers. *Lancet 339*, 23–25.

Robson, M., Phillips, L.G., Thomason, A., et al. (1992). Recombinant human growth factor-bb for the treatment of chronic pressure ulcers. *Ann Plast Surg 29*, 193–201.

Rodeheaver, G. (1988). Controversies in topical wound management. *Ostomy/Wound Management Fall*, 59–68.

Stotts, N. (1995). Determination of bacterial burden in wounds. *Adv Wound Care 8*(3, Suppl.), 28–46.

Van Rijswijk, L. (1993). Full-thickness pressure ulcers: Patient and wound healing characteristics. *Decubitus 6*(1), 16–30.

Van Rijswijk, L., & Polansky, M. (1994). Predictors of time to healing deep pressure ulcers. *Wounds 6*(5), 159–165.

Additional Recommended References

Bergstrom, N., Bennett, M.A., Carlson, C.E., et al. (1994). *Treatment of Pressure Ulcers: Clinical Practice Guideline, No. 15* (AHCPR Publ. No. 95-0652) Rockville, MD: Agency for Health Care Policy and Research.

Bryant, R.A. (ed.). (1992). *Acute and Chronic Wounds: Nursing Management.* St. Louis: Mosby–Year Book.

Jeter, J.F., Faller, N., & Norton, C. (eds.). (1990). *Nursing for Continence.* Philadelphia: W.B. Saunders Co.

Krasner, D., & Kane, D. (eds.). (1990). *Chronic Wound Care* (2nd ed.). King of Prussia, PA: Health Management Publications, Inc.

Maklebust, J., & Sieggreen, M. (1996). *Pressure Ulcers: Guidelines for Prevention and Nursing Management* (2nd ed.). Springhouse, PA: Springhouse Corporation.

Panel for the Prediction and Prevention of Pressure Ulcers in Adults. (1992). *Pressure Ulcers in Adults: Prediction and Prevention: Clinical Practice Guideline, No. 3* (AHCPR Publ. No. 92-0047). Rockville, MD: Agency for Health Care Policy and Research.

Panel on Urinary Incontinence in Adults. (1992). *Urinary Incontinence in Adults: Clinical Practice Guidelines.* (AHCPR Publ. No. 92-0038). Rockville, MD: Agency for Health Care Policy and Research.

Parish, L.C., Witkowski, J.A., & Crissey, J.T. (eds.). *The Decubitus Ulcer in Clinical Practice.* Berlin: Springer.

COMMON DERMATOLOGIC DISORDERS

Adverse Cutaneous Drug Eruptions

DEFINITION

An adverse cutaneous drug eruption is a skin eruption caused by any *systemically* administered drug or medication; medications could include vitamins, laxatives, or "tonics." Reactions tend to occur more rapidly with drugs administered by parenteral routes. An eruption occurring from a *locally* applied drug is a contact dermatitis.

ETIOLOGY/INCIDENCE

1. Two to 3% of all hospitalized patients experience an adverse drug reaction.
2. The reaction may present as a rash, urticaria, angioedema, skin pain or pruritus, mucous membrane erosions, blisters, or skin necrosis.
3. The majority of reactions are mild and resolve quickly after the offending drug is stopped.

SIGNS AND SYMPTOMS

1. A measles-like pattern (morbilliform), with symmetric bright red macules and papules.
2. Papules, vesicles in an annular configuration in a "bull's-eye" or target shape, commonly on the palms and soles (sometimes called erythema multiforme minor).
3. Hives, angioedema, anaphylaxis.

4. Severe systemic symptoms: fever, hepatitis, arthralgias, lymphadenopathy along with a rash, vesicles, or blisters.
5. Fixed solitary bulla/erosion at *identical* site within hours of ingestion of a drug.
6. Reactions can occur immediately, as the drug is being administered, or can be delayed as long as several weeks.

PHYSICAL FINDINGS

1. Bright red macules and/or papules developing within 2 or 3 days after the administration of the offending drug.
   A. The distribution is symmetric and usually is found on the trunk and extremities.
   B. The rash may spare surgical scars, the face, and periareolar areas.
   C. *Drugs with highest probability of reaction:* Penicillin and related antibiotics, anticonvulsives, and antihypertensives.
2. Urticarial wheals, commonly known as hives, can appear suddenly and resolve within minutes to several hours.
   A. The wheals can have white central areas surrounded by a red halo.
   B. The size may vary from a few millimeters to large lesions >22 cm in diameter.
3. Angioedema is often pronounced on the face, lips, and tongue.
   A. The condition may be life-threatening if the tissue swelling extends to airway obstruction.
   B. *Drugs with highest probability of reaction:* Penicillin, sulfonamides, and their derivatives; calcium-channel blockers; phenytoin drugs releasing histamines (morphine, radiographic contrast material, hydralazine).
4. A fixed drug eruption can present as a single, well-demarcated macule that progresses within a few hours to an edematous, painful lesion that can then evolve into a bulla.
   A. The color is bright red to violaceous and fades to brownish when healing.
   B. *Drugs with the highest probability of reaction:* Phenolphthalein, tetracyclines, sulfonamides, aspirin, and barbiturates.
5. Stevens-Johnson syndrome (also known as erythema multiforme major) and toxic epidermal necrolysis (TEN) are the most severe forms of mucocutaneous drug reactions.
   A. Oral, nasal, ocular, urethral, and genital mucosa are often involved with blisters, weeping, and erosions.
   B. A positive Nikolsky's sign: Lateral pressure on the blister causes the blister to enlarge or the skin to slough.
   C. Constitutional symptoms include cough, high fever, vomiting and diarrhea, and arthralgias.
   D. Patients can be ill enough to require hospitalization to combat severe dehydration, fluid and electrolyte imbalances secondary to loss of the skin barrier.
   E. TEN is a true dermatologic emergency, with a high percentage of fully developed cases dying.
      1) Rapid identification and removal of the causative agent is prime.
      2) Individuals are often given supportive care in an ICU or burn unit.
   F. *Commonly implicated medication for both conditions:* Sulfonamides, allopurinol, penicillin, and tetracycline.

DIFFERENTIAL DIAGNOSIS

1. Viral exanthems
2. Widespread allergic dermatitis
3. Secondary syphilis
4. Serum sickness
5. Insect bites
6. Cellulitis
7. Herpes simplex virus
8. Vasculitis
9. Graft-versus-host disease.
10. With blistering lesions: herpes simplex, bullous pemphigoid

DIAGNOSTIC TESTS/FINDINGS

1. The diagnosis is normally based on clinical findings.
2. A skin biopsy may be helpful in determining the type of reaction; it does not help in identifying the drug triggering the reaction.
3. Laboratory testing may show abnormal liver functions tests and a very high eosinophil count ($>1000/\mu L$).

MANAGEMENT/TREATMENT

1. Identify and discontinue the drug through careful patient history, especially the drug history and physical examination.
2. Epinephrine for airway emergencies: Initial adult dose is 0.3–0.5 mg (1:1000) SC or IM repeating prn every 20 minutes to 4 hours. Important to follow the protocols established in the individual ACNP's facility!
3. Use of oral antihistamines and/or H_2 antihistamine (e.g., ranitidine).
4. Topical corticosteroids, if intense pruritis and subsequent scratching has occurred. Consult with physician concerning potency levels.
5. Consult with collaborating physician regarding possible transfer to an ICU or burn unit if the condition is life-threatening.

PATIENT EDUCATION

Instruct the patient to:
1. Inform all subsequent health care providers of the reaction.
2. Wear a medical alert bracelet.
3. Never take the drug again.
4. Be aware of cross-reactions to "similar drugs."

References

American Academy of Pediatrics. (1997). *1997 Red Book: Report of the Committee on Infectious Diseases* (24th ed.). Elk Grove, IL: American Academy of Pediatrics

Cohen, B.A. (1993). *Atlas of Pediatric Dermatology*. London: Wolfe.

Drug facts and comparisons (50th ed.). (1996). St. Louis, MO: Facts and Comparisons.

du Vivier, A. (1993). *Atlas of Clinical Dermatology* (2nd ed.). London: Mosby-Wolfe.

Fitzpatrick, T.B., Johnson, R.A., Wolff, K., et al. (1997). *Color Atlas and Synopsis of Clinical Dermatology: Common and Serious Diseases* (3rd ed.). New York: McGraw-Hill.

Reizner, G.T. (1996). *Dermatology Essentials*. Madison: University of Wisconsin, Department of Medicine, Department of Dermatology.

Sauer, G.C., & Hall, J.C. (1996). *Manual of Skin Diseases* (7th ed.). Philadelphia: Lippincott-Raven.

ALLERGIC AND CONTACT DERMATITIS

Overview

ALLERGIC CONTACT DERMATITIS VERSUS IRRITANT CONTACT DERMATITIS

1. The immune response for *allergic contact dermatitis* represents the classical expression of delayed (cellular) hypersensitivity—a new antigen is created. It *requires prior exposure* with the offending material to cause a reaction. This delayed reaction needs only small amounts of antigen to trigger the reaction.
2. Two effects separate irritant contact dermatitis from allergic dermatitis.
   A. In irritant contact dermatitis large qualities of the substance are needed to produce the reaction, while allergic contact dermatitis requires only miniscule amounts of material.
   B. The initial irritant does not require prior exposure.
3. Most people will react to the chemical if the concentration is strong enough or the exposure is long enough.
4. Poison ivy and skin of the mango are examples of allergic contact dermatitis, while dishwashing soap, alkalis, organic solvents, and detergents are examples of noxious agents that can cause irritant contact dermatitis. Other common agents include neomycin, benzocaine gel, nickel sulfate in jewelry, and formalin in disinfectants and plastics.

DIAGNOSTIC TEST

Patch testing can be done, especially in chronic cases.

PATIENT EDUCATION

Instruct the patient to:

1. Avoid the offending substances by wearing protective gear, gloves, and the like if working with irritants or allergenic (for the particular individual) material.
2. Consult with primary care physician; generally will refer to dermatologist or allergist.

References

Marks, J.G., Jr., & DeLeo, V.A. (1997). *Contact and Occupational Dermatology* (2nd ed.). St. Louis: Mosby–Year Book.

Reizner, G. (1997). *Dermatology Essentials*. Madison: University of Wisconsin, Department of Medicine, Division of Dermatology.

Poison Ivy (Rhus Dermatitis)

DEFINITION

Rhus dermatitis is an acute inflammatory reaction in the skin triggered by direct contact with the colorless oil (urushiol) of poison ivy, poison oak, or poison sumac plants. *Requires prior exposure* to material to induce reaction.

ETIOLOGY/INCIDENCE

1. Generally a seasonal dermatitis occurring when the plant is growing.
2. Recurrent or persistent dermatitis may indicate contact with fomites (golf balls, pets, tools, etc.) that are contaminated with urushiol.

SIGNS AND SYMPTOMS

1. History of exposure by outdoor activities or contact with animals, tools, or clothing of individuals in contact with the oil from a broken plant.
2. Pruritus and "rash" appearing 12–72 hours after contact.

PHYSICAL FINDINGS

1. Linear group of erythematous papules
2. Vesicles, edema, and bullae subsequently develop

DIFFERENTIAL DIAGNOSIS

Allergic/contact dermatitis—dozens of common allergens.

DIAGNOSTIC TESTS/FINDINGS

Rhus dermatitis is usually a clinical diagnosis.

MANAGEMENT/TREATMENT

1. Wash exposed skin with copious amounts of water as soon as possible (within 15 minutes is best).
2. Scrub underneath fingernails, especially if gardening without gloves.
3. Apply cold, wet compresses with astringents (Domeboro) for 15–20 minutes three to four times a day during the blistering stage.
4. Take cool tub baths with colloidal oatmeal to decrease inflammation.
5. Wash the clothing worn when exposed to the allergenic resin.
6. Use medications to control pruritus.
   A. Hydroxyzine 25 mg PO three to four times daily *or*
   B. Clorpheniramine 4 mg PO three times daily
7. Consult the primary care physician if the lesions are extensive, involving the eyes, face, genitalia, or mucous membranes. An oral corticosteroid may be prescribed: prednisone 40 to 60 mg daily with taper closing. Consult with physician for regimen tailored to patient's condition.

PATIENT EDUCATION

Instruct the patient to:
1. Follow up in 2–3 days for severe reactions.
2. Prevent subsequent exposures by using an over-the-counter (OTC) medication called Ivy Block when working or exercising in areas where poison ivy foliage is common.
3. Wear long pants and shirts if entering a high-risk area.
4. Wash exposed skin with copious amounts of water as soon as possible (within 15 minutes is best).
5. Apply cold, wet compresses with astringents (Domeboro) for 15–20 minutes three to four times a day during the blistering stage.
6. Take cool tub baths with colloidal oatmeal to decrease inflammation.
7. Be aware that new lesions can continue to appear during the entire duration of the eruption; new lesions to *do not* mean that the rash is spreading.
8. Avoid the use of OTC-strength hydrocortisone because it is rarely effective.

References

American Academy of Dermatology. (1991). *Poison Ivy, Sumac & Oak* (Form TPAM11). Schaumburg, IL: American Academy of Dermatology.

Cohen, B.A. (1993). *Atlas of Pediatric Dermatology*. London: Wolfe.

Epstein, W.L., Guin, J.D., & Maibach, H.I. (1997). It's always poison ivy time. *Patient Care June 15*, 31–52.

Graham, M.V., & Uphold, C.R. (1994). *Clinical Guidelines in Child Health*. Gainesville, FL: Barmarrae Books.

Sauer, G.D., & Hall, J.C. (1997). *Manual of Skin Diseases* (7th ed.). Philadelphia: Lippincott-Raven.

AUTOIMMUNE DISORDER—SYSTEMIC LUPUS ERYTHEMATOSUS (CUTANEOUS MANIFESTATIONS)

DEFINITION

SLE is a serious multisystem disorder involving the immune system. It is difficult to predict which systems will be affected for each individual. After arthritis, the most common clinical findings are dermatologic.

ETIOLOGY/INCIDENCE

1. Average age at diagnosis is 30 for females and 40 for males.
2. Female/male ratio is 8:1.

SIGNS AND SYMPTOMS

1. Duration of lesions can be from weeks to months.
2. Pruritus common with papular lesions.
3. Photosensitivity.
4. Fatigue and fever.
5. Oral ulcers.
6. Arthralgias.

Physical Findings (from Revised Criteria for Classification of SLE [Tan et al, 1982])

1. Malar rash: Fixed erythema, flat or raised over the malar area; tends to spare nasolabial folds; "butterfly pattern"
2. Discoid rash: Red raised patches with adherent keratotic scaling; follicular plugging
3. Painless oral ulcers

DIFFERENTIAL DIAGNOSIS

1. Secondary syphilis
2. Psoriasis
3. Tinea corporis

DIAGNOSTIC TESTS/FINDINGS

SLE is diagnosed by serologic markers: ANA, C3 and C4, anti-RNP, others

MANAGEMENT/TREATMENT

1. Refer to rheumatologist or primary care physician comfortable with treating disease, especially if there is active renal disease, a central nervous system disorder, or an infection.
2. Hydroxychloroquine is drug of choice: 200 mg twice a week.

PATIENT EDUCATION

The ACNP will:

1. Instruct the patient to use sun protection factor (cSPF) so sunscreen.
2. Recommend an eye exam within 60 days of initiating therapy and then every 6 months.

References

Fitzpatrick, T.B., Johnson, R.A., Wolff, K., et al. (1997). *Color Atlas and Synopsis of Clinical Dermatology: Common and Serious Diseases* (3rd ed.). New York: McGraw-Hill.

Peck, B. (1995). Systemic lupus erythematosus. *ADVANCE Nurse Practit October*, 24–29.

Tan, E.M., Cohen, A.S., Fries, J.F., et al. (1982). The 1982 revised criteria for the classification of systemic lupus erythematous (SLE). *Arthritis Rheum 25*, 1271–1277.

COMMON CUTANEOUS MALIGNANT NEOPLASMS

The most common malignant neoplasms of the skin are basal cell carcinoma, squamous cell carcinoma, melanoma, and Kaposi's sarcoma. Table 11–16 presents the incidence, physical findings, diagnostic methods, and types of treatment for each.

MANAGEMENT/TREATMENT

1. Curettage and electrodesiccation: Good cures rates for small basal cell carcinoma (<2 cm)
2. Excision: Permits histologic diagnosis of margins; preferred for squamous cell carcinoma.
3. Topical fluorouracil: An option for very superficial basal cell carcinoma.
4. Mohs' surgery (micrographic): Best cure rates with lowest reoccurrence; avoids removal of healthy tissue; preferred for recurrent basal or squamous cell carcinoma
5. Radiation therapy: Possible for medically compromised individuals; numerous sessions needed

PATIENT EDUCATION

Instruct the patient to:

1. Schedule an appointment with a dermatologist for evaluation and possible biopsy.
2. Seek care from an infectious disease specialist if KS is suspected.

TABLE 11-16. **Common Cutaneous Malignant Neoplasms**

Type	Incidence	Findings	Diagnosis	Treatment
Basal cell carcinoma	Most common: 600,000 cases/yr	Waxy, semitranslucent nodule with pearly rolled borders with overlying telangiectasias; develops central ulcerations eventually	Shave, punch or excisional biopsy	Excision; curettage and electrodessication; topical fluorouracil; Mohs' surgery
Squamous cell carcinoma	Second most common: 200,000 cases/yr; 2100 deaths	Slow-growing red plaques with scales, crusts, and focal erosion	As above	Excision; Mohs' surgery; radiation
Melanoma	Third most common: 38,000–80,000 cases/yr; most deadly: 7300 deaths	Dark brown to black with admixture of pink, gray, bluish hues; lesion growing over 6 cm; asymmetric with irregular or notched borders; can proceed to bleeding, eroding lesion	Excisional biopsy	Wide excision; elective regional lymph node dissection is controversial; survival rates can depend on thickness of lesion
Kaposi's sarcoma (KS)	Immuno-compromised individuals: renal transplant, HIV (58% of HIV-positive men have KS)	Initially oval, firm, palpable lesion; violaceous to purple-brown	Biopsy; positive serologic markers for HIV	Local radiotherapy for classic non-HIV KS; chemotherapy to control symptoms—no cure

References

Battling the skin cancer epidemic. (1994). *Clinician Rev 4,* 60–70.

Fitzpatrick, T.B., Johnson, R.A., Wolff, K., et al. (1997). *Color Atlas and Synopsis of Clinical Dermatology: Common and Serious Diseases* (3rd ed.). New York: McGraw-Hill.

Marghoob, A.A. (1997). Basal and squamous cell carcinomas: What every primary care physician should known. *Postgrad Med 102,* 139–159.

McEldowney, S. (1997). Malignant melanoma: Familial, genetic and psychosocial risk factors. *Clinician Rev 7,* 65–82.

COMMON DERMATOSES

Acute Sun Damage (Sunburn)

DEFINITION

Sunburn is a delayed, transient inflammatory skin response following exposure to ultraviolet radiation. It is the first acute sign of solar damage. Chronic damage can result in early wrinkling, mottled pigmentation, small "spider" blood vessels, and coarseness and atrophy of the skin.

ETIOLOGY/INCIDENCE

A history of "blistering" sunburns in childhood is a risk factor for developing any one of the three most common types of skin cancers in later years.

SIGNS AND SYMPTOMS

1. Pain and tenderness on exposed areas
2. Pruritus
3. Headache, chills, feverishness

PHYSICAL FINDINGS

1. Erythema, edema
2. Vesicles, bullae
3. Never any "rashes" in normal sunburn
4. Resolves with peeling (desquamation)

DIFFERENTIAL DIAGNOSIS

1. SLE can cause a sunburn-like reaction.
2. Obtain history of recent medications: Sulfonamides, naproxen, tetracyclines (especially doxycycline)can cause an exuberant "overresponse" to a sunburn.

DIAGNOSTIC TESTS/FINDINGS

Sunburn is a clinical diagnosis.

MANAGEMENT/TREATMENT

1. Prophylactic treatment
   A. Most sunscreens of SPF over 15 will protect against 93% of ultraviolet B (UVB) rays.
   B. Shade UVA Guard is the only sunscreen that protects against UVB and ultraviolet A (UVA) radiation. UVA rays are longer and may have more carcinogenic potential.
2. Moderate sunburn
   A. Cool wet dressings, topical hydrocortisone (OTC)
   B. Aspirin or OTC NSAIDs
   C. Severe burns can be treated with silver sulfadiazene (Silvadene) cream

PATIENT EDUCATION

Instruct the patient to:

1. Use sunscreens and lip balm (with SPF over 15) on a daily basis for all individuals particularly those with skin photo types 1 and 2.
   A. Type 1: Always burns, never tans (blond, redhead)
   B. Type 2: Always burns, sometimes tans
   C. Type 3: Sometimes burns, always tans
   D. Type 4: Never burns, always tans
   E. Type 5: African American skin
   F. Type 6: Never burns
2. Apply sunscreen 15–30 minutes before entering the sun and apply the sunscreen every 1–2 hours if swimming or excessively perspiring.

3. Wear sunscreen clothing such as Solumbra (catalog available from Sun Precautions; 1-800-882-7860)
4. Use sunglasses capable of blocking 99–100% of UVA and UVB rays.
5. Avoid the use of sunscreen on infants younger than 6 months. Use protective clothing or umbrella/canopy.
6. Avoid artificial tanning devices.
7. Examine skin for redness or blistering and for new or changing moles.

References

du Vivier, A. (1993). *Atlas of Clinical Dermatology* (2nd ed.). London: Mosby-White.

Fitzpatrick, T.B., Johnson, R.A., Wolff, K., et al. (1997). *Color Atlas and Synopsis of Clinical Dermatology: Common and Serious Diseases* (3rd ed.). New York: McGraw-Hill.

Kim, H.J., Ghali, F.E., & Tunnessen, W.W. (1997). Here comes the sun. *Contemp Pediatr, 14*, 41–69.

Atopic Dermatitis (Eczema)

DEFINITION

Atopic dermatitis is a pruritic inflammation of the skin, often occurring in association with a family or personal history of hayfever, allergic rhinitis, asthma, or "eczema."

ETIOLOGY/INCIDENCE

1. Etiology is unknown; the skin of the atopic individuals is very sensitive and has a greater than normal tendency to develop "itching," which then leads to rubbing and scratching, causing vicious cycle to emerge.
2. Most individuals show evidence of the condition from early infancy to the age of 2.
3. Only 10% will develop the disorder after the age of 6.
4. More males are affected.
5. Incidence has been estimated at 7:100 individuals in the United States.
6. Condition improves in the summer, worsens in winter.

SIGNS AND SYMPTOMS

1. Pruritus, moist abrasions on cheeks, forehead, etc.
2. Skin appears "puffy."

PHYSICAL FINDINGS

1. Dry skin: Patches and large areas of minute dry scale on trunk and extremities while the palms may show fine wrinkles, especially along the finger pads.
2. Extra crease in the lower lid: "Atopic pleat."
3. Skin exhibits "white dermographism": The skin blanches a minute after stroking (i.e., with a tongue blade) instead of demonstrating the normal red line reaction to the strokes.
   A. In infants: Acute condition with exudation and crusting on the face, neck, and flexural surface of extremities. Weeping skin is susceptible to bacterial infections.
   B. In adults: More dermatitis with lichenification, fissuring on the face, neck, and upper extremities.

DIFFERENTIAL DIAGNOSIS

1. Seborrheic dermatitis
2. Irritant or allergic dermatitis

DIAGNOSTIC TESTS/FINDINGS

1. History in infancy
2. Clinical findings regarding typical distribution sites, shape of lesions, and "white dermographism"

MANAGEMENT/TREATMENT

1. Wet compresses of Burrow's solution.
2. Hydration of the skin through bathing with immediate application of an emollient cream (Eucerin).
3. Avoid hot water and use mild, high-fat soaps.
4. Humidification of dry air in the winter and use of air conditioner in summer to avoid perspiration, a pruritic stimulus.
5. Topical corticosteroids using the lowest potency levels to control the symptoms (class V or Vi).

PATIENT EDUCATION

Instruct the patient regarding:

1. The chronic nature of the condition can be controlled with consistent care.
2. Exacerbations can occur related to unknown precipitants or stress.
3. Calling a primary care provider if the patient has herpes or develops honey-colored discharge from an open atopic lesions (may indicate a superimposed staphylococcal infection; acyclovir or antibiotics are prescribed).
4. The disease is not scarring or contagious.
5. Condition is often outgrown by adolescence.
6. Diet may *not* play a significant part of treatment.

References

Cohen, B.A. (1993). *Atlas of Pediatric Dermatology*. London: Wolfe.

du Vivier, A. (1993). *Atlas of Clinical Dermatology* (2nd ed.). London: Mosby-White.

Fitzpatrick, T.B., Johnson, R.A., Wolff, K., et al. (1997). *Color Atlas and Synopsis of Clinical Dermatology: Common and Serious Diseases* (3rd ed.). New York: McGraw-Hill.

Singleton, J.K. (1997). Pediatric dermatoses: Three common skin disruptions, *Nurse Pract 22*(6), 32–50.

Psoriasis

DEFINITION

Psoriasis is a chronic benign disorder characterized by well-defined red plaques with a thick, dry, white-silvery scale. It runs a variable course over a lifetime, with exacerbations and remissions.

ETIOLOGY/INCIDENCE

1. Etiology is unknown; the condition has both environmental and hereditary components.

2. Affects both sexes equally and is seen in 1–2% of the population.
3. More common in Caucasians.
4. Evident at any age, but adolescence to middle adulthood is the most usual time.

SIGNS AND SYMPTOMS

1. Slow-growing lesions can be present for months or small, drop-like lesions (guttate psoriasis) may appear suddenly.
2. Pruritus is common, especially on the scalp and genital regions.

PHYSICAL FINDINGS

1. "Salmon pink," sharply marginated plaques and papules covered with a silvery-white scale.
2. Lesions are normally symmetric and bilateral and may vary from small coin-sized lesions to large coalescing lesions.
3. Scale removal results in small bleeding points, referred to as the Auspitz sign.
4. Psoriatic lesions can develop in skin trauma sites.
5. A recent B-streptococcal infection may cause spot-size psoriatic lesions in a small percentage of young adults.
6. Favored sites are elbows, knees, scalp, and intertriginous areas, including the genitals and nails.

DIFFERENTIAL DIAGNOSIS

1. Seborrheic dermatitis
2. Lichen simplex chronicus
3. Secondary syphilis (small papule size)
4. *Candida* if in the genital area

DIAGNOSTIC TESTS/FINDINGS

1. Diagnosis is usually made by clinical impression.
2. If unsure, obtain a biopsy.
3. Throat culture for streptococcus if lesions appeared suddenly.

MANAGEMENT/TREATMENT

1. Difficult and complex: Refer to dermatologist for treatment of this chronic condition.
2. Coal tar compounds alone or with acetylsalicylic acid.
3. Ultraviolet B light treatments.
4. Potent topical steroids (class I and II).
5. Calcipotriene ointment (vitamin D analog) and tazarotene gel (a retinoid) are new topical medications.

PATIENT EDUCATION

Instruct the patient to schedule an appointment with a dermatologist or dermatologic nurse practitioner for ongoing management.

References

Cohen, B.A. (1993). *Atlas of Pediatric Dermatology*. London: Wolfe.

Reizner, G.T. (1996). *Dermatology Essentials*. Madison: University of Wisconsin, Department of Medicine, Department of Dermatology.

Sauer, G.C., & Hall, J.L. (1996). *Manual of Skin Diseases* (7th ed.). Philadelphia: Lippin-cott-Raven.

Scheman, A.J., & Severson, D.L. (1997). *Pocket Guide to Medications Used in Dermatology* (5th ed.). Baltimore: Williams & Wilkins.

Seborrheic Dermatitis

DEFINITION

Seborrheic dermatitis is a common erythematous scaling disorder occurring where sebaceous glands are most active: face, scalp, in skin folds, and on the upper trunk. In an infant the condition is known as "cradle cap," while mild form in the scalp of an adult is called "dandruff." Adolescents may exhibit the dermatitis in the eyebrows, nasolabial folds, and postauricular areas.

ETIOLOGY/INCIDENCE

1. Although the cause is unknown, *Pityrosporum ovale* and *Candida* species are implicated.
2. A genetic predisposition is common, and immunocompromised individuals have an increased incidence.
3. Two to 5% of the population.

SIGNS AND SYMPTOMS

1. Symmetric red scaling eruption.
2. Scales may appear greasy salmon to yellow colored.
3. Nonpruritic.

PHYSICAL FINDINGS

1. Ill-defined sticky, greasy, yellow to salmon-colored plaques.
2. Arrangement is scattered, discrete on the face and trunk; diffuse involvement of scalp.

DIFFERENTIAL DIAGNOSIS

1. Atopic dermatitis, contact dermatitis
2. Tinea corporis, capitis
3. Psoriasis

DIAGNOSTIC TESTS/FINDINGS

Diagnosis is usually made on clinical findings.

MANAGEMENT/TREATMENT

1. Antiseborrheic shampoos containing selenium sulfide, zinc, or salicylic acid for the scalp.
2. Ketoconazole shampoo 2% for scalp and face; ketoconazole cream for face and trunk.
3. Low-potency corticosteroid lotion or gel for more severe cases; monitor for steroid atrophy.

PATIENT EDUCATION

Instruct the patient regarding:
1. The chronicity of seborrheic dermatitis, with recurrences and remissions; improves in the summer and flares in the fall.

2. That maintenance therapy is often needed after the initial treatment.
3. That the condition may disappear with age, especially if seen initially in young children.
4. Making a follow-up appointment, if there is no response to therapy in 2–4 weeks.

INFESTATIONS AND INFECTIOUS DISEASES

Dermatophytoses (Superficial Fungal Infections)

DEFINITION

Dermatophytoses are superficial fungal infections that survive only on the soft keratin of the skin and the hard keratin of the nails and hair. Dermatophyte infections are normally referred to by their anatomic location; the word *tinea* is used in front of the infected site. For example, "tinea corporis" refers to a dermatophyte infection of the body, while "tinea pedis" is a dermatophytic infection of the feet. Many people continue to call the infection "ringworm."

ETIOLOGY/INCIDENCE

Microsporum, Trichophyton, and *Epidermophyton* are the most common organisms of clinical importance. Predisposing factors include age of the patient, living in tropical climate, contact with infected individuals or animals, and whether the person is immunocompromised. Infections of the nails, palms, and soles are more common in adults, while scalp and hair infections are more common in children.

SIGNS AND SYMPTOMS

1. Pruritus in site of infection, reddened skin
2. Hair loss in tinea capitis
3. Thickening and yellowing of the nail plate in tinea unguium

PHYSICAL FINDINGS

1. Capitis
   A. Hair loss: "Salt and pepper" appearance; the broken short hairs resemble black dots on scalp.
   B. Diffuse fine scaling, scaly pustular bald areas.
   C. Presence of a "kerion": a boggy lesion that represents a hypersensitivity reaction to the dermatophyte.
2. Corporis
   A. Well-demarcated annular lesions with raised red, scaly border.
   B. Central area clears and is less scaly as the active border expands outward.
   C. May coexist with tinea pedis.
3. Cruris:
   A. Known as "jock itch."
   B. Large, scaling raised red plaques on medial thighs and groin; scrotum and penis rarely involved.
   C. May coexist with tinea pedis.
4. Pedis
   A. Fine white scaling and hyperkeratosis on heels, soles, and lateral sides of feet.
   B. Maceration, fissuring, and peeling of the toe webs.

5. Unguium or toenails
   A. Gradually developing chalky opacity of nail plate: More than one nail can be involved
   B. Nail can become thickened, cracked, and raised by underlying hyperkeratotic debris under the nail bed.

DIFFERENTIAL DIAGNOSIS

1. Impetigo
2. Eczema
3. Seborrheic, contact, or allergic dermatitis
4. Psoriasis

DIAGNOSTIC TESTS/FINDINGS

1. Performing a KOH examination:
   A. Scale from lesions are placed on a slide: collected by a #15 blade scalpel or edge of microscope slide.
   B. KOH (10% potassium hydroxide) is added and a cover slip is added.
   C. Observe under low magnification for the hyphae of the fungus.
2. Culturing infected scrapings of the nails, hair, or skin.

MANAGEMENT/TREATMENT

1. Capitis
   A. Griseofulvin (microsize) 20 mg/kg/day for 8 weeks.
   B. Topical antifungals are ineffective—do not penetrate the hair shaft to the fungus.
   C. Selenium sulfide 2.5% shampoo twice a week to reduce infectivity; other members of the household should also use selenium shampoo.
2. Corporis, pedis, and cruris
   A. Topical antifungals are appropriate (i.e., OTC clotrimazole 1% cream *or* econazole nitrate 1% cream bid for 14–28 days.
   B. Check with primary care provider for additional medication choices.
3. Unguium
   A. Refer to a dermatologist, dermatologic nurse practitioner, or primary care physician for treatment.
   B. New medications include "pulse-dosing" of itraconazole and terbinafine. Liver function tests are performed at intervals over the course of treatment.

PATIENT EDUCATION

Instruct the patient to:
1. Take medication with a fatty meal (ice cream or whole milk), if treating tinea capitis, to enhance absorption.
2. Avoid "over-the-counter" medications for tinea capitis because there is no noticeable improvement in the condition, which then may become more widespread and passed to other family members.
3. Have household contacts checked, including a family pet (veterinarian would treat).
4. Not to share combs, brushes, or headgear.
5. Make a 4-week follow-up appointment with primary care provider to evaluate effectiveness of therapy; longer intervals are needed to assess the treatment of toenail dermatophytosis.

References

Brosell, R.T., & Elewski, B. (1997). Superficial fungal infections: Errors to avoid in diagnosis and treatment. *Postgrad Med 101*, 279–287.

Cohen, B.A. (1993). *Atlas of Pediatric Dermatology.* London: Wolfe.

Fitzpatrick, T.B., Johnson, R.A., Wolff, K., et al. (1997). *Color Atlas and Synopsis of Clinical Dermatology: Common and Serious Disease* (3rd ed.). New York: McGraw-Hill.

Graham, M.V., & Upham, C.R. (1994). *Clinical Guidelines in Child Health.* Gainesville, FL: Barmarrae Books.

Parkinson, R.W., & Griffin, G.C. (1997). Dermatitis of the feet: A common yet often misdiagnosed problem. *Postgrad Med 101*, 95–110.

Vasiloudes, P., Morelli, J.G., & Weston, W.L. (1997). Bald spots: Remember the "big three." *Contemp Pediatr 14,* 76–91.

Lyme Disease

DEFINITION

Lyme disease is an infectious disease transmitted through infected ticks. The initial disorder affects the skin but has potential joint, cardiac, and neurologic sequelae. The pathognomonic "rash" is called erythema migrans.

ETIOLOGY/INCIDENCE

The disease is caused by the spirochete *Borrelia burgdorferi*. The main vectors are deer ticks and white-footed mice. Over 13,000 cases were reported in 1994, with the majority occurring from late May until early fall. The disease is endemic in the northeastern states.

SIGNS AND SYMPTOMS

1. Prodrome of malaise, headache, arthralgia, typically flu-like symptoms 7–12 days after a tick bite.
2. Initial single papule that expands within days.

PHYSICAL FINDINGS

1. Enlarging red plaque with central clearing. Center may become indurated, necrotic, or vesicular.
2. New lesions may arise. Average diameter is 15 cm (range 4–69 cm).
3. Later manifestations (cardiac, arthritis, neurologic) range from several weeks to months after the bite.

DIFFERENTIAL DIAGNOSIS

1. Urticaria
2. Viral exanthems
3. Insect bites
4. Fixed drug eruption
5. Tinea corporis or secondary syphilis

DIAGNOSIS TESTS/FINDINGS

1. History of a tick bite and the erythema migrans rash permit a clinical diagnosis.
2. PCR can detect *B. burgdorferi* in lesional skin biopsies, blood, or joint fluid; expensive to date.

3. Serologic testing can be unreliable if performed improperly. Consult with an infectious disease specialist.

MANAGEMENT/TREATMENT

1. Erythema migrans
   A. Doxycycline 100 mg PO bid for 14–21 days *or*
   B. Amoxicillin 500 mg PO tid for 14–21 days *or*
   C. Cefuroxime axetil 500 mg PO bid for 14–21 days
2. Arthritis, cardiac, and neurologic disease treatment: Consult an infectious disease specialist.

PATIENT EDUCATION

Instruct the patient to:

1. Wear long-sleeved shirts and pants when hiking or working where ticks are endemic.
2. Perform body checks, especially in the hairline and scalp. The deer tick is small (3 mm), transmission of Lyme disease occurs only after 18 hours of attachment and feeding.

References

Cohen, B.A. (1994). *Atlas of Pediatric Dermatology.* London: Wolfe.

du Vivier, A. (1993). *Atlas of Clinical Dermatology* (2nd ed.). London: Mosby-White.

Fitzpatrick, T.B., Johnson, R.A., Wolff, K., et al. (1997). *Color Atlas and Synopsis of Clinical Dermatology: Common and Serious Diseases* (3rd ed.). New York: McGraw-Hill.

Treatment of Lyme disease (1997). *Med Lett Drugs Ther 30,* pp. 47–48.

Pediculosis

DEFINITION

Pediculosis is an infestation of the hair or skin caused by two species of blood-sucking lice:

1. Pediculosis capitis (head louse) or corporis (body louse)
2. *Phthirus pubis* (crab or pubic louse)

ETIOLOGY/INCIDENCE

1. Capitis: More common in children but found in all ages. Transmission through shared hats, combs, and brushes. Louse dies if off host over 55 hours. Six to 10 million cases a year in the United States.
2. Corporis: People with poor hygiene. Increases where crowding and unsanitary living conditions are common. Louse dies within 4–10 days, but nits survive over 30 days.
3. Pubis: Young, sexually active adults. More extensive infestation in males. Louse die in less than 24 hours when separated from the host.

SIGNS AND SYMPTOMS

1. Intense pruritus at site of infestation
2. Occipital or cervical lymphadenopathy (capitis)

3. Purpuric papules and parallel linear excoriations on shoulder, trunk, and buttocks (corporis)

PHYSICAL FINDINGS

1. Capitis: Eggs (nits) that resemble pearly oval dewdrops and/or a live louse. Sometimes scratches and crusting pustules are found behind the ears and neck.
2. Corporis: Nits and lice in the seams of clothing in contact with axillae, belt-line, neck, and groin area.
3. Pubis: Live louse or nits. Sometimes blue-gray pinpoint macules on the lower abdomen that represent minute hemorrhages cause by the louse.

DIFFERENTIAL DIAGNOSIS

1. Scabies
2. Dandruff
3. Impetigo

DIAGNOSTIC TESTS/FINDINGS

Finding a nit or live louse is diagnostic of pediculosis.

MANAGEMENT/TREATMENT (See Table 11–17)

PATIENT EDUCATION

Instruct the patients to:

1. Launder all clothing, bedding in hot water.
2. Wash all combs, brushes, and hair accessories in very hot water for 15 minutes.
3. Remove nits (capitis) by saturating the hair with a mixture of 50% vinegar and 50% water, then using a fine-tooth comb.
4. Seal nonwashables items in plastic bags for 35 days.
5. Carefully vacuum car seats, upholstered furniture, and mattresses.
6. Discourage the sharing of caps and hats.
7. Return for evaluation of treatment in 1 week.

TABLE 11–17. **Products Used to Treat Pediculosis**

Trade Name	Active Agents	Indications	Contact Time
A200 shampoo (OTC)	Pyrethrum extract 0.33% with piperonyl	Head, body lice	10 min; repeat in 7–10 days
Pronto shampoo (OTC)	As for A200	Head, pubic, body lice	10 min; repeat in 7–10 days
Rid shampoo (OTC)	As for A200	Head, pubic, body lice	10 min; repeat in 7–10 days
NIX cream rinse (OTC)	Permethrin 0.5%	Head lice	10 min; repeat in 7–10 days
Kwell shampoo (Rx)	Lindane 1%	Head, pubic lice	4 min; may repeat—7 days
Rid spray (OTC)	Permethrin 0.5%	Inanimate objects	3 sec/sq ft
A200 spray (OTC)	Permethrin 0.5%	Inanimate objects	As for A200

8. Contact the National Pediculosis Association if more information is desired (P.O Box 149, Newton, MA 02161; 1-617-449-6487).

References

American Academy of Pediatrics. (1997). *1997 Red Book: Report of the Committee on Infectious Diseases* (24th ed.). Elk Grove, IL: American Academy of Pediatrics.

du Vivier, A. (1993). *Atlas of Clinical Dermatology* (2nd ed.). London: Mosby-Wolfe.

Newland, J.A. (1995). Excerpted from Newland, J.A. & Rich, E. (eds.), *Clinical Protocols Manual* (2nd ed.). Pleasantville, NY: Pace University, 1995. Pediculosis, *American Journal of Nursing*, (Nurse Practitioner Edition) September 1995, 16a.

Witkowski, J.A., & Parish, C. (1997). What's new in the management of lice. http://medscape. com/SCP/IIM/1997v14.witkowski/m19477.witkowskii.html#Tab1.

Scabies

DEFINITION

Scabies is a cutaneous infestation with the mite *Sarcoptes scabiei.*

ETIOLOGY/INCIDENCE

1. Scabies knows no geographical or socioeconomic limits.
2. Young adults usually acquire the mite through sexual contact; children through personal contact with family and other children at day care settings.
3. Health care workers can pick up the infestation through contact with mite-infested sheets from bedridden patients.
4. Scabies is also very common in homeless populations.
5. In temperate climates, the condition is more prevalent during the winter, when individuals spend more time indoors and in closer contact with other people.
6. Eruptions occur 4–6 weeks after initial contact.

SIGNS AND SYMPTOMS

1. Generalized intense pruritus often beginning on the thighs; initial diagnosis can be easily missed.
2. The itching can interfere with sleep.
3. Widespread small urticarial edematous papules ("id," or autosensitization reaction) on anterior trunk, thighs, forearms, and buttocks.

PHYSICAL FINDINGS

1. Serpiginous burrows 1–10 mm in length (skin-colored to gray ridges with a tiny vesicle or papule located at the end of the lesion).
2. Burrows located where skin is thin and soft and has fewer hair follicles: Wrists; finger webs; beltline; genitalia, including the shaft of the penis; and the flexor surfaces, especially elbows.
3. Infants can also have burrows on the hands and feet.

DIFFERENTIAL DIAGNOSIS

1. Pediculosis
2. Atopic dermatitis
3. Insect bites: Round and blister-like, located on exposed areas
4. Poison ivy and acute contact dermatitis: Elongated linear vesicles found in areas of the body not covered by clothing

DIAGNOSTIC TESTS/FINDINGS

How to perform a scabies preparation:

1. Place mineral oil on several suspected burrows using a cotton-tipped applicator.
2. Vigorously scrape skin with #15 scalpel blade and place material on slide.
3. Examine slide under microscope using low power (presence of a mite is diagnostic; if eggs or fecal material is observed, it is sensible to treat for scabies).
4. If no microscope available, make a clinical diagnosis on identification of the shape of the burrows and a suggestive history.

MANAGEMENT/TREATMENT

1. Permethrin 5% cream (Elimite): Massage into skin from the head down; leave on for 8–14 hours, then wash off in the shower. May need to use in the scalp of infants, young children and the elderly.
2. Alternative regimen: Apply crotamiton cream 10% to entire body below the neck for two consecutive nights; wash off 24 hours after the second application
3. Retreat only if continued evidence of mites is unmistakable.
4. A tapered course of prednisone (1–2 weeks) is used for severe "id" reactions; consult with physician prn.
5. Antihistamines are often use to control pruritus; secondary bacterial infections are treated with topical mupirocin or systemic antibiotics.

PATIENT EDUCATION

Inform the patient regarding:

1. The contagiousness of scabies; all family or household members need to be treated.
2. That all bedding and clothing needs to be machine washed, machine dried on hot or dry cleaned.
3. The need to store nonwashable items for 3–4 days (without skin contact, the mite cannot survive off the host this length of time).

References

Cohen, B.A. (1993). *Atlas of Pediatric Dermatology*. London: Wolfe.

Cohen, B.A. (1993). When to think scabies. *Contemp Pediatr 10*, 1–20.

du Vivier, A. (1993). *Atlas of Clinical Dermatology* (2nd ed.). London: Mosby-Wolfe.

VIRAL DISEASES

Herpes Simplex

DEFINITION

Herpes simplex is a viral infection characterized by grouped vesicles on the skin and mucous membranes. The initial infection can include regional adenopathy, fever, and malaise. Reoccurrences are common and appear at the same site.

ETIOLOGY/INCIDENCE

1. Most commonly seen in young adults; range from infancy to old age.
2. Caused by two types of herpes simplex virus (HSV-1 and HSV-2).
3. Transmission is skin-to-skin or mucosal surfaces by direct contact with active lesions.

SIGNS AND SYMPTOMS

1. A sudden onset of grouped lesions that progress to painful vesicles that have an erythematous base; typically located on the lips, facial area, buccal mucosa, or genitals.
2. With the primary infection, individuals may have fever, myalgia, malaise, or lymphadenopathy.
3. Recurrent infections may be triggered by sun exposure, menses, fatigue, fever, or localized trauma.

PHYSICAL FINDINGS

1. Vesicles at the site of inoculation; these rupture, leaving crusted erosions. Healing may take over 2 weeks.
2. Recurrent herpes can begin with a tingling or discomfort under the skin that proceeds to a typical vesicular appearance.

DIFFERENTIAL DIAGNOSIS

1. Aphthous ulcers
2. Herpangina
3. Hand-foot-and-mouth disease
4. Erythema multiforme

DIAGNOSTIC TESTS/FINDINGS

1. Tzanck smear
2. Viral culture (may take 3–7 days for results and is more expensive)

MANAGEMENT/TREATMENT

1. Refer or consult with primary physician if patient is immunocompromised.
2. Medications
   A. First episodes
      1) Acyclovir 400 mg PO 5 times daily for 7–10 days *or*
      2) Famciclovir 250 mg PO tid for 5–10 days *or*
      3) Valacyclovir 1 gm PO bid for 7–10 days
   B. Recurrences
      1) Acyclovir 400 mg PO tid for 5 days *or*
      2) Famciclovir 125 mg PO bid for 5 days *or*
      3) Valacyclovir 500 mg PO bid for 5 days
   C. Recurrent Orolabial HSV: Penciclovir 1% cream (Denavir)—apply every 2 hours while awake for 4 days

PATIENT EDUCATION

Instruct the patient to:

1. Use cool compresses, Burrow's solution soaks, and oral/topical analgesics.
2. Complete the course of prescription medication.
3. Discuss how to avoid transmission of the virus to others by frequent handwashing and/or avoiding sexual activity until lesions have healed.

4. Offer educational literature/resources: National Herpes Hotline (1-919-361-8488 weekdays, 9:00 A.M. to 7:00 P.M. EST); American Social Health Association (P.O. Box 13827, Research Triangle Park, NC 27709); Glaxo Wellcome Inc. Herpes Resource Center (1-800-230-6039).
5. Inform her health care practitioner if she has had HSV when she is pregnant; there is a risk of transmission from a pregnant woman to her neonate (includes devastating sequelae).

References

Drugs for non-HIV viral infections. (1997). *Med Lett Drugs Ther 39,* 69–76.

Fitzpatrick T.B., Johnson, R.A., Wolff, K., et al. (1997). *Color Atlas and Synopsis of Clinical Dermatology: Common and Serious Diseases* (3rd ed.). New York: McGraw-Hill.

New hope for oral herpes. (1997). *Emerg Med Oct,* 78–79.

Reizner, G.T. (1996). *Dermatology Essentials.* Madison: University of Wisconsin, Department of Medicine, Department of Dermatology.

Sauer, G.C., & Hall, J.C. (1996). *Manual of Skin Diseases* (7th ed.). Philadelphia: Lippincott-Raven.

Topical penciclovir for herpes labialis. (1997). *Med Lett Drugs Ther 39,* 57–58.

Herpes Zoster (Varicella-Zoster Virus)

DEFINITION

Herpes zoster, or "shingles," is an acute viral infection characterized by *unilateral* pain with grouped vesicular lesions appearing along one to three sensory dermatomes.

ETIOLOGY/INCIDENCE

1. Herpes zoster represents the reactivation of the dormant varicella-zoster virus ("chicken pox").
2. The virus remained latent in the basal ganglia after the initial infection.
3. More than 60% of the cases are in individuals over the age of 50, while 5% of the cases are in children under the age of 15.
4. Herpes zoster occurs in 25% of HIV-positive individuals.

SIGNS AND SYMPTOMS

1. Prodromal symptoms: Unilateral paresthesia or neuritic pain normally precedes 3–5 days before the cutaneous eruptions.
2. Active vesiculation: Neuritic pain of the involved skin, headache, fever, and malaise
3. Chronic "burning" or "shooting" pain after the lesions have healed may indicate postherpetic neuralgia.

PHYSICAL FINDINGS

1. Papules progressing to vesicles within 48 hours.
2. Arranged in herpetiform clusters distributed in a unilateral dermatomal pattern (two or three dermatomes); rarely noncontiguous.
3. Sites: Thoracic, over 50%; trigeminal, 10–15%.
4. More than ten lesions outside the primary dermatomes suggests the possibility of an immunodeficiency state.

DIFFERENTIAL DIAGNOSIS

1. Prodromal stage: Back pain, cardiac pain, migraines, or lung disease
2. Skin/vesicular eruption: Herpes simplex, poison ivy, "chicken pox," and contact dermatitis.

DIAGNOSTIC TESTS/FINDINGS

Herpes zoster is diagnosed by culture of the fluid in a vesicle.

MANAGEMENT/TREATMENT

1. Antiviral medications
   A. Valacyclovir 1 gm PO tid for 7 days *or*
   B. Famciclovir 500 mg PO tid for 7 days *or*
   C. Acyclovir 800 mg PO five times a day for 7–10 days
2. Use NSAIDs of health care facility's choice for pain and fever.
3. Use wet compresses of water or Burrow's solution for 30 minutes several times a day.
4. Use mupirocin tid if lesions are secondarily infected; consult with primary care physician if unsure if skin is bacterially infected.
5. Trigeminal nerve involvement (eye, nose, and forehead) *requires an immediate referral to an ophthalmologist!*
6. Referral to a specialist if individual is immunocompromised.

PATIENT EDUCATION

Instruct the patient to:
1. Complete the medications as prescribed.
2. Make a follow-up appointment in 1 week.

References

Drugs for treatment of viral infections. (1997). *Med Lett Drugs Ther 39,* 69–76.

du Vivier, A. (1993). *Atlas of Clinical Dermatology* (2nd ed.). London: Mosby-Wolfe.

Fitzpatrick, T.B., Johnson, R.A., Wolff, K., et al. (1997). *Color Atlas and Synopsis of Clinical Dermatology: Common and Serious Diseases* (3rd ed.). New York: McGraw-Hill.

Graham, M.V., & Uphold, C.R. (1994). *Clinical Guidelines in Child Health.* Gainesville, FL: Barmarrae Books.

Review Questions

11.34 Which of the following is not a bacterial infection?
  A. Impetigo
  B. Cellulitis
  C. Tinea corporis
  D. Folliculitis

11.35 Malignant melanoma:
  A. Is the second most common skin cancer

    B. Can metastasize early and widely
    C. Is frequently difficulty to recognize because it has regular symmetric borders
    D. All of the above

11.36 Which of the following treatments would the ACNP recommend for a moderate case of seborrheic dermatitis?
    A. Gentle scrubbing with an antiseborrheic shampoo two to three times a week
    B. Cleocin-T lotion A.M. and P.M.
    C. Using a NIX rinse whenever symptoms arise
    D. Monistat cream tid

11.37 Skin aging:
    A. Is a natural process
    B. Is accelerated by exposure to ultraviolet light
    C. May be seen sooner in people with lighter complexions
    D. All of the above

11.38 An elderly "street person" has been admitted to your unit in congestive heart failure. The nightshift staff reports that he has been extremely restless. During your rounds, you observe that he has a vesicular rash between his fingers, around his waist, on his genitals, and in his axilla. The excoriation seems to exhibit a J-shaped pattern. You suspect that he has:
    A. Tinea
    B. Scabies
    C. Koplik's spots on the throat
    D. Trichotillomania

11.39 A 28-year-old woman with a urinary tract infection has been taking genetic Bactrim for the past 6 days. Suddenly she becomes acutely ill with a very high fever, accompanied by an extreme weakness, a purulent conjunctivitis, thick hemorrhagic crusts of lips, buccal mucosal ulcers, and a vesicular target-like rash on her trunk. Similar target lesions, fewer in number, begin to develop on the soles and palms. She does not have a cough or coryza, and has not been traveling outside her local urban area. While she is being admitted to the unit, your most likely diagnosis would be:
    A. Staphylococcal scalded skin syndrome
    B. Rocky mountain spotted fever
    C. Rubeola
    D. Stevens-Johnson syndrome

11.40 A 20-year-old woman presents in the emergency room with a 3-day history of increasingly painful sores in the genital area, malaise, and bilateral inguinal adenopathy. Your clinical diagnosis is HSV and you prescribe an appropriate oral antiviral. Which is the most cost-effective test in the diagnosis of HSV?
    A. A Pap smear
    B. A Tzanck smear
    C. A blood test
    D. A rapid immunosorbent assay

Answers and Rationales

11.34 **C** Tinea is a fungal infection; the other presentations are caused by bacteria.

11.35 **B** Basal cell and squamous cell carcinomas are the first and second most common skin cancers. Melanoma is characterized by an *irregular border* and/or an *asymmetric lesion*.

11.36 **A** Using an antiseborrheic shampoo two to three times weekly is the preferred treatment.

11.37 **E** All of the statements are true of skin aging.

11.38 **C** Small serpiginous burrows commonly located on the genital area, finger and toe webs, waistline, and flexor surfaces characterize scabies. Tinea is one of the superficial fungal infections of the skin. It presents as erythematous scaling plaques and has a tendency toward central clearing—essentially "ringworm"-shaped lesions. Koplik's spots on the throat are blue-white spots that appear on the buccal surfaces of the mouth during the prodome of measles, a viral infection. Trichotillomania is a condition of self-induced hair loss. Individuals pull or twist out their own hair. It may represent a simple habit or a deeper emotional problem.

11.39 **D** Stevens-Johnson syndrome (erythema multiforme major) frequently follows treatment with sulfonamide medications. The illness begins abruptly with prostration, a high fever, and an extensive skin eruption with blister formation and severe involvement of mucosal membranes. The basic skin lesions are urticarial and vesicular and have a target-like configuration. Staphylococcal scalded skin syndrome occurs almost without exception in toddlers and infants. The rash in Rocky Mountain spotted fever first appears on the wrists and ankles, then spreads to the trunk within hours. Although the rash initially is red and macular, it often becomes petechial. Measles is an acute disease characterized by fever, cough, coryza, conjunctivitis, and a morbilliform rash that begins at the hairline and spreads cephalocaudally over 3 days. The rash does not usually appear until the third or fourth day of illness.

11.40 **B** The Tzanck smear is a test in use for rapid detection of multinucleated giant cells; these cells are pathognomonic for all herpetic infections. The Tzanck smear takes 2 minutes to perform and costs much less than other diagnostic tests. The Pap test has a low sensitivity for HSV detection; blood testing requires paired samples collected 4 weeks apart. An immunosorbent assay shows nonspecific reactivity with cellular antigens.

CHAPTER 12

Mental Health Disorders

Suzanne Clark, RN, MSN, MA, NP

Anxiety

DEFINITION

Anxiety is a state of apprehension in response to a real or perceived threat. It is a painful emotional experience characterized by feelings of uneasiness, tension, apprehension, and worry. The subjective experience of anxiety is often accompanied by a physiologic response mediated by neural and endocrine pathways.

ETIOLOGY/INCIDENCE

1. Can occur in 70–90% of critically ill patients.
2. Anxiety is a complex behavioral pattern that can be the result of widely differing causes.
   A. *Inability to cope with the perceived threat:* The individual either perceives the threat as too large or the coping resources available as too limited to meet the challenge.
   B. *Changing physiologic status:* Many disease states or an imbalance in homeostasis result in the complex behaviors of anxiety. A partial list includes:
      1) Hypoglycemia
      2) Hypovolemia
      3) Hypoxia
      4) Electrolyte imbalance
      5) Pneumothorax/pulmonary embolus
      6) Lack of pain relief
      7) Sleep deprivation
      8) Medications/drugs
         a. Sympathomimetics
         b. Anticholinergics
         c. Caffeine
         d. Cocaine
      9) Withdrawal from nicotine, alcohol, barbiturates, amphetamines, cocaine
   C. *An underlying psychiatric disorder:* Phobias, panic attacks, generalized anxiety disorder, adjustment disorder with anxiety and posttraumatic

859

stress syndrome are five primary psychiatric disorders that are manifested by anxiety.

1) A phobia is a persistent fear of a specific stimulus, such as needles or enclosed spaces. Exposure to the stimulus causes an immediate anxiety response.

2) A panic attack is an acute, severe anxiety response that occurs without warning and that may be unrelated to an identified threat.

3) An adjustment disorder with anxiety is excessive anxiety that is more than a natural response to a specific stressful situation.

4) Generalized anxiety disorder is present when anxiety persists and is present for at least 6 months, and the anxiety is difficult to control and is associated with at least three of the following:

a. Restlessness

b. Easy fatigability

c. Difficulty in concentrating or mind going blank

d. Irritability

e. Muscle tension

f. Sleep disturbance

5) Posttraumatic stress disorder occurs in response to an event that is outside the range of normal experience, such as a rape, kidnapping, or natural disaster. The patient re-experiences the trauma through recurrent and intrusive memories and dreams.

3. Mediator of anxiety, irrespective of the underlying cause, is the humoral response to stress identified as the "fight-or-flight" response, which is activated by interaction of the hypothalamus-pituitary-adrenal axis and the sympathetic nervous system. Increased levels of catecholamines, cortisol, and antidiuretic hormone are released and result in a wide variety of signs and symptoms.

4. Effective interventions interfere with the sympathetic response and the release of catecholamines.

SIGNS AND SYMPTOMS

1. Number and intensity of symptoms depends on the intensity of the anxiety, which can range from mild to panic levels.

A. Mild: Some discomfort that heightens attention, stimulates problem solving.

B. Moderate: Symptoms are intrusive, decreased ability to discriminate between realistic and unrealistic threats, can still respond to reassurance.

C. Severe: Information is not heard or it is misinterpreted, thinking is simplistic, very limited problem solving.

D. Panic: Feeling of impending death, agitated, out of control, unresponsive to realistic interventions.

2. Cognitive indicators: Disruption of perceiving, thinking, and conceptualizing.

A. Feelings of self-consciousness

B. Hypervigilence

C. Confusion

D. Difficulty concentrating

3. Physiologic indicators:

A. Cardiovascular: Palpitations, chest pain, tachycardia

B. Respiratory: Shortness of breath, gasping, bronchial spasm, choking sensation

C. Neuromuscular: Increased startle reaction, tremors, rigidity, generalized weakness, lightheadedness, dizziness

D. Gastrointestinal: Anorexia, nausea, vomiting, abdominal discomfort, diarrhea

E. Genitourinary: Urgency, frequency, hesitancy

F. Skin: Flushing, blanching, increased perspiration, hot and cold flashes, cold hands/feet, paresthesias

4. Behavioral indicators are individualized and reflect the individual's coping style (i.e., aggressive behavior, avoident behavior, unrealistic demands for attention, attempts to control the environment, refusal of medical treatment).

PHYSICAL FINDINGS

Physical findings depend on level of anxiety. Physical findings intensify as the level of anxiety increases.

1. Increased heart rate
2. Increased blood pressure
3. Increased respiratory rate
4. Hypertonic reflexes
5. Dilated pupils
6. Cardiac dysrhythmias
7. Altered mental status

DIFFERENTIAL DIAGNOSIS

1. Organic conditions (e.g., endocrine, cardiac, neurologic problems; unrelieved pain)
2. Delirium
3. Side effects of pharmacologic agents (i.e., antihistamines, steroids)
4. Drug-induced anxiety: Substance abuse or withdrawal

DIAGNOSTIC TESTS/FINDINGS

If anxiety is psychogenic in origin, diagnostic tests will in general be normal. If anxiety is a symptom of an underlying physiologic problem, this will be reflected in the specific tests (i.e., hypoglycemia, hypoxia, etc.).

1. Complete blood count (CBC): Normal
2. Electrolytes, blood urea nitrogen (BUN), creatinine, glucose: Normal
3. Urinalysis: Normal
4. Arterial blood gases/oxygen saturation, chest x-ray: Normal
5. Toxic drug screen: Negative
6. Mental status exam: Oriented to time, place, person, situation; no hallucinations (mental status exam may be abnormal in cases of severe anxiety)

MANAGEMENT/TREATMENT

1. Institute appropriate diagnostic tests to identify and treat underlying etiology.

2. Select and institute appropriate symptomatic management.
   A. Nonpharmacologic treatments can be instituted independently.
      1) Psychological
         a. Brief relaxation
         b. Hypnosis; guided imagery
         c. Therapeutic touch
         d. Cognitive restructuring
         e. Distraction
         f. Development of therapeutic relationship
      2) Environmental
         a. Flexible visitor policy
         b. Restore sleep-wake cycles
         c. Decrease noise
         d. Provide orientation to time, date, etc.
   B. Pharmacologic treatments, depending on state or institutional regulations, may be instituted independently or only under protocol.
      1) First line for patients who are agitated and whose behavior is immediate threat to safety or who require physical restraints and frequent verbal reinforcing of limits; adjunctive for milder levels of anxiety
      2) Benzodiazepines: diazepam (Valium), midazolam (Versed), lorazepam (Ativan) (see Table 12–1)
         a. All work equally well.
         b. Can have prolonged effect on sleep patterns.
         c. Can depress respirations, lorazepam the least.
         d. Metabolism may be impaired by age, cirrhosis. Use with caution in liver disease.
         e. Lorazepam has shortest terminal half-life, less affected by exogenous influences, forms inactive metabolites rapidly excreted by kidney.
         f. When used continuously for >2 weeks, discontinue by slow titration to avoid withdrawal (10%/day over 10 days)
         g. May exacerbate delirium
      3) Titrate to clinical endpoints
         a. Decrease purposeless activity.
         b. Stop life-threatening movements.
         c. Allow control of mechanical ventilation.
         d. Promote sleep.
         e. Subjectively more relaxed.
3. Consult with physician for patients whose symptoms are beyond one's expe-

TABLE **12–1. Selected Anxiolytics**

Drug	Route	Initial Dose	Onset of Action (min)	Half-life (hr)	Dosing Interval (hr)
Diazepam	PO	2–10 mg	15–45	60	6–12
(Valium)	IV	2–10 mg	1–5	60	3–4
Lorazepam	PO	0.5–2 mg	15–20	15	8–12
(Ativan)	IV.	1.0–4 mg			
Midazolam	IV	0.5–2 mg initially, then 1–4 mg/hr infusion	1–3	1–12	—

rience and expertise or cannot be managed within the protocols instituted within one's practice setting.

4. Refer to psychiatrist, psychologist, advanced psychiatric–mental health nurse practitioner, or other mental health professional regarding patients with underlying anxiety disorder who could benefit from ongoing treatment.

PATIENT EDUCATION

1. Prepare patients for procedures by telling them what is going to happen as well as how it will feel.
2. Anticipatory guidance for the course of illness and recovery.
3. Teach deep breathing and relaxation techniques.
4. Educate patients regarding the physical symptoms of anxiety and differentiate from underlying medical conditions with similar symptoms.

Review Questions

12.1 The symptom least likely to be seen in a highly anxious person is:
   A. An increased decision-making capacity
   B. Restlessness
   C. Increased heart rate
   D. Dilated pupils
   E. Increased perspiration

12.2 The one laboratory test used to confirm the diagnosis of anxiety is:
   A. Complete blood count
   B. The differential portion of the white blood cell count
   C. Urinalysis
   D. Liver enzymes
   E. Serum electrolytes
   F. None of these tests confirms the diagnosis of anxiety

12.3 Anxiety is least likely to be a concomitant symptom of:
   A. Hypoxia
   B. Hyperglycemia
   C. Pulmonary embolus
   D. Hypoglycemia
   E. Hypovolemia

12.4 Mrs. W. is a 48-year-old woman who began to experience chest pain at her mother's funeral. She is admitted to the coronary care unit to rule out a myocardial infarction. She is very tearful and visibly upset. She exhibits thought stopping and tremulousness. The ACNP decides to treat her anxiety with a benzodiazepine. Which of the following principles should guide the prescribing of this class of drugs?
   A. Normal sleep is promoted if used in appropriate doses
   B. They should not be stopped abruptly if they have been used continuously for >2 weeks
   C. Because of their short half-life, there is little danger in discontinuing their use immediately in patients who have needed them for longer than 2 weeks for sedation.

    D. Of all the benzodiazepines used, lorazepam has the longest half-life and for this reason should be avoided in the elderly.

    E. Benzodiazepines should never be considered first-line treatment for anxiety. Behavioral interventions should always be given an opportunity to work first.

12.5 Mrs. B. is a 35-year-old woman who is waiting to go to the operating room for repair of an atrial septal defect. She is crying and clinging to you, yelling that she is afraid she is going to die. She is tachypnic and tachycardic, and her blood pressure is elevated. Which intervention(s) could be used to interrupt the fight-or-flight response and help the patient regain some control?

    A. Teaching the patient deep breathing

    B. Using guided imagery

    C. Using therapeutic touch

    D. Guiding the patient through a progressive muscle relaxation exercise

    E. All of the above

Answers and Rationales

12.1   **A**   One of the cardinal cognitive signs present in anxiety is a disruption in the ability to perceive, think, and conceptualize, making it more difficult to make decisions.

12.2   **F**   Although laboratory tests might be useful to rule out other medical conditions that might mimic anxiety (i.e., electrolytes to rule out hyponatremia or blood gases to rule out hypoxia), there is no one lab test that would confirm the presence of anxiety.

12.3   **B**   Anxiety may be the first sign of hypoxia, pulmonary embolus, low blood sugar, or volume depletion. Hyperglycemia is more likely to present with increased drowsiness.

12.4   **B**   The abrupt withdrawal of benzodiazepines may result in the recurrence of anxiety, often beyond baseline symptoms, or withdrawal symptoms.

12.5   **E**   All of the interventions invoke the relaxation response, which is the opposite of the stress response and can negate the fight-or-flight response.

References

Bone, R.C. (1995). Recognition, assessment, and treatment of anxiety in the critical care patient. *Dis Mon 41*, 293–360.

Higgins, T.L. & Coyle, J.P. (1995). Sedation, pain relief and neuromuscular blockade in the critically ill. In E.D. Sivak, T.L. Higgins, & A. Seiver (eds.). *The High Risk Patient: Management of the Critically Ill*. Baltimore: Williams & Wilkins, pp. 1278–1290.

Keltner, N.L., & Folks, D.G. (1993). *Psychotropic Drugs*. St. Louis: C.V. Mosby Co., pp. 108–138.

Additional Recommended References

American Psychiatric Association. (1994). *Diagnostic and Statistical Manual of Mental Disorders* (4th ed.). Washington, DC: American Psychiatric Press.

Mejo, S.L. (1990). Post-traumatic stress disorder: An overview of three etiologic variables and psychopharmacologic treatment. *Nurse Pract 15*(8), 41–45.

Valente, S.M. (1996). Diagnosis and treatment of panic disorder and generalized anxiety in primary care. *Nurse Pract 21*(8), 26–47.

Depression

DEFINITION

Depression is a mood state characterized by feelings of sadness, lowered self-esteem, and pessimistic thinking and guilt; term is used to describe a normal response to life events as well as the psychiatric syndrome of "major depression."

ETIOLOGY/INCIDENCE

1. Incidence in the medically ill ranges from 6% to 72%. This wide range is due to the differing definitions of depression used, the specific medical population studied, and the wide variety of tools used to measure depression.
2. Causes of depression depends on theoretical framework.
   A. Psychodynamic
      1) Anger not directly acknowledged or expressed is directed inward.
      2) Partial or complete loss of self-esteem related to feelings of not having lived up to one's expectations.
      3) Reaction to loss and deprivation.
   B. Cognitive
      1) Individuals possess a learned worldview that influences their perceptions of all new experiences.
      2) Depression develops in response to negative beliefs and dysfunctional thinking.
      3) Three beliefs likely to lead to depression
         a. "It will *always* be like this" (stable causality)
         b. "*Everything* is ruined" (global thinking)
         c. "It's *my* fault" (internal vs. external causes)
   C. Biochemical (partial list)
      1) Neurotransmitter imbalance: Dopamine/serotonin/epinephrine/norepinephrine
      2) Abnormalities of cortisol metabolism
      3) Thyroid dysfunction
      4) Vitamin deficiencies: B_{12}
      5) Hypo/hypercalcemia
      6) Medication side effects
   D. Social: Lack of adequate quality social support

SIGNS AND SYMPTOMS

1. Criteria from the American Psychiatric Association's *Diagnostic and Statistical Manual of Mental Disorders, Fourth Edition* (DSM-IV). Five or more of the following symptoms for the same 2-week period and represent a change in previous functioning (one of the symptoms marked with an asterisk (*) must be present).

    A. *Depressed mood most of the day nearly every day

    B. *Markedly diminished interest or pleasure in almost all activities (anhe-donia)

    C. Significant weight loss or weight gain (a change in more than 5% of body weight in a month without conscious effort)

    D. Insomnia or hypersomnia

    E. Psychomotor agitation or retardation

    F. Fatigue or loss of energy

    G. Diminished ability to think or concentrate or indecisiveness nearly every day

    H. Feelings of worthlessness or excessive or inappropriate guilt nearly every day

    I. Recurrent thoughts of death, recurrent suicidal ideation without a plan or a suicide attempt

2. Diagnosing depression in the medically ill is challenging and relates to the difficulty of distinguishing between major depression and less severe reactions involving sadness, as well as distinguishing those symptoms that are manifestations of a physical illness.

DIFFERENTIAL DIAGNOSIS

1. Grief reaction
2. Mood disorder secondary to a general medical condition
   A. May involve depressed mood
   B. May involve markedly diminished interest or pleasure
   C. Depending on the physiologic disturbance, may see
      1) weight loss or weight gain (i.e. diabetes, congestive heart failure [CHF], hyper- or hypothyroidism, cancer)
      2) Fatigue, weakness (i.e., diabetes, hypothyroidism, anemia, postviral syndrome)
      3) Sleep disturbance (i.e., pulmonary edema, urinary tract infection, CHF)
   D. Common medications/drugs known to cause depression
      1) Antihypertensives—reserpine, methyldopa, thiazides, spironolactone, clonidine HCl
      2) Oral contraceptives
      3) Steroids
      4) Cimetidine
      5) Benzodiazepines
      6) β-blockers, especially propranolol
      7) Digitalis toxicity
      8) Cocaine withdrawal
      9) Amphetamine withdrawal
      10) Alcohol
   E. Common metabolic factors presenting as depression
      1) Acidosis
      2) Alkalosis
      3) Anemia
      4) Hypoxia
      5) Hypercapnia
      6) Uremia

7) Hypokalemia
8) Lack of sleep
3. Organic brain syndrome: Delirium, dementia; can look like depression: apathy, flat affect, slow response

DIAGNOSTIC TESTS/FINDINGS

1. Diagnostic questions
   A. Is the patient's depressed mood part of the normal despondency that can follow a serious illness?
   B. Is the patient's depressed mood an indication that the patient is suffering from a major depression?
   C. Are the patient's symptoms related to some biologic factor related to the illness and treatment?
   D. Is the patient currently a danger to him/herself because of the inability to care for self or escalating suicidal ideation?
2. Diagnostic tests: As with anxiety, diagnostic tests may be abnormal if they reflect that a physiologic problem is the etiology of the depressive symptoms. In general, lab tests will be normal if depression is psychogenic in origin.
   A. CBC, urinalysis, electrolytes, thyroid function, blood sugar, BUN, creatinine, arterial blood gases, toxic drug screen, Venereal Disease Research Laboratory test all normal
   B. Mini-mental status exam to rule out delirium
   C. Depression screening instruments (i.e., Beck Depression Inventory; Zung Self-rating Depression Scale, Hamilton Depression Scale)
      1) Screening instruments include somatic items such as weight loss, lack of appetite, and difficulty sleeping and may not be useful in identifying depression in a hospitalized medically ill patient in whom there would be a physiologic or environmental basis for the symptoms.
      2) Helpful discriminators for depression in a medically ill patient are:
         a. Cognitive indicators
            i. Feeling like a failure
            ii. Loss of interest in people
            iii. Feeling punished
            iv. Suicidal ideation
            v. Dissatisfaction
            vi. Difficulty with decisions
            vii. Crying
         b. Items i–iv: Helpful discriminators for marked depression
         c. Items v–vii: Common in mild levels of depression and grief in the medically ill but if pronounced are good discriminators for severe depression in the medically ill

MANAGEMENT/TREATMENT

1. Screen for possible physiologic syndromes or disease that could present as or with depression and treat underlying cause.
2. Symptomatic management of depression includes:
   A. Mild depression: Symptoms are not disabling; person is still able to participate in medical treatment plan and has hope for improvement; low suicide risk

1) Develop a supportive relationship.
2) Provide information:
   a. About depression, its self-limiting nature
   b. The specific course of the medical illness, the medical treatment plan, the steps needed to move toward wellness
3) Allow for expression of feelings.
4) Provide alternatives to negative thoughts, correct errors in thinking.
5) Incorporate supportive family members in treatment.
6) Reinforce positive behaviors.
7) Teach relaxation, guided imagery.
8) Consider alternative therapies (i.e., music, touch).
9) Appropriate referrals to mental health consultant for therapy or psychiatrist for medication evaluation. Criteria for referral depend on:
   a. Patient preference: Some patients refuse intervention from a psychiatric-mental health professional, while others request it.
   b. Availability of affordable psychiatric professionals, including psychiatrist, advanced practice nurse, social worker, or marriage and family counselor.
B. Severe depression: Lasting longer than 2 weeks; symptoms disabling; individual no longer concerned about getting well
   1) Evaluate for suicide intent and take appropriate precautions, such as providing 24-hour surveillance.
   2) Consider antidepressant medications (see Table 12–2).
      a. Most take 7–14 days to show some effect, and full effect can sometimes take 4–6 weeks.
      b. Needs initial close monitoring for side effects.
   3) Psychiatric evaluation
   4) Depending on availability, electroconvulsive shock treatment may be considered. Often more effective than medications in patients with complicating medical illness.

TABLE 12–2. Selected Antidepressant Medications

| Drug | Side Effect | | | | Dose Range (mg/day) | Average Half-life (hr) | Potentially Fatal Drug Interactions |
	Anti-cholinergic*	Orthostatic hypotension	Cardiac dysrhythmia	GI distress			
Tricyclics							
Amitriptyline (Elavil)	+ + + +	+ + + +	+ + +	0	75–300	16–46	Antiarrythmics MAOIs
Doxepin (Sinequan)	+ + +	+ +	+ +	0	75–300	10–47	Antiarrythmics MAOIs
Heterocyclic							
Trazadone (Desyrel)	0	+	+	+	150–600	4–14	—
Selective Serotonin Reuptake Inhibitors							
Fluoxetine (Prozac)	0	0	0	+ + +	10–40	72–360	MAOIs
Sertraline (Zoloft)	0	0	0	+ + +	50–150	10–30	MAOIs

* Dry mouth, blurred vision, urinary hesitancy, constipation.
GI, gastrointestinal; MAOIs, monoamine oxidase inhibitors.

PATIENT/FAMILY EDUCATION

1. Discuss usual course of depression, possible underlying factors as it relates to this particular patient, planned treatment, and expected outcomes.
2. If medications are used, expected effects and onset of action, possible side effects.
3. Alternative coping skills, such as relaxation techniques, guided imagery, therapeutic touch, and distraction.

Review Questions

12.6 Out of the following list, select the most useful indicator of depression in the hospitalized patient.
 A. Insomnia
 B. Hypersomnia
 C. Feeling like a failure
 D. Crying
 E. Loss of appetite

12.7 The criterion that marks a mood disorder as major depression is:
 A. The mood fluctuates over time.
 B. The patient is disoriented as to time and place but oriented to situation and person.
 C. The patient alternates sad mood with irritability.
 D. The symptoms must have been present consistently for 2 weeks.
 E. Laboratory results will demonstrate electrolyte imbalance.

12.8 Mr. W is a 48-year-old married man who was admitted for an inferior wall myocardial infarction. As you are assessing his progress, he expresses many of his thoughts and feelings about his situation to you. Which of the following should alert you that he may be depressed?
 A. Now that I've had a heart attack, I'll never be able to have sex again.
 B. I should be able to get better faster.
 C. I'm never going to get well.
 D. What's the point of trying anyway—I'll never walk again since my heart attack so I might as well curl up and die.
 E. All of the above.

12.9 The most common depressive experience in the hospitalized patient is:
 A. Delirium
 B. Major depression
 C. Digitalis toxicity
 D. Alcohol withdrawal
 E. Grief

12.10 Mrs. C, a 38-year-old woman with aplastic anemia, is recovering from a bone marrow transplant and is facing a long hospital stay away from her family. She began to experience the symptoms of a major depression and was placed on an antidepressant. Now when she gets out of bed she begins to complain of dizziness. Her blood pressure lying down is 120/

76 and when standing it is 90/62. Which of the following antidepressants is most likely to cause this problem?

A. Trazodone
B. Amitriptyline
C. Doxepin
D. Fluoxetine

Answers and Rationales

12.6   **C**   Somatic symptoms are not helpful in distinguishing depression in the hospitalized patient. More useful are the cognitive symptoms such as feeling like a failure. Although crying is an indicator of depression if pronounced, it may not distinguish depression from a grief response.

12.7   **D**   The DSM-IV lists as mandatory criteria for major depression that the symptoms must be present for 2 weeks and must be consistently present during that time. Unless the depression is so severe as to include psychotic symptoms, depressed patients are oriented.

12.8   **E**   Depressed people think in global terms—the illness colors all aspects of life, not just the affected part. They think in all-or-none terms and tend to blame themselves for their state rather than the circumstances.

12.9   **E**   Grief is the experience of loss. All illness and hospitalization represent some form of loss—loss of independence, family, role, former health status. Most patients experience this loss to some degree.

12.10   **B**   Tricyclic antidepressants have the greatest potential for causing orthostatic hypotension, and amitriptyline is more potent in this regard than trazadone.

References

American Psychiatric Association. (1994). *Diagnostic and Statistical Manual of Mental Disorders* (4th ed.). Washington DC: American Psychiatric Press.

Davis, T., & Jensen, L. (1988). Identifying depression in medical patients. *Image J Nurs Scholarship 20*(4), 191–195.

Rodin, G., Crave, J., & Littlefield, C. (1991). *Depression in the Medically Ill: An Integrated Approach*. New York: Brunner/Mazel.

Additional Recommended References

Clark, S. (1990). Nursing interventions for the depressed cardiovascular patient. *J Cardiovasc Nurs 5*(1), 54–64.

Rush, A.J. (Panel chair). (1993). *Depression in Primary Care: Vol. I. Detection and Diagnosis: Clinical Practice Guideline* (AHCPR Publ. No. 93–0550). Washington, DC: Agency for Health Care Policy and Research.

Rush, A.J. (Panel chair). (1993). *Depression in Primary Care: Vol. 2: Treatment of Major Depression Clinical Practice Guideline* (AHCPR Publ. No. 93–0551). Washington, DC: Agency for Health Care Policy and Research.

The Suicidal Patient

DEFINITION

Suicide is the intentional taking of one's own life either by active measures or passive, ongoing consciously or unconsciously motivated behaviors that are self-destructive and will eventually lead to one's own death.

ETIOLOGY/INCIDENCE

1. Over 30,000 Americans per year successfully suicide.
2. It is the eighth leading cause of death in all age groups.
3. In the acute care setting, the suicidal patient presents in three major ways:
   A. The patient who has unsuccessfully attempted suicide and is in the emergency department awaiting stabilization and referral.
   B. The patient who is admitted to the hospital because of actual or anticipated medical complications of the attempt.
   C. A patient who may or may not have made a prior suicide attempt who either directly threatens self-harm or offers verbal indications that he/she has been having suicidal thoughts. It is a myth that patients who talk about suicide intent will not carry out the act.

SIGNS AND SYMPTOMS

Factors that should alert the nurse practitioner to the high risk of suicide are:

1. Severe anxiety
2. Severe depression
3. Few coping strategies or strategies that are destructive
4. Very few, if any, active and available support systems
5. Alcohol or substance abuse
6. Giving possessions away or making a will
7. Sudden lifting of mood in a patient who has been depressed or started on antidepressant medication
8. Marked disorientation or confusion
9. A clear suicide plan (i.e., knows when, how, and has the means; thinks about it frequently)
10. Previous suicide attempts
11. Family history of suicide
12. Current life crisis

PHYSICAL FINDINGS

Physical findings vary widely and are related to the method used in the case of a suicide attempt. Common agents used in attempted suicide include acetaminophen, salicylates, antidepressants, theophylline, digoxin, ethylene glycol and methanol (used in solvents or antifreezes), cyanide, iron, pesticides, and carbon monoxide, as well as substances of abuse and miscellaneous pharmacologic agents such as insulin and nonsteroidal anti-inflammatory drugs. The following is a partial listing:

Associated Finding	Examples of Type of Agent
Increased heart rate	Anticholinergics, amphetamine
Decreased heart rate	Digoxin, β-blockers
Increased respirations	Salicilates, cyanide
Decreased respirations	Barbiturates, opiates, tricyclic antidepressants
Increased temperature	Amphetamines, anticholinergics
Decreased temperature	Ethanol, barbiturates
Dilated pupils	Sympathomimetics, amphetamines
Constricted pupils	Opioids

Other findings would vary depending on the method used in the suicide attempt (i.e., the type of weapon used and the part of the body injured).

DIFFERENTIAL DIAGNOSIS

1. From a mental health standpoint, differential diagnosis includes:
    1. Suicidal ideation associated with grief or despondency with little or no risk of being carried out
    2. Suicide threat with high likelihood of being carried out
    3. Unintentional action related to altered mental status or physical handicap (i.e., visual impairment leading to ingestion of wrong dose or substance)
    4. Child, elder, or spousal abuse
2. From a physiologic standpoint, differential diagnosis will depend on the means used and the organ system affected. For example, the comatose patient creates a different set of possibilities (suicide attempt, head injury, increased intracranial pressure, substance abuse, etc.) than the patient who presents with cardiac dysrhythmias (electrolyte imbalance, myocardial infarction, suicide attempt with cardiotoxic agents, etc.)

DIAGNOSTIC TESTS/FINDINGS

1. Physiologic evaluation
    A. Blood gases: Metabolic acidosis with salicylates, methanol; respiratory acidosis with barbiturates, benzodiazepines and opioids
    B. Electrolytes: Hyperkalemia in digitalis poisoning, acid-base evaluation to identify metabolic acidosis and alkalosis
    C. Specific organ function studies: Liver function tests in acetaminophen overdose, warfarin overdose
    D. Hypoglycemia: Insulin overdose
    E. Drug screens of urine, blood, gastric contents
2. Psychiatric evaluation
    A. The clinical interview that assesses suicide risk is the best way to identify those at high risk for a suicide attempt.
    B. Patients who have attempted suicide should be considered at risk for at least 3 months after the attempt.
    C. Nurse practitioners should become comfortable with asking patients about their suicidal thoughts and plans.
    D. Questions to assess risk include:
        1) "Do you ever feel so (bad/depressed/hopeless) that you have thought about killing yourself?" Many patients may answer yes to this ques-

tion; it is important to pursue the topic further to rule out mild suicidal ideation.

2) "Have you thought about how you would go about it?" Assess the lethality of the plan. Does patient actually have the means (i.e. possess the gun, knife, poison)?

3) "How likely is it that you would actually carry out this plan?"

4) "Have you been able to tell anyone how badly you are feeling? Would you consider getting some help for how you are feeling?"

5) If a patient has already made an attempt, try to determine method and lethality:

    a. "Did you expect that you would die?"

    b. "How do you feel about still being alive?"

    c. If the suicide attempt was made to try and manipulate another's behavior, ask if the patient feels that the attempt was successful in achieving that goal.

6) Is there an active support system present?

7) Is the patient willing to make a contract with you that he/she will not make another attempt until he/she can be put in contact with a mental health professional?

E. Often it is the clinician's intuition that guides the compiling of the information gleaned from the interview along with the patient's behavior and willingness to engage in a helpful dialogue, added to the lethality and clarity of the patient's intent, that leads to the determination of risk.

MANAGEMENT/TREATMENT

Management and treatment depend on patient presentation.

1. For patients stabilized in the emergency department and admitted for observation of potential complication:

  A. Provide an atmosphere that will permit the patient to talk about thoughts of hopelessness and suicide.

  B. If risk is high for suicide attempt, provide for protection in the form of constant observation.

  C. Activate procedures for mental health consultation.

2. For patients who are unresponsive or stuporous:

  A. Maintain cardiopulmonary status.

  B. Call for immediate physician backup and consultation.

  C. Institute treatment specific to toxin ingested or wound inflicted. (See the chapter by Brass listed in the References for an excellent review of specific toxins and management.)

PATIENT EDUCATION

1. Provide information about treatment services and support services available.

2. Provide illness-specific support services (i.e., the American Cancer Society, the Multiple Sclerosis Society, the American Heart Association, etc.).

3. Provide 24-hour suicide prevention hotline phone number.

Review Questions

12.11 A patient on your service has just found out that he will require a triple coronary artery bypass graft procedure. He states that he might as well be dead as to have the surgery. The best response would be:

A. Tell him that you have a film describing the surgery and the recovery period and that he should feel much more hopeful after seeing it.

B. Realize that many patients feel that way on hearing such sudden news and that the feelings are normal and will pass.

C. Ask the patient to tell you more about his feelings.

D. Describe other patients you have cared for who felt the same way and are now back doing everything they were prior to the surgery.

E. Tell the patient that you will call the social worker to come and talk to him.

12.12 Mr. B is the husband of one of your patients who is on ventilator support and is unlikely to be weaned. He tells you that, if his wife dies, he will probably take his own life because he does not think that he can go on without her. The nurse practitioner should realize that:

A. Mr. B is just expressing normal grief and the likelihood of his killing himself is actually very low.

B. Mr. B is very likely to carry out this plan and needs to be hospitalized.

C. Mr. B is severely depressed and should be considered for antidepressant medications.

D. Mr. B needs an opportunity to talk at length with someone about his suicidal thoughts.

E. Mr. B needs an opportunity to participate in his wife's care because this will make him feel more useful and less depressed.

12.13 A patient who had been feeling quite discouraged greets you with a big smile and tells you that all of a sudden the world seems to be a better place. Your best response would be:

A. To recognize that the patient has finally worked through the problem and come to a new understanding.

B. To recognize that the patient may have come to a decision to kill him/herself and that the indecision that was contributing to the depression is gone.

C. Tell the patient how glad you feel that he/she is feeling better.

D. Tell the patient that you do not believe that he/she could be feeling better so quickly.

E. Cancel the referral to the mental health professional.

12.14 A patient you are working with acknowledges that she has thoughts of killing herself. Which piece of information would be most useful in assessing suicide risk?

A. If the patient has family or friends she can talk to.

B. If she has thought about how she would kill herself.

C. If she uses alcohol or drugs.

D. If she has ever had psychiatric help in the past.

E. If she has tried to kill herself in the past.

Answers and Rationales

12.11 **C** Although the patient's reaction is not that unusual and he probably would be helped by knowing about the procedure and others who have recovered, it is also important to give the message that it is all right to feel discouraged. It is also an opportunity to learn how hopeless the patient is and whether he would, in fact, think about killing himself. Once this is known, then a plan can be devised.

12.12 **D** Suicidal thoughts need to be explored to understand intensity, and to assess suicidal risk. It is a myth that people who talk about suicide will not actually carry out the threat. However, it is also possible that, with an opportunity to discuss their situations, people will find other resources, either internal or external, that help to sustain them through the crisis.

12.13 **B** Although, in fact, a patient may work through his/her problems, it is important for nurse practitioners to be mindful that a sudden lifting of depression often comes when the patient has decided to take action to end his/her life. The agony of not being able to decide is lifted and he/she feels better. Also, antidepressant medications may modify the symptoms of depression, and the patient may now have the energy to kill him/herself. It is important to explore this concern with the patient openly.

12.14 **B** Although all of the information would be helpful, the most important information to assess current risk is if the patient has a well-thought-out plan and the means to carry it out.

References

Brass, E.P. (1995). Toxins and poisons. In E. Sivak, T. Higgins, & A. Seiver (eds.). *The High Risk Patient: Management of the Critically Ill*. Baltimore: Williams & Wilkins, pp. 1454–1472.

Gorman, L.M., Sultan, D., & Luna-Raines, M. (1989). *Psychosocial Nursing Handbook for the Non-psychiatric Nurse*. Baltimore: Williams & Wilkins, pp. 95–107.

Maurer, R. (1996). Suicide assessment. In R. Rakel (ed.). *Saunders Manual of Medical Practice*. Philadelphia: W.B. Saunders Co., pp. 1114–1115.

Additional Recommended References

Hacket, T.P., & Stern, T.A. (1987). Suicide and other disruptive states. In T. Hackett & N. Casem (eds.). *Massachusetts General Hospital Handbook of General Hospital Psychiatry*. Littleton, MA: PSG Publishing Co., pp. 268–274.

Kulig, K. (1992). Initial management of ingestions and toxic substances. *N Engl J Med 126*, 1677–1681.

Grief

DEFINITIONS

The grief reaction is the emotional response to a loss in which something valued is changed or altered so that it no longer has its previously valued traits.

ETIOLOGY/INCIDENCE

1. Grief is the most common depressive experience in patients who are medically ill. Grief is experienced by almost everyone who is seriously ill themselves or has a loved one who is seriously ill.
2. Grief is experienced by people reacting to death or the anticipation of death or to the losses created by illness, such as the loss of an important part of one's self-definition (i.e., body image, health, role, financial security, etc.).
3. The degree of grief experienced is moderated by the meaning of the loss to the individual, the adequacy of coping responses, and the support systems available.

SIGNS AND SYMPTOMS

1. Emotional responses
   A. Shock and disbelief, denial of the event or meaning of the loss, emotional numbness
   B. Angry, hostile response or intense suffering, sobbing, depression as the impact of the loss enters awareness
   C. Anxiety or fear related to the anticipated changes that the loss represents
   D. Calm acceptance of the loss, a sense of peace and calm as the reality of the loss is accepted (usually experienced if the person has had a chance to work through the loss, such as during a long illness)
2. Physical symptoms
   A. Initial response may include hyperventilation, chest pain, syncope
   B. Insomnia, extreme fatigue
   C. Weight loss or gain
   D. Gastrointestinal problems—anorexia, diarrhea, constipation, epigastric pain
   E. Chest pressure, palpitations
   F. Increased illness related to immunosuppression
3. Cognitive responses
   A. Idealizing the way things "used to be"
   B. Guilt over actions taken or omitted prior to the loss (i.e., not maintaining diet, noncompliance with medications, smoking, substance abuse, etc.)
   C. Ruminating over how loss could have been prevented
   D. Dreaming about the person who has died
   E. Thoughts of wanting to join the deceased
   F. Delusions or hallucinations where the deceased is seen or heard
   G. Abnormal thoughts that need attention
      1) Guilt about things other than actions taken or not taken prior to the loss
      2) Thoughts of death other than the survivor feeling that he/she would be better off dead or should have died with the deceased
      3) Feelings of worthlessness
      4) Hallucinations other than thinking he/she has heard or seen the image of the deceased
4. Course of response
   A. Culturally influenced.
   B. If response is to losses created by illness, should expect resolution of the symptoms as healing takes place.

    C. Intense symptoms lasting longer than 2 months should be reassessed and depression ruled out.

DIFFERENTIAL DIAGNOSIS

1. Major depression
2. Mood disorder secondary to general medical condition

DIAGNOSTIC TESTS/FINDINGS

1. No specific diagnostic tests; refer to section on "Depression."
2. Important to explore suicidal ideation and suicide risk.

MANAGEMENT/TREATMENT

1. Accept wide variations in expressions of grief; many are culturally determined.
2. Expect variability in response in any given individual. Individuals may be accepting at one time and then later react with denial and anger. Grief work is highly individual and symptoms wax and wane.
3. Encourage but don't demand expression of feelings.
4. Provide support and insight into the process as appropriate.
5. Help develop personal control through use of alternative measures such as relaxation, guided imagery, music therapy.
6. Involve support systems.
7. Make appropriate referrals: mental health professional, illness-specific support groups, grief groups, etc.
8. Identify individuals who seem to be experiencing a major depression rather than a grief reaction and make appropriate referrals.
9. Consider a short course of anxiolytics to assist with symptoms of anxiety, insomnia, etc., recognizing that eventually the feelings must be experienced in order to be resolved.

PATIENT/EDUCATION

1. Provide information regarding the illness and expected recovery and the steps needed to achieve healing.
2. Discuss normal grief responses and validate the individual's own experience.
3. Provide information related to community resources.

Review Questions

12.15 A family member confides in you that, since the death of her husband last month, she has ongoing conversations with him and has actually seen him working in their garden. The best response would be:
    A. To have her evaluated for acute psychotic reaction
    B. Refer her for antipsychotic medication evaluation
    C. Do nothing; this is a normal grief reaction
    D. Ask her to tell more about her experience
    E. Tell her this is to be expected and many people have this happen

12.16 The most common depressive experience in patients who are medically ill is:
A. Grief
B. Major depression
C. Mood disorder related to medical condition
D. Suicidal ideation
E. Fatigue

12.17 Many of the symptoms experienced by those who are grieving are identical to those in people experiencing major depression. One major differentiating factor is:
A. Anorexia and weight loss
B. Extreme irritability
C. Feelings of self-loathing
D. Auditory hallucinations of hearing the deceased
E. Sobbing

12.18 Mrs. C's husband of 42 years died 3 weeks ago. She shares with you some of her feelings. Which of the following statements should alert you that you might need to refer her to a mental health professional?
A. "I can hear John calling to me as I lay quietly in bed at night."
B. "I can't believe that he would leave me alone like this!"
C. "I keep thinking that there was something I could have done to keep him alive."
D. "I feel like nothing without John. Why would anyone even want to sit here and talk to me; I'm nothing but a burden."
E. "I look forward to being able to join John in heaven."

Answers and Rationales

12.15 **D** Although this is a normal grief reaction and experienced by others, it would be important to know what the conversations are about and how she is feeling about them. She may be considering suicide to join him or hearing him ask her to join him. It is always prudent to take opportunities to assess suicide risk.

12.16 **A** Grief, or the reaction to the losses created by serious illness, is experienced to some degree by almost everyone who has a serious illness.

12.17 **C** Lowered self-esteem is a common finding in depression but is not a characteristic of the grief response.

12.18 **D** Feelings of worthlessness are not an expected reaction to the experience of grief or loss. The person may be experiencing a major depression underneath the grief reaction.

References

American Psychiatric Association. (1994). *Diagnostic and Statistical Manual of Mental Disorders* (4th ed.) Washington, D.C.: American Psychiatric Press, pp. 684–685.

Gorman, L.M., Sultan, D., & Luna-Raines, M. (1989). *Psychosocial Nursing Handbook for the Non-psychiatric Nurse.* Baltimore: Williams & Wilkins, pp. 107–117.

Kubler-Ross, E. (1969). *On Death and Dying.* Toronto: Macmillan Co.

Additional Recommended References

Patel, C.T.C. (1996). Hope-inspiring strategies of spouses of critically ill adults. *J Holist Nurs 14* (1), 44–65.

Alterations in Mental Status: Confusion, Delirium, and Dementia

DEFINITIONS

> *Confusion:* A loss of intellectual ability in one or more areas, including memory, concentration, attention, orientation, comprehension, and interpretation of the environment. It is an isolated symptom that requires investigation as to the underlying cause.
>
> *Delirium:* An organic mental *syndrome* of symptoms, not a diagnosis. It is an *acute, reversible* state not caused by enduring changes in the brain. It is characterized by a range of symptoms that can vary from a slight clouding of consciousness to global impairment and psychosis. Hallmarks are a waxing and waning of the symptoms, a decrease in the ability to attend and concentrate, and disorientation to time, place, and person.
>
> *Dementia:* An organic mental *syndrome* that is characterized by a *slow decline in intellectual functioning over time* severe enough to interfere with social or occupational functioning. Some of the causes of dementia are reversible while others are not.

INCIDENCE

1. Incidence of delirium in hospitalized patients has been estimated to be as high as 15–30%. Can occur in as many as 50% of intensive care unit (ICU) patients.
2. Of elderly living in long-term care environments, 50–75% have some cognitive impairment. Of these, 10–33% have a potentially reversible cause.

ETIOLOGY

Confusion and organic mental syndromes are caused by (1) a brain cell metabolism that is altered by systemic problems, (2) mechanical problems that deprive the brain of nutrients, or (3) actual destruction of brain cells.

1. Common causes of delirium include:
   A. Physiologic problems (partial list)
      1) Hypoxia; hypercapnia
      2) Organ failure: Renal, cardiac, liver
      3) Electrolyte imbalance
      4) Hypo/hyperglycemia
      5) Withdrawal from drugs/alcohol
      6) Infection
      7) Vascular: Cerebrovascular accident, transient ischemic attack
   B. Pharmacologic (partial list)
      1) Steroids
      2) Anesthetics

        3) Analgesics
        4) Anticholinergics
        5) Cardiac medications
        6) Sedatives
    C. Environmental
        1) Lack of sleep
        2) Altered circadian rhythms
2. Common causes of dementia
    A. Reversible (20% of cases)
        1) Nutritional disorders such as vitamin deficiency; B_{12}, folate, thiamin
        2) Metabolic disorders such as hypothyroidism
        3) Trauma: Subdural hematoma
        4) Infections
        5) Drug reaction
    B. Irreversible causes
        1) Alzheimer's disease (50% of cases)
        2) Multi-infarct dementia
        3) Parkinson's disease
        4) Jakob-Creutzfelt disease (race generative brain disease caused by infective agent)
        5) Neurodegenerative disorders such as Pick's disease
        6) Acquired immunodeficiency syndrome
        7) Korsakoff's syndrome (chronic amnestic disorder secondary to alcohol abuse)
        8) Chronic inflammatory disorders such as lupus, multiple sclerosis

SIGNS AND SYMPTOMS

1. Delirium
    A. Reduced ability to maintain attention to external stimuli
    B. Disorganized thinking
    C. At least two of the following:
        1) Reduced level of consciousness
        2) Perceptual disturbances (illusions, hallucinations, delusions)
        3) Sleep-wake cycle disturbance
        4) Increased or decreased motor activity
           a. The hypoactive, hypoalert form
           b. The hyperactive, hyperalert form
        5) Disorientation to time, place, person
        6) Memory impairment
2. Dementia
    A. Symptoms vary in intensity from mild to severe.
    B. Memory impairment is usually the first, most prominent symptom.
        1) Initially, affects most recent events
        2) In later stages, only fragments remain
    C. Gradual disorientation to time, place, and finally person.
    D. Impairment in judgment and ability to function independently.
    E. In later stages:
        1) Loss of coordination and ability to carry out motor activities (apraxia)
        2) Speech difficulties, including aphasia
    F. Personality changes

DIFFERENTIAL DIAGNOSIS

1. Delirium
   A. Dementia
   B. Functional psychiatric disorder
      1) Anxiety disorder
      2) Depression
      3) Acute psychotic disorder
      4) Schizophrenia
2. Dementia
   A. Delirium
   B. Pseudodementia: Severe depression in the elderly
   C. Factitious disorder
   D. Schizophrenia
3. Factors that can lead to misdiagnosis of alteration in mental status:
   A. Similarity between some of the symptoms of dementia and delirium.
   B. The first sign of medical illness in the elderly may be confusion.
   C. Belief that confusion and memory problems are "just a normal part of the aging process."
   D. Belief that confusion/memory deficits are always indicators of Alzheimer's disease.
   E. Delirium can occur in the setting of dementia.

DIAGNOSTIC TESTS/FINDINGS

1. Delirium
   A. Abnormal mental status examination using published reliable tests (i.e., Folstein Mini-Mental Status Exam)
   B. Diagnostic and laboratory tests specific to suspected underlying problem
      1) CBC, electrolytes, blood sugar, urinalysis, blood gases, liver function, toxicology screen, blood levels of pharmacologic agents, etc.
      2) Head computed tomography (CT)
      3) Electroencephalogram: Helps differentiate organic and psychiatric disorders; generalized slowing in delirium
      4) Chest x-ray
      5) Electrocardiogram (ECG)
2. Dementia
   A. Abnormal mental status examination
   B. Dementia rating scales
   C. Reversible causes
      1) CBC: Rule out anemia, infection
      2) Thyroid-stimulating hormone: Rule out thyroid disease
      3) Iron studies: Rule out iron-deficiency anemia
      4) B_{12}, folate, thiamine: Rule out vitamin deficiency
      5) Erythrocyte sedimentation rate: Rule out inflammatory disease
      6) Fluorescent treponemal antibody absorption test: Rule out tertiary syphilis
      7) Human immunodeficiency virus (HIV): Rule out in high-risk individuals
      8) Lumbar puncture: Rule out central nervous system (CNS) infections, normal pressure hydrocephalus

9) CT scan, head: Rule out mass lesions, subdural hematoma, multi-infarct dementia

10) Magnetic resonance imaging: brain scan: Rule out tumor, brain scan, arteriovenous (AV) malformation

MANAGEMENT/TREATMENT

1. Delirium
   A. Identify most likely causative factors and correct underlying problem, discontinue medication, provide adequate pain relief, or provide for adequate rest.
   B. Provide frequent orientation to time, place, person, situation.
   C. Enlist family members to stay with patient.
   D. Protect patient and others from injury.
   E. Treat agitation with benzodiazepines or haloperidol alone or in combination.
      1) Lorazepam is preferred benzodiazepine when used in combination with haloperidol.
         a. Can be given IV and IM
         b. Short acting
      2) Usual dose of lorazepam is 0.5–4.0 mg IV bolus.
      3) Haloperidol IV
         a. Not approved by United States Food and Drug Administration *Needs institutional protocol
         b. Well suited to the agitated ICU patient
         c. Onset of action 15–20 min
         d. Usual dose of haloperidol is:
            1. Mild agitation: 0.5–2.0 mg IV
            2. Moderate agitation: 0.5–10.0 mg IV
            3. Severe agitation: 10.0 mg or more IV
         e. May be bolused but if patient is hypotensive or volume depleted should be given over 5 minutes.
         f. Precipitates with phenytoin and heparin.
      4) Benzodiazepines may worsen delirium, especially in the elderly.
   F. Consider referral to psychiatrist or appropriate physician according to protocol, or when the underlying source of the delirium is not clear, or if the delirium does not resolve with appropriate management as listed above.
2. Dementia
   A. Rule out reversible causes.
   B. Protect patient and others from injury by modifying environment. Consider short-acting anxiolytics and low anticholinergic neuroleptic medications to manage anxiety and agitation.
   C. Newer drug to augment acetylcholine: tetrahydroaminoacridine (tacrine HCl), which may augment memory in some cases. Suggested dose is 40 mg to start and then increase by 40 mg every 6 weeks until 160 mg is reached. Liver enzymes are increased in 30% of patients and drug should be discontinued if alanine aminotransferase level reaches five times normal. Nausea, vomiting, and diarrhea can be problems, as well.
   D. Simplify medication regimen to avoid increased risks of side effects.
   E. Rule out overlying delirium, depression, which can worsen confusion.

F. Referral to neurologist or psychiatrist according to protocol, when patient's symptoms are beyond nurse practitioner's scope of practice or experience, or to evaluate and treat complex cases.

PATIENT/FAMILY EDUCATION

1. Delirium
   A. Define delirium and reassure as to the temporary nature of the condition.
   B. Describe assessment measures being taken and update progress.
   C. Reassure that the patient is not responsible for his/her behavior if he/she is combative or verbally aggressive.
   D. Teach patient and family relaxation measures to promote relaxation and sleep.
2. Dementia
   A. Explain diagnosis, behavioral syndromes, and treatment.
   B. Refer for caregiver support.
   C. Anticipate legal and ethical issues and make appropriate referrals.

Review Questions

12.19 The cardinal sign of mental status changes seen in delirium is:
   A. Agitation
   B. Consistent, persistent alterations in mental status
   C. Somnolence
   D. Decreased ability to attend and concentrate
   E. Hallucinations

12.20 Pseudodementia is a term used to describe:
   A. Elderly patients who are malingering
   B. Severe depression in the elderly
   C. Delirium that mimics dementia
   D. A side effect of anticholinergic medications
   E. None of the above

12.21 Reversible causes of dementia include:
   A. Infection, hypothyroidism, subdural hematoma
   B. Depression, acute psychotic disorder, schizophrenia
   C. Hypothyroidism, B_{12} deficiency, multi-infarct dementia
   D. AV malformation, inflammatory disease, Jakob-Creutzfeldt disease
   E. All of the above

12.22 Mrs. V is worried about her 72-year-old mother because she is more irritable than she used to be. Mrs. V thinks her mother is becoming demented. In order to address her concerns and help with the diagnosis, the nurse practitioner should ask:
   A. "How irritable has she been?"
   B. "Does your mother know the date and who she is?"
   C. "Is your mother still able to dress herself?"

D. "Does your mother have trouble forming sentences?"

E. "Is your mother showing signs of memory loss?"

12.23 An elderly patient is brought to the hospital in a confused state that began about 3 days ago after her cat died. The family states that the patient could no longer recognize them, was restless and agitated, and was incontinent. The most likely diagnosis is:

A. Dementia, Alzheimer's type

B. Dementia due to a reversible cause

C. Pseudodementia

D. Delirium

E. Depression

Answers and Rationales

12.19 **D** Delirious patients may present as withdrawn or agitated; the symptoms wax and wane and hallucinations may or may not be present.

12.20 **B** Pseudodementia is depression in the elderly, manifesting symptoms that appear to be dementia.

12.21 **A** Depression, acute psychotic disorder, and schizophrenia may all mimic dementia and are considered rule outs before the diagnosis of dementia can be made. Multi-infarct dementia and Jakob-Creutzfeldt disease are irreversible.

12.22 **E** Memory impairment, initially of most recent events, is usually the first, most prominent symptom of dementia. Other changes occur later.

12.23 **D** An important distinction between dementia and delirium is the rapidity of onset. Dementia is usually slow to develop, while the onset of delirium is sudden. Although the patient may be depressed over the loss of the cat, depressed patients are less likely to be incontinent than patients with delirium.

References

Harvey, M.A. (1996). Managing agitation in critically ill patients. *Am J Crit Care 5*, 7–16.

Inaba-Roland, K.E., & Maricle, R.A. (1992). Assessing delirium in the acute care setting. *Heart Lung 21*, 48–54.

Tesar, G.E. & Stern, T.A. (1995). Neuropsychiatric disturbance in the critically ill patient. In E.D. Sivak, T.L. Higgins, & A. Seiver (eds.). *The High Risk Patient: Management of the Critically Ill*. Baltimore: Williams & Wilkins, pp. 29–50.

Additional Recommended References

Gorman, L.M., Sultan, D., & Luna-Raines, M. (1989). *Psychosocial Nursing Handbook for the Non-psychiatric Nurse*. Baltimore: Williams & Wilkins, pp. 128–161.

Mateo, M. (1990). Confusion in older adults: Assessment and differential diagnosis. *Nurse Pract 15*(9), 32–46.

Sleep Deprivation in the Intensive Care Unit

DEFINITION

Sleep deprivation in the ICU patient includes a decrease in the amount of sleep that is achieved in a 24-hour period as well as decreases in the consistency and quality of that sleep.

Sleep fragmentation occurs when patients are prevented from achieving a complete 90-minute average sleep cycle that includes non–rapid eye movement (NREM) as well as rapid eye movement (REM) sleep. Signs and symptoms of sleep deprivation can occur even though the total sleep time may be within normal limits.

ETIOLOGY/INCIDENCE

In order to understand sleep deprivation, it is important to understand the basics of normal sleep.

1. There are two distinct stages of sleep:
    A. REM sleep, or dreaming sleep, promotes emotional healing, brain restoration, and growth.
        1) Blood flow to cerebral gray matter nearly doubles during REM sleep.
        2) Heart rate, blood pressure, respirations, intracranial pressure, and MVO_2 are all increased
    B. NREM promotes physical healing and growth; stages I–IV
        1) Seventy percent of growth hormone is secreted during stages III and IV.
        2) Growth hormone stimulates protein anabolism for cell growth, repair, and replication.
2. Normal adult sleep occurs in distinct cycles:
    A. The average adult has a sleep cycle of 90 minutes, with four to six sleep cycles over a 6- to 8-hour period.
    B. Sleep begins with NREM stage I, progresses through stages II, III, and IV, then moves back through stages III and II, culminating in REM sleep.
    C. Duration of REM sleep lengthens as the night progresses.
    D. Stages III and IV disappear in the latter sleep cycles.
    E. Sleep patterns change throughout the life cycle, with infants and neonates having a predominance of REM sleep and the elderly have increased periods of wakefulness and reduction of stage NREM IV sleep.
3. Sleep in the ICU: Results of research. (Refer to References at end of section for review of literature.)
    A. Small studies with selected patient populations demonstrate loss of total sleep time in patients with respiratory failure, noncardiac and cardiac surgery (as reported by Evans and French).
    B. Fragmentation of sleep was also shown in these patient populations, with loss of stages II, III, REM sleep and increases in the percentage of stage I and wakefulness. Mean total sleep time was 285.5 minutes, with a mean of 50 awakenings.
4. Causes of sleep deprivation:
    A. Degree of illness: The sicker the patient, the less sleep
    B. Sophisticated invasive and noninvasive monitoring

    C. Medications used in the treatment of the illness
       1) Opiates reduce REM activity.
       2) Repeated use of benzodiazapines can completely abolish stage IV sleep.
    D. The ICU environment
       1) Conversations among staff
       2) Artificial lighting that denies day-night orientation
       3) Equipment noise and alarms

SIGNS AND SYMPTOMS

1. REM deprivation
   A. Decreased alertness
   B. Irritability—aggressive behavior
   C. Mental status changes—confusion, delusions, hallucinations
2. NREM deprivation
   A. Physiologic symptoms—headache, dizziness, neck muscle weakness, nausea, diarrhea, constipation
   B. Delayed healing
   C. Decreased pain tolerance
   D. Exhaustion, restlessness, anxiety

PHYSICAL FINDINGS

There are no findings specific to sleep deprivation that would be identified in the average ICU setting.

DIFFERENTIAL DIAGNOSIS

1. Lack of adequate pain control
2. Anxiety
3. Delirium due to other causes

DIAGNOSTIC TESTS/FINDINGS

1. There are no specific diagnostic tests to identify sleep deprivation.
2. Careful attention to actual time set aside for rest and sleep would give specific information for a given patient; the mean duration of uninterrupted sleep for a patient in the adult ICU has been found to be 8 minutes.

MANAGEMENT/TREATMENT

1. Ensure adequate pain relief.
2. Provide support and education to reduce anxiety.
3. Develop relationship that assures patients of competency to promote their willingness to place themselves in another's hands.
4. Consider including provision of adequate sleep times in critical pathway documentation. Try to include at least two 90-minute periods of uninterrupted sleep in a 24-hour period.
5. Prioritize activities and delay making routine assessments in patients who are stable.

6. Collaborate with others to change the noise levels in the ICU, which is some studies equal those of the cafeteria at noon or the boiler room.
7. Recognize barriers to providing adequate sleep:
    A. Action-oriented subculture of the ICU that demands constant activity
    B. Lack of system supports that allow nurses to make independent judgments or take the necessary latitude to ensure adequate rest
8. Judicious use of pharmacologic agents to assist in sleep.
    A. Benzodiazepines
        1) General guidelines
            a. Alter normal sleep cycles by prolonging latency to REM sleep, reducing state I, increasing stage II, and disrupting stage IV possibly lessening the release of growth hormone normally released during stage IV.
            b. Become ineffective if given continuously for a period of 2 weeks.
        2) Temazepam (Restoril)
            a. Dose: 15–30 mg PO
            b. Causes little residual impairment.
            c. Relatively rapid elimination with half-life of about 8 hours.
        3) Triazolam (Halcion)
            a. Dose: 0.125–0.250 mg (0.125 mg in elderly).
            b. Ultrarapid elimination with half-life of about 3 hours.
            c. Abrupt withdrawal after long-term use may cause severe rebound symptoms of drug withdrawal.
        4) Fluazepam (Dalmane)
            a. Dose: 15–30 mg PO (15 mg in elderly).
            b. Rapid onset of action.
            c. Extremely long half-life of about 100 hours *can lead to accumulation of the drug.*
    B. Other medications
        1) Diphenhydramine (Benadryl), antihistamine
        2) Sedating antidepressants
            a. Trazadone (Desyrel): Increases total sleep time, decreases nighttime awakenings, does not decrease stage IV sleep. Dose: 50–100 mg PO hs.
            b. Amitriptyline (Elavil): 25 mg PO hs.
            c. Doxepin (Sinequan): 10 mg PO hs.

PATIENT EDUCATION

1. Inform patient, family, and visitors of the importance of sleep and of the commitment to provide uninterrupted rest periods.
2. Teach patient and family relaxation techniques to promote rest and sleep.

Review Questions

12.24 Dreaming occurs in:
    A. All phases of sleep
    B. Only in the deepest sleep, stage IV
    C. In stage III as well as stage IV

      D. During rapid eye movement sleep
      E. During REM sleep but only in the early part of the total sleep cycle

12.25 NREM sleep is associated with increased:
      A. Heart rate
      B. Metabolic rate
      C. Cerebral blood flow
      D. Secretion of growth hormone
      E. Blood pressure

12.26 Benzodiazepines, when given repeatedly:
      A. Have not been shown to influence sleep patterns
      B. Eliminate REM sleep
      C. Increase periods of wakefulness
      D. Abolish stage IV sleep
      E. Increase REM sleep

12.27 Mr. B is a 48-year-old man who has been in the ICU for 1 week after a motor vehicle accident. He has required suctioning every hour to manage copious secretions. As the nurse practitioner overseeing his care, you become concerned that he may be sleep deprived. The symptom(s) that should alert you that this is becoming a problem is (are):
      A. A decreased level of attention
      B. Agitation and aggressiveness
      C. Lethargy
      D. Delusions and hallucinations
      E. All of the above

12.28 Mrs. D is an 80-year-old woman who is in the hospital for a fractured hip. She also has atherosclerotic heart disease, stable angina, and high blood pressure for which she is taking a long-acting nitrate and a β-blocker. She complains that she is unable to sleep. You decide to offer a hypnotic as a sleep aid. Out of the following choices, which would be the optimal one for this patient?
      A. Amitriptyline (Elavil) 25 mg hs
      B. Fluazepam (Dalmane) 15 mg hs
      C. Trazodone (Desyrel) 25 mg hs
      D. Temazepam (Restoril) 30 mg hs
      E. Temazepam (Restoril) 15 mg hs

Answers and Rationales

12.24 **D** Rapid eye movement is the hallmark of the stage of sleep in which dreaming occurs.

12.25 **D** Seventy percent of the growth hormone secretion occurs during stages III and IV.

12.26 **D** Benzodiazepines can abolish stage IV sleep if given over time.

12.27 **E** Patients who are sleep deprived have a range of symptoms from lethargy to agitation, delirium, and psychosis. Given the likelihood that ill patients who have long ICU stays are sleep deprived, this should be part of a differential diagnosis for all behavior and mental status changes.

12.28 **E** Restoril is a benzodiazepine and will have the least cardiovascular side effects. It has a relatively short half-life and causes little residual effects the next day. Fifteen milligrams is the correct dose. Fluazepam has too long a half-life, and amitriptyline and trazodone both have cardiotonic side effects.

References

Evans, J.C., & French, D.G. (1995). Sleep and healing in intensive care settings. *Dimensions Crit Care Nurs 14*(4), 189–199.

Keltner, N.L., & Folks, D.G. (1993). *Psychotropic Drugs*. St. Louis: C.V. Mosby Co., pp. 170–199.

Krachman, S.L., D'Alonzo, G.E., & Criner, G.J. (1995). Sleep in the intensive care unit *Chest 107*, 1713–1720.

Aggression and Violence

DEFINITION

Aggression is forceful physical or verbal behavior that may or may not cause harm to others. Violence is the ultimate maladaptive coping response and is the acting out of aggression that results in injury to others or destruction of property.

ETIOLOGY/INCIDENCE

1. Aggression and violent behavior can be present in:
    A. Personality disorders
        1) Antisocial personality
        2) Borderline personality
    B. Organic illness
        1) Stroke
        2) Alzheimer's disease
        3) Brain tumor
        4) Head injury
        5) Delirium
    C. Psychiatric illness
        1) Schizophrenia
        2) Brief reactive psychosis
        3) Manic episode
        4) Adjustment disorder
    D. Substance abuse or withdrawal
2. Violence is often triggered by a specific incident or an accumulation of stressors that triggers feelings of desperation, and lack of effective coping skills to resolve the situation by other means.
3. In a psychiatric emergency service during a 6-month period, 7% of the patients had violent behavior. The majority of patients were either schizophrenic or had a substance abuse problem.
4. Of patients on the medical-surgical services, 4.4% of patients were evaluated as violent. The majority of those patients had an underling organic disorder or a personality disorder.

5. Patients who have a past history of violence, escalating irritability, paranoia, and substance abuse should be considered at high risk for aggression and violence.

SIGNS AND SYMPTOMS

1. Anger as evidenced by yelling, use of profanity
2. Pacing, agitation
3. Verbal threatening
4. Impulsivity
5. Limited tolerance for anxiety
6. Confusion, delusions, paranoia, hallucinations
7. Evidence of substance abuse

PHYSICAL FINDINGS

1. Increased muscle tension
2. Increased heart rate, respirations, blood pressure

DIFFERENTIAL DIAGNOSIS

See possible etiologies. It is important for the treatment plan to identify, as soon as possible, the most likely underlying cause.

DIAGNOSTIC TESTS/FINDINGS

1. Mental status exam to assess level of consciousness and rule out organic origins of behavioral change.
2. Toxic drug screen.
3. Appropriate laboratory tests to rule out possible organicity: random blood sugar, BUN, creatinine, liver enzyme studies, electrolytes.
4. Review medications and potential side effects and interactions.

MANAGEMENT/TREATMENT

1. Interventions are based on the understanding that:
   A. Violence in the presence of a neurologic disorder or physiologic damage must be viewed as beyond the person's control.
   B. Violence is often the endpoint of unmanaged anger and hostility, and interventions are most effective in the early stages before all control is lost.
   C. Interventions involve a choice of verbal, chemical, and physical restraint.
   D. Some settings have a higher potential for violent behavior than others. Emergency rooms and hospitals that receive victims of gang violence, psychiatric emergencies, or high numbers of patients with substance abuse are examples of settings where there should be a high level of preparedness for violence, not only from patients but from visitors and family members.
2. Allow the patient to ventilate verbally, uninterrupted.
3. Speak in a soft tone of voice, with care to assume a nonthreatening posture; sitting down is often helpful.

4. Make sure that you allow yourself an avenue of escape from the area. Keep door open to give the patient the sense of freedom as well.
5. Respect a wider body-boundary zone and do not touch the patient.
6. Focus on the particular incident at hand rather than exploration of underlying dynamics.
7. Set clear limitations on what will and will not be tolerated as well as outlining consequences of behavior.
8. Evaluate who is best suited to calm the patient down: Would a male or female be best, someone who has more or less authority?
9. Assure patient that the goal is to help the patient get back in control.
10. In settings with a high likelihood for violence, security should be a constant presence or readily available.
11. When violence seems imminent, step in with appropriate physical or chemical restraints. Criteria for the use of restraint include:
    A. The prevention of harm to others or to the patient when other means have been ineffective
    B. The prevention of serious damage to the environment
    C. A request from the patient
    D. To decrease the amount of sensory stimulation
12. Chemical restraints include:
    A. Anxiolytics
       1) May prevent the escalation of violence in a patient who is anxious and who is potentially violent.
       2) May result in disinhibition or further loss of control over feelings and should be used cautiously in patients who have a history of violent outbursts or assaultive behavior.
       3) Commonly prescribed medications:
          a. Lorazepam 0.5–2 mg parenterally, 1–2 mg PO; maximum daily dose 8 mg
          b. Diazepam 5–10 mg IV or IM, 5–10 mg PO; maximum daily dose 40 mg
    B. High-potency neuroleptics (i.e., Haloperidol)
       1) Reserved for wildly agitated or psychotic patients.
       2) Goal is to calm patient; relief of psychotic symptoms may not occur for days.
       3) Dose: 2–5 mg PO or IM every 30–60 minutes to a total daily dose of 100 mg.
          a. Medicate every 4 hours for a low-dose strategy.
          b. Medicate every 30–60 minutes for high-dose strategy.
          c. Note response every 20 minutes after a dose.
          d. Document levels of consciousness and vital signs before each dose.
          e. Observe for signs of tardive dyskinesia or extrapyramidal symptoms (EPS) after each dose
             i. Tardive dyskinesia: Lip smacking, grinding of teeth, rolling of tongue
                • Very rarely can occur after one dose
                • No effective treatment
                • Discontinue medication
             ii. EPS: Abnormal involuntary movement disorders; treatment includes:

- Lorazepam 1 mg tid
- Clonazepam 1 mg bid

13. Physical restraints require an order that must be renewed on a daily basis. In order to apply restraints:
    A. Have a cohesive plan.
    B. Have the personnel necessary to carry out the plan.
    C. Calmly and without being punitive, explain that restraint are going to be used until the patient can regain control.
    D. Check and reposition the patient frequently.
14. After the violence or aggression has subsided, have conference with patient to develop a plan of care to avoid future episodes.
15. Psychiatric consultation is very helpful has violent behavior escalates in order to provide a neutral party to help diffuse the situation, give the individual an opportunity to discuss underlying issues at length, and plan for long-term treatment, if necessary.

PATIENT EDUCATION

1. Do not try to educate patient regarding aggression and violence while the aggression is escalating.
2. If violence is due to organicity, patient's significant others need to understand the difference between behavior that is under one's control versus that which is not.
3. Provide information about outpatient treatment for appropriate problem (i.e., support groups for the mentally ill, caregivers for Alzheimer's patients; substance abuse programs; anger management groups).

Review Questions

12.29 Violence is almost always unexpected.
   A. True
   B. False

12.30 One of the primary conditions underlying violent behavior is:
   A. Substance abuse
   B. Electrolyte imbalance
   C. Dislike of rules and regulations
   D. Reaction to authority figures
   E. Feelings of dominance

12.31 Mrs. E has been waiting to be seen in the urgent care clinic for 30 minutes. Her husband begins to be agitated, raising his voice, demanding to be seen immediately. The best intervention to make at this point is to:
   A. Call security to demonstrate a show of force
   B. Ask calmly and softly, "What has happened to make you so upset?"
   C. Take the husband into a private space, close the door so that you can calmly evaluate the situation
   D. Try to demonstrate to the husband that you are more powerful than he is by standing over him and not being out-shouted
   E. Try to distract the husband from the situation until he calms down

12.32 The use of physical restraint requires:
1. A prearranged plan
2. Adequate personnel
3. An order, renewable on a daily basis
4. Careful monitoring of the patient afterward
5. An explanation to the patient
A. 1,2,4
B. 1,2,3
C. 1,2,4,5
D. 2,3,4,5
E. 1,2,3,4,5

Answers and Rationales

12.29 **B** In most situations, violent behavior can be anticipated because of the past history of the patient, presence of substance abuse, organic mental disease, or escalating aggression.

12.30 **A** In one study, 66% of patients with violent behavior had history of alcohol or substance abuse.

12.31 **B** Calmness is often contagious as well as demonstrating that you are in control. Also, being calm and quite avoids potential power struggles. This option also gives the patient a chance to air the grievance and be heard, the first step in de-escalating aggression.

12.32 **E** All of these elements are necessary when restraints are applied.

References

Menninger, W.W. (1993). Management of the aggressive and dangerous patient. *Bull Menninger Clin 57*, 208–217.

Turnbull, J., Aitkin, I., Black, L., et al. (1990). Turn it around: Short-term management for aggression and anger ... training for nurses. *J Psychosocial Nurs Ment Health Serv 28* (6), 7–10, 13.

Additional Recommended References

Gorman, L.M., Sultan, D., & Luna-Raines, M. (1989). *Psychosocial Nursing Handbook for the Non-psychiatric Nurse.* Baltimore: Williams & Wilkins, pp. 72–77.

Runyon, N., Allen, C.L., & Ilnicki, S.H. (1988). The borderline patient on the med-surg unit. *Am J Nurs 88*, 1644–1650.

Alcohol Abuse and Withdrawal

DEFINITION

Alcohol abuse: The continued use of alcohol despite negative consequences in family relationships or the workplace, or recurrent use in hazardous situations, over a 12-month period, without meeting the criteria for physical dependence.

Alcohol dependence: Requires at least three of the following symptoms:
1. Continued drinking despite physical or psychological consequences caused or worsened by alcohol
2. Neglect of activities other than drinking
3. Inordinate time spent drinking and recovering
4. Drinking more or over a longer period of time than intended
5. Inability to control drinking
6. Increased amounts needed for the same effects (tolerance)
7. Withdrawal symptoms without drinking, or drinking to avoid withdrawal

Alcohol intoxication: A diminished state of physical and mental control caused by the ingestion of alcohol

Alcohol withdrawal syndrome (delirium tremens [DTs]): The physiologic reaction that can occur following the cessation of alcohol use that has been heavy or prolonged.

ETIOLOGY/INCIDENCE

1. Ten percent of the adult population is alcoholic.
2. Ninety-seven percent of alcoholics are employed; of these, 37% have a high school education, 25% are in white-collar jobs, 30% are manual laborers, and 45% are in managerial or professional jobs. Three percent of alcoholics fit the stereotypical "skid row type."
3. Forty percent of admissions to general medical-surgical wards are related to alcohol abuse; 20% of patients have alcohol dependence.
4. Alcohol is the most common drug intoxication and is a component in 70% of drug overdoses.
5. Causes are multifactorial and not well understood:
   A. Genetic: Sons of alcoholics are four times as likely to be alcoholics as are sons of nonalcoholics, whether raised by biologic or adoptive parents.
   B. Psychosocial: Individuals fixed in a lower level of psychosocial development, poor impulse control, low self-esteem, and low frustration tolerance.
   C. High comorbidity with depression.

SIGNS AND SYMPTOMS

1. Alcohol intoxication
   A. Initially euphoria and then sedation
   B. Decreased inhibitions
   C. Visual impairment, diplopia, nystagmus
   D. Muscular incoordination
   E. Slurred speech
   F. Ataxia
   G. Slowing of reaction time
   H. Blackouts
   I. Palpitations
   J. Odor of alcohol on the breath
2. Alcohol withdrawal syndrome
   A. Mild to moderate dependency
      1) Signs and symptoms most likely to occur 8–24 hours after cessation of alcohol ingestion.

2) Early signs of withdrawal are:
   a. Psychomotor agitation
   b. Tremors
   c. Anxiety
   d. Weakness
   e. Nausea and vomiting
B. Moderate to severe dependency
   1) Onset of symptoms 12–24 hours after early signs appear
   2) Signs of withdrawal in this phase include:
      a. Severe tremors
      b. Fever and diaphoresis
      c. Muscle cramps
      d. Tachycardia
      e. High blood pressure
      f. Extreme agitation
      g. Shift from metabolic acidosis to respiratory alkalosis
C. Signs indicative of physical dependence
   1) Occur 2–4 days after cessation of drinking
   2) Symptoms include:
      a. Confusion and disorientation
      b. Delusions
      c. Paranoia
      d. Hallucinations
      e. Myoclonic jerks that can progress to seizures
      f. Insomnia, restlessness, agitation
      g. Cognitive impairment, disorientation
      h. Nausea and vomiting
      i. Myalgias
      j. Systolic hypertension (without prior history of hypertension)
      k. Hallucinations (may occur in the presence of an otherwise normal mental status exam)

PHYSICAL FINDINGS

1. Alcohol intoxication
   A. May be no specific findings or may be related to the conditions commonly associated with substance abuse:
      1) Upper respiratory tract infections
      2) Hepatitis, mononucleosis
      3) Malnutrition
      4) Pancreatitis
      5) Sexually transmitted diseases
   B. Pupil constriction
   C. Nystagmus
   D. Spider nevi
   E. Facial angiomas
   F. Altered mental status exam—disorientation, memory impairment, hallucination (predominantly visual), delusions
2. Alcohol withdrawal (Refer to "Signs and Symptoms"): The importance of recognizing alcohol withdrawal be overestimated. The withdrawal syndrome increases oxygen consumption and, if comorbity exists (i.e., cardiovascular conditions), the oxygen demand be met, resulting in death.

DIFFERENTIAL DIAGNOSIS

1. Alcohol intoxication
   A. Intoxication with other substances
   B. Severe hypoglycemia
2. Alcohol withdrawal: Any other potential cause of illness–induced delirium

DIAGNOSTIC TESTS/FINDINGS

1. Screen for alcoholism: The CAGE questionnaire

   C—Have you ever felt the need to *cut* down on your drinking?
   A—Have people *annoyed* you by criticizing your drinking?
   G—Have you ever felt bad or *guilty* about your drinking?
   E—Have you ever had a drink first thing in the morning to steady your
      nerves or get rid of a hangover? (*Eye-opener*)

2. Other useful questions:
   A. When was your last drink?
   B. Have you ever had withdrawal symptoms if you did not have anything
      to drink? For example, feelings of anxiety or shakiness, seeing things
      that were not there, etc.?
3. Laboratory tests
   A. Blood alcohol level (BAL)
      1) BAL >300 mg/dL at any time
      2) BAL >150 mg/dL if not obviously intoxicated
      3) BAL >100 mg/dL on a routine visit
   B. GGTP (gamma-glutamyl transpeptidase) screening for progressive liver
      disease. Mean corpuscular volume (increased in 40–60% of chronic alco-
      holics).
   C. Urine toxicology screen to rule out presence of other substance of abuse
   D. In alcohol withdrawal: Liver function tests, prothrombin time, partial
      thromboplastin time, electrolytes, Mg^+, Ca^+, CBC
4. Use of Severity Assessment Scale or Clinical Institute Withdrawal Assessment for Alcohol (CIWA-A) scale to quantify severity of withdrawal and
   guide treatment (Lohr, 1995; Watling et al., 1995)

MANAGEMENT/TREATMENT

1. Alcohol intoxication
   A. Unless there is a risk of alcohol withdrawal syndrome, does not usually
      require hospitalization.
   B. Observation for 4–6 hours is usually sufficient.
   C. Admission is usually reserved for those with apparent trauma, persis-
      tent CNS depression, abnormal vital signs, pulmonary aspiration, fulmi-
      nating hepatic failure, or sepsis.
   D. Communication techniques:
      1) Alert security before starting interview.
      2) Assume nonthreatening manner.
      3) Avoid direct eye contact for longer than 1–2 seconds (can be seen as
         threatening or challenging).

      4) Offer food/coffee.

      5) See management/treatment in section on "Aggression and Violence."

   E. Sedation with benzodiazepines:

      1) IM lorazepam is used to manage alcohol-induced agitation.

      2) Start with lower dose (i.e., 1–2 mg) to avoid negative drug interaction.

      3) Wait 30–60 minutes before giving a second dose.

2. Alcohol withdrawal

   A. Benzodiazepines are drug of choice, short acting best.

      1) Give based on scores from CIWA-A or Severity Assessment Scale.

      2) Titrate medications to effect, reassessing score every 15–30 minutes; repeat dose as necessary.

      3) IV or oral route preferred because of erratic IM absorption.

   B. Adjunctive treatment:

      1) Thiamine 100 mg IV push over 2 minutes, then 100 mg PO for 3 days

      2) Folate 1 mg PO for 3 days

      3) Multivitamins PO qd

3. Referral to long-term treatment program (outpatient or inpatient)

PATIENT EDUCATION

1. Discuss alcohol abuse/dependence in nonjudgmental manner.
2. A trial of controlled drinking with careful follow-up may be appropriate for alcohol *abuse*. Would require referral to therapist who would guide treatment and follow-up.
3. Abstinence is the only treatment for alcohol *dependence*.
4. Strongly recommend 12-step program such as Alcoholics Anonymous; provide with literature.
5. Family members should be referred to Alanon or Alateen.
6. Discuss mental health referral to rule out or treat underlying depression.

Review Questions

12.33 Mr. R is a 32-year-old man who is admitted for severe cellulitis of his right leg. During your history and physical exam, he tells you that he normally drinks 3–4 gin and tonics a night and he has done so for 3 years. You would anticipate signs of withdrawal to occur in:

   A. 8–24 hours

   B. 3–4 days

   C. 1–3 days

   D. 1 week

   E. None of the above

12.34 Out of the following questions, select those that are part of the CAGE assessment tool.

   1. Have you ever tried to *C*ut down your drinking?

   2. Have you ever been *A*rrested for driving under the influence?

   3. Have others been *A*nnoyed with you because of your drinking?

   4. Has your liver enzyme test (*G*GT) ever been elevated?

   5. Have you ever felt *G*uilty over your drinking?

   6. Do you ever have an *E*ye-opener drink as soon as you get up in the morning?

7. Have you *E*ntered an alcohol treatment program in the past and quit?
8. Have you ever lost *C*onsciousness because of your drinking?
   A. 1,2,4,6
   B. 8,3,4,7
   C. 1,3,5,6
   D. 1,2,5,6
   E. 8,3,5,6

12.35 Mrs. W is a 45-year-old woman admitted for aortic valve replacement. On taking her history, you learn that she normally drinks every day, at least 4–5 oz of hard liquor daily. You anticipate that she might be a candidate for alcohol withdrawal syndrome. The most effective treatment regimen would be to:
   A. Treat with fixed dosing schedules
   B. Give high doses of IM benzodiazepines to control DTs
   C. Begin with higher than usual doses of benzodiazepines to control concomitant anxiety
   D. Titrate benzodiazepines to severity of symptoms
   E. None of the above

12.36 A patient admitted as a result of a work accident, who has a normal mental status exam (MSE), had a routine BAL drawn that came back 155 mg/dL.
   A. This is confirmatory for a diagnosis of alcoholism
   B. This is an incidental finding and not indicative of alcoholism
   C. The patient's normal MSE rules out a diagnosis of alcoholism
   D. Although this finding is significant, further assessment, such as the CAGE, would have to be performed before a diagnosis of alcoholism could be made
   E. None of the above

12.37 Alcohol withdrawal should be a consideration in which of the following patients?
   A. An 80-year-old nursing home resident who develops delirium 2 days postoperatively
   B. A 25-year-old motorcycle rider admitted with a fractured femur who, after 1 day in the hospital, becomes belligerent
   C. A 45-year-old business executive who, after 2 days in the coronary care unit, begins to exhibit mild tremor of his hands
   D. A 17-year-old homeless teenager, admitted for pelvic inflammatory disease
   E. All of the above

Answers and Rationales

12.33 **A** Although some patients develop symptoms 1 week after the last drink, the more common time frame for early withdrawal is 8–24 hours.

12.34 **C** C = tried to cut down; A = annoyed by others regarding your drinking; G = guilt over drinking; E = eye-opener.

12.35 **D** Some patients with mild symptoms may not require any treatment, while those with high scores on assessment tools may require frequent dosing with high doses.

12.36 **A** A normal MSE in combination with a BAL >150 mg/dL is indicative of a high level of tolerance and is a criterion for alcoholism.

12.37 **E** Given the high prevalance of alcoholism in our society, and the high number of admissions to the general hospital that are alcohol related, the potential for alcohol withdrawal should be a consideration in any patient with mental status changes or associated risk factors.

References

Dougherty, J., & Heiselman, D. (1995). Substance abuse and overdose. In E. Sivak, T. Higgins, & A. Seiver (eds.). *The High Risk Patient: Management of the Critically Ill*. Baltimore: Williams & Wilkins, pp. 1424–1453.

Hackett, T.P. (1987). Alcoholism: Acute and chronic states. In T. Hackett & N. Cassem (eds.). *Massachusetts General Hospital Handbook of General Hospital Psychiatry*. Littleton, MA: PSG Publishing Co., pp. 14–28.

Lohr, R.H. (1995). Treatment of alcohol withdrawal in hospitalized patients. *Mayo Clin Proc 70*, 777–782.

Thompson, W.G. (1996). Alcoholism. In R. Rakel (ed.). *Saunders Manual of Medical Practice*. Philadelphia: W.B. Saunders Co., pp. 1131–1133.

Watling, S.M., Fleming, C., Casey, P., et al. (1995). Nursing based protocol for treatment of alcohol withdrawal in the intensive care unit. *Am J Crit Care 4*(1), 66–70.

Additional Recommended Reference

American Psychiatric Association. (1994). *Diagnostic and Statistical Manual of Mental Disorders* (4th ed.). Washington, DC: American Psychiatric Press.

Psychoactive Substance Abuse

DEFINITION

Psychoactive substance abuse involves the use of a substance to modify or control mood or state of mind in a manner that is illegal or harmful to oneself or others. In the acute care setting, the associated problems are:

1. *Intoxication:* A diminished state of physical and/or mental control
2. *Withdrawal syndromes:* A predictable syndrome following the abrupt withdrawal of a psychoactive substance on which an individual has become dependent. Withdrawal syndromes are often characterized by hyperactivity in physiologic functions that were suppressed by the drug or, conversely, depression of the activities that were stimulated by the drug.

ETIOLOGY/INCIDENCE

1. The etiology of substance abuse is multifactorial. Common theories include:
   A. Biologic predisposition

   B. Psychodynamic theories involving inadequate ego development or inef-
       fective coping skills
   C. System theories involving dysfunctional families or societal conflicts
2. In a 1992 survey, 11% of the population surveyed admitted to using illicit
   drugs in the past year.
3. Persons between the ages of 18 and 25 are the most likely to use illicit drugs.
4. Excluding alcohol, the most abused drugs fall into the categories of:
   A. Stimulants—cocaine, dextroamphetamines, caffeine, tobacco
   B. Depressants—heroin, opiates, benzodiazepines, antidepressants
   C. Hallucinogens—lysergic acid diethylamide (LSD), phencyclidine (PCP)
       cannabis

SIGNS AND SYMPTOMS

1. Problems common to drug abusers
   A. Infectious
       1) Septic arthritis
       2) Osteomyelitis
       3) Hepatitis B
       4) Endocarditis
       5) HIV
       6) Sexually transmitted diseases
       7) Tuberculosis
   B. Psychiatric
       1) Paranoia
       2) Psychosis
       3) Anxiety
       4) Depression
       5) Suicidal ideation
       6) Flashbacks
   C. Multisystem trauma
2. Signs and symptoms that may serve as clues
   A. Disheveled appearance
   B. Agitated or altered mental status
   C. Rapid mood shifts
   D. Manipulative behavior
   E. Evasive, inconsistent history
   F. Needle marks, nasal septal perforation
3. Signs and symptoms related to abuse of depressants
   A. Drowsiness, psychomotor retardation
   B. Mood swings
   C. Constricted pupils
   D. Lack of coordination
   E. Impaired mental status
   F. Hallucinations
   G. Signs and symptoms of narcotic withdrawal
       1) Occur 8–10 hours after last dose
       2) Include yawning, lacrimation, rhinorrhea, sweating
   H. Signs and symptoms of sedative-hypnotic withdrawal
       1) Appear 12–16 hours after last dose
       2) Include apprehension, weakness, tremors, insomnia, diaphoresis
       3) Severe withdrawal includes orthostatic hypotension, seizures

4. Signs and symptoms related to abuse of stimulants
   A. Agitation
   B. Headache
   C. Increased heart rate, blood pressure, temperature, respiratory rate
   D. Dysrhythmias
   E. Anxiety, sense of doom, paranoia, insomnia
   F. Diaphoresis
   G. Dilated pupils
5. Signs and symptoms related to use of hallucinogens
   A. Hallucinations, primarily visual
   B. Ego dissolution and detachment
   C. Diminished sense of reality
   D. Subjective slowing of time
   E. Increased sense of meaning of experience
   F. Vertical and horizontal nystagmus
   G. Marked anxiety, paranoia
   H. Flashbacks
   I. Insensitivity to pain

PHYSICAL FINDINGS

1. Pupillary changes, nystagmus
2. Accelerated or depressed vital signs
3. Needle marks, track marks: May be under tongue or in between toes
4. Bruises, burns, scars, ulcers, cellulitis
5. Tender abdomen with organomegaly
6. Dysrhythmias, cardiac ischemia
7. Altered mental status exam
8. Lack of coordination, decreased pain perception, ataxia

DIFFERENTIAL DIAGNOSIS

1. Any other condition that would mimic the signs and symptoms of specific drug abuse: Head injury, thyroid storm, hypoglycemia, CNS infection, coronary artery disease, acute psychotic reaction, panic attack, major depression, etc.
2. Always consider the possibility of polysubstance abuse.

DIAGNOSTIC TESTS/FINDINGS

1. Urine and drug screens to identify substance(s) used
2. CBC, electrolytes, random blood sugar, BUN, creatinine, liver enzymes to rule out associated diseases or differential diagnoses
3. ECG

MANAGEMENT/TREATMENT

1. Criteria for admission to acute care facility include:
   A. Chest pain not explained by musculoskeletal source (cocaine abuse)
   B. Cardiac dysrhythmia
   C. Persistently abnormal vital signs after 4–6 hours of observation
   D. Suspected CNS, cardiovascular, or neuropsychiatric complication

2. Specific drug overdoses or withdrawal syndromes are primarily treated in emergency room settings and are beyond the scope of this section. The reader is referred to material in the References for complete discussion.
3. Withdrawal syndromes may appear as a surprise syndrome in any patient who has not been forthright in his/her history of substance abuse.
    A. Specific treatment of withdrawal states includes replacing the substance with a short- or long-acting barbiturate and then tapering the dose.
    B. Narcotic withdrawal is treated symptomatically and is seldom life threatening: Phenothiazines for nausea and vomiting; nonnarcotic pain medication, nonnarcotic antidiarrheal agents, and clonidine.
4. Narcotic overdose with obtundation can be treated with naloxone 2 mg IV, IM, sublingually, or via endotracheal tube. May repeat once.
5. Hallucinogens: Adverse reactions range from psychotic reactions and panic attacks to milder anxiety reactions.
    A. Patients using PCP may exhibit inordinate amounts of physical strength because of sympathomimetic activity. Protection of the patient and others is a priority.
    B. Treatment of anxiety symptoms ranges from reassurance to benzodiazepines.
    C. If psychotic reactions are the predominant symptom, haloperidol is the drug of choice.
    D. Phenothiazine neuroleptics should be avoided because they can enhance the anticholinergic effects of PCP.

PATIENT EDUCATION

1. Short- and long-term effects of substance abuse can be discussed in a nonjudgmental atmosphere.
2. Referral to appropriate mental health or substance abuse resources should be made.

***

Review Questions

12.38 As you examine a patient who is exhibiting signs and symptoms of anxiety and paranoid delusions, you note nystagmus. A probable diagnosis is:
    A. Panic attack
    B. Schizophrenia
    C. Acute psychotic reaction
    D. Withdrawal from opiates
    E. PCP abuse

12.39 Naloxene can be used as a diagnostic tool as well as treatment for:
    A. PCP overdose
    B. Marijuana overdose
    C. Amphetamine withdrawal
    D. Morphine overdose
    E. Alcohol intoxication

12.40 Which pharmacologic agent is contraindicated in treating patients who have ingested PCP?
A. Lorazepam (Ativan)
B. Chlorpromazine (Thorazine)
C. Diazepam (Valium)
D. Morphine
E. None of the above

12.41 A patient who was experiencing withdrawal from diazepam dependence would be:
A. Hallucinating
B. Tearing, perspiring, and blowing his/her nose frequently
C. Anxious, tremulous, and having trouble sleeping
D. Complaining of flashback experiences
E. All of the above

12.42 In all patients experiencing effects of substance abuse, it is important to look for:
A. Multiple substances that could be involved
B. Suicidal ideation
C. Underlying depression
D. Sexually transmitted diseases
E. All of the above

Answers and Rationales

12.38 **E** A distinguishing characteristic of PCP use is nystagmus, which is not seen in mental health problems or opiate withdrawal.

12.39 **D** Naloxene is an agonist that can reverse 10–100 times the amount of opioids.

12.40 **B** Phenothiazines may exacerbate the anticholinergic effects of PCP.

12.41 **C** Symptoms of withdrawal are often a mirror of the effects of the substance. Diazepam is a depressant; consequently withdrawal consists of rebound symptoms of anxiety.

12.42 **A** Many people abuse several drugs or the drug they use may have been cut with other substances. Many people self-medicate depression with drugs, or the side effect of the drug or drug withdrawal is depression. Suicidal ideation is common in substance abusers, either as part of the depressive syndrome resulting from the drug or as a pre-existing condition. Because inhibitions may be loosened with drug use, people may act on sexual impulses that are usually contained. In some populations sexual activity is a method of payment for substance abuse.

References

Bevans, D. (1996). Chemical and drug overdose. In J. Clochesy, C. Bren, S. Cardin, A. Whittaker & E. Rudy (eds.). *Critical Care Nursing* (2nd ed.). Philadelphia: W.B. Saunders Co., pp. 1413–1428.

D'Lugoff, B., & Hawthorne, J. (1991). Use and abuse of illicit drugs and substances. In L.R. Barker, J.R. Burton, & P.D. Zieve (eds.). *Principles of Ambulatory Medicine*. Baltimore: Williams & Wilkins, pp. 232–250.

Tractenberg, A.I. & Fleming, M.F. (1994). Diagnosis and treatment of drug abuse in family practice. *Am Family Physician (Summer):* 1–24.

Additional Recommended References

Dougherty, J., & Heiselman, D. (1995). Substance abuse and overdose. In E. Sivak, T. Higgins, & A. Seiver. (eds.). *The High Risk Patient: Management of the Critically Ill*. Baltimore: Williams & Wilkins, pp. 1424–1453.

Harrington, A.M., & Clifton, D. (1995). Toxicology and management of acute drug ingestions in adults. *Pharmacotherapy 15*, 183–200.

CHAPTER 13

Health Promotion and Health Protection

Nancy M. Oldham, RN, MN, FNP

This chapter provides guidelines for preventive health services within the activities of health promotion and health protection to be used by the acute care nurse practitioner (ACNP). Services for health promotion and health protection include periodic history and physical examination, routine screening tests, immunizations, and health counseling. More specifically, health promotion refers to interventions that increase well-being, human health, and quality of life. Health protection is a general term within the classically known concepts of primary and secondary preventive services, and is defined as interventions that either prevent illness, provide early detection of illness, or maintain function within the constraints of illness.

Even though the ACNP is generally involved in the care of acutely and critically ill patients, the role of health promotion and health protection cannot be understated. Each patient encounter should be considered as an opportunity to deliver preventive health care and health promotion. An understanding of the basic tenets of health promotion and protection will lay the groundwork for invoking these concepts when the opportunity arises.

This area of medicine is filled with controversy and is constantly evolving. Each professional medical organization has its own set of recommendations and guidelines, and there are often no universally accepted recommendations. The organizations pooled for general recommendations include the U.S. Preventive Services Task Force (USPSTF), the American Cancer Society (ACS), the American Heart Association (AHA), American College of Physicians (ACP), and the American Diabetes Association (ADA). In this chapter, an attempt is made to present a well-rounded set of guidelines that does not contradict the various recommendations made by these expert panels and that complies with common practice standards. It is important to understand that, when accepted recommendations are not specific or do not apply to a particular patient group, the clinician must utilize judgment to make specific recommendations.

Periodic Health Evaluation: General Adult Population

HEALTH HISTORY

1. Past medical history
   A. Previous significant illnesses and surgeries
   B. Hospitalizations
   C. Immunizations
2. Family history: List of diseases/illnesses in family members. Especially important are familial and genetic disorders such as coronary artery disease, diabetes mellitus, cancer, hypertension, alcoholism, and mental illness.
3. Drug allergies: List the drug and the reaction
4. Medications: List all prescription and over-the-counter drugs.
5. Review of systems: Focused inventory of major organ systems
6. Social history
   A. Identify social network/support—family, friends, co-workers
   B. Identify resources—financial, spiritual, emotional
   C. Living situation
   D. Occupation
7. Occupational/environmental history
   A. Exposure to toxic substances (e.g., asbestos)
   B. Possible occupational cause of illness/injury
   C. Occupational Safety and Health Administration (OSHA): 1-800-321-OSHA
   D. National Institute of Occupational Safety and Health (NIOSH): 1-800-356-4674
8. Nutritional assessment
   A. Assess for well-balanced intake: 24-hour dietary recall may be useful.
   B. Identify undernutrition (malnutrition) or overnutrition (obesity).
   C. Inquire about anorexia or weight loss.
9. Physical activity assessment
   A. Regular physical activity
   B. Sedentary lifestyle
10. Substance use inventory and pattern of use
    A. Alcohol: CAGE instrument or Michigan Alcoholism Screening Test
    B. Tobacco: Inhaled, chewed
    C. Drugs: Illicit and prescription (sedatives/pain medications)
11. Sexual practices

PERIODIC PHYSICAL EXAMINATION

The annual comprehensive physical examination has been replaced by the periodic physical exam. The word "periodic" is meant to imply that this type of exam may be done *as necessary* or at the discretion of the health care provider. The frequency may be individualized according to the individual's health history, risk factors, and clinical suspicion. The entire exam may be completed over a number of visits or during one extended visit.

1. Height and weight
2. Blood pressure for hypertension screening

3. Carotid artery auscultation for peripheral vascular disease
4. Clinical breast examination for breast cancer—ACS: Every 3 years for women ages 20–40; annually thereafter
5. Clinical skin examination for skin cancer—ACS: Annual screening all adults
6. Clinical testicular examination for testis cancer—ACS: Every 1–3 years for men ages 20–40, annually thereafter
7. Digital rectal examination for prostate cancer—ACS: Age ≥40, annually
8. Oral cavity examination for oral cancer—ACS: Every 3 years for men and women ages 20–40, annually thereafter
9. Pelvic examination for gynecologic cancer—ACS: Every 1–3 years for women ages 18–40, annually thereafter
10. Thyroid examination for thyroid cancer—ACS: Every 3 years for men and women ages 20–40, annually thereafter

PERIODIC SCREENING TESTS

1. Bone mineral analysis for osteoporosis
   A. USPSTF: No recommendations for routine screening; however, selective screening may be appropriate for high-risk women who would consider hormone replacement therapy if their risk for osteoporosis or fracture were known.
   B. ACP: Selective postmenopausal women considering hormone replacement therapy.
2. Cervical cytologic screening: Papaniculoaou test
   A. USPSTF: Age ≥20, every 1–3 years or annually if high risk
   B. ACS: Age ≥18 or first intercourse; repeat annually until three consecutive normal exams, then every 1–3 years at discretion of health care provider
3. Chest radiography for lung cancer
   A. USPSTF: No recommendation
   B. ACS: No recommendation
4. Colonoscopy for colon cancer
   A. USPSTF: No recommendation for routine screening
   B. ACS: No recommendation for routine screening
5. Exercise stress test for coronary artery disease—USPSTF: Age ≥40, if high risk or beginning an exercise program
6. Fasting plasma glucose for diabetes mellitus type 2
   A. USPSTF: No recommendations for or against routine screening; however, selective screening may be appropriate for high risk individuals.
   B. ADA: Consider screening asymptomatic undiagnosed individuals at age 45 years. If normal, repeat every 3 years.
7. Hematocrit for iron-deficiency anemia
8. Human immunodeficiency virus (HIV) serologic screening
9. Intraocular pressure for glaucoma
10. Mammography for breast cancer
    A. USPSTF: Age ≥50, annually; age ≥35 if breast cancer in premenopausal first-degree relative
    B. ACS: Annual screening for all women age 40 and older
11. Prostate-specific antigen (PSA) for prostate cancer
    A. USPSTF: No recommendation
    B. ACS: Age ≥50, annually

12. Resting electrocardiography (ECG) for coronary artery disease
    A. USPSTF: No recommendation for routine screening
    B. AHA: Baseline testing for men and women over 40 years of age
13. Serum cholesterol for coronary artery disease—USPSTF: Periodic screening for all men ages 35–65 and all women ages 45–65
14. Sigmoidoscopy for colon cancer
    A. USPSTF: Age ≥40, if high risk (refer to section) on "Special Circumstances"
    B. ACS: Age ≥50, then every 3–5 years thereafter
15. Stool for occult blood for colon cancer
    A. USPSTF: Age ≥40, if high risk
    B. ACS: Annual screening for all men and women over age 50
16. Thyroid testing for thyroid disease

Health Promotion via Patient Education and Counseling: Primary Prevention

Primary prevention refers to the prevention of disease or injury *prior to* its development. Successful intervention is incumbent on appropriately timed preventive health education and requires patient behavioral changes.

IMMUNIZATIONS: CENTERS FOR DISEASE CONTROL AND PREVENTION ADULT IMMUNIZATION SCHEDULE

1. Tetanus and diphtheria toxoids combined (Td)
    A. Primary series if no previous history of vaccination.
    B. Primary series schedule: Two doses 4–6 weeks apart and a third dose 6–12 months after the second dose.
    C. Td booster: One dose every 10 years.
    D. Td for wound management: One dose of Td for clean, minor wounds only if more than 10 years since last dose; for other wounds give Td if over 5 years since the last dose.
    E. Dose: 0.5 mL IM
    F. Major contraindications: Neurologic or severe hypersensitivity reaction to any prior dose.
2. Measles and mumps vaccine
    A. Indicated for all adults born after 1956 without written documentation of immunization on or after the first birthday, health care personnel born after 1956 who are at risk of exposure to patients with measles or mumps without written documentation of two doses of vaccine on or after the first birthday or of measles seropositivity, HIV-infected persons, travelers to foreign countries, and persons entering college
    B. Dose: 0.5 mL SC
    C. Major contraindications: Immunosuppressive therapy or immunodeficiency (except HIV infection), anaphylactic allergy to eggs or neomycin, pregnancy, immune globulin preparation or blood/blood product received during the previous 3–11 months
3. Rubella vaccine
    A. Indicated for all adults born after 1956 without written documentation of immunization on or after the first birthday or of seropositivity. Health care personnel who are at risk of exposure to patients with rubella and

who may have contact with pregnant patients should have at least one dose on or after the first birthday.

B. Dose: 0.5 mL SC

C. Major contraindications: Pregnancy; immunosuppressive therapy or immunodeficiency (except HIV infection), immune globulin preparation or blood/blood products received during the previous 3–11 months.

D. Special consideration: Women should avoid pregnancy for 3 months after immunization.

4. Poliovirus vaccine: IPV (inactivated virus); OPV (oral live vaccine)

A. Indicated for health care/laboratory personnel who are at risk of exposure to patients who are excreting live poliovirus or who handle specimens from such patients, members of communities with current disease caused by wild poliovirus, and travelers to developing countries.

B. Primary schedule for unimmunized adults: IPV (dose: 0.5 mL SC), two doses at 4- to 8-week intervals with a third dose given 6–12 months after the second dose

C. Schedule for partially immunized adults: Complete primary series with IPV as above or with OPV scheduled as two doses 6–8 weeks apart and a third dose at 6–12 months after the second dose, with no need to repeat doses if schedule is interrupted

D. Booster
   1) OPV: None needed
   2) IPV: Possibly one dose every 5 years; however, the need is unclear

E. Major contraindications
   1) IPV: Pregnancy, anaphylactic allergy to neomycin or streptomycin
   2) OPV: Pregnancy is relative contraindication (OPV may be used if immediate protection is needed); anaphylactic allergy to neomycin or streptomycin; or vaccine recipient or household contact is immunodeficient or immunosuppressed (including HIV infection)

5. Varicella vaccine

A. Indicated for adults of any age without a reliable history of varicella disease or seronegative for varicella, all susceptible health care personnel, all susceptible family contacts for immunocompromised persons, all susceptible persons who belong in the following groups and are at high risk of exposure (where transmission is likely or can occur): teachers of young children, day care employees, college students, military personnel, international travelers, and nonpregnant women of childbearing age

B. Schedule: Two doses 4–8 weeks apart with no need to repeat the first dose if the second dose is administered >8 weeks from the first dose

C. Dose: 0.5 mL SC

D. Major contraindications: Pregnancy, anaphylactic allergy to gelatin or neomycin, immunosuppressive therapy or immunodeficiency (including HIV infection), immune globulin preparation or blood/blood product received during the previous 5 months, or family history of congenital or hereditary immunodeficiency in first-degree relative (unless the immune competence of the potential vaccine recipient has been clinically substantiated or verified by a laboratory)

E. Special consideration: Women are to avoid pregnancy for 1 month following each dose of the vaccine

6. Influenza vaccine

A. Indicated for all adults 65 years of age and older; adults of any age with chronic diseases or disorders: cardiovascular or pulmonary disorders (including asthma), metabolic diseases (e.g., diabetes mellitus), renal dysfunction, hemoglobinopathies, immunosuppressive/immunodeficiency disorders; residents of chronic care facilities or nursing homes; health care/laboratory personnel and family/close contact persons caring for high-risk individuals

  B. Schedule is one dose to be given annually each fall prior to the influenza season

  C. Dose: 0.5 mL IM

  D. Major contraindications: Anaphylactic allergy to eggs

7. Pneumoccocal vaccine

  A. Indicated for all adults 65 years of age and older; adults of any age with chronic diseases/disorders (same as for influenza vaccine as above); adults of any age with splenic dysfunction, asplenia, Hodgkin's disease, multiple myeloma, cirrhosis, alcoholism, renal failure, and cerebrovascular fluid leaks.

  B. Revaccination 6 years after initial dose is indicated for those persons with functional or anatomic asplenia, transplant patients, patients with chronic kidney disease, immunodepressed or immunodeficient persons and any adult at highest risk of fatal pneumococcal infection.

  C. Dose: One dose only of 0.5 mL IM or SC polyvalent pneumococcal vaccine.

  D. Major contraindications: None listed.

  E. Special consideration: If elective splenectomy or immunosuppressive therapy is planned, give vaccine 2 weeks ahead if possible.

8. Hepatitis B vaccine (HBV)

  A. Indicated for persons with occupational risk of exposure to blood or blood-contaminated body fluids, clients and staff of institutions for the developmentally disabled, hemodialysis patients, recipients of clotting factor concentrates, household contacts and sex partners of HBV carriers, adoptees from countries where HBV infection is endemic, injection drug users, sexually active homosexual and bisexual men, sexually active heterosexual men and women with multiple sex partners or recent episodes of a sexually transmitted disease, inmates of long-term correctional facilities.

  B. Scheduled series of three doses: First and second doses 1 month apart with the third dose given 6 months after the first dose (no need to start series over if schedule is interrupted or if different manufacturer's vaccine is used).

  C. Dose: 1.0 mL IM.

  D. Booster: Need is unclear, not presently recommended.

  E. Major contraindications: Anaphylactic allergy to yeast.

  F. Special considerations: Persons with serologic markers of prior or continuing HBV infection (carrier state) do not need immunization; vaccine is doubled (or special preparation is used) for hemodialysis patients and other immunosuppressed or immunodeficient patients; pregnant patients should be screened for HbsAg and, if positive, their infants should be given postexposure prophylaxis.

  G. Postexposure phrophylaxis: Consult the Advisory Committee on Immunization Practices or local health department.

9. Report adverse events following vaccinations: Department of Health and Human Services, P.O. Box 1100, Rockville, MD 20849 (1-800-822-7967).

PREVENTIVE DRUG THERAPIES/CHEMOPROPHYLAXIS

1. Vitamin and mineral supplements: Not routinely recommended if the patient maintains adequate nutritional intake.
2. Estrogen replacement for postmenopausal women.
3. Calcium supplementation for women with inadequate dietary intake: Adolescents and young adults, 1200–1500 mg/day; adult women, 1000 mg/day; postmenopausal women, 1000–1500 mg/day; pregnant or nursing women, 1200–1500 mg/day.
4. Pregnancy: Daily multivitamin containing folic acid at a dose of 0.4–0.8 mg beginning at least 1 month prior to conception and continuing through at least the first trimester.
5. Consider iron supplementation for menstruating women.
6. Consider supplementation of vitamin D and zinc for homebound/institutionalized elderly.

NUTRITION: MAJOR DIETARY GUIDELINES

1. Maintain proper nutrition by eating a variety of foods from each of the five food groups. The U.S. Department of Health and Human Services and the U.S. Department of Agriculture have published nutrition guidelines for the five groups of the "Food Guide Pyramid."
   A. Milk group: 2–3 servings/day
   B. Meat group: 2–3 servings/day
   C. Vegetable group: 3–5 servings/day
   D. Fruit group: 2–4 servings/day
   E. Breads/cereals group: 6–11 servings/day
2. Achieve caloric balance to maintain ideal body weight.
   A. Established standards for weight according to height and gender based on the 1959 Metropolitan Life Insurance Tables
   B. Body Mass Index (BMI): Body weight in kilograms divided by the square of height in meters
      1) BMI of 18–25 defines normal nutrition.
      2) BMI of 28 or more defines significant obesity.
3. Reduce overall consumption of fat.
   A. Total fat: <30% of total caloric intake
   B. Saturated fat: <10% of total caloric intake
   C. Cholesterol: <300 mg/day
4. Increase consumption of complex carbohydrates to 50–55% of total caloric intake.
5. Increase consumption of fiber to 25–35 gm/day.
6. Reduce salt intake to <6 gm/day.

EXERCISE

Regular physical activity is a significant component of a healthy lifestyle.
1. Emphasize the role of exercise in the prevention of disease.
   A. Heart disease: Reduces elevated systolic and diastolic blood pressure, raises high-density lipoprotein, cholesterol and reduces triglycerides.
   B. Diabetes: Increases muscle glucose uptake and insulin sensitivity.
   C. Cancer: May provide health protection against breast and colon cancer.

D. Osteoporosis: Weight-bearing exercise will maintain bone mineral density and reduce the decline in bone mass in postmenopausal women.

E. Weight control: Increases caloric expenditure and increases metabolic rate.

F. Mental health: May reduce anxiety and depression.

2. Promote an active lifestyle: Incorporate intermittent, moderate-intensity activities in daily life

3. Provide an exercise prescription.

A. Traditional medical advice: 20 minutes or more of continuous aerobic exercise at a frequency of at minimum three times per week.

B. Stretching exercises improve joint flexibility.

C. Resistance exercises develop and maintain muscle strength.

D. Aerobic exercise facilitates cardiovascular fitness.

SMOKING CESSATION

1. Define the dangers of tobacco use and tobacco-related illness.
   A. Cardiovascular disease
   B. Pulmonary disease
   C. Cancer risk
   D. Environmental hazards of second-hand smoke
   E. Ulcer disease
   F. Osteoporosis
   G. Fetal growth retardation
   H. Psychoactive substance addiction

2. Clearly and directly advise all smokers or smokeless tobacco user to quit.
   A. Education and counseling.
   B. Self-help materials.
   C. Nicotine replacement medications.
   D. Arrange regular follow-up to encourage maintenance of nonsmoking status.

3. Referral to community resources:
   A. American Cancer Society: 1-800-ACS-2345
   B. American Lung Association: 1-800-LUNG USA
   C. SmokeEnders: 1-800-828-4357

ALCOHOL

1. Educate regarding the hazardous effects of regular and excessive use of alcohol.
   A. Addiction/dependence
   B. Liver disease
   C. Cerebral atrophy
   D. Cardiovascular disease
   E. Nutritional deficiencies
   F. Intentional/unintentional injury

2. Recommend abstinence from alcohol.
   A. Until patient reaches legal drinking age
   B. During pregnancy
   C. While operating any motor vehicle or equipment
   D. If history of substance abuse

3. Advise use of alcohol in moderation.

A. Moderate use for men: 2 drinks or less/day.

B. Moderate use for women: 1 drink or less/day.

C. A standard drink is defined as 0.5 oz of alcohol.

D. Approximate standard drink equivalencies: 12 oz beer, 4 oz wine, 1.5 oz liquor.

ILLICIT DRUG USE

1. Advise abstinence.
2. Dangers of use while driving, swimming, or operating equipment.

SEXUAL BEHAVIOR

1. Sexually transmitted disease (STD) and HIV prevention
   A. Abstinence
   B. Male condoms
   C. Female barrier contraceptives
2. Unintended pregnancy prevention
   A. Abstinence
   B. Effective contraceptive techniques and clear directions regarding their proper use

SAFETY PROMOTION AND INJURY PREVENTION

1. Auto safety
   A. Lap/shoulder safety belts: Driver and all passengers
   B. Airbags
2. Safety helmets: Bicycle, motorcycle, all-terrain vehicle (ATV), roller/inline skates
3. Fire safety
   A. Smoke detectors: Proper operation, correct installation, and periodic testing
   B. Hazards of smoking in bed or near upholstery
4. Firearm safety: Proper storage and use
5. Hot water heater: Reduce temperature to 125°F

PERSONAL VIOLENCE AND INJURY

1. Raise the issues of family violence as an epidemic in our country and a public health issue.
   A. Child abuse
   B. Spousal abuse
   C. Elder abuse
2. Identify resources in the community and make available this information.
   A. Community shelters
   B. Telephone "hotlines": Local advocacy or "batterers" groups
   C. Law enforcement

STRESS REDUCTION AND MANAGEMENT

1. Relationship between stress and disease
2. Relaxation techniques

    A. Meditation
    B. Yoga
    C. Music therapy
3. Alternative therapies
    A. Acupuncture
    B. Massage
4. Exercise

DENTAL/ORAL HEALTH

1. Recommend regular visits to dental health care providers: Annual evaluation is minimum.
2. Brush teeth at least twice daily with fluoride toothpaste.
3. Floss teeth daily.
4. Dietary recommendations:
    A. Avoid cariogenic foods.
    B. Abstain from regular alcohol use.
5. Abstain from tobacco product use.

Special Circumstances: Patients with Special Needs and/or Identified Risk Factors—Secondary Prevention

Secondary prevention refers to the early detection and treatment of subclinical disease in asymptomatic patients. Additional laboratory and/or diagnostic screening tests may be utilized in selected patients for whom there is a special concern. The concern has been identified in the periodic health examination and as such labels the patient as a high-risk individual.

SEXUAL BEHAVIOR—HIGH RISK

1. Early age at first intercourse (age 20 or earlier).
2. Multiple sexual partners.
3. Anal intercourse.
4. Sex for money or drugs.
5. Inconsistent use of or failure to use barrier protection.
6. Provide appropriate patient education focused on reducing high-risk sexual practices.
7. Screen for diseases:
    A. Chlamydia
    B. Gonorrhea culture
    C. Rapid plasma reagin, Venereal Disease Research Laboratory tests
    D. HIV

ALCOHOL

1. High-risk alcohol use.
    A. Problem drinking: Has been defined as five drinks/day for men and three drinks/day for women and/or if there are any social, legal, or health consequences associated with drinking.
    B. Frequent intoxication.

    C. Any history of blackout related to alcohol consumption.

    D. Family history of alcoholism.

2. Direct advice to limit or cease drinking.

    A. Medically supervised detoxification.

    B. Referral to rehabilitation program: Alcoholics Anonymous.

    C. Encourage active participation of family, friends.

DRUG USE

1. High-risk drug use.

    A. Any illicit drug use

    B. Improper use of prescription sedatives/narcotics

    C. Denial or minimization of use

2. Patterns of abuse and appropriate treatment for each type of drug used: Sedatives, stimulants, opioids, cannabis (marijuana), hallucinogens, and inhalants.

3. Direct advice to cease using drug and treat drug dependency.

    A. Acknowledge the problem.

    B. Medically supervised detoxification to limit adverse effects.

    C. Provide appropriate treatment and pharmacotherapy to minimize withdrawal syndrome.

    D. Referral to rehabilitation services that specialize in the treatment of drug abuse: Narcotics Anonymous.

    E. Mental/behavioral services: Individual, group, or family counseling.

4. Information to reduce abuse-related risk of infection.

    A. Use new and sterile syringes.

    B. Risks of sharing injection equipment/drug paraphernalia.

    C. Cleaning/sterilization of injection equipment.

    D. Safe disposal of needles, syringes, and other drug paraphernalia.

    E. Indiscriminate sexual practices or sex with past or present IV drug users.

5. Educate regarding the harmful effects of drug abuse.

    A. Physical illness

    B. Behavioral/mood problems

    C. Social problems: Work, home, legal

6. Screen for diseases.

    A. HIV

    B. STD

    C. Hepatitis B

DEPRESSION

1. High risk

    A. Recent divorce or separation

    B. Unemployment

    C. Alcohol/drug abuse

    D. Serious medical illness

    E. Recent bereavement

    F. Social isolation: Living alone, inadequate social support

2. Identification of depression

    A. Zung self-rating depression scale (Zung, 1965)

    B. Geriatric Depression Scale (Yesavage, 1992)

    C. Clinical evaluation

3. Treatment
   A. Encourage healthy lifestyle: Appropriate diet, rest, and exercise prescription.
   B. Discontinue any alcohol or drug use.
   C. Counseling.
   D. Pharmacotherapy to reduce symptoms.
4. Suicide potential/risk
   A. Depressive illness
   B. Previous suicide attempt
   C. Substance abuse
   D. Adolescents: Family turmoil, doing poorly in school
   E. Elderly: Vision loss, hearing loss

CARDIOVASCULAR DISEASE

1. High risk
   A. Family history
   B. Tobacco use
   C. Hypertension (HTN)
   D. Diabetes mellitus (DM)
   E. Hypercholesterolemia
   F. Obesity
   G. Physical inactivity
2. Screening: Based on patient history and physical examination
   A. Baseline ECG
   B. Treadmill stress test
3. Risk factor modification
   A. Smoking cessation
   B. Treatment of HTN
   C. Treatment of DM
   D. Treatment of hypercholesterolemia
   E. Weight loss and/or maintenance of ideal body weight
   F. Regular physical activity or exercise regimen
4. Prevention—Aspirin therapy to reduce myocardial infarction in asymptomatic people with risk factors for coronary artery disease: No consensus recommendation

DIABETES MELLITUS

1. High risk
   A. Positive family history
   B. Women with a history of gestational DM or large-for-gestational-age babies
   C. Obesity
   D. Impaired glucose tolerance
   E. Elderly
   F. Higher risk populations: African American, Latinos, Native Americans
2. Screening
   A. Fasting serum glucose
   B. Oral glucose tolerance test
3. Risk factor modification
   A. Weight loss and/or maintenance of ideal body weight

   B. Well-balanced nutrition program
   C. Adoption of a healthy lifestyle that is physically active and regular exercise program

CEREBROVASCULAR DISEASE

1. High risk
   A. Hypertension
   B. Smoking
   C. Heavy alcohol consumption and binge drinking
   D. Cardiovascular disease
   E. Diabetes mellitus
   F. Obesity
2. Screening
   A. Neurologic exam
   B. Auscultation for carotid bruit
3. Risk factor modification
   A. Treatment of HTN
   B. Treatment of DM
   C. Treatment of cardiovascular disease
   D. Weight loss and maintenance of ideal body weight
   E. Abstinence or reduction of alcohol consumption
   F. Lower cholesterol

OSTEOPOROSIS

1. High risk
   A. Estrogen deficiency: Postmenopausal, bilateral oophrectomy, or early menopause not on estrogen therapy
   B. Genetic factors: Female gender and white race
   C. Environmental factors: Slender build and fair skinned
2. Screening: Bone mineral analysis
3. Risk factor modification
   A. Estrogen replacement
   B. Maintenance of adequate calcium intake: 1000 mg/day on estrogen replacement; 1500 mg/day not on estrogen
   C. Weight-bearing exercise
   D. Smoking cessation.
4. Resources: National Osteoporosis Foundation, 1150 17th Street N.W., Washington, DC 20036

TUBERCULOSIS

1. High risk
   A. Health care/laboratory personnel
   B. Close contacts of persons with known or suspected tuberculosis
   C. Recent immigrants from countries with high prevalence of tuberculosis: Asia, Africa, South America, Pacific Islands
   D. Medically underserved or poverty-stricken individuals
   E. Immunocompromised individuals
   F. Residents of chronic care facilities or nursing homes

2. Screening
   A. Purified protein derivative (PPD).
   B. Mantoux test is the preferred method: 0.1 mL PPD intradermally on forearm; read for induration 48 hours later.
   C. Chest radiograph: Persons with history of positive skin test or vaccination.

HUMAN IMMUNODEFICIENCY VIRUS

1. High risk
   A. Anal intercourse and/or orogenital contact
   B. Multiple sexual partners
   C. Sexual contact with parenteral drug users
   D. Prostitution
   E. Sexual activity associated with vaginal or rectal mucosal injury and trauma
   F. Previous history of other STDs
   G. Recipients of blood products between 1975 and 1985
2. Prevention
   A. Abstinence from high-risk sexual practice and parenteral drug use
   B. Condom use with anal/vaginal intercourse
   C. Nonoxynol-9 spermicide combined with condom use
   D. Avoidance of shared needles/drug paraphernalia
   E. Universal precaution guidelines published by the Centers for Disease Control and Prevention (CDC)
3. Education
   A. Latex condoms are preferred to natural skin condoms because of increased durability and decreased permeability to infectious agents.
   B. Avoidance of petroleum-based lubricants, which may interfere with the condom integrity.
   C. Water-based lubricants are acceptable.
   D. Proper placement and removal of condom.
   E. Condoms should be used only once for each act of intercourse.
   F. Disinfecting of drug paraphernalia with 1:100 diluted chlorine bleach solution if new/sterile equipment not available.

RISK OF TRAVEL-RELATED ILLNESSES

1. High risk
   A. Developing countries
   B. South America
   C. Africa
   D. Asia
   E. India
2. CDC resources
   A. International travelers hotline: 1-404-332-4559
   B. *Health Information for International Travel* (Available from U.S. Government Printing Office; revised annually)
3. Prevention with vaccines indicated for the immunization of international travelers: The choice of vaccine is dependent on travel destination, current recommendations, and risk/benefit evaluation.

    A. Hepatitis A/B

    B. Typhoid

    C. Yellow fever

    D. Meningococcus

    E. Rabies

    F. Japanese encephalitis

    G. Cholera

    H. Tetanus and diphtheria

    I. Malaria

    J. Traveler's diarrhea

    K. Poliomyelitis

4. Other preventive measures

    A. All adult immunizations should be up to date.

    B. Follow food and water precautions.

    C. Only eat foods served piping-hot if sanitation and hygiene practices of food handlers are in question.

BREAST CANCER

1. High risk

    A. Family history of breast cancer in a primary relative

    B. Bilateral disease or diagnosed prior to menopause

    C. Early menarche and late menopause

    D. Nulliparity

    E. First pregnancy after age 30

    F. Excessive alcohol consumption

2. Screening

    A. Monthly breast self-examination

    B. Annual clinical breast examination by a health care provider

    C. Annual mammography to commence at age 40 or 10 years prior to the age when the diagnosis was made in primary relative

COLORECTAL CANCER

1. High risk

    A. Family history

    B. Personal history of familial polyposis

    C. Chronic ulcerative colitis

    D. Family cancer syndrome

2. Screening

    A. Digital rectal exam

    B. Fecal occult blood test

    C. Flexible sigmoidoscopy

    D. Colonoscopy

LUNG CANCER

1. High risk

    A. Tobacco smoker

    B. Asbestos exposure

2. Screening: Chest x-ray is controversial and generally not recommended.

SKIN CANCER

1. High risk
    A. Familial history of melanoma
    B. Increased exposure to sun: Occupational or recreational
    C. Personal history of precancerous skin lesions
2. Prevention
    A. Avoid excessive or midday sun exposure: Between the hours of 11 A.M. and 3 P.M.
    B. Use of sunscreen: Sun protection factor (SPF) 15
    C. Protective clothing—hats, long sleeves, sunglasses
3. Screening
    A. Annual clinical integument examination.
    B. Skin self-inspection: Teach ABCD's (*a*symmetry, *b*order irregularity, *c*olor variety, *d*iameter)

ORAL CANCER

1. High risk
    A. Tobacco use: Inhaled or chewed
    B. Regular alcohol use
2. Screening—Clinical exam: Inspection and palpation of oral cavity.
3. Prevention: Discontinue tobacco product and regular alcohol use.

TESTIS CANCER

1. High risk
    A. Young adult (average patient age 32)
    B. Cryptorchism
    C. Testicular atrophy
    D. Orchiopexy
2. Screening
    A. Physical exam
    B. Self-palpation: testis self-exam

PROSTATE CANCER

1. High risk: Age 50
2. Screening
    A. Digital rectal examination: Commence at age 50, then annually
    B. PSA: Controversial; however, ACS recommends annual screening commencing at age 50

CERVICAL CANCER

1. High risk
    A. Onset of sexual activity before age 20
    B. Multiple sexual partners
    C. Personal history of infection of human papillomavirus and herpes simplex virus type 2
2. Screening
    A. Commence screening at age 18 or onset of sexual activity.
    B. Annual Pap smear.
    C. Colposcopic examination if screening smear is "atypical."

ENDOMETRIAL CANCER

1. High risk
    A. Postmenopausal women with unopposed estrogen therapy
    B. Family history
    C. Obesity
    D. History of infertility or failure to ovulate
    E. Tamoxifen history
2. Screening: Endometrial biopsy at menopause with frequency thereafter at discretion of health care provider

OVARIAN CANCER

1. High risk
    A. Women with 40 ovulation years and more
    B. Nulliparity
    C. Pregnancy after age 30
    D. Family history
2. Screening
    A. Physical exam: Pelvic examination
    B. Carcinoembryonic antigen serum tumor marker: Not recommended
    C. Pelvic ultrasonography: Not recommended
3. Prevention: Oral contraceptive use

Health Promotion and Health Protection for the Frail Elderly

The approach one must take in order to meet the unique needs of the frail elderly is grounded in a solid foundation and understanding of the biologic changes associated with the aging process. Most recommendations for younger adults apply to elderly persons as well. However, there is additional information to consider when selecting preventive health services for the frail elderly population.

FUNCTIONAL STATUS

Assessment of functional status provides data about self-care activities, general physical health, and overall quality of life. Identification of the patient's functional status will help predict health care needs, potential costs, and the individual's propensity for serious illness or injury. Routine evaluation of functional status is recommended and may be performed through the clinical health history or by formal questionnaires and functional assessment tools. The information obtained enables the ACNP to monitor a patient's response to treatment and changes in function over time. The Katz Index of Activities of Daily Living provides assessment in the following areas:

1. Bathing
2. Continence
3. Dressing
4. Eating
5. Toileting
6. Transferring

FALL RISK ASSESSMENT

Older adults are often at risk for falls as a result of common changes in balance and gait caused by normal aging, illness, pain, or deconditioning.

1. Fall assessment and identification of individuals at risk of falling
   A. Level of consciousness and mental status
   B. Previous history of falls
   C. Ambulation: Independent, needs assistant to walk or uses assistive devices, chair/bed bound
   D. Vision/hearing defects
   E. Gait/balance impairment
   F. Systolic blood pressure
   G. Medications: Polypharmacy with potential for drug interactions and/or medications that may pose a risk (narcotics, sedatives/hypnotics, antihistamines, diuretics, antihypertensives and hypoglycemics, etc.)
   H. Predisposing diseases: Parkinson's disease, postural hypotension, syncope, vertigo, amputation, arthritis, cognitive impairment/confusion, cerebrovascular accident, osteoporosis or fractures
   I. Predisposing symptoms: Dizziness, weakness
2. Fall prevention
   A. Environmental safety changes: Keep all floors free from clutter; apply skid-proof backing to carpets and rugs; maintain well-lit stairwells; install grab bars on bathroom walls near tub, shower, and toilet; wear supportive, low-heeled shoes at home and avoid walking around in socks, slippers, or stockings.
   B. Gait retraining.
   C. Strengthening exercises.
   D. Use of ambulatory assist devices.
   E. Treatment of disorders that predispose an individual to falls.

COGNITIVE FUNCTION

1. High risk for cognitive decline
   A. Persons 85 years of age and older
   B. Those demonstrating functional decline
   C. Those entering long-term care facilities
2. Screening—Folstein's Mini-Mental State Examination: this is a well-known, highly utilized, practical tool used to grade the patient's cognitive state

Conclusion

In summary, the ACNP should remember the adage, "an ounce of prevention is worth a pound of cure."

Review Questions

13.1 Nutritional counseling of major dietary guidelines for the general adult population includes the recommendation to reduce overall consumption of fat, including the specific reduction of cholesterol to less than:

A. 350 mg/day
B. 300 mg/day
C. 275 mg/day
D. 200 mg/day

13.2 Influenza vaccination is recommended as a primary preventive strategy for all adults age 65 years and older. Which of the following groups of high-risk individuals also need vaccination?
A. Residents of chronic care facilities or nursing homes
B. Patients practicing high-risk sexual behavior
C. Parenteral illicit drug users
D. Patients diagnosed with thyroid disease

13.3 Breast cancer screening for high-risk women includes monthly breast self-examination, annual clinical breast examination, and annual evaluation with which one of the following tests?
A. Magnetic resonance imaging
B. Computed tomography scan
C. Mammography
D. Biopsy

13.4 Mr. D is an 80-year-old male who recently lost his wife of 62 years to ovarian cancer. He has a history of clinical depression and feels he may again be exhibiting signs of depression. He lives alone, cannot drive because of visual impairment, and is hard of hearing. As your top priority, your clinical evaluation must include which one of the following assessments?
A. Functional assessment
B. Cognitive assessment
C. Self-rating depression scale
D. Assessment for suicidal potential or risk

13.5 As an ACNP, you are caring for a 52-year-old woman admitted to the hospital because of a motor vehicle accident resulting in a right hip fracture. The hip fracture has been repaired and stabilized. You remember that, during the health history, it was noted the patient has a positive family history of colon cancer in a first-degree relative. As part of your daily evaluation of the patient, you may want to perform which of the following tests?
A. Flat-plate radiologic evaluation of the abdomen
B. Sedimentation rate
C. Digital rectal examination and fecal occult blood test
D. Fecal fat test

Answers and Rationales

13.1 **B** The U.S. Department of Health and Human Services and the U.S. Department of Agriculture have published nutrition guidelines that recommend reducing cholesterol intake to less than 300 mg/day.

13.2 **A** Residents of chronic care facilities and nursing homes should have an annual influenza vaccination regardless of age or medical condition.

13.3   **C**   Mammography should be done annually for all women of this age.

13.4   **D**   Assessment of suicidal potential or risk is essential in the clinical evaluation of this patient.

13.5   **C**   The digital rectal examination and fecal occult blood testing may be done in this situation.

References

American Cancer Society: (1997). *Cancer Facts and Figures*. Atlanta: American Cancer Society.

American Nurses Association and American Association of Critical Care Nurses. (1995). *Standards of Clinical Practice and Scope of Practice for the Acute Care Nurse Practitioner*. Washington, DC: American Nurses Publishing.

Bennett, J.C., & Plum, F. (eds.). (1996). *Cecil Textbook of Medicine* (20th ed.) Philadelphia: W.B. Saunders Co.

Centers for Disease Control and Prevention. (1996). Vaccine recommendations for travelers—health-care provider information. In *Health Information for International Travel*. Atlanta: Centers for Disease Control and Prevention.

Ewing, J.A. (1984). Detecting alcoholism: The CAGE questionnaire. *JAMA 252*, 1905–1907.

Hayward, R.S.A. Steinberg, E.P., Ford, D.E., et al. (1991). Preventive care Guidelines: 1991. *Ann Intern Med 114*, 758–783. [Erratum, *Ann Intern Med 115*, 332, 1991]

Holleb, A.I., Fink, D.J., & Murphy, G.P. (1996). *American Cancer Society Textbook of Clinical Oncology*. Atlanta: American Cancer Society.

Scheitel, S.M., Fleming, K.C., Chutka, D.S., et al. (1996). Geriatric health maintenance. Symposium on Geriatrics–Part IX. *Mayo Clinic Proc 71*, 289–302.

Sox, H.C. (1994). Preventive health services in adults. *N Engl J Med 330*, 1584–1595.

The Expert Committee on the Diagnosis and Classification of Diabetes Mellitus: Report of the Expert Committee on the Diagnosis and Classification of Diabetes Mellitus (1997). *Diabetes Care 20*, 1183–1197.

U.S. Preventive Services Task Force. (1996). *Guide to Clinical Preventive Services* (2nd ed.). Baltimore: Williams & Wilkins.

Yesavage, J.A. (1992). Depression in the elderly: How to recognize masked symptoms and choose appropriate therapy. *Postgrad Med 91*, 1–5.

Zung, W.W.K. (1965). A self-rating depression scale. *Arch Gen Psychiatry 12*, 63–70.

CHAPTER 14

Ethical and Legal Issues

Mary K. Shook, RN, BSN, NP

Ethical Issues

Continued advances in modern technology and the complexity of modern health care are certain to intensify the ethical dilemas of the future. Just as the challenges of past ethical dilemmas have tested the values and assumptions believed in, nurses will continue to be confronted with moral conflicts in various areas of their professional lives. The acute care nurse practitioner (ACNP) plays a major role in health care, being sensitive to the issues and policies of the present and those that will develop in the future. Recent changes in legislation, the American Nurses Association Code for Nurses, the caregiver role of the nurse, and the emergence of nursing ethics committees all enhance the role of the professional ACNP as patient advocate and educator in the clinical settings of health care. The revised Code of Nursing, as well as the Standards of Clinical Practice and Scope of Practice for the Acute Care Nurse Practitioner, outline an active role for ACNPs in ethical issues.

ADVANCE DIRECTIVES

Definition

An advance directive is a formal document prepared prior to an incapacitating illness or injury by a competent adult individual, documenting interventions, choices, and medical treatment decisions in the event he/she can no longer represent him/herself.

Legislative History

1. 1976: *Statutory living wills* were developed to provide instructions to physicians and empower individuals to accept or reject life-sustaining treatment in certain situations. Issues such as advances in modern technology that provide the means to save and prolong lives, prolonging the moment of death and excluding quality-of-life issues, led to the first legislation regarding living wills by the state of California.
2. 1983: *Durable Powers of Attorney for Health Care* (DPAHCs) were developed by various states. These documents further empowered individuals by permitting them to name a surrogate decision maker to make decisions for

them when they were no longer able to speak for themselves. Every state now has laws giving legal standing to such documents in that particular state.

3. 1990: *The Patient Self-Determination Act (PSDA) of 1990* became law in October as part of the Omnibus Budget Reconciliation Act, requiring health care facilities receiving Medicare and Medicaid funds to comply. The act has the legal intent of assuring patients' rights to participate in and direct their health care decisions (patient autonomy). This law makes it mandatory for health care facilities to provide patients with written information about their rights under state law to make decisions concerning their medical care. These rights include the right to accept or refuse treatment and the right to prepare an advanced directive. Every state must comply with the PSDA, a federal law, and each state is responsible for developing guidelines and descriptions of the laws of that state, whether statutory or as recognized by the courts of that state (case law).
   A. Who must comply:
      1) Hospitals
      2) Skilled nursing facilities
      3) Home health agencies
      4) Hospices
      5) Health maintenance organizations
   B. Written information must be provided describing the right to refuse treatment and prepare an advanced directive. Documentation of an advanced directive (yes or no) must be contained in the medical record. Written policies and procedures in compliance with state laws and educational materials are to be made available.
   C. Health care facilities and plans must provide information on advanced directives at the time of admission or enrollment.
   D. The PSDA requirement is to provide persons with information about their rights. It does not require anyone to complete an advance directive.
   E. The beneficial aspects of PSDA include increasing communication between patient and physician, fostering family discussions of death and dying, encouraging persons to complete advance directives, and increasing the awareness of treatment options and outcomes.

LIVING WILLS AND THE DURABLE POWER OF ATTORNEY FOR HEALTH CARE

1. Living wills (directives or declarations to physicians)
   A. Have legal status in every state. Laws change from state to state and each state's laws must be observed.
   B. Do not provide for the naming of an agent, a person to speak for the patient when the patient cannot.
   C. Are directed solely to the health care provider, the physician.
   D. Become effective when:
      1) The declaration is communicated to the physician.
      2) The declarant is diagnosed and declared in writing to be in a terminal condition or a permanent unconscious state.
      3) Diagnosis is confirmed by a second physician who has examined the patient.
      4) The patient is no longer able to speak for him/herself regarding the administration of life-sustaining treatment.

      5) The declaration is not effective while a declarant is pregnant and the physician is aware of this.

      6) The laws of the state determine the restrictions of life-sustaining treatment. Clarification of issues regarding the withholding or withdrawing of medications, artificially administered food and fluid must be done at the state level.

      7) Is not as effective and comprehensive as the Durable Power of Attorney for Health Care.

2. Durable power of attorney for health care

    A. A form of advance directive allowing individuals 18 years or older to appoint an agent to make decisions for them when they become unable to make decisions for themselves. It must be signed, dated, and witnessed by two individuals, one unrelated to the person, or notarized.

    B. Control of health care is maintained by clearly stating what treatment modalities are wanted or not wanted and conveying to the agent sufficient knowledge about values and preferences.

    C. It provides clear evidence of wishes regarding medical treatments, surgery, artificially administered food and fluids, etc.

    D. DPAHCs have legal standing in all states. States have their own specific laws and forms that must be observed and used.

    E. It becomes effective when the individual can no longer speak for him/herself.

    F. The PSDA requires all above-named facilities to comply with the federal law regarding advance directives in the manner stated above, in compliance with state laws.

    G. Beginning in 1992 the Joint Commission on Accreditation of Healthcare Organizations developed the "Patients Rights Standards," addressing the use of advance directives. The standards are now part of the accreditation process and needed for accreditation.

3. Durable powers of attorney for health care is the preferred document.

    A. It is a communication tool to one's own value system; to the chosen agent, family, physician, ACNP, and friends; to anyone at bedside involved in the decision-making process.

    B. It increases the awareness of physicians and ACNPs to patients' rights and autonomy. Recent court decisions and the PSDA have aided this.

    C. It decreases legal risks and ethical conflicts.

    D. The difference between the DPAHC and financial durable powers of attorney (DPAs) is highlighted.

    E. It has fewer restrictions and is the most flexible advance directive, covering most circumstances.

    F. It encourages health care consumers to be informed, to question physicians and ACNPs about treatment options and risks, to ask for information regarding health care, and to know what is in an individual's "best interests."

THE ADVANCE DIRECTIVE PROCESS

The ACNP should be familiar with the advance directive process because it enhances the role of the knowledgeable professional as a patient advocate and educator in assisting clients in the end-of-life decision-making process. Some key points for the ACNP to be knowledgeable about include:

1. Who can fill out an advance directive? Any competent adult 18 years or older, sick or well, may complete either the living will or a DPAHC. State laws vary for minors.
2. Does the patient need a lawyer? In general a lawyer is not needed to complete an advance directive. It is suggested in special circumstances: when patient is a minor, when competency may be questioned, if there is family dissension, in situations regarding guardianship.
3. Can changes be made if circumstances or wishes change?
   A. Changes can be made orally or in writing. Verbal changes to physicians take priority over previously written directions as long as the person can speak for him/herself.
   B. Changes must always be communicated to the physician and noted in the medical record when treatment is in progress.
4. How effective is the document of one state in another state?
   A. The value of each state's documents are generally recognized by other states. Advance directives are considered legal in all states.
   B. Each state has its own laws and the laws of another state will not supersede those laws.
   C. However, a written advance directive expressing a person's intentions can be influential in the decision-making process in another state.
5. Who makes health care decisions for incompetent individuals who no longer speak for themselves? Generally, if there is no advance directive, and the person can no longer speak for him/herself, physicians consult family members and close friends. Acting in the "best interests" of the patient, consensus is usually reached. Turning to the courts should be a last resort.
6. What options are available in times of conflict in making difficult health care decisions?
   A. Bioethics committees are available in many health care facilities.
   B. Patient care conferences between the ACNP, nurses, physicians, family members, pastoral care staff, and patient representatives are valuable in assisting and reviewing difficult cases. These individuals play a consulting role and can make recommendations.
7. Does the presence or absence of an advance directive affect the providing of health care? No, discrimination in the providing of care is prohibited by state and federal law. The PSDA expressly states care cannot be determined by the presence or absence of one of these documents.

HEALTH CARE WISHES AND VALUES
(End-of-Life Decisions)

1. End-of-life decisions are made in conjunction with a person's perception of him/herself in daily life.
2. Values supporting the self-identity and self-concept of the individual play a major role.
3. Some of these values are feelings about activities of daily living (walking, talking, driving, bathing, etc.), pain and suffering, living independently, decreased mental and physical abilities. Consideration is given to fears concerning death, economics, and unwanted medical treatment.
4. Physician- and/or ACNP-patient dialogue provides information concerning treatment options and alternatives, medical conditions, risks, benefits and burdens of medical treatment, and side effects of treatments in varying situations. It ensures sharing complete and pertinent information and corrects any misinformation or misperceptions.

5. The role of the ACNP as patient advocate and educator
    A. Can encourage dialogue among the patient, family, physicians, and the health care team.
    B. Can be supportive of decisions made by the patient.
    C. Is knowledgeable about the types of documents available and the significance of completing them.
    D. Is aware of the PSDA and is a source of information concerning state and federal laws.
    E. May participate in the writing of policies and procedures concerning the withholding and withdrawal of medical care.
    F. Is aware of the bioethical issues revolving around end-of-life decision making and the sources of conflict.
    G. May be a member of the nursing bioethics or hospital bioethics committees.
6. Religious concerns
    A. Respect for the religious beliefs and spirituality of patients, family, and caregivers must be maintained.
    B. Pastoral care departments and outlying religious sources can serve as resources for patients and caregivers.
7. Cultural issues and concerns
    A. Culturally sensitive care of the patient is meaningful when the patient's history, family, and socioeconomic status are included in the assessment, as well as race and ethnic background.
    B. There is a range of variation in response to illness, behavior when in pain, expressions of grief, death in the home versus hospice or hospital, autopsy, organ donation, and other culturally patterned situations. These can be a source of conflict in the absence of knowledge and the lack of respect for cultural diversity.
    C. It is important for the ACNP to recognize, especially in the bioethical area of end-of-life decision making, that many of the practices, values, and beliefs entertained are those of western philosophy and legal traditions.
    D. Things for the ACNP to consider include the degree and openness in discussing the illness and its prognosis, whom the primary decision maker in the family may be, fears of treatment limitation, religious beliefs and the meaning of death, generational interrelationships of the family, and past experiences related to access to care, poverty, and immigration status.
    E. Implications for the ACNP
        1) Be culturally aware that not all cultures are in accord with western bioethics practices relating to end-of-life decision making, patient rights, and individual autonomy.
        2) All verbal and nonverbal health care directives are as legally valid as statutory directives.
        3) Do not assume an individual who writes an advance directive does not want aggressive treatment.

Review Questions

14.1 What advance directive(s) are commonly used in most states?
    A. Patient self-determination document

    B. Handwritten, unsigned, and undated living will
    C. DPA
    D. DPAHC or medical power of attorney and living will (directive to physicians)

14.2 What is the purpose of the Patient Self-Determination Act of 1990?
    A. To prevent patients from making their own decisions about treatment they can receive
    B. To continue the paternalistic patterns in medicine
    C. To assure patients' right to participate in health care and direct their health care decisions
    D. To keep health care facilities from providing information about patients' rights

14.3 Mrs. J, age 68, is seriously ill. She has a history of diabetes mellitus and cardiac disease and has recently been diagnosed with carcinoma of the lung. She has one younger brother who visits her frequently, no spouse or children. She faces a limited and poor quality of life. Her request is for "everything to be done, I want to live, no matter what." What is an important consideration for using the Durable Power of Attorney for Health Care in this case?
    A. It is the less flexible document and has more restrictions
    B. To deter health care consumers from interfering in the decision-making process by less questioning and not asking for information
    C. To highlight differences between the DPAHC and the DPA
    D. To encourage conversation about health care with family and friends and using one's own value system to assist in the decision-making process and decrease the risk of legal and ethical conflicts

14.4 A 37-year-old male, unconscious, unresponsive, and bleeding, is brought to the emergency room by paramedics unaccompanied by family or friends. The electrocardiogram shows various dysrhythmias. Life-sustaining medical treatment is begun, and the patient is stabilized and admitted to the intensive care unit. History is unavailable. A family member is not located until several days after admission. There is no advance directive to anyone's knowledge. Who makes decisions for this patient, who can no longer make decisions for himself?
    A. The physician unilaterally makes these decisions
    B. The surrogate decision maker if a valid DPAHC is completed
    C. A family member or close friend in conjunction with the physician acting in the "best interests" of the patient
    D. No one

14.5 You are admitting a 71-year-old male to a medical-surgical unit with a history of cerebrovascular accident left-sided weakness, congestive heart failure (CHF), and difficulty breathing. What part of the admitting process would determine if he is aware of his rights and would ensure his wishes being carried out?
    A. Questioning the patient about his health care insurance contract
    B. Requesting a deposit for the hospital stay
    C. Asking the patient if he has an advance directive or would like additional information concerning his rights to make end-of-life medical care decisions and fill out an advance directive

D. Informing the patient it is not necessary to have a copy of the advance directive on the medical record

---

Answers and Rationales

14.1 **D** The two most common statutory advance directives in use in most states are the DPAHC and the living will (directive to physicians). Most states have both documents; however, some states offer a living will document solely.

14.2 **C** The Patient Self-Determination Act of 1990 has the legal intent of assuring the patient be given information concerning his/her right to participate in health care treatment decisions, to make decisions for him/herself, and to fill out an advance directive. It does not demand that everyone have an advance directive.

14.3 **D** Important reasons for encouraging patients to fill out a DPAHC are to use it as a communication tool with family and friends, to make known one's personal preferences and wishes regarding end-of-life medical treatment, to ensure one's medical care decisions and wishes are carried out in accordance with one's own value system, and to help decrease legal risks and ethical conflicts. It is especially important that accurate information concerning diagnosis and prognosis is given to the patient and/or surrogate decision maker to make a decision that provides comfort and serenity to the patient.

14.4 **C** In the absence of an advance directive, consultations between the physician, the ACNP, and family members or friends are used to make decisions and act in the "best interests" of the patient. Every effort must be made to contact family in their absence. Hospital administration, ethicists and ethics committees, and legal counsel are resources in difficult cases involving unidentified and/or homeless individuals. In some situations the courts may become involved.

14.5 **C** The PSDA requires the patient be asked if he has an advance directive or if he would like information concerning the document if one has not been completed. If the patient has filled a document out, a copy is placed in the medical record to protect his decisions regarding life-sustaining treatment and medical care. It is the responsibility of the patient to provide a copy of the document.

References

American Nurses Association and the American Association of Critical Care Nurses. (1995). *Standards of Clinical Practice and Scope of Practice for the Acute Care Nurse Practitioner*. Washington, DC: American Nurses Publishing.

Badzek, L.A. (1992). What you need to know about Advance Directives. *Nursing '92 June*, 58–59.

California Consortium on Patient Self-Determination. (1991). *The PSDA Handbook: Guidance for Hospitals on Policies, Procedures, and California Law Related to Fulfilling their Obligations under the Patient Self-Determination Act (OBRA '90)*. Los Angeles: Pacific Center for Health Policy and Ethics, University of Southern California Law Center.

Emanuel, L.L. (1995). Advance Directives: Do They work? *J Am Coll Cardiol 25*, 35–38.

Koenig, B., & Gates-Williams, J. (1995). Understanding cultural difference in caring for dying patients. *West J Med 163*, 244–248.

O'Connell, L.J. (1995). Religious dimensions of dying and death. *West J Med 163*, 231–235.

Intensity of Care Issues

The role of the ACNP in the acute care arena is a critical, responsible position. Expectations are the ACNP will be an intelligent observer and interpreter of changes in the patients' physiological and psychosocial status. The ACNP role of patient advocate and educator is crucial and enhanced by the circumstances and environment he/she is working in. Quick diagnosis of changes in condition and treatment of the patient is foremost. The prompt detection of early signs and changes in the patient's condition signals the nurse to initiate treatment in many circumstances, preventing further deterioration. One of the primary objectives of acute care units is to prevent a health care crisis by observing and treating the early signs of impending arrest.

The Scope of Practice includes a core body of knowledge derived from the full spectrum of high-acuity patient care needs with specialty determined by patient characteristics. Facets of the ACNP's assessment of the complex acutely ill patient include a complete health history, physical and mental status examination, and health risk appraisal. Inherent components also include diagnostic reasoning, advanced therapeutic interventions, and consultations and referrals to other nurses, physicians, and other health care providers as needed. The theories of nursing regarding functional and psychosocial assessments are incorporated and applied to the care provided by the ACNP. Individualized patient care is provided by the culturally competent ACNP.

The Standards of Clinical Practice and Scope of Practice for the ACNP states that the ACNP practices in any setting in which patient care requirements include complex monitoring and therapies, high-intensity nursing intervention, or continuous nursing vigilance within the full range of high-acuity care. Advanced acute care practitioners are optimally suited for managing the more complex, uncertain, and resource-limited situations characteristic of high-acuity coverage. This section discusses intensity of care issues the ACNP may be faced with. These include (1) withholding and withdrawal of medical care, (2) Do-Not-Resuscitate orders, (3) administration of artificial food and fluids, and (4) palliative care, hospice care, and futile treatment.

WITHHOLDING AND WITHDRAWING OF MEDICAL CARE

1. The right to make personal health care choices has long been a fundamental right of U.S. citizens and supported by federal and state courts.
   A. Justice Cardoza in 1914 emphasized the individual's right to self-determination.
   B. The concept of personal privacy and the right to refuse treatment was clarified by Supreme Court Justice Brandeis, and became the basis of court decisions regarding these rights.
2. The American Nurses Association (ANA) Code for Nurses supports and recognizes the moral and ethical imperatives reflected in patient self-determination.

3. The decision to withdraw or withhold medical care, including life-sustaining treatment, is a fundamental right and personal decision of an individual in an effort to maintain control over health care based upon personal values and wishes.
   A. The consent of a competent adult or surrogate decision maker is required for any medical or surgical therapeutic intervention, including diagnostic tests, and artificially administered food and fluids. The laws of the state determine the extent of what can be legally withheld and withdrawn.
   B. The health care provider does not have to agree with the patient's decision, or comply with it, if it conflicts with the moral and ethical principles of health care providers.
      1) The physician, discussing matters of death and dying in advance, can be cognizant of and have a clear understanding of the patient's wishes.
      2) The option of the physician is to transfer the patient to the care of another physician whose views are compatible with the patient's.
      3) The ACNP plays an advocate role, educating the patient about risks, benefits, alternatives, and outcomes while supporting the patient's right to accept or refuse treatment and helping provide understanding of the necessity of patient transfer.
4. There is no legal or ethical difference between withholding and withdrawing care.
   A. Circumstances may determine the final outcome of any decision based on clinical changes, changes in perspective, or evolution of situations.
   B. Confirmation of the medical diagnosis and prognosis should be followed by careful deliberation and consideration of the decision.
   C. Adequate time should be given to the decision-making process, even in emergency situations, though it may be brief in these circumstances.
   D. Life-sustaining treatment, once initiated, may be withdrawn as circumstances change.
5. The laws regarding the withholding and withdrawing of medical care differ from state to state. In some states it is against state law to withhold or withdraw artificially administered food and fluids.
6. The ACNP will work with the primary care physician in determining the diagnosis and prognosis, identifying the risks and benefits of treatment, and providing information necessary for evaluation to make the decision to withhold or withdraw treatment.
7. In any area of doubt or disagreement concerning the withholding or withdrawing of treatment, the ACNP should consult hospital administration and the institution's legal counsel.
8. Ethicists, ethics committees, pastoral care departments, and patient advocates are other resources of information for the ACNP.

DO-NOT-RESUSCITATE ORDERS

Definition

Do-Not-Resuscitate (DNR) orders can be written by the ACNP in collaboration with the physician to suspend the automatic initiation of cardiopulmonary resuscitation (CPR). They are written in the medical record, co-signed by the physician within 24 hours, as determined by the policies and procedures of the institution. CPR is defined to include chest compression, ventilation and intubation for respiratory assistance, and modalities related to the procedure, including defibrillation and cardiopulmonary medications.

Historical Perspective

1. In the absence of a DNR order, CPR administration has become a routine emergency procedure in health care settings, attempted with and without consent, performed on individuals suffering cardiac or respiratory arrest, including many in the dying process, possibly doing harm rather than good in some patients (violating the principle of nonmalfeasance).
2. The broad use of CPR on terminally ill and dying patients and the questionable success rate of CPR prompted concern in the medical and nursing communities.
3. Guidelines to assist the medical community in writing appropriate Do-Not-Resuscitate orders and the use of CPR were first developed in 1987 by the American Medical Associations's Council on Ethical and Judicial Affairs.
4. DNR orders have not been generally addressed by law in most states.
   A. The legality of DNR orders has been upheld by the courts and the rights of patients or surrogates have been affirmed.
   B. In 1994 only New York and Georgia had passed laws providing physicians with guidelines for writing DNR orders, granting protection from prosecution if the orders followed the statutory guidelines.

General Considerations For DNR Orders

It is essential the ACNP be aware of the following general considerations when writing a DNR order.

1. A DNR order in a strict interpretation means no CPR.
   A. Additional appropriate treatment may be continued in accordance with specific patient needs.
   B. Assessments are done to determine the expected benefits versus burdens of other life-sustaining treatment.
2. The patient or surrogate decision maker, in consultation with the physician and/or ACNP, makes the decision to write a DNR order.
   A. The end-of-life decision to have a DNR order written is generally based on ethical, religious, and cultural beliefs, as well as physiologic, psychosocial, and medical reasons. Considering all of these aspects ensures a more appropriate decision.
   B. DPAHCs and directives to physicians (living wills), when completed, signed, and dated, should be obtained and placed in the medical record.
3. The guidelines for withholding CPR and writing DNR orders are based on:
   A. The competent patient's preferences and desires. Early discussion between the patient and the physician and/or the ACNP concerning the procedure, outcomes, patient preferences and values, and alternatives ensures active patient participation and decisions based on accurate knowledge.
   B. The decision of a surrogate decision maker in the absence of patient capacity, acting in the "best interests" of the patient if wishes and desires are not previously known.
   C. The patient's quality of life prior to CPR being administered.

    D. Circumstances that would indicate a futile outcome inconsistent with patient goals, be of no benefit to the patient, or where the moment of death may be prolonged. The personal values of the physician regarding quality of life must not transcend the interests and desires of the patient.

4. DNR orders should be written clearly and specifically, especially in the event of other life-sustaining treatment being provided.
   A. The order should clarify what has been agreed upon, and what treatment is appropriate or inappropriate.
   B. The DNR order should direct the care in the absence of the primary physician and/or ACNP.

5. "Partial Code" orders must be clearly written and discussed with the patient and family to avoid confusion, deception, and the imposition of physicians values on the patient (i.e., CPR with No Intubation).
   A. The ACNP may initiate patient care conferences, which facilitate discussion among the persons involved and usually result in resolution of many disagreements. Social workers, chaplains, patient advocates, physicians, nursing staff, family members, and significant other may be included to discuss and clarify the issues.
   B. When the ACNP identifies difficult ethical situations that cannot be resolved, referrals to ethics committees or a hospital ethicist, or withdrawal from the case, are options.

6. The labeled "slow code" is a covert procedure that denies the patient or his/her surrogate information about resuscitation and prognosis.
   A. According to Mark Ebell, M.D., it is unethical and deceptive and is to be discouraged.
   B. Lack of discussion with the patient about the true status of the situation may lead to liability risks resulting in part from a violation of patient rights.

7. The patient's right to consent to or refuse treatment must be respected. The Patient Self-Determination Act supports patient autonomy and the right to write an advance directive directing his/her care.
   A. Physicians and/or the ACNP must discuss medical care with patients in a caring and compassionate manner.
   B. Not discussing a DNR order with patients is no longer an option.
   C. Institutional policies and procedures are to be written governing patient autonomy.

8. The ACNP maintains the role of patient advocate and educator in an organized and professional manner in ethical situations where conflicts may arise.
   A. The ACNP often has knowledge and insights the physician is unaware of, reflecting the special nurse-patient relationship.
   B. The patient's fear of abandonment and the fear of pain are important factors for the ACNP to be aware of and to consider when resuscitation decisions are being made.

Role of the Nurse Practitioner and Patient Autonomy

1. It is imperative that the ACNP be aware of what the patient is communicating when discussing life-sustaining measures and rights to make his/her own decisions.
2. Providing accurate information concerning therapy, outcomes, and other options may help to diminish ethical conflicts.

    A. Use of the advance directive as a communication tool may assist in discussing the desired options.

    B. The role of the ACNP may be to alert the physician to the need for discussing the issues with the patient. The ACNP may recognize the need for a DNR order before the physician.

3. The ACNP plays a major role in upholding the standard of care for DNR patients.

    A. DNR orders must not decrease aggressiveness or level of care.

    B. It is the responsibility of the ACNP to ensure appropriate treatments are ordered for the dying patients.

4. The ACNP recognizes the benefits of advance planning and early discussion of DNR orders for certain patients. These patients may include:

    A. Those suffering from any terminal illness

    B. Those with a severe and disabling condition or illness that is considered irreversible

    C. Those at increased risk of cardiac or respiratory arrest

    D. Patients likely to lapse into a persistent vegetative state (irreversible unconsciousness)

    E. Those whose prognosis is poor because of other end-stage disease processes, in whom CPR may be futile

    F. If there is a question of presumed consent for CPR

ADMINISTRATION OF ARTIFICIAL FOOD AND FLUIDS

1. Artificial administration of food and fluids is a complex issue in the realm of long-term nursing care.

    A. Conflict arises in the definition—is it comfort care or a life-sustaining measure?

    B. Opinions vary based on what may be an inaccurate assumption of the suffering and indignity of "starving to death" or "dying of thirst."

    C. Many states prohibit, by law, the withdrawal or withholding of nourishment under any circumstances.

    D. State law variability in part reflects the lack of clear definition of artificial food and fluid as a life-sustaining technology.

        1) It is a widely used life-sustaining technology for persons of all ages and in particular for the elderly.

        2) It is used as a restorative measure and in custodial care as a medical intervention.

    E. The use of artificial nutrition and hydration is questioned in cases of persistent vegetative states and bedfast persons whom it may not benefit other than to prolong life. In some situations adding additional years may be unwelcome and unwanted by institutionalized persons.

    F. Because of the variability of state laws and opinions of the experts, this issue must be dealt with on an individual basis.

2. The laws regarding the withholding and withdrawing of medical care differ from state to state. In some states it is against state law to withhold or withdraw artificially administered nutrition and hydration.

    A. It is imperative that primary caregivers check the laws of the state and federal guidelines in reference to DNR orders and withholding and withdrawing of food and fluids.

    B. In some states artificially administered food and fluid is not considered life-sustaining treatment.

C. The policies and procedures of a particular health care facility must also be adhered to.

3. Legal precedents have developed following the Karen Ann Quinlan case supporting the removal of feeding tubes when spontaneous respirations occur after the removal of a ventilator.

   A. In a 1986 opinion, the American Medical Association stated that removal of a feeding tube is ethically no different from the termination of any life-sustaining treatment.

   B. Controversy continues, however, with some believing in the concept of comfort, others stating the treatment is an invasive procedure causing discomfort, as does mechanical life support.

4. The Supreme Court decision in the Nancy Cruzan case of 1990 concluded that competent patients have a constitutional right to refuse life-sustaining medical treatment, including lifesaving hydration and nutrition. Justice Rehnquist stated in the majority opinion, "the principle that a competent person has a constitutionally protected liberty interest in refusing unwanted medical treatment may be inferred from our prior decision."

PALLIATIVE CARE, HOSPICE CARE, AND FUTILE TREATMENT

Palliative Care

DEFINITION

Palliative care is supportive or comfort care. It is care given to a dying person to keep them comfortable physically, emotionally, and spiritually. Aggressive treatment is not undertaken. There is recognition the person is dying and the prolongation of life is not the goal. The ACNP needs to review care options with the goal of enhancing patient comfort and making present life meaningful.

CANDIDATES FOR PALLIATIVE CARE

1. Patients with a progressive disease (e.g., acquired immunodeficiency syndrome), who have no curative care options
2. Those suffering from advanced neuromuscular disease (e.g., amyotrophic lateral sclerosis), pulmonary and malignant processes
3. Any person ill with a terminal or irreversible condition who may choose to refuse treatment

Hospice Care

1. Hospices have been established for the care of the dying patient to augment services for those who cannot be cared for in the home.

   A. Lack of denial of death permits open, reassuring conversations and questions about death.

   B. The atmosphere is one of acceptance.

   C. Professional staff are able to assist the dying person to validate feelings of anger and pain, and acknowledge the grieving that accompanies death.

   D. While it is important to be aware of the physiologic aspect of the dying process, the psychosocial and spiritual aspects of death are equally important.

    E. Loss of control is one aspect of illness the professional can address by allowing the individual as much control as possible over his/her life.

    F. Developing the art of listening is an excellent way to provide insight into the needs of the patient so they may be satisfied.

    G. Providing good information and assistance helps a patient maintain his/her goals.

2. Personal autonomy is to be respected in the hospice environment as in any other health care agency.

    A. The consent or refusal of treatment by the patient or the surrogate decision maker is governed by the process of decision making established by the Patient Self-Determination Act.

    B. The wishes and preferences of the patient should be known and careful planning should be done by the physician, ACNP, and family. Decision making at the time of crisis can thus be alleviated. Advance planning prevents the technological entrapment.

    C. Honesty, support, and willingness are the principles on which palliative care is built.

3. Palliative care is not limited to those in a hospice unit or other unit established for that purpose. It is provided for the dying patient wherever the person may be. The principles of palliative care are the significant hallmarks to follow.

4. Family members and friends assisting in the care of the dying offer a special dimension of care and should be allowed to participate.

    A. Staff members, lay ministers, and spiritual leaders offer support to patient and family.

    B. Counseling family members and friends regarding the purposes and goals of palliative care assists their understanding of the care.

5. Being able to live and die in a caring community benefits those receiving care and the caregivers. It is a mutual relationship based on service and accepting care. Fidelity and trust are the foundation.

Futile Treatment

DEFINITION

The ongoing debate about futility has not finalized a definition of the concept of futile treatment.

1. It can be thought of in a bioethical way as treatment that should not be provided because the risks exceed the benefits.

2. Another theory addresses appropriate versus inappropriate treatment.

3. Others question if it is definable and able to be achieved. It may be an "elusive concept."

    A. If treatment has not worked in a specified number of cases, can it then be called futile?

    B. Is treatment futile if persons remain in a persistent vegetative state following treatment or become confined to an ICU without the hope of achieving other life goals?

4. The futility debate began when the concept of patient autonomy and the right to refuse or accept treatment collided with physician decision making.

    A. Was it the obligation of the physician to provide any treatment a patient or surrogate decision maker requested against his/her medical judgment?

B. How are the goals of medicine to be interpreted, and who interprets whether or not treatment meets the goals or what the goals are?

GENERAL INFORMATION FOR THE ACNP REGARDING FUTILE TREATMENT

1. The ACNP must consult with the physician when informing a patient treatment will not be offered.
2. Exceptions can be made for special requests or wishes of the patient (i.e., CPR to allow time for a last visit with family or friends).
3. The focus reverts to comfort and supportive care, allowing the person a peaceful death with dignity.
4. Encourage clarity of thinking by distinguishing futility (no therapeutic benefit) from rationing (are the benefits worth the cost).
5. The ACNP needs to educate the public about intensity of care issues and the meaning of futile treatment.
6. The ACNP should ensure the place of employment has policies and procedures regarding futile care.
    A. There may be a variation in policies based on institutional standards and/or mission.
    B. Ethics committees are a resource to ensure a lack of discrimination.
    C. Communication related to not providing treatment that might be wanted by the patient must be developed, and the values of all concerned must be considered.
7. Education and collaboration with the medical community and the public can be a thoughtful way of developing guidelines and communicating the valid reasons for withholding futile treatment.
    A. Ethics committees can play an invaluable role in this dialogue.
    B. Justification for withholding treatment must be part of any guideline.
    C. Clearly stated and articulated professional guidelines for not offering treatment have been suggested as a way to inform society and letting the public respond.
    D. The religious and cultural concerns of physicians, patients, and caregivers must be considered as in other areas of providing sensitive, compassionate care.

Review Questions

14.6   In what way may DNR orders cause conflict in an acute care setting?
    A. DNR orders are always clear and concise and understood by all professionals caring for a patient
    B. DNR orders are frequently misinterpreted by various members of the physician and nursing staff
    C. Therapeutic interventions not included in the DNR order may be withheld or withdrawn, leading to confusion and misunderstandings
    D. The loss of patient autonomy and neglect of patient rights in the intensive care environment as a result of critical circumstances is very possible

14.7   Intensity of care issues include which of the following?
    A. Palliative care

B. Cultural issues and personal autonomy
C. Futile treatment
D. All of the above

14.8   Mrs. G, a 38-year-old mother of three children, was diagnosed with carcinoma of the breast 3 years ago. She had a radical mastectomy and three courses of chemotherapy followed by radiation. One year ago she was told it had metastasized to her right lung. Her mother died of cancer. Mrs. G was formerly a heavy smoker. Mrs. G has chosen to forego any further treatment. She has discussed this at length with her family and physician, ACNP, and members of the health care team. Mrs. G has been assured her children will be cared for and is comfortable with her decision. Which of the following statements is true about a patient's right to accept or refuse medical treatment, including life-sustaining technology?
A. States vary in the determination of patients rights and what they may accept or refuse
B. Physicians do not have to consult or communicate with patients concerning these rights
C. The Patient Self-Determination Act supports patient autonomy and the right to enact an advance directive of his/her choice
D. The patient's right of self-determination and to write an advance directive is not supported by any state or federal law

14.9   A healthy 60-year-old man had just remarried and traveled from California to Illinois to visit his new wife's family. Six hours after his arrival, he fell forward, striking his head, and became unconscious. He was rushed to a local trauma center and, following a detailed work-up for head trauma in the emergency room, underwent a craniotomy for hematoma evacuation. After surgery he was placed on a ventilator and transferred to the critical care unit. His level of consciousness continued to deteriorate. What intensity of care issues will be addressed in the care of this patient?
A. Determination of a surrogate decision maker to act in the "best interests" of the patient
B. Guidelines to be used to continue ventilator support and other life-sustaining medical treatment
C. When a DNR order will be appropriate
D. All of the above

14.10   An 87-year-old female has been admitted to the intensive care unit. Diagnosis is dysphagia S/P percutaneous endoscopic gastrostromy insertion with complications, end-stage CHF, renal failure, and atrial tachycardia. She is being maintained on nitroglycerin and renal dopamine and has not responded to treatment for atrial tachycardia. On admission she was made a "Chemical Code Only." Which of the following is a guideline to consider for writing a DNR order? She is responsive. There is no advance directive.
A. Knowing the wishes and preferences of a patient capable of decision-making capacity and obtaining accurate information concerning the patient's diagnosis and prognosis that can influence his/her decision to request or accept a DNR order

    B. Not discussing outcomes, risks of treatment, values, and alternatives with the patient

    C. Fears of addressing these issues with the patient because of underestimation of her ability to understand

    D. Consultation with the surrogate decision maker to act in the "best interests" of the incapacitated patient

Answers and Rationales

14.6   **C**   Strictly interpreted a DNR order means no cardiopulmonary resuscitation. DNR orders written in the critical care area can be the cause of conflict because of the complexity and broad array of interventions used in life-sustaining treatment. DNR orders must be written in a clear and concise manner to avoid misinterpretation by various members of the health care team. Therapeutic interventions not included in the DNR may be withheld or withdrawn, creating conflict. Treatments that meet a patient's specific needs may be continued if appropriate, providing the goals of treatment have not changed from curative to palliative. Accurate assessment of the patient's needs is done to determine the benefits versus burdens of other life-sustaining treatment.

14.7   **D**   The advances in modern technology have prolonged many lives and created a continuum of care that extends through many stages and requires different decisions in many different areas. From the time a critical patient is brought to an intensive care unit until the time of death, the patient may experience various levels of care. The decision-making process, who makes the decisions, what treatment is accepted or refused, and what is the final outcome are all issues of patient autonomy to be addressed, either by the patient or the surrogate decision maker. Included in this panorama are personal autonomy, cultural and religious issues, palliative care, and futile treatment.

14.8   **C**   The Patient Self-Determination Act supports patient autonomy, and these rights are protected by the laws of the state and federal government. Policies and procedures written by individual health care facilities govern and protect patient autonomy. It is up to the health care team to openly communicate with the patient concerning the quality of life and the possible outcomes of treatment. The patient's decision may not always be agreed with, and it is not necessary that anyone do so. It is only necessary that physicians, ACNPs, family members, and supportive relationships respect the rights of the patient to make his/her own decisions.

14.9   **D**   The intensity of care issues began in the emergency room with the decision made by someone to consent to surgical treatment following the initial work-up. The patient was in an unconscious state and it is presumed his wife made the decision to go forward with treatment. After his admission to a special care unit with life-sustaining measures being provided, further decisions must be made to determine how long to maintain him, what determines the intensity and continuation of care, and who makes the decisions if there is no advance directive. It is possible that, for support and discussion, the wife would enlist the opinions and wishes of other family members. Consideration must be given to the laws of the state he is in and that he is being treated by physicians who do not know him or his preferences.

14.10 **A**   A useful guideline when discussing or writing a DNR order is obtaining accurate information concerning the patient's diagnosis and prognosis. What are the patient's goals of treatment? Nothing surpasses an honest dialogue with the patient and/or the surrogate decision maker. Patients are very capable of understanding and have a need to discuss end-of-life decisions. The ACNP caring for the patient may approach the competent adult patient and family with information concerning the current course of treatment and its effect on outcome. The physician can be informed by the ACNP of the patient's deteriorating condition. The physician, ACNP, nursing staff, and family meet to discuss what is in the "best interests" of the patient. In the case of an incompetent patient, the named surrogate decision maker would be part of the consultation process. A decision can then be made to write a DNR order and to maintain the patient as comfortably as possible, providing palliative care. The patient can be transferred to a medical floor with a DNR order and cared for there.

References

American Nurses Association and the American Association of Critical Care Nurses. (1995). *Standards of Clinical Practice and Scope of Practice for the Acute Care Nurse Practitioner.* Washington, DC: American Nurses Publishing.

Annas, G.J. (1976). The legal aspects of a patient care classification system. *Hosp Med Staff February*, 12–18.

Blackhall, L.J., Murphy, S.T., Frank, G., et al. (1995). Ethinicity and attitudes toward patient autonomy. *JAMA 274*, 820–825.

Cohen, L.M., Woods, A., & McCue, J. (1991). The Challenge of advance directives and ESRD. *Dialysis Transplant 20*, 593–594, 614.

Council on Ethical and Judicial Affairs. (1991). Guidelines for the appropriate use of Do-Not-Resuscitate orders. *JAMA 265*, 1868–1875.

Davila, F. (1996). The impact of Do-Not-Resuscitate orders and patient care category policies on CPR and ventilator support rates. *Arch Intern Med 156*, 405–408.

Ebell, M.M. (1994). Practical guidelines for Do-Not-Resuscitate orders. *Am Fam Physician 50*, 1293–1299.

Gumbiner, C.H. (1995), "Do-Not-Resuscitate" orders for children. *Nebraska Med J January*, 5–7.

Haddad, A.M., & Kapp, M.B. (1991). Withholding and withdrawing treatment. In *Ethical and Legal Issues in Home Health Care: Case Studies and Analyses.* Norwalk, CT: Appleton & Lange, pp. 79–99.

Henneman, E.A., Baird, B., Bellamy, P.E., et al. (1994). Effect of Do-Not-Resuscitate orders on the nursing care of critically ill patients. *Am J Crit Care 3*, 467–472.

Klessig, J. (1992). Cross cultural medicine, a decade later: The effect of values and culture on life-support decisions. *West J Med 157*, 316–322.

Lagerlof, J. (1989). Prolonging death: medical ethicists struggle with dilemma. *California Nurs Rev January/February*, 26–27.

Marsee, V. (1994). Ethical dilemmas in the delivery of intensive care to critically ill oncology patients. *Semin Oncol Nurs 10,* 156–164.

Medical Intensive Care Unit. (1997). *Medical Intensive Care Unit Resuscitation Plan.* Los Angeles: UCLA Medical Center.

Oppenheimer, E.A. (1996). Palliative care and the bioethics committee. *Ethical Currents 45,* 3.

Ross, J.W. (1990). Arrests, pre-arrest interventions, and DNR orders. *Ethical Currents 22,* 1–2.

Ross, J.W. (1993). Futile treatment: Where are we? *Ethical Currents 35,* 1–3, 7.

Shoemaker, W.C. (1975). Problems in the classification of prognosis for purposes of disengagement of therapy in the critically ill patient. *Linacre Q May,* 105–109.

Tomlinson, T., Howe, K., Notman, M., et al. (1990). An empirical study of proxy consent for elderly persons. *Gerontologist 30,* 54–64.

Wetle, T., Levkoff, S., Cwikel, J., et al. (1988). Nursing home resident participation in medical decisions: Perceptions and preferences. *Gerontologist 28*(Suppl.), 32–38.

Van Stralen, D., & Perkin, R.M. (1995). Do not resuscitate, but do not forget comfort. *Am J Emerg Med 13,* 93–94.

Legal/Ethical Issues

DEFINITION

Ethics is a moral philosophy concerned with right and wrong and the dynamics of decision making. Making a moral decision invovles the common good and the rights and obligations of individuals. Law and ethics have been developed from the same historical, cultural, social, and philosophical beliefs and can be in basic agreement. The law is based on legal principles and ethics on the principles of ethics. However, they may disagree and/or overlap in different ways. Some actions can be legal and ethical or legal and unethical. Other actions are ethical but illegal or unethical and illegal. It is the conflicts that arise between ethical and lawful areas that can be the cause of difficulties. Knowledge and awareness of these issues provides the ACNP with tools to avoid conflicts and assist in the avoidance of ethical dilemmas.

Bioethics, or medical ethics, began as a discipline about 30 years ago with the focus primarily on medicine and the physician. In the intervening years social, cultural, and legal factors have been integrated with the change of focus in medicine from the disease entity to concern for the patient. Moral decision making has become part of the scientific aspects of medicine. The principles of autonomy and justice play a prominent role in the developing philosophy.

Nursing ethics has evolved to meet the unique needs of the nursing profession. A personal ethical framework is necessary in making professional nursing judgments. A firm foundation in the knowledge of nursing ethics is a primary requirement for the ACNP to be an adequate clinical advocate promoting the well-being of patients, family, and society. The Standards of Clinical Practice and Scope of Practice for the Acute Care Nurse Practitioner provides counsel; the ACNP serves as an advocate for the patient and is obliged to demonstrate nonjudgmental and nondiscriminatory attitudes and behaviors that are sensitive to patient diversity. Ethical behavior decreases patient vulnerability. ACNPs work to promote an ethical practice environment and embrace meaningful patient decision making.

REASONS FOR ETHICAL AWARENESS

Health care professionals in the world of modern medicine encounter ethical issues unknown in the past, calling for an increased awareness of ethical principles and guidelines.

1. Advances in modern technology assist not only in healing and saving lives, but also in prolonging lives and delaying the moment of death.
2. The patients' rights movement has given new impetus to who has the right to make health care decisions and the responsibility of health care professionals to respect those rights.
3. Ethical dilemmas arising out of conflicting values and differences of opinion have given rise to an increased number of malpractice cases and court involvement.
4. Ethical dilemmas have not always been solved in the court system but have brought attention to the protection of patients' legal rights and the ethical issues involved. A related issue is that of focusing on medical practice to avoid lawsuits rather than on the best interests of the patient.
5. Institutional goals in the changing health care environment may conflict with the professional goals and values of the caregivers, whose purpose is to provide quality patient care. The change in focus and pace of the hospital environment is necessitating a new approach to care that is multidisciplinary and collaborative and the cause of ethical conflicts and dilemmas.

PRINCIPLES OF APPROACH TO ETHICAL DILEMMAS FOR THE ACNP

The ACNP, as the moral agent in the nurse-patient relationship, can in a systematic way approach ethical situations by reasoning, analyzing, and conceptualizing the various health care dilemmas.

1. Listening, careful assessment, and education are helpful actions in prevention of repeated ethical dilemmas and finding solutions to new ones.
2. The ACNP acknowledges the importance of knowing his/her own personal ethical beliefs and values and their effect on situations and behaviors, knowing everyone wants to act in an ethically appropriate manner.
3. The ACNP should be aware that emotional reaction to a situation, rather than reasoning from an ethical viewpoint, clouds the ethical position.
4. It is important for the ACNP to articulate clearly his/her ethical position and the ethical issues in a conflict situation.

ETHICAL THEORIES

Ethical theories provide data and differing ways to support decision making in circumstances needing alternative solutions in areas of rights and obligations.

1. Theories provide structures needed for discussions leading to choices of action or nonaction, not specific solutions.
2. Several ethical theories, traditional and contemporary, present different perspectives, strengths, and limitations when applied to health care and ethical dilemmas in nursing.
3. Knowledge of these various theories provides the ACNP with information

to respond to questions revolving around the moral issues of what is a right or wrong moral judgment or action.

4. Conflicts between the bioethical standards of nursing and some of the traditional ethical theories do exist. In the development of nursing ethics, some traditional ethical theories will be discarded in favor of theories related to the nursing profession upholding the integrity of the role of the nurse.

5. The professional nurse acts efficiently and with awareness of bioethical standards in the context of nursing.

NURSING ETHICS

1. Nursing ethics is evolving from a background of professional conventions and ethical theories based on duty, goals, rights, and institution to one founded on the unique field of nursing.

2. Some nursing theorists advocate an ethical theory grounded in the nurse-patient relationship.
   A. The concept of care is central to this relationship and has a moral dimension bonding it to the moral and social role of the nursing profession.
   B. Focus on the nurse-patient relationship frees nursing from justifying decisions based on other bioethical theories or codes.
   C. Advanced practice nurses are looking for realistic solutions to problems in practice and how different ethical theories may affect them.

3. The Standards of Clinical Practice and Scope of Practice for the Acute Care Nurse Practitioner states that the ACNP bases decisions and actions on behalf of acutely ill patients consistent with the ANA Code for Nurses with Interpretive Statement (ANA, 1995). The ACNP acknowledges the patients' rights of self-determination. The ACNP respects the patients' dignity, autonomy, cultural beliefs, and privacy.

THE ACNP AS PATIENT ADVOCATE

1. Giving authentic care to patients allows them the freedom to act in a self-determinate way and care for themselves.
   A. The ACNP, as advocate and educator, encourages patients to take responsibility for their health care and supports the decisions they make regarding health care.
   B. Providing information about the nature of the illness and the meaning of treatment assists patients in assessing their situation and helping them be the best they can be.

2. The art of ministering to those wanting care involves the relinquishment of personal control and beliefs and becoming aware of wants of others when respecting another's autonomy.
   A. It does not mean the ACNP must agree with the decisions made by others or that he/she gives up personal beliefs; the nurse also has rights.
   B. The ACNP must have a firm ethical foundation in the role of the nurse practitioner to make sound, justifiable decisions.
   C. In an interpersonal patient relationship, the ACNP will focus on the individual, be open to his/her personal values, and treat him/her appropriately to help fulfill his/her wishes.

3. The ACNP performs a unique role in response to the ethical issues and dilemmas concerned with end-of-life decisions and the role of autonomy.

A. Many of these are major legal issues created in part by advances in modern technology and the doctrine of self-determination.

B. The approach in the ethical inquiry will revolve around the four ethical principles of autonomy, nonmaleficence, beneficence, and justice.

4. ACNPs have a well-defined challenge and evolving role necessitating becoming consciously aware of what they do to others and what others are doing to them. Knowledge of value systems, clinical situations, and expected outcomes affect the decisions made and the approaches taken to problem solving.

5. Nursing ethics must become an integral part of professional nursing to foster effective ethical decision making.

EUTHANASIA AND LEGAL ISSUES

1. Euthanasia has become an openly debated issue in recent years and is not to be confused with other issues and decisions about foregoing life-sustaining treatment or pain relief.

2. The concept of euthanasia is not new, and the renewed interest may be due to the evolving right of self-determination movement prevalent in our present society. According to Peter B. Terry, M.D., several other influential factors include our aging population, fears generated by the uncontrolled use of modern technology in end-of-life situations, patient autonomy and participation in decision making, and an increasing distrust in professional medicine.

3. The pre-Socratic definition of euthanasia was the preparation of a patient for a peaceful death by the physician, to relieve the psychological suffering accompanying the dying process. The current definition of euthanasia followed the discovery of hemlock and other chemicals that became means of causing death.

4. Confusion of the issue results from the many words added to the original concept. These include active and passive, voluntary and involuntary, direct and indirect.

A. A dictionary definition of the word *euthanasia* is an act or way of causing death painlessly, to prevent suffering.

B. The addition of any of the above words changes this original definition and general assumptions are made, increasing the confusion.

5. "Assisted suicide" means one person helping another by providing the means or assisting someone, to kill themselves. Confusion frequently arises when an accurate distinction is not made between the definition of this term and euthanasia. This is seen many times in legislation.

6. Several states have proposed initiatives regarding euthanasia and assisted suicide. Knowledge of current state laws regarding this issue is important. Presently, (1997) they are being constitutionally debated at the Supreme Court level.

7. The American Medical Association, in June 1996, reaffirmed its opposition to "physician-assisted suicide."

ORGAN DONATIONS

1. New proposals to increase organ donations are being considered to enhance the efforts to increase the donation of organs. Education and awareness-of-need strategies have not been successful in increasing the altruistic donation of organs.

2. Two strategies being proposed raise ethical issues and may affect nurses involved in the procuring and transplantation process.
    A. One proposal suggests lifestyle choice be a criterion for selecting candidates for transplant.
    B. The second uses financial incentives rather than continuing the current altruistic plan.
    C. Both concepts at present have raised many questions to which no reasonable or acceptable answers have been found.
3. ACNPs working within this arena are certain to be involved in the strategic discussions concerning organ donation and transplantation.
    A. ACNPs can be helpful in a positive way by documenting the factors that seem to influence and increase the number of families who would be willing to donate organs of loved ones.
    B. ACNPs can also help giving assistance to local organ procurement organizations in their efforts to increase the number of donations.
    C. By continuing to respect the dignity and rights of dying patients and their families, nurses can play a significant role in solving a difficult situation in an ethical manner.

Review Questions

14.11 Which of the following situations describes an ethical behavior or action by an ACNP?
    A. A nurse presenting herself for duty inappropriately dressed and using unprofessional language
    B. It may be against the law *in some states* to withhold or withdraw artificially administered nutrition and hydration, but the ACNP encourages the family to request it
    C. A family member may disagree with the preferences of a loved one but respects the personal health care treatment decisions of the individual and supports his/her right to make them; the ACNP provides comfort and support to the patient and family
    D. An ACNP neglects to keep abreast of ethical issues and has a decreased awareness and ability to reason through situations of ethical conflicts

14.12 The ACNP must be actively involved in ethical decision making because:
    A. Ethical awareness is not important because these issues are taken care of by ethics committees and pastoral representatives
    B. Consumers of health care are more aware of patients rights and the right to make decisions for themselves; ethical dilemmas and conflict will increase in intensity in the future and the ACNP will encounter them with increasing frequency
    C. The advances in medical technology have not created situations unexperienced in the past (i.e., saving lives previously lost, reviving persons from unexpected accidents)
    D. Consumers of health care are less aware of patients rights and the right to make decisions for themselves

14.13 Mr. S, a 52-year-old male, has a family history of extensive heart disease and has suffered two recurrent myocardial Infarctions. He is in medical retirement and describes himself as a cardiac cripple. He is married, with three children. Following his last cardiac arrest and resuscitation in the hospital, he requested nothing further be done in the future. He has discussed this with his family and physician. What role does the ACNP play in this time of changing health care demands and increasing ethical situations?

A. The ACNP may not agree with the decisions of the patient and neglects to support them or recognize the patient's right to make them, having a firm foundation in her role as an ACNP

B. The ACNP is not involved in the ethical decision-making process because it is in the realm of the physician

C. Patients are not educated by the ACNP or given information about the nature of illness and the meaning of treatment

D. The ACNP acts in collaboration with the physician and family and plays a role in encouraging patients to take responsibility for their health care, respecting personal values, focusing on the individual, and helping patients fulfill personal wishes and preferences; the ACNP is supportive of the patient's decisions and a resource for the family for comfort and support

14.14 Mrs. M, age 80, is in long-term care and has no advance directive. She has been maintained on artificial nutrition and hydration for approximately 6 years. Her diagnosis is persistent vegetative state and prognosis is poor. She is unable to make decisions for herself. What ethical principles would the ACNP, in collaboration with the physician, use to help make an end-of-life decision on behalf of this patient?

A. The values and preferences of the patient, if known, are not considered part of the decision-making process

B. This is an easy decision to make; it is a tragedy to continue feeding this patient because there is no hope for her future and no one to speak for her

C. The courts must *always* be involved in the absence of an advance directive, when considering the withholding or withdrawal of food and fluids

D. The four ethical principles to be considered in a case of possible ethical conflicts are autonomy, nonmaleficence, beneficence, and justice

14.15 The 60-year-old out-of-state man in critical care following a craniotomy (described in Review Question 14.9) continued to deteriorate, and he was pronounced "brain dead" on the third day. Children from the first marriage were notified of their father's condition and came to his bedside. End-of-life decisions were imminent. Which of the following describes a solution made in the "best interests" of the patient?

A. Let the ACNP, in collaboration with the physician, make the necessary end-of-life decision to terminate treatment

B. Ask the children and current wife individually what they think the patient would want

C. Schedule a patient care conference including all family members and members of the health care team, ACNP, physician, social worker, and pastoral care to discuss the diagnosis, prognosis, and possible outcomes of the current situation

D. Ignore the situation and hope no legal or ethical conflicts arise

Answers and Rationales

14.11 **C** Confusion may be experienced regarding ethical actions and attitudes. The areas of conflict include the law, value clarification, unprofessional behavior or dress, and using the ethical guidelines of another profession. The law and ethics overlap in various ways and there may be disagreement; however, what is ethical may not be against the law and what is lawful may be unethical. The patient has the legal right to make personal health care choices regarding medical treatment. Ethical actions by the ACNP ensure respect and protection of a patient's rights. ACNPs have responsibility to the patient, relative to the nurse-patient relationship, to be a loyal advocate for him/her. Comfort and support may be provided to the family members in a compassionate manner.

14.12 **B** Modern technology advances have increased situations and occasions for ethical and legal conflicts. The patients' right movement has increased the health care consumer's knowledge of patients rights and the responsibility of health care providers to respect them. Nurses have encountered and will continue to encounter ethical dilemmas of increasing intensity in the future. An increased awareness of ethical guidelines and principles and knowledge of nursing ethics are tools the professional nurse will use to identify ethical issues in nursing and justify decisions in an intelligent manner.

14.13 **D** The role of patient advocate mandated by the nurse-patient relationship obligates the nurse to provide authentic care to promote self-determination and freedom to act. Advocating and encouraging patients to take personal responsibility for health care is an integral part of the education process. Open, truthful, and continuous communication concerning relevant facts, risks, and benefits provides a firm base for self-determination and well-being. A patient who has sufficient knowledge of the risks and outcomes of treatment is better prepared to make health care decisions. The role of the ACNP includes respecting these decisions and assisting the patient in the fulfillment of personal wishes and preferences. A firm foundation in the ACNP role supports loyalty to one's own rights and the patient's own rights to make decisions.

14.14 **D** Common sense is a hallmark of good decisions. Caution is to be exercised when the end-of-life decision-making process is unfolding. The ACNP, in collaboration with the physician, family member, or proxy, will play a unique role in the decision-making process for a patient without an advance directive using the standard of substituted judgment or "best interest." The advances in medical technology and patient autonomy present a challenge that encourages ACNPs to become consciously aware of what they do to others. Knowledge of a patient's value systems, clinical situations, and expected outcomes affects the decision-making process. Awareness of the laws of the state and the policies of the institution concerning the withholding and withdrawing of life-sustaining measure is imperative. There may be no satisfactory outcome. Making an ethical decision is not always easy. The ACNP, in collaboration with the physician in consultation with family members or friends, appoints a spokesperson for the individual to act in the "best interests" of the individual.

14.15 **C** The presence of an advance directive in this case would provide the guidelines for the care and treatment the man desired. It would outline the wishes and preferences in the event of incapability to make decisions. If there is no advance directive, a surrogate decision maker will be chosen from among family members. The laws of the state of Illinois will supersede those of the state of California, especially in the area of artificial administration of food and fluid. The professional staff, to decrease the possibility of legal and ethical conflicts, will give consideration, comfort, and support to the wishes of the spouse and children. Thoughtfulness regarding their cultural and religious beliefs and a systematic way of approaching ethical issues can be attained by listening, careful assessment, and education. Good communication and documentation are the essence of avoiding ethical and legal conflicts in any situation involving end-of-life decisions.

References

American Nurses Association and the American Association of Critical-Care Nurses. (1995). *Standards of Clinical Practice and Scope of Practice for the Acute Care Nurse Practitioner.* Washington, DC: American Nurses Publishing, p. 15.

Bandman, E.L., & Bandman, B. (1990). *Nursing Ethics Through the Life Span* (3rd ed.). Norwalk, CT: Appleton & Lange.

Benjamin, M., & Curtis, J. (1992). *Ethics in Nursing.* New York: Oxford University Press.

Bishop, A.H., & Scudder, J.R., Jr. (1996). *Nursing Ethics.* Boston: Jones and Bartlett Publishers.

Davis, A.J., & Aroskar, M.A. (1991). *Ethical Dilemmas and Nursing Practice* (3rd ed.). Norwalk, CT: Appleton & Lange.

Deloughery, G.L. (1991). *Ethical influences on nursing.* In G.L. Deloughery (ed.). *Issues and Trends in Nursing.* St. Louis: Mosby/Year Book, (pp. 177–216).

Husted, G.L., & Husted, J.H. (1995). *Ethical Decision Making in Nursing.* St. Louis: C.V. Mosby Co.

Singer, P.A., & Siegler, M. (1990). Euthanasia—a critique. *N Engl J Med 26,* 1881–1883.

Terry, P.B. (1995). Euthanasia and assisted suicide. *Mayo Clin Proc 70,* 189–192.

Additional Recommended References

Almgren, G. (1993). Living will legislation, nursing home care, and the rejection of artificial nutrition and hydration: An analysis of bedside decision-making in three states. *J Health Social Policy 4* (3), 43–63.

Davis, A.J. (1982). Helping your staff address ethical dilemmas. *J Nurs Admin February* 9–12.

Dupre, L. (1990) Ethical dilemmas in the health care trenches. *Bioethics Rationing, May/June* 11–13, 15, 17.

Emanuel, E.J. (1988). A review of the ethical and legal aspects of terminating medical care. *Am J Med 84,* 291–301.

Emanual, E.J., & Emanual, L.L. (1992). Proxy decision making for incompetent patients. *JAMA 267,* 2067–2071.

Jecker, N.S. (1990). The role of intimate others in medical decision making. *Gerontologist 30*, 65–71.

Sachs, G.A., Stocking, C.B., & Miles, S.H. (1992). Empowerment of the older patient? A randomized, controlled trial to increase discussion and use of advance directives. *J Am Geriatr Soc 40*, 269–273.

Siwek, J. (ed.). (1994). Decision-making in terminal care: four common pitfalls. *Am Fam Physician 50*, 1207–1211.

Richter, K.P., Langel, S., Fawcett, S.B., et al. (1993). Promoting the use of advance directives. An empirical study. *Arch Fam Med 4*, 609–615.

CHAPTER 15

Roles, Issues, Policies, and Trends

Diana I. G. Lithgow, RN, MSN, FNP
Ruth M. Kleinpell, RN, PhD, CS-ACNP, CCRN

Acute Care Nurse Practitioner Role

DEFINITION

The Acute Care Nurse Practitioner (ACNP) is skilled, knowledgeable, and proficient in a designated area of advanced nursing practice. Professional activities that promote the ACNP as an expert include advanced skills in clinical practice and participation in aspects of education, collaboration, and research. Additional activities such as publishing, public speaking, involvement in professional nursing organizations, and interdisciplinary consultation provide the ACNP with many avenues for achieving recognition as a professional in advanced practice.

The American Nurses Association (ANA) defines advanced clinical practice as that which includes graduate education with expanded knowledge in a specialty area of practice. The mission of advanced practice nursing is to provide expert-quality comprehensive care to clients. Identified roles in advanced practice nursing include nurse practitioners, clinical nurse specialists, certified nurse midwifes, and certified registered nurse anesthetists. The ACNP functions in a nurse practitioner role in caring for acute and chronically ill clients.

ACNP ROLE DEVELOPMENT

History of the Role

The evolution of advanced nursing practice was based on the need for expert nursing care in the clinical setting. The role of the nurse practitioner developed in the early 1960s as a result of physician shortages in the area of pediatrics. The first nurse practitioner program was a pediatric nurse practitioner program begun in 1964 by Dr. Loretta Ford and Dr. Henry Silver at the University of Colorado Health Sciences Center in Denver, Colorado.

Growth of nurse practitioner programs soon ensued, with distribution of nurse practitioners in various practice settings with an emphasis on ambulatory and outpatient care. The historical service of nurse practitioners in primary care resulted in part from the availability of federal funding for preventative and primary care nurse practitioner education. Movement of nurse practitioners to the inpatient setting resulted from collaborative partnerships and the need for advanced practitioners to focus on direct patient care.

Neonatal nurse practitioners, who care for acute and critically ill neonates, were a prototype for the ACNP in the critical care arena. The ACNP role evolved to meet the need for an advanced practitioner to care for clients in acute and critical care settings in the hospital setting. The role has expanded as a result of managed care, hospital restructuring, and decreases in medical residency programs. The ACNP now practices in a variety of settings, including tertiary and secondary health care centers.

Growth of ACNP Programs

In 1993, the first Acute Care Nurse Practitioner Consensus Conference was held in Boston to draft standards for educational programs preparing ACNPs. Nine ACNP college- and university-affiliated programs existed, with an additional four in development. In 1994, there were 11 programs with an additional 7 in development. Currently, there are over 63 educational programs nationwide that prepare ACNPs either at the master's or postmaster's level (American Association of Critical Care Nurses, 1996; American College of Nursing, 1997).

Types of Roles

Four distinct roles for the ACNP include expert clinician, consultant/collaborator, educator, and researcher.
1. ACNP as clinician: Provides direct care, manages care, interprets and integrates data for directing patient care.
   A. Clinical expertise—The ACNP:
      1) Integrates care across acute care continuum
      2) Has accountability and authority for patient outcomes
      3) Performs interventions that are restorative, rehabilitative, or maintenance
      4) Performs all aspects of health assessment:
         a. Health history and risk appraisal
         b. Physical and mental status examination
         c. Interpretation of diagnostic studies
         d. Psychosocial assessment
         e. Disease prevention
         f. Discharge planning
         g. Family assessment
      5) Integrates data to make clinical judgments and decisions about appropriate treatments in managing acute and chronic illness and promote wellness
      6) Prescribes interventions to achieve expected outcomes
      7) Utilizes organizational resources to formulate a multidisciplinary plan of care
      8) Maintains current knowledge in advanced nursing practice
   B. Clinical protocols: The ACNP utilizes clinical practice protocols to structure patient care. The ACNP:
      1) Follows established protocols and guidelines in providing patient care

2) Is involved in revising existing protocols/guidelines to reflect accepted changes in patient care management

3) Develops new protocols to address emerging care problems

C. Clinical privileges: Seeking practice privileges to perform independent advanced medical skills enables ACNPs to expand their practice base within a designated setting. Issues for the ACNP to consider include:

1) Individual state practice acts may dictate the realm of independent practice for the ACNP.

2) Levels of supervision (the degree of supervision required from physician/other practitioner for clinical functions performed) may need to be established for the ACNP.

3) Existing policies may designate which clinical procedures/functions the ACNP may perform.

4) A collaborating physician is usually needed when applying for medical practice privileges.

5) A log demonstrating successful completion of procedures and established technique may be required when petitioning for privileges.

6) Annual competencies may need to be performed to ensure proficiency in privileged skills.

7) Audits of compliance to practice standards may be conducted and evaluated for renewal of practice privileges.

2. ACNP as consultant/collaborator: Engages in shared planning and action to attain desired patient goals. As a consultant/collaborator, the ACNP:

A. Utilizes professional knowledge, experience, and skills

B. Effectively communicates

C. Participates in patient care decision making

D. Enlists other health care professionals in planning and evaluating patient care

E. Makes referrals, including provisions for continuity of care, as needed

F. Consults/collaborates with the patient, significant others, and other health care providers to provide coordinated, multidisciplinary care

G. Engages in both informal (giving advise/providing knowledge based on personal and professional expertise) and formal (contracted services) consultation

H. Can participate in internal (within the work setting) and external (outside the work environment) consultation

I. Provides direction for a variety of consultive services ranging from advocate to information expert

3. ACNP as educator: Teaches in many capacities to a variety of audiences. The ACNP:

A. Participates in the education of clients and their family members, nursing staff, and other members of the health care team

B. Performs teaching activities to promote, maintain, and improve health and prevent illness and injury

C. Fosters a learning environment when mentoring and precepting students and medical residents

D. Utilizes knowledge of the learning process/learning theories in assessing the learner and developing teaching strategies

E. Evaluates teaching effectiveness and aims to improve teaching skills based on feedback

F. Acquires and maintains current knowledge in advanced practice nursing

4. ACNP as researcher: Uses the research process to create improvement in patient care. Knowledge of the steps in the research process facilitates participation in and critique of research.
   A. Major steps in the research process
      1) Formulating the research problem
      2) Reviewing related literature
      3) Formulating the hypotheses
      4) Selecting the research design
      5) Identifying the population to be studied
      6) Specifying methods of data collection
      7) Designing the study
      8) Conducting the study
      9) Analyzing the data
      10) Interpreting the results
      11) Communicating the findings
   B. Types of research
      1) Nonexperimental: Includes two broad categories: descriptive research and ex post facto/correlational research. Descriptive research aims to describe situations, experiences, and phenomena as they exist. Ex post facto or correlational research examines relationships among variables.
      2) Experimental: Includes experimental manipulation of variables utilizing randomization and a control group to test the effects of an intervention or experiment. Quasi-experimental research involves manipulation of variables but lacks a comparison group or randomization.
      3) Qualitative: Includes case studies, open-ended questions, field studies, participant observation, and ethnographic studies, where observations and interview techniques are used to explore phenomena through detailed descriptions of people, events, situations, or observed behavior.
   C. The role of the ACNP in research includes:
      1) Identifies research problems
      2) Participates in the research process, including serving as investigator, project manager, data collector, or consultant
      3) Critically evaluates research for use in practice, including establishing clinical relevance, scientific merit, and implementation potential
      4) Uses the research utilization process to evaluate and integrate research into practice
      5) Uses research findings in the development of policies, procedures, and guidelines for client care
      6) Participates in research dissemination

PROMOTING PROFESSIONAL PRACTICE

1. Publishing in nursing: The communication of information through writing advances the profession and establishes the ACNP as an expert clinician and advanced practice professional. Opportunities for publishing include:
   A. Nursing journal articles
   B. Medical journal articles
   C. Interdisciplinary journal articles
   D. Lay publications

    E. Association newsletters
    F. Education materials
    G. Books and periodicals
    H. Newspapers, other print and electronic media
2. Public speaking: The ACNP can further communicate clinical expertise via oral and written presentations. Opportunities include:
    A. Poster presentations at professional meetings/conferences
    B. Oral presentations at professional meetings/conferences
    C. Speaking engagements for interdisciplinary, community, and public events
    D. Participation in education days, health fairs
    E. Testimony at public/government hearings
3. Professional organizations: The ACNP can advance in a career trajectory through involvement in professional organizations. Opportunities include:
    A. Holding office
    B. Committee work
    C. Advisory groups
    D. Expert panels
4. Outcomes analysis: The ACNP:
    A. Evaluates the effectiveness of the role, including:
        1) Patient outcomes (may include but not limited to achieving goals of therapy, decreasing morbidity/mortality, decreasing complications, increasing patient satisfaction, increasing functional status—as described below)
        2) Nursing staff and physician satisfaction
        3) Peer review
        4) Patient variance analysis
        5) Performance appraisal/self-audit
    B. Monitors the outcomes of care, including:
        1) Length of stay
        2) Morbidity/mortality statistics
        3) Rehospitalizations
        4) Physical functioning
        5) Health status
        6) Psychosocial status
        7) Return to work
        8) Quality of life
        9) Patient satisfaction
        10) Costs of care
        11) Side effects
        12) Complication rates
        13) Patient safety
        14) Symptom management and control

Review Questions

15.1 Advanced clinical nursing practice:
    A. Includes nurses with advanced knowledge and skill
    B. Is defined as the provision of expert-quality nursing care

C. Incorporates a variety of practice settings where advanced nursing care is given
D. Is designated as care provided by a nurse with graduate education and expertise in a specialty area of practice

15.2 Practice arenas for the ACNP:
A. Are primarily in hospital ICU settings
B. Have expanded to include tertiary and secondary settings
C. Involve collaborative arrangements with physician groups
D. Are restricted to acute and critically ill areas

15.3 The ACNP as clinician:
A. Performs all aspects of health assessment and management
B. Provides substitutive care traditionally given by physicians
C. Is required to obtain clinical privileges before practicing
D. Must be supervised by a physician

15.4 The ACNP's role in research:
A. Is primarily involved in assisting with data collection, for practical reasons
B. Involves both identifying potential research problems and evaluating research use in practice
C. Is limited because patient care concerns are a priority
D. Involves only the process of research utilization practice

15.5 The focus of outcomes analysis for the ACNP:
A. Should be on tracking survival and costs of treatment
B. Should be compared to physician care to establish the effectiveness of the role
C. Includes both performance appraisal and patient outcomes of care
D. Should be predominantly concerned with complications that occur during treatment

---

Answers and Rationales

15.1   **D**   Advanced practice nursing is defined as that which includes graduate education with expanded knowledge in a specialty area of practice. Identified roles in advanced practice nursing include nurse practitioners, clinical nurse specialists, certified nurse midwifes, and certified registered nurse anesthestists.

15.2   **B**   ACNP practice settings have expanded to include a variety of settings, such as acute and critical care, ambulatory settings, subacute care, emergency, collaborative practice, and numerous other settings where advanced skills and knowledge in care of acute and chronic illness is needed.

15.3   **A**   The ACNP provides all aspects of health assessment in the management of acute and chronic illness. Obtaining clinical privileges enables the ACNP to independently perform a variety of advanced skills and procedures, but clinical privileges are not required for all practice settings.

15.4 **B** The ACNP's role in research includes participating in all phases of the research process, research evaluation and critique, research utilization, and research dissemination.

15.5 **C** Measuring the outcome of care given by the ACNP involves assessing the performance of the ACNP and the effect of care on patients. Monitoring outcomes such as survival and costs are just one facet of outcomes analysis.

References

Acute Care Consensus Conference. (1993). Standards for educational programs: Preparing students as acute care nurse practitioners. *AACN Clin Issues Crit Care Nurs 4,* 593–589.

American Association of Critical Care Nurses. (1995). *Advanced Practice Nursing: Key Messages and Action Strategies.* Aliso Viejo, CA: American Association of Critical Care Nurses.

American Association of Critical Care Nurses. (1996). *Graduate Nursing Programs.* Aliso Viejo, CA: American Association of Critical Care Nurses.

American College of Nursing. (1997). *Peterson's Guide to Nursing Programs: Baccalaureate and Graduate Nursing Education in the U.S. and Canada.* Princeton, NJ: Peterson's Guides Inc.

American Nurses Association. (1995). *Standards of Clinical Practice and Scope of Practice for the Acute Care Nurse Practitioner.* Washington, DC: American Nurses Publishing.

American Nurses Association. (1996). *Scope and Standards of Advanced Practice Registered Nursing.* Washington, DC: American Nurses Association.

Champagne, M., Tornquist, E., & Funk, S. (1996). Research use in advanced practice nursing. In J. Hickey, R. Ouimette, & S. Venegon (eds.). *Advanced Practice Nursing—Changing Roles and Clinical Applications.* Philadelphia: Lippincott-Raven, 213–224.

Clancy, G., & Maguire, D. (1995). Advanced practice nursing in the neonatal intensive care unit. *Crit Care Nurs Clin North Am 7*(1), 71–76.

Gawlinski, A. (1995). Practice protocols development and use. *Crit Care Nurs Clin North Am 7*(1), 17–23.

Hampton, J., & Snyder, M. (1995). Research. In M. Snyder, & M. Mirr (eds.). *Advanced Practice Nursing—A Guide to Professional Development.* New York: Springer-Verlag, pp. 241–252.

Hickey, J. (1996). Reformation of healthcare and implications for advanced nursing practice. In J. Hickey, R. Ouimette, & S. Venegoni (eds.). *Advanced Practice Nursing—Changing Roles and Clinical Applications.* Philadelphia: Lippincott-Raven, pp. 3–21.

Hilgart, C., & Karl, M. (1995). Developing clinical protocols and guidelines for APN practice. In M. Snyder & M. Mirr (eds.). *Advanced Practice Nursing—A Guide to Professional Development.* New York: Springer-Verlag, 93–102.

Hravnak, M., Rosenzweig, M., & Baldisseri, M. (1996). Current questions with regard to acute care nurse practitioner preparation and role implementation. *AACN Clin Issues Adv Pract Acute Crit Care 7,* 289–299.

Ingersoll, G. (1995). Evaluation of the advanced practice nurse role in acute and specialty care. *Crit Care Nurs Clin North Am 7*(1), 25–34.

Keane, A., Richmond, T., & Kaiser, L. (1994). Critical care nurse practitioners: Evolution of the advanced practice nursing role. *Am J Crit Care 3,* 232–237.

King, K., Parrinello, K., & Baggs, J. (1996). Collaboration and advanced practice nursing. In J. Hickey, R. Ouimette, & S. Venegoni (eds.). *Advanced Practice Nurs-*

ing—Changing Roles and Clinical Applications. Philadelphia: Lippincott-Raven, pp. 146–162.

Kleinpell, R. (1996). A new role for critical care nursing: The acute care nurse practitioner. *Dimensions Crit Care Nurs 15*(3), 168.

Kleinpell, R. (1997). Acute care nurse practitioners: Roles and practice profiles. *AACN Clin Issues Adv Pract Acute Crit Care, 8,*(1), 156–162.

Kleinpell, R. (in press). Acute care nurse practitioners. Reports from the practice setting. In R. Kleinspell, M. Piano (eds). *Practice Issues for the Acute Practitioner.* New York: Springer.

Kyle, M. (1995). Collaboration. In M. Snyder & M. Mirr (eds.). *Advanced Practice Nursing—A Guide to Professional Development.* New York: Springer-Verlag, pp. 169–182.

Mirr, M. (1993). Advanced clinical practice: A reconceptualized role. *AACN Clin Issues Crit Care Nurs 4*, 599–602.

Mirr, M. (1995). Evaluation the effectiveness of advanced practice. In M. Snyder & M. Mirr (eds.). *Advanced Practice Nursing—A Guide to Professional Development.* New York: Springer-Verlag, pp. 153–168.

Monicken, D. (1995). Consultation in advanced practice nursing. In M. Snyder & M. Mirr (eds.). *Advanced Practice Nursing—A Guide to Professional Development.* New York: Springer-Verlag, pp. 197–214.

Parrinello, K. (1995). Advanced practice nursing. *Crit Care Nurs Clin North Am 7*(1), 9–16.

Polit, D., & Hungler, B. (1995). *Nursing Research: Principles and Methods.* Philadelphia: J.B. Lippincott Company.

Snyder, M. (1995). Professional communication: Publishing and public speaking. In M. Snyder & M. Mirr (eds.). *Advanced Practice Nursing—A Guide to Professional Development.* New York: Springer-Verlag, pp. 215–218.

Additional Recommended References

Ackerman, M., Norsen, L., Martin, B., et al. (1996). Development of a model of advanced practice. *Am J Crit Care 5*, 68–73.

Clochesy, J., Daly, B., Idemoto, B., et al. (1994). Preparing advanced practice nurses for acute care. *Am J Crit Care 3*, 255–259.

DeNicola, L., Kleid, D., Brink, L., et al. (1994). Use of pediatric physician extenders in pediatric and neonatal intensive care units. *Crit Care Med 22*, 1856–1865.

El-Sherif, C. (1995). Nurse practitioners—where do they belong within the organizational structure of the acute care setting? *Nurse Pract 20*(1), 62–65.

Frik, S., & Pollock, S. (1993). Preparation for advanced nursing practice. *Nurs Health Care 14*, 190–195.

Gaedeke, M., & Blount, K. (1995). Advanced practice nursing in pediatric acute care. *Crit Care Nurs Clin North Am 7*(1), 61–70.

Genet, C., Brennan, P., Ibbotson-Wolff, S., et al. (1995). Nurse practitioners in a teaching hospital. *Nurse Pract 20*(9), 47–54.

Giacalone, M., Mullaney, D., DeJoseph, D., et al. (1995). Development of a nurse-managed unit and the advanced practitioner role. *Crit Care Nurs Clin North Am 7*(1), 35–41.

Hravnak, M., Kovert, S., Risco, K., et al. (1995). Acute care nurse practitioner curriculum: Content and development process. *Am J Crit Care 4*, 179–188.

Kelso, L., & Massaro, L. (1994). Implementation of the acute care nurse practitioner role. *AACN Clin Issues Crit Care Nurs 5*, 404–407.

Keough, V., Jennrich, J., Holm, K., et al. (1996). A collaborative program for advanced practice in trauma/critical care nursing. *Crit Care Nurse 16*, 120–127.

Kindig, D., & Libby, D. (1994). How will graduate medical education reform affect specialties and geographic areas? *JAMA 272*, 37–42.

King, K., & Ackerman, M. (1995). An educational model for the acute care nurse practitioner. *Crit Care Nurs Clin North Am 7*(1), 1–8.

Piano, M., Kleinpell, R., & Johnson, J. (1996). The acute care nurse practitioner and management of common health problems: A proposal. *Am J Crit Care 5*, 289–292.

Richmond, T., & Keane, A. (1992). The nurse practitioner in tertiary care. *J Nurs Admin 22*(11), 11–12.

Richmond, T., & Keane, A. (1996). Acute care nurse practitioners. In J. Hickey, R. Ouimette, & S. Venegoni (eds.). *Advanced Practice Nursing—Changing Roles and Clinical Applications.* Lippincott-Raven.

Rudissil, P. (1995). Unit-based advanced practice nurse in critical care. *Crit Care Nurs Clin North Am 7*(1), 53–59.

Shah, H., Sullivan, D., Lattanzio, J., et al. (1993). Preparing acute care nurse practitioners at the University of Connecticut. *AACN Clin Issues Crit Care Nurs 4*, 625–629.

Snyder, J., Sirio, C., Angus, D., et al. (1994). Trial of nurse practitioners in intensive care. *New Horizons 2*, 296–304.

Vaska, P. (1993). The clinical nurse specialist in cardiovascular surgery: A new twist. *AACN Clin Issues Crit Care Nurs 4*, 637–644.

Watts, R., Hanson, M., Burke, K., et al. (1996). The critical care nurse practitioner: An advanced practice role for the critical care nurse. *Dimensions Crit Care Nurs 15*(1), 48–56.

Professionalism in Advanced Practice

THE NURSE PRACTITIONER ROLE

1. A nurse practitioner is:
   A. A registered nurse with advanced skills, education, and training in a health care specialty
   B. Responsible for the outcomes of her/his practice as an independently licensed provider
   C. Prepared with training and competency standards that include the diagnosis and management of common acute illnesses, disease prevention, health promotion, and management of stable, chronic illness
2. Specialty certifications as a nurse practitioner are growing, with acute care nurse practitioner as the most recent addition to the list.
3. What distinguishes nurse practitioners from other primary care providers is a focus on wellness and illness prevention from a holistic perspective and within the context of family and community.
4. Working with families and people of all ages, acute care nurse practitioners provide many of the same overlapping health care services as physicians:
   A. Performing physical examinations
   B. Performing routine procedures (i.e., insertion or placement of venous/arterial access ports and tubes, wound suturing, etc.)
   C. Ordering diagnostic tests and evaluations
   D. Treating illnesses
   E. Prescribing medications and therapies
   F. Patient education

5. Numerous studies conclude that nurse practitioners perform as well as physicians in diagnosis, management of specific conditions, and health care outcomes within their scope of practice (Safriet, 1992).
6. In 1991, the ANA defined advanced nursing practice:

> *Nurses in advanced clinical nursing practice have a graduate degree in nursing. They conduct comprehensive health assessments and demonstrate a high level of autonomy, they . . . integrate education, research, management, leadership and consultation into their clinical role. . . .*

NURSE PRACTITIONER KNOWLEDGE BASE

The 1996 American Association of Colleges of Nursing's *The Essentials of Master's Education for Advanced Practice Nursing* was developed by a national task force to establish consistency and professional standards for nurse practitioner education.

1. Core curriculum content for all nurse practitioner (NP) programs includes:
   A. Research: To prepare for the utilization of new knowledge to provide high-quality health care, initiate change, and improve nursing practice.
   B. Health Care Policy, Financing and Organization: In an environment with ongoing changes in the organization and financing of health care, it is imperative that all graduates of master's degree nursing programs have a keen understanding of this area.
   C. Ethics: Expanding health technologies and increasing demands for cost containment have emphasized the need for ethical decision making by all health care professionals.
   D. Professional Role Development: To provide the student with a clear understanding of the nursing profession, advanced practice nursing roles, the requirements for and regulation of these roles.
   E. Theoretical Foundations of Nursing Practice: The graduate should be prepared to critique, evaluate, and utilize appropriate theory within his/her practice.
   F. Human Diversity and Social Issues: Global awareness is necessary to provide culturally sensitive care. The social issues of domestic violence, abuse, drugs, and racism, among others, must be part of the health care providers' concerns and awareness for holistic care.
   G. Health Promotion and Disease Prevention: Personal, clinical, community-based interventions that influence the goal of achieving health and preventing illness.
   H. Advanced Practice Nursing Core: Advanced health/physical assessment, advanced physiology and pathophysiology, advanced pharmacology.
   I. Clinical Experiences: Direct client care to individuals, families, and/or communities.
2. Elements of nurse practitioner competencies
   A. Domain 1: Management of client health illness status (e.g., provides health promotion, disease prevention, anticipatory guidance and counseling regarding wellness, lifestyle, and disease risks; diagnoses and manages acute and chronic diseases while attending to the illness experience)

B. Domain 2: Nurse-client relationship (e.g., creates a relationship that acknowledges the client's strengths and assists the client in addressing his/her needs; applies principles of self-efficacy/empowerment in promoting behavior change in clients and their families)

C. Domain 3: The teaching-coaching function (e.g., assesses client's motivation for learning and maintenance of health-related activities using principles of change theory; assists clients in learning specific information or skills by designing a learning plan that is composed of sequential, cumulative steps)

D. Domain 4: Professional role (e.g., functions in a variety of role dimensions—health care provider, consultant, educator, administrator, researcher; interprets and markets the nurse practitioner role to the public and other health care professions)

E. Domain 5: Managing and negotiating health care delivery systems (e.g., provides case management services to meet multiple client health care needs; acts as a community consultant in the planning, development, and implementation of public and community health programs)

F. Domain 6: Monitoring and ensuring the quality of health care practice (e.g., incorporates professional/legal standards into practice; develops a base for personal ethics in practice as related to client issues and the professional code)

CREDENTIALING

1. Licensure

   A process by which an agency of the state government grants permission to individuals accountable for the practice of a profession to engage in the practice of that profession and prohibits all others from legally doing so. It permits use of a particular title. Its purpose is to protect the public by ensuring a minimum level of professional competence. (ANA, 1979)

2. Certification

   A process by which a non-governmental agency or association certifies that an individual licensed to practice as a professional has met certain predetermined standards specified by that profession for specialty practice. Its purpose is to assure the public that an individual has mastered a body of knowledge and acquired skills in a particular specialty. (ANA, 1979)

3. Certifying bodies
   A. The American Nurses Credentialing Center (ANCC) has offered certification exams for nurses since 1973. Certification is reserved for those nurses who have met requirements for clinical or functional practice standards. The nurse practitioner certification is offered in seven specialties:
      1) Adult nurse practitioner
      2) Family nurse practitioner
      3) School nurse practitioner
      4) Pediatric nurse practitioner
      5) Gerontological nurse practitioner
      6) Clinical specialist in psychiatric and mental health nursing
      7) Acute care nurse practitioner

B. The ANCC now offers certification exams for acute care nurse practitioners.
C. Other certifying bodies of nurse practitioners do not offer the acute care nurse practitioner specialty as yet.

PROFESSIONAL ORGANIZATIONS

1. Purpose of professional organizations
   A. Enhance the profession through education and improving the health care system through involvement in legislative issues
   B. Promote a strong nurse practitioner communication system
   C. Strengthen the public image of nurse practitioners
   D. Support legislative action that encourages the development of the nurse practitioner role and makes the health care system more responsive to the needs of the consumer
   E. Provide a collective voice for promoting and supporting key health care issues
   F. Monitor and influence laws and regulations that affect nurse practitioner practice and scope of care
   G. May design and coordinate studies of practice issues
   H. Establish standards for practice by which others are measured
2. Multiple-level organizational membership will give depth to acute care nurse practitioner knowledge of practice issues.
   A. National professional organizations (e.g., American Academy of Nurse Practitioners, American College of Nurse Practitioners, American Nurses Association)
   B. State nurse practitioner professional organizations
   C. Specialty nurse practitioner professional organization (e.g., American Association of Critical Care Nurses)

Review Questions

15.6 The primary distinction between advanced practice nurses and other primary care providers is:
   A. The ability to care for the entire family
   B. The focus on wellness and illness prevention
   C. Prescriptive authority
   D. The ability to integrate education, research, management leadership, and consultation into their clinical role

15.7 Documented benefits of acute care nurse practitioners functioning in the inpatient setting include all of the following *except:*
   A. Decreased medical complications
   B. Increased patient/family satisfaction
   C. Fewer hospital admissions
   D. Decreased lengths of hospital stay

15.8 The first nurse practitioner program was developed in Colorado and focused on:
   A. Rural health care of the poor
   B. Pediatric well-child care

    C. Expanding the knowledge base of traditional nursing to the master's level

    D. Overlapping with medical care in an independent role

15.9 Licensure refers to:

    A. Granting permission to use a specific title

    B. Prohibiting those not licensed from engaging in the practice of that profession

    C. The process by which a governmental agency ensures minimum levels of professional competence

    D. All of the above

15.10 Certification is:

    A. Basically the same as licensure

    B. Not necessary in all states to practice as a nurse practitioner

    C. The process by which a governmental agency evaluates individuals to be sure they have mastered the body of knowledge in that particular specialty

    D. All of the above

Answers and Rationales

15.6 **B** The focus on wellness and illness prevention are the hallmark characteristics of nurse practitioners as opposed to other providers.

15.7 **C** Fewer hospital admissions is not a documented outcome of acute care nurse practitioner interventions.

15.8 **B** Pediatric well-child care was in short supply in the 1960s, when it was suggested that specially trained nurses could fill the void.

15.9 **D** All of these characteristics apply to licensure.

15.10 **B** Certification is not mandatory in all states to practice as a nurse practitioner; however, the majority do require this.

References

American Association of Colleges of Nursing. (1996). *The Essentials of Master's Education for Advanced Practice Nursing.* Washington, DC: American Association of Colleges of Nursing.

American Nurses Association. (1991). *Nursing's Agenda for Health Care Reform. Advanced Practice Nurses: An Innovation for Primary Care.* Kansas City, MO: American Nurses Association.

American Nurses Association. (1979). *The Study of Credentialing in Nursing: A New Approach.* Kansas City, MO: American Nurses Association.

Safriet, B.J. (1992). Health care dollars and regulatory sense: The role of advanced practice nursing. *Yale J Regulation 9,* 417–487.

Health Policy

National and international health policy affects the roles of advanced practice nurses. Many organizations and institutions synthesize trends, data, and practice standards to formulate our country's health policy. The actions and published works of some of those organizations influence the nurse practitioner role in our country's health care system. This section reviews pertinent actions and publications in the 1990s.

1990: HEALTHY PEOPLE 2000

1. The World Health Organization put forward the objective of all persons to obtain a level of health by the year 2000 that will allow them to live socially and economically productive lives.
2. The objectives focused on care: Equal access, acceptability, availability, continuity, cost, and quality.

1991: NURSING'S AGENDA FOR HEALTH CARE REFORM

1. In this American Nurses Association document, advanced practice nurses were identified and supported as the innovative provider of primary care that needed to be promoted.
2. The agenda content included:
    A. Primary care and how advanced practice nurses (APNs) fit the qualifications
    B. Studies reflecting lower costs when utilizing advanced practice nurses
    C. Categories of advanced practice nurses, with educational requirements, salary ranges, areas of specialization in practice, and the number currently in active practice
    D. Comparisons and studies documenting advance practice nurses' high quality of care
    E. APNs' practice setting flexibility and availability in schools, hospitals, corporate/industrial sites, community health centers, correctional facilities, health maintenance organizations, hospices, private practices, and homes

1991: HEALTHY AMERICA: PRACTITIONERS FOR 2005, AN AGENDA FOR ACTION FOR U.S. HEALTH PROFESSIONAL SCHOOLS

The Pew Commission (Shugars et al., 1991) stated that access to primary care was limited or nonexistent because of:

1. Patients' lack of health insurance and/or ability to pay for themselves
2. Reduced provider availability in rural areas
3. Lack of choice of providers

These issues could be addressed by increased numbers of nurse practitioners, increased funding to educate primary care providers more economically, and increased NP programs offering incentives to rural locations after graduation.

1992: "HEALTH CARE DOLLARS AND REGULATORY SENSE: THE ROLE OF ADVANCED PRACTICE NURSING"

As an attorney outside the health care system, Barbara Safriet's (1992) article had tremendous impact. She outlined three areas of barriers and restrictions of the nurse practitioner's practice that prevented the effective utilization of the profession in the health care system.

1. Scope of practice barriers were primarily due to the wide variety of laws and regulations in the many states' nurse practice acts.
   A. Limitations of practice setting.
   B. Frequent dependence on physicians.
   C. Improper compositions of the nursing regulatory bodies.
   D. Frequent direct restrictions on the scope of practice was widespread from state to state.
2. Common practice barriers to prescribing were identified.
   A. Authority to prescribe drugs, devices, and treatments varied greatly from state to state.
   B. Inconsistent site restrictions.
   C. Limitations on types and class of drugs.
   D. Physician and pharmacist resistance.
3. Third-party reimbursement restrictions.
   A. Inconsistent reimbursement rules apply for different specialties.
   B. Practice setting limitations on ability to be reimbursed.
   C. State and federal regulations often do not match in the area of reimbursement.
   D. No mandate requires private insurance companies to recognize the nurse practitioner as a provider.

Safriet called for national and state legislation and regulatory changes that would remove the above barriers to practice for advanced practice nurses and thereby immediately improve the efficiency of the health care system and utilization of the health care dollar.

1992: HEALTH CARE REFORM AGENDA

The 1992 elections set off a national debate about health care reform and the role of the government in health care policy. Nurse practitioners were mentioned in the news, more often than any other time in history, as a source of cost-effective, high-quality care providers.

1. The media
   A. Terms such as "managed competition" and "managed care" began to surface in the professional literature and the public sector.
   B. The topic of a single-payer national health care system was much debated.
2. The American Medical Association (AMA)
   A. Heightened its efforts to prevent advanced practice nurses' expansion of scope, role, or power by blocking legislation and financially supporting candidates of public office against advanced practice nurses' roles (e.g., prescriptive authority, direct reimbursement, and increased scope of practice).
   B. The AMA House of Delegates (AMA, 1991) distributes resolutions to:
      1) "Work to eliminate federal funding for training of further numbers of mid level practitioners"
      2) "Recommend to all hospital staffs that admission history and physicals be performed only by physicians,"

1995: PRIMARY CARE: AMERICA'S HEALTH IN A NEW ERA

The Institute of Medicine (IOM) is a private, nonprofit organization providing health policy advice under a congressional charter granted to the National Academy of Sciences. In this 1995 publication, the IOM made recommendations regarding primary care in contemporary practice.

1. New IOM measures
   A. Redefined primary care:

   Primary care is the provision of integrated, accessible health care services by clinicians who are accountable for addressing a large majority of personal health care needs, developing a sustained partnership with patients and practicing in the context of family and community.

   B. Refined the definition of primary care provider to include a broader range of health care providers.
      1) Defined clinicians as physicians, nurse practitioners, and physician assistants.
      2) The new definition stresses the importance of the patient and family, the community, an integrated delivery system, and the relationship between patient and primary care provider.
   C. Encouraged provision of universal coverage for primary care.
   D. Encouraged using capitation payment methods instead of fee for service to promote primary care.
   E. Promoted creating an all-payer system to fund education and training in health professions, and moving that teaching into more non-hospital-based ambulatory care facilities.
2. Advanced practice nurses are educated to focus on primary health care.

   Primary Health Care is the product of a collaborative effort among many health care professionals. Taking into account the needs and strengths of the whole person, it includes the identification, management, and/or referral of health problems, as well as guidance toward health-maintaining behavior. Continuous and comprehensive, Primary Health Care entails co-ordination of all the services necessary for health promotion, maintenance, rehabilitation and the prevention of disease and disability. (ANA, 1991)

3. The acute care nurse practitioner does well to incorporate aspects of primary health care emphasis in rendering care to acutely ill clients. The ACNP can work to bridge health restoration care and health promotion as he/she cares for the client at the beginning of an illness in the acute setting, through the discharge planning phase, and back to the family and community. The acute care setting is any environment where intervention for the acutely ill is delivered and encompasses hospitals, extended care facilities, and home care.

Review Questions

15.11 The 1990 World Health Organization's *Healthy People 2000* was a statement of national health policy that put forward all of the following care objectives EXCEPT:

    A. Equal access to care
    B. Availability and continuity of care
    C. Free access to care for all
    D. Reasonable cost and high-quality care

15.12 In 1991, the ANA published *Nursing's Agenda for Health Care Reform*, in which advanced practice nurses were identified and supported as the innovative providers of care that:
    A. Focused on primary care
    B. Had documented studies reflecting high quality of care
    C. Had diversity of practice settings, with availability in schools, hospitals, community health centers, hospices, private practices, and homes
    D. All of the above

15.13 National and international health policy is predominantly influenced by which of the following groups?
    A. Consumers, government agencies, and health care providers
    B. Insurance plans, employers, and professional organizations
    C. Congress, the president, and the judicial system
    D. A and B only

15.14 In 1992–1994, health care reform was a national agenda item. What changes occurred in our health care system as a result of the focus and attention?
    A. All patients have equal access to care now.
    B. Managed care has continued to slowly evolve to incorporate a greater share of the health care market in all parts of the country and all forms of health care delivery.
    C. The AMA has realized the need for more health care providers in the system and is working to support all primary care provider roles.
    D. Nurse practitioners are now guaranteed recognition as official health care providers in the system.

15.15 The 1995 Institute of Medicine report *Primary Care: America's Health in a New Era* supports which of the following measures?
    A. Using capitation payment methods instead of fee-for-service methods for primary care in a universal coverage system that would include physicians, nurse practitioners, and physician assistants
    B. Continuing the fee-for-service method of payment with the government as the primary payer in a single-payer system like that of Canada
    C. Redefining primary care while encouraging a shift to a universal coverage of all and a physician-dominated provider system
    D. None of the above

Answers and Rationales

15.11 **C** The World Health Organization did not promote free access to health care for all—only high-quality, low-cost, available, continuous health care with equal access.

15.12 **D** The ANA supported all of the stated variables.

15.13 **D** The Congress, the president, and the judicial system play a less predominant role in the formation of health policy; but rather, they are more responsive role to prevailing market influences.

15.14 **B** The continued growth of managed care systems was the only result of the much-discussed health care reform of the early 1990s. It was the end result of the drive to decrease health care costs on the part of the insurance plans. Managed care is therefore the result of health care reform only by privatization and not by national policy change.

15.15 **A** The IOM encouraged a capitated system with the inclusion of a wide variety of clinicians providing universal care.

References

American Medical Association House of Delegates. (1991). Cut federal funds for advanced nurse training.

American Nurses Association. (1991). *Nursing's Agenda for Health Care Reform. Advanced Practice Nurses: An Innovation for Primary Care.* Kansas City, MO: American Nurses Association.

Institute of Medicine. (1995). *Primary Care: America's Health in a New Era.* Washington, DC: Institute of Medicine, Division of Health Care Services.

Safriet, B.J. (1992). Health care dollars and regulatory sense: The role of advanced practice nursing. *Yale J Regulation 9,* 417–487.

Shugars, D.A., Bader, J.D., O'Neil, E.H., et al. (1991). *Pew Health Professions Commission. Healthy America: Practitioners for 2005, an Agenda for Action for U.S. Health Professional Schools.*

World Health Organization. (1990). *Healthy People 2000.* Geneva: World Health Organization.

Practice Issues

SCOPE OF PRACTICE AND STANDARDS OF PRACTICE

1. The scope of nursing practice has overlapped with that of medical practice over the years. As technology and practice patterns evolve, so must the scope of practice. The general guidelines for defining the two scopes of practice are threefold:
   A. Independent practice: Those functions that are independent of the medical scope and fall completely within the scope of common nursing practice.
   B. Interdependent practice: Those functions that overlap with the arena of medicine and fall in the collaborative scope of practice.
   C. Dependent practice: Those functions that can only be done with the direct assistance and guidance of the medical practitioner.
2. Standards of practice
   A. The ANA defines a standard of practice as an "authoritative statement by which the quality of practice, service or education can be judged."
   B. Standards reflect minimum levels of acceptable performance and are tools by which to measure the quality of care given.
   C. They are consumer and legal yardsticks by which to assess individual nursing care rendered.

PROTOCOLS AND STANDARDIZED PROCEDURES

These are the legal mechanisms by which some states' nurse practice acts allow registered nurses to amplify their practice into areas traditionally considered to be within the realm of medical practice.

1. Disease-specific protocols are descriptions of the steps to be taken for a specific presenting condition.
   A. Some authorities believe that they are cumbersome, unwieldy, and unnecessarily restrictive while providing a false sense of security in fostering the belief that a recipe for care is all that is needed.
   B. Others think the disease-specific protocols control for misinterpretation and loose application of protocols and offer measurable legal protection in a court of law.
2. Process protocols are descriptions of the steps to be taken in performing a given function (e.g., management of chronic diseases or acute illnesses). Protocols that are based upon the functions performed specify requirements for care without mandating medical content.
   A. Supporters of process protocols feel that parameters of action may be delineated without unnecessarily restricting management options or encumbering the practitioner with multiple disease-specific protocols. Within these parameters, the registered nurse can evaluate and treat patients according to practice standards.
   B. Detractors state that the process protocols are too loose and offer insufficient protection from overlapping practice with medicine.
   C. The supporters of process protocols are more prevalent, and the support documents extend to state boards of nursing in some states (e.g., California Board of Registered Nurses states either protocol is acceptable).

EVALUATION OF PRACTICE: CONTINUOUS QUALITY IMPROVEMENT AND TOTAL QUALITY MANAGEMENT

1. Continuous quality improvement (CQI) and total quality management are quality standard terms that are used at various locations in the country and in different settings. The concepts and application processes are essentially equivalent.
2. Objectives of having a CQI system in place:
   A. Provides a system of accountability for individual providers to practice high standards of care
   B. Reduces facility and practitioner liability risks
   C. Improves documentation practices in patient records
   D. Can be used as input for practitioner work at annual evaluations of practice
   E. Offers a tool for evaluating and measuring patient outcomes of care
3. Work site CQI committee and peer review
   A. Provides opportunity to evaluate adherence to standards and establishes support for the quality of the acute care nurse practitioner's practice.
   B. Peers enforce practice standards of care in the community by limiting practice beyond the scope of legal and commonly accepted standards.
   C. Ensures that multiprovider settings have consistency in quality and continuity of care.

    D. Work site CQI committee uses a multidisciplinary approach and evaluates care across the CQI continuum.
4. Quality organizations and systems
    A. The Joint Commission on the Accreditation of Healthcare Organizations (JCAHO) defines continuous quality improvement as a system to evaluate and monitor the quality of patient care and the quality of the facility management.
        1) Licensed independent provider (LIP) is a new term that encompasses advanced practice nurses. JCAHO has new regulations addressing the practice of LIPs.
        2) Written policies regarding CQI processes, committee work, and records are reviewed for industry standards.
    B. Professional Standards Review Organizations (PSROs)
        1) They were conceived as a quality assurance program by means of which physicians might control the quality and cost of federally funded health care through a peer review process in each state.
        2) They were created by Congress in amending the Social Security Act in 1972.
        3) They approve or deny payments for care provided in the Medicare and Medicaid programs by determining the medical necessity, appropriateness, and quality of care.
    C. Audits (by U.S. Department of Health and Human Services, health insurance plans, grant-offering institutions, and other reimbursement entities)
    D. Patient satisfaction surveys or tools
    E. Utilization review evaluations

LEGAL LIABILITY

Ours is becoming an ever more litigious society, and there is always the possibility that even the most innocent of actions will be taken by someone as grounds for a lawsuit.

(Bullough, 1980)

It may seem a strange principle to enunciate as the very first requirement in a Hospital that it should do the sick no harm.

(Florence Nightingale, *Notes on Hospitals*, 1859)

1. Standards of care
    A. Standards of care are the criteria to measure against to determine whether or not negligence occurred.
    B. Negligence is defined as a failure to meet the standard of care that is equal to the care provided by similar providers with similar training and similar experience under similar circumstances.
    C. Knowledge of the community standard of care helps prevent malpractice suits.
2. Good Samaritan statutes
    A. Good Samaritan statutes have been passed in all of the states, with the first one enacted in 1959 in California.
    B. The purpose of the statutes was to protect from malpractice suits medical professionals who stop at the scene of an emergency to offer their medical expertise.

C. Skilled professionals are therefore encouraged to offer assistance without being held liable for acts that they did or did not do.

3. "Confidentiality" versus "A Duty to Warn"

A. If a patient's condition constitutes a danger to others, a duty to warn someone (police, public health department, social services, etc.) takes precedence over the right to confidentiality.

B. The duty to protect the public supersedes the right to confidentiality—a judicial standard.

C. The duty to protect the patient from harming him/herself supersedes the right to confidentiality and necessitates using a 72-hour hold or some sort of conservatorship. The practitioner must be familiar with specific state statutes dealing with circumstances such as these should the immediate need arise.

4. Invasion of privacy

A. Invasion of privacy occurs when medical information is given out to a third party without consent of the patient and the dissemination of that information causes damage to a person's reputation.

B. This charge cannot be made if it can be shown that the information is true and was given out in good faith, and the receiver had a valid reason to receive it (e.g., the next care provider of the patient has a valid reason to receive medical information).

C. Specific statutes regarding sensitive types of medical information (e.g., human immunodeficiency virus status) vary from state to state, and the practitioner must be familiar with these to ensure proper handling of the medical record and information entrusted to them.

5. "Reporting" statutes

A. These statutes require the health care provider to report a medical finding—they take precedence over confidentiality.

B. These statutes vary from state to state, and the practitioner must be familiar with them to ensure proper reporting to protect public health.

C. Common reporting statutes involve injury from a dangerous weapon, criminal acts, certain infectious diseases, animal bites, domestic violence, child abuse (all states), conditions involving lapses in consciousness, pesticide poisoning, some newborn conditions, and attempted suicide.

D. The statutes protect practitioners from liability in suits alleging defamation, and many carry penalties for not reporting.

6. Risk management

Risk Management includes systems and activities which are designed to recognize and intervene to reduce the risk of injury to patients and consequent claims against health care providers. It is based on the assumption that many injuries to patients are preventable.

(Edmunds. 1991)

A. Managing medical risk is controlling for practice issues involving procedures, quality indicators, medical records, administrative practices, and patient care.

B. Two types of practice surveys can assess for risk:

1) The self-directed survey is where the practitioner is evaluating his/her own practice and taking whatever steps may be necessary to correct problems. Medical risk management companies have forms and tools to assist the practitioner assess their practice.

2) The external survey uses the same basic process, enhanced by the on-site presence of professional risk management specialists. The surveyor will review policies and procedures, patient relations, scheduling, telephone protocols, follow-up tracking methods, and other areas of the practice. The costs of such a process could be outweighed by the benefit of any litigation aversion.

7. Malpractice/liability insurance
   A. Errors in judgment do occur.
   B. Malpractice insurance will not protect the nurse practitioner from charges of practicing outside of his/her legal scope of practice (i.e., practicing medicine without a license).
   C. It is universally recommended and standard for nurse practitioners to carry their own malpractice insurance over and above any coverage from the institution of employment. Too often, the employer's coverage is not adequate, is too general in scope, or is not supportive of advanced practice nurses.
   D. The National Practitioner Data Bank tracks all information regarding adverse actions taken against health care practitioners. All hospitals are required to check the data bank every 2 years to identify health care providers on their staff or who may be granted clinical privileges.
   E. There are two general types of insurance contracts for liability policy options.
      1) "Occurrence coverage" covers events of alleged malpractice that have occurred during the specified policy period only, regardless of when the claim was filed.
      2) "Claims-made coverage" covers only those claims filed during the policy coverage period, regardless of when they occurred. Usually an optional "tail coverage" contract is available to extend the coverage of claims-made policies into the future to cover all possible claims to be filed in the future.

PRESCRIPTIVE AUTHORITY

1. Prescriptive authority is central to advanced practice nurses' effective practice.
2. Historically:
   A. The authority to prescribe drugs and devices to patients was only within the scope of medical practice.
   B. Organized medicine has played a central role in shaping the states' current advanced practice nurses' prescriptive authority.
   C. Consistently, medical associations have lobbied against any legislative efforts to acknowledge or expand prescriptive authority for advanced practice nurses.
3. The first state to recognize limited prescriptive authority for nurse practitioners, in 1975, was North Carolina.
4. Currently, 45 states authorize nurse practitioner prescriptive authority, ranging from full authority to limited. There is also variation in the types of drugs and devices they permit advanced practice nurses to use.
5. Many states limit prescriptive authority by:
   A. Imposing requirements for written protocols
   B. Requiring physician supervision
   C. Requiring use of formularies specifying which drugs may be prescribed
   D. Limiting authority to certain geographic areas or practice settings

6. The above limitations that exist are incrementally being removed. There is growing support for the movement of full prescriptive authority in the nature of statutorial change or through regulations promulgated by state boards of nursing.

7. Studies of prescriptive practice patterns of advanced practice nurses have consistently demonstrated dramatically less use of prescriptive drugs and controlled substances than physician counterparts.

8. A national nursing task force (The National Council of State Boards of Nursing in collaboration with the National Organization of Nurse Practitioner Faculties) has outlined a standard pharmacology curriculum for nurse practitioner education programs in an attempt to standardize the information being taught and position nursing to promote full prescriptive authority without restrictions.

9. Advanced practice nurses are rapidly expanding their educational preparation, including pharmacology—which is experiencing dynamic growth in itself. Nurse practitioners' practice capabilities are continually growing, especially in the area of increased technology-based care, thereby making it unwise to rigidly restrict their ability to prescribe and therefore practice effectively.

INFORMATION AND RESOURCE SYSTEMS FOR PRACTITIONERS

1. "Telemedicine" or "telehealth" is the use of remote electronic equipment for consultations and referrals not available in the local area.
   A. The concept of "telemedicine" was primarily initiated by the military to care for the members of the armed forces stationed at great distances. It was expanded to rural health care systems and is now becoming more common in urban centers for specialty consultation.
   B. To date, all telehealth transactions must be initiated and received by a physician. Nurse practitioners can make referrals to the system but are currently not permitted to negotiate telecommunications.
   C. The Federal Communications Commission (FCC) is implementing the Telecommunications Act of 1996 and is investigating the role nursing will be allowed to play in the area of telemedicine. The Joint Interagency Work Group on Telemedicine is advising the FCC about implementation issues of telehealth projects, including barriers to practice.
   D. The Internet has grown to serve as a tool for health care providers. Current uses being promoted are:
      1) Online hospital registration
      2) Use of a "Home Page" to provide clients with information about scheduled diagnostic procedures
      3) Dissemination of clinical practice guidelines at a specific practice setting
      4) Provision of continuing education (CE) programs
      5) Sending prescription requests from the client's home directly to the prescriber's office
   E. Dr. Larry Weed, Professor Emeritus of the University of Vermont, considered by many to be the father of medical informatics, states that knowing where to go for information is more crucial than memorizing it.

F. As public Internet access improves, and the use of the World Wide Web increases, advanced practice nurses, whether student, educator, researcher, or seasoned clinician, will have to be able to use the web for the most current information and resources.

2. Journals: Contain current research and practice applications within the various specialties.

3. Conferences and CE: Offer networking with peers, presentations by specialty experts, and the opportunity to discuss education and practice issues. An example is the "Annual Consensus Conference on Acute Care Nurse Practitioners," hosted each year by an Acute Care Nurse Practitioner Program college.

NEGOTIATING AN EMPLOYMENT CONTRACT

1. A contract is an exchange of promises of actions that, but for the agreement, the parties would not be legally obligated to perform. It should have the following general items:
   A. A mutual exchange of promises
   B. The duration of the contract
   C. The capacity to contract (can each party signing the agreement legally bind the actual parties to the contract?)
2. Types of items that may be included in the employment contract:
   A. Scope of services: Employee services, employer supervision, employee authority, exclusive service
   B. Compensation for services: Salary, malpractice insurance, disability insurance, facility and supplies, additional expenses like professional dues or CE
   C. Duration of contract: Renewal and termination stipulations
   D. Signatures and date

Review Questions

15.16 The scope of practice of a nurse practitioner has some overlapping roles with that of medical practice. The three functions that best describe the scope of nurse practitioner practice in relation to that of medical practice are:
   A. Independent, interdependent, and dependent
   B. Exclusive, overlapping, and nonexclusive
   C. Binding, nonbinding, and independent
   D. Primary care, specialty care, and hospital care

15.17 Objectives of continuous quality improvement systems include all of the following except:
   A. Reducing practitioner liability risks
   B. Ensuring proper diagnosing and treatments at the facility
   C. Offering a tool for evaluating and measuring patient outcomes of care
   D. Improving documentation practices in patient records

15.18 What are standards of care?
   A. Community expectations of care, given the current technology available
   B. Do no harm
   C. Community care criteria to measure against to determine whether or not negligence occurred
   D. The most recent text written on the subject

15.19 Risk management is the term used to describe a system:
   A. Designed to decrease patient risk of illness
   B. Designed to decrease risk of malpractice suits against the provider
   C. Of controlling for practice issues involving procedures, quality indicators, medical records, administrative practices, and patient care
   D. B and C only

15.20 Liability insurance has two options of coverage. If a patient were to sue you for a negligent event that they claim happened 7 years ago, and you retired 2 years ago, what type of coverage would you want to have?
   A. Claims-made coverage
   B. Occurrence coverage with a tail coverage
   C. Occurrence coverage
   D. Negligence coverage

Answers and Rationales

15.16 **A** Independent, interdependent, and dependent functions with medicine are the best description of the overlapping roles.

15.17 **B** CQI does not ensure proper diagnosis and treatment judgments by the provider, but rather attempts to encourage a provider's best practice patterns and documentation, and thereby decrease liability and better patient outcomes.

15.18 **C** They are the community care criteria against which to compare practice.

15.19 **D** Risk management is designed to control the variables of practice procedures, medical records, and other aspects of health care in order to decrease provider risk of malpractice liability suits.

15.20 **C** Occurrence coverage covers the event of alleged malpractice that occurred during the specified policy period, regardless of when the claim is filed.

References

Bullough. (1980). The Nation's Health, San Francisco: Boyd & Fraser Publishing Co.

Edmunds, M.W. (1991). NPs who replace physicians: Role expansion or exploitation? *Nurse Pract 16*(9), 46, 49.

Woodham-Smith, C. (1951). *Florence Nightengale, 1890–1910. Los Altos: Lange Medical Publications.*

Political Activism

Health care legislation and regulation are continually changing. As the evolution proceeds, nurse practitioners need to be politically savvy to stay in a position to be able to continue to care for their patients and be recognized as health care professionals.

A HISTORY LESSON FOR NPs: THE CANADIAN NURSE PRACTITIONER EXPERIENCE

The late 1960s and early 1970s brought national health care funding reform to Canada. It evolved without nursing's input and the nurse practitioner was not listed as a reimbursable health care provider. The year 1972 was the last year any province in Canada legally had advanced practice nurses working. By 1983, the last Canadian nurse practitioner program was discontinued. This is slowly changing back, province by province, with local work and input from politically active nurse practitioners and motivated nurses. The original elimination of the role of nurse practitioner in that country stands as a reminder that nursing's diligence and political activism is critical to survival and progress.

THE LEGISLATIVE PROCESS

1. The federal level
   A. An issue of interest is formulated into a bill and introduced into Congress.
   B. Committee hearings with House and Senate review and vote.
   C. If the bill passes both floors, it goes to the president for signature or veto.
   D. After it becomes a law, appropriate regulatory agencies draft rules and regulations to implement the law.
   E. There ensues a public comment period and process.
   F. Then the law is implemented via the regulations.
2. The state level
   A. This varies from state to state, but the basic committee, House, and Senate process is the same.
   B. The process culminates with a governor's signature.
3. The lobbyist
   A. A professional who disseminates information to the policy makers and legislators to influence policy formation.
   B. They are employed by interest groups or professions to know who and how to influence the process of passing or blocking a bill's progress.
   C. Health specialist lobbyists are employed to help influence health profession and policy bills.
4. Grassroots legislative efforts
   A. These efforts start at the basic individual or small-group level and mobilize upward to the legislator and the legislative process.
   B. The process protects nurse practitioners from legislation that may be detrimental to the profession and supports legislation that enhances the ability to practice.
   C. Local grassroots nurse practitioner group activities include:
      1) Monitoring legislation introduced into the state or federal legislature

      2) Working closely with a lobbyist to assess the political climate and best course of action

      3) Determining the impact a bill may have on nurse practitioners, nurses, and health consumers

      4) Deciding to actively support or oppose or watch key bills of interest

5. Interviews with a legislator
   A. Make an appointment—do not drop in unannounced.
   B. Legislative aids are often well informed on health care issues and frequently are the source of information for the legislator to rely upon.
   C. Know as much as possible about the person you are trying to influence.
   D. Relay actual stories of your practice and patient care situations that will educate the legislator about the issue.
   E. Try to avoid any prolonged controversial arguments. It will be remembered in a negative light against your issue.
   F. Whenever possible, make a specific request of the legislator. This gives them something tangible to respond to.
   G. Be sure to express your appreciation for any support and thank the legislator for the interview.
   H. Write a follow-up letter summarizing the key points of your issue and any commitments the legislator made to "think about" or to "vote" a certain way—and thank the legislator for his/her time again.

6. Letter writing, faxing, or e-mailing a legislator
   A. A letter from each member of a group makes more impact than a single letter with 20 signatures on it.
   B. Summarize the issue.
   C. Make a specific request.
   D. Personalize the issue as to how it affects your practice and their constituents.
   E. Have a patient or family member of a patient write a letter to the legislator describing how your care and the issue are related—for example, blocked access to care if you are not able to be listed as a primary care provider on the patient's health maintenance organization directory because of state regulations disallowing it.
   F. Thank them for their time and offer to be a resource on any future nurse practitioner issues to be considered.

7. Influencing local health care issues
   A. Local issues can be influenced by working on:
      1) A health task force
      2) An action group
      3) A health board
      4) A regulatory board
      5) A local coalition organized around a specific community issue
      6) A professional organization committee
   B. Nurse practitioners need to become visible in these roles to promote the profession and protect their scope of practice

MARKETING THE ACNP ROLE TO NURSING COLLEAGUES, THE PUBLIC, HEALTH POLICY MAKERS, AND LEGISLATORS

1. Identify yourself by the nurse practitioner title:
   A. To your patients
   B. On business cards

C. On name tags

D. At speaking engagements

E. To other health professional colleagues

F. During public interviews with newspapers, radio, and television

2. Generate and distribute educational brochures and materials about who acute care nurse practitioners are and why they are effective to:

A. Patients

B. Patient waiting areas

C. Other health care professional colleagues

D. Legislators

E. Health policy makers

F. Local community groups

3. Volunteerism generates good will toward you and the profession as a whole. Volunteer at:

A. Health fairs

B. Schools

C. Community centers (e.g., senior centers)

D. Public events (e.g., the local Fourth of July parade or volleyball tournament)

E. Political campaigns

F. Local boards or health authorities

G. Professional committee work

4. Establish a Nurse Practitioner subheading in the local telephone directory and encourage regional nurse practitioners to become listed.

5. Attempt to focus local media on the deeds of local community acute care nurse practitioners and their unique practice outcomes.

6. Generate networks of colleagues to refer patients to and to consult with in other nurse practitioner specialty areas.

Review Questions

15.21 Given the Canadian nurse practitioners' experiences, U.S. NPs would do best to rely upon which group to represent and look out for their profession?

A. The governmental agencies and commissions

B. The legislators

C. The consumers

D. Their professional organizations—local, state, and national

15.22 The legislative process is complex, yet offers which of the following checks and balances?

A. An issue of interest is formulated, a bill is introduced into Congress, committee hearings review and vote, and then it may go to the president or governor for signature or veto

B. An issue of interest is formulated, a bill is introduced into the judiciary branch, committees review and vote, and then it goes to Congress and the president/governor for signature or veto

C. A bill is written by a congressional member, it is reviewed by his/her House or Senate, then it goes to the president/governor for signature or veto, then the committees review how it should be implemented after public input

D. Public hearings determine if an issue is even worth introducing to the Congress and the president/governor for consideration, then the process begins if worth is determined

15.23 In letters or interview with a legislator, a nurse practitioner should be sure to include the following points:

A. Personal stories of his/her patients' experiences with the practice issue being discussed and how it affected them positively or negatively

B. Professional barrier problems and how the impending legislation would help improve the situation, thereby allowing nurse practitioners to provide better care for their patients

C. Your political party affiliation and if you voted for the legislator or not

D. A and B only

15.24 Influencing local health care issues may be accomplished by:

A. Participating on task forces, boards, action groups, and coalitions organized around a local issue

B. Speaking to other nurse practitioners at regional professional organizations' meetings

C. Voting

D. All of the above

15.25 Variables involved in marketing the acute care nurse practitioner role may include which of the following?

A. Avoiding volunteerism at local community events or groups to protect yourself from liability and any negative publicity

B. Educational brochures explaining why nurse practitioners are better than any other care providers

C. Always identifying yourself as a nurse practitioner to your patients, on business cards, on name tags, at speaking engagements, to other health professional colleagues, and during interviews with newspapers, radio, and television

D. All of the above

Answers and Rationales

15.21 **D** Professional advocacy and involvement is the best approach to protecting the nurse practitioner role—do not depend on others to look after you.

15.22 **A** The process as outlined is the correct process for state and federal legislation to progress through the system.

15.23 **D** You should not discuss your nurse practitioner issues in the context of a political party. If you are in the district of the legislator, you could mention that you voted for him or her, but if you did not do so, do not mention it.

15.24 **D** All of these methods are valid for influencing local health care issues.

15.25 **C** Marketing involves getting the message out about who you are and what you do. Always identifying yourself as a nurse practitioner can aid in this. (*Note:* You should not avoid volunteerism; on the contrary, it is an excellent method of putting the role forward to the public. Also, you should never claim you are any better than other health care providers.)

Health Care Delivery Systems

The United States does not have a single health care system; rather, health care is made up of four major systems: private, local government, active military, and veterans. Between the first two years systems, namely private and local government, some of the lines are becoming blurred.

THE PRIVATE SYSTEM

1. The "private system" of health care delivery is the system most frequently described as the American health care system and is said to represent the best medical care available in the United States and possibly anywhere else in the world.
2. It is typically utilized by the middle-class, middle-income individuals and families because this system is supported as an "employee benefit" by the working class.
3. It is coordinated by the physician (e.g., private practice) or the plan (e.g., a health maintenance organization).
4. It is financed by personal, nongovernmental funds that are paid either by the consumer or through private health insurance plans.
5. It has two general system structures:
   A. Private practice or fee-for-service system
      1) Where the individual or family puts together a network of care providers and facilities that meet their own needs.
      2) Few or no restrictions are placed on provider choice, facility choice, or types of services sought.
      3) The traditional private medical office, hospitals, specialists, and ancillary services are all participants.
   B. Managed care system
      1) A health care system that integrates the financing and delivery of health care services to covered individuals, most often by arrangements with selected providers.
      2) This system's hallmark is coordinating services through a designated primary care provider and "managing" access to specialty care based on evaluated need.
      3) It is usually a prepaid or capitated payment mechanism, which means that a stipulated dollar amount is established to cover the cost of health care delivered for a person and is paid periodically, usually monthly, to a health care provider/plan.
      4) In 1980, 12% of the insured population of the United States was in some form of managed health care. By 1992, that number had grown to 60%.
      5) There are many service systems and "alphabet soup" terms floating around in the managed health care arena, as discussed below. All health care providers need to be savvy in this ever-expanding market.

6. Alphabet soup
  A. Health maintenance organization (HMO)
     1) An organized system of care that provides a specified range of comprehensive health services to an enrolled set of members that focuses on health promotion and maintenance.
     2) Providers are either salaried employees or contracted groups of the system.
     3) Reimbursement is prepaid per capita and the HMO is both the insurer and provider of care.
     4) Patients have a choice of providers and facilities within the HMO.
  B. Independent practice association (IPA)
     1) A type of HMO in which providers participate in a prepaid medical plan by joining an association that negotiates on their behalf.
     2) IPA providers charge agreed-upon rates and bill the plan on either a capitated or fee-for-service basis.
     3) Patients have a choice of providers and facilities only within the network.
  C. Preferred provider organization (PPO)
     1) A group of providers and hospitals that contract with insurers, employers, or other sponsoring groups to provide services to covered persons at agreed-upon rates.
     2) Providers negotiate lower fees or capitated payments in anticipation of a greater patient volume and agree to basic managed care principles.
     3) These systems are marketed to purchasers as opposed to consumers.
  D. Preferred provider arrangement (PPA): A program in which payers such as insurance companies offer their insured members financial incentives to obtain services from a panel of providers under contract at discounted rates.
  E. Integrated delivery system (IDS)
     1) Hybrids of integration that range from provider-based to payer-provider-based
     2) Examples are group practice without walls (GPWW), physician-hospital organization (PHO), and medical service organization (MSO)
  F. Point of service (POS): This option allows the patient to go outside the plan's provider panel if they are willing to pay a percentage of the outside fee.
  G. Other terms common in these systems: Prepaid health plan (PHP), primary care case management (PCCM), and health insuring organization (HIO).

THE LOCAL GOVERNMENT HEALTH CARE SYSTEM

1. This system generally serves the poor, inner-city populations.
2. It is not an organized system, but rather a safety-net system assembled by various federal, state, and county government agencies and funding sources.
3. City or county hospitals and the local health department are the hub of this safety-net system.
4. Continuity of services or care is not usually a characteristic element.
5. Acute episodic care is common, with little or no emphasis placed on health promotion or prevention.
6. It is almost entirely composed of public, government-sponsored services.

THE MILITARY MEDICAL CARE SYSTEM

1. This system has the responsibility of protecting the health of all active-duty military personnel wherever their military duty may take them.
2. It provides them with all the services that they may eventually need for any service-connected problem.
3. It covers the participant immediately upon entering the service—no probationary time.
4. Emphasis is on keeping personnel well with preventing illness, injury and on finding health problems early while they are still amenable to treatment.
5. Great stress is placed on preventive approaches such as vaccination, regular physical exams and tests, and education programs for improved lifestyle and health.

VETERANS ADMINISTRATION HEALTH CARE SYSTEM

1. The Veterans Administration health care system is for retired and disabled veterans of previous U.S. military service.
2. It is not as complete, well integrated, or extensive as the active military system.
3. It is primarily hospital oriented and not "health" oriented.
4. It is lifetime coverage.

Review Questions

15.26 The PPO is characterized as:
  A. A group of providers that contract for a fee-for-service payment and negotiate lower fees in anticipation of a very healthy patient volume
  B. A group of providers that contract with insurers and others to provide services to covered persons at agreed-upon rates; providers negotiate lower fees or capitated payments in anticipation of a greater patient volume
  C. A program in which payers such as insurance companies offer their insured members financial incentives to obtain services from a panel of providers that will charge them fee-for-service
  D. None of the above

15.27 Managed care systems are:
  A. Stabilizing at 50% of the population enrolled in such a system
  B. Another name for health maintenance organizations
  C. Growing across the country; it is estimated that 60% of the population is enrolled in some form of managed care system
  D. Created to manage the illnesses of an individual and coordinate appropriate and low-cost specialty care

15.28 A small community clinic cares for indigent, Medicaid, and low-income patients. It collects small donations whenever it can from the clients and obtains foundational grants, private donations, and county program money for vaccine and prenatal projects as its funding source. It is considered what type of health care delivery system?

A. A private system
B. Veterans Administration system
C. Military medical care system
D. Local government system

15.29 The military medical care system is designed for providing care for active-duty military personnel. The emphasis of care is:
A. Acute episodic intervention
B. Wellness promotion and illness prevention
C. Vaccinations and foreign country illness treatments
D. A and C only

15.30 The Veterans Administration health care system is for retired and disabled veterans of previous military service. It can be characterized as:
A. Primarily hospital, acute, and chronic illness care oriented
B. One of the best health promotion systems in the country
C. Effective for 20 years after discharge from the service
D. A complete integrated system of primary care

Answers and Rationales

15.26 **B** PPOs anticipate a larger patient volume, not a healthy patient volume, to be able to contract for lower fees.

15.27 **C** Managed care is still growing and is currently at about 60% of the U.S. population. HMOs are only one type of managed care system.

15.28 **D** Local government systems are those that receive county and state monies and are publicly funded.

15.29 **B** Wellness promotion and illness prevention are the focus to keep the military personnel in good health to perform their duties.

15.30 **A** It is primarily a system of acute care for episodic illnesses—focusing on inpatient care. There is lesser focus on the chronic illness clinics of hypertension and the like and nearly a complete lack of wellness promotion, full women's health services, and patient education services focusing on disease prevention.

Types of Reimbursement

Nurse practitioners are reimbursed differently under the various types of provider reimbursement mechanisms. Some systems are very complex, with multiple barriers for the nurse practitioner to overcome before reimbursement is possible. Other systems are nurse practitioner friendly, with recognition of their provider status.

THIRD-PARTY PAYER DIRECT REIMBURSEMENT

1. This is the traditional form of payment where the provider receives payment from a third-party insurer for each service that is provided.
2. Nurses are mandated by state statute to receive direct reimbursement from third-party private insurance in 25 states. (This is increased from the 15 states that required this in 1988.)

3. Variable levels of reimbursement are paid in relation to physician reimbursement rates (e.g., some states outline pay schedules for nurse providers at 80% of the physician rate).
4. Advantages to receiving direct reimbursement include:
   A. Decreased costs involved in nurse practitioner practice patterns
   B. Increased consumer choice of health care providers
   C. More professional autonomy for nursing

MEDICAID

1. This program is authorized by Title XIX of the Social Security Act, which is a federal-state matching program providing medical assistance to low-income people who are aged, blind, disabled, or members of families with dependent children.
2. The federal funds are at a fixed percentage of the total program expenditures, but conversion to a "block grant" system is possible in the future, where only a set amount of dollars would come from the federal part of the program.
3. Each state is responsible for designing and administering their own type of program within federal guidelines. Each state sets eligibility and coverage standards.
4. Federal oversight of the Medicaid program is the responsibility of the Health Care Financing Administration (HCFA).
5. Free-for-service reimbursement of Medicaid-covered services has been the standard, but most states plan to shift or have already shifted care to a Medicaid managed care reimbursement system.
6. The 1989 federal Omnibus Budget Reconciliation Act (OBRA 89) currently mandates direct Medicaid reimbursement for certified nurse midwives, pediatric nurse practitioners, and family nurse practitioners only.
7. States may pass regulations authorizing Medicaid direct reimbursement to other nurse practitioner specialties (e.g., acute care nurse practitioners could bill directly for their Medicaid services if the state had passed a regulation authorizing it.)
8. The levels of reimbursement payments are determined by the state Medicaid agency and range from 60% to 100% of the physician rate in various states.
9. Within managed care Medicaid systems, nurse practitioners are finding difficulty becoming designated as primary care providers to allow their inclusion in the system and thereby allow them to care for and receive reimbursement for caring for patients.

MEDICARE

1. This program provides health insurance protection to the aged and disabled population.
2. It covers hospital, physician, and other medical services regardless of income.
3. The program is administered by the HCFA in the federal Department of Health and Human Services.
4. Medicare is divided into two parts:
   A. "Part A" is hospital insurance that covers inpatient hospital and related institutional care. All people over age 65 are eligible to enroll and all are entitled to receive Part A benefits.

B. "Part B" is supplemental medical insurance that covers physician and other related medical services and supplies. This is a voluntary program and individuals who enroll pay a premium to receive benefits.

5. The Omnibus Budget Reconciliation Act of 1989 (OBRA 89) enacted a payment system to providers based on a fee schedule that uses a resource-based relative value scale. Payments are determined according to the resources and effort needed to perform a service, instead of a percentage of fees charged. This fee schedule began implementation in 1992 and was to be phased in over 5 years.

6. Nurse practitioner reimbursement for services provided to Medicare-insured patients has many prerequisites.

   A. Must be a licensed registered nurse and satisfy nurse practitioner qualifications in the state where services are provided.
   B. Must meet specific requirements about primary care certification, education, and experience.
   C. The nurse practitioner must work in collaboration with a physician.
   D. Nurse practitioner services are covered under four basic situations:
      1) Services were furnished incident to a physician's services.
      2) Services were furnished under contract to an HMO.
      3) Services were furnished in a skilled nursing facility.
      4) Services were furnished in a rural area (specific definition).

CIVILIAN HEALTH AND MEDICAL PROGRAM OF THE UNITED STATES

1. The Civilian Health and Medical Program of the United States (CHAMPUS) is the federal health plan that provides coverage to military personnel and their families.
2. It shares the cost of covered health care obtained by eligible members when they seek care from civilian sources. This may occur when they live too far from a military hospital or clinic.
3. The program reimburses at 80% of allowable charges.
4. CHAMPUS reimburses nurse practitioners for services provided, independent of physician referral or supervision.

FEDERAL EMPLOYEES HEALTH BENEFITS PROGRAM

1. The Federal Employees Health Benefits Program (FEHBP) is a voluntary program open to all employees of the federal government. Through the various plans, employees are offered an opportunity to acquire for themselves and their families protection against the cost of health care services.
2. The program reimburses at 80–90% of allowable charges, depending upon the plan chosen.
3. Nurse practitioners are recognized as designated health care providers under the FEHBP system.

Review Questions

15.31 Third-party reimbursement is the traditional method of health care provider payment in the United States. Advantages of the system are the following, *with the exception of*:

    A. Increased consumer choice of health care provider and facility

    B. More professional autonomy for nurse providers

    C. Decreased personnel in the billing and collections infrastructure

    D. Decreased costs involved in practitioner care because of practice patterns

15.32 Medicaid is a federal-state matching program providing medical assistance to low-income people who are aged, blind, disabled, or members of families with dependent children. It is characterized by all of the following EXCEPT:

    A. Each state is responsible for designing and administering its own type of program within federal guidelines.

    B. The HCFA is responsible for federal oversight of the program.

    C. The nurse practitioner levels of reimbursement range from 60% to 100% of the physician rates, depending on the state.

    D. Nurse practitioners are not allowed to be reimbursed for care provided.

15.33 You are caring for a 66-year-old woman who had been hospitalized for pulmonary edema. She is ready to be discharged home and you find her crying over her concern about the bill. She states she has never been sick before and could not afford the extra premiums for her Medicare insurance and had opted not to buy it. Now she does not know what she is going to do. What do you advise her?

    A. She can buy the extra insurance now and it can be effective retroactively 1 month.

    B. She has misunderstood the system. She is over 65 and entitled to Medicare Part A, which covers inpatient hospital care without extra premiums. She is needs to contact social services to aid her with this.

    C. She is entitled to Supplemental Part B coverage whether or not she can pay the premiums and needs to contact social services.

    D. She needs to file for bankrupcy and get a good lawyer to protect her assets from the hospital bill collectors.

15.34 Nurse practitioners can be reimbursed for services furnished to Medicare patients provided:

    A. They are licensed as registered nurses, meet nurse practitioner qualifications in their state, meet primary care certification and education with experience, and work in collaboration with a physician

    B. The services are furnished incident to a physician's services or under contract to an HMO or in a skilled nursing facility or in a rural health area

    C. Nurse practitioners cannot be reimbursed for Medicare services

    D. A and B only

15.35 CHAMPUS is the insurance coverage of your patient. It is a plan that covers military personnel and their families. Your patient was visiting his family in town and became ill. He asks you to explain the CHAMPUS system to him. What things do you tell him?

    A. This insurance is for when military personnel need to seek care from civilian sources; it is a federal program that reimburses nurse practitioner services.

    B. This insurance is for when military personnel are discharged; because he is currently in active service, he needs to transfer to a military hospital as soon as possible.

C. CHAMPUS does not cover nurse practitioner services and he will have to pay for his care.

D. B and C only.

Answers and Rationales

15.31 **C** The expensive personnel involved in the billing and collections aspect of third-party reimbursement has been a major focus of criticism of this system.

15.32 **D** Federal law allows family and pediatric nurse practitioners to be reimbursed for care provided to Medicaid patients, and states may pass their own laws allowing other nurse practitioners to be reimbursed as well.

15.33 **B** After 65 years of age, you are entitled to Medicare Part A without any extra premiums.

15.34 **D** All of the provisions in A and B are correct. Nurse practitioners are allowed to be reimbursed for services to Medicare patients.

15.35 **A** CHAMPUS covers military personnel when they are ill and away from any military services. Nurse practitioner services are reimbursable at 80% of physician rates.

Emerging Trends

MANAGED CARE

The coast-to-coast tidal wave of managed care is changing the patient care message in the sand forever. The gatekeeper's role is to control patient care *costs*. The designated primary care provider controls the patient's *care*. Too often the primary care provider has the pressure of the gatekeeper focus and must learn to ethically integrate the two roles simultaneously without a decrease in quality of care.

1. Managed care systems focus on the provider of the care and closely evaluate the provider by many criteria. Increasingly, some areas of interest are the provider's:
   A. Practice patterns:
      1) Frequency of consultations, diagnostic tests
      2) Frequency of injections used as therapy
      3) Use of ancillary services
      4) Referral patterns
      5) Tracking patient outcomes (do they get well or return for more visits?)
   B. Contract compliance:
      1) Failure to obtain preauthorizations
      2) Patient admissions to noncontracted facilities
      3) Unnecessary hospitalizations
      4) Readmission rates
      5) Emergency room (ER) usage

    C. Quality review commitments:
      1) Attendance on the usage review or CQI committee
      2) Peer review
      3) Chart completion
    D. Pharmacy control:
      1) Number of prescriptions written by each clinician
      2) Notation of incompatible drugs prescribed
      3) Frequency of use of generics
      4) Inappropriate or unnecessary drugs prescribed
      5) Costs of drugs prescribed

2. According to the Physician Payment Review Commission (Buppert, 1995), 57% of nurse practitioners practicing in HMOs in 1992 had primary responsibility for a specific group of patients, compared with 69% of nurse practitioners overall. Nurse practitioner participation in the managed care system could take on one of three forms:
    A. The traditional approach: Patients are assigned to physicians, who delegate tasks of care to the nurse practitioners with whom they work.
    B. The team approach: Patients are assigned to teams of physicians and nurse practitioners and their care is managed in a collaborative manner.
    C. The panel approach: Patients may be assigned directly to a nurse practitioner or a physician, selected from a panel of care providers, who then assumes full responsibility for the their care.

3. The current barrier being experienced by nurse practitioners across the country is that of not being allowed to contract and care for patients as their designated primary care provider. Without this designation, nurse practitioners are invisible to the patient for access and choice. This must be addressed state by state.

NURSE PRACTITIONER SECOND LICENSURE ISSUE

Currently, the use of the term *nurse practitioner* does not require that a second license be obtained prior to a registered nurse being allowed to function in an advanced practice role. There is a national debate that perhaps the equivalent of a second license should be required to ensure a national standard competancy of a nurse practitioner.

1. In 1995, the National Council of State Boards of Nursing (NCSBN) began a process to ensure the legal defensibility of the different states' regulatory systems for advanced nursing practice.
2. At this point in time, each state establishes statutory authority for licensure of registered nurses through its nurse practice act. This authority includes the use of title, authority to practice within a defined scope of practice, standards of practice, and disciplinary actions.
3. Nurse practitioners engage in practice that is determined to be beyond the usual and prevailing scope of nursing practice, and therefore legal authorization must be established to do so. This legal authority is granted by the state statutes and administered through the state boards of nursing. The state boards of nursing must recognize any nursing title for it to be used legally and given full legal authority.
4. Currently, 39 states have national certification (by a national professional body such as the ANCC) as a requirement for legal recognition as a nurse practitioner.

5. The NCSBN has stated that, if national certification is to be used as a prerequisite to legal recognition as a nurse practitioner, then it is the responsibility of that state's board of nursing to ensure that the certification exam is legally defensible, psychometrically sound, and sufficient for regulatory purposes. The issue is whether or not the examinations are suitable to measure entry into practice.

6. A study is in process by the NCSBN to evaluate all the national certifying bodies for suitability. Concurrently, a job analysis is being performed by the NCSBN to determine a comprehensive picture of current nurse practitioner practice. This job analysis may be the measure by which minimum entry into practice standards are developed.

7. This "second licensure" issue has sparked national debate on both sides; however, the NCSBN contends that the national legal defensibility of the title "Nurse Practitioner" is at the heart of the matter. They also state that the quality of the exam must measure minimum standards of safe entry into practice.

SHIFTING TRENDS IN THE NURSE PRACTITIONER SPECIALTY NEEDS

1. Acute care nurse practitioners are filling needed positions where health care changes and restructuring mandate the need for an advanced practitioner to comprehensively manage patient care. In addition to the inpatient setting, acute care nurse practitioners are practicing in a variety of settings (outpatient, subacute care, urgent care) and in a variety of roles (direct care providers, case managers, care coordinators, and collaborative practice). The void of hospital physician training programs has established one role for the ACNP.

2. With the aging baby boom population, there will be an increasing need for geriatric care, care of the menopausal woman, and other nursing specialists predominantly caring for the aging (e.g., cardiology).

3. Currently in the United States, fewer than 33% of physicians practice primary care. In other industrialized countries, 50–70% of physicians practice primary care. In 1992, only 14.6% of graduating U.S. medical students chose primary care as their specialty. Primary care is the nurse practitioners' focus, whether in the community or acute care setting.

SIGNIFICANT PATTERNS IN SALARY TRENDS

1. Health care administration roles were the most highly compensated.
2. Males earn 16–20% more than females across specialty and years of experience as nurse practitioners.

TELEMEDICINE, TELEHEALTH, TECHNOLOGY-BASED PATIENT CARE

1. The health care industry's progressive shift toward high-tech care has paved the way for innovation, entrepreneurial endeavors, and creative patient care.
2. Politically savvy leadership for nurse practitioners is keeping the role on the cutting edge for the next generation of advanced practice nurses.

3. Consumer use of the Internet and other high-tech sources of health information has created the need for providers to have rapid access to data bases of current research and information.

4. FCC regulations regarding telemedicine provider use are under consideration, and nursing professional organizations are promoting the nurse practitioner as an appropriate user.

CONSUMER MARKET-DRIVEN HEALTH CARE CHOICES

1. The current health care system is implemented with the employer and the insurer controlling where the consumer seeks care, what care they can seek, and whom they can seek their care from.

2. Typically, employers shop for health plans that offer the most economical mix of costs and services. Then this option is given to the employee. The new plan or plans are the only employee choices, regardless of previously established patient-provider relationships.

3. New consumer driven systems are being experimented with in the midwest that place the decisions of provider choice back into the hands of the patient.

   A. Vouchers of health care dollars are being provided to employees at fixed amounts. The employees/consumers/patients then make their own choice of where to seek care. If savings are generated, they may keep them. If they choose to seek a plan or provider that exceeds the voucher amount, they pay the difference.

   B. In consumer-driven voucher systems, patient-provider relationships are valued and can be built without arbitrary shifts in the workplace causing them to be broken. This system rewards providers who nurture health promotion, patient education, and strong patient relationships. This is the opposite of the current system.

   C. Historically, nurse practitioner education and training promotes preventive health, patient education, and holistic approaches to care of the patient, family, and community. Education of the ACNP focuses on management of health care problems as well as acute exacerbations of chronic diseases.

4. Consumer frustration with the lack of health care provider choice and continuity of care is driving the market shift to a new system that values these choices. Nurse practitioners, therefore, would be well positioned to market themselves and any practice they were associated with in a consumer-driven system.

Review Questions

15.36 The emergence of managed care has created a new set of provider review indicators that are being utilized by the plans and employing entities to oversee provider practice patterns and contractual compliance. Some of these include:

A. Frequency of consultations and referrals, ER usage, number of prescriptions by each clinician, readmission rates, and failure to obtain preauthorization for procedures

B. Frequency of use of generics, patient admissions to noncontracted facilities, number of staff employed in office, and frequency of patient illnesses

C. Inappropriate or unnecessary drugs prescribed, chart completion, readmission rates, use of family support systems, and patient complaints

D. None of the above

15.37 Prescriptive authority is an integral tool for the nurse practitioner and is still not universal in the United States, although most states allow it in some form. Identify the statement below that is not an accurate reflection of the trends emerging in prescriptive authority.

A. More categories of controlled substances are being added.

B. Less restriction on settings and sites in which nurse practitioners may prescribe.

C. Nurse practitioners are prescribing more and more medications per patient encounter.

D. Fewer rigid restrictions are being attached to the prescriptive authority of nurse practitioners.

15.38 The concept of second licensure or universal certification for nurse practitioners is:

A. Being investigated by the National Council of State Boards of Nursing

B. Welcomed by all nurse practitioners and organizations

C. Not applicable to all because 39 states already have certification as a requirement for entry into nurse practitioner practice

D. Where nurse practitioners get the right to their title, role, and authority to function within a defined scope of practice

15.39 The trend toward telemedicine and telehealth may affect the nurse practitioner role in what manner?

A. Consumer use of the Internet has increased the need for the nurse practitioner to be able to identify current research in a time-efficient manner with access to quality information systems.

B. The availability of telemedicine will decrease the need for nurse practitioners in the rural community, because now the patient can have access to care and consultations via satellite.

C. The increased use of telemedicine will increase the need for nurse practitioners comfortable with the medium to bring specialty consultations and referrals to the rural community where the patient lives.

D. A and D only.

15.40 The lack of patient choice in health care providers and facilities has stimulated the phenomenon of a consumer-driven voucher system. This system is different from the current employer-obtained health care coverage system and has which of the following characteristics?

A. Supplementing the voucher out of pocket or using it as full coverage, the employee now can choose any provider or health system with the voucher dollars provided by the employer.

B. The employee now has to pay more.

C. The nurse practitioner cannot function in such a system because patients will not be able to choose him/her.

D. Employers will not support such a system because the costs will be prohibitive to them.

Answers and Rationales

15.36 **A** Number of staff employed, frequency of patient illness, family support systems, and patient complaints are not indicators.

16.37 **C** Research indicates that nurse practitioners prescribe fewer medications than physician counterparts in states with full prescriptive authority.

15.38 **A** The NCSBN states that, if certification is being used as a prerequisite to legal recognition as a nurse practitioner, then it is the responsibility of that state's board of nursing to ensure that the certification exam is legally defensible, psychometrically sound, and sufficient for regulatory purposes.

15.39 **D** The advent of telemedicine will not decrease the need for nurse practitioners in rural areas because the specialty physicians do not practice in the rural areas, and their expertise will need to be coordinated by the providers of rural health.

15.40 **A** The voucher system will benefit the employee (because of increased choice), the employer (with stabilized and standardized employee health benefits), and the nurse practitioner (because the nurse practitioner has a long history of high patient satisfaction with care provided).

References

Brown, S.A., & Grimes, D.E. (1993). *A Meta-analysis of the Process of Care, Clinical Outcomes and Cost-effectiveness of Nurses in Primary Care Roles: Nurse Practitioners and Certified Nurse-Midwives.* Washington, DC: American Nurses Association.

Buppert, C.K. (1995). Justifying nurse practitioner existence: Hard facts to hard figures. *Nurse Pract 20*(8), 43–48.

Callan, E. (1992). Nurse practitioner management of hospital-affiliated primary care center. *Nurse Pract 17*(8), 71–47.

El-Sherif, C. (1995). Nurse practitioners—where do they belong within the organizational structure of the acute care setting? *Nurse Pract 29*(1), 62–65.

Ford, L.C., & Silver, H.K. (1967). The expanded role of the nurse in child care: The pediatric nurse practitioner at Colorado. *Am J Nurs 167,* 1443.

Francis, A. (1996). Changes in medicaid mean changes for NPs. *NP News 4*(2), 1–4.

Griffin, G. (1993). Your "family doctor" may be a nurse! *Postgrad Med 94,* 23–26.

Harkless, G.E. (1989). Prescriptive authority: Debunking common assumptions. *Nurse Pract 14*(8), 57–61.

Hooker, R.S., & McCaig, L. (1996). Emergency department uses of physician assistants and nurse practitioners: A national survey. *Am J Emerg Med 14,* 245–249.

Hravnak, M., Kobert, S.N., Risco, K.G., et al. (1995). Acute care nurse practitioner curriculum: Content and development process. *Am J Crit Care 4,* 179–188.

Kearnes, D. (1992). A productivity tool to evaluate NP practice: monitoring clinical time spent in reimbursable, patient-related activities. *Nurse Pract 17*(6), 55–67.

Mahoney, D.F. (1992). Nurse practitioners as prescribers: Past research trends and future study needs. *Nurse Pract 17*(1), 44–51.

Mahoney, D.F. (1994). Appropriateness of geriatric prescribing decisions made by nurse practitioners and physicians. *Image 26,* 41–46.

McGrath, J. (1990). The cost effectiveness of nurse practitioners. *Nurse Pract 15*(7), 41–42.

Mittelstadt, P. (1993). *The Reimbursement Manual: How to Get Paid for Your Advanced Practice Nursing Services*. Washington, DC: American Nurses Association.

Mundinger, M. (1994). Advanced-practice nursing—good medicine for physicians? *N Engl J Med 330*, 211–214.

Nichols, L. (1992). Estimating costs of underusing advanced practice nurses. *Nurs Econ 10*, 343–351.

Office of Technology Assessment. (1986). *Nurse Practitioners, Physician Assistants, and Certified Nurse Midwives: A Policy Analysis* (Health Technology Case Study 37). Washington, DC: Office of Technology Assessment.

Pearson, L. (1997). Annual update of how each state stands on legislative issues affecting advanced nursing practice. *Nurse Pract 22*(1), 18–86.

Petty, A. (1993). Nurse practitioners fight job restrictions. *The Wall Street Journal, September 3, B1,* p. 1.

Scott, A. (1995). Critical care nurse practitioners: Evolution of the advanced practice role. *Am J Crit Care 4*, 88.

Scudder, L. (1996). Update on NP second licensure issue. *Nurse Pract World News, 1*(5), 1, 18.

Sharp, N. (1992). The issue of reimbursement. *Nurs Manage 23*(6), 17.

Sharp, N. (1992). Legislation introduces equal pay for nonphysician providers. *Nurs Manage 23*(2), 30.

Van Der Horst, M. (1992). Canada's health care system provides lessons for NPs. *Nurse Pract 17*(8), 44–60.

Ventura, M.R., & Crosby, F. (1991). An information synthesis to evaluate nurse practitioner effectiveness. *Mil Med 156*, 286–291.

Watts, Hanson, M.J., Burke, K.G., et al. (1996). The critical care nurse practitioner: An advanced practice role for the critical care nurse. *Dimensions Crit Care Nurs 15*(1), 48–56.

Wilkens, M. (1995). Providers: How regulations affect availability and access to care. *Nurs Policy Forum 1*(2), 29–37.

Index

Note: Page numbers in *italics* indicate figures; page numbers followd by t indicate tables.